Antitumor Activity of Natural Products and Related Compounds

Antitumor Activity of Natural Products and Related Compounds

Editors

Barbara De Filippis
Alessandra Ammazzalorso
Marialuigia Fantacuzzi

MDPI

Basel • Beijing • Wuhan • Barcelona • Belgrade • Novi Sad • Cluj • Manchester

Editors
Barbara De Filippis
"G. d'Annunzio" University
Chieti-Pescara
Chieti, Italy

Alessandra Ammazzalorso
"G. d'Annunzio" University
Chieti-Pescara
Chieti, Italy

Marialuigia Fantacuzzi
"G. d'Annunzio" University
Chieti-Pescara
Chieti, Italy

Editorial Office
MDPI
St. Alban-Anlage 66
4052 Basel, Switzerland

This is a reprint of articles from the Topic published online in the open access journals *International Journal of Molecular Sciences* (ISSN 1422-0067), *Cancers* (ISSN 2072-6694), *Biomolecules* (ISSN 2076-328X), *Molecules* (ISSN 1420-3049), *Marine Drugs* (ISSN 1660-3397), and *Scientia Pharmaceutica* (ISSN 2218-0532) (available at: https://www.mdpi.com/topics/AntitumorActivityofNaturalProductsandRelatedCompounds).

For citation purposes, cite each article independently as indicated on the article page online and as indicated below:

Lastname, A.A.; Lastname, B.B. Article Title. *Journal Name* **Year**, *Volume Number*, Page Range.

ISBN 978-3-0365-9746-1 (Hbk)
ISBN 978-3-0365-9747-8 (PDF)
doi.org/10.3390/books978-3-0365-9747-8

Contents

About the Editors

Barbara De Filippis

Dr Barbara De Filippis obtained her degree in Pharmaceutical Chemistry and Technology and her Ph.D. in Pharmaceutical Sciences at the University of Chieti–Pescara (Italy) and is currently an assistant professor of medicinal chemistry. Her research work is focused on the design and synthesis of small molecules with anticancer and antimicrobial activities. Her studies are related to derivatives of natural phenols involved in neurodegenerative diseases. She is the author/co-author of 82 international papers in peer-reviewed journals and serves as a guest editor and editorial board member of international journals. She is a reviewer for many medicinal chemistry journals.

Alessandra Ammazzalorso

Alessandra Ammazzalorso is an associate professor of medicinal chemistry at the Department of Pharmacy, "G. d'Annunzio" University of Chieti–Pescara (Italy). She obtained her degree in Pharmaceutical Chemistry and Technology and her Ph.D. in Pharmaceutical Sciences from the same university. Her research activities address the synthesis of small molecules endowed with biological activity. In detail, her studies are focused on compounds targeting peroxisome proliferator-activated receptors, with special attention paid to the antitumor potential of their agonists and antagonists. She is also involved in the identification of enzyme inhibitors as anticancer agents.
Her research activity is documented by 82 papers in international, peer-reviewed journals, several contributions to scientific meetings, and participation in international and national research projects. She is also a reviewer for several high-ranked medicinal chemistry journals, and she serves as an editorial board member of international journals.

Marialuigia Fantacuzzi

Marialuigia Fantacuzzi is an assistant professor of medicinal chemistry at the Department of Pharmacy, "G. d'Annunzio" University of Chieti–Pescara (Italy). She received her degree in Pharmaceutical Chemistry and Technology cum laude and her Ph.D. in Pharmaceutical Sciences from the same university. Her research interests are mainly focused on the design, synthesis, biological evaluation, and docking study of compounds of pharmaceutical interest useful for the treatment of inflammatory pathology, metabolic syndrome, neurodegenerative diseases, and cancer.
Her scientific activity is certified by 68 papers in international, peer-reviewed journals and different communications in scientific meetings. Her commitment to pharmaceutical chemistry is highlighted by her role as a reviewer for major international medicinal chemistry journals as well as her participation as an editorial board member and a special issue guest editor.

International Journal of
Molecular Sciences

MDPI

Editorial

Anticancer Activity of Natural Products and Related Compounds

Barbara De Filippis, Marialuigia Fantacuzzi * and Alessandra Ammazzalorso

Department of Pharmacy, G. d'Annunzio University of Chieti-Pescara, Via dei Vestini 31, 66100 Chieti, Italy; barbara.defilippis@unich.it (B.D.F.); alessandra.ammazzalorso@unich.it (A.A.)
* Correspondence: marialuigia.fantacuzzi@unich.it

Citation: De Filippis, B.; Fantacuzzi, M.; Ammazzalorso, A. Anticancer Activity of Natural Products and Related Compounds. *Int. J. Mol. Sci.* **2023**, *24*, 16507. https://doi.org/10.3390/ijms242216507

Received: 13 November 2023
Accepted: 15 November 2023
Published: 20 November 2023

Nature has always been a precious source of bioactive molecules which are used for the treatment of various diseases [1]. Natural compounds such as dietary phytochemicals, nutritional herbs, and their constitutive bioactive agents possess a great variety of chemical scaffolds and distinct bioactivity profiles, which make them suitable for applications in therapy or as valuable lead compounds to obtain novel potent bioactive compounds [2]. Significant advances in natural source isolation and extraction techniques have led to the identification of novel compounds as useful starting points for the generation of optimized molecules with enhanced therapeutic potential via semi-synthetic or synthetic processes [3].

The application of natural products in the field of chemotherapy and chemoprevention is a valuable research topic, leading to the extensive use of plant-derived compounds as potent antitumor molecules [4]. In addition, marine-based pharmaceuticals have been extensively studied for their applications in the anticancer field, providing useful compounds such as cytarabine and trabectedin [5]. Alternative treatments in complement with traditional methods (radiotherapy, chemotherapy, and surgery) have been shown to be helpful and offer very reasonable alternatives to current medicines for cancer [6]. Much effort has also been directed towards the discovery of novel targets [7–9] in an attempt to obtain anticancer effects via multiple mechanisms, overcoming the resistance phenomena developed by most cancers.

Natural products effectively inhibit cell proliferation, regulate the cell cycle, and interfere with several tumorigenic signaling pathways [10,11]. The anticancer properties of polyphenols, found abundantly in plants, as flavonoids [12], terpenoids [13], and alkaloids [14], have been extensively reported [15]. However, important research efforts are necessary to fully understand the mechanisms of action of natural compounds by which these agents affect cell proliferation, differentiation, apoptosis, angiogenesis, and metastasis; in addition, there is a need to overcome major problems such as toxicity, poor selectivity, and unfavorable pharmacokinetics [16].

Currently, many plant-based antitumor drugs are in clinical use, such as taxanes, vinblastine, vincristine, and podophyllotoxin analogues. The combined use of phytochemicals like resveratrol, curcumin, and thymoquinone with other antitumor agents has shown significant success in preclinical studies, allowing enhanced efficacy and mitigation of side effects [17,18]. Emerging nanotechnology applications for anticancer drug formulations have been revolutionizing cancer therapy. Tissue-specific nanomedicines play a key role in advanced cancer diagnostic techniques by using liposomes, micelles, and nanoparticles as effective delivery vehicles [19]. Moreover, medicinal plant extracts have proven most effective in various cancers, paving the way for developing novel therapeutic strategies [20]. Many studies have been based on crude aqueous and ethanol extracts, with few explorations of their mechanisms [21].

In this Topic, 30 original articles and 3 reviews have been collected, with a particular focus on the isolation of bioactive compounds from natural sources, the mechanisms of action of anticancer compounds at the cellular level, and the application of active molecules against a panel of solid and hematological cancers, including melanoma, breast, lung, colorectal, prostate, bladder, and gastric cancer. Most of the analyzed compounds were from natural sources, whereas some semi-synthetic derivatives were also identified and discussed.

The most recent findings on the effects of extracts and their constituents in treating various cancers are discussed. Most works focus on the effect of water or ethanolic extracts from natural plants or fungi, such as *Viscum album* var. *coloratum*, *Drimia Maritima*, *Trichosanthes*, *Lupinus albus*, *Bryopsis plumosa*, *Elephantus scaber* L., *Paejangsan*, *Coix Seed*, *Lupinus albus*, *Ocimum sanctum* Linn., *Euphorbia fischeriana*, *Moldavian dragonhead*, *Streptomyces ardesiacus*, *Cichorium intybus*, and *Trichosanthes*.

The extracts and the isolated components have proven effective against breast, colorectal, lung, bladder, myeloma, and prostate cancer through several mechanisms, including decreased tumor cell viability, modulation of cytokines, secretion of chemokines, modulation of ROS, reduction of specific MMP subtypes, apoptosis, cell cycle inhibition, or by downregulating MAPK.

Table 1 schematically illustrates the content of this Topic, with all the contributions published in the six participating journals.

Table 1. Original articles and reviews collected in the six journals participating in the Topic.

Title	Author	Journal	Year	DOI
Fermented Mangosteen (*Garcinia mangostana* L.) Supplementation in the Prevention of HPV-Induced Cervical Cancer: From Mechanisms to Clinical Outcomes	Kharaeva, Z.	*Cancers*	2022	https://doi.org/10.3390/cancers14194707
Scabertopin Derived from *Elephantopus scaber* L. Mediates Necroptosis by Inducing Reactive Oxygen Species Production in Bladder Cancer In Vitro	Gao, Y.	*Cancers*	2022	https://doi.org/10.3390/cancers14235976
Therapeutic Potential of Deflamin against Colorectal Cancer Development and Progression	Silva, S.	*Cancers*	2022	https://doi.org/10.3390/cancers14246182
Design, Synthesis and Biological Evaluation of Neocryptolepine Derivatives as Potential Anti-Gastric Cancer Agents	Ma, Y.	*IJMS*	2022	https://doi.org/10.3390/ijms231911924
FOXO1 Is a Key Mediator of Glucocorticoid-Induced Expression of Tristetraprolin in MDA-MB-231 Breast Cancer Cells	Jeon, D.	*IJMS*	2022	https://doi.org/10.3390/ijms232213673
New Angucycline Glycosides from a Marine-Derived Bacterium *Streptomyces ardesiacus*	Anh, C.	*IJMS*	2022	https://doi.org/10.3390/ijms232213779
Flavones, Flavonols, Lignans, and Caffeic Acid Derivatives from *Dracocephalum moldavica* and Their In Vitro Effects on Multiple Myeloma and Acute Myeloid Leukemia	Jöhrer, K.	*IJMS*	2022	https://doi.org/10.3390/ijms232214219
Anti-Cancer Effects of a New Herbal Medicine PSY by Inhibiting the STAT3 Signaling Pathway in Colorectal Cancer Cells and Its Phytochemical Analysis	Han, S.	*IJMS*	2022	https://doi.org/10.3390/ijms232314826
Combination Therapy of Curcumin and Disulfiram Synergistically Inhibits the Growth of B16-F10 Melanoma Cells by Inducing Oxidative Stress	Fontes, S.	*Biomolecules*	2022	https://doi.org/10.3390/biom12111600
Efficient Synthesis for Altering Side Chain Length on Cannabinoid Molecules and Their Effects in Chemotherapy and Chemotherapeutic Induced Neuropathic Pain	Raup-Konsavage, W.	*Biomolecules*	2022	https://doi.org/10.3390/biom12121869
Ent-Abietane Diterpenoids from *Euphorbia fischeriana* and Their Cytotoxic Activities	Zhu, Q-F.	*Molecules*	2022	https://doi.org/10.3390/molecules27217258

Table 1. *Cont.*

Title	Author	Journal	Year	DOI
Lactucin, a Bitter Sesquiterpene from *Cichorium intybus*, Inhibits Cancer Cell Proliferation by Downregulating the MAPK and Central Carbon Metabolism Pathway	Imam, K.	*Molecules*	2022	https://doi.org/10.3390/molecules27217358
Anticancer Activity of Mannose-Specific Lectin, BPL2, from Marine Green Alga *Bryopsis plumosa*	Lee, J.	*Marine Drugs*	2022	https://doi.org/10.3390/md20120776
Ethanolic Extract of *Ocimum sanctum Linn.* Inhibits Cell Migration of Human Lung Adenocarcinoma Cells (A549) by Downregulation of Integrin $\alpha v\beta 3$, $\alpha 5\beta 1$, and VEGF	Kustiati, U.	*Scientia Pharmaceutica*	2022	https://doi.org/10.3390/scipharm90040069
Libertellenone T, a Novel Compound Isolated from Endolichenic Fungus, Induces G2/M Phase Arrest, Apoptosis, and Autophagy by Activating the ROS/JNK Pathway in Colorectal Cancer Cells	Gamage, C.	*Cancers*	2023	https://doi.org/10.3390/cancers15020489
New Affordable Methods for Large-Scale Isolation of Major Olive Secoiridoids and Systematic Comparative Study of Their Antiproliferative/Cytotoxic Effect on Multiple Cancer Cell Lines of Different Cancer Origins	Papakonstantinou, A.	*IJMS*	2023	https://doi.org/10.3390/ijms24010003
Synthesis and Anti-Proliferative Evaluation of Arctigenin Analogues with C-9′ Derivatisation	Paulin, E.	*IJMS*	2023	https://doi.org/10.3390/ijms24021167
Trichosanthin Promotes Anti-Tumor Immunity through Mediating Chemokines and Granzyme B Secretion in Hepatocellular Carcinoma	Wang, K.	*IJMS*	2023	https://doi.org/10.3390/ijms24021416
Camptothecin Effectively Regulates Germline Differentiation through Bam-Cyclin A Axis in *Drosophila melanogaster*	Zhang, J.	*IJMS*	2023	https://doi.org/10.3390/ijms24021617
JI017 Induces Cell Autophagy and Apoptosis via Elevated Levels of Reactive Oxygen Species in Human Lung Cancer Cells	Ku, J.	*IJMS*	2023	https://doi.org/10.3390/ijms24087528
α-Tocotrienol and Redox-Silent Analogs of Vitamin E Enhances Bortezomib Sensitivity in Solid Cancer Cells through Modulation of NFE2L1	Ishii, K.	*IJMS*	2023	https://doi.org/10.3390/ijms24119382
Modulation of the Endomembrane System by the Anticancer Natural Product Superstolide/ZJ-101	Sanchez, P.	*IJMS*	2023	https://doi.org/10.3390/ijms24119575
Mitochondria-Targeting 1,5-Diazacyclooctane-Spacered Triterpene Rhodamine Conjugates Exhibit Cytotoxicity at Sub-Nanomolar Concentration against Breast Cancer Cells	Heise, N.	*IJMS*	2023	https://doi.org/10.3390/ijms241310695
Phytochemical Analysis and Anticancer Properties of *Drimia maritima* Bulb Extracts on Colorectal Cancer Cells	Al-Abdallat, K.	*Molecules*	2023	https://doi.org/10.3390/molecules28031215
Synthesis of Oleanolic Acid-Dithiocarbamate Conjugates and Evaluation of Their Broad-Spectrum Antitumor Activities	Tang, L.	*Molecules*	2023	https://doi.org/10.3390/molecules28031414
Genistein Inhibits Proliferation and Metastasis in Human Cervical Cancer Cells through the Focal Adhesion Kinase Signaling Pathway: A Network Pharmacology-Based In Vitro Study in HeLa Cells	Chen, T.	*Molecules*	2023	https://doi.org/10.3390/molecules28041919
Anti-Proliferative and Pro-Apoptotic vLMW Fucoidan Formulas Decrease PD-L1 Surface Expression in EBV Latency III and DLBCL Tumoral B-Cells by Decreasing Actin Network	Saliba, J.	*Marine Drugs*	2023	https://doi.org/10.3390/md21020132
A Novel Aldisine Derivative Exhibits Potential Antitumor Effects by Targeting JAK/STAT3 Signaling	Wang, D.-P.	*Marine Drugs*	2023	https://doi.org/10.3390/md21040218

Table 1. *Cont.*

Title	Author	Journal	Year	DOI
Light-Mediated Transformation of Renieramycins and Semisynthesis of 4′-Pyridinecarbonyl-Substituted Renieramycin-Type Derivatives as Potential Cytotoxic Agents against Non-Small-Cell Lung Cancer Cells	Sinsook, S.	*Marine Drugs*	2023	https://doi.org/10.3390/md21070400
Immuno-Modulatory Effects of Korean Mistletoe in MDA-MB-231 Breast Cancer Cells and THP-1 Macrophages	Lim, W.-T.	*Scientia Pharmaceutica*	2023	https://doi.org/10.3390/scipharm91040048
Molecular Mechanism of Tanshinone against Prostate Cancer	Li, W.	*Molecules*	2022	https://doi.org/10.3390/molecules27175594
Can Natural Products Targeting EMT Serve as the Future Anticancer Therapeutics?	Anwar, S.	*Molecules*	2022	https://doi.org/10.3390/molecules27227668
Natural Products and Small Molecules Targeting Cellular Ceramide Metabolism to Enhance Apoptosis in Cancer Cells	Afrin, F.	*Cancers*	2023	https://doi.org/10.3390/cancers15184645

Author Contributions: Writing—review and editing, B.D.F., M.F. and A.A. All authors have read and agreed to the published version of the manuscript.

Conflicts of Interest: The authors declare no conflict of interest.

References

1. Cragg, G.M.; Newman, D.J. Natural products: A continuing source of novel drug leads. *Biochim. Biophys. Acta* **2013**, *1830*, 3670–3695. [CrossRef] [PubMed]
2. Atanasov, A.G.; Zotchev, S.B.; Dirsch, V.M.; the International Natural Product Sciences Taskforce; Supuran, C.T. Natural products in drug discovery: Advances and opportunities. *Nat. Rev. Drug Discov.* **2021**, *20*, 200–216. [CrossRef] [PubMed]
3. Astrain-Redin, N.; Sanmartin, C.; Sharma, A.K.; Plano, D. From Natural Sources to Synthetic Derivatives: The Allyl Motif as a Powerful Tool for Fragment-Based Design in Cancer Treatment. *J. Med. Chem.* **2023**, *66*, 3703–3731. [CrossRef]
4. Naeem, A.; Hu, P.; Yang, M.; Zhang, J.; Liu, Y.; Zhu, W.; Zheng, Q. Natural Products as Anticancer Agents: Current Status and Future Perspectives. *Molecules* **2022**, *27*, 8367. [CrossRef]
5. Nigam, M.; Suleria, H.A.R.; Farzaei, M.H.; Mishra, A.P. Marine anticancer drugs and their relevant targets: A treasure from the ocean. *Daru* **2019**, *27*, 491–515. [CrossRef]
6. Lin, S.R.; Chang, C.H.; Hsu, C.F.; Tsai, M.J.; Cheng, H.; Leong, M.K.; Sung, P.J.; Chen, J.C.; Weng, C.F. Natural compounds as potential adjuvants to cancer therapy: Preclinical evidence. *Br. J. Pharmacol.* **2020**, *177*, 1409–1423. [CrossRef]
7. Zhong, L.; Li, Y.; Xiong, L.; Wang, W.; Wu, M.; Yuan, T.; Yang, W.; Tian, C.; Miao, Z.; Wang, T.; et al. Small molecules in targeted cancer therapy: Advances, challenges, and future perspectives. *Signal Transduct. Target. Ther.* **2021**, *6*, 201. [CrossRef]
8. Franzese, O.; Graziani, G. Role of PARP Inhibitors in Cancer Immunotherapy: Potential Friends to Immune Activating Molecules and Foes to Immune Checkpoints. *Cancers* **2022**, *14*, 5633. [CrossRef]
9. Ammazzalorso, A.; Agamennone, M.; De Filippis, B.; Fantacuzzi, M. Development of CDK4/6 Inhibitors: A Five Years Update. *Molecules* **2021**, *26*, 1488. [CrossRef]
10. Li, W.; Chen, H.; Xu, B.; Wang, Y.; Zhang, C.; Cao, Y.; Xing, X. Research progress on classification, sources and functions of dietary polyphenols for prevention and treatment of chronic diseases. *J. Future Foods* **2023**, *3*, 289–305. [CrossRef]
11. Memarzia, A.; Saadat, S.; Asgharzadeh, F.; Behrouz, S.; Folkerts, G.; Boskabady, M.H. Therapeutic effects of medicinal plants and their constituents on lung cancer, in vitro, in vivo and clinical evidence. *J. Cell Mol. Med.* **2023**, *27*, 2841–2863. [CrossRef] [PubMed]
12. Dhyani, P.; Quispe, C.; Sharma, E.; Bahukhandi, A.; Sati, P.; Attri, D.C.; Szopa, A.; Sharifi-Rad, J.; Docea, A.O.; Mardare, I.; et al. Anticancer potential of alkaloids: A key emphasis to colchicine, vinblastine, vincristine, vindesine, vinorelbine and vincamine. *Cancer Cell Int.* **2022**, *22*, 206. [CrossRef] [PubMed]
13. Fantacuzzi, M.; Gallorini, M.; Gambacorta, N.; Ammazzalorso, A.; Aturki, Z.; Balaha, M.; Carradori, S.; Giampietro, L.; Maccallini, C.; Cataldi, A.; et al. Design, Synthesis and Biological Evaluation of Aromatase Inhibitors Based on Sulfonates and Sulfonamides of Resveratrol. *Pharmaceuticals* **2021**, *14*, 984. [CrossRef] [PubMed]
14. Kopustinskiene, D.M.; Jakstas, V.; Savickas, A.; Bernatoniene, J. Flavonoids as Anticancer Agents. *Nutrients* **2020**, *12*, 457. [CrossRef]
15. Gozari, M.; Alborz, M.; El-Seedi, H.R.; Jassbi, A.R. Chemistry, biosynthesis and biological activity of terpenoids and meroterpenoids in bacteria and fungi isolated from different marine habitats. *Eur. J. Med. Chem.* **2021**, *210*, 112957. [CrossRef]

16. Estrela, J.M.; Mena, S.; Obrador, E.; Benlloch, M.; Castellano, G.; Salvador, R.; Dellinger, R.W. Polyphenolic phytochemicals in cancer prevention and therapy: Bioavailability versus bioefficacy. *J. Med. Chem.* **2017**, *60*, 9413–9436. [CrossRef]
17. Blanco-Vaca, F.; Cedó, L.; Julve, J. Phytosterols in Cancer: From Molecular Mechanisms to Preventive and Therapeutic Potentials. *Curr. Med. Chem.* **2019**, *26*, 6735–6749. [CrossRef]
18. De Filippis, B.; De Lellis, L.; Florio, R.; Ammazzalorso, A.; Amoia, P.; Fantacuzzi, M.; Giampietro, L.; Maccallini, C.; Amoroso, R.; Veschi, S.; et al. Synthesis and cytotoxic effects on pancreatic cancer cells of resveratrol analogs. *Med. Chem. Res.* **2019**, *28*, 984–991. [CrossRef]
19. Dhupal, M.; Chowdhury, D. Phytochemical-Based Nanomedicine for Advanced Cancer Theranostics: Perspectives on Clinical Trials to Clinical Use. *Int. J. Nanomed.* **2020**, *15*, 9125–9157. [CrossRef]
20. Greenwell, M.; Rahman, P.K. Medicinal Plants: Their Use in Anticancer Treatment. *Int. J. Pharm. Sci. Res.* **2015**, *6*, 4103–4112. [CrossRef]
21. Radošević, K.; Ćurko, N.; Gaurina Srček, V.; Cvjetko Bubalo, M.; Tomašević, M.; Kovačević Ganić, K.; Radojčić Redovniković, I. Natural deep eutectic solvents as beneficial extractants for enhancement of plant extracts bioactivity. *LWT* **2016**, *73*, 45–51. [CrossRef]

cancers

MDPI

Article

Fermented Mangosteen (*Garcinia mangostana* L.) Supplementation in the Prevention of HPV-Induced Cervical Cancer: From Mechanisms to Clinical Outcomes

Zaira Kharaeva [1], Pavel Trakhtman [2], Ilya Trakhtman [3], Chiara De Luca [4], Wolfgang Mayer [4], Jessie Chung [5], Galina Ibragimova [6] and Liudmila Korkina [3,6,*]

1 Microbiology, Immunology, and Virology Department, Berbekov's Kabardino-Balkar State Medical University, Chernishevskiy Str. 176, 360000 Nalchik, Russia
2 Blood Bank, Dmitry Rogachev National Medical Research Center of Pediatric Hematology, Oncology and Immunology, Samora Mashela Str. 1, 117988 Moscow, Russia
3 R&D Department, Swiss Dekotra GmbH, Badenerstrasse 549, CH-8048 Zurich, Switzerland
4 R&D Department, Medena AG, Industriestrasse 16, CH-8910 Affoltern-am-Albis, Switzerland
5 Natural Health Farm Ltd., 39 Jalan Pengacara U1/48, Temasya Industrial Park, Shah Alam 40150, Selangor, Malaysia
6 Centre for Innovative Biotechnological Investigations Nanolab (CIBI-NANOLAB), Vernadskiy Pr. 97, 117437 Moscow, Russia
* Correspondence: korkina@cibi-nanolab.com or korkina@dekotra.com; Tel.: +39-3497364787

Citation: Kharaeva, Z.; Trakhtman, P.; Trakhtman, I.; De Luca, C.; Mayer, W.; Chung, J.; Ibragimova, G.; Korkina, L. Fermented Mangosteen (*Garcinia mangostana* L.) Supplementation in the Prevention of HPV-Induced Cervical Cancer: From Mechanisms to Clinical Outcomes. *Cancers* **2022**, *14*, 4707. https://doi.org/10.3390/cancers14194707

Academic Editor: Lingzhi Wang

Received: 15 July 2022
Accepted: 21 September 2022
Published: 27 September 2022

Simple Summary: Human papillomavirus (HPV) is connected with virtually all cases of cervical cancer. The viral infection-associated chronic inflammation, oxidative stress, and alterations in apoptosis have been considered as leading risk factors for carcinogenesis in humans. In an observational clinical study, we identified oxidative markers and the cervical/circulating ligands of TNF-alpha-induced apoptosis involved in HPV-associated cervical carcinogenesis. In the following clinical trial, 250 females infected with high-cancer-risk HPV16/18 (healthy and pre-cancerous) were recruited into a placebo-controlled clinical study of supplementation with fermented mangosteen (FM, 28g/day, daily) for three months. Our findings indicate that FM, and not a placebo, in combination with routine anti-viral therapy, could prevent, slow down, or even interrupt HPV-associated cervical carcinogenesis, mainly through the suppression of leukocyte recruitment into infected tissue, through anti-inflammatory effects, and through the restoration of nitric oxide metabolite-initiated TRAIL-dependent apoptosis.

Abstract: In the observational clinical study, we identified the oxidative markers of HPV-associated cervical carcinogenesis and the local/circulating ligands of TNF-alpha-induced apoptosis. Cervical biopsies of 196 females infected with low-cancer-risk HPV10/13 or high-cancer-risk HPV16/18 (healthy, pre-cancerous CIN I and CIN II, and CIN III carcinoma) were analysed for OH radical scavenging, catalase, GSH-peroxidase, myeloperoxidase (MPO), nitrate/nitrite, nitrotyrosine, and isoprostane. Ligands of TNF-alpha-dependent apoptosis (TNF-alpha, TRAIL, IL-2, and sFAS) were determined in cervical fluid, biopsies, and serum. Cervical MPO was highly enhanced, while nitrotyrosine decreased in CIN III. Local/circulating TRAIL was remarkably decreased, and higher-than-control serum TNF-alpha and IL-2 levels were found in the CIN I and CIN III groups. Then, 250 females infected with HPV16/18 (healthy and with CIN I and CIN II) were recruited into a placebo-controlled clinical study of supplementation with fermented mangosteen (FM, 28g/day, daily) for three months. Post-trial colposcopy revealed normal patterns in 100% of the FM group versus 62% of the placebo group. Inflammatory cells in cervical fluid were found in 21% of the FM group versus 40% of the placebo group. Locally, FM drastically diminished MPO and NO_2/NO_3, while it remarkably increased TRAIL. Additionally, FM supplementation normalised serum TRAIL, TNF-alpha, and IL-2.

Keywords: apoptosis; cervical carcinogenesis; fermented mangosteen; HPV; IL-2; myeloperoxidase; nitric oxide metabolites; sFAS; TRAIL; TNF-alpha

1. Introduction

Human papillomavirus (HPV) is connected with virtually all cases of cervical cancer. The viral infection-associated chronic inflammation has been considered as a leading risk factor for carcinogenesis in humans [1–3]. It has been estimated that 15–20% of cancers worldwide are attributable to virus, bacteria, or parasite infections causing chronic inflammation [4]. One of the characteristic features of chronic inflammation is the long-lasting overproduction of reactive oxygen and nitrogen species (ROS and RNS, respectively) released by inflammatory, epithelial, and endothelial cells [5–7]. From one side, ROS and RNS play multiple essential roles in the innate immune response to infectious agents [8,9], as well as in metabolism and the elimination of mediators of inflammation [10]. On the other hand, their excess could negatively affect the normal structure and functions of host cells and tissues, thus creating conditions for endogenous mutagen formation [11] and/or carcinogenic transformations [11–13]. For example, oxidative and nitration/nitrosylation metabolites that are formed upon the interaction of DNA with ROS and RNS are either mutagenic [11] factors causing tumour progression [14] or can induce carcinogenesis through the activation of proto-oncogenes and the inactivation of tumour suppressor genes [15–17].

Oxidative imbalance has been clearly recognised as a promoting factor in HPV-initiated carcinogenesis [18]. For example, while the expression of thioredoxin reductase 2 and glutathione-S-transferase peaked, inducible nitric oxide synthase (iNOS) was progressively reduced in dysplastic and neoplastic cervical tissue. Applying a redox proteomic approach, De Marco et al. came to the conclusion that the HPV16 neoplastic progression of cervical cancer is associated with the oxidative modifications (carbonylation) of DNA and proteins involved in cell morphogenesis and terminal differentiation in dysplastic tissues. In contrast, cancer tissues were characterised by the selective reduction of carbonyl adducts on detoxifying/pro-survival proteins that reflected an improved control of oxidative alterations [18].

The cytokines of the tumour necrosis factor (TNF) ligand family, such as the cell surface death receptor (sFAS), TNF, and TNF-related apoptosis-inducing ligand (TRAIL), are well-known regulators of apoptosis through their corresponding receptors [Ryu]. TRAIL was first identified as an inducer of p53-independent apoptosis in a variety of tumour cell lines and in cervical cancer patients (reviewed in [19]).

There are several evolving preventive strategies that could substantially reduce the burden from cervical carcinoma by the elimination of etiological factors and the inhibition of its development. First of all, they include HPV vaccines, diets enriched in fruits and vegetables [20–23], food supplements [23,24], and other chemopreventive agents [25–30]. Major molecular and cellular pathways for non-medicinal anti-cervical carcinoma preparations target the elimination/diminishing of the load of existing high-risk HPV infection [30–32], the restoration of normal non-viral microbiota [33] and redox balance [25,31,34–38], anti-inflammatory action [21,39], cell cycle influencers, and pro-apoptotic effects towards infected tumour transformed cells [40,41].

One of the most promising candidates, possessing several of the indicated activities, is fermented mangosteen (*Garcinia mangostana* Linn., Guttiferae), a popular botanical food supplement sold in large quantities around the world. Although well-known in ethnopharmacology since ages past, mangosteen-based products have been only recently studied for their phytochemical content and biological activities. Thus, the widely claimed cancer chemopreventive and anti-cancer effects of fermented mangosteen (FM) have been mainly attributed to the xanthons, tannins, and polyphenols of this health dietary additive [42–45]. These biological actives are mainly concentrated in the pod (synonyms: pericarps or rinds) [46] and seeds, non-edible parts of this delicious fruit usually referred to as "the queen of fruits". The blue and purple colours of the rape mangosteen skin are associated with anthocyanines, resveratrol, quercetin, rutin, and ellargic acid, all of them known for numerous biological activities, including chemopreventive anti-cancer effects [26–28,40,41,47,48]. The white colour of the seed placenta, characteristic of the mangosteen pod, indicates the presence of beta-glucans and lignans with specific immunomodulating and anti-cancer actions, while the seed shells contain large amounts of lignins, which possess anti-cancer, anti-viral, and anti-microbial properties (reviewed in [49,50]). To increase the bioavailability of secondary plant metabolites encaged into the fibrous skin, mesopericarp, and seeds, they are subjected to a long-lasting controlled microbial and/or yeast fermentation.

Fermentation is the most ancient and the most natural way of plant food processing and preservation. During the fermentation (or external digestion) of plant parts, high molecular weight molecules, such as polysaccharides, glycolipids/glycoproteins, and nucleic acids of plant cell walls, seeds, peels, or pods, are decomposed to low molecular weight units (molecular moieties) that are readily absorbed through the gastrointestinal barrier and immediately available for a variety of metabolic processes [51]. Fermentation significantly enhances the cancer chemopreventive properties of non-fermented plants [52]. Moreover, fermented fruit preparations are enriched with the membrane fragments, lipoglycopeptide complexes, and exometabolites of fermenting yeasts and lactobacilli, probiotics that contribute to their immuno-modulating, nutritional, and physiological value [53,54]. Unfortunately, practically all research on the bioactivity of FM has been carried out in in vitro and ex vivo experiments, while clinical data are lacking.

The primary goal of the present study was the search for oxidative markers of HPV16- and HPV18-related cervical carcinogenesis and their possible connection with local and circulating ligands of TNF-alpha-induced apoptosis. In the first stage of the study, we found that the content of nitric oxide metabolites (nitrotyrosine and nitrates/nitrites) was significantly enhanced in the dysplastic cervical intraepithelial neoplasia (CIN) of different grades (CIN I and CIN II) groups, and the activity of MPO peaked in the invasive cervical cancer (CIN III) group.

Based on the results obtained, the placebo-controlled clinical trial on the clinical efficacy (the prevention and/or slowing down of carcinogenesis) of standardised FM gel, taken orally, was carried out. The secondary outcomes of the trial were oxidative and TNF-alpha-induced apoptosis ligand markers at systemic and cervical tissue levels in the practically healthy and the pre-cancerous CIN I and CIN II groups of female patients infected with HPV16/18, and in healthy females infected with low-risk HPV10/13.

2. Materials and Methods

2.1. Ethics Statement

All experiments with human material (blood, cervical biopsies, and cervical fluid) were carried out in accordance with the Helsinki Declaration, and the protocols of two clinical studies were reviewed and approved by the Ethical Committee of Berbekov's Kabardino-Balkar State Medical University, Nal'chik, Russia (Protocol No. 133-2/2018 of 21st November 2018). The recruited patients and the healthy age-matched female donors signed an informed consent form.

2.2. Clinical Study Design and Recruitment Criteria

Two clinical studies were conducted. The first was an observational trial aimed at identifying local tissue oxidative markers of papillomavirus (HPV)-connected cervical carcinogenesis and their possible connection with local and circulating ligands of TNF-alpha-induced apoptosis. During the period from January 2019 to December 2019, 196 women attending the Gynaecology Department of Kabardino-Balkar Berbekov's State University, Nal'chik, Russia, and presenting HPV infections of low (HPV10 and HPV13, n = 42; age range: 21-44 years) and high (HPV16 and HPV18, n = 154; for age range see Table 1) risk of cervical carcinogenesis, were recruited into the study after obtaining their informed consent. Fifteen age-matched females, not infected with HPV or other common viruses, such as cytomegalovirus (CMV) or herpes virus (HV1 and HV2), were invited to participate in the study as healthy controls. The demographic features, HPV infections, and clinical diagnoses of the participants in the first stage of the clinical observational study are collected in Table 1.

Table 1. Demographic and clinical data of women—participants in the observational study on the oxidative markers and TNF-alpha apoptosis ligands in HPV infections associated with cervical carcinogenesis.

Group	Number of Subjects	Age Range
HPV10, HPV13, healthy	42	21–44 year
HPV16, HPV18, CIN I + CIN II	75	24–45 year
HPV16, HPV18, CIN III	45	28–53 year
Healthy female controls	15	25–47 year

Women infected with HPV16 and HPV18 were diagnosed colposcopically and histologically on the basis of dysplastic lesions of different histological grades (n = 75; age range: 24–45 years; the pre-cancerous well-differentiated CIN I and moderately differentiated CIN II groups) or with clinically, histologically, and immunologically confirmed invasive cervical cancer (n = 45; age range: 28–53 years; the poorly differentiated CIN III group). The inclusion criteria were as follows: (a) patients older than 18 years; (b) not pregnant; (c) not infected with any other common viruses; (d) not bearing or have had any tumour apart from invasive cervical cancer in order to be included in the CIN III group; (e) not treated with any immune response-modulating or anti-viral drug for the last three months.

At the first visit, all participants were subjected to a full gynaecological examination. Cervical fluid containing ectopic cervical cells was collected and processed for cytological, immunological, and virological analyses. Biopsies were taken for standard histological evaluation, as well as for oxidative marker and apoptosis ligand assays. Of note, in the cases of dysplastic and neoplastic lesions, biopsies were taken from the area in a close vicinity (5 mm from the lesion border). All participants donated their venous blood for immunological analyses, as well. Any decision about the diagnostic procedures, treatment protocols, and follow-up period was based exclusively on the objective clinical picture, irrespective of any need of the observational trial.

Taking into account the outcome that several definite oxidative markers and TRAIL levels (in plasma and cervical fluid) corresponded to the severity of HPV-associated cervical dysplasia/neoplasia, we proceeded with a randomised, double-blind, placebo-controlled single-centre trial on the clinical efficacy and effects towards redox and apoptosis parameters of the FM food supplementation on HVP-infected patients with cervical dysplasia (CIN I and CIN II). A 5% honey solution in mineral water was used as the placebo. Females infected with HPV16 and HPV18 without clinical and colposcopic evidence of dysplasia (n = 152; age range: 25–45 years; practically healthy controls) and presenting clinical/colposcopic features of cervical dysplasia of different grades (CIN I or CIN II, n = 98; age range: 25–52 years) were invited to participate in the trial and signed informed consent forms. The inclusion criteria (a)–(c) and (e) were similar to those for the first observational clinical study. The criteria (d) were re-formulated as "not bearing or have had any tumour". One more criterium was added: (f) no antioxidant and mineral supplementation for at least three months before entry to the trial. During the period from January 2019 to November 2019, two hundred and fifty women were enrolled and randomly placed into four groups: Group 1—practically healthy, placebo (n = 70); Group 2—practically healthy, FM supplementation (n = 82); Group 3—CIN I and CIN II, placebo (n = 48); Group 4—CIN I and CIN II, FM supplementation (n = 50). All patients with clinical symptoms of dysplasia received surgical removal of lesions. All the participants were prescribed conventional anti-viral therapy per os and in vaginal lavages. The patients' demographic distribution and clinical data are summarised in Table 2.

Table 2. Demographic and clinical data of women—participants in placebo-controlled trial on the clinical efficacy, oxidative markers, and TNF-alpha ligand levels of fermented mangosteen (FM) supplementation.

Group	Number of Subjects	Age Range
HPV16, HPV18, no dysplasia	152	
Group 1—placebo	70	25–45 year
Group 2—fermented mangosteen (FM)	82	
HPV16, HPV18, CIN I + CIN II	98	
Group 3—placebo	48	25–52 year
Group 4—fermented mangosteen (FM)	50	
Healthy controls without viral infections	30	27–42 year

In addition, patients from Groups 2 and 4 received FM supplementation as a standardised syrup (14 mL × 2 times a day at meal time for three months). The patients assigned to Groups 1 and 3 received 5% honey diluted in mineral water (14 mL × 2 times a day at mealtime for three months). FM was kindly provided free of charge by Carica Ltd., Manila, the Philippines.

As positive controls, the serum and cervical fluid of 30 healthy age-matching females without serum antibodies to HPV, herpes simplex types I and II, and cytomegalovirus (CMV), as well as free of HPV and CNV DNA in the cervical fluid, were used.

2.3. Food Supplement in Question

Standardised syrup of fermented mangosteen (FM) manufactured by Carica Ltd. (Manila, the Philippines), approved as a food supplement and distributed locally and abroad, was a kind gift of the manufacturer. The FM was produced from fruits collected from wild (non-cultivars and non-genetically modified) species of tropical *Garcinia mangostana* Linn. grown in remote, non-industrial parts of the Philippines. In brief, pods of rape fruit were separated from the edible flesh, washed, and mashed. The mash underwent the process of controlled fermentation by a food-quality culture of *Saccharomyces cerevisia* yeasts and *Lactobaccilus casei* within a 6-month period. Controlled enzymatic splitting was reached due to the strictly regulated temperature, oxygen, and nutrient supply, as well as frequent in-process quality tests. The fermentation process was stopped by adding the honey of wild bees (5%), followed by pasteurisation at 55 °C and filtration under pressure. The final FM product was a sour-sweet thick gel that was reddish-brown in colour. Post-fermentation analyses showed a high concentration of phenolics, fruit acids (pH 5.2), unsaturated fatty acids, sitosterols, macroelements, such as calcium, magnesium, and potassium, and microelements, such as copper, zinc, and iron. The ready FM product was free from pathogenic microorganisms and toxic elements, i.e., Sr, As, and Pb.

2.4. Clinical Diagnosis

All participants were subjected to a scrupulous gynaecological examination. The extended colposcopy with a magnification ×15 was carried out by a Letsegang colposcope (Germany) with video registration in order to identify and register the state of cervical epithelia. The cytological screening of cells that were collected from eczo- and endo-cervices by a spatula was performed by a conventional Papanicolaou smear test (Pap smear test).

2.5. Viral Analyses

Different types of HPV were determined by a type-specific PCR assay, using corresponding primers [55–57]. Total RNA was isolated using the GenElute Mammalian Total RNA kit (Sigma-Aldrich, Milan, Italy) and was reverse-transcribed using the iScript cDNA Synthesis kit (Bio-Rad, Hercules, CA, USA). cDNA was amplified with IQ SYBR green Supermix (Bio-Rad, Hercules, CA, USA), using the MiniOpticon Real-Time PCR Detection System (Bio-Rad, Hercules, CA, USA).

Herpes (HSV1 and HSV2) and cytomegalovirus (CMV) infections were assessed by real-time PCR, using the following primers: HSV1 fwd: CCT-TCG-AAC-AGC-TCC-TGG; rev: ATG-ACG-CCG-ATG-TAC-TTT-TTC-TT. HSV2 fwd: TCC-ATT-TTC-GTT-TTG-TGC-CGG; rev: ATG-ACG-CCG-ATG-TAC-TTT-TTC-TT. CMV fwd: ATG-ACG-CCG-ATG-TAC-TTT-TTC-T; rev: 5′-ACT-GGT-CAG-CCT-TGC-TTC-TAG-TCA-CC [Fax].

2.6. Biological Material Sampling and Processing

2.6.1. Blood Sampling and Processing

Venous blood (6 mL) was taken into two hermetically sealed tubes and left for 1 h at room temperature for blood cell sedimentation. Serum was collected, aliquoted, and stored at −70 °C until the ELISA and PCR assays.

2.6.2. Cervical Tissue Sampling and Processing

Biopsies were taken for standard histological pathological evaluation, as well as for oxidative marker and apoptosis ligand assays, in a colposcopy-guided manner. Of note, in the cases of dysplastic and neoplastic lesions, biopsies were taken from the area in a close vicinity (5 mm from the lesion border). The biopsies were placed in an ice-cold 0.1 M potassium phosphate buffer (pH 7.4) and thoroughly homogenised. The homogenates were centrifuged at 900× *g* and +4 °C for 40 min. The supernatants were collected and stored at −80 °C until they were analysed. The protein content in the supernatants was determined by Lowry's method, which is described elsewhere.

2.6.3. Cervical Fluid Collecting and Processing

Fluid containing ectopic cervical cells was collected from the walls of the cervical channel after its opening by a spatula, was centrifuged at 230× *g* for 10 min, and then the supernatant was stored for immunological analyses. The cervical cell sediment was washed twice with a potassium phosphate buffer and used for differential counting with an automatic Coulter counter (Beckman Coulter Inc., High Wycombe, UK) and for the HPV type-specific PCR assay.

2.7. Assays for Oxidative Markers

2.7.1. Enzymatic Activities

The activities of pro- and antioxidant enzymes were measured by spectrophotometric methods: for MPO, the absorbance at 560 nm was recorded after the reaction with ortho-dianizidine; for catalase, the absorbance at 240 nm was recorded during the reaction with hydrogen peroxide; and for glutathione peroxidase, the absorbance at 412 nm was measured after the reaction with GSH in the presence of t-butyl peroxide. Homogenates were added to the reaction mixture at a concentration of 1 mg protein per mL, and the results were expressed in % of the control mixtures without homogenates.

2.7.2. Hydroxyl Radical Scavenging

Hydroxyl radical scavenging capacity was assessed by luminol-dependent chemiluminescence in a Fenton reaction. In brief, the reaction was initiated by the addition of 17.7 μM $FeSO_4$ to 0.01 M potassium phosphate buffer containing 17.7 μM hydrogen peroxide and 0.2 mM luminol. The integral square under the chemiluminescence spike was calculated and plotted against the value obtained in the absence of homogenate. The data were expressed in arbitrary units.

2.7.3. Nitrotyrosine Determination

The levels of nitrotyrosine were measured in accordance with methods described previously [58,59]. The supernatants were assayed for 3-nitrotyrosine using a Nitrotyrosine ELISA kit (Northwest/AMS Biotechnology, Manchester, UK), following the manufacturer's instructions. Briefly, the samples were incubated in the wells coated with a captured nitrotyrosine antibody and a biotinylated secondary tracer antibody. The addition of streptavidine-peroxidase, followed by tetra-methyl benzidine, resulted in colour development proportional to the nitrotyrosine levels, which were quantified spectrophotometrically at 450 nm. Total nitrate/nitrite levels were measured by Griess reaction using the analytical kit "Nitrate/nitrite Assay Kit Colorometric" (Sigma Co., Milan, Italy).

2.7.4. Isoprostane Determination

The isoprostane content in the cervical tissue was determined as described in [60]. The homogenates were prepared on ice and the supernatants were diluted with distilled and de-ionised water. The solutions were acidified to below pH 4.0 and used for the further determination of free 15-F2t-IsoP by enzyme immunoassay (EIA) (Northwest NWLSSTM). Briefly, 15-F2t-IsoP in the samples or standards was allowed to compete with 15-isoprostane F2t conjugated to horseradish peroxidase (HRP) for binding to a polyclonal antibody specific for 15-isoprostane F2t coated on a micro plate. Subsequent tetra-methyl benzidine additions resulted in a blue colour development that was inversely proportional to the quantity of 15-isoprostane F2t in the original samples or standards. After the addition of a stop solution, the absorbance was read at 450 nm.

2.8. Assays for Ligands of Apoptosis

The ligands of TNF-dependent apoptosis were quantitatively determined in serum, circulating leukocytes, cervical fluid, and cervical wall cells. The protein levels of sFAS, TRAIL, TNF-alpha, and IL-2 were measured by the ELISA method, using corresponding kits and following the manufacturer's instructions (BCM Diagnostics, Woodland, CA, USA).

Gene expression for sFAS and TRAIL in cervical biopsies was determined by quantitative real-time PCR, using TaqMan technology in accordance with the protocols of the European Anti-Cancer Program (EAC 2003). In brief, cervical tissue was soaked in an RNA-stabilising solution (RNA-later, Ambion, Austin, TX, USA) and stored at −20 °C for a period of not more than 3 months. The samples were homogenised on ice, and total RNA was isolated using an iPrepPureLink TM Total RNA kit (Invitrogen, Waltham, MA, USA). The primers for sFAS were: fwd: AAGCGGTTTACGAGTGACT; rev: TG-GTTCCAGGTATCTGCTTC [Itoh]. Primers for TRAIL were: fwd: TGAAATCGAAAGTAT-GTTTGGGAATAGATG; rev: TGACGAAGAGAGTATGA ACAGCCCCTGCTG [61,62].

2.9. Statistics

Statistical analysis was performed using the STATISTICA 6.0 program from StatSoft Inc. The reported values were treated as continuous. The normality of the data was checked using the Shapiro–Wilk test. Since the distribution of the data was significantly different from normal, non-parametric statistics were used. The results were expressed as the mean ± SD. In some cases, values were presented as median, lower and upper quartiles, and minimum and maximum. The Mann–Whitney U test was employed for comparison between independent groups of data. To evaluate the difference between connected data, the two-tailed Student's t-test was applied, and p values < 0.05 were considered to be significant.

Correlations between different oxidative markers, as well as between oxidative markers and ligands of TNF-alpha-induced apoptosis, were evaluated by the Pearson linear correlation coefficient. A p value < 0.05 was considered to be statistically significant. If necessary (comparison among three groups or more), p-values were adjusted for multiple comparisons, using the Bonferroni adjustment.

3. Results

3.1. Local Cervical Oxidative and Nitrosative Markers in HPV-Infected Female Patients at Different Stages of Cervical Carcinogenesis

The measurement of selected markers of oxidative and nitrosative stress in the cervical biopsies (Figure 1) revealed a significant increase in MPO activity in the CIN III group as compared to the CIN I-II HPV16/18 group, and to the low oncogenic HPV10/13 non-dysplastic group. The levels of nitrotyrosine were significantly reduced in the CIN III group as compared to the CIN I-II and the HPV10 and HPV13 groups.

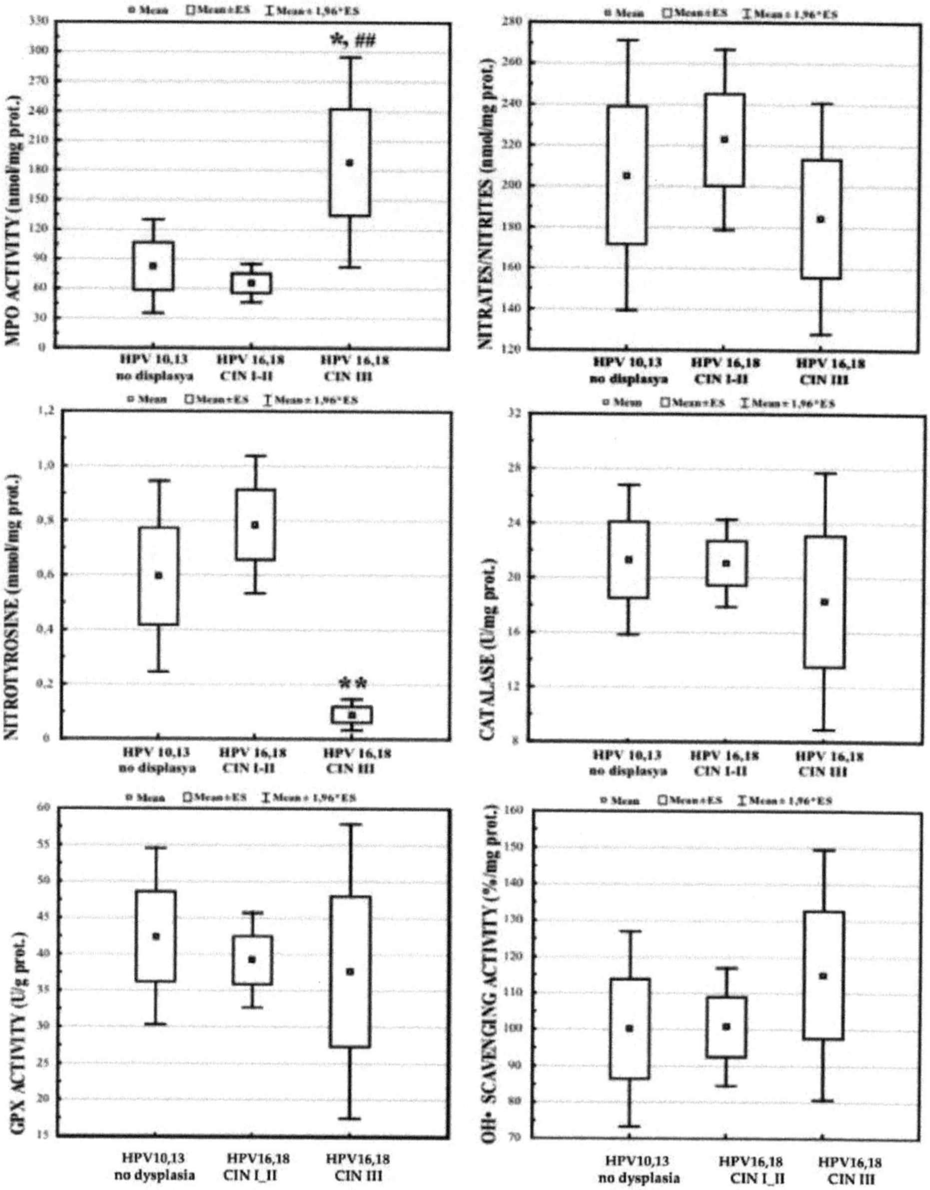

Figure 1. Markers of oxidative stress and antioxidant defence in cervical tissue of females infected with different types of human papillomavirus and at different stages of the disease. Sample size of groups: HPV10/13, n = 42; HPV16/18 CIN I and CIN II, n = 75; HPV16/18 CIN III, n = 45. * $p < 0.05$ versus HPV10/13 group; ## $p < 0.05$ versus HPV16/18 CIN I-II group; ** $p < 0.01$ versus HPV10/13 and HPV16/18 CIN I-II groups.

In the CIN I-II group, a strongly significant ($p < 0.01$) negative correlation between nitrotyrosine and MPO activity levels was found, as well as a positive significant ($p < 0.05$) correlation between nitrate/nitrite levels and nitrotyrosine, as shown in Figure 2.

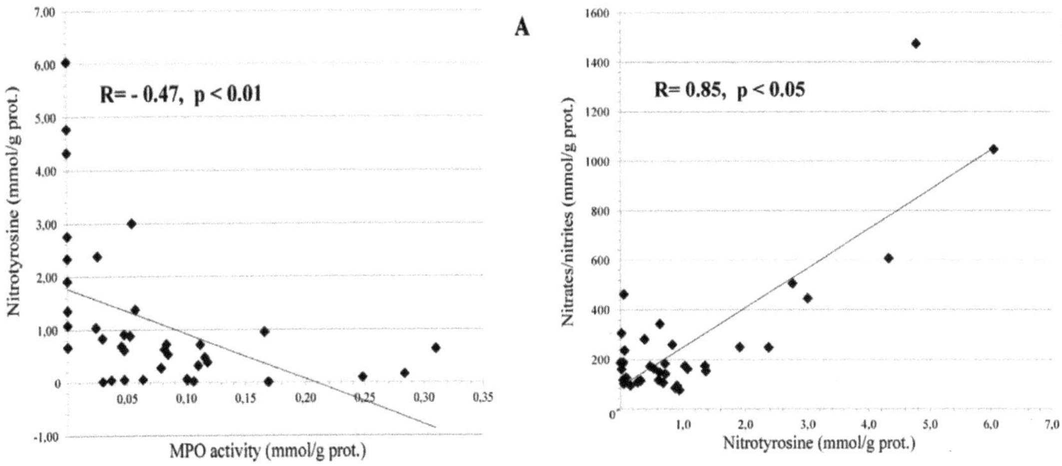

Figure 2. Correlations between redox parameters in cervical tissue of HPV-infected females with CIN I and CIN II (n = 75). (**A**) Correlation between MPO activity and nitrotyrosine content; (**B**) correlation between nitrotyrosine and nitrate/nitrite levels.

3.2. Cervical and Circulating Ligands of TNF-Alpha Apoptosis in HPV-Infected Female Patients at Different Stages of Cervical Carcinogenesis

The data on TNF-alpha-induced apoptosis ligands in the serum and the cervical fluid are shown in Figure 3. The TRAIL levels were found significantly ($p < 0.01$) reduced in the cervical fluid of the HPV16 and HPV18 groups, both with CINI-II dysplasia and with CIN III cancerous lesions. Non-significant changes could be observed among the study groups for the TNF-alpha and sFAS ligands. The analysis of the serum levels of the circulating ligands of TNF-alpha-induced apoptosis revealed significant differences between the CIN I-II dysplastic group and both the healthy donors and the low oncogenic HPV-infected groups for sFAS, IL-2, and TRAIL ($p < 0.05$), and even more marked ($p < 0.01$) in the case of TNF-alpha. The difference versus healthy donors was highly significant ($p < 0.01$) for all ligands in the CIN III group.

At the same time, the analysis of the mRNA expression of sFAS and TRAIL in cervical tissue (biopsies) showed a significant ($p < 0.01$) decrease in the expression of sFAS in the groups infected with high oncogenic HPV strains, both without dysplasia and with CIN I-II, as well as a marked ($p < 0.01$) reduction in TRAIL mRNA expression in the CIN I-II pre-cancerous group (Figure 4).

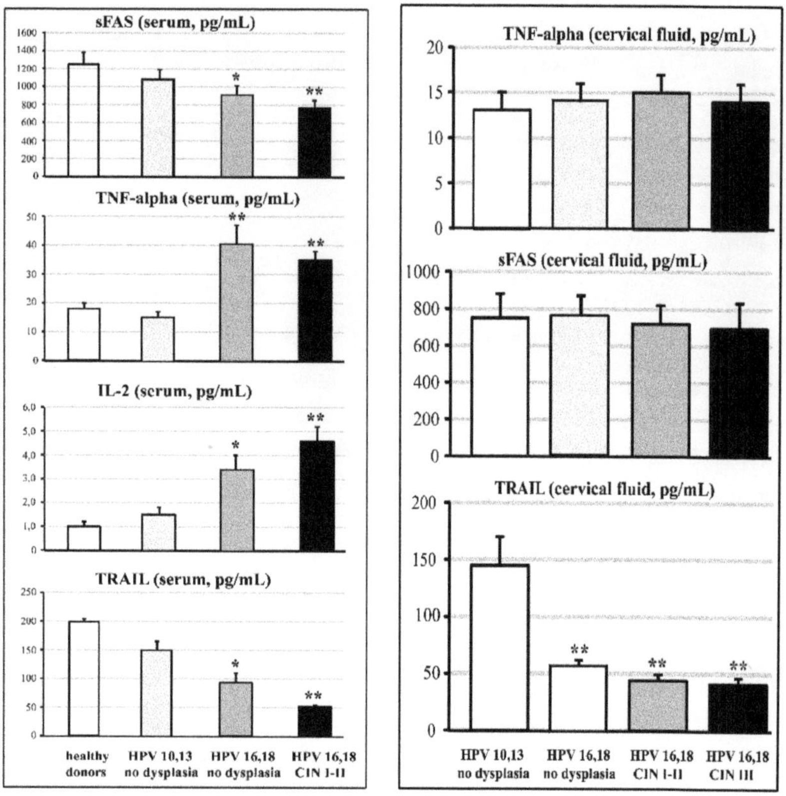

(a) (b)

Figure 3. Serum (**a**) and cervical (**b**) ligands of TNF-alpha-induced apoptosis in females at different stages of HPV-associated carcinogenesis. Sample size of groups: HPV 10/13, n = 42; HPV 16/18 and healthy, n = 152; HPV 16/18 CIN I and CIN II, n = 75; healthy donors, n = 15. * $p < 0.05$ vs. healthy donors and low oncogenic HPV infection; ** $p < 0.01$ vs. healthy donors and low oncogenic HPV infection.

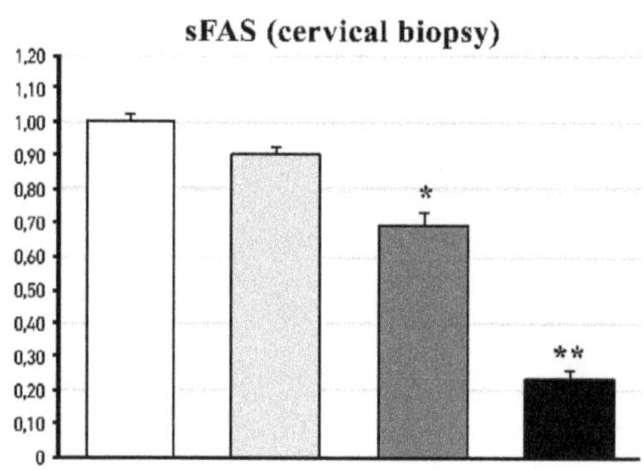

Figure 4. *Cont.*

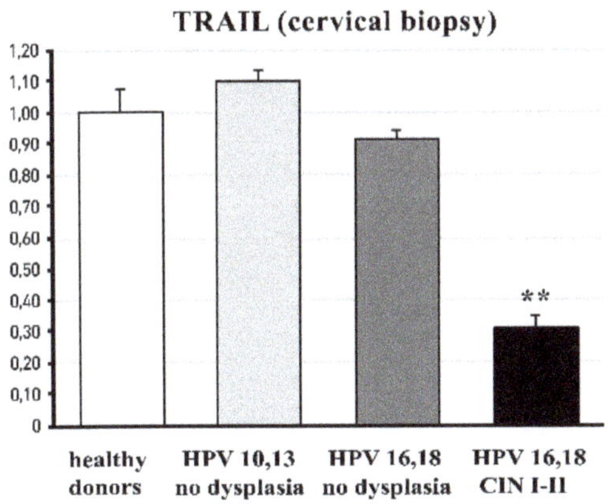

Figure 4. sFAS and TRAIL mRNA expression (arbitrary units) in cervical biopsies of females with HPV infection and of healthy donors. Sample size of groups: HPV 10/13, n = 42; HPV 16/18 and healthy, n = 152; HPV 16/18 CIN I and CIN II, n = 75; healthy donors, n = 15. * $p < 0.05$ ** $p < 0.01$ vs. healthy donors, and low and highly oncogenic HPV infection.

3.3. *Effects of FM Supplementation on Macro-Histological Symptoms of Cervical Dysplasia*

The post-trial colposcopic examination revealed normal patterns in 100% of the FM group versus 62% of the placebo group. A sample of macro-histological effects of FM supplementation is shown on Figure 5, where the (a) panel photos were taken in the beginning of the trial, and the panel (b) photos were taken at the cessation of it. Before the administration of FM, ectopic transformed areas, squamous cell metaplasia, and mosaics marked by the iodine-negative areas were evident. After a three-month course of FM, we observed normal tissue basis, the shrinkage of iodine-negative areas, and cervical coagulation. Inflammatory cells in cervical fluid were found in 21% of the FM group versus 40% of the placebo group.

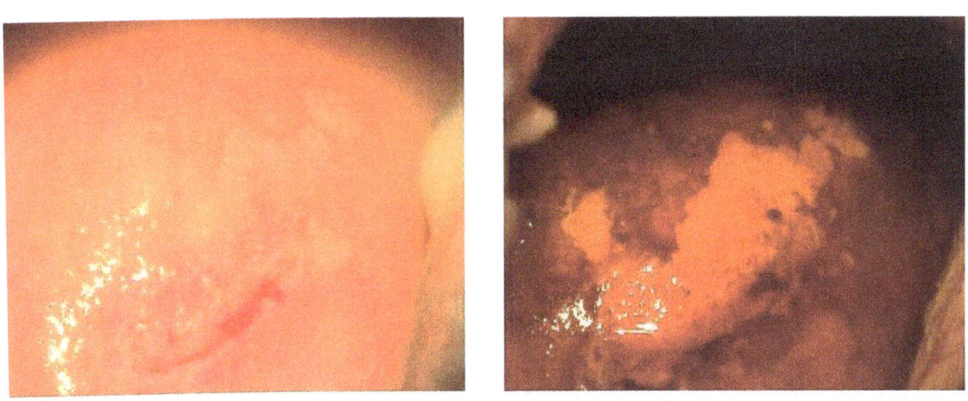

(a)

Figure 5. *Cont.*

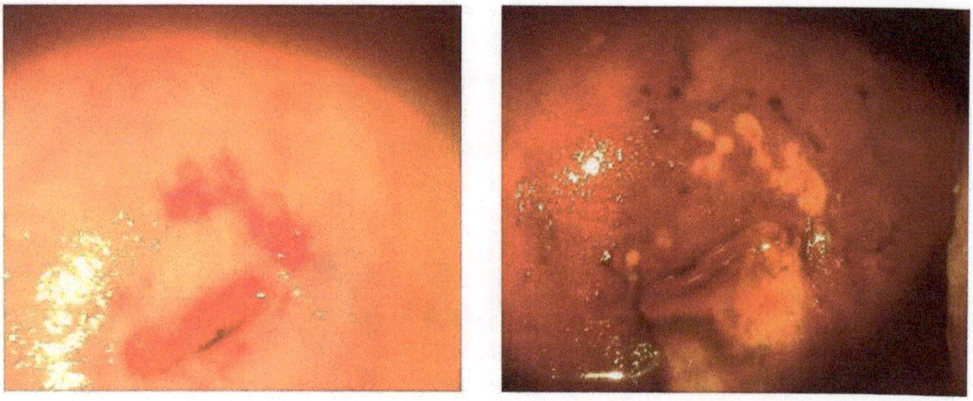

(b)

Figure 5. Typical colposcopy of CIN I and CIN II lesions before (**a**) and after (**b**) administration of antioxidants. (**a**) Before administration of antioxidants (ectopic transformed areas, squamous cell metaplasia, and mosaics marked by the iodine-negative areas). (**b**) After a three-month course of antioxidants (normal tissue basis, shrinkage of iodine-negative areas, and cervical coagulation). **Left** panels are colposcopic images without iodine staining. **Right** panels are colposcopic images after iodine staining.

3.4. Effects of FM Supplementation on Oxidative and Nitrosative Markers in Cervical Tissue

The cervical tissue markers of oxidative and nitrosative stress appeared to be selectively modified by the FM treatment of the CIN I-II patients (Table 3). After 3 months, MPO activity was significantly ($p < 0.01$) decreased, as well as nitrate/nitrite and nitrotyrosine levels ($p < 0.05$). Catalase activity showed a trend toward reduction, whilst isoprostane and GSH-peroxidase differences, before and after FM treatment, were not detected at the cervical level.

Table 3. Oxidative markers in cervical tissue of CIN I and CIN II patients (n = 50) treated with fermented mangosteen for 3 months. * $p < 0.05$; ** $p < 0.01$.

Marker	Before Treatment	After Treatment
Myeloperoxidase, nmol/mg	76 ± 12	5.9 ± 1.3 **
Nitrates/Nitrites, nmol/mg	207 ± 18	147 ± 30 *
Catalase, U/mg	20 ± 1.8	15 ± 3
Isoprostanes, ng/mg	1.1 ± 0.2	0.9 ± 0.2
Nitrotyrosine, nmol/mg	1.1 ± 0.2	0.5 ± 0.3 *

3.5. Effects of Fermented Mangosteen Supplementation on Systemic and Topical (Cervical) Ligands of TNF-Alpha Apoptosis

The results of the three-month-long course of FM supplementation are collected in Figures 6 and 7. The FM treatment remarkably affected circulating ligands of TNF-alpha-induced apoptosis in both experimental groups with HPV16- and HPV18-infected females, with or without clinical features of cervical carcinogenesis. In these groups, highly enhanced serum levels of TNF-alpha and IL-2 went down to normal values (Figure 6B,C).

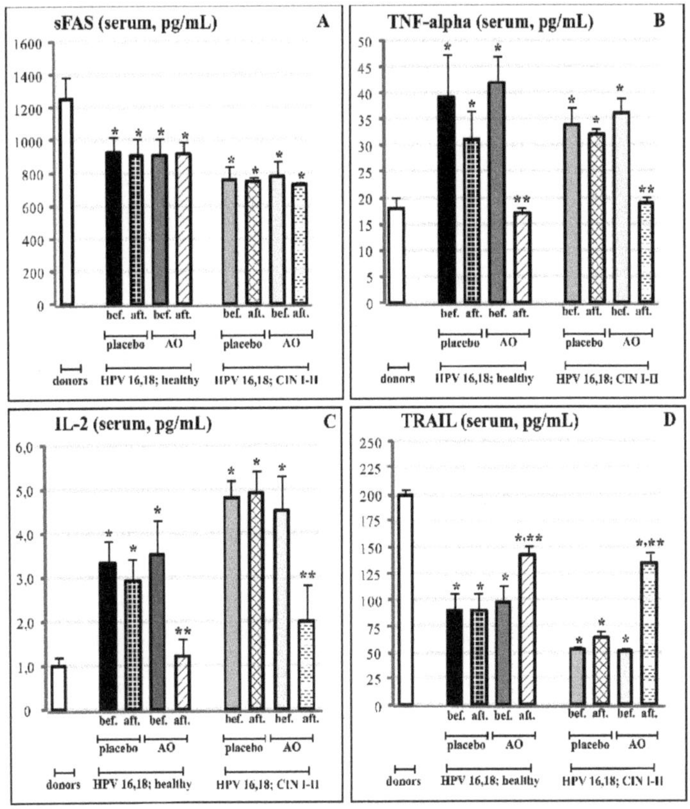

Figure 6. Effects of FM supplementation (AO) or placebo on serum content of the apoptosis ligands (**A**—sFAS; **B**—TNF-alpha; **C**—IL-2; **D**—TRAIL) in groups of practically healthy HPV16- and HPV18-infected females (n = 152), and in groups of HPV16- and HPV18-infected females with pre-cancerous cervical lesions (CIN I and CIN II) (n = 98). * $p < 0.05$ vs. donors; ** $p < 0.05$ vs. before treatment.

At the same time, strongly suppressed serum content of TRAIL was statistically significantly restored, although TRAIL levels did not reach the normal values (Figure 6D). The FM supplementation did not induce any significant change in circulating sFAS ligands; we also did not observe any effects on circulating ligands in both placebo groups (Figure 6A).

Regarding the cervical levels of the same ligands, the course of FM, and not of the placebo, led to the statistically significant enhancement of TRAIL, while, again, it did not affect suppressed levels of sFAS (Figure 7A,D). At the cervical level, the background concentrations of TNF-alpha and IL-2 did not differ in HPV-infected females with and without pre-cancerous lesions. They remained within the background range after the cessation of the clinical trial with FM (Figure 7B,C).

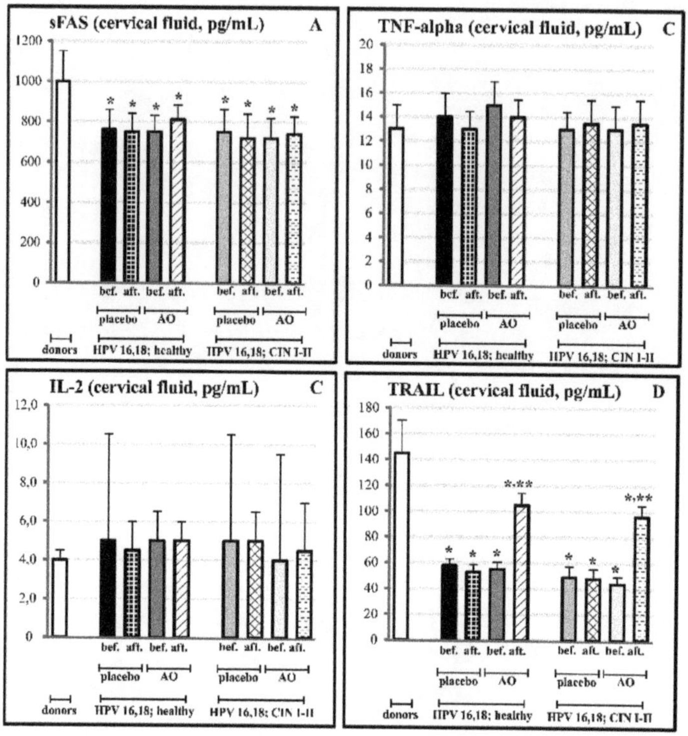

Figure 7. Effects of fermented mangosteen (FM) supplementation on cervical fluid content of the apoptosis ligands (**A**—sFAS; **B**—TNF-alpha; **C**—IL-2; **D**—TRAIL) in groups of practically healthy HPV16- and HPV18-infected females (n = 152) and in groups of HPV16- and HPV18-infected females with pre-cancerous cervical lesions (CIN I and CIN II) (n = 98). * $p < 0.05$ vs. donors; ** $p < 0.05$ vs. before trial.

4. Discussion

Clinical and epidemiological studies have revealed that certain pathogens causing persistent infections and chronic inflammation were associated with cancer [1,9,63]. The oncogenic action seems to be induced, maintained, and mediated by chronic inflammation and/or by alterations in host cells caused by the microbial genome [9,64]. Here, we observed (Figure 1) two molecular markers of chronic inflammation, MPO and nitrotyrosine, which were significantly changed in the cervical fluid of the females with cervical cancer (CIN III). As expected, there was a strong positive correlation between NO_2^-/NO_3^- and nitrotyrosine, the latter being formed under nitration of the amino acid by these nitrative species (Figure 2A). At the same time, we found a quite significant negative correlation between MPO and nitrotyrosine (Figure 2B). Human granulocytes release MPO from intra-cytoplasmic granules being challenged by microbes or viruses [17]. At the same time, they contain very low levels of inducible nitric oxide synthase [14]. Hence, they do not generate reactive nitrogen species intracellularly [65]. Instead, human granulocytes are likely to use nitrite (NO_2^-) from other sources, thus forming nitrating oxidants and, as a consequence, nitrotyrosine in the extracellular environment [13]. Nitrating oxidants are implicated in the host defence and pathogenesis of many diseases [13,15,16]. Nitrative stress contributes to asbestos-induced carcinogenesis [10] through myeloperoxidase (MPO), which plays a crucial role in the asbestos-derived inflammatory response and following asbestos-induced carcinogenesis [11–13]. In the cystic fibrosis airways, MPO acts as a phagocyte-derived NO oxidase that diminishes NO bioavailability and, consequently, its immune protective (anti-bacterial and anti-viral) and anti-inflammatory properties [66]. On these grounds, it has been suggested that MPO could be a target for therapeutic intervention to attenuate the oxidative burden and preserve essential physiological functions of NO. The inflammatory environment in HPV-infected cervical tissue provides all the factors necessary for the generation of nitrating agents by MPO, granulocyte invasion, and a high local level of NO_2^- [13,15,16].

Irreversible tyrosine modifications by inflammatory oxidants such as peroxynitrite include the formation of characteristic markers 3-nitrotyrosine and 3,3′-dityrosine [67,68]. These modifications of critical tyrosine residues in proteins inactivate a variety of enzymes [67] and affect their structures [69]. Of great importance, tyrosine nitration may interfere with signal transduction pathways involving both the kinase-dependent and auto-phosphorylation of tyrosine. Thus, in epidermoid carcinoma cells, tyrosine nitration altered the epidermal growth factor receptor (EGFR) activation through irreversible dimerisation [70]. An alteration of EGFR-mediated signalling pathways in epithelial cells would inevitably affect cell proliferation or differentiation, which may bear implications on carcinogenesis [71–73].

Solid tumours (human gastric, colorectal, cervical, and bronchoalveolar carcinomas, as well as epithelial ovarian cancer) frequently contain inflammatory cells, such as neutrophils, macrophages, and T-lymphocytes [74–77]. Their recruitment is mainly explained by C-X-C chemokines, namely IL-8 (a potent chemoattractant for neutrophils) or C-C chemokines (MCP-1) [63]. The inflammatory cells recruited to tumours become an important additional source of the chemokines [14]; thus, a vicious cycle is formed. It is well-established that activated neutrophils induce prolonged DNA damage in neighbouring cells [78], mainly through the genotoxic effects of ROS and RNS [79,80]. These species are widely recognised as key carcinogenic agents, causing tumour transformation, progression, and metastasis.

As per comprehensive review [81], HPV-encoded intracellular proteins can reshape signalling pathways in a mode that facilitates carcinogenesis through escaping immune surveillance and the impairment of TRAIL-mediated apoptosis. In the present study, we found that circulating levels of two cytokines (TNF-alpha and IL-2) and two ligands (sFAS and TRAIL) contributing to TRAIL-mediated apoptosis were significantly compromised versus normal values in females infected by highly oncogenic HPV forms without any symptoms of cervical pre-cancerous lesions as yet (Figure 3A). The impairment was aggravated in females with pre-cancerous CIN I and CIN II stages, while no differences were seen between healthy non-infected HPV females and those infected by low-risk HPV 10,13. When TNF-alpha, sFAS, and TRAIL proteins were measured in the cervical fluid, there were no differences between groups in the content of sFAS and TNF-alpha; however, local levels of TRAIL were dramatically diminished in all HPV16/18-infected groups of females (with no lesions, CIN I-II, and CIN-III stages) (Figure 3B). At the level of mRNA for sFAS and TRAIL in cervical tissue, the remarkable suppression of both was observed in the group with pre-cancerous states (CIN I-II). In the groups with no dysplasia, infected either by low- or high-risk HPV, mRNA expression was practically at normal levels.

A new approach to target and kill circulating tumour cells has been proposed recently [82]. The method is based on the coating of circulating leukocytes with liposomes loaded by TRAIL. The coated leukocytes could be considered as "un-natural killer cells", because they resemble natural killers activated by IL-2, which overexpresses TRAIL to attack and induce apoptosis in cancer cells. Applying the immunohistochemical approach, Carrero and co-authors [77] showed that in the advanced stage of pre-malignant lesions of the cervix, a progressive stage-dependent CD3/VEGF-positive lymphocyte infiltration correlated with the increased number of superoxide-producing cells, while tissue levels of nitrites and nitrates remained unchanged. However, in this work, only 16% of patients with CIN were infected with HPV; hence, one cannot estimate the impact of oxidative stress on virus-associated carcinogenesis.

Nutritional paradigms and dietary active components in the chemoprevention of carcinogenesis and in the potentiation of anti-cancer therapies have drawn a lot of attention recently (reviewed in [9,20–25]). Resveratrol has been shown to potentiate the apoptotic effects of TRAIL and other death cytokines, as well as chemotherapeutic agents and gamma irradiation [47,83,84]. On these grounds, a novel strategy to enhance the efficacy of TRAIL-targeting chemoprevention/therapies has been suggested. However, recent publications raised serious concerns about the feasibility of resveratrol in anti-cancer therapy and possibly in cancer chemoprevention due to its poor pharmacokinetics, low potency, and nephrotoxicity [84]. The publication of our group [85] clearly showed the strong phototoxicity of resveratrol, which is widely promoted for the prevention of UV-induced skin tumours. The anti-proliferative effect of the dietary anti-carcinogenic compound phenyl ethyl isothiocyanate in human cancer stem cells, derived from the human cervical tumour-derived HeLa cell line, partially resulted from the up-regulation of death receptors DR4 and DR5 of the TRAIL-mediated apoptotic pathway [86]. The dietary substances cucurbitacins, glycosylated triterpenes [87], luteolin [88], and epigallocatechin gallate [89] have been shown to regulate DNA repair systems and TRAIL-driven signalling in a number of cancer cells.

FM has been suggested as an effective chemopreventive/anti-cancer dietary product on the basis of phytochemical analyses [42], the in vitro and in vivo experiments [40,43–45] showing that its active components, such as polyphenols, terpenes, and xanthons, acted by different mechanisms, i.e., mTOR, deranged cell cycle, autophagy, and p53-dependent apoptosis. Direct antioxidant effects have been shown, as well [44,45]. Clinical data on the anti-cancer or cancer chemopreventive efficacy are completely lacking. In the present placebo-controlled clinical study, we showed, for the first time, that a 3-month-long supplementation with FM in females infected by HPV16/18 of high oncogenic risk, with the first symptoms of cancerous dysplasia (CIN I-II), resulted in the normalisation of macro-histological patterns in cervical tissue (100% of patients) and diminished the invasion of inflammatory neutrophils into the cervix (Figure 5). Along with the observed clinical efficacy, FM supplementation significantly suppressed the MPO presence, nitrative agents NO_2^-/NO_3^-, and nitrotyrosine in cervical tissue (Table 3). All these species are known for their carcinogenic action (see above). The most impressive findings were on the effects of FM supplementation on the TRAIL protein, circulating as well as localised, in the cervical fluid (Figures 6 and 7). This TNF-alpha-related apoptosis-inducing ligand, an inducer of cancer cell apoptosis through death receptors [84], was initially greatly suppressed in HPV16/18-infected females without symptoms of dysplasia; gradually, its suppression became deeper in HPV16/18-induced cervical dysplasia (CIN I and CIN II) and cervical cancer (CIN III) (Figure 4). Supplementation with FM, and not with the placebo, led to the significant restoration of circulating and local TRAIL levels. Unusually low TRAIL levels in the cervical fluid in the beginning of the study were not accompanied by any significant change in the three other cytokines and ligands (TNF-alpha, IL-2, and sFAS), while the circulating TNF-alpha and IL-2 in serum were highly increased in all HPV16/18-infected females with or without signs of pre-cancer. That, in our opinion, could reflect the generalised chronic inflammatory response to viral infection. Of great importance, FM supplementation completely normalised the circulating levels of both pro-inflammatory cytokines, thus diminishing the burden from chronic inflammation.

On the grounds of the results described here and the literature data, we assumed that FM could exert preventive effects on HPV-induced cervical cancer through several pathways, where one or another of its numerous active ingredients could:

- theoretically diminish the load of high-risk HPV [28];
- regulate neutrophil chemotaxis and the degranulation of MPO-containing granules at sites where the virus is harboured;
- increase the bioavailability of NO to fight viruses that would also lead to diminished levels of potentially carcinogenic nitrative agents and nitrotyrosine;
- down-regulate the overexpression of inflammatory cytokines involved in chronic general inflammation;
- deeply affect TRAIL-related events, such as the apoptosis of HPV-infected cells, preventing them from cancerous transformation;

- the presence of numerous active compounds derived from the plant and fermenting microbes in the natural matrix of FM could attenuate their potential individual toxicity, increase bioavailability, and exhibit a synergy between them.

5. Conclusions

Our findings indicate that FM, in combination with anti-viral therapy, could prevent or slow down HPV-associated cervical carcinogenesis, mainly through the suppression of leukocyte recruitment into infected tissue, suppression of general virus-associated chronic inflammation, and restoration of nitric oxide metabolite-initiated TRAIL-dependent apoptosis.

Much more research is needed to elucidate the mechanism(s) of FM's cancer-preventive effects. There are still many critical issues in the wide acceptance of fermented fruits as remedies for health problems, such as the lack of reliable clinical evidence, as well as scarce data on individual active components in fermented fruits and on the molecular mechanisms of their cancer chemopreventive effects. There is also an urgent need to optimise/standardise technologies of fermentation and to develop drugs based on the actives of fermented products.

Author Contributions: Conceptualization, Z.K., P.T. and L.K.; methodology, Z.K., I.T., G.I. and J.C.; software, P.T. and W.M.; validation, Z.K., C.D.L. and I.T.; formal analysis, P.T. and C.D.L.; investigation, I.T., G.I. and J.C.; resources, W.M. and L.K.; data curation, P.T. and J.C.; writing—original draft preparation, L.K.; writing—review and editing, W.M. and J.C.; visualization, C.D.L., P.T. and I.T.; supervision, L.K.; project administration, Z.K.; funding acquisition, I.T. and L.K. All authors have read and agreed to the published version of the manuscript.

Funding: This research received no external funding. The APC was shouldered by Fame Team Internat., Hong Kong, PRC.

Institutional Review Board Statement: The study was conducted in accordance with the Declaration of Helsinki and was approved by the Local Ethics Committee (Berbekov's Kabardino-Balkar State Medical University, Nal'chik, Russia), Protocol No. 133-2/2018 of 21 November 2018 for studies involving humans.

Informed Consent Statement: Informed consent was obtained from all subjects involved in the study.

Data Availability Statement: The data can be shared upon request.

Acknowledgments: The authors are grateful to Fame Team Ltd. (Hong Kong, PRC) for covering the publication costs and to Carica Ltd., Manila, the Philippines, for providing fermented mangosteen syrup (BioRex Mangosteen) free of charge.

Conflicts of Interest: The authors declare no conflict of interest.

References

1. Coussens, L.M.; Werb, Z. Inflammation and cancer. *Nature* **2002**, *420*, 860–867. [CrossRef]
2. Kawanishi, S.; Hiraku, Y. Oxidative and nitrative DNA damage as biomarker for carcinogenesis with special reference to inflammation. *Antioxid. Redox Signal.* **2006**, *8*, 1047–1058. [CrossRef] [PubMed]
3. Murata, M.; Thanan, R.; Ma, N.; Kawanishi, S. Role of nitrative and oxidative DNA damage in inflammation-related carcinogenesis. *J. Biomed. Biotechnol.* **2012**, *2012*, 623019. [CrossRef] [PubMed]
4. IARC. Chronic infections. In *World Cancer Report*; Stewart, B.W., Kleihues, P., Eds.; IARC Press: Lyon, France, 2008; pp. 128–135.
5. Schetter, A.J.; Heegaard, N.Y.; Harris, C.C. Inflammation and cancer: Interweaving microRNA, free radical, cytokine and p53 pathways. *Carcinogenesis* **2010**, *31*, 37–49. [CrossRef]
6. Ohnishi, S.; Ma, N.; Thanan, R.; Pinloar, S.; Hammam, O.; Murata, M.; Kawanishi, S. DNA damage in inflammation-related carcinogenesis and cancer stem cells. *Oxid. Med. Cell. Longev.* **2013**, *2013*, 387014. [CrossRef] [PubMed]
7. Lala, P.K.; Chakraborty, C. Role of nitric oxide in carcinogenesis and tumour progression. *Lancet Oncol.* **2001**, *2*, 149–156. [CrossRef]
8. Fukumura, D.; Kashiwagi, S.; Jain, R.K. The role of nitric oxide in tumour progression. *Nat. Rev. Cancer* **2006**, *6*, 521–534. [CrossRef]
9. De Luca, C.; Kharaeva, Z.; Korkina, L. Is there a role for antioxidants in the prevention of infection-associated carcinogenesis and in the treatment of infection-driven tumors? *Curr. Top. Med. Chem.* **2015**, *15*, 120–135. [CrossRef]

10. Haegens, A.; Van Der Vliet, A.; Butnor, K.J.; Heintz, N.; Taatjes, D.; Hemenway, D.; Vacek, P.; Freeman, B.A.; Hazen, S.L.; Brennan, M.L.; et al. Asbestos-induced lung inflammation and epithelial cell proliferation are altered in myeloperoxidase-null mice. *Cancer Res.* **2005**, *65*, 9670–9677. [CrossRef]
11. Eiserich, J.P.; Hristova, M.; Cross, C.E.; Jones, A.D.; Freeman, B.A.; Halliwell, B.; van der Vliet, A. Formation of nitric oxide-derived inflammatory oxidants by myeloperoxidase in neutrophils. *Nature* **1998**, *39*, 393–397. [CrossRef]
12. Van Der Vliet, A.; Eiserich, J.P.; Shigenaga, M.K.; Cross, C.E. Reactive nitrogen species and tyrosine nitration in the respiratory tract: Epiphenomena or a pathobiologic mechanism of disease? *Am. J. Respir. Crit. Care Med.* **1999**, *160*, 1–9. [CrossRef] [PubMed]
13. Gaut, J.P.; Byun, J.; Tran, H.D.; Lauber, W.M.; Carroll, J.A.; Hotchkiss, R.S.; Belaaouaj, A.; Heinecke, J.W. Myeloperoxidase produces nitrating oxidants in vivo. *J. Clin. Investig.* **2002**, *109*, 1311–1319. [CrossRef] [PubMed]
14. Sandhu, J.K.; Privora, H.F.; Wenckebach, G.; Birnboim, H.C. Neutrophils, nitric oxide synthase, and mutations in the mutatect murine tumor model. *Am. J. Pathol.* **2000**, *156*, 509–518. [CrossRef]
15. Nathan, C.; Shiloh, M.U. Reactive oxygen and nitrogen intermediates in the relationship between mammalian hosts and microbial pathogens. *Proc. Natl. Acad. Sci. USA* **2000**, *97*, 8841–8848. [CrossRef]
16. Ishiropoulos, H. Biological tyrosine nitration: A pathophysiological function of nitric oxide and reactive oxygen species. *Arch. Biochem. Biophys.* **1998**, *356*, 1–11. [CrossRef]
17. Klebanoff, S.J.; Nathan, C.F. Nitrite production by stimulated human polymorphonuclear leukocytes supplemented with azide and catalase. *Biochem. Biophys. Res. Commun.* **1993**, *197*, 192–196. [CrossRef]
18. De Marco, F.; Bucaj, E.; Foppoli, C.; Fiorini, A.; Blarzino, C.; Filipi, K.; Giorgi, A.; Schinina, M.E.; Di Domenico, F.; Coccia, R.; et al. Oxidative stress in HPV-driven viral carcinogenesis: Redox proteomics analysis of HPV-16 dysplastic and neoplastic tissues. *PLoS ONE* **2012**, *7*, e34366. [CrossRef]
19. Ryu, H.S.; Chang, K.H.; Chang, S.J.; Kim, M.S.; Joo, H.J.; Oh, K.S. Expression of TRAIL (TNF-related apoptosis-inducing ligand) receptors in cervical cancer. *Int. J. Gynecol. Cancer* **2000**, *10*, 417–424. [CrossRef]
20. Chih, H.J.; Lee, A.H.; Colville, L.; Binns, C.W.; Xu, D. A review of dietary prevention of human papillomavirus-related infection of the cervix and cervical intraepithelial neoplasia. *Nutr. Cancer* **2013**, *65*, 317–328. [CrossRef]
21. Patra, S.; Pradhan, B.; Nayak, R.; Behera, C.; Das, S.; Patra, S.K.; Efferth, T.; Jena, M.; Bhutia, S.K. Dietary polyphenols in chemoprevention and synergistic effect in cancer: Clinical evidences and molecular mechanisms of action. *Phytomedicine* **2021**, *90*, 153554. [CrossRef]
22. Ono, A.; Koshiyama, M.; Nakagawa, M.; Watanabe, Y.; Ikuta, E.; Seki, K.; Oowaki, M. The Preventive Effect of Dietary Antioxidants on Cervical Cancer Development. *Medicina* **2020**, *56*, 604. [CrossRef]
23. Park, S.-H.; Kim, M.; Lee, S.; Jung, W.; Kim, B. Therapeutic potential of natural products in treatment of cervical cancer: A review. *Nutrients* **2021**, *13*, 154. [CrossRef]
24. Koshiyama, M. The effects of the dietary and nutrient intake on gynecological cancers. *Healthcare* **2019**, *7*, 88. [CrossRef]
25. Di Domenico, F.; Foppoli, C.; Coccia, R.; Perluigi, M. Antioxidants in cervical cancer: Chemopreventive and chemotherapeutic effects of polyphenols. *Biochim. Biophys. Acta* **2012**, *1822*, 737–747. [CrossRef]
26. Morosetti, G.; Criscuolo, A.A.; Santi, F.; Perno, C.F.; Piccione, E.; Ciotti, M. Ellagic acid and Annona muricata in the chemoprevention of HPV-related pre-neoplastic lesions of the cervix. *Oncol. Lett.* **2017**, *13*, 1880–1884. [CrossRef]
27. Einbond, L.S.; Zhou, J.; Wu, H.; Mbazor, E.; Song, G.; Balik, M.; DeVoti, J.A.; Redenti, S.; Castellanos, M.R. A novel cancer preventative botanical mixture, TriCurin, inhibits viral transcripts and the growth of W12 cervical cells. harbouring extrachromosomal or integrated HPV16 DNA. *Br. J. Cancer* **2021**, *124*, 901–913. [CrossRef]
28. Polansky, H.; Itzkovitz, E.; Javaherian, A. Human papillomavirus (HPV): Systemic treatment with Gene-Eden-VIR/Novirin safely and effectively clears virus. *Drug Des. Dev. Ther.* **2017**, *11*, 575. [CrossRef]
29. Dretcanu, G.; Iuhas, C.I.; Diaconeasa, Z. Involvement of natural polyphenols in the chemoprevention of cervical cancer. *Int. J. Mol. Sci.* **2021**, *22*, 8812. [CrossRef]
30. Rock, C.L.; Michael, C.W.; Reynolds, R.K.; Ruffin, M.T. Prevention of cervix cancer. *Crit. Rev. Oncol. Hematol.* **2000**, *33*, 169–185. [CrossRef]
31. Williams, V.M.; Filippova, M.; Filippov, V.; Payne, K.J.; Duerlsen-Hughes, P. Human papillomavirus type 16 E6* induces oxidative stress and DNA damage. *J. Virol.* **2014**, *88*, 6751–6761. [CrossRef]
32. Cherry, J.J.; Rietz, A.; Malinkevich, A.; Liu, Y.; Xie, M.; Bartolowitz, M.; Jo Davisson, V.; Jo Davisson, V.; Baleja, J.D.; Androphy, E.J. Structure based identification and characterization of flavonoids that disrupt human papillomavirus-16 E6 function. *PLoS ONE* **2013**, *8*, e84506. [CrossRef] [PubMed]
33. Läsche, M.; Urban, H.; Gallwas, J.; Gründker, C. HPV and Other Microbiota; Who's Good and Who's Bad: Effects of the Microbial Environment on the Development of Cervical Cancer—A Non-Systematic Review. *Cells* **2021**, *10*, 714. [CrossRef]
34. Preci, D.P.; Almeida, A.; Weiler, A.L.; Mukai Franciosi, M.L.; Cardoso, A.M. Oxidative damage and antioxidants in cervical cancer. *Int. J. Gynecol. Cancer* **2021**, *31*, 265–271. [CrossRef]
35. Calaf, G.M.; Urzua, U.; Termini, L.; Aguaio, F. Oxidative stress in female cancers. *Oncotarget* **2018**, *9*, 23824–23842. [CrossRef]
36. Foppoli, C.; De Marco, F.; Cini, C.; Perluigi, M. Redox control of viral carcinogenesis: The human papillomavirus paradigm. *Biochim. Biophys. Acta* **2015**, *1850*, 1622–1632. [CrossRef] [PubMed]
37. Cruz-Gregorio, A.; Manzo-Merino, J.; Lizano, M. Cellular redox, cancer and human papillomavirus. *Virus Res.* **2018**, *246*, 35–45. [CrossRef]

38. Lin, H.Y.; Fu, Q.; Kao, Y.H.; Tseng, T.S.; Reiss, K.; Cameron, J.E.; Ronis, M.J.; Su, J.; Nair, N.; Chang, H.-M.; et al. Antioxidants Associated with Oncogenic Human Papillomavirus Infection in Women. *J. Infect. Dis.* **2021**, *224*, 1520–1528. [CrossRef]
39. Georgescu, S.R.; Mitran, C.I.; Mitran, M.I.; Caruntu, C.; Sarbu, M.I.; Matei, C.; Nicolae, I.; Tocut, S.M.; Popa, M.I.; Tampa, M. New Insights in the Pathogenesis of HPV Infection and the Associated Carcinogenic Processes: The Role of Chronic Inflammation and Oxidative Stress. *J. Immunol. Res.* **2018**, *2018*, 5315816. [CrossRef]
40. Khan, F.; Pandey, P.; Upadhyay, T.K.; Jafri, A.; Jha, N.K.; Mishra, R.; Singh, V. Anti-cancerous effect of rutin against HPV-C33A cervical cancer cells via G0/G1 cycle arrest and apoptotic induction. *Endocr. Metab. Immune Drug Targets* **2020**, *20*, 409–418. [CrossRef] [PubMed]
41. Clemente-Soto, A.F.; Salas-Vidal, E.; Milan-Pacheco, C.; Sanchez-Carranza, J.N.; Peralta-Zaragoza, O.; Gonzalez-Maya, L. Quercetin induces G2 phase arrest and apoptosis with the activation of p53 in an E6 expression-independent manner in HPV-positive human cervical cancer-derived cells. *Mol. Med. Rep.* **2019**, *19*, 2097–2106. [CrossRef]
42. Gutierrez-Orozco, F.; Failla, M.L. Biological activities and bioavailability of mangosteen xanthons: A critical review of the current evidence. *Nutrients* **2013**, *5*, 3163–3183. [CrossRef]
43. Liu, Z.; Antalek, M.; Nguyen, L.; Li, X.; Tian, X.; Le, A.; Zi, X. The effect of gartanin, a naturally-occurring xanthone in mangosteen juice, on the mTOR pathway, autophagy, apoptosis and the growth of human urinary bladder cancer cell lines. *Nutr. Cancer* **2013**, *65*, 68–77. [CrossRef]
44. Shan, T.; Ma, Q.; Gui, K.; Liu, J.; Li, W.; Wang, F.; Wu, E. Xanthones from mangosteen extracts as natural chemopreventive agents: Potential anticancer drugs. *Curr. Mol. Med.* **2011**, *11*, 666–677. [CrossRef]
45. Chin, Y.-W.; Kinghorn, A.D. Structural characterization, biological effects, and synthetic studies on xanthones from mangosteen (*Garcinia mangostana*), a popular botanical dietary supplement. *Mini Rev. Org. Chem.* **2008**, *5*, 355–364. [CrossRef]
46. Karim, A.A.; Azlan, A. Fruit pod extracts as a source of nutraceuticals and pharmaceuticals. *Molecules* **2012**, *17*, 11931–11946. [CrossRef]
47. Sun, X.; Fu, P.; Xie, L.; Chai, S.; Xu, Q.; Zeng, L.; Wang, X.; Jiang, N.; Sang, M. Resveratrol inhibits the progression of cervical cancer by suppressing the transcription and expression of HPV E6 and E7 genes. *Int. J. Mol. Med.* **2021**, *47*, 335–345. [CrossRef]
48. Shin, S.-A.; Moon, S.Y.; Kim, W.-Y.; Paek, S.-M.; Park, H.H.; Lee, C.S. Structure-based classification and anti-cancer effects of plant metabolites. *Int. J. Mol. Sci.* **2018**, *19*, 2651. [CrossRef]
49. Korkina, L.G.; Pastore, S.; De Luca, C.; Kostyuk, V.A. Metabolism of plant polyphenols in the skin: Beneficial versus deleterious effects. *Curr. Drug Metab.* **2008**, *9*, 710–729. [CrossRef]
50. Korkina, L.G.; De Luca, C.; Kostyuk, V.A.; Pastore, S. Plant polyphenols and tumors: From mechanisms to therapies, prevention, and protection against toxicity of anti-cancer treatments. *Curr. Med. Chem.* **2009**, *16*, 3943–3965. [CrossRef]
51. Chilton, S.N.; Burton, J.P.; Reid, G. Inclusion of fermented foods in food guides around the world. *Nutrients* **2015**, *7*, 390–404. [CrossRef]
52. Vuong, T.; Mallet, J.-F.; Ouzounova, M.; Rahbar, S.; Hernandez-Vargas, H.; Herceg, Z.; Matar, C. Role of a polyphenol-enriched preparation of chemoprevention of mammalian carcinoma through cancer stem cells and inflammatory pathways modulation. *J. Trans. Med.* **2016**, *14*, 13. [CrossRef]
53. Swain, M.R.; Anandharaj, M.; Ray, R.C.; Rani, P.R. Fermented fruits and vegetables of Asia: A potential source of probiotics. *Biotechnol. Res. Int.* **2014**, *2014*, 250424. [CrossRef] [PubMed]
54. Pessione, E.; Cirrincione, S. Bioactive molecules released in food by lactic acid bacteria: Encrypted peptides and biogenic amines. *Front. Microbiol.* **2016**, *7*, 876. [CrossRef]
55. Cuzick, J.; Beverley, E.; Ho, L.; Terry, G.; Sapper, H.; Mielzynska, I.; Lorincz, A.; Chan, W.K.; Krausz, T.; Soutter, B. HPV testing in primary screening of older women. *Br. J. Cancer* **1999**, *8*, 554–558. [CrossRef]
56. Franco, E.L.; Duarte-Franco, E.; Ferenczy, A. Cervical cancer: Epidemiology, prevention, and role of human papillomavirus infection. *J. Can. Med. Assoc.* **2001**, *164*, 1017–1025.
57. Franco, E.L. Chapter 13: Primary screening of cervical cancer with human papilloma virus tests. *J. Natl. Cancer Inst. Monogr.* **2003**, *31*, 89–96. [CrossRef]
58. Kowluru, R.A.; Kanwar, M. Effects of curcumin on retinal oxidative stress and inflammation in diabetes. *Nutr. Metab.* **2007**, *4*, 8. [CrossRef]
59. Saidel-Sulkowska, E.M.; Lipinski, B.; Windom, H.; Audhya, T.; McGinnis, W. Oxidative stress in autism: Elevated cerebellar 3-nitrotyrosine levels. *Am. J. Biochem. Biotechnol.* **2008**, *4*, 73–84.
60. Walsh, S.W.; Vaughan, J.E.; Wang, Y.; Roberts, L.J., II. Placental isoprostane is significantly increased in preeclampsia. *FASEB J.* **2000**, *14*, 1289–1296. [CrossRef]
61. Takahashi, T.; Tanaka, M.; Inazawa, J.; Abe, T.; Suda, T.; Nagata, S. Human Fas ligand: Gene structure, chromosomal location and species specificity. *Int. Immunol.* **1994**, *6*, 1567–1574. [CrossRef]
62. Itoh, N.; Yonehara, S.; Ishii, A.; Yonehara, M.; Mizushima, S.-I.; Hase, A.; Seto, Y.; Nagata, S. The polypeptide encoded by the cDNA for human cell surface antigen Fas can mediate apoptosis. *Cell* **1991**, *66*, 233–234. [CrossRef]
63. Fernandes, J.V.; De Medeiros Fernandes, T.A.; De Azevedo, J.C.; Cobucci, R.N.; De Carvalho, M.G.; Andrade, V.S.; De Araujo, J.M.G. Link between chronic inflammation and human papillomavirus-induced carcinogenesis (Review). *Oncol. Lett.* **2015**, *9*, 1015–1026. [CrossRef]

64. Akagi, K.; Li, J.; Broutian, T.R.; Padilla-Nash, H.; Xiao, W.; Jiang, B.; Rocco, J.W.; Tecnos, T.N.; Kumar, B.; Wangsa, D.; et al. Genome-wide analysis of HPV integration in human cancers reveals recurrent, focal genomic instability. *Genome Res.* **2014**, *24*, 185–199. [CrossRef]
65. Jiang, Q.; Hurst, J.K. Relative chlorinating, nitrating, and oxidizing capabilities of neutrophils determined with phagocytosable probes. *J. Biol. Chem.* **1997**, *272*, 32767–32772. [CrossRef]
66. Chapman, A.L.; Morrissey, B.M.; Vasu, V.T.; Juarez, M.M.; Houghton, J.S.; Li, C.S.; Cross, C.E.; Eiserich, J.P. Myeloperoxidase-dependent oxidative metabolism of nitric oxide in the cystic fibrosis airway. *J. Cyst. Fibros.* **2010**, *9*, 84–92. [CrossRef]
67. Beckman, J.S. Oxidative damage and tyrosine nitration from peroxynitrite. *Chem. Res. Toxicol.* **1996**, *9*, 836–844. [CrossRef]
68. Van Der Vliet, A.; Eiserich, J.P.; Kaur, H.; Cross, C.E.; Halliwell, B. Nitrotyrosine as biomarker for reactive nitrogen species. *Methods Enzymol.* **1996**, *269*, 175–184.
69. Denisov, E.T.; Afanas'ev, I.B. *Oxidation and Antioxidants in Organic Chemistry and Biology*; CRC Press, Taylor & Francis Group: Boca Raton, FL, USA, 2005.
70. Van Der Vliet, A.; Hristova, M.; Cross, C.E.; Eiserich, J.P.; Goldcorn, T. Peroxynitrite induces covalent dimerization of epidermal growth factor receptors in A431 epidermoid carcinoma cells. *J. Biol. Chem.* **1998**, *273*, 31860–31866. [CrossRef]
71. Potapovich, A.I.; Lulli, D.; Fidanza, P.; Kostyuk, V.A.; De Luca, C.; Pastore, S.; Korkina, L. Plant polyphenols differentially modulate inflammatory responses of human keratinocytes by interfering with activation of transcription factors NFκB and AhR and EGFR-ERK pathway. *Toxicol. Appl. Pharmacol.* **2011**, *255*, 138–149. [CrossRef]
72. Pastore, S.; Lulli, D.; Maurelli, R.; Dellambra, E.; De Luca, C.; Korkina, L.G. Resveratrol induces long-lasting IL-8 expression and peculiar EGFR activation/distribution in human keratinocytes: Mechanisms and implications for skin administration. *PLoS ONE* **2013**, *8*, e59632. [CrossRef]
73. Korkina, L.G.; Pastore, S.; Dellambra, E.; De Luca, C. New molecular and cellular targets for chemoprevention and treatment of skin tumors by plant polyphenols: A critical review. *Curr. Med. Chem.* **2013**, *20*, 852–868.
74. Bellocq, A.; Antoine, M.; Flahault, A.; Philippe, C.; Crestani, B.; Bernaudin, J.F.; Mayaud, C.; Milleron, B.; Baud, L.; Cadranel, J. Neutrophil alveolitis in bronchioloalveolar carcinoma: Induction by tumor-derived interleukin-8 and relation to clinical outcome. *Am. J. Pathol.* **1998**, *152*, 83–92.
75. Brew, R.; Southern, S.A.; Flanagan, B.F.; McDicken, I.W.; Christmas, S.E. Detection of interleukin-8 mRNA and protein in human colorectal carcinoma cells. *Eur. J. Cancer* **1996**, *32*, 2142–2147. [CrossRef]
76. Negus, R.P.; Stamp, G.W.; Hadley, J.; Balkwill, F.R. Quanitative assessment of the leukocyte infiltrate in ovarian cancer and its relationship to the expression of C-C chemokines. *Am. J. Pathol.* **1997**, *150*, 1723–1734.
77. Carrero, Y.; Callejas, D.; Alaña, F.; Silva, C.; Mindiola, R.; Mosquera, J. Increased vascular endothelial growth factor expression, CD3-positive cell infiltration, and oxidative stress in premalignant lesions of the cervix. *Cancer* **2009**, *115*, 3680–3688. [CrossRef]
78. Shacter, E.; Beecham, E.J.; Covey, J.M.; Kohn, K.W.; Potter, M. Activated neutrophils induce prolonged DNA damage in neighbouring cells. *Carcinogenesis* **1988**, *9*, 2297–2304. [CrossRef]
79. Tamir, S.; Tannenbaum, S.R. The role of nitric oxide (NO) in the carcinogenic process. *Biochim. Biophys. Acta Rev. Cancer* **1996**, *1288*, F31–F36. [CrossRef]
80. Felley-Bosco, E. Role of nitric oxide in genotoxicity: Implication for carcinogenesis. *Cancer Metastasis Rev.* **1998**, *17*, 25–37. [CrossRef]
81. Halim, T.A.; Farooqi, A.A.; Zaman, F. Nip the HPV encoded evil in the cancer bud: HPV reshapes signaling landscapes. *Cancer Cell Int.* **2013**, *13*, 61. [CrossRef]
82. Mitchell, M.J.; Wayne, E.; Rana, K.; Schaffer, C.B.; King, M.R. TRAIL-coated leukocytes that kill cancer cells in the circulation. *Proc. Natl. Acad. Sci. USA* **2014**, *111*, 930–935. [CrossRef]
83. Fulda, S.; Debatin, K.M. Sensitization for tumor necrosis factor-related apoptosis-inducing ligand-induced apoptosis by the chemopreventive agent resveratrol. *Cancer Res.* **2004**, *64*, 337–346. [CrossRef]
84. Ren, B.; Kwah, M.X.Y.; Liu, C.; Ma, Z.; Shanmugam, M.K.; Ding, L.; Xian, X.; Ho, P.C.L.; Wang, L.; Ong, P.S. Resveratrol for cancer therapy: Challenges and future perspectiveas. *Cancer Lett.* **2021**, *515*, 63–72. [CrossRef]
85. Pastore, S.; Lulli, D.; Pascarella, A.; Maurelli, R.; Dellambra, E.; Potapovich, A.; Kostyuk, V.; De Luca, C.; Korkina, L. Resveratrol enhances solar UV induced responses in normal human epidermal keratinocytes. *Photochem. Photobiol.* **2012**, *88*, 1522–1530. [CrossRef]
86. Wang, D.; Upadhyaya, B.; Liu, Y.; Knudsen, D.; Dey, M. Phenetyl isothiocyanate upregulates death receptors 4 and 5 and inhibits proliferation in human cancer stem-like cells. *BMC Cancer* **2014**, *14*, 591. [CrossRef]
87. Lin, X.; Farooqui, A.A. Cucurbitacin mediated regulation of deregulated oncogenic signaling cascades and non-coding RNAs in different cancers: Spotlight on JAK/STAT, Wnt/β-catenin, mTOR, TRAIL-mediated pathways. *Semin. Cancer Biol.* **2021**, *73*, 302–309. [CrossRef] [PubMed]
88. Farooqi, A.A.; Butt, G.; El-Zanaby, S.A.; Attar, R.; Sabitaliyevich, U.Y.; Jovic, J.J.; Tang, K.F.; Naureen, H.; Xu, B. Luteolin mediated targeting of protein network and microRNAs in different cancers: Focus on JAK-STAT, NOTCH, mTOR and TRAIL-mediated signaling pathways. *Pharmacol. Res.* **2020**, *160*, 105188. [CrossRef] [PubMed]
89. Farooqi, A.A.; Pinheiro, M.; Granja, A.; Farabegoli, F.; Reis, S.; Attar, R.; Sabitalievich, U.Y.; Xu, B.; Ahmad, A. EGCG Mediated Targeting of Deregulated Signaling Pathways and Non-Coding RNAs in Different Cancers: Focus on JAK/STAT, Wnt/β-Catenin, TGF/SMAD, NOTCH, SHH/GLI, and TRAIL Mediated Signaling Pathways. *Cancers* **2020**, *12*, 951. [CrossRef] [PubMed]

cancers

Article

Scabertopin Derived from *Elephantopus scaber* L. Mediates Necroptosis by Inducing Reactive Oxygen Species Production in Bladder Cancer In Vitro

Yuanhui Gao [1,†], Zhenyu Nie [1,†], Hui Cao [1], Denggao Huang [1], Mei Chen [1], Yang Xiang [1], Xiaolong Yu [2,*] and Shufang Zhang [1,*]

1 Central Laboratory, Affiliated Haikou Hospital of Xiangya Medical College, Central South University, Haikou 570208, China
2 School of Materials Science and Engineering, Hainan University, Haikou 570228, China
* Correspondence: yuxiaolong@hainanu.edu.cn (X.Y.); zsf66189665@126.com (S.Z.)
† These authors have contributed equally to this work.

Simple Summary: Scabertopin is one of the major sesquiterpene lactones from *Elephantopus scaber* L. Sesquiterpene lactones are thought to have fairly strong anti-cancer efficacy. However, there has not been any research report on the efficacy and mechanism of Scabertopin in the treatment of bladder cancer. The aim of this study is to evaluate the antitumor activity of scabertopin in bladder cancer and its potential molecular mechanism in vitro. In this study, we found that scabertopin can induce necroptosis in bladder cancer cells by promoting the production of mitochondrial reactive oxygen species, and also inhibit the migration and invasion ability of bladder cancer cells. At the same time, we also demonstrated that the half-inhibition rate of scabertopin on various bladder cancer cell lines is much lower than that on human ureteral epithelial immortalized cells. This shows that scabertopin is a safe and effective anti-bladder cancer drug.

Abstract: Bladder cancer remains one of the most common malignant tumors that threatens human health worldwide. It imposes a heavy burden on patients and society due to the high medical costs associated with its easy metastasis and recurrence. Although several treatment options for bladder cancer are available, their clinical efficacy remains unsatisfactory. Therefore, actively exploring new drugs and their mechanisms of action for the clinical treatment of bladder cancer is very important. Scabertopin is one of the major sesquiterpene lactones found in *Elephantopus scaber* L. Sesquiterpene lactones are thought to have fairly strong anti-cancer efficacy. However, the anticancer effect of sesquiterpenoid scabertopin on bladder cancer and its mechanism are still unclear. The aim of this study is to evaluate the antitumor activity of scabertopin in bladder cancer and its potential molecular mechanism in vitro. Our results suggest that scabertopin can induce RIP1/RIP3-dependent necroptosis in bladder cancer cells by promoting the production of mitochondrial reactive oxygen species (ROS), inhibit the expression of MMP-9 by inhibiting the FAK/PI3K/Akt signaling pathway, and ultimately inhibit the migration and invasion ability of bladder cancer cells. At the same time, we also demonstrated that the half-inhibition concentration (IC50) of scabertopin on various bladder cancer cell lines (J82, T24, RT4 and 5637) is much lower than that on human ureteral epithelial immortalized cells (SV-HUC-1). The above observations indicate that scabertopin is a potential therapeutic agent for bladder cancer that acts by inducing necroptosis and inhibiting metastasis.

Keywords: scabertopin; bladder cancer; reactive oxygen species; necroptosis; *Elephantopus scaber* L.

Citation: Gao, Y.; Nie, Z.; Cao, H.; Huang, D.; Chen, M.; Xiang, Y.; Yu, X.; Zhang, S. Scabertopin Derived from *Elephantopus scaber* L. Mediates Necroptosis by Inducing Reactive Oxygen Species Production in Bladder Cancer In Vitro. *Cancers* **2022**, *14*, 5976. https://doi.org/10.3390/cancers14235976

Academic Editors: Barbara De Filippis, Alessandra Ammazzalorso and Marialuigia Fantacuzzi

Received: 30 September 2022
Accepted: 1 December 2022
Published: 2 December 2022

1. Introduction

Bladder cancer is one of the most common malignant tumors of the urinary system. The cancer statistics released in 2022 state that, in the United States, bladder cancer has an estimated incidence of 81,800 cases and a mortality rate of 17,100 cases [1]. These rates are slightly lower than those reported in 2021 [2]. In China, bladder cancer had an incidence of approximately 80,500 and a mortality rate of 32,900 in 2015 [3]. Uroepithelial cancer is the main pathological type of bladder cancer. Approximately 75% and 25% of the cases of this type of cancer are non-muscle-invasive bladder cancer (NMIBC) and muscle-invasive bladder cancer (MIBC), respectively. The current clinical treatment of bladder cancer remains based on surgery combined with postoperative radiotherapy [4,5]. Mitomycin C, epirubicin, adriamycin, methotrexate, vincristine, pirarubicin, and cisplatin are used as the first-line chemotherapeutic agents for bladder cancer in clinical practice [6]. However, the use of these drugs is greatly limited by their unsatisfactory efficacy, the widely reported drug tolerance of bladder cancer, and their adverse effects. Although the rapid development of molecular biology and genetics research has provided new therapeutic tools for the clinical development of immunotherapy, gene therapy, and targeted therapy, these approaches fail to exert an ideal treatment effect on bladder cancer because they use a large number of chemically synthesized drugs. This approach results in high treatment costs, drug side effects, hepatotoxicity, and drug resistance. Therefore, the search for new drugs with low toxicity and side effects has been a hot issue in tumor treatment.

In recent years, many natural compound products have played an important role in the treatment of tumors. Finding compounds with significant tumor-inhibiting activity from natural products is an important approach and means for the research and development of anticancer drugs [7]. Scabertopin is a sesquiterpene lactone compound that is mainly derived from the chemical constituents of *Elephantopus scaber* L. It is a kind of herbaceous plant belonging to the phylum Angiosperm, class Dicotyledonous, order Campanulaceae, family Asteraceae, and genus Elephantopus [8], which is widely distributed worldwide, particularly in East Asia, Southeast Asia, Africa, Australia, India, and South America, and has been reported to have various pharmacological properties, such as anti-bacterial, anti-diabetic, anti-inflammatory, and anti-cancer efficacy [9,10]. An increasing number of studies have shown that the antitumor activity of *Elephantopus scaber* L. is attributed to sesquiterpene lactones, which execute significant antitumor activities in nasopharyngeal [11,12], cervical [13], breast [14], colon [15,16], and hepatocellular carcinomas [17]. For example, in HCT116 and RKO cells, deoxyelephantopin (DET), another sesquiterpene lactone compound derived from *Elephantopus scaber* L. can significantly increase reactive oxygen species (ROS) levels, thereby activating the JNK signaling pathway and triggering cell death. In the mouse breast cancer cell line TS/A, DET can inhibit TNF-α-induced NF-κB activity and down-regulate the NF-κB regulated gene products of matrix metalloproteases (MMP)-2 and MMP-9, thereby inhibiting the migration and invasion in vitro and in vivo [14]. In addition, sesquiterpenoids exhibit different cytotoxicities toward tumor cells and normal cells, whereby they selectively target tumor cells and show little systemic toxicity [18,19]. However, the research on the anticancer effect and mechanism of scabertopin in bladder cancer has not been reported.

Necroptosis is a unique form of programmed cell death, which is characterized by caspase-independent activation and is morphologically accompanied by the swelling of organelles and the rupture of cell membranes, resulting in the spillage of the cellular contents into the surrounding cells and, consequently, triggering inflammatory response [20,21]. Various drugs and active sites of traditional Chinese medicine have been confirmed to exert their anticancer activity through necroptosis [22,23]. Receptor-interacting protein (RIP)1, RIP3, and mixed lineage kinase-like (MLKL) are three key factors in the regulation of necroptosis; RIP3 has been well-established to recruit MLKL and induce its phosphorylation. Phosphorylated-MLKL (p-MLKL) then undergoes oligomerization and translocates to the plasma membrane to execute cellular necrosis [24–26]. However, the pathway through which RIP1 undergoes autophosphorylation remains controversial. ROS have been recently reported to act as upstream cell signaling molecules to activate and drive necroptosis [27]. RIP1 can sense ROS by modifying three key cysteine residues (C257, C268, and C586) and, subsequently, induces their autophosphorylation at the S161 site, which in turn results in the recruitment of RIP3 to form a necrosome [28]. Previous studies have also shown a correlation between necroptosis and drug-induced ROS. For example, artesunate can inhibit the proliferation of renal cancer cell lines in vitro by inducing elevations in ROS levels and, thus, promoting RIP1-dependent necrotic apoptosis [29]. In addition, emodin promotes the occurrence of necrotic apoptosis in renal cell carcinoma (RCC) cell lines, thereby restricting tumor development by inducing the production of ROS that promote increases in the levels of RIP1 and MLKL phosphorylation [30]. In conclusion, the positive correlation of necroptosis with ROS implies that regulating ROS to induce necroptosis in tumor cells is a potential strategy for cancer therapy.

In this study, we aimed to evaluate the inhibitory effects and potential molecular mechanisms of scabertopin on bladder cancer cells in vitro. Scabertopin is one of the four sesquiterpene lactones with the highest content in *Elephantopus scaber* L. Since DET has shown a good anti-tumor effect in a variety of tumor cell lines, we speculated that scabertopin would also have similar efficacy. Therefore, we determined our research objective was to study the effect of scabertopin on bladder cancer cell lines and explore its way to promote the death of bladder cancer cell lines. Our results showed that scabertopin with antitumor properties inhibited the growth, migration, and invasion of the bladder cancer cell line J82. Further in-depth studies demonstrated that the above effects of scabertopin may be related to the promotion of ROS generation, the induction of focal adhesion kinase (FAK) phosphorylation, and the activation of necroptotic signaling pathways.

2. Materials and Methods

2.1. Main Reagents

Scabertopin (PS1863-0010) was purchased from Chengdu Push Biotechnology Co., Ltd. (Chengdu, China). DMEM basal medium (10569010) and trypsin-EDTA (25200056) were purchased from Gibco (Grand Island, NY, USA). RPMI 1640 (PM150110) was purchased from Procell Life Science & Technology Co., Ltd (Wuhan, China). Fetal bovine serum (FBS) (1907301) was purchased from Biological Industries (BI) (Kibbutz Beit Haemek, Israel). Cell Counting Kit-8 (CK04) was purchased from Dojindo Laboratories (Kumamoto, Japan). LIVE/DEAD cell viability assay kit (L3224) was purchased from Invitrogen (Carlsbad, CA, USA). The cell cycle assay kit (KGA512) and the apoptosis assay kit (KGA1018) were purchased from KeyGen BioTECH (Shanghai, China). ROS detection kit (S0033S) was purchased from Beyotime Biotechnology (Shanghai, China). B cell lymphoma-2 (Bcl-2, ab182858), Bcl-2-associated X (Bax, ab32503), phospho-PI3K (Y607, ab182651), AKT (ab179463), phospho-AKT (S472, S473, S474, ab192623), and GAPDH (ab181602) antibodies were purchased from Abcam (Cambridge, MA, USA). Gasdermin D (97558), GPX4 (59735), FAK (71433), phospho-FAK (Y397, 8556), MMP-9 (13667), PI3K (4257S), caspase-3 (14220), caspase-8 (9746), caspase-9 (9508), MLKL (14993), phospho-MLKL (S358, 91689), RIP1 (3493), phospho-RIP1 (Ser166, 65746), RIP3 (13526), and phospho-RIP3 (Ser227, 93654) antibodies were purchased from Cell Signaling Technology (Danvers, MA, USA).

2.2. Material Preparation

Scabertopin (10 mg) was dissolved in 1 ml of dimethyl sulfoxide DMSO (Beyotime Biotechnology, ST2335-100 mL) and configured into a master batch with a concentration of 40 μM such that the maximum concentration of DMSO in the cell culture medium was 0.143%. In the subsequent experiment, in order to exclude the effect of DMSO on cells, 0.143% DMSO was contained in all negative control group media as control. A total of 10 μL of scabertopin and deoxyelephantopin solution was applied evenly on KBr-pressed plates, evaporated and dehydrated using an infrared lamp, and analyzed using a Fourier-transform infrared (FTIR) spectroscopy and KBr-pressed plates. KBr (P116274-100 g) was purchased from Aladdin Biochemical Technology Co., Ltd. (Shanghai, China).

2.3. Infrared Spectroscopy

A Fourier-transform infrared tester (Nexus-670 produced by Nexus, Madison, WI, USA) was used to conduct IR spectrum test on the scabertopin powder: the wavelength range was 400–4000 cm^{-1}, the number of scans was 32, and the resolution was 4 cm^{-1}. The operation was as follows: grind KBr dried under vacuum for 8 h at 140 °C, take 10 mg and press into tablets to obtain background tablets, and grind another 10 mg of KBr and 1 mg of scabertopin powder in an agate mortar evenly. The IR spectroscopy was performed on the obtained background pieces (only KBr) and the samples (KBr and scabertopin powder).

2.4. UV Absorption Assay

The mixed solution of scabertopin and DMEM medium was tested using an UV-Vis spectrophotometer (UV9100B from Beijing LabTech Instrument Co., Ltd., Beijing, China), with a wavelength range of 200–360 nm and a resolution of 2 nm.

If the chemical structure of the substance were stable, its UV maximum absorption wavelength would not change. It could be seen from the UV spectrum that the UV maximum absorption peak of scabertopin is around 214 nm, which is consistent with the UV spectrum of the α,β-unsaturated carbonyl moiety. There was no change at 0, 24, and 48 h, and it could be inferred from the Beer–Lambert law that, when the length of the absorption cell, the light source, and the type of the substance to be tested are the same, the absorbance is strictly proportional to the substance concentration.

$$Abs = \lg\left(\frac{1}{T}\right) = Kcl \tag{1}$$

Abs: Absorbance; *T*: transmittance; *K*: molar extinction coefficient, $cm^2 \cdot mol$; *c*: molar concentration, mol/L; and *l*: the length of the absorption cell, cm.

2.5. Cell Lines and Culture

Human bladder cancer cell lines (J82 and T24) and human ureteral epithelial immortalized cells (SV-HUC-1) were purchased from the ATCC cell bank, and 5637 and RT4 cell lines were purchased from the China Centre for Type Culture Collection (Shanghai, China). All cell culture media and FBS (30044333) were obtained from Gibco. J82 cells were cultured in DMEM (10% FBS) medium, T24 and 5637 cells were cultured in RPMI 1640 (10% FBS), RT4 cells were cultured in McCoy's 5A (Gibco, 16600082) (10% FBS) medium, and SV-HUC-1 cells were cultured in F-12K (Gibco, 21127022) (10% FBS) medium. All cell lines were grown in a cell culture incubator at 37 °C and 5% CO_2 to maintain cell growth. The cells were revived and passaged two times for subsequent experiments.

2.6. CCK-8 Assay

The human bladder cancer cells (J82 and T24) and human ureteral epithelial immortalized cells (SV-HUC-1) were inoculated into 96-well plates (100 µL per well). Subsequently, after being added with different concentrations of drugs, the plates were incubated in an incubator at 37 °C and 5% CO_2 for 24–48 h. A total of 10 µL of CCK-8 reagent (Dojindo Laboratories, CK04) was added to each well, and incubation was continued in the incubator for 1–4 h. Finally, absorbance was detected at 450 nm by using an enzyme marker (Bio-Rad, Hercules, CA, USA). The experimental data (mean ± standard deviation) were plotted in the form of histograms. Dose–response curves were generated using GraphPad Prism 7 (GraphPad Software, San Diego, CA, USA) software, and the absolute 50% inhibitory concentration (IC50) was determined.

2.7. LIVE/DEAD Cell Activity Assay

The J82 cells were inoculated at a density of 1×10^4 cells/mL into 96-well plates and treated with gradient concentrations of scabertopin for 24–48 h. Subsequently, the cells were washed with phosphate buffered saline (PBS) in accordance with the instructions of the LIVE/DEAD cell vitality assay kit (Invitrogen), and each group was incubated for 30 min at room temperature with 5 µL of the supplied 4 mM calcein AM stock solution to the 10 mL ethidium dimers (EthD-1). The cells were observed and photographed with an inverted fluorescence microscope, which showed live cells in green (AM) and dead cells in red (EthD-1).

2.8. Scanning and Transmission Electron Microscopy

The human bladder cancer J82 cells were inoculated at a density of 2×10^4 cells/mL on slides attached to a 24-well plate, and then treated with the drug at a concentration of 10 μM. After being cultured in the incubator for 24 h, the cells were taken out and washed with precooled PBS twice. The scabertopin-treated cells were fixed with 4% paraformaldehyde (Beyotime Biotechnology, P0099-500 mL) at room temperature and dehydrated with alcohol. Then, their morphology was observed using a scanning electron microscope (SEM) (Regulus8100, HITACHI, Tokyo, Japan).

The J82 cells were inoculated into 6-well plates and then treated with gradient concentrations of scabertopin for 24 h. The culture medium was discarded. The cells were treated with an electron microscope fixative (Servicebio Technology, Wuhan, China, G1102-100 mL) for 2–4 h at 4 °C, collected, and then centrifuged at low speed until green bean-sized clumps of cells could be seen at the bottom of the tubes. After further wrapping, postfixation, dehydration, permeabilization, embedding, sectioning, and staining, the cells were observed under a transmission electron microscope (TEM) and images were collected for analysis.

2.9. Measurement of Reactive Oxygen Species

Intracellular ROS levels were measured using an intracellular ROS assay kit (Solarbio Science & Technology, Beijing, China, CA1420). The J82 cells were treated with gradient concentrations of scabertopin for 24–48 h. In the rescue experiments, the cells were incubated with scabertopin for 2 h with 5 mM of ROS scavenger *N*-acetylcysteine (NAC) (MedChemExpress, Monmouth Junction, NJ, USA, HY-B0215). The cells were washed three times with PBS and treated with 10 μM of dichlorofluorescein diacetate probe for 20–30 min. Subsequently, the cells were washed three times with a serum-free medium, and their fluorescence intensity was measured using a fluorescence microplate reader (BioTek, Winooski, VT, USA, Synergy H1).

In order to determine the type of ROS, the J82 cells were treated with gradient concentrations of scabertopin and then loaded with dihydroethidium (DHE) probe (KeyGEN BioTECH, KGAF019) at a concentration of 25 μM and incubated at 37 °C for 60 min in the darkness. After the incubation, the cells were washed with a fresh culture medium and their fluorescence intensity was measured using a fluorescence microplate reader (BioTek, Winooski, VT, USA, Synergy H1). The cells were then imaged under an inverted fluorescence microscope.

2.10. Mitochondrial Membrane Potential Assay

The effect of scabertopin on mitochondrial membrane potential ($\Delta\Psi$) was detected using the Mitochondrial membrane potential assay kit JC-1 (Beyotime Biotechnology, C2006). The cells were treated with gradient concentrations of scabertopin, washed with PBS, added to a cell culture medium, mixed with the JC-1 solution, and incubated at 37 °C for 20 min according to the manufacturer's instructions. The fluorescence intensity of the cells was measured using a fluorescence microplate reader (BioTek, Winooski, VT, USA, Synergy H1), and the cells were imaged under an inverted fluorescence microscope. Whereas green fluorescence is an indicator of depolarized mitochondria, intact mitochondria produce red fluorescence.

When $\Delta\Psi$ is at higher levels, JC-1 aggregates in the matrix of mitochondria to form polymers and produce red fluorescence. When $\Delta\Psi$ is at a lower level, JC-1 cannot aggregate in the mitochondrial matrix. At this time, JC-1 is monomer and can produce green fluorescence. The ratio of monomer/polymer represents the ratio of green fluorescence/red fluorescence, which can be used to measure the proportion of mitochondrial depolarization

2.11. GSH Assay

The GSH (reduced glutathione) and GSSG (oxidized glutathione disulfide) assay kit (Beyotime Biotechnology, S0053) is a simple and easy-to-use assay that can detect the contents of GSH and GSSG, respectively. Briefly, total GSH and GSSG levels were measured at a wavelength of 412 nm after the cells were treated with gradient concentrations of scabertopin. The level of reduced GSH was calculated according to the following formula:

$$GSH = total\ glutathione\ (GSH + GSSG) - 2 \times GSSG \quad (2)$$

2.12. Wound Healing Assay

A total of 70 μL of J82 cells were inoculated at a density of 8×10^5 cells/mL into each insert of a Culture-Insert 2 Well (ibidi, Grafelfing, Germany, 80206) in the middle of a dish. After the cells were attached, the insert was removed with forceps and the old medium was aspirated off. The cells were washed gently 1–2 times with PBS, treated with different concentrations of the drugs, placed in the incubator for further incubation, and removed at 0 and 24 h for fluorescent inverted microscopy (IX71, Olympus, Tokyo, Japan) to observe whether the peripheral cells had migrated to the central scratch area. The cells were photographed and recorded. The percentage of wound healing was analyzed using ImageJ software and calculated as the ratio of the initial scratch area minus the partially healed area that had healed at a certain time to the initial area, according to the following formula.

$$initial\ area - \frac{area\ at\ a\ certain\ time\ point}{initial\ area} \quad (3)$$

2.13. Transwell Assay

The J82 cells treated with different concentrations of drugs for 24 h were collected and their density was adjusted to 5×10^4 cells/well. The cells were inoculated into the upper chamber of a transwell plate and the lower chamber was supplemented with 10% FBS medium. The plate was placed in the incubator for 24 h, washed twice with PBS, and fixed with methanol. Then, the cells were treated with 0.1% Giemsa staining solution, washed three times with PBS, and allowed to air dry. The number of migrated cells was recorded by photography under multiple high-magnification fields using a microscope (Etaluma, Inc., San Diego, CA, USA, LS720) and by counting the number of migrated cells.

2.14. Cell cycle Assays

The J82 cells were treated with different concentrations of drugs for 24 h, digested with tryspin, collected, and washed 1–2 times with PBS. The cells were fixed by adding precooled 70% ethanol and then washed with PBS to remove the fixative. The cells were administered with a RNase/propidium iodide (PI) staining working solution and incubated for 30 min at room temperature under protection from light. The samples were subjected to flow cytometry (FACSCanto, Becton, Dickinson and Company, Franklin Lakes, NJ, USA), and Modfit software was used to analyze the results.

2.15. Cell Apoptosis Analysis

The J82 cells were treated with different concentrations of drugs for 24 h, digested by using EDTA-free trypsin, collected, washed and resuspended with PBS, and centrifuged to collect cell precipitates. The precipitates were resuspended again with a small amount of a binding buffer, mixed with an Annexin-V-FITC working solution, incubated for 5 min at room temperature under protection from light, and mixed with a PI reagent and PBS. The samples were analyzed using flow cytometry and the results were analyzed using Modfit software.

2.16. Western Blot Analysis

A total of 10 μL of ProteinSafe™ Phosphatase inhibitor cocktail (DI201, TransGen Biotech, Beijing, China) and ProteinSafe™ Protease inhibitor cocktail (DI101, TransGen Biotech, Beijing, China) was added to every 1 ml of ProteinExt® Mammalian total protein extraction kit (TPEB) (DE101, TransGen Biotech, Beijing, China). The TPEB mixed reagents were made by mixing the above three reagents according to the protocols. The cells were mixed with the TPEB mixed reagents on ice after 24 h of scabertopin treatment. The lysates were collected and centrifuged at 14,000× *g* for 10 min at 4 °C. Protein concentrations were analyzed using a Bicinchoninic acid (BCA) kit (P0010, Beyotime Biotechnology). Equal amounts of protein samples were separated through electrophoresis on a 10% precast gel (M00664, GenScript Biotech, Nanjing, China). The proteins were then transferred to PVDF membranes. The membranes were blocked with 5% skimmed milk at 4 °C overnight. Afterward, the membranes were incubated for 2 h at room temperature with different primary antibodies, including Bax (1/10,000), Bcl-2 (1/10,000), caspase-9 (1/1000), caspase-3 (1/1000), caspase-8 (1/1000), GAPDH (1/10,000), MMP-9 (1/500), PI3K (1/1000), p-PI3K (1/1000), AKT (1/1000), p-AKT (1/1000), glutathione peroxidase 4 (GPX4, 1/1000), gasdermin-D (GSDMD, 1/1000), RIP (1/1000), p-RIP (1/1000), MLKL (1/1000), p-MLKL (1/1000), RIP3 (1/1000), and p-RIP3 (1/1000). The membranes were washed three times with TBST and incubated with the secondary antibodies (1/2000–1/20,000) for 1 h at room temperature. The target protein lane was imaged using an iBright 1500 (Invitrogen) with enhanced chemiluminescent substrates (Merck Millipore, Darmstadt, Germany, WBKLS0500). Original blots see Supplementary File S1.

2.17. Statistical Analysis

Statistics and bar graphs were analyzed using the Xiantao Academic Online Tools (https://www.xiantao.love/products) (accessed on 30 August 2022), which is based on R and the ggplot2 R package. The means of two groups were considered significantly different if * $p < 0.05$, ** $p < 0.01$, and *** $p < 0.001$.

3. Results

3.1. Bladder Cancer Cells Are Sensitive to Scabertopin

The chemical structure of scabertopin is shown in Figure 1A. The two boxes show the α-methylene-γ-lactone and butenolide moieties that confer the drug activity. The FTIR spectrum of scabertopin is shown in Figure 1B, and the UV absorption peaks of scabertopin in the DMEM medium at 0, 24, and 48 h are shown in Figure 1C. According to the Beer–Lambert law, when the length of the absorption cell, the light source, and the type of the substance to be measured are the same, the absorbance is strictly proportional to the concentration of the substance. Since the intensity of the UV maximum absorption peaks of scabertopin at 0, 24, and 48 h were all around 0.55, the concentration of scabertopin did not change. In conclusion, it can be considered that scabertopin can maintain stability in a DMEM medium. The viability of scabertopin-treated bladder cancer cells (T24, J82, RT4, and 5637) and human ureteral epithelial immortalized cells (SV-HUC-1) was determined using the CCK-8 assay. The results showed that scabertopin significantly inhibited the viability of the human bladder cancer cells (J82, T24, RT4, and 5637) in a dose-dependent manner (Figure 1D). The 24 h IC50 of scabertopin for the bladder cancer cell lines was approximately 20 μM, and the 48 h IC50 was even lower (approximately 18 μM). However, the IC50 values of scabertopin for the SV-HUC-1 cells at 24 and 48 h were 59.42 and 55.84 μM, which were considerably higher than those for the bladder cancer cells (Figure 1D). Next, the J82 cell line was arbitrarily selected for further study. In the following section, if the treatment time of scabertopin is not explicitly mentioned, it defaults to 24 h.

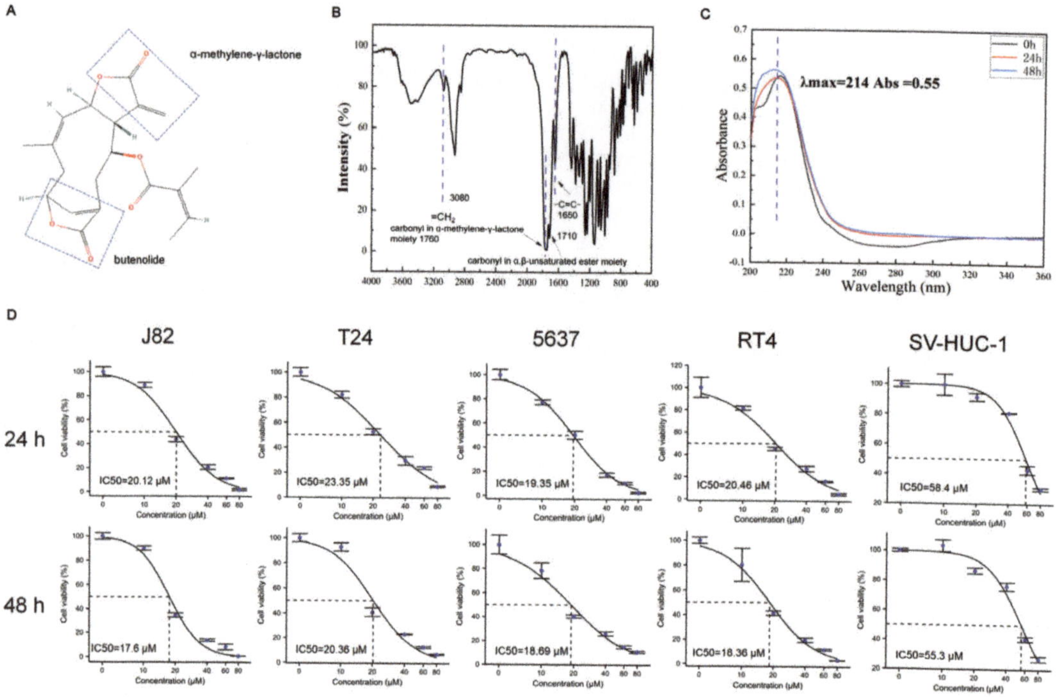

Figure 1. Chemical structure, stability, and efficacy of scabertopin against bladder cancer cells. (**A**). Chemical structure scabertopin. The two boxes show the structure of the molecule with the drug activity of α-methylene-γ-lactone and butenolide. (**B**). Infrared spectrum of scabertopin. The stretching vibration of $=CH_2$ exists at 3080 cm^{-1}, and the carbonyl stretching vibration of α-methylene-γ-lactone structure exists at 1760 cm^{-1}. The peak at 1710 cm^{-1} is the carbonyl stretching vibration of another non-lactone α,β-unsaturated ester, and the C=C stretching vibration exists at 1650 cm^{-1}. (**C**). The UV absorption peak of scabertopin in the DMEM medium at 0, 24, and 48 h. (**D**). 24 and 48 h IC50 of bladder cancer cell lines (J82, T24, 5637, and RT4) and human ureteral epithelial immortalized cells (SV-HUC-1) (n = 4).

3.2. *Increased Mitochondrial ROS Levels in J82 Cells Treated with Scabertopin*

We detected the cells treated with scabertopin for 24 and 48 h using a DCF fluorescent probe and found that scabertopin treatment could significantly increase the content of intracellular ROS (Figure 2A). To determine the mechanism of ROS production caused by scabertopin, we used a JC-1 assay to observe the changes of ΔΨ in the J82 cells treated with scabertopin. The results showed that ΔΨ decreased (red fluorescence decreased while green fluorescence increased) after scabertopin treatment (Figure 2C,D). In conclusion, the ΔΨ of the scabertopin treatment group decreased significantly compared to the control group.

The ROS in mitochondria are usually in the form of hydrogen peroxide (H_2O_2) and superoxide anions (O_2^-). However, H_2O_2 is hardly able to escape through the mitochondrial membrane and be detected in the cytoplasm, and, thus, superoxide anion produced in the mitochondria and transported to the cytoplasm has become a key signaling factor for mitochondrial ROS [31]. Therefore, we used a DHE fluorescent probe to detect the content of superoxide anion in the cells treated with scabertopin. The results showed that the level of superoxide anion in the scabertopin treatment group was significantly higher than that in the control group (Figure 2B).

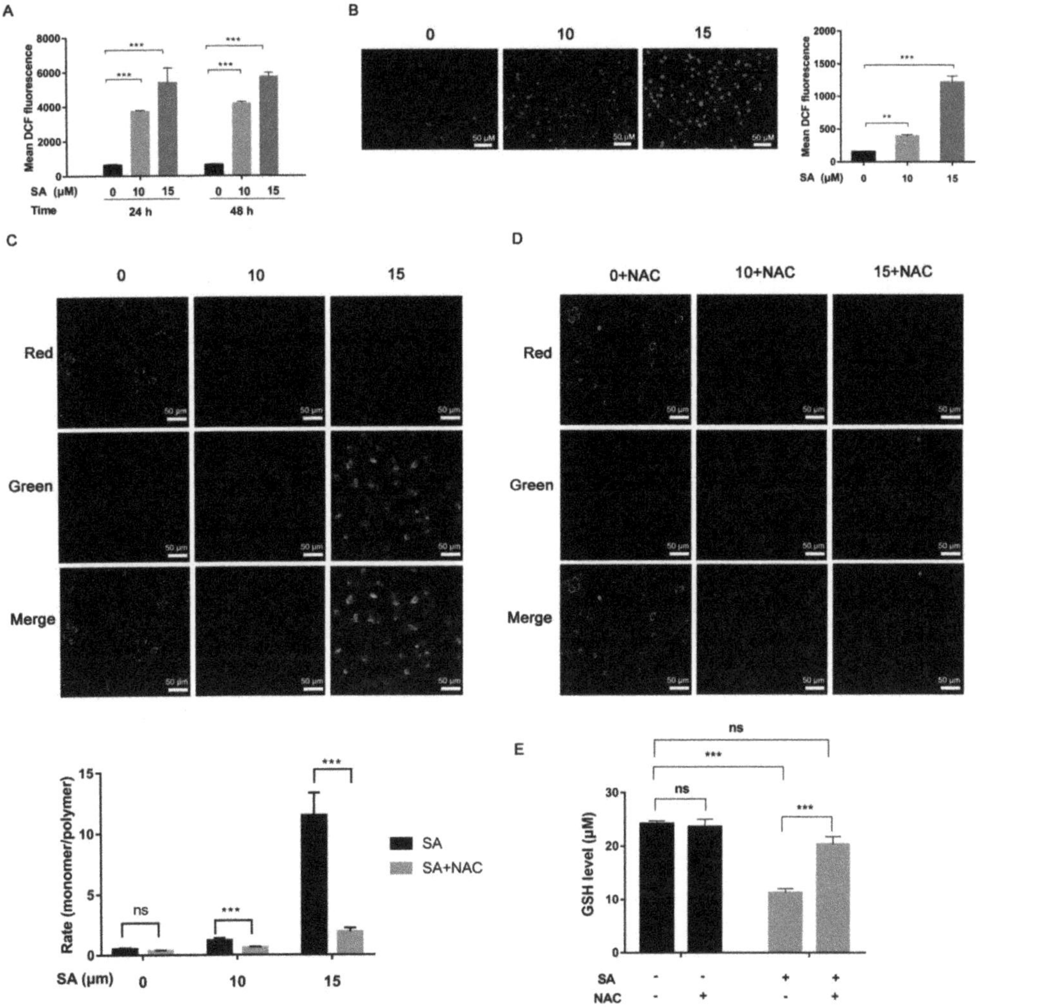

Figure 2. Increased mitochondrial ROS and reduced mitochondrial membrane potential in J82 cells treated with scabertopin. (**A**) Scabertopin induces ROS production in a dose- and time-dependent manner. (**B**) The DHE probe assay shows that superoxide anion is positively correlated with the scabertopin dose. (**C**) The JC-1 assay shows that, after 24 h treatment, scabertopin decreases the mitochondrial membrane potential in J82 cells in a dose-dependent manner. (**C**) The JC-1 assay shows that NAC treatment can restore the mitochondrial membrane potential reduced by 24 h treatment of scabertopin to some extent. (**D**) The DHE probe assay shows that superoxide anion is positively correlated with the scabertopin dose. (**E**) A 24 h treatment with 10 μM of scabertopin is efficient in depleting GSH through a dose-dependent mechanism in J82 cells, which can be reversed with NAC treatment. A total of 5 μM of NAC was used in the experiments. Data represent the mean ± standard error of mean (s.e.m.) of the three independent experiments. ** $p < 0.01$, *** $p < 0.001$, ns: no significance vs. 0 μM scabertopin-treated group. NAC: *N*-acetylcysteine; SA: scabertopin.

In addition, GSH is an important antioxidant in cells, and we also detected the changes in intracellular GSH after scabertopin treatment (Figure 2E). The results showed that scabertopin treatment could deplete GSH, which is one of the reasons for the accumulation of intracellular ROS, and the efficacy of scabertopin depleting GSH could be blocked by NAC (Figure 2E).

3.3. Cell Death Induced by Scabertopin Treatment Was Not Apoptosis and Ferroptosis

We utilized a scanning electron microscope to observe the effects of scabertopin treatment on cell morphology. The results showed that the cells without scabertopin treatment had strong three-dimensionality and thick and long pseudopodia; after scabertopin treatment, the cell spreading area increased and the pseudopodia shortened and thinned out (Figure 3A). To preliminarily elucidate the potential mechanism of scabertopin cytotoxicity in bladder cancer cells, we analyzed the effect of scabertopin treatment on the potential disruption of cell cycle phases using flow cytometry. The results showed that scabertopin treatment induced a significant increase in the percentage of cells both in the S and G2/M phases in a concentration-dependent manner (Figure 3B). Meanwhile, we detected the effect of scabertopin on the apoptosis and necrosis of J82 cells using the AnnexinV-FITC/PI double-staining method. The transfer of the cell membrane phospholipid phosphatidylserine from the inner to the outer layer of the plasma membrane is one of the early features of apoptosis. A single positive for AnnexinV-FITC is considered a typical cell in early apoptosis, i.e., the fourth quadrant (Q4), whereas AnnexinV-FITC and PI double-positive cells are considered to be in the end stage of apoptosis, necrosis, or are already dead, i.e., the second quadrant (Q2). The results in Figure 3C showed that, under the treatment with gradient concentrations of scabertopin, the number of early apoptotic cells was relatively small. Under scabertopin treatment, the number of necrosis cells significantly increased in a dose-dependent manner. In addition, water-soluble tetrazolium salts and green-fluorescent calcein-AM were deployed to determine whether scabertopin had an effect on the viability of bladder cancer cells. The results showed that, in contrast to the control treatment, scabertopin increased cytotoxicity in a concentration- and time-dependent manner, thus resulting in cell death (Figure 3D). However, scavenging of ROS with NAC significantly rescued scabertopin-induced cell death (Figure 3E). To reveal the mechanism of scabertopin-induced J82 cell death, we verified apoptosis-related caspase proteins Bcl-2 and Bax (Figure 3F), on the one hand, and ferroptosis-related GPX4 and pyroptosis-related GSDMD, on the other hand, using WB (Figure 3G). The results showed that scabertopin-treated J82 cells did not die by apoptosis, ferroptosis, or pyroptosis.

3.4. Necroptosis Is a Type of Cell Death Induced by Scabertopin and can Be Inhibited by NAC

To further investigate the extent to which cell organelles were altered by scabertopin treatment and to further determine the manner in which scabertopin induces death in bladder cancer cells, we performed TEM. The results showed that, in contrast to the control group cells, the scabertopin-treated cells were swollen with vacuolated cytoplasm, had severely swollen mitochondria, had a lack of membrane blebbing, had partially dissolved or absent organelles, and showed perforation of cell membranes (Figure 4A). These morphological changes are consistent with the characteristics of necroptosis [32]. We examined the expression of necroptosis-related proteins using Western blotting, and the expressions of phosphorylated RIP1, RIP3 and MLKL significantly increased in the J82 cells treated with scabertopin (Figure 4B). NAC significantly inhibited the expressions of phospho-RIP1, phospho-RIP3, and phospho-MLKL (Figure 4C).

3.5. Scabertopin Inhibits the Migration and Invasion of Bladder Cancer Cells

We performed wound healing and transwell assays to characterize how scabertopin affected the migratory and invasive abilities of bladder cancer cells. To this end, 24 h treatment with scabertopin inhibited the wound healing ability of J82 cells in a dose-dependent manner (Figure 5A). Similarly, the results of the transwell assays also showed that, after scabertopin treatment, the invasive ability of cells significantly reduced. This effect was negatively correlated with the concentration of scabertopin (Figure 5B). In addition, we further detected the expressions of motor-related molecules p-FAK, FAK, p-PI3K, PI3K, p-AKT, AKT, and MMP-9 after scabertopin treatment by performing Western blot analysis. The results showed that the expressions of phospho-FAK (Tyr397), phospho-PI3K (Tyr607), phospho-AKT (Ser472, Ser473, Ser474), and MMP-9 decreased significantly after scabertopin treatment in a dose-dependent manner (Figure 5C). Therefore, we suggest that scabertopin can downregulate the expression of MMP-9 by inhibiting the activation of the FAK/PI3K/Akt signaling axis and, ultimately, inhibit the invasiveness of bladder cancer cells. Similarly, we sought to understand the role of ROS in this process. We found that the expressions of phospho-FAK, phospho-PI3K, phospho-Akt, and MMP-9 were significantly inhibited by NAC (Figure 5D). This indicated that ROS played a very important role in scabertopin-mediated invasion and metastasis of J82 cells. These results suggested that scabertopin may be a multifunctional inhibitor for the treatment of bladder cancer.

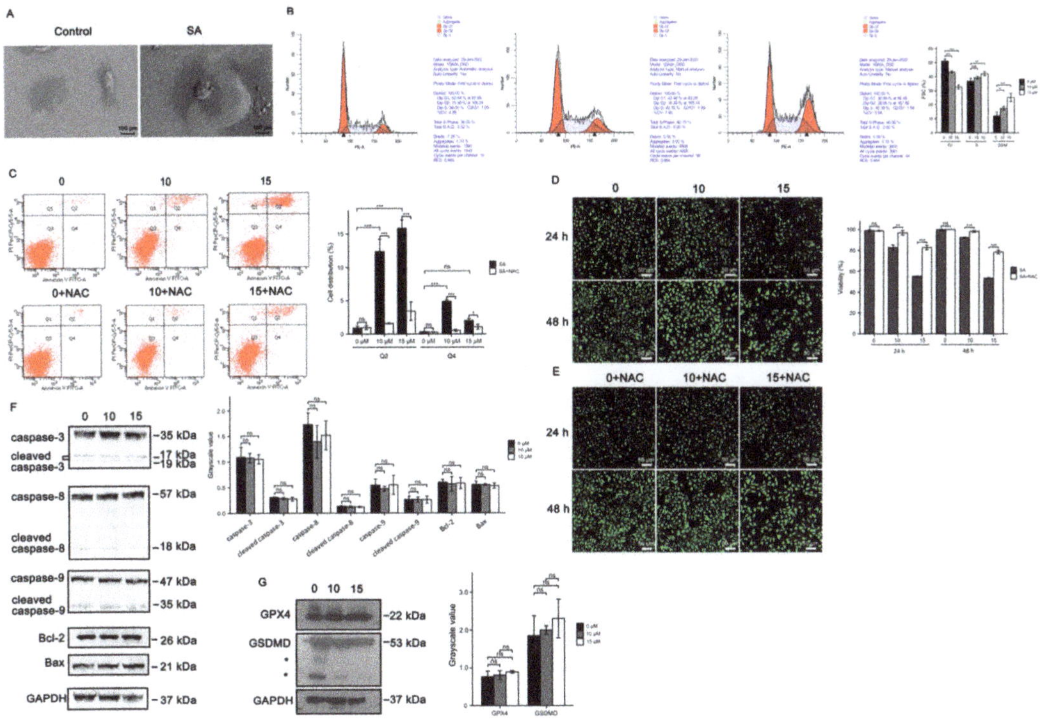

Figure 3. Cell death induced by scabertopin treatment can be rescued by NAC. (**A**) SEM images show that, in J82 cells treated for 24 h with 10 μM of scabertopin, the cell spreading area increases and the cell pseudopods shorten and thin out. The 24 h scabertopin treatment induces cell cycle arrest (**B**) and death (**C**) in J82 cells in a concentration-dependent manner (the black arrowheads in Figure 3B indicate the values of the peaks). The live/death cell assay shows scabertopin inhibits the viability of J82 cells after 24 and 48 h of treatment (**D**), and this effect can be reduced by NAC treatment (**E**,**F**). The expression levels of the apoptosis-related proteins caspase-9, caspase-8, caspase-3, Bax, and Bcl-2 in J82 cells do not significantly change after 24 h of scabertopin treatment. (**G**). Scabertopin does not significantly alter the expression of the ferroptosis- and pyroptosis-related proteins GPX4 and GSDMD, respectively, in J82 cells after 24 h treatment. A total of 5 μM of NAC was used in the experiments, * means nonspecific bands. Data represent the mean ± s.e.m. of the three independent experiments. * $p < 0.05$; ** $p < 0.01$; *** $p < 0.001$, ns: no significance vs. 0 μM scabertopin-treated group. The grayscale values are normalized to GAPDH. Bax: Bcl-2-associated X; Bcl-2: B cell lymphoma-2; GPX4: glutathione peroxidase 4; GSDMD: Gasdermin-D; NAC: *N*-acetylcysteine; PE-A: phycoerythrin area; PerCP-Cy5-5-A: Peridinin-Chlorophyll-Protein Complex-Cyanine5.5 area; SA: scabertopin.

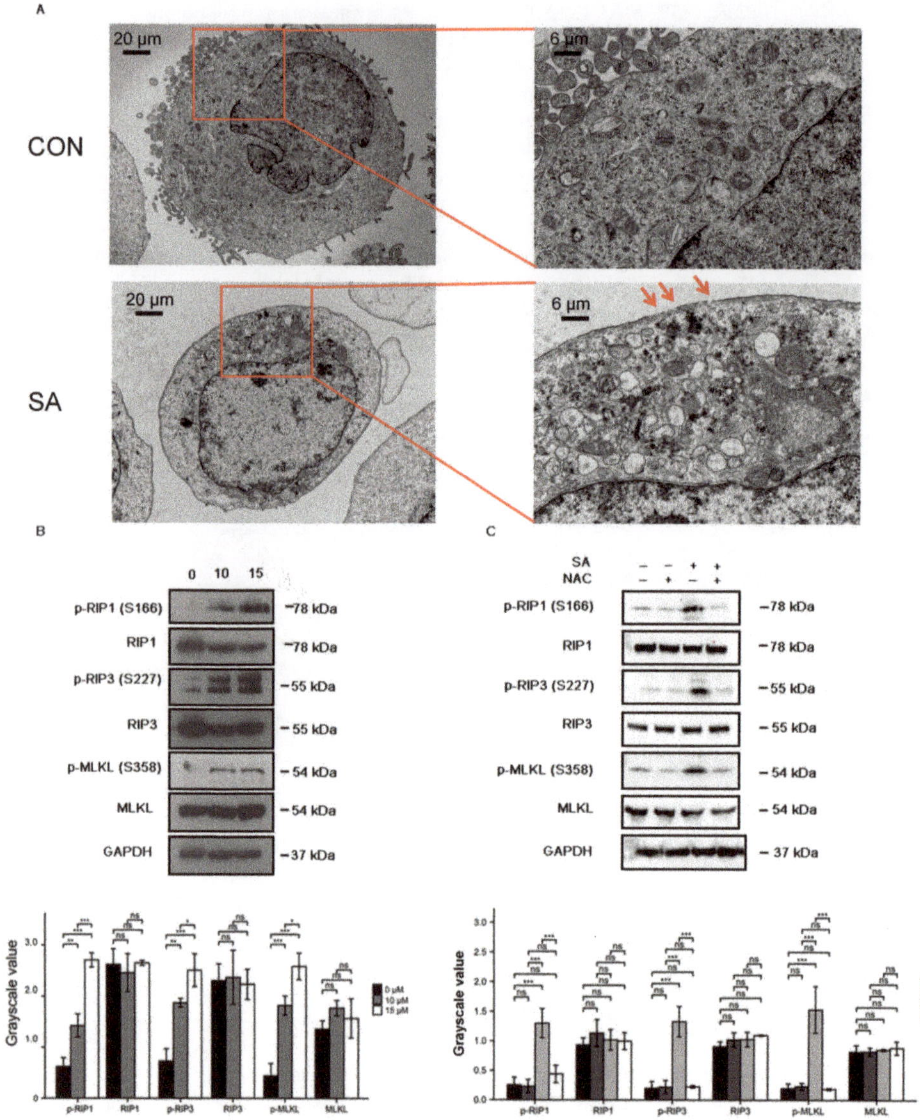

Figure 4. Scabertopin-treated J82 cells undergo necroptosis, which can be rescued by NAC. (**A**) TEM images are shown for the control group (CON) and the J82 cells treated with 10 μM of scabertopin (SA) for 24 h. The image on the right is an enlarged image of the left image, and the red arrow points to the perforation on the cell membrane during necroptosis; at least three independent samples were observed in each group. (**B**) Scabertopin can significantly increase the phosphorylation of the necroptosis-related proteins RIP1, RIP3, and MLKL (n = 3) after 24 h of treatment; (**C**) Scabertopin-induced phosphorylation of RIP1, RIP3, and MLKL can be reversed by NAC in the group treated with 10 μM of scabertopin for 24 h. A total of 5 μM of NAC was used in the experiments. The grayscale values are normalized to GAPDH. Data represent the mean ± s.e.m. of the three independent experiments. * $p < 0.05$, ** $p < 0.01$, *** $p < 0.001$, ns: no significance vs. 0 μM scabertopin-treated group. MLKL: mixed lineage kinase like; NAC: N-acetylcysteine; p-: phosphorylated; RIP1: receptor-interacting protein.

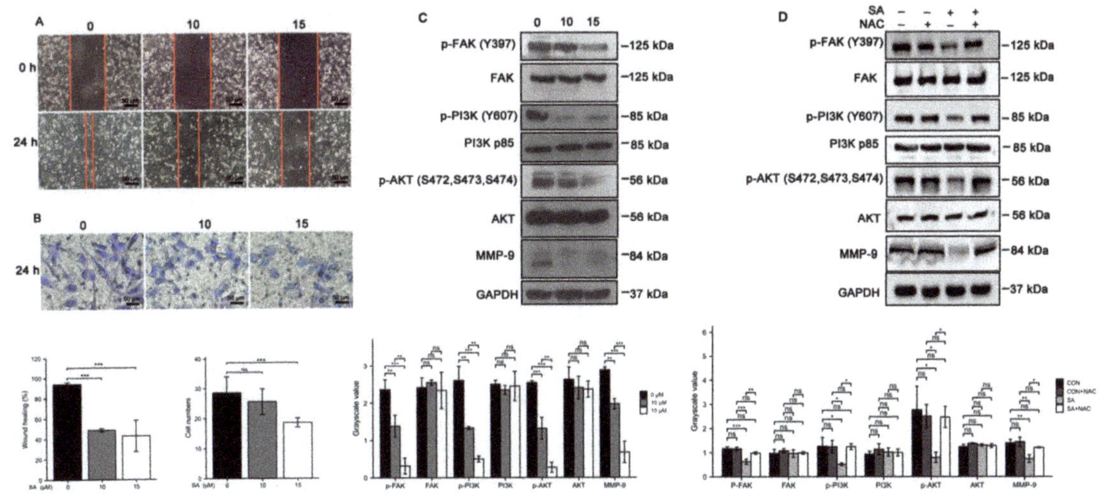

Figure 5. Scabertopin treatment inhibits the migratory and invasive ability of J82 cells by inhibiting the FAK/PI3K/Akt/MMP-9 signaling pathway, which can be rescued by NAC. Scabertopin significantly inhibits the migration ability (difference in area reduction between red lines) (n = 3) (**A**) and invasion of (n = 5) (**B**) of J82 cells treated with gradient concentrations of scabertopin for 24 h. (**C**) Phospho-FAK, phospho-PI3K, phospho-Akt, and MMP-9 expression levels significantly decrease in J82 cells after 24 h of scabertopin treatment. (**D**) Scabertopin-induced phosphorylation of p-FAK, p-PI3K, p-Akt, and MMP-9 expression can be reversed by NAC. A total of 5 μM of NAC was used in the experiments. The grayscale values are normalized to GAPDH. Data are presented as the mean ± s.e.m. of the three independent experiments (n = 3). * $p < 0.05$, ** $p < 0.01$, *** $p < 0.001$, ns: no significance vs. 0 μM scabertopin-treated group. AKT: Akt-protein kinase B; CON: control group; FAK: focal adhesion kinase; MMP-9: matrix metalloprotease-9; NAC: N-acetylcysteine; p-: phosphorylated; PI3K: phosphoinositide 3-kinase; SA: scabertopin.

4. Discussion

Despite extensive advances in the treatment of bladder cancer, it remains one of the most recurring and life-threatening tumors. Natural herbs are an important source of potential anticancer compounds in the field of drug discovery and development [33]. Natural compounds themselves contain unique structurally diverse molecules with multiple targets, making them ideal candidates for drug discovery and development.

Scabertopin, a sesquiterpene compound extracted from *E. scaber L*, has attracted interest because of its promising antitumor effects. In the present study, the anti-proliferative ability of scabertopin against various bladder cancer cell lines and human ureteral epithelial immortalized cells (SV-HUC-1) was assessed using the CCK-8 assay. Our results showed that scabertopin significantly inhibited the viability of bladder cancer cells in a dose-dependent manner but had a weak effect on the viability of noncancerous SV-HUC-1 cells. The above results suggested that scabertopin may be a potentially useful agent for bladder tumor treatment. In addition, we also found that J82 cells treated with scabertopin displayed a decrease in ΔΨ and an increase in superoxide anion production. ROS are a different class of molecular oxygen derivatives produced during normal aerobic metabolism. They include peroxides, superoxides, singlet oxygen, and free radicals. ROS levels are higher in different types of cancer cells than in normal cells. However, further elevation of ROS levels increases the susceptibility of cancer cells to oxidative stress-induced cell death [34,35]. Natural active ingredients and their derivatives are one of the main sources of antitumor drugs [7], and studies have shown that natural products can exert antitumor effects by increasing ROS levels. For example, isoalantolactone induces the elevation of

ROS levels in human pancreatic ductal epithelial carcinoma PANC-1 cells, arrests these cells in the S phase, thereby inhibiting cell proliferation and inducing apoptosis [36]. We used flow cytometry to detect the effect of scabertopin on the cell cycle of J82 cells. Our results demonstrated that scabertopin could induce cell cycle arrest at the S and G2/M phases in a concentration-dependent manner. In addition, ROS can act as signaling molecules and play a key role in the drug-induced inhibition of tumor invasion and metastasis. In the present study, we likewise observed that scabertopin significantly inhibited cell migration and invasive ability. Cell migration and invasion are key phenotypes that affect the metastasis of tumors. FAK is a cytoplasmic nonreceptor protein tyrosine kinase, a member of the adhesion patch complex family, and an important regulator that mediates cell adhesion to the extracellular matrix (ECM) [37]. The upregulation and hyperphosphorylation of FAK expression have been shown to increase the invasive capacity of several malignancies, including gastric and breast cancers, whereas the inhibition of FAK activity significantly reduces the migration capacity of breast cancer cells [38]. Tyr397 is the major phosphorylation site of FAK and phosphorylation of FAK leads to tumor metastasis and disease progression by promoting migration and invasion [39]. We found that scabertopin could inhibit the expression of MMP-9 in J82 cells by inhibiting the FAK/PI3K/Akt signaling pathway, and the inhibition could be rescued by NAC. MMP-9 is a member of the MMP family and a key enzyme necessary for the degradation of the ECM. The ECM is the first barrier that restricts tumor cells from undergoing migration. Activated MMP-9 can degrade the ECM and basement membrane components, allowing tumor cells to break through the primary site and become invasive and metastatic [40]. Therefore, we propose that scabertopin inhibits the pathway of FAK/PI3K/Akt/MMP-9 axis, which in turn inhibits cell migration and invasion.

In the present study, we found that scabertopin could induce the production and accumulation of ROS in J82 cells, which was identified as superoxide anion-dominated mitochondrial ROS (Figure 2). ROS is one of the important mechanisms that cause ferroptosis in cells, and the level of intracellular ROS accumulation is often positively correlated with the severity of ferroptosis [41]. However, in this study, although we found an increase in ROS, there was no difference in the expression of ferroptosis-related molecules (Figure 3). This phenomenon may be related to the type of ROS. They can cause cell death by damaging DNA, RNA, and lipid molecules [42]. During ferroptosis, the accumulation of lipid peroxides, especially phospholipid peroxides, is considered to be a landmark event of ferroptosis and also a prerequisite for ferroptosis [43]. Accordingly, some scholars refer to lipid peroxides that can specifically cause ferroptosis, such as arachidonoyl (AA)-phosphatidylethanolamine (PE) and adrenoyl (AdA)-PE, as ferroptosis-specific lipid peroxidation [44]. However, this is not rigid, because hydrogen peroxide in the presence of iron ions can be converted into hydroxyl radicals through the Fenton reaction, which in turn oxidizes lipids to form lipid peroxides [45]. While levels of iron, iron-containing proteins [46], and lipid peroxides [47] also promote necroptosis, GPX4 can prevent RIP3-dependent necroptosis in erythroid precursor cells by avoiding lipidic ROS accumulation [48]. Another major difference between ferroptosis and necroptosis is that the cellular morphology of ferroptosis is very unique. Unlike apoptosis or necroptosis, the morphological features of ferroptosis are mainly changes in mitochondrial structure without the shrinkage, rupture, and perforation of the plasma membrane [32]. In tumor cells, the original level of ROS is higher than that of ordinary cells, but abnormally high levels of ROS can also induce different forms of cell death [49]. The occurrence of necroptosis is closely related to the overproduction of ROS [44]. Although the mechanism of ROS in necroptosis is not fully understood, there is a lot of evidence that ROS play a crucial role in many drugs-induced necroptosis [50,51], which is accompanied by mitochondrial injury and decreased expression of MMPs [52]. The key molecules in necroptosis, RIP1 and RIP3, are most closely related to mitochondrial ROS. For example, mitochondrial ROS can mediate the autophosphorylation of RIP1, which subsequently induces necroptosis by recruiting and promoting the phosphorylation of RIP3, suggesting that mitochondrial

ROS are the initiators of necroptosis [28]. On the other hand, it has been observed in hepatic stellate cells that the activation of RIP1/RIP3 not only promotes necroptosis, but also increases ROS production via a positive feedback loop [22]. Mediating necroptosis by drug-induced ROS has emerged as a potential approach for tumor therapy because the occurrence of necroptosis not only bypasses apoptosis [53,54], but also causes death in apoptosis-resistant cancer cells. Second, this mechanism of necroptosis induced by ROS can occur in most common cancers. This is consistent with the phenomena we observed, such as membrane perforation and mitochondrial shrinkage, in the scabertopin-treated J82 cells using TEM. Flow cytometry showed that the treatment of scabertopin could increase the number of late apoptotic, necrotic, and dead J82 cells in the Q2 region. However, the expression of apoptosis-related caspase protein, Bcl-2, and Bax displayed no significant difference, which was the same as for ferroptosis. However, necroptosis-related phospho-RIP1, phospho-RIP3, and phospho-MLKL were significantly upregulated by scabertopin treatment and could be inhibited by NAC. Therefore, we believe that scabertopin can promote the increase of mitochondrial ROS by causing a decrease in mitochondrial membrane potential, thereby stimulating the phosphorylation and activation of RIP1/RIP3/MLKL and, finally, triggering necroptosis (Figure 6).

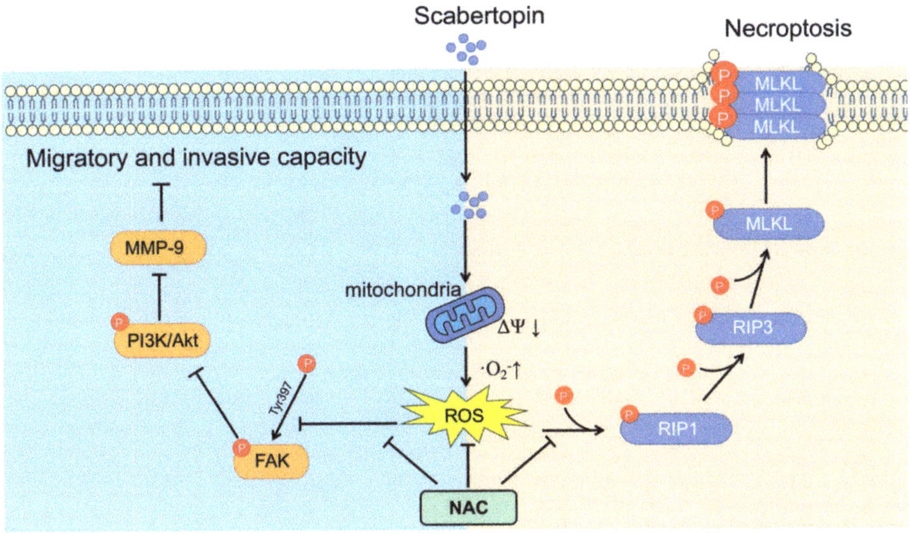

Figure 6. Mechanism of scabertopine inhibiting invasion and promoting necroptosis in human bladder cancer J82 cells. Scabertopin can reduce mitochondrial membrane potential and stimulate mitochondrial ROS production, thereby activating RIP1/RIP3/MLKL phosphorylation, mediating J82 cell necroptosis, and inhibiting the FAK/PI3K/Akt/MMP-9 signaling pathway. This in turn inhibits the migration and invasive potential of J82 cells. Akt: Akt-protein kinase B; FAK: focal adhesion kinase; MLKL: mixed lineage kinase like; MMP-9: matrix metalloprotease 9; NAC: *N*-acetylcysteine; PI3K: phosphoinositide 3-kinase; p-: phosphorylated; RIP: receptor-interacting protein.

In fact, previous studies have reported the phenomenon of sesquiterpenoid-induced ROS increase. For example, Verma et al. found that isodeoxyelephantopin and deoxyelephantopin can inhibit the activation of NF-κB by inducing the production of ROS and inhibit the growth of breast cancer [55]. Xanthatin, a sesquiterpenoid derived from Xanthium strumarium L, may induce the elevation of ROS, mitochondrial injury, and apoptosis in non-small cell lung cancer (NSCLC) [56]. The ability of sesquiterpenes to induce ROS generation may stem from the fact that they both have α-methylene-γ-lactone and [57] a cyclopentenone ring-like structure (butenolide in scabertopin) (Figure 1A) [58]. The most direct mechanism of sesquiterpenoid-induced ROS elevation may be related to its ability to change the mitochondrial $\Delta\Psi$ [59]. In fact, there are a variety of ROS inducers that directly act on the mitochondrial voltage-dependent anion channel, resulting in a change in $\Delta\Psi$, a decrease in glycolysis, and an increase in ROS [60,61]. From this, we speculate that these unique structures of sesquiterpenes, namely α-methylene-γ-lactone and cyclopentenone ring-like structures, may affect the changes in mitochondrial $\Delta\Psi$ and cause the increase in ROS. Scabertopin not only has the capacity to trigger this mechanism owing to its unique structure but also meets the rules of five in terms of pharmacokinetics. Since the molecular weight (MW) of SA is 358.4 Da, the logarithm of lipid water partition coefficient (LogP) is 2.6, the hydrogen bond donor count is 0, the hydrogen bond acceptor count is 6, and the rotatable bond count is 3 [62]. These characteristics of SA well meet the Lipinski rules, which requires the MW to be less than 500 Da, the LogP to be between -2 and 5, the hydrogen bond donor count to be less than 5, and the count of hydrogen bond acceptor and the rotatable bond to be less than 10 [63]. In our study, we found that scabertopin significantly reduced $\Delta\Psi$, promoted ROS generation, and increased intracellular ROS accumulation by depleting GSH in J82 cells. ROS-induced necroptosis is likely to be associated with decreased GSH [64]. The decrease in GSH, the most important antioxidant-reduction factor in cells, is the result of ROS-induced GSH oxidation, and ROS production is further enhanced by depleting GSH [65]. NAC can supplement GSH by donating cysteine, thereby exerting anti-ROS effect [66]. NAC-treated cells also promote mitochondrial integrity through multiple mechanisms, maintain mitochondrial function, and reduce ROS production, thereby protecting cells from necroptosis [67].

However, we did not evaluate the therapeutic efficacy of scabertopin in vivo, and its pharmacokinetics and pharmacodynamics in vivo remain unclear. Therefore, further studies are needed to provide additional evidence for the use of scabertopin as a chemotherapeutic agent or adjuvant in the chemotherapy of bladder cancer.

5. Conclusions

We demonstrate that scabertopin can deplete GSH in bladder cancer cells and cause ROS elevation and accumulation by reducing $\Delta\Psi$. It also inhibits bladder cancer cell migration and invasion by targeting the FAK/PI3K/Akt/MMP-9 axis. Furthermore, scabertopin can mediate necroptosis of bladder cancer cells by activating the RIP1/RIP3/MLKL pathway through phosphorylation and inhibit the proliferation and viability of bladder cancer cells. Using the ROS scavenger NAC can not only reduce cell death caused by scabertopin but also rescue J82 cells from scabertopin-mediated necroptosis and limit their invasive and migratory ability by inhibiting the phosphorylation activation of the two abovementioned signaling pathways. In conclusion, our study provides new insights into the anti-bladder cancer mechanisms of scabertopin, suggesting that scabertopin may be a potential alternative drug for bladder cancer therapy.

Supplementary Materials: The following supporting information can be downloaded at: https://www.mdpi.com/article/10.3390/cancers14235976/s1, File S1: Original blots.

Author Contributions: Experiments and data collection were performed by Y.G., Z.N. and H.C. Data analysis was performed by Y.G., Z.N., H.C., M.C., Y.X. and D.H. The study was designed by Y.G., Z.N., X.Y. and S.Z. The manuscript was written by Y.G. and Z.N. All authors revised the previous versions of the manuscript. Y.G. and Z.N. contributed equally to this work. All authors have read and agreed to the published version of the manuscript.

Funding: This work was supported by the Finance Science and Technology Project of Hainan Province (grant numbers 820QN423, 821QN424, and ZDYF2021SHFZ096), the National Nature Science Foundation of China (grant No. 82160531), and the Health Industry Scientific Research Project of Hainan Province (grant numbers 21A200412 and 21A200149).

Institutional Review Board Statement: Not applicable.

Informed Consent Statement: Not applicable.

Data Availability Statement: The data can be shared upon request.

Conflicts of Interest: The authors declare no conflict of interest.

References

1. Siegel, R.L.; Miller, K.D.; Fuchs, H.E.; Jemal, A. Cancer statistics, 2022. *CA A Cancer J. Clin.* **2022**, *72*, 7–33. [CrossRef] [PubMed]
2. Siegel, R.L.; Miller, K.D.; Fuchs, H.E.; Jemal, A. Cancer Statistics, 2021. *CA A Cancer J. Clin.* **2021**, *71*, 7–33. [CrossRef] [PubMed]
3. Chen, W.; Zheng, R.; Baade, P.D.; Zhang, S.; Zeng, H.; Bray, F.; Jemal, A.; Xue, Q.Y.; Jie, H. Cancer statistics in China, 2015. *CA A Cancer J. Clin.* **2016**, *66*, 115–132. [CrossRef] [PubMed]
4. Saluja, M.; Gilling, P. Intravesical bacillus Calmette-Guérin instillation in non-muscle-invasive bladder cancer: A review. *Int. J. Urol.* **2017**, *25*, 18–24. [CrossRef]
5. Motzer, R.J.; Jonasch, E.; Boyle, S.; Carlo, M.I.; Motter, A.D. NCCN Guidelines Insights: Kidney Cancer, Version 1.2021. *J. Natl. Compr. Cancer Netw.* **2020**, *18*, 1160–1170. [CrossRef]
6. Campodonico, A.; Crocellà, A.; Fresu, I. Influence of glucose and saline solutions on biliary secretion, in relation to hepatic elimination of biligrafin. Experimental study on cholecystectomized dogs. *IL Fegato* **1965**, *11*, 219–225.
7. Safe, S.; Kasiappan, R. Natural Products as Mechanism-based Anticancer Agents: Sp Transcription Factors as Targets. *Phytother. Res.* **2016**, *30*, 1723–1732. [CrossRef]
8. Xu, G.; Liang, Q.; Gong, Z.; Yu, W.; He, S.; Xi, L. Antitumor activities of the four sesquiterpene lactones from *Elephantopus scaber* L. *Exp. Oncol.* **2006**, *28*, 106–109.
9. Anitha, V.T.; Marimuthuantonisamy, J.; Jeeva, S. Anti-bacterial studies on Hemigraphis colorata (Blume) H.G. Hallier and *Elephantopus scaber* L. *Asian Pac. J. Trop. Med.* **2012**, *5*, 52–57. [CrossRef]
10. Tahir, M.; Amara, M.; Hamed, G.; Muhammad, K.; Ma, T. Deoxyelephantopin and Isodeoxyelephantopin as Potential Anticancer Agents with Effects on Multiple Signaling Pathways. *Molecules* **2017**, *22*, 1013.
11. Su, M.; Chung, H.Y.; Li, Y. Deoxyelephantopin from *Elephantopus scaber* L. induces cell-cycle arrest and apoptosis in the human nasopharyngeal cancer CNE cells. *Biochem. Biophys. Res. Commun.* **2011**, *411*, 342–347. [CrossRef] [PubMed]
12. Yan, G.R.; Tan, Z.; Wang, Y.; Xu, M.L.; Yu, G.; Li, Y.; He, Q.Y. Quantitative proteomics characterization on the antitumor effects of isodeoxyelephantopin against nasopharyngeal carcinoma. *Proteomics* **2013**, *13*, 3222–3232. [CrossRef] [PubMed]
13. Beeran, A.A.; Maliyakkal, N.; Rao, M.C.; Udupa, N. The enriched fraction of Elephantopus scaber Triggers apoptosis and inhibits multi-drug resistance transporters in human epithelial cancer cells. *Pharmacogn. Mag.* **2015**, *11*, 257–268. [PubMed]
14. Huang, C.C.; Lo, C.P.; Chiu, C.Y.; Shyur, L.F. Deoxyelephantopin, a novel multifunctional agent, suppresses mammary tumour growth and lung metastasis and doubles survival time in mice. *Br. J. Pharmacol.* **2010**, *159*, 856–871. [CrossRef]
15. Hong, L.; Chen, J.; Wu, F.; Wu, F.; Xia, Y. Isodeoxyelephantopin Inactivates Thioredoxin Reductase 1 and Activates ROS-Mediated JNK Signaling Pathway to Exacerbate Cisplatin Effectiveness in Human Colon Cancer Cells. *Front. Cell Dev. Biol.* **2020**, *8*, 580517. [CrossRef] [PubMed]
16. Kabeer, F.A.; Rajalekshmi, D.S.; Nair, M.S.; Prathapan, R. Molecular mechanisms of anticancer activity of deoxyelephantopin in cancer cells. *Integr. Med. Res.* **2017**, *6*, 190–206. [CrossRef]
17. Mehmood, T.; Maryam, A.; Zhang, H.; Li, Y.; Khan, M.; Ma, T. Deoxyelephantopin induces apoptosis in HepG2 cells via oxidative stress, NF-κB inhibition and mitochondrial dysfunction. *BioFactors* **2017**, *43*, 63–72. [CrossRef]
18. Geetha, B.S.; Nair, M.S.; Latha, P.G.; Remani, P. Sesquiterpene Lactones Isolated from *Elephantopus scaber* L. Inhibits Human Lymphocyte Proliferation and the Growth of Tumour Cell Lines and Induces Apoptosis In Vitro. *J. Biomed. Biotechnol.* **2012**, *2012*, 721285. [CrossRef]
19. Koe, X.F.; Lim, E.L.; Seah, T.C.; Amanah, A.; Wahab, H.A.; Adenan, M.I.; Sulaiman, S.F.; Tan, M.L. Evaluation of in vitro cytochrome P450 induction and inhibition activity of deoxyelephantopin, a sesquiterpene lactone from *Elephantopus scaber* L. *Food Chem. Toxicol.* **2013**, *60*, 98–108. [CrossRef]
20. Galluzzi, L.; Kroemer, G. Necroptosis: A Specialized Pathway of Programmed Necrosis. *Cell* **2009**, *135*, 1161–1163. [CrossRef]
21. Berghe, T.V.; Linkermann, A.; Jouan-Lanhouet, S.; Walczak, H.; Vandenabeele, P. Regulated necrosis: The expanding network of non-apoptotic cell death pathways. *Nat. Rev. Mol. Cell Biol.* **2014**, *15*, 135–147. [CrossRef] [PubMed]
22. Jia, Y.; Wang, F.; Guo, Q.; Li, M.; Wang, L.; Zhang, Z.; Jiang, S.; Jin, H.; Chen, A.; Tan, S.; et al. Curcumol induces RIPK1/RIPK3 complex-dependent necroptosis via JNK1/2-ROS signaling in hepatic stellate cells. *Redox Biol.* **2018**, *19*, 375–387. [CrossRef] [PubMed]
23. Liu, X.; Zhang, Y.; Gao, H.; Hou, Y.; Lu, J.J.; Feng, Y.; Xu, Q.; Liu, B.; Chen, X. Induction of an MLKL mediated non-canonical necroptosis through reactive oxygen species by tanshinol A in lung cancer cells—ScienceDirect. *Biochem. Pharmacol.* **2019**, *171*, 113684. [CrossRef] [PubMed]
24. Chen, X.; Li, W.; Ren, J.; Huang, D.; He, W.T.; Song, Y.; Chao, Y. Translocation of mixed lineage kinase domain-like protein to plasma membrane leads to necrotic cell death. *Cell Res.* **2014**, *24*, 105–121. [CrossRef] [PubMed]
25. Wang, H.; Sun, L.; Su, L.; Rizo, J.; Liu, L.; Wang, L.F.; Wang, F.S.; Wang, X. Mixed Lineage Kinase Domain-like Protein MLKL Causes Necrotic Membrane Disruption upon Phosphorylation by RIP3. *Mol. Cell* **2014**, *54*, 133–146. [CrossRef] [PubMed]

26. Dondelinger, Y.; Declercq, W.; Montessuit, S.; Roelandt, R.; Goncalves, A.; Bruggeman, I.; Hulpiau, P.; Weber, K.; Sehon, C.A.; Marquis, R.W.; et al. MLKL comprises plasma membrane integrity by binding to phosphatidylinositol phosphates. *Cell Rep.* **2014**, *7*, 971–981. [CrossRef] [PubMed]
27. Hsu, S.K.; Chang, W.T.; Lin, I.L.; Chen, Y.F.; Chiu, C.C. The Role of Necroptosis in ROS-Mediated Cancer Therapies and Its Promising Applications. *Cancers* **2020**, *12*, 2185. [CrossRef]
28. Zhang, Y.; Su, S.; Zhao, S.; Yang, Z.; Zhong, C.; Chen, X.; Cai, Q.; Yang, Z.; Huang, D.; Wu, R.; et al. RIP1 autophosphorylation is promoted by mitochondrial ROS and is essential for RIP3 recruitment into necrosome. *Nat. Commun.* **2017**, *8*, 14329. [CrossRef]
29. Chauhan, A.K.; Min, K.J.; Kwon, T.K. RIP1-dependent reactive oxygen species production executes artesunate-induced cell death in renal carcinoma Caki cells. *Mol. Cell. Biochem.* **2017**, *435*, 15–24. [CrossRef]
30. Wang, K.J.; Meng, X.Y.; Chen, J.F.; Wang, K.Y.; Ma, Q. Emodin Induced Necroptosis and Inhibited Glycolysis in the Renal Cancer Cells by Enhancing ROS. *Oxid. Med. Cell. Longev.* **2021**, *2021*, 8840590. [CrossRef]
31. Pak, V.; Ezeriņa, D.; Lyublinskaya, O.; Pedre, B.; Tyurin-Kuzmin, P.; Mishina, N.; Thauvin, M.; Young, D.; Wahni, K.; Martínez Gache, S.; et al. Ultrasensitive Genetically Encoded Indicator for Hydrogen Peroxide Identifies Roles for the Oxidant in Cell Migration and Mitochondrial Function. *Cell Metab.* **2020**, *31*, 642–653.E6. [CrossRef] [PubMed]
32. Nie, Z.; Chen, M.; Gao, Y.; Huang, D.; Cao, H.; Peng, Y.; Guo, N.; Zhang, S. Regulated Cell Death in Urinary Malignancies. *Front. Cell Dev. Biol.* **2021**, *9*, 789004. [CrossRef] [PubMed]
33. Millimouno, F.M.; Dong, J.; Yang, L.; Li, J.; Li, X. Targeting apoptosis pathways in cancer and perspectives with natural compounds from mother nature. *Cancer Prev. Res.* **2014**, *7*, 1081. [CrossRef] [PubMed]
34. Zhang, J.; Wang, X.; Vikash, V.; Ye, Q.; Dong, W. ROS and ROS-mediated cellular signaling. *Oxid. Med. Cell. Longev.* **2016**, *2016*, 4350965. [CrossRef] [PubMed]
35. De Sá Junior, P.L.; Dias, C.D.A.; Saj, P.A.; Moreira, F.P.M.; Doria, J.S.O.; Pinheiro, A.R.; Kleber, F.A. The Roles of ROS in Cancer Heterogeneity and Therapy. *Oxid. Med. Cell. Longev.* **2017**, *2017*, 2467940. [CrossRef] [PubMed]
36. Khan, M.; Ding, C.; Rasul, A.; Fei, Y.; Ma, T. Isoalantolactone Induces Reactive Oxygen Species Mediated Apoptosis in Pancreatic Carcinoma PANC-1 Cells. *Int. J. Biol. Sci.* **2012**, *8*, 533–547. [CrossRef] [PubMed]
37. Murphy, J.M.; Jeong, K.; Lim, S. FAK Family Kinases in Vascular Diseases. *Int. J. Mol. Sci.* **2020**, *21*, 3630. [CrossRef]
38. Mclean, G.W.; Carragher, N.O.; Avizienyte, E.; Evans, J.; Brunton, V.G.; Frame, M.C. The role of focal-adhesion kinase in cancer—a new therapeutic opportunity. *Nat. Rev. Cancer* **2005**, *5*, 505–515. [CrossRef]
39. Lai, I.R.; Chu, P.Y.; Lin, H.S.; Liou, J.Y.; Jan, Y.J.; Lee, J.C.; Shen, T.L. Phosphorylation of Focal Adhesion Kinase at Tyr397 in Gastric Carcinomas and its Clinical Significance. *Am. J. Pathol.* **2010**, *177*, 1629–1637. [CrossRef]
40. Jang, H.; Hong, O.; Youn, H.; Kim, M.; Kim, C.; Jung, S.; Kim, J. 15d-PGJ2 inhibits NF-κB and AP-1-mediated MMP-9 expression and invasion of breast cancer cell by means of a heme oxygenase-1-dependent mechanism. *BMB Rep.* **2020**, *53*, 212–217. [CrossRef]
41. Yang, W.; Stockwell, B. Synthetic lethal screening identifies compounds activating iron-dependent, nonapoptotic cell death in oncogenic-RAS-harboring cancer cells. *Chem. Biol.* **2008**, *15*, 234–245. [CrossRef]
42. Yang, W.; Stockwell, B. Ferroptosis: Death by Lipid Peroxidation. *Trends Cell Biol.* **2016**, *26*, 165–176. [CrossRef] [PubMed]
43. D'Herde, K.; Krysko, D. Ferroptosis: Oxidized PEs trigger death. *Nat. Chem. Biol.* **2017**, *13*, 4–5. [CrossRef] [PubMed]
44. Florean, C.; Song, S.; Dicato, M.; Diederich, M. Redox biology of regulated cell death in cancer: A focus on necroptosis and ferroptosis. *Free. Radic. Biol. Med.* **2019**, *134*, 177–189. [CrossRef]
45. Reczek, C.; Chandel, N. ROS-dependent signal transduction. *Curr. Opin. Cell Biol.* **2015**, *33*, 8–13. [CrossRef] [PubMed]
46. Xie, C.; Zhang, N.; Zhou, H.; Li, J.; Li, Q.; Zarubin, T.; Lin, S.; Han, J. Distinct roles of basal steady-state and induced H-ferritin in tumor necrosis factor-induced death in L929 cells. *Mol. Cell. Biol.* **2005**, *25*, 6673–6681. [CrossRef] [PubMed]
47. Vandenabeele, P.; Galluzzi, L.; Vanden Berghe, T.; Kroemer, G. Molecular mechanisms of necroptosis: An ordered cellular explosion. Nature reviews. *Mol. Cell. Biol.* **2010**, *11*, 700–714. [CrossRef]
48. Canli, Ö.; Alankuş, Y.; Grootjans, S.; Vegi, N.; Hültner, L.; Hoppe, P.; Schroeder, T.; Vandenabeele, P.; Bornkamm, G.; Greten, F. Glutathione peroxidase 4 prevents necroptosis in mouse erythroid precursors. *Blood* **2016**, *127*, 139–148. [CrossRef]
49. Galadari, S.; Rahman, A.; Pallichankandy, S.; Thayyullathil, F. Reactive oxygen species and cancer paradox: To promote or to suppress? *Free. Radic. Biol. Med.* **2017**, *104*, 144–164. [CrossRef]
50. Zhang, Z.; Zhang, Z.; Li, Q.; Jiao, H.; Chong, D.; Sun, X.; Zhang, P.; Huo, Q.; Liu, H. Shikonin induces necroptosis by reactive oxygen species activation in nasopharyngeal carcinoma cell line CNE-2Z. *J. Bioenerg. Biomembr.* **2017**, *49*, 265–272. [CrossRef]
51. Liu, T.; Sun, X.; Cao, Z. Shikonin-induced necroptosis in nasopharyngeal carcinoma cells via ROS overproduction and upregulation of RIPK1/RIPK3/MLKL expression. *OncoTargets Ther.* **2019**, *12*, 2605–2614. [CrossRef] [PubMed]
52. Huangfu, M.; Wei, R.; Wang, J.; Qin, J.; Yu, D.; Guan, X.; Li, X.; Fu, M.; Liu, H.; Chen, X. Osthole induces necroptosis via ROS overproduction in glioma cells. *FEBS Open Bio.* **2021**, *11*, 456–467. [CrossRef]
53. Su, Z.; Yang, Z.; Xie, L.; DeWitt, J.; Chen, Y. Cancer therapy in the necroptosis era. *Cell Death Differ.* **2016**, *23*, 748–756. [CrossRef]
54. Moriwaki, K.; Bertin, J.; Gough, P.; Orlowski, G.; Chan, F. Differential roles of RIPK1 and RIPK3 in TNF-induced necroptosis and chemotherapeutic agent-induced cell death. *Cell Death Dis.* **2015**, *6*, e1636. [CrossRef] [PubMed]
55. Verma, S.; Rai, V.; Awasthee, N.; Dhasmana, A.; Rajalaksmi, D.; Nair, M.; Gupta, S. Isodeoxyelephantopin, a Sesquiterpene Lactone Induces ROS Generation, Suppresses NF-κB Activation, Modulates LncRNA Expression and Exhibit Activities Against Breast Cancer. *Sci. Rep.* **2019**, *9*, 17980. [CrossRef] [PubMed]

56. Xie, Y.; Zhu, X.; Liu, P.; Liu, Y.; Geng, Y.; Zhang, L. Xanthatin inhibits non-small cell lung cancer proliferation by breaking the redox balance. *Drug Dev. Res.* **2022**, *83*, 1176–1189. [CrossRef] [PubMed]
57. Ghantous, A.; Gali-Muhtasib, H.; Vuorela, H.; Saliba, N.; Darwiche, N. What made sesquiterpene lactones reach cancer clinical trials? *Drug Discov. Today* **2010**, *15*, 668–678. [CrossRef]
58. Woerdenbag, H.; Merfort, I.; Passreiter, C.; Schmidt, T.; Willuhn, G.; van Uden, W.; Pras, N.; Kampinga, H.; Konings, A. Cytotoxicity of flavonoids and sesquiterpene lactones from Arnica species against the GLC4 and the COLO 320 cell lines. *Planta Med.* **1994**, *60*, 434–437. [CrossRef]
59. Armstrong, J. The role of the mitochondrial permeability transition in cell death. *Mitochondrion* **2006**, *6*, 225–234. [CrossRef]
60. Chang, Y.; Kim, C. Molecular Research of Glycolysis. *Int. J. Mol. Sci.* **2022**, *23*, 5052. [CrossRef]
61. Yagoda, N.; von Rechenberg, M.; Zaganjor, E.; Bauer, A.; Yang, W.; Fridman, D.; Wolpaw, A.; Smukste, I.; Peltier, J.; Boniface, J.; et al. RAS-RAF-MEK-dependent oxidative cell death involving voltage-dependent anion channels. *Nature* **2007**, *447*, 864–868. [CrossRef] [PubMed]
62. National Library of Medicine (US), National Center for Biotechnology Information. PubChem Compound Summary for CID 93959111. 2004. Available online: https://pubchem.ncbi.nlm.nih.gov/compound/93959111 (accessed on 10 August 2022).
63. Lipinski, C.; Lombardo, F.; Dominy, B.; Feeney, P. Experimental and computational approaches to estimate solubility and permeability in drug discovery and development settings. *Adv. Drug Deliv. Rev.* **2001**, *46*, 3–26. [CrossRef] [PubMed]
64. D'Alessio, M.; Cerella, C.; De Nicola, M.; Bergamaschi, A.; Magrini, A.; Gualandi, G.; Alfonsi, A.; Ghibelli, L. Apoptotic GSH extrusion is associated with free radical generation. *Ann. N. Y. Acad. Sci.* **2003**, *1010*, 449–452. [CrossRef]
65. Moloney, J.; Cotter, T. ROS signalling in the biology of cancer. *Semin. Cell Dev. Biol.* **2018**, *80*, 50–64. [CrossRef]
66. Kavčič, N.; Pegan, K.; Vandenabeele, P.; Turk, B. Comparative study of the differential cell death protecting effect of various ROS scavengers. *Biol. Chem.* **2019**, *400*, 149–160. [CrossRef] [PubMed]
67. Li, C.; Sun, L.; Pang, C. Synergistic protection of N-acetylcysteine and ascorbic acid 2-phosphate on human mesenchymal stem cells against mitoptosis, necroptosis and apoptosis. *Sci. Rep.* **2015**, *5*, 9819. [CrossRef] [PubMed]

cancers

MDPI

Article

Therapeutic Potential of Deflamin against Colorectal Cancer Development and Progression

Sara Silva [1,†], Ana Cavaco [1,†], Bianca Basso [1], Joana Mota [2,3], Raquel Cruz-Duarte [1], Miguel Costa [1], Lara Carvalho [1], Ana Lima [2,3,*], Luis Costa [1,4], Ricardo Ferreira [3,‡] and Marta Martins [1,*,‡]

1 Instituto de Medicina Molecular—João Lobo Antunes, Faculdade de Medicina, Universidade de Lisboa, 1649-028 Lisbon, Portugal
2 Faculty of Veterinary Medicine, Lusófona University, 1749-024 Lisbon, Portugal
3 LEAF—Linking Landscape, Environment, Agriculture and Food, Instituto Superior de Agronomia, Universidade de Lisboa, Tapada da Ajuda, 1349-017 Lisbon, Portugal
4 Oncology Division, Hospital de Santa Maria, Centro Hospitalar Lisboa Norte, 1649-028 Lisbon, Portugal
* Correspondence: agusmaolima@gmail.com (A.L.); marta.martins@medicina.ulisboa.pt (M.M.)
† These authors contributed equally to this work and share first authorship.
‡ These authors contributed equally to this work and share last authorship.

Simple Summary: We have previously identified deflamin, an oligomeric protein isolated from the white lupine seeds (*Lupinus albus*) with anti-MMPs and anti-inflammatory properties. Given the involvement of MMPs and inflammation in the carcinogenesis process, we aimed to assess deflamin's role in cancer development and progression. Using colorectal cancer cell lines and zebrafish xenotransplant models, we found that deflamin exhibits anti-MMP-2 and anti-MMP-9 activity, being able to reduce tumor size and metastasis formation in vivo. Deflamin was shown to impair cancer cell migration and invasion, as well as collagen remodeling and angiogenesis in the tumor microenvironment, highly impacting cancer behavior. Overall, our results unravel the nutraceutical potential of deflamin in colorectal cancer treatment.

Abstract: Matrix metalloproteinases (MMPs) are proteolytic enzymes that play a crucial role in tumor microenvironment remodeling, contributing to inflammatory and angiogenic processes, and ultimately promoting tumor maintenance and progression. Several studies on bioactive polypeptides isolated from legumes have shown anti-migratory, anti-MMPs, and anti-tumor effects, potentially constituting novel strategies for both the prevention and progression of cancer. In this work, we investigated the anti-tumor role of deflamin, a protein oligomer isolated from white lupine seeds (*Lupinus albus*) reported to inhibit MMP-9 and cell migration in colorectal cancer (CRC) cell lines. We found that deflamin exerts an inhibitory effect on tumor growth and metastasis formation, contributing to increased tumor apoptosis in the xenotransplanted zebrafish larvae model. Furthermore, deflamin resulted not only in a significant reduction in MMP-2 and MMP-9 activity but also in impaired cancer cell migration and invasion in vitro. Using the xenograft zebrafish model, we observed that deflamin inhibits collagen degradation and angiogenesis in the tumor microenvironment in vivo. Overall, our work reveals the potential of deflamin as an agent against CRC development and progression.

Keywords: deflamin; colorectal cancer; MMP-2; MMP-9

Citation: Silva, S.; Cavaco, A.; Basso, B.; Mota, J.; Cruz-Duarte, R.; Costa, M.; Carvalho, L.; Lima, A.; Costa, L.; Ferreira, R.; et al. Therapeutic Potential of Deflamin against Colorectal Cancer Development and Progression. *Cancers* **2022**, *14*, 6182. https://doi.org/10.3390/cancers14246182

Academic Editors: Barbara De Filippis, Alessandra Ammazzalorso and Marialuigia Fantacuzzi

Received: 8 November 2022
Accepted: 7 December 2022
Published: 14 December 2022

1. Introduction

Colorectal cancer (CRC) is the third most common and the second leading cause of death by cancer worldwide [1]. As CRC patients die of metastatic disease, prevention of the development of metastasis is essential to improve cure rates.

To metastasize, a tumor cell has to invade the surrounding tissue, enter the bloodstream, survive in circulation, and extravasate and colonize the distant organ, a process that requires multiple interactions between the malignant cell and its microenvironment [2].

Matrix metalloproteinases (MMPs) comprise a large family of homologous zinc-dependent endoproteases, several of which play critical roles in this process, not only by degrading the extracellular matrix (ECM), allowing tumor dissemination and seeding but also by promoting angiogenesis and inflammation [3]. Therefore, increased MMP expression was detected in malignant tissues and was correlated with metastatic spread and unfavorable prognosis in multiple types of cancer [4,5]. Expectedly, MMPs were seen as ideal pharmacological targets for cancer therapy with preclinical studies of synthetic MMP inhibitors (MMPIs) holding great promise [6,7]. However, clinical trials developed during the late 1990s and early 2000s were unsuccessful in showing MMPIs effect in reducing tumor burden or improving overall survival, in addition to demonstrating severe side effects [8–10]. Further studies led to the conclusion that some MMPs, such as MMP-8, have anti-tumor effects, therefore the broad-spectrum of MMPIs was shown to be counter-productive, ultimately resulting in tumor progression and overall intense toxicity [11]. Thereby, it has now become apparent that to successfully target MMPs in the setting of cancer therapy, in situ inhibition of specific MMPs is essential. In particular, inhibition of the gelatinases MMP-2 and MMP-9 is envisaged, given their involvement in the degradation of the ECM and basement membrane, but also due to their role in the proteolysis of cell adhesion molecules and other bioactive proteins. In this context, old drugs and common natural products are now being explored for their potential to inhibit MMP-2 and MMP-9. Importantly, compounds derived from foods have been showing encouraging results in this regard, for example, curcumin, a component of the South Asian spice turmeric, has been shown to decrease MMP-2, -9, and -14 expression in various cancers, leading to decreased MMP activity and decreased cancer cell migration and invasion [12–14]. Similarly, antioxidant polyphenols in common foods, such as trans-resveratrol and quercetin from grapes and wine, as well as oleuropein and hydroxytyrosol from olive oil have also been shown to decrease the expression and activity of MMP-9 and decrease cancer cell migration, invasion, and angiogenesis [15–17]. Experimental studies of animal models fed with legume seeds have shown to reduce both the incidence and the number of colon tumors by 50% [18] and clinical studies have now started to provide evidence that legume consumption can decrease the risk of CRC [19]. In agreement with these reports, the World Cancer Research Fund/American Institute for Cancer Research recognized the potential of legume consumption in CRC prevention, supporting the need for additional research in this area.

We have recently discovered deflamin (patent WO/2018/060528), an oligomeric polypeptide isolated from the edible seeds of white lupin (*Lupinus albus*), that reduces MMP-2 and MMP-9 activity in CRC cell lines, in a dose-dependent manner and with an IC50 of 10 μg/mL. Being of food origin, and an oligomer of two storage proteins in legume seeds, deflamin isolated from white lupine was found to be safe for consumption, without impairing gene expression nor exerting cytotoxicity [20–23]. Its gelatinase inhibitory features suggested that it can be used in pathologies related to enhanced gastrointestinal MMP-9 activity, namely cancer, and inflammatory diseases. So far, deflamin was only successfully tested as a nutraceutical in inflammatory bowel disease models. In mice models of colitis, it significantly inhibited colonic MMP-9 activities, whilst reducing inflammation and colitis-induced lesions, when administered orally as a lupin seed extract or as a food additive to wheat cookies [21,24]. These works showed that deflamin is not only an efficient MMP-9 and MMP-2 inhibitor, but it also is highly resistant to digestion and not absorbed by the digestive tract (our unpublished results). These features infer that deflamin holds the potential to act locally in the intestinal path, bypassing the problem of systemic toxicity associated with common MMPIs [20–24]. Moreover, since it is water-soluble and rather effortlessly isolated [20], deflamin can easily become a novel nutraceutical for pathologies related to aberrant MMP-9 activities, particularly in the digestive system, such as CRC [22]. However, despite its potential against this disease, deflamin has never been tested in more realistic cancer models. In this context, we sought to explore the nutraceutical anti-tumor potential of this polypeptide in CRC progression. Not only this is the first report of deflamin in CRC models, but it also opens a door to novel approaches to tackle this disease.

2. Materials and Methods

2.1. Cell Lines

The following colorectal carcinoma cell lines were used in this work: HT-29 (ECACC, no. 91072201), HCT116 (ATCC® CCL-247), and SW480 (ATCC® CCL-228). All cell lines were cultivated in DMEM media supplemented with 10% (*v*/*v*) FBS and 1% penicillin/streptomycin at 37 °C and 5% CO_2, in a humidified atmosphere. Cells were maintained at a low passage and routinely tested for mycoplasma contamination by qPCR. Cell lines were validated by short tandem repeat (STR) profile.

2.2. Lentiviral Infection

For transduction of HCT116, SW480 and HT29 with tdTomato fluorescent protein, cells were infected with lentiviral particles containing FUdtTW plasmid. 2×10^5 cells were seeded in 6-well plates and incubated overnight at 37 °C. The next day, a mixture containing complete growth medium with 5 µg/mL polybrene, and lentiviral particles was added to the cells. The medium was replaced 24 h after infection and cells were expanded and then sorted in BD FACSAria III with a 98% purity.

2.3. Deflamin Purification

Deflamin was isolated from mature and dried white lupin seeds (*Lupinus albus*) as described previously [20] Briefly, lupin seeds were milled to a fine powder and extracted using 50 mM of Tris-HCl buffer, pH 7.5 (1:10, *w*/*v*). The homogenate was centrifugated at 12,000× *g* for 30 min at 4 °C. The supernatant was collected, boiled for 10 min, and centrifugated at 12,000× *g* for 20 min at 4 °C. The supernatant was then made to pH 4.0 and centrifugated at 12,000× *g* for 20 min at 4 °C. The resulting pellet was resuspended in 40% (*v*/*v*) ethanol containing 0.4 M NaCl, and centrifugated at 13,500× *g*, 30 min, 4 °C. The supernatant was made to 90% (*v*/*v*) ethanol and left overnight at −20 °C. The following day, the mixture was centrifugated at 13,500× *g* for 30 min at 4 °C and the pellet, containing isolated deflamin, was resuspended in the smallest possible volume of milli-Q water. Desalting was performed with PD-10 Columns (GE Healthcare Life Science, Uppsala, Sweden) according to manufacturer recommendations and the final solution was collected, frozen at −20 °C, and lyophilized. The obtained deflamin reached 98% purity and the integrity of the protein was detected by polyacrylamide gel electrophoresis and subsequent Coomassie brilliant blue staining [20]. Deflamin was diluted in PBS for in vitro and in vivo experiments.

2.4. Cellular Viability Assay

CRC cells were seeded at a density of 1–2 × 10^4 cells in 96-well plates. A total of 24 h after seeding, cells were treated with 0, 25, 50, or 75 µg/mL of deflamin. Every day, for 5 consecutive days, 1:10 of AlamarBlue reagent (Invitrogen, Waltham, MA, USA) was added to each well, and fluorescence was measured 2 h after (excitation 560 nm; emission 590 nm) in Infinite M200 Plate Reader (Tecan).

2.5. Cellular Apoptosis Assay

For apoptosis analysis, cells were seeded at a density of 1–2 × 10^4 cells in 96-well plates. 24 h after seeding, cells were treated with 0, 25, 50, or 75 µg/mL of deflamin for 48 h. The measurement of caspase 3/7 activity was performed using the Apo-ONE® Homogeneous Caspase-3/7 Assay kit (G7790, Promega, Madison, WI, USA) following manufacture instructions.

2.6. Zymography

In order to determine the anti-MMP role of deflamin in cancer cells, a zymographic analysis was performed as previously described [22]. Briefly, 12.5% polyacrylamide-SDS gels (*v*/*v*) were co-polymerized with 1% gelatin (*w*/*v*). CRC cell lysates (without and with deflamin treatment at 20 µg/mL, 40 µg/mL, 80 µg/mL) were treated with a nonreducing buffer containing 62.6-mM Tris–HCl pH 6.8, 2% (*w*/*v*) SDS, 10% (*v*/*v*) glycerol and 0.01% (*w*/*v*) bromophenol blue were loaded into each well of the SDS-gel. Electrophoresis was carried out vertically at 100 V and 20 mA per gel. Subsequently, gels were washed three times in 2.5% (*v*/*v*) Triton X-100 for 90 min each, to remove the SDS and incubated with a solution of 50-mM Tris–HCl pH 7.4, 5-mM $CaCl_2$, 1-μM $ZnCl_2$, and 0.01% *w*/*v* sodium azide, for 48 h at 37 °C. After incubation, gels were stained with Coomassie Brilliant Blue G-250 0.5% (*w*/*v*) in 50% (*v*/*v*) methanol and 10% (*v*/*v*) acetic acid, for 30 min, and destained with a solution of 50% (*v*/*v*) methanol, 10% (*v*/*v*) acetic acid. The gelatin degradation bands (white bands against a blue background), denoting relative MMP gelatinolytic activity, were analyzed according to their intensity with UN-SCAN-IT gelTM 6.1 software (Silk Scientific Corporation, Orem, UT, USA) and the relative values expressed in % of untreated lysate control.

2.7. Wound Healing Migration Assay

The effect of deflamin on cancer cell migration was analyzed by the wound healing assay. CRC cell lines were seeded in a 24-well plate at a density of 1×10^5 cells/well and cultured until a monolayer of ~85% confluence was reached. A central scratch-like gap was created with a pipette tip and a medium containing increasing concentrations of deflamin (0, 20, 40, or 80 μg/mL) was added to each well. The migration ability of the cancer cells was assessed by the capacity to close the "wound" after 48 h of deflamin treatment. The cell-free area in the well was calculated with the Fiji/ImageJ software, and the relative values were calculated in percentage of control condition area values.

2.8. 3D Cell Invasion Assay

The 3D invasion assay was performed as previously described [25]. Briefly, for the generation of spheroids, we combined 1/4 of the final volume of methylcellulose (6 mg/mL), 10% (*w*/*v*) FBS, 20 to 40 μg/mL collagen, 1 μg/mL mitomycin in DMEM medium. Five hundred cancer cells were then suspended in 50 μL of this spheroid formation medium and plated into a non-adherent 384-well plate. Cells were incubated for 24 h to allow the formation of an individual spheroid per well. The medium was then replaced by 50 μL of collagen matrix composed of two parts of collagen (3 mg/mL), 15% (*w*/*v*) FBS, 1 μg/mL mitomycin, 2% (*w*/*v*) NaOH (1 M) and DMEM. Deflamin, at a concentration of 50 μg/mL and 100 μg/mL, was added to the treated cells. After 1 h incubation, imaging of the spheroids was performed by fluorescence microscopy in a Zeiss LSM710 confocal microscope. This time point was accounted as 0 h. The next images were taken at the time points of 24, 48, and 72 h. Images were analyzed using the FIJI/ImageJ software. Invasive cells were counted between the inner perimeter (spheroid external border at 0 h) and the outer perimeter (the furthest invasive cell at each time point).

2.9. Cell Labeling

CRC cell lines at 70% confluence were stained with lipophilic dye Vybrant™ DiI cell labeling solution (V22885 from Invitrogen) at 4 μL/mL in PBS 1X for 10 min at 37 °C.

2.10. In Vivo Zebrafish Xenograft Model

Wild-type and transgenic Tg(kdrl:EGFP) zebrafish (*Danio rerio*) [26] embryos were provided by the zebrafish facility of Instituto de Medicina Molecular (iMM). For husbandry, adult zebrafish were maintained at 28.5 °C in a 10/14 h dark-light cycle, according to standard protocols of the European Animal Welfare Legislation, Directive 2010/63/EU (European Commission, 2016), following the Federation of European Laboratory Animal Science Associations (FELASA) guidelines and recommendations. All procedures in this study were performed in early life forms of zebrafish development, with embryos up to 120 h post-fertilization (hpf), that do not yet show the ability to feed themselves and are, therefore, considered unprotected under the European Animal Welfare Legislation, Directive 2010/63/EU (European Commission, 2016).

For zebrafish injection, HCT116 cells expressing dTomato fluorescent protein or labeled with DiI were used as indicated. 2.5×10^5 cells/mL (approximately 800 cells per injection) were microinjected into the perivitelline space (PVS) of 48 hpf larvae previously anesthetized with tricaine 1.5% (*w*/*v*; Pharmaq), as described before [27]. Microinjections were performed under a stereo microscope (Leica S8 APO) using borosilicate glass microcapillaries attached to a microinjector (World Precision Instruments, Pneumatic Pico pump PV820) coupled with a micromanipulator (Narishige MN-153). At 24 h post-injection, successfully injected xenografts were treated with 100 µg/mL deflamin in E3 medium or E3 with PBS (controls) and incubated at 34 °C. The medium was replaced daily for three days. After this period, animals were fixed in 4% (*w*/*v*) paraformaldehyde overnight and stored at −20 °C in 100% (*v*/*v*) methanol.

2.11. Immunofluorescence

Frozen xenografts were re-hydrated in methanol series (75% > 50% > 25%) and then permeabilized in acetone at −20 °C. Xenografts were then washed in a buffer containing 1x PBS, 0.5% (*v*/*v*) Tween 20, 0.5% TritonX-100, and 100 mM glycine for 1 h at room temperature (RT), followed by blocking in 1x PBS, 1% *w*/*v* BSA, 1% *v*/*v* DMSO, 1% *v*/*v* TritonX-100 and 1.5% *w*/*v* FBS, for 1 h at RT. Next, xenografts were incubated with primary antibodies: rabbit monoclonal anti-cleaved caspase-3 (Asp175) (1:100, #9661 from Cell Signaling); and mouse monoclonal anti-GFP (1:100, #11814460001 from Roche) for 1 h at RT and overnight at 4 °C. The following day, secondary antibody incubation with goat Anti-rabbit IgG H&L Alexa Fluor® 488 (1:400, #A-11008 from Invitrogen) and 50 µg/mL DAPI was performed for 1 h at RT and then overnight at 4 °C. Xenografts were mounted with Vectashield® mounting media between two coverslips and stored at 4 °C for subsequent analysis.

Xenografts were imaged in a confocal microscope Zeiss LSM 710 with a Z-stack interval of 5 µm. Images were analyzed in FIJI/ImageJ software using the plugin cell counter. For tumor size calculation, three representative slices of the tumor from the top (Zfirst), the middle (Zmidle), and the bottom (Zlast) were analyzed and the number of cells calculated as the sum of cells in Zfirst, Zmidle, Zlast/total number of Z stacks × 1.5. The 1.5 correction number was estimated for these CRC cells that have nuclei with an average of 10–12 µm of diameter. The number of mitotic figures and activated caspase-3 were counted in every slice of the tumor (from Zfirst to Zlast) and the percentage was obtained by dividing the value by the total number of cells in tumor size.

Metastasis was counted in the caudal hematopoietic tissue and in the gills of zebrafish larvae.

For the analysis of angiogenesis, all images were obtained with a 7 µm interval Z-stack and two parameters were measured: vessel density (VD) and vessel infiltration (VI). Vessel density and vessel infiltration were assessed through Z-projections of corresponding images using the ImageJ Z-Projection tool and the area of eGFP fluorescent signal per tumor was quantified. To analyze the vessel infiltration, the superficial slices of the images were not considered (about 20% of total stacks).

$$VD = \frac{\text{eGFP area}}{\text{Tumour area}} \times 100,\ VI = \frac{\text{eGFP area in tumour core}}{\text{core of the tumour area}} \times 100$$

For degraded collagen analysis, the 5-FAM fluorescence area corresponding to collagen degradation points per tumor was measured, using Z-projections of corresponding images with ImageJ Z-projection tool. The value was normalized by the total tumor area.

$$\text{Degraded collagen} = \frac{\text{eGFP area}}{\text{Tumour area}} \times 100$$

2.12. Statistical Analysis

GraphPad Prism 8 software (Dotmatics, San Diego, USA) was used for the statistical analysis of in vivo experiments. Pared, unpaired t-test and one-way ANOVA were used to analyze in vitro and in vivo data, as indicated in figure legends. Results are presented as average ± standard error of the mean (SEM). The level of statistical significance was set as non-significant (NS); *, $p < 0.05$; **, $p < 0.01$; ***, $p < 0.001$; and ****, $p < 0.0001$. For all the statistical analysis p value as a confidence interval of 95%.

3. Results

3.1. Deflamin Exhibits Anti-Tumor Activity in Zebrafish CRC Xenotransplanted Tumors

In previous studies, we found that deflamin had anti-MMP-2 and -MMP-9 activities in CRC cell line HT-29, as well as anti-inflammatory role in mouse models of induced-intestinal colitis [21]. Therefore, we sought to investigate deflamin's role in cancer development using the zebrafish larvae CRC xenograft model. This is a well-established tumorigenesis model that displays several advantages: it is a quick assay with cellular resolution and allows the evaluation of crucial hallmarks of cancer, such as tumor proliferation, and metastatic and angiogenic potentials [27]. Therefore, CRC cell line HCT116 was labeled with a lipophilic dye (DiI) and injected into the periviteline space (PVS) of 48 hpf zebrafish embryos (Figure 1A). The day after injection (1 dpi), xenotransplanted zebrafish larvae were either treated with 100 μg/mL deflamin (the highest tolerable dose) or left untreated. Deflamin was extracted, isolated, purified, and concentrated from dry Lupinus albus seeds as previously described [20]. E3 medium, containing or not containing deflamin was refreshed every day for a total of 3 days of treatment. At 4 dpi, animals were fixed and stained, and analyses of tumor size, apoptosis (activated caspase3), and proliferation (mitotic figures) were performed by confocal microscopy (Figure 1A). Results showed that deflamin treated tumors were on average four times smaller than untreated tumors (Figure 1B,C, *** $p < 0.001$). Importantly, analysis of cell death suggests that deflamin induces approximately a four-fold increase in apoptosis when compared to untreated tumors (Figure 1B,D, **** $p < 0.0001$). Tumor proliferation was not significantly affected by deflamin treatment (Figure 1B,E).

Moreover, this zebrafish xenograft model provides the opportunity to analyze metastasis formation given that at 4 dpi human fluorescently labeled tumor cells can be found in distant sites such as the brain, optic cup, gills, and caudal hematopoietic tissue (CHT). To assess the value of deflamin in metastasis formation, the number of xenografted zebrafish with micrometastasis was assessed. Results revealed that under deflamin treatment, HCT116 tumors had a reduced capacity to colonize secondary tissues (about 40% reduction in micrometastasis formation, Figure 1F,G).

Taken together, these results indicate that deflamin has an anti-tumor and anti-metastatic role in CRC development, suggesting important applications for cancer therapy.

3.2. Deflamin Does Not Play a Direct Role in Cancer Cell Proliferation or Apoptosis

To further investigate the mechanism of action of deflamin, we explored the direct effect of this molecule on cancer cell proliferation and apoptosis in vitro. To accomplish this, we treated HCT116, HT-29, and SW480 CRC cell lines with increased concentrations of deflamin (25 μg/mL, 50 μg/mL, and 75 μg/mL) for 5 days. The results showed no effect of this oligomeric protein on cancer cell proliferation rates, suggesting that deflamin does not play a direct role in cell cycle regulation (Figure 2A). Moreover, deflamin did not induce apoptosis of the HCT116, HT-29, and SW480 cells when caspase 3/7 activity was measured in vitro (Figure 2B), indicating that it does not hold a direct cytotoxic effect on cancer cells either. To further validate the absence of toxicity of deflamin in live organisms, we treated 72 hpf zebrafish larvae for three days with increased concentrations of deflamin (50 μg/mL and 100 μg/mL). Figure S1 shows no mortality associated with zebrafish treatments under the conditions tested.

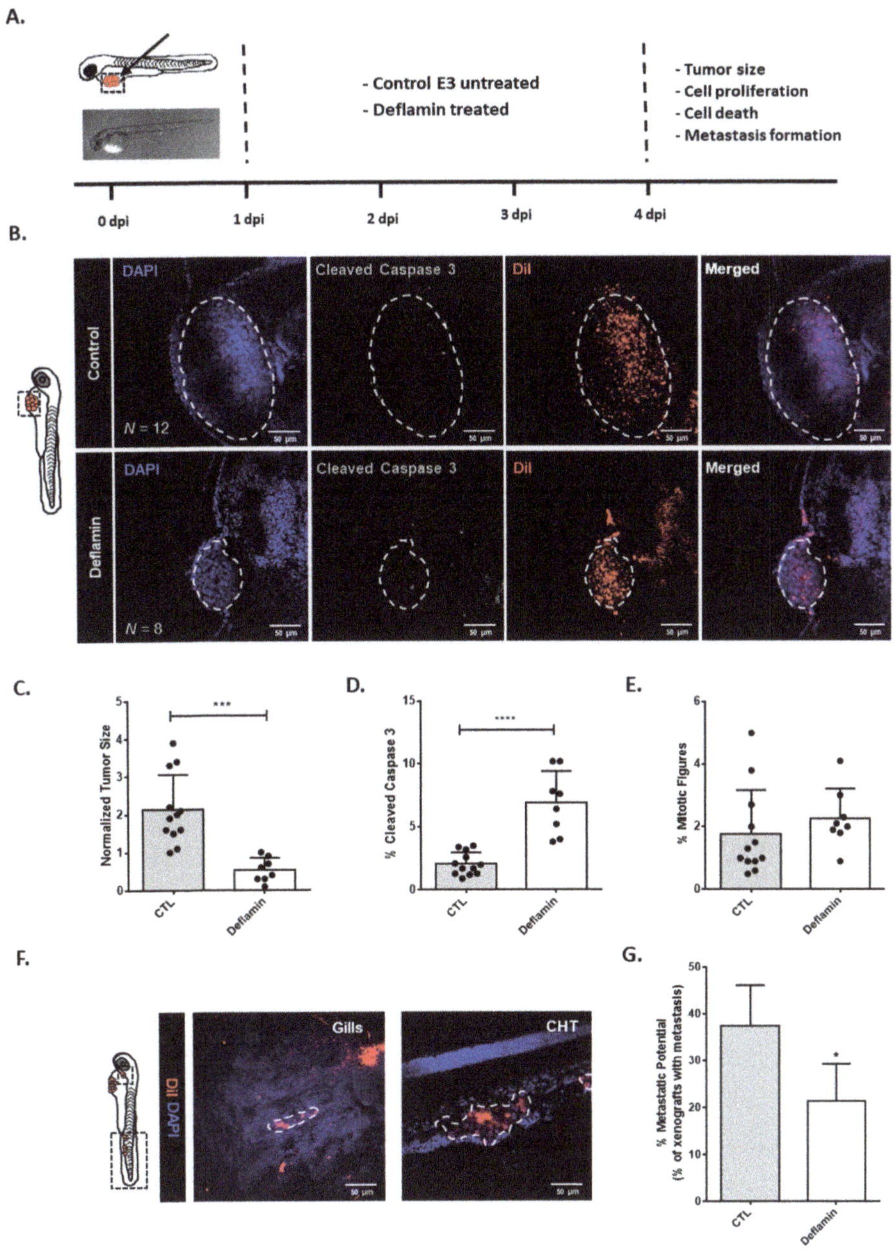

Figure 1. Zebrafish xenotransplant model of HCT116 cells exposed to deflamin: (**A**) Human cancer cell line HCT116 was fluorescently labeled with DiI (red) and injected into the perivitelline space (PVS) 2 days post-fertilization (dpf) nacre/casper zebrafish larvae. Zebrafish xenografts were treated in vivo with deflamin for 72 h and compared with untreated controls regarding tumor size, cell death, cell proliferation, and metastasis formation; (**B**) At 4 days post-injection (dpi), zebrafish xenografts were imaged on PVS by confocal microscopy; (**C**) Analysis of tumor size (***, $p \leq 0.001$); (**D**) Analysis of activated caspase 3 (apoptosis, ****, $p \leq 0.0001$); (**E**) Analysis of mitotic figures (proliferative cells,

(ns); **F**) Zebrafish xenografts were also imaged over the entire body by confocal microscopy. Representative images of HCT116 micrometastasis in gills and caudal hematopoietic tissue (CHT); (**G**) % of zebrafish exhibiting metastasis. The number of xenografts analyzed is indicated in the representative images. In the graphs, each dot represents one zebrafish xenograft. Statistical analysis was performed as described in the Statistical Analysis section (*, $p \leq 0.05$, ***, $p \leq 0.001$, ****, $p \leq 0.0001$). Scale bars represent 50 µm. All images are anterior to the left, posterior to the right, dorsal up, and ventral down.

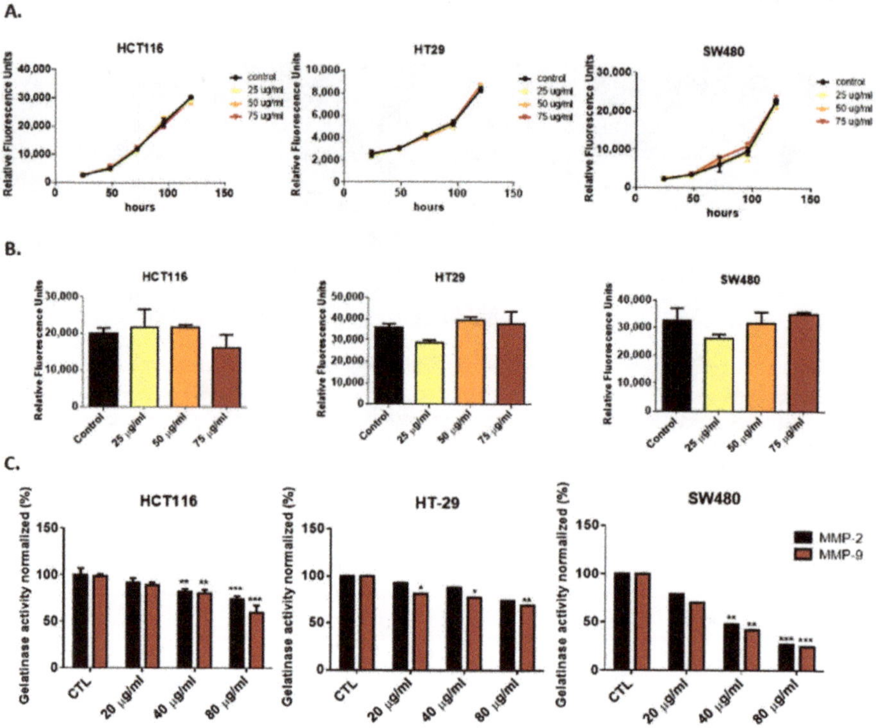

Figure 2. Effect of Deflamin on viability and MMPs of CRC cell lines HCT116, HT-29, and SW480: (**A**) Viability of human CRC cell lines when exposed to deflamin; (**B**) Analysis of cell death by apoptosis of human CRC cell lines treated with deflamin; (**C**) Zymographic analysis of the anti-gelatinases activity of deflamin. Statistical analysis was performed as described in the Statistical Analysis section (*, $p \leq 0.01$; **, $p \leq 0.01$, ***, $p \leq 0.001$).

Overall, deflamin appears as a safe polypeptide oligomer to be administered in vivo. Furthermore, these results suggest that the increased apoptosis seen in the zebrafish model, was not caused by a direct effect of deflamin on cancer cells, but rather an indirect role, possibly through MMPs inhibition.

3.3. *Deflamin Inhibits MMP-2 and MMP-9, Contributing to Impaired Cancer Cell Migration and Invasion*

Although deflamin was not found to have a direct effect on cancer cell viability, gelatinases MMP-2 and MMP-9 are known to be critical for the ability of cancer cells to migrate and invade since they act not only on the degradation of the ECM (contributing to the rearrangement of the matrix and release of growth factors) but also on the degradation of cell–cell and cell–matrix adhesion molecules [3]. Zymographic analysis of MMPs from HCT116, HT-29, and SW480 CRC cell lines showed that deflamin exerts an inhibitory role on the activity of both MMP-2 and MMP-9 in all cell lines tested, displaying the greatest effect on SW480 cell line (a reduction of about 75% of MMPs activity at a deflamin concentration of 80 μg/mL, *** $p < 0.001$, Figure 2C). Therefore, we investigated the effect of deflamin on cancer cell migration using the wound healing in vitro assay (Figure 3A). Migration of cancer cells was shown to be impaired by the addition of deflamin to all cell lines tested, with the SW480 cell line showing the highest inhibition of cellular migration (about 77% reduction in migration at 80 μg/mL of deflamin concentration upon 72 h of treatment, ** $p < 0.01$, Figure 3A). We further tested the role of deflamin on cancer cell invasion using a 3D matrix of collagen (Figure 3B). MMP-2 and MMP-9 degrade collagen types III and I, respectively, being both able to cleave collagen types IV and V [28]. Therefore, analysis of 3D spheroids of the same cell lines showed a dose-dependent inhibition of invasion of 3D spheroids on a collagen matrix, being once more SW480 the cell line with the highest inhibition of invasive cells (reduction of about 40% invasiveness after 72 h of exposure to deflamin, *** $p < 0.001$, Figure 3B).

Overall, these results indicate that deflamin exerts an inhibitory effect on the activity of both MMP-2 and -9, as well as on cancer cell migration and invasion, with important implications for cancer development and progression.

3.4. *Deflamin Inhibits Collagen Degradation and Angiogenesis In Vivo*

For a tumor to continue to grow and start migrating/invading, two processes need to occur: (1) elimination of the physical barriers by ECM degradation; (2) generation of pro-angiogenic factors to allow the formation of new blood vessels. MMP-2 and MMP-9 are particularly important for both these processes since they increase the bioavailability of important factors such as vascular endothelial growth factor (VEGF), basic fibroblast growth factor (bFGF) and transforming growth factor β (TGF-β) by degrading ECM components such as collagen type IV and perlecan [29]. Thus, we investigated the role of deflamin in both of these processes through analysis of the extracellular collagen degradation and tumor angiogenesis in the zebrafish xenotransplant model. For that, HCT116 cells were stably transduced with a fluorescent dtTomato expressing vector and xenotransplanted into the PVS of wild type AB and Tg(kdrl:EGFP) zebrafish larvae (Figure 4A). For the analysis of collagen degradation in vivo, we used the collagen hybridizing peptide (CHP) which is a 5-FAM conjugated synthetic peptide that specifically binds to denatured collagen strands through hydrogen bonding (Figure 4B). CHP is an extremely specific probe for unfolded collagen molecules, while showing negligible affinity for intact collagen molecules due to a lack of binding sites [30]. In order to investigate blood vessel formation in the tumor area, the zebrafish Tg(kdrl: EGFP) model, which has the vessels labeled with GFP, was used [31] (Figure 4C). Using these models, our results show an inhibitory role of deflamin on collagen degradation when compared to control tumors in vivo (about 85% reduction in collagen degraded area, * $p < 0.05$, Figure 4D). Furthermore, analysis of tumor blood vessel formation showed about an 80% reduction in infiltrating vessels per tumor area (*** $p < 0.001$, Figure 4F).

Overall, our results indicate that, by inhibiting MMP-2 and -9 functions, deflamin impairs ECM remodeling through inhibition of collagen degradation and tumor angiogenesis, important processes for cancer progression, rather than having a direct action on cancer cell proliferation and apoptosis.

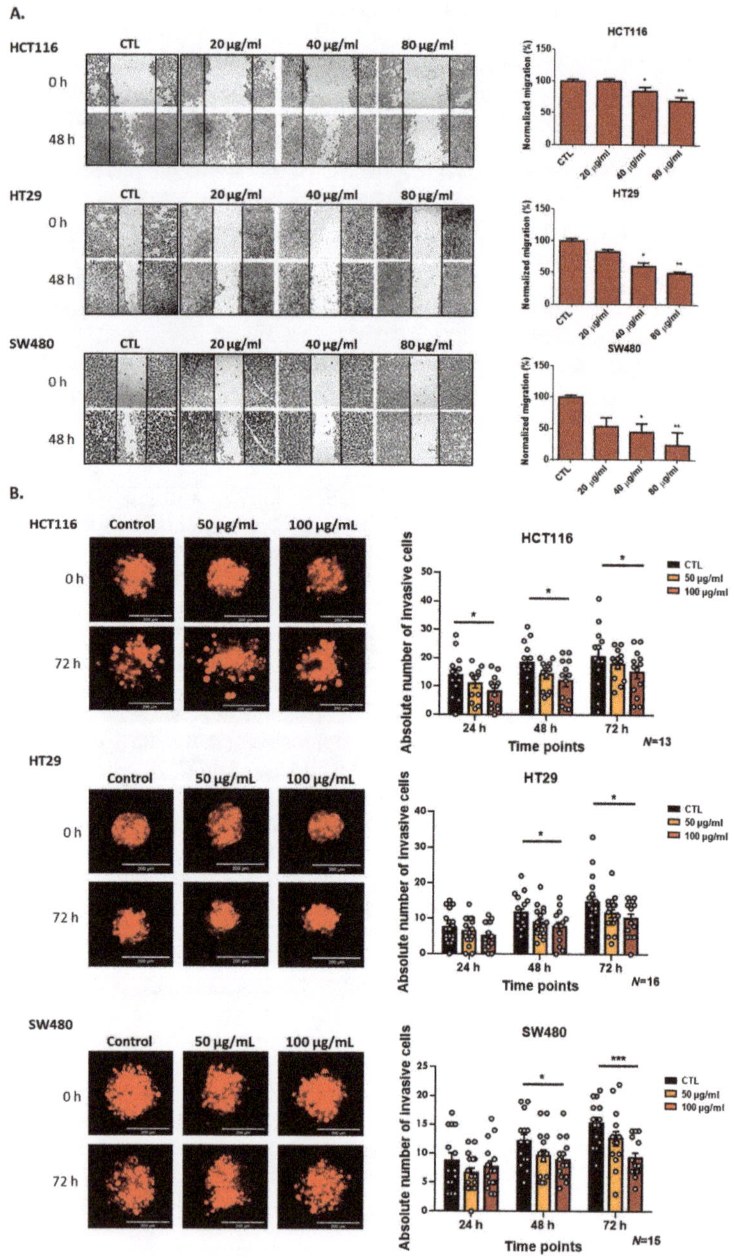

Figure 3. Migration and invasion of CRC cell lines HCT116, HT-29, and SW480 upon treatment with deflamin: (**A**) Analysis of migration by the wound healing assay of human CRC cell lines HCT116, HT-29 and SW480 treated with deflamin for 48 h and its corresponding quantification (%) ($n = 3$). (**B**) 3D spheroid invasion assay of human CRC cell lines HCT116, HT-29, and SW480 treated with deflamin and the corresponding quantification (number of absolute invasive cells). The number of spheroids analyzed is indicated in the graphs. Statistical analysis was performed as described in the Statistical Analysis section (*, $p \leq 0.05$; **, $p \leq 0.01$; ***, $p \leq 0.001$).

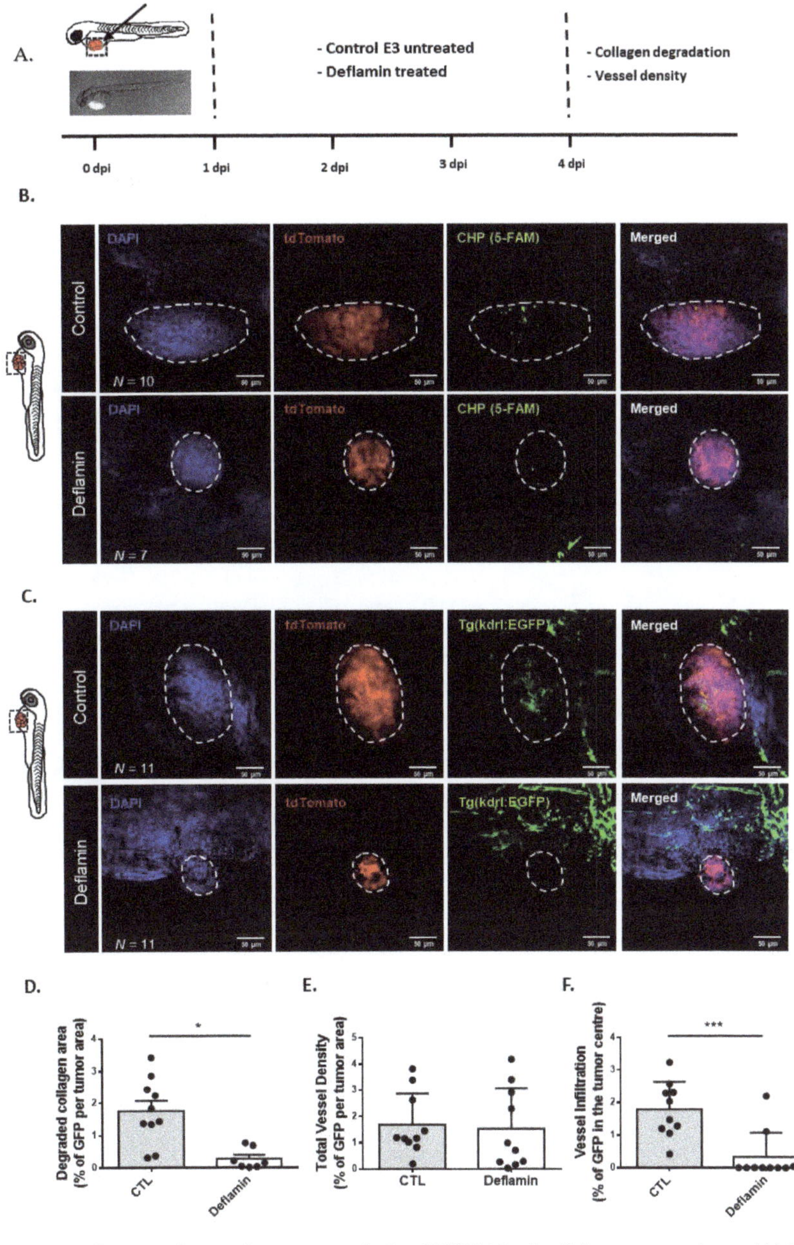

Figure 4. Cancer microenvironment analysis of HCT116 zebrafish xenotransplants: (**A**) Human cancer cell line HCT116 was stably transduced with FUdtTW plasmid (tdTomato expression marker) and injected into the perivitelline space (PVS) of 2 days post-fertilization (dpf) nacre/casper zebrafish larvae. Zebrafish xenografts were treated in vivo with deflamin for 72 h and compared with untreated controls regarding collagen degradation and vessel density; (**B**,**C**) At 4 days post-injection (dpi), zebrafish xenografts were imaged on PVS by confocal microscopy; (**D**) Quantification of degraded collagen area by analysis of CHP staining (5-FAM stained area); (**E**) Total vessel density analysis by EGFP marker; (**F**) Tumor vessel infiltration analysis by EGFP marker. The number of

xenografts analyzed is indicated in the representative images. In the graphs, each dot represents one zebrafish xenograft. Statistical analysis was performed as described in the Statistical Analysis section (*, $p \leq 0.05$; ***, $p \leq 0.001$). Scale bars represent 50 μm. All images are anterior to the left, posterior to the right, dorsal up, and ventral down.

4. Discussion

Over the past decade, cancer pharmaceutics has been facing the challenge of maximizing the effectiveness and specificity of treatments, as well as minimizing the toxicity and resistance of therapeutic regimens. The increase in MMPs activity detected in a wide range of cancers has been taken as evidence for their implication in the cancer invasive and metastatic potential, therefore marking MMPs as important targets for both diagnostic and therapeutic purposes [5]. This feature has been well demonstrated in several works, comprising selective inhibition and MMP-9-deficient mice, all of which pointed to MMP-9 as an important target of neoplastic diseases [32]. Indeed, in recent years a substantial amount of research has been made, attempting to develop synthetic, low-molecular-weight inhibitors of MMPs (MMPIs) for the potential treatment of diseases in which they play a major role. However, technical difficulties, side effects, and dose-dependent toxicity have greatly limited the success of these anti-MMP drugs [8–11]. Nevertheless, interesting results have been obtained with natural compounds with anti-inflammatory and anti-tumoral activity. Currently, studies on molecules of natural origin have shown promise in inhibiting MMPs, especially MMP-9, in inflammatory and oncogenic pathological processes [12–17]. Deflamin is a natural food component extracted from white lupine seeds (*Lupinus albus*) that shows anti-MMP-2 and MMP-9, as well as anti-inflammatory activities [20–23]. Importantly, deflamin has the advantage of being a water-soluble molecule easily extracted and isolated in vitro, that shows resistance to boiling and to digestive enzymatic reactions and has the potential to act locally in the intestinal system (without being absorbed into circulation), likely bypassing the problem of systemic toxicity associated with common MMPIs [20–23]. In this sense, this work aimed to explore deflamin therapeutic potential, using 3D cellular systems and zebrafish larvae models. Even though drug pharmacodynamics in zebrafish may differ from mammals, many compounds have been shown to block disease in a similar way in both organisms [33]. Therefore, this work corroborated that deflamin does not hold a cytotoxic effect on the CRC cell lines and zebrafish embryos, providing evidence for its safety as a potential therapeutic strategy. Moreover, deflamin showed inhibitory activity of the invasive process both in cellular systems and in zebrafish cancer models. Importantly, deflamin was effective in inhibiting MMP-2, MMP-9, and general ECM remodeling, favoring spatial constraints of tumor growth/progression and limited nutrient/oxygen supply, due to decreased angiogenesis. In agreement with this work, our previous studies have suggested that deflamin's mode of action involves direct inhibition of MMP-9 and -2, due to its biochemical features [21]. Hence, rather than inhibiting any of the regular pathways of MMP activation or expression, deflamin reduces gelatinase activity, without inducing direct alterations in the cell cycle or in gene expression. However, by limiting ECM remodeling, deflamin prevents the angiogenic process, as well as the degradation of the physical barriers necessary for tumor growth. In this context, physical constraint renders tumors unable to proliferate and metastasize, finishing by becoming apoptotic. Thus, by reducing gelatinase activities in situ, deflamin provides a simple manner to restrict the tumor and render it unable to progress.

Although the present work has some limitations as the zebrafish model is limited in terms of its similarity to mammal models, our results, paired with our previous findings on deflamin, bring a novel view on the use of MMP-2 and -9 inhibitors in cancer models. Indeed, despite MMP-9 being known for decades as an attractive target for anticancer therapies, the development of effective and safe MMP9 inhibitors as anticancer drugs has been shown to be extremely difficult. Recently, therapies have been aiming at more specificity through blocking antibodies that selectively inactivate MMP9, and these are currently in clinical trials [34]. It seems however that the feature of being able to reduce gelatinolytic activity directly and in situ by a food component such as deflamin might be a similar and simpler approach for tackling cancer disease via MMP inhibition.

Overall, although MMP9 has been well established as an important target in anticancer treatments, there is still a need for selective, safe, and effective MMP-9 inhibitors. This is the first report on an effective food protein gelatinase inhibitor that reduces cancer development via a constriction of the tumor's 3D space distribution. Added to the fact that it is of food origin and easy to isolate, this work revealed the nutritional potential of deflamin as a co-adjuvant therapeutic agent in the treatment of CRC, as a nontoxic dietary supplement. Further work using more complex animal models of cancer and pre-clinical trials will, with no doubt, bring novel insights into the effectiveness of deflamin against CRC.

5. Conclusions

The work presented here demonstrated that deflamin was able to impair CRC angiogenesis and tumor microenvironment remodeling, via gelatinase inhibition, which led to a constriction and limitation of the tumor's spatial distribution and nutrient and oxygen supply. This type of mechanism seems to be a good depiction of what a specific MMP inhibitor should attain by reducing gelatinase activity, angiogenesis is efficiently impaired limiting tumor growth and inducing cancer cell apoptosis.

Our results suggest that being a natural compound, non-toxic, and resistant to digestion, deflamin holds the potential to be a novel nutraceutical, adjuvant or even a functional food to be used in treating and preventing CRC via a specific, in situ, gelatinase inhibition. Further studies of the use of this oligomeric protein are needed to assess its clinical and commercial value, but it seems plausible to infer that using this type of gelatinase inhibition could be a novel and effective approach to tackling gastrointestinal cancer disease.

Supplementary Materials: The following supporting information can be downloaded at: https://www.mdpi.com/article/10.3390/cancers14246182/s1, Figure S1: Zebrafish lethality curves of the acute toxicity assay. At 72 hpf zebrafish embryos were exposed to increased concentrations of deflamin (n = 20) and mortality was evaluated during 72 h of treatment.

Author Contributions: S.S. was involved in in vitro and in vivo research models; B.B., J.M., A.L. were involved in deflamin purification and in vitro and in vivo research models; A.C. was involved in in vitro 3D models and supervision; R.C.-D. developed in vitro and in vivo research models and supervision; M.C. was involved in in vitro and in vivo models; L.C. (Lara Carvalhoand) zebrafish housing management, zebrafish model and supervision; L.C. (Luis Costa), R.F. and A.L. were involved in funding acquisition and supervision; R.F. project conceptualization, resources and supervision; M.M. project conceptualization, supervision, writing the manuscript. All authors have read and agreed to the published version of the manuscript.

Funding: This work was supported by national funds from Fundação para a Ciência e a Tecnologia (Lisbon, Portugal) through the research unit UID/AGR/04129/2020 (LEAF), Project PTDC/BAA-AGR/28608/2017 and Project PTDC/OCE-ETA/4836/2021. Joana Mota was funded by Fundação para a Ciência e Tecnologia SFRH/BD/132832/2017. Raquel Cruz-Duarte was funded by SFRH/BD/139138/2018.

Institutional Review Board Statement: Not applicable.

Informed Consent Statement: Not applicable.

Data Availability Statement: The data presented in this study are available on request from the corresponding author.

Acknowledgments: The authors acknowledge the support of IMM Fish facility and Bioimaging.

Conflicts of Interest: The authors declare no conflict of interest.

References

1. Bray, F.; Ferlay, J.; Soerjomataram, I.; Siegel, R.L.; Torre, L.A.; Jemal, A. Global Cancer Statistics 2018: GLOBOCAN Estimates of Incidence and Mortality Worldwide for 36 Cancers in 185 Countries. *CA Cancer J. Clin.* **2018**, *68*, 394–424. [CrossRef] [PubMed]
2. Fares, J.; Fares, M.Y.; Khachfe, H.H.; Salhab, H.A.; Fares, Y. Molecular Principles of Metastasis: A Hallmark of Cancer Revisited. Signal Transduct. *Target. Ther.* **2020**, *5*, 28. [CrossRef]
3. Gialeli, C.; Theocharis, A.D.; Karamanos, N.K. Roles of Matrix Metalloproteinases in Cancer Progression and Their Pharmacological Targeting. *FEBS J.* **2011**, *278*, 16–27. [CrossRef] [PubMed]
4. Coussens, L.M.; Fingleton, B.; Matrisian, L.M. Matrisian Matrix Metalloproteinase Inhibitors and Cancer—Trials and Tribulations. *Science* **2002**, *295*, 2387–2392. [CrossRef]
5. Yang, B.; Tang, F.; Zhang, B.; Zhao, Y.; Feng, J.; Rao, Z. Matrix Metalloproteinase-9 Overexpression Is Closely Related to Poor Prognosis in Patients with Colon Cancer. *World J. Surg. Oncol.* **2014**, *12*, 24. [CrossRef]
6. Wylie, S.; MacDonald, I.C.; Varghese, H.J.; Schmidt, E.E.; Morris, V.L.; Groom, A.C.; Chambers, A.F. The Matrix Metalloproteinase Inhibitor Batimastat Inhibits Angiogenesis in Liver Metastases of B16F1 Melanoma Cells. *Clin. Exp. Metastasis* **1999**, *17*, 111–117. [CrossRef]
7. Giavazzi, R.; Garofalo, A.; Ferri, C.; Lucchini, V.; Bone, E.A.; Chiari, S.; Brown, P.D.; Nicoletti, M.I.; Taraboletti, G. Batimastat, a Synthetic Inhibitor of Matrix Metalloproteinases, Potentiates the Antitumor Activity of Cisplatin in Ovarian Carcinoma Xenografts. *Clin. Cancer Res.* **1998**, *4*, 985–992.
8. Bramhall, S.R.; Schulz, J.; Nemunaitis, J.; Brown, P.D.; Baillet, M.; Buckels, J.A.C. A Double-Blind Placebo-Controlled, Randomised Study Comparing Gemcitabine and Marimastat with Gemcitabine and Placebo as First Line Therapy in Patients with Advanced Pancreatic Cancer. *Br. J. Cancer* **2002**, *87*, 161–167. [CrossRef]
9. Hirte, H.; Vergote, I.B.; Jeffrey, J.R.; Grimshaw, R.N.; Coppieters, S.; Schwartz, B.; Tu, D.; Sadura, A.; Brundage, M.; Seymour, L. A Phase III Randomized Trial of BAY 12-9566 (Tanomastat) as Maintenance Therapy in Patients with Advanced Ovarian Cancer Responsive to Primary Surgery and Paclitaxel/Platinum Containing Chemotherapy: A National Cancer Institute of Canada Clinical Trials Group Study. *Gynecol. Oncol.* **2006**, *102*, 300–308. [CrossRef]
10. Sparano, J.A.; Bernardo, P.; Stephenson, P.; Gradishar, W.J.; Ingle, J.N.; Zucker, S.; Davidson, N.E. Randomized Phase III Trial of Marimastat versus Placebo in Patients with Metastatic Breast Cancer Who Have Responding or Stable Disease after First-Line Chemotherapy: Eastern Cooperative Oncology Group Trial E2196. *J. Clin. Oncol.* **2004**, *22*, 4631–4638. [CrossRef]
11. López-Otín, C.; Palavalli, L.H.; Samuels, Y. Protective Roles of Matrix Metalloproteinases: From Mouse Models to Human Cancer. *Cell Cycle* **2009**, *8*, 3657–3662. [CrossRef] [PubMed]
12. Lin, S.S.; Lai, K.C.; Hsu, S.C.; Yang, J.S.; Kuo, C.L.; Lin, J.P.; Ma, Y.S.; Wu, C.C.; Chung, J.G. Curcumin Inhibits the Migration and Invasion of Human A549 Lung Cancer Cells through the Inhibition of Matrix Metalloproteinase-2 and -9 and Vascular Endothelial Growth Factor (VEGF). *Cancer Lett.* **2009**, *285*, 127–133. [CrossRef] [PubMed]
13. Hong, J.H.; Ahn, K.S.; Bae, E.; Jeon, S.S.; Choi, H.Y. The Effects of Curcumin on the Invasiveness of Prostate Cancer in vitro and in vivo. *Prostate Cancer Prostatic Dis.* **2006**, *9*, 147–152. [CrossRef] [PubMed]
14. Yodkeeree, S.; Chaiwangyen, W.; Garbisa, S.; Limtrakul, P. Curcumin, Demethoxycurcumin and Bisdemethoxycurcumin Differentially Inhibit Cancer Cell Invasion through the down-Regulation of MMPs and UPA. *J. Nutr. Biochem.* **2009**, *20*, 87–95. [CrossRef]
15. Tang, F.Y.; Chiang, E.P.I.; Sun, Y.C. Resveratrol Inhibits Heregulin-B1-Mediated Matrix Metalloproteinase-9 Expression and Cell Invasion in Human Breast Cancer Cells. *J. Nutr. Biochem.* **2008**, *19*, 287–294. [CrossRef]
16. Scoditti, E.; Calabriso, N.; Massaro, M.; Pellegrino, M.; Storelli, C.; Martines, G.; De Caterina, R.; Carluccio, M.A. Mediterranean Diet Polyphenols Reduce Inflammatory Angiogenesis through MMP-9 and COX-2 Inhibition in Human Vascular Endothelial Cells: A Potentially Protective Mechanism in Atherosclerotic Vascular Disease and Cancer. *Arch. Biochem. Biophys.* **2012**, *527*, 81–89. [CrossRef]
17. Banerjee, S.; Bueso-Ramos, C.; Aggarwal, B.B. Suppression of 7,12-Dimethylbenz(a)Anthracene-Induced Mammary Carcinogenesis in Rats by Resveratrol: Role of Nuclear Factor-KB, Cyclooxygenase 2, and Matrix Metalloprotease 9. *Cancer Res.* **2002**, *62*, 4945–4954.
18. Bennink, M.R. Consumption of Black Beans and Navy Beans (*Phaseolus vulgaris*) Reduced Azoxymethane-Induced Colon Cancer in Rats. *Nutr. Cancer* **2002**, *44*, 60–65. [CrossRef]
19. Aune, D.; De Stefani, E.; Ronco, A.; Boffetta, P.; Deneo-Pellegrini, H.; Acosta, G.; Mendilaharsu, M. Legume Intake and the Risk of Cancer: A Multisite Case-Control Study in Uruguay. *Cancer Causes Control* **2009**, *20*, 1605–1615. [CrossRef]
20. Mota, J.; Figueira, M.E.; Ferreira, R.B.; Lima, A. An Up-Scalable and Cost-Effective Methodology for Isolating a Polypeptide Matrix Metalloproteinase-9 Inhibitor from *Lupinus albus* Seeds. *Foods* **2021**, *10*, 1663. [CrossRef]
21. Mota, J.; Direito, R.; Rocha, J.; Fernandes, J.; Sepodes, B.; Figueira, M.E.; Raymundo, A.; Lima, A.; Ferreira, R.B. *Lupinus albus* Protein Components Inhibit MMP-2 and MMP-9 Gelatinolytic Activity in vitro and in vivo. *Int. J. Mol. Sci.* **2021**, *22*, 13286. [CrossRef] [PubMed]
22. Mota, J.; Lima, A.; Ferreira, R.B.; Raymundo, A. Technological Potential of a Lupin Protein Concentrate as a Nutraceutical Delivery System in Baked Cookies. *Foods* **2021**, *10*, 1929. [CrossRef] [PubMed]
23. Lima, A.I.G.; Mota, J.; Monteiro, S.A.V.S.; Ferreira, R.M.S.B. Legume Seeds and Colorectal Cancer Revisited: Protease Inhibitors Reduce MMP-9 Activity and Colon Cancer Cell Migration. *Food Chem.* **2016**, *197*, 30–38. [CrossRef]

24. Mota, J.; Casimiro, S.; Fernandes, J.; Hartmann, R.M.; Schemitt, E.; Picada, J.; Costa, L.; Marroni, N.; Raymundo, A.; Lima, A.; et al. Lupin Protein Concentrate as a Novel Functional Food Additive That Can Reduce Colitis-Induced Inflammation and Oxidative Stress. *Nutrients* **2022**, *14*, 2102. [CrossRef] [PubMed]
25. Cavaco, A.C.M.; Rezaei, M.; Caliandro, M.F.; Lima, A.M.; Stehling, M.; Dhayat, S.A.; Haier, J.; Brakebusch, C.; Eble, J.A. The Interaction between Laminin-332 and A3β1 Integrin Determines Differentiation and Maintenance of Cafs, and Supports Invasion of Pancreatic Duct Adenocarcinoma Cells. *Cancers* **2019**, *11*, 14. [CrossRef] [PubMed]
26. Matsuoka, R.L.; Marass, M.; Avdesh, A.; Helker, C.S.M.; Maischein, H.M.; Grosse, A.S.; Kaur, H.; Lawson, N.D.; Herzog, W.; Stainier, D.Y.R. Radial Glia Regulate Vascular Patterning around the Developing Spinal Cord. *Elife* **2016**, *5*, e20253. [CrossRef]
27. Fior, R.; Póvoa, V.; Mendes, R.V.; Carvalho, T.; Gomes, A.; Figueiredo, N.; Ferreira, M.G. Single-Cell Functional and Chemosensitive Profiling of Combinatorial Colorectal Therapy in Zebrafish Xenografts. *Proc. Natl. Acad. Sci. USA* **2017**, *114*, E8234–E8243. [CrossRef]
28. Okada, Y. *Proteinases and Matrix Degradation*, 10th ed.; Elsevier Inc.: Amsterdam, The Netherlands, 2017.
29. Quintero-Fabián, S.; Arreola, R.; Becerril-Villanueva, E.; Torres-Romero, J.C.; Arana-Argáez, V.; Lara-Riegos, J.; Ramírez-Camacho, M.A.; Alvarez-Sánchez, M.E. Role of Matrix Metalloproteinases in Angiogenesis and Cancer. *Front. Oncol.* **2019**, *9*, 1370. [CrossRef]
30. Li, Y.; Foss, C.A.; Summerfield, D.D.; Doyle, J.J.; Torok, C.M.; Dietz, H.C.; Pomper, M.G.; Yu, S.M. Targeting Collagen Strands by Photo-Triggered Triple-Helix Hybridization. *Proc. Natl. Acad. Sci. USA* **2012**, *109*, 14767–14772. [CrossRef]
31. Choe, C.P.; Choi, S.-Y.; Kee, Y.; Kim, M.J.; Kim, S.-H.; Lee, Y.; Park, H.-C.; Ro, H. Transgenic Fluorescent Zebrafish Lines That Have Revolutionized Biomedical Research. *Lab. Anim. Res.* **2021**, *37*, 26. [CrossRef]
32. Vandooren, J.; Van den Steen, E.; Opdenakker, G. Biochemistry and molecular biology of gelatinase B or matrix metalloproteinase-9 (MMP-9): The next decade. *Crit. Rev. Biochem. Mol. Biol.* **2013**, *48*, 222–272. [CrossRef] [PubMed]
33. MacRae, C.A.; Peterson, R.T. Zebrafish as Tools for Drug Discovery. *Nat. Rev. Drug Discov.* **2015**, *14*, 721–731. [CrossRef] [PubMed]
34. Augoff, K.; Hryniewicz-Jankowska, A.; Tabola, R.; Stach, K. MMP9: A Tough Target for Targeted Therapy for Cancer. *Cancers* **2022**, *14*, 1847. [CrossRef] [PubMed]

International Journal of
Molecular Sciences

MDPI

Article

Design, Synthesis and Biological Evaluation of Neocryptolepine Derivatives as Potential Anti-Gastric Cancer Agents

Yunhao Ma [1,†], Yanan Tian [1,†], Zhongkun Zhou [1], Shude Chen [2], Kangjia Du [1], Hao Zhang [1], Xinrong Jiang [1], Juan Lu [1], Yuqing Niu [1], Lixue Tu [1], Jie Wang [1], Huanxiang Liu [1], Hongmei Zhu [1], Peng Chen [1,*] and Yingqian Liu [1,*]

1 School of Pharmacy, Lanzhou University, Lanzhou 730000, China
2 The Second Clinical Medical College, Lanzhou University, Lanzhou 730000, China
* Correspondence: chenpeng@lzu.edu.cn (P.C.); yqliu@lzu.edu.cn (Y.L.); Tel./Fax: +86-931-8915686 (P.C. & Y.L.)
† These authors contributed equally to this work.

Abstract: Natural products play an important role in drug development and lead compound synthesis. Neocryptolepine is a polycyclic quinoline compound isolated from *Cryptolepis sanguinolent*. The cytotoxicity of neocryptolepine to gastric cancer cells AGS, MKN45, HGC27, and SGC7901 was not very strong, and it also had certain toxicity to gastric mucosa cells GES-1. Therefore, a series of neocryptolepine derivatives were synthesized by the modification of the structure of neocryptolepine, and their cytotoxicity was evaluated. The results showed that compounds **C5** and **C8** exhibited strong cytotoxicity to AGS cells. The cell colony formation and cell migration experiments suggested that compounds **C5** and **C8** could inhibit the proliferation and cell migration of AGS and HGC27 cells. Cell cycle and apoptosis experiments showed that compounds **C5** and **C8** did not cause the apoptosis of AGS and HGC27 cells but, mainly, caused cell necrosis. Compound **C5** had no significant effect on AGS and HGC27 cell cycles at low concentration. After treatment with AGS cells for 24 h at high concentration, compound **C5** could significantly arrest the AGS cell cycle in the G2/M phase. Compound **C8** had no significant effect on the AGS and HGC27 cell cycles. The results of molecular docking and Western blot showed that compounds **C5** and **C8** might induce cytotoxicity through the PI3K/AKT signaling pathway. Therefore, compounds **C5** and **C8** may be promising lead compounds for the treatment of gastric cancer.

Keywords: neocryptolepine derivatives; AKT; AGS cell; HGC27 cell; PI3K/AKT signaling pathway

Citation: Ma, Y.; Tian, Y.; Zhou, Z.; Chen, S.; Du, K.; Zhang, H.; Jiang, X.; Lu, J.; Niu, Y.; Tu, L.; et al. Design, Synthesis and Biological Evaluation of Neocryptolepine Derivatives as Potential Anti-Gastric Cancer Agents. *Int. J. Mol. Sci.* **2022**, *23*, 11924. https://doi.org/10.3390/ijms231911924

Academic Editors: Marialuigia Fantacuzzi, Barbara De Filippis and Alessandra Ammazzalorso

Received: 18 September 2022
Accepted: 5 October 2022
Published: 7 October 2022

1. Introduction

Cancer is the second leading cause of human death after cardiovascular disease, and cancer of the digestive system accounts for about 50% of all cancers [1]. According to the global cancer statistics in 2018, gastric cancer is the most common cancer of digestive system tumors, with about 1.03 million new cases of gastric cancer worldwide, ranking fifth in the incidence of malignant tumors and becoming the third leading cause of cancer death [2]. The five-year survival rate of gastric cancer is less than 25%, and we are often powerless for patients with advanced gastric cancer [3,4]. The methods of cancer treatment mainly include radiotherapy, chemotherapy, surgery, and gene therapy, but chemotherapy is a necessary means to treat solid tumors at present. Compared with other cancer treatments, oral chemotherapy drugs have the advantages of low cost and strong patient compliance. However, chemical drugs have large side effects, and drug resistance is difficult to solve [5,6]. Therefore, in order to overcome these obstacles, it is very necessary to develop new and less toxic chemical drugs to treat gastric cancer.

Among natural products, alkaloids are one of the main natural products. Alkaloids were discovered and used as early as 4000 years ago, and alkaloids and their derivatives have been used as drug sources to treat various diseases around the world, including the development of anticancer drugs [7]. Traditional alkaloids extracted from plants have played a huge role in the past [8], and more than 5000 alkaloids have been reported since the discovery of the first alkaloid, morphine, in 1805 [9]. A large number of studies have also shown that alkaloids performed excellent cytotoxicity to different cancers, including human melanoma, breast cancer, pancreatic cancer, colorectal cancer, oral cancer, liver cancer, and gastric cancer [10–15]. *Cryptolepis sanguinolenta* is a vine that grows in some African countries, and the roots of this plant have proven to be a rich source of indoline-quinoline alkaloids [16]. In recent years, neocryptolepine, a promising natural quinoline indole alkaloid, has attracted much attention. Some neocryptolepine derivatives have strong cytotoxicity to leukemia cells MV4-11, with an IC_{50} of 42 nM and also to lung cancer cells with an IC_{50} of 197 nM [17]. Neocryptolepine and its derivatives have a wide range of biological activities, and compounds containing this ring system have antifungal, antibacterial, antiviral, and cytotoxic activity [18–21]. In fact, indolequinoline alkaloids have good anticancer activities, and semi-synthetic analogues of these neocryptolepine can be prepared, which have shown great potential effects of cytotoxic agents [22]. Therefore, indolequinoline alkaloids are considered as a promising framework for drug development and can be further developed as effective anticancer drugs [8,22].

Due to the complex structure of natural products, different chemical components have different anticancer mechanisms [23]. Studies have shown that some alkaloids can induce apoptosis and cell cycle arrest [24]. The activation of cancer signaling pathways is common in the occurrence of cancer [25]. Multiple signaling pathways are involved in the occurrence of gastric cancer [26]. Phosphatidylinositol 3-kinase (PI3K)/protein kinase B (AKT) is an important signaling pathway in cells. When the PI3K/AKT signaling pathway is abnormally activated, it may cause the activation of downstream signaling molecules, thus affecting the development of gastric cancer, lung cancer, and other malignant tumors [27–29]. Studies have shown that the development of gastric cancer is related to excessive cell proliferation and inhibition of apoptosis, and activation of the PI3K/AKT cell signaling pathway often prevents programmed cell death [30]. The PI3K/AKT cell signaling pathway plays an important role not only in tumor development but also in tumor therapy, and many new targeted agents are realized by acting on relevant targets of the PI3K/AKT signaling pathway [31,32].

In the previous studies, in addition to numerous activity tests and mechanistic studies on the parent structure of neocryptolepine, a great deal of work has been done on the derivatives with the **C11** position substitution of neocryptolepine. Some studies have found that neocryptolepine derivatives have good antibacterial, anti-proliferative, and antifungal activities [33–35]. For example, in 2009, Ibrahim El Sayed et al. introduced a long amino-alkyl chain substitution at the **C11** position of neocryptolepine. A series of derivatives were prepared and further tested for their inhibitory activity against Plasmodium. Among them, the IC_{50} of the most active compound was 0.043 μM [36]. In 2012, Li Wang et al. reported the effects of derivatives obtained by modifying the **C11** position with a variety of amino alkyl chains on the human leukemia MV4-11 cell line in anti-proliferation experiments. The experimental results showed that most of the derived molecules had good anti-proliferation activity, but they also had high cytotoxicity [35,37]. Therefore, after performing the cytotoxicity study of 8-chloroneocryptolepine, the substitution at **C11** might be ideal to improve the inhibitory activity of 8-chloroneocryptolepine on cancer cells.

As a result, we aimed to perform the modification of the **C11** position of 8-chloroneocryptolepine, and a series of neocryptolepine derivatives were synthesized. The cytotoxic effects of neocryptolepine derivatives on liver cancer SMMC7721 and gastric cancer AGS cells were evaluated in vitro. The results showed that compounds **C5** and **C8** exhibited strong cytotoxicity against gastric cancer cells and may be promising lead compounds in the treatment of gastric cancer.

2. Results and Discussion

2.1. Chemistry

As shown in Scheme 1, in previous work, the structure of neocryptolepine was optimized by structural modification, and 8-chloroneocryptolepine performed good anti-fungal effects. The active functional group piecing strategy has been widely used in the field of derivative synthesis and structure optimization of antitumor compounds [24]. Moreover, the introduction of amino long-chain alkanes at the **C11** position of neocryptolepine could improve the cytotoxic effect of the compound [36,37]. Therefore, the cytotoxicity evaluation of a series of derivatives, by introducing an active functional group to **C11** of 8-chloroneocryptolepine, is a promising strategy for the development of a lead compound with anti-tumor drugs.

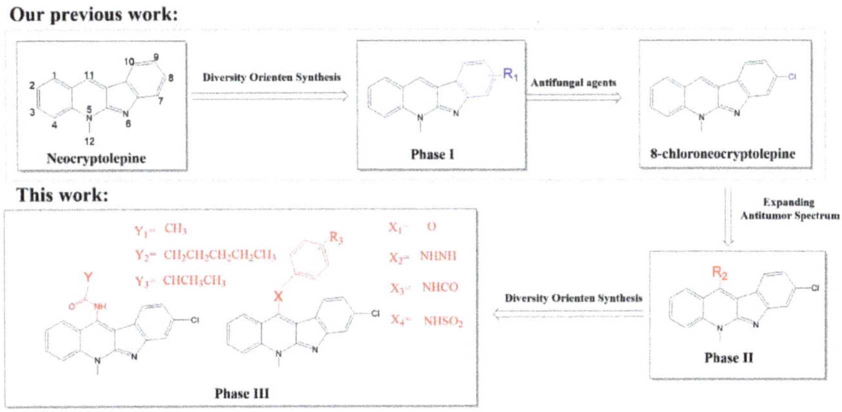

Scheme 1. Design strategy of target compounds in this study.

The synthesis of neocryptolepine derivatives and intermediates was shown in Scheme 2. Intermediate I was easily obtained with a yield of more than 80%. Indoles, trichloroacetyl chloride, and tetrahydrofuran were acylated to obtain intermediate I. Subsequently, intermediate II was obtained with the reaction of intermediate I and *N*-methylaniline, and the yield was more than 60%. Intermediate III was obtained by the reaction of intermediate II with diphenyl ether, and intermediate IV was obtained by the interaction with phosphorus oxychloride, with a yield of more than 60%. Intermediate IV reacted with the corresponding alcohol hydroxyl compound in N, N-dimethylformamide (DMF) to obtain the corresponding compounds **A1–A10**, and with the corresponding phenylhydrazine compound to obtain compounds **B1–B9**, with the corresponding amide compound to obtain compounds **C1–C10**, **D1–D6**. The structures of these compounds can be found in Table 1. It is important to note that the commercially available raw materials were obtained through the synthesis of intermediates and final products with a good yield. The structures of the target compounds were confirmed by ^{1}H and ^{13}C NMR and MS.

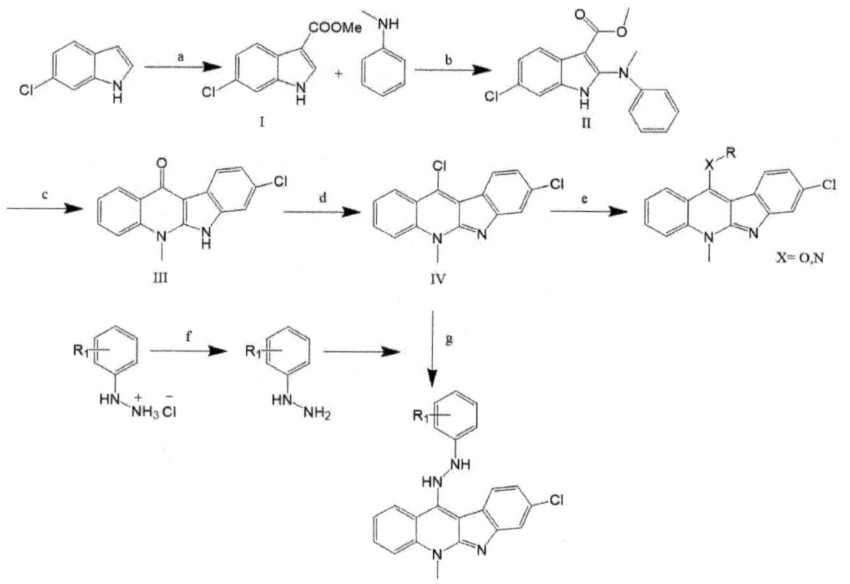

Scheme 2. Synthetic route of a series of neocryptolepine derivatives. Reagents and conditions: (a) trichloroacetyl chloride, pyridine, KOH, 85% (b) N-chlorosucccinimide, 1,4-dimethylpiperazine, CH_2Cl_2, 0 °C, 2 h; trichloroacetic acid, RT, 2 h, 64%; (c) diphenyl ether, reflux, 1.3 h; (d) $POCl_3$, toluene, reflux, 6–12 h, 70%; (e) amino derivatives or hydroxyl, DMF; (f) KOH; (g) ethanol, heat.

Table 1. Chemical structures of neocryptolepine derivatives.

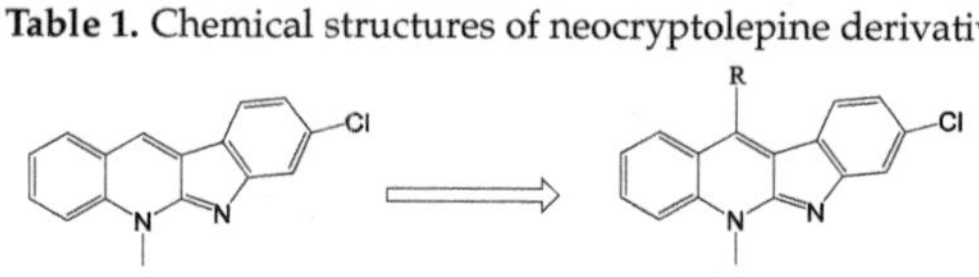

Compound	R	Compound	R	Compound	R
A1	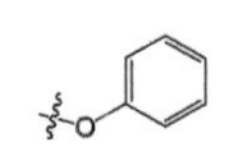	**B3**	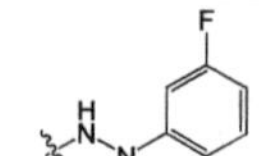	**C6**	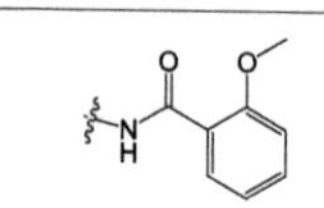
A2	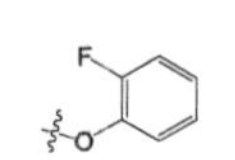	**B4**	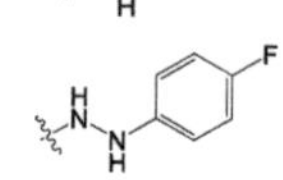	**C7**	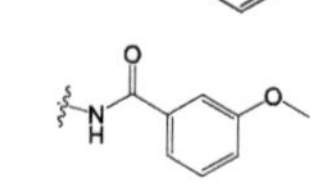
A3	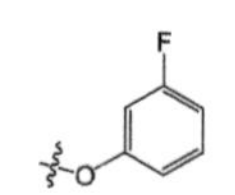	**B5**	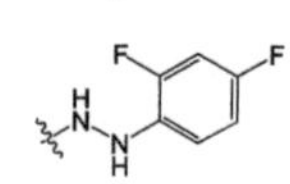	**C8**	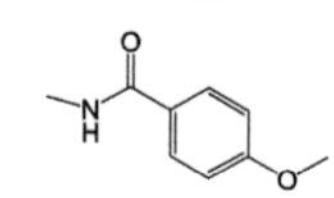
A4	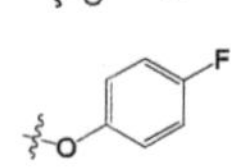	**B6**	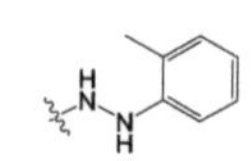	**C9**	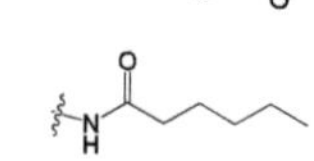
A5	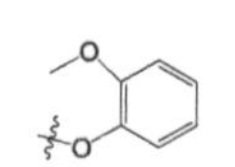	**B7**	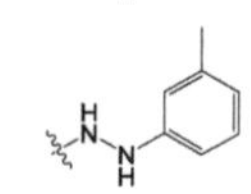	**C10**	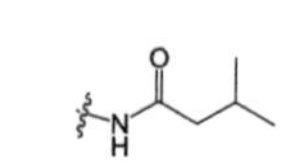

Table 1. *Cont.*

Compound	R	Compound	R	Compound	R
A6	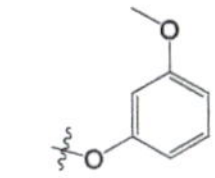	**B8**	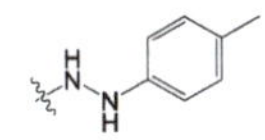	**D1**	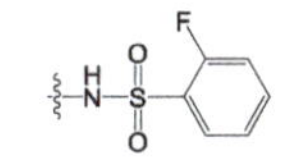
A7	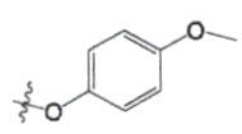	**B9**	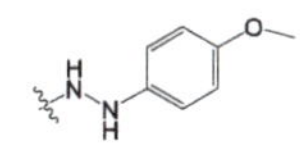	**D2**	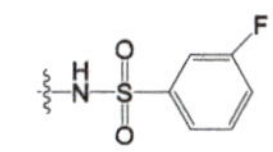
A8	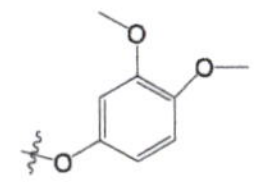	**C1**	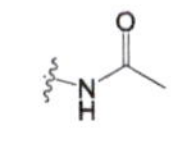	**D3**	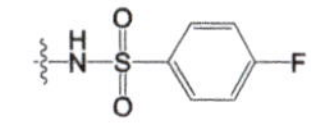
A9	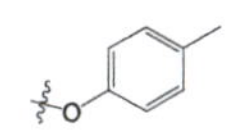	**C2**	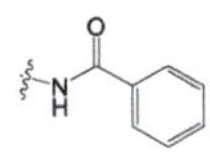	**D4**	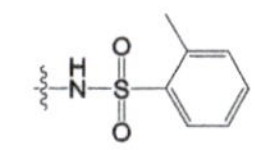
A10	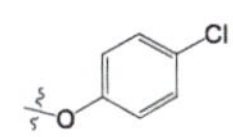	**C3**	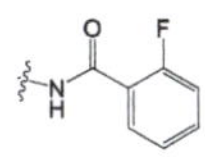	**D5**	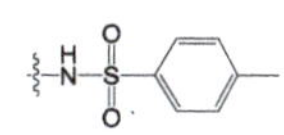
B1	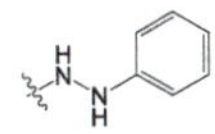	**C4**	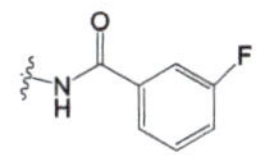	**D6**	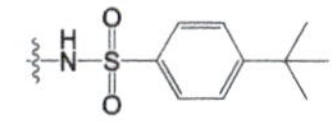
B2	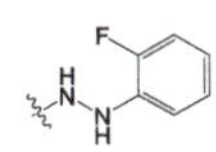	**C5**	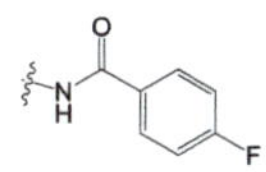	**E1**	

2.2. Cytotoxic Activity In Vitro and Structure-Activity Relationship (SAR)

The cytotoxicity of intermediate IV and neocryptolepine derivatives on gastric cancer AGS cells and hepatoma SMMC7721 cells was determined by MTT assay. Based on our results of cytotoxicity, the structure–activity relationship was studied for neocryptolepine derivatives (as shown in Figure 1). Firstly, the **C11** position of 8-chloroneocryptolepine was substituted with ether groups. However, in Table 2, the results suggest that the IC_{50} of compounds **A1–A10** was greater than 50 μM for SMMC7721, but some of the compounds had a strong cytotoxicity on AGS cells. According to the cytotoxicity results, the *para*-site substitution of F atom (**A4**) is better than the *meta*-site (**A3**) and *ortho*-site (**A2**) substitution, and the methoxy *ortho*-site (**A5**) substitution is more cytotoxic than the *meta* (**A6**) and *para*-site (**A7**) substitution, as well as the dimethoxy (**A8**) substitution, on benzene ring.

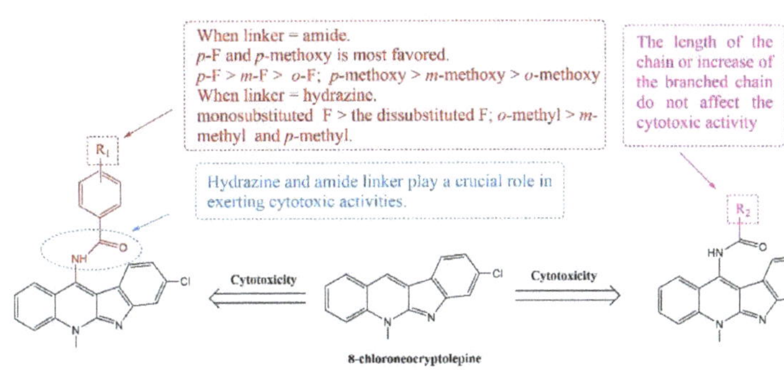

Figure 1. Structure-activity relationship analysis of neocryptolepine derivatives. Different colours indicated different substituted functional groups, and different arrows indicated different cytotoxic activities after functional group substitution.

Table 2. Antiproliferative activities (IC_{50}, μM) of compounds **A1–A10** on SMMC7721 and AGS cells for 48 h.

Compound	IC_{50} (μM)	
	SMMC7721	AGS
A1	>50	>50
A2	>50	14.7 ± 6.7
A3	>50	26.1 ± 0.7
A4	>50	12.6 ± 7.0
A5	>50	8.9 ± 0.6
A6	>50	29.6 ± 5.6
A7	>50	27.8 ± 0.0
A8	>50	>50
A9	>50	9.3 ± 0.6
A10	>50	14.3 ± 4.7

In 2016, Masashi Okada et al. performed an anti-proliferative activity assay on breast cancer MDA-MB-453 cells, colorectal cancer WiDr Cells, and ovarian cancer SKOv3 cells by introducing amino long-chain alkanes at the **C11** position. The experimental results showed that the introduction of amino long-chain alkanes at the **C11** position was beneficial to the improvement of anti-proliferative activity [38]. Based on the above structural modification and cytotoxicity, the **C11** position of 8-chloroneocryptolepine was substituted by hydrazine group to obtain compounds **B1–B9**. According to the cytotoxicity results in Table 3, the substitution of hydrazine group (**B1–B9**) was more cytotoxic than that of ether group (**A1–A10**). The results show that, in hydrazine group substitution, the substitution of F or methyl group increased its activity. Moreover, mono-substituted (**B2–B4**) F atom on benzene rings was more cytotoxic than disubstituted (**B5**) F atoms, and *meta*-substituted (**B3**) F atom was more cytotoxic than *para*-substituted (**B4**) F atom. The substitution of *ortho* (**B6**) methyl groups on benzene rings was better than that of *meta* (**B7**) and *para* (**B8**) groups.

Table 3. Antiproliferative activities (IC_{50}, μM) of compounds **B1–B9** on SMMC7721 and AGS cells for 48 h.

Compound	IC_{50} (μM)	
	SMMC7721	AGS
B1	38.7 ± 13.46	4.5 ± 0.6
B2	23.3 ± 1.90	1.5 ± 1.4
B3	14.7 ± 6.24	2.2 ± 0.3
B4	27.1 ± 5.83	3.5 ± 0.7
B5	28.9 ± 7.60	26.5 ± 17.6
B6	15.2 ± 1.23	3.3 ± 1.6
B7	38.3 ± 12.54	7 ± 0.6
B8	>50 (898.4)	9.9 ± 0.0
B9	40.9 ± 9.19	16.4 ± 0.0

Compounds **C1–C10** were synthesized by substituting **C11** sites with amide groups through electron iso-arrangement. In Table 4, by comparison and verification of experimental results, compounds **C5** and **C8** were found to be more active against AGS cells, and their possible mechanisms were studied at the cellular level. Moreover, as shown in Table 5, the cytotoxic effects of compounds **C5** and **C8** were significantly better than the positive drug cisplatin and the parent nucleus 8-chloroneocryptolepine. According to the cytotoxicity results in Table 4, the *para*-F (**C5**) atomic substitution of benzene ring was more cytotoxic than the *ortho* (**C3**) and *meta*-position (**C4**), and the *meta*-position (**C7**) and *para*-methoxy (**C8**) substitution were better than the *ortho*-substitution (**C6**). The increase in alkyl side chain (**C9** and **C10**) showed better cytotoxicity against AGS cells than compounds **A1–A10**. The structure–activity relationship of compounds **C1–C10** can also be found in Figure 1.

Table 4. Antiproliferative activities (IC_{50}, μM) of compounds **C1–C10** on SMMC7721 and AGS cells for 48 h.

Compound	IC_{50} (μM)	
	SMMC7721	AGS
C1	>50	5.1 ± 0.0
C2	>50	7.3 ± 4.4
C3	>50	>50
C4	>50	4.2 ± 3.1
C5	40.4 ± 18.08	2.9 ± 0.1
C6	>50	>50
C7	151.2 ± 90.86	4.7 ± 0.5
C8	12.2 ± 0.51	4.5 ± 2.5
C9	>50	5.7 ± 1.2
C10	>50	6.4 ± 0.0

Table 5. Antiproliferative activities (IC_{50}, μM) of compounds **D1-D6** and E1 on SMMC7721 and AGS cells for 48 h.

Compound	IC_{50} (μM)	
	SMMC7721	AGS
D1	>50	15.0 ± 0.0
D2	>50	3.9 ± 0.0
D3	>50	4.7 ± 0.0
D4	>50	10.4 ± 2.0
D5	>50	>50
D6	>50	>50
Intermediate **IV**	>50	>50
8-chloroneocryptolepine	27.0 ± 0	>50
CIS	>50	22.4 ± 3.8

Further evaluation of the cytotoxicity of 8-chloroneocryptolepine on gastric cancer AGS and liver cancer SMMC7721 cells revealed that its cytotoxicity was not ideal (as shown in Table 5). Finally, the **C11** position of 8-chloroneocryptolepine was substituted with a sulfonamide group to obtain compounds **D1–D6**. However, in Table 5, the cytotoxicity results suggested that the cytotoxicity for SMMC7721 cells was very weak. Therefore, the substitution of the sulfonamide group at the **C11** position was not an ideal choice. However, in the cytotoxicity results of AGS cells, the *meta*-positional (**D2**) substitution of F atom was less potent (or less cytotoxic) than *ortho*- (**D1**) and *para*-substitutions (**D3**). The *ortho*-methyl substitution (**D4**) in benzene ring was more cytotoxic than the *para*-methyl (**D5**) substitution.

2.3. *Preliminary Cytotoxic Mechanism of Compounds **C5** and **C8** against AGS and HGC27 Cells*

2.3.1. The Cytotoxic Effect of Compounds **C5** and **C8** on Gastric Cancer Cells

The cytotoxicity of compounds **C5** and **C8** were systematically evaluated by an MTT assay. As shown in Figure 2, we performed cytotoxicity experiments on five gastric cancer cell lines—AGS, HGC27, MKN45, MGC803, and SGC7901—using neocryptolepine and cisplatin as the control. The results showed that the IC_{50} values of neocryptolepine were 20, 18, 19, 40, and 37 μM on AGS, HGC27, MKN45, MGC803, and SGC7901 cells, after 48 h, respectively. Compared with the cytotoxicity of the parent nucleus of neocryptolepine, we found that compounds **C5** and **C8** had stronger cytotoxicity by structural modification. The IC_{50} values of compound **C5** on AGS, HGC27, MKN45, MGC803, and SGC7901 cells, for 48 h, were 9.2, 6.6, 5.9, 13, and 8.7 μM, respectively. The IC_{50} values of compound **C8** on AGS, HGC27, MKN45, MGC803, and SGC7901 cells, after 48 h treatment, were 6.9, 4.3, 3.5, 10, and 10 μM, respectively. Compared with the positive drugs, compounds **C5** and **C8** showed significantly stronger cytotoxicity than cisplatin.

In Figure 2G, it was found that the cytotoxic effects of compounds **C5** and **C8** to normal cells (IC_{50} = 12.8 and 12.6 μM, respectively) were relatively weaker than gastric cancer cells. We also performed concentration-dependent and time-dependent experiments on the cytotoxicity of compound **C8** and cisplatin to AGS, and the results showed (Figure 2) that compound **C8** and cisplatin could inhibit the growth of gastric cancer cell lines AGS, HGC27, and MKN45 in a concentration-dependent and time-dependent manner. Moreover, compound **C8** showed strong cytotoxicity to gastric cancer cells at 5 μM, while cisplatin was weak. Therefore, the results of the MTT assay showed that we improved the cytotoxicity of the parent nuclear structure of neocryptolepine by structural modification, and compounds **C5** and **C8** showed stronger cytotoxicity effects compared with the positive drug cisplatin.

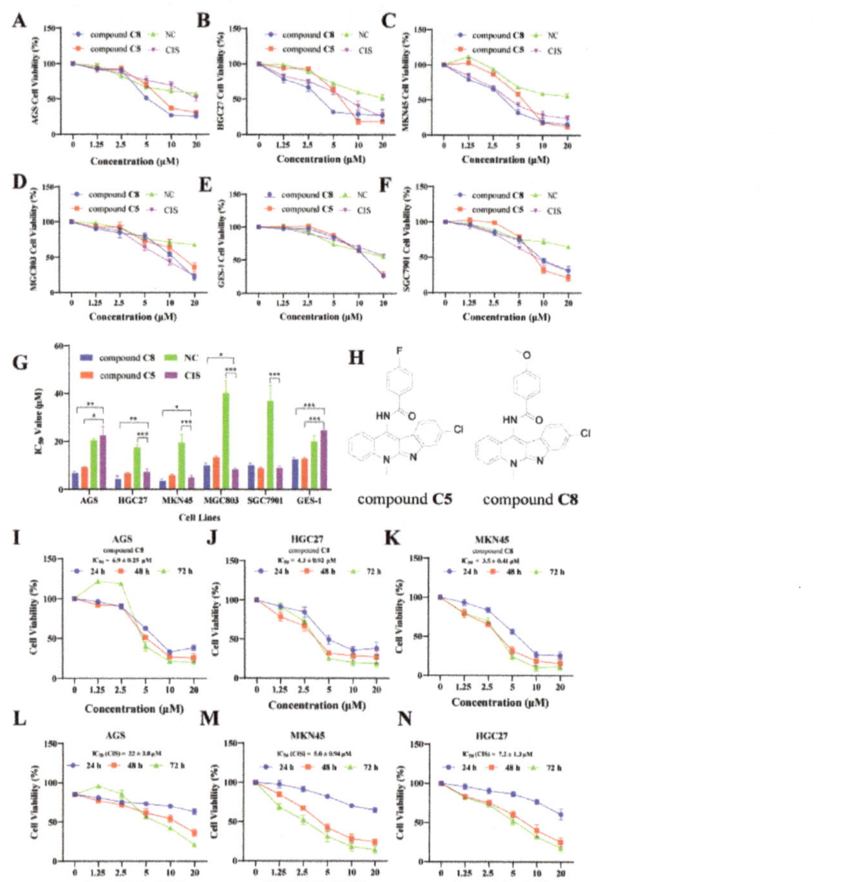

Figure 2. Cytotoxicity evaluation of neocryptolepine (NC), compounds **C5**, **C8**, and CIS on gastric cancer cell lines. (**A–F**) The cytotoxic effects of NC, compound **C5**, compound **C8**, and CIS at different concentrations on AGS, HGC27, MKN45, MGC803, GES-1, and SGC7901 cells, at 48 h, respectively. (**G**) IC_{50} comparison of NC, compound **C5**, compound **C8**, and CIS on gastric cancer cell lines at 48 h. (**H**) Chemical structure of compounds **C5** and **C8**. (**I–K**) The cytotoxic effects of compound **C8** with different concentrations on AGS, HGC27, and MKN45 cells at 24 h, 48 h, and 72 h, respectively. (**L–N**) Cytotoxic effects of CIS at different concentrations on AGS, HGC27, and MKN45 cells at 24 h, 48 h, and 72 h. Values are shown as the means ± standard, n = 3. * $p < 0.05$, ** $p < 0.01$, *** $p < 0.001$ compared to negative DMSO control group.

2.3.2. Compounds **C5** and **C8** Inhibited the Proliferation and Migration of AGS and HGC27 Cells

To study the effects of compounds **C5** and **C8,** on the proliferation of AGS and HGC27 cells, the colony formation assays were performed. The results showed that, as shown in Figure 3A, compound **C8** at 1 μM and 2 μM, as well as compound **C5** at 2 μM and 4 μM, could inhibit the proliferation of AGS HGC27 cells. When the concentration of compound **C8** was 4 μM and compound **C5 was** at 6 μM, the proliferation of AGS and HGC27 cells was completely inhibited, and no cell clones were formed. Therefore, our results showed that compounds **C5** and **C8** had a certain inhibitory effect on the proliferation of AGS and HGC27 cells, and the proliferation of AGS and HGC27 cells could be completely inhibited when compounds **C5** and **C8** reached a certain concentration.

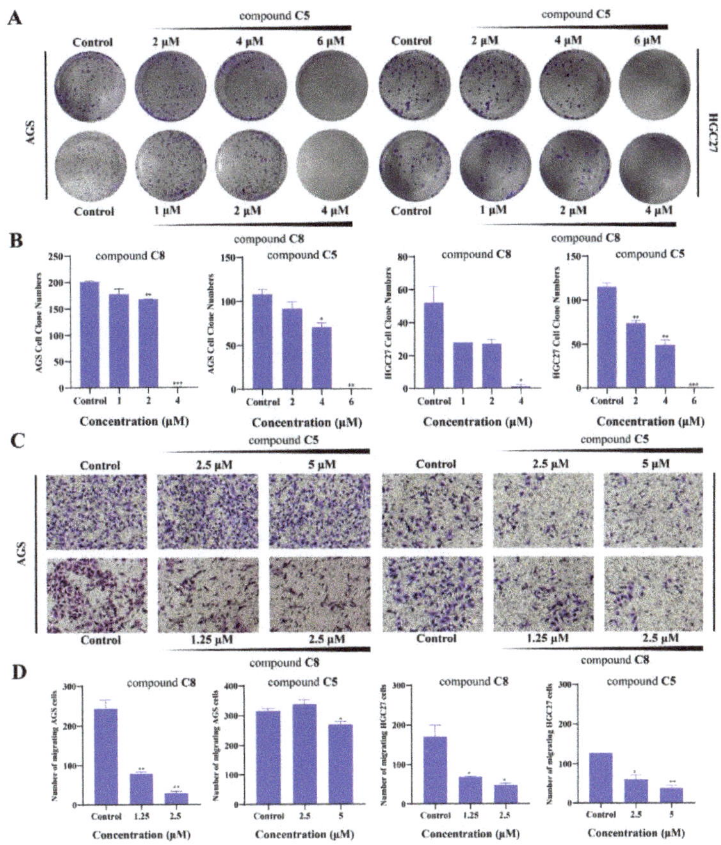

Figure 3. The proliferation and migration of AGS and HGC27 cells were inhibited after treatment compounds **C5** or **C8** for 48 h. (**A**) The proliferation of AGS and HGC27 cells were inhibited for treatment of different concentrations of compounds **C5** or **C8** for 48 h. (**B**) Statistical analysis of AGS and HGC27 cell migration numbers. (**C**) The proliferation of AGS and HGC27 cells was inhibited after the treatment of compounds **C5** and **C8** for 8–10 days. (**D**) Statistical analysis of AGS and HGC27 cell proliferation numbers. Values are shown as the means ± standard. * $p < 0.05$, ** $p < 0.01$, *** $p < 0.001$ compared to negative DMSO control group.

The migration of tumor cells is an important embodiment of the lethal effect of tumor. Therefore, cell migration experiments were performed to study the effects of compounds **C5** and **C8** on the migration ability of AGS and HGC27 cells. Results are shown in Figure 3C, after treatment with compound **C8** at 1.25 μM for 48 h, and the migrating ability of AGS and HGC27 cells was significantly inhibited. As the concentration of compound **C8** increased, the number of AGS cells decreased from 243 to 28, and the number of HGC27 cells decreased from 170 to 47. Similarly, compound **C5** inhibited the migration of HGC27 cells in a concentration-dependent manner. However, our results showed that compound **C5** did not have an obvious effect on the migration of AGS cells. It may be that the tumor specificity caused the different inhibitory effect of compounds on AGS and HGC27 cells. In conclusion, different concentrations of compound **C8** inhibited the migration of AGS and HGC27 cells, and compound **C5** also inhibited the migration of HGC27 cells at certain concentrations.

2.3.3. The Effects of Compounds **C5** and **C8** on AGS and HGC27 Cell Cycle

Cell cycle regulation plays an important role in anti-tumor drugs. Therefore, to evaluate the effect of neocryptolepine derivatives on cell cycle, flow cytometry was used to test the changes of AGS and HGC27 cell cycle after neocryptolepine derivatives treatment. Results are shown in Figure 4A, AGS cells were treated with 2.5 μM and 5 μM compound **C8** for 24 h, and there was no significant change in AGS and HGC27 cell cycles. After the AGS and HGC27 cells were treated with different concentrations of compound **C5** for 24 h, it was found that HGC27 cells died when treated with 10 μM of compound **C5**. Therefore, we reduced the concentration of compound **C5**. The results showed that compound **C5** had no significant change in the HGC27 cell cycle when treated with 2.5 μM and 5 μM. However, the AGS cells were treated with 10 μM compound **C5** for 24 h, the AGS cells were mainly arrested in the G2/M phase. In the apoptosis experiment, although compound **C5** caused the necrosis of most AGS cells after treatment for 48 h, AGS cells did not die completely after treatment with compound **C5** for 24 h in the cell cycle. The cell cycle experiments suggested that compounds **C5** and **C8** had no significant effect on the cell cycles of AGS and HGC27 cells at low concentration, while compound **C5** could significantly block AGS cells in G2/M phase at high concentration.

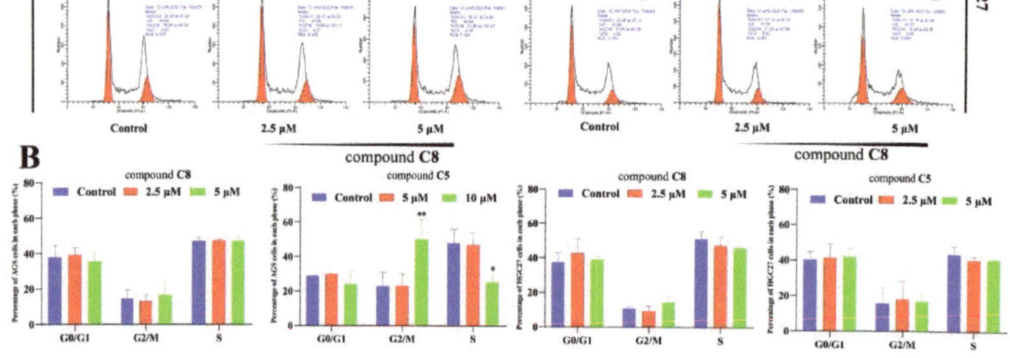

Figure 4. *Cont.*

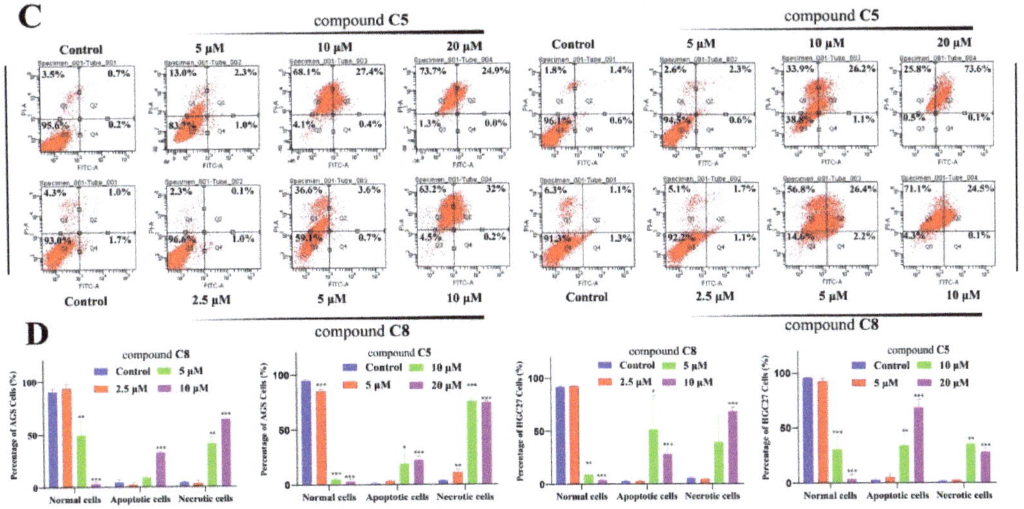

Figure 4. Effects of different concentrations of compounds **C5** or **C8** on AGS cell cycle and cell apoptosis after treatment for 24 h or 48 h. (**A**) Effects of different concentrations of compounds (**C5**) and **C8** on AGS and HGC27 cell cycle after 24 h treatment. (**B**) Analysis of the proportion of AGS and HGC27 cells, at different cell stages, before and after treatment with compounds **C5** or **C8**. (**C**) Statistical analysis of apoptosis percentage of AGS and HGC27 cells. (**D**) Treatment of AGS or HGC27 cells, with different concentrations of compound **C5** or **C8** for 48 h, caused cell necrosis.

2.3.4. The Effects of Compounds **C5** and **C8** on Apoptosis of AGS and HGC27 Cells

Apoptosis is a common characteristic of most chemotherapeutic drugs that can exert antitumor effects. To investigate whether the neocryptolepine derivatives exert cytotoxic effects by cell apoptosis, we detected the effects of compounds **C5** and **C8** on the apoptosis of AGS and HGC27 cells by flow cytometry. The results (Figure 4C) showed that, when the concentration of compound **C8** was 2.5 µM, it did not cause the apoptosis or necrosis of AGS and HGC27 cells, but when the concentration reached 5 µM, compound **C8** had caused the necrosis of AGS and HGC27 cells, and when the concentration reached 10 µM, all AGS and HGC27 cells had apoptosis or necrosis. Similarly, compound **C5** showed the same effect in AGS and HGC27 cells, but it should be noted that, after treatment with 10 µM compound **C5** for 48 h, most AGS cells died. Moreover, cell cycle results also showed that compound **C5** treatment of AGS cells, at a concentration of 10 µM for 24 h, did not completely cause the death of AGS. Therefore, it can be concluded that compound **C5** and **C8** do not exert cytotoxic effects, mainly, through apoptosis but directly lead to cell necrosis.

2.3.5. Molecular Docking of Compounds **C5** and **C8** with AKT Protein

The activation of carcinogenic signaling pathway is very frequent in the occurrence of cancer, and multiple signaling pathways are involved in the development of gastric cancer [25,26]. To find the cause of cytotoxicity of neocryptolepine derivatives to gastric cancer cell lines, that is, the intracellular targets of compounds **C5** and **C8**, a series of proteins related to cancer cell signaling pathways were docked with compounds **C5** and **C8** by molecular docking experiments. The results (Figure 5) showed that both compounds **C5** and **C8** had the best scores with the AKT protein. Its scores with the AKT protein were −8.529 and −8.359 kcal/mol, respectively. The side of the benzene ring in the small molecule is close to the hydrophobic region consisting of LEU210, TYR263, LEU264, VAL270, and TYR272, forming hydrophobic interactions with the receptor. The benzene ring of the small molecule forms a Π–Π interaction with the pyrrole of tryptophan 80. Therefore, the molecular docking results suggested that AKT may be a potential intracellular target of compounds **C5** and **C8**.

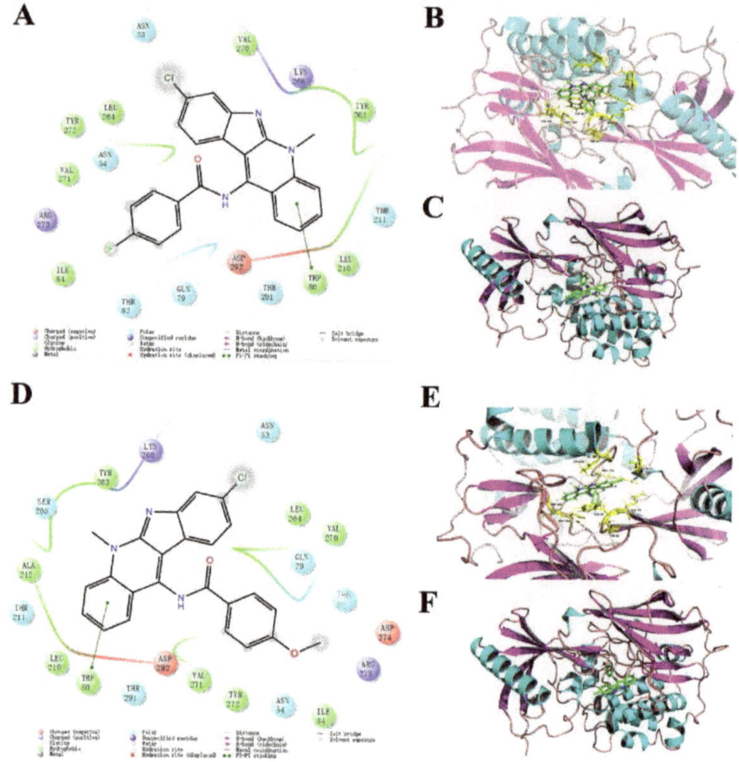

Figure 5. Molecular docking between compounds **C5** or **C8** and AKT proteins. Different colours in **A** and **D** indicated different types of amino acids, and different colours in B, C, E and F indicated different structures of the protein. (**A**) 2D diagram of AKT interacting with small molecule ligand compound **C5**. (**B**) Diagram of compound **C5** binding interaction with AKT protein. (**C**) Overall view of compound **C5** binding to the AKT protein. (**D**) A 2D diagram of AKT interacting with small molecule ligand compound **C8**. (**E**) Diagram of compound **C8** binding interaction with AKT protein. (**F**) Overall view of compound **C8** binding to the AKT protein.

2.3.6. Compounds **C5** and **C8** Inhibited AGS and HGC27 Cell Growth by Regulating PI3K/AKT Signaling Pathway

A variety of cell signaling pathways are involved in the occurrence of gastric cancer [26]. PI3K/AKT is an important signaling pathway, and when this pathway is abnormally activated, it affects the expression of downstream related proteins, thus affecting the occurrence and development of gastric cancer [39]. To further verify the results of molecular docking, Western blot experiments were performed to study the effects of compounds **C5** and **C8** on PI3K/AKT signaling pathway-related proteins in AGS and HGC27 cells. Results are shown in Figure 6, after AGS and HGC27 cells were treated with 5 μM compounds **C5** and **C8** for 48 h, and the expression levels of PI3KCA, AKT, and p-Akt proteins in the PI3K/AKT signaling pathway were down-regulated. The results further confirmed the molecular docking results: compounds **C5** and **C8** may act as AKT inhibitors to play an anti-proliferation role in gastric cancer. In conclusion, compounds **C5** and **C8** may inhibit the proliferation of gastric cancer AGS and HGC27 cells through the PI3K/AKT signaling pathway.

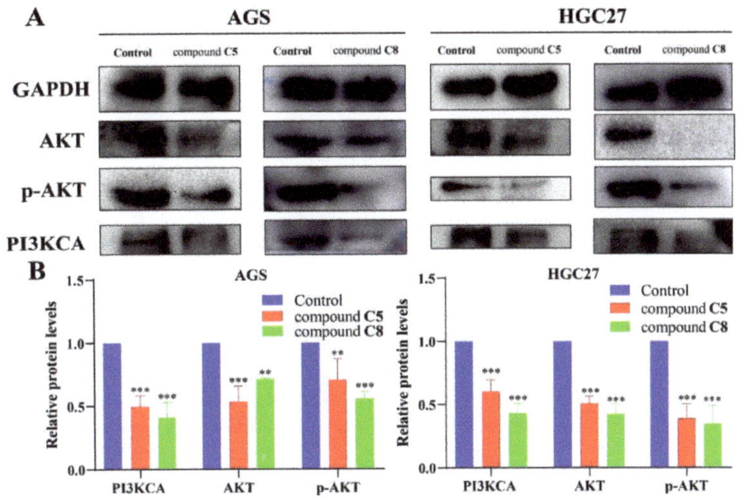

Figure 6. Changes of PI3K/AKT signaling pathway related proteins in AGS and HGC27 cells treated with compounds **C5** or **C8** for 48 h. (**A**) The expression of PI3KCA, AKT, and p-AKT of AGS or HGC27 cells was inhibited after treatment with compound **C5** or **C8** for 48 h at 5 μM. (**B**) Changes of PI3KCA, AKT, and p-AKT protein expression levels on AGS and HGC27 cells, after treatment with 5 μM of compounds **C5** and **C8**, for 48 h. ** $p < 0.01$, *** $p < 0.001$ compared to negative DMSO control group.

3. Materials and Methods

3.1. Reagents

All chemical reagents and solvents were of reagent grade or purified according to standard methods before use. The ^{1}H NMR and ^{13}C NMR spectra were recorded using JNM-ECS-400 MHz and 100 MHz. Mass spectrometry was performed using a Bruker Micro TOF ESI-TOF mass spectrometer. During the experiment, all pH values were measured by PH-10C pH meter. The purity of the synthesized derivatives was characterized by a purity test (as shown in Figures S1–S42).

3.2. Synthesis

3.2.1. Synthesis Method of Intermediate I

The indole (10.88 mmol) was added to the mixture of pyridine (14.2 mmol) and tetrahydrofuran (40 mL) at 0 °C, and the reaction was stirred at 0 °C for 0.5 h. Then, the mixed solution of trichloroacetyl chloride (14.2 mmol) and tetrahydrofuran (30 mL) was added slowly. After the reaction was raised to room temperature and stirred continuously for 16 h, 10% HCl solution was added to the reaction system at 0 °C, and the organic phase was extracted with ethyl acetate (300 mL), washed with salt water, and dried with anhydrous magnesium sulfate. The solvent was removed on the rotary evaporator, and the solid product was directly dissolved in anhydrous methanol (150 mL). Then, 10% KOH solution (20 mL) was added, the reaction mixture was heated and reflux for 5 h, and, then, concentrated in the rotary evaporator, the solvent was removed, and the large solid product was extracted with ethyl acetate (200 mL). The organic phase was washed with salt water, dried with anhydrous magnesium sulfate, and the solvent was removed. The crude product was purified by silica gel column chromatography with the eluent of n-hexane/ethyl acetate (4/1). Finally, Intermediate I was obtained.

Methyl 6-chloro-1H-indole-3-carboxylate (Intermediate I)

Yield, 85%; white solid, m.p. 182–185 °C (DMSO); ^{1}H NMR (400 MHz, DMSO-d_6) δ 12.05 (s, 1H), 8.14 (d, J = 3.0 Hz, 1H), 7.99 (d, J = 8.5 Hz, 1H), 7.55 (d, J = 2.0 Hz, 1H), 7.22 (d, J = 8.5 Hz, 1H), 3.82 (s, 3H). ^{13}C NMR (100 MHz, DMSO-d_6) δ 164.89, 137.24, 133.90, 127.51, 124.86, 122.20, 122.09, 112.51, 107.03, 51.25. MS-ESI m/z: calcd for $C_{10}H_8ClN_2O$[M + H]+: 210.0244; found: 210.1683.

3.2.2. Synthesis Method of Intermediate II

Under the protection of inert gas, intermediate I (2.5 mmol) was dissolved in dichloromethane (5 mL) and N-chlorosuccinimide (NCS, 2.75 mmol), and N, N-dimethylpiperazine (1.25 mmol) dichloromethane (1 mL) solution was added drop-by-drop at 0 °C. The reaction system was stirred continuously at 0 °C for 2 h. Then, a mixed solution of trichloroacetic acid (0.63 mmol) and N-methylaniline (5 mmol) dichloromethane (2 mL) was added. The reaction was then heated to room temperature and stirred continuously for 3.5 h at room temperature. At the end of the reaction, the reaction mixture was washed with saturated sodium bicarbonate aqueous solution, 1N concentration of hydrochloric acid, and salt water, and then, the separated organic phase was dried by anhydrous magnesium sulfate and condensed under pressure on a rotary evaporator. Finally, the solid product was purified by column chromatography with the eluent of n-hexane/ethyl acetate (7/1), and the intermediate II was finally obtained.

Methyl 6-chloro-2-(methyl(phenyl)amino)-1H-indole-3-carboxylate (Intermediate II)

Yield, 64%; white solid, m.p. 154–156 °C (DMSO); ^{1}H NMR (400 MHz, DMSO-d_6) δ 12.08 (s, 1H), 7.92 (d, J = 8.5 Hz, 1H), 7.34 (d, J = 1.9 Hz, 1H), 7.28–7.20 (m, 2H), 7.17 (d, J = 8.5 Hz, 1H), 6.86 (t, J = 7.3 Hz, 1H), 6.83–6.77 (m, 2H), 3.65 (s, 3H), 3.37 (s, 3H). ^{13}C NMR (100 MHz, DMSO-d_6) δ 163.77, 148.66, 147.76, 133.48, 129.46 (2C), 126.94, 125.51, 122.26, 121.79, 120.10, 115.75 (2C), 111.38, 97.10, 50.93, 40.15. MS-ESI m/z: calcd for $C_{17}H_{15}ClN_2O_2$[M + H]+: 315.0822; found: 315.1015.

3.2.3. Synthesis Method of Intermediate III

An appropriate amount of diphenyl ether was added to the round bottom flask, and then, the reactor temperature was heated to about 60 °C, until the diphenyl ether was in the molten state, and then, intermediate II was added to the diphenyl ether. Then, the temperature increased to 250 °C reflux for 1–3 h, the end of the reaction, until the temperature was reduced to room temperature, and reactants were dumped into a large quantity of petroleum ether. The intermediate III was obtained by collecting precipitated precipitation.

3.2.4. Synthesis Method of Intermediate IV

Under nitrogen protection, Dry intermediates III was added to the phosphorus oxychloride, reflux, under 110 °C for about 12 h of reaction. After the reaction is cooled to room temperature, phosphorus oxychloride was removed on the rotary evaporator. Then, ice water was added to the residue, the pH was adjusted to 9.0 with sodium bicarbonate, and the temperature during the period did not exceed 40 °C. The organic phase was extracted with dichloromethane, and the crude product was concentrated on a rotary evaporator. The crude product was first purified by silica gel column chromatography with the eluent of petroleum ether/ethyl acetate (2/1) to remove other impurities and, then, purified with the eluent of dichloromethane/methanol (40/1) to obtain orange–red product Intermediate **IV**.

8,11-dichloro-5-methyl-5H-indolo[2,3-b]quinoline (Intermediate IV)

Yield, 64%; white solid, m.p. 227–229 °C (DMSO); ^{1}H NMR (400 MHz, Chloroform-d) δ 8.29 (d, J = 8.2 Hz, 1H), 8.11 (d, J = 8.2 Hz, 1H), 7.75 (t, J = 7.8 Hz, 1H), 7.61 (d, J = 8.6 Hz, 1H), 7.52 (d, J = 1.8 Hz, 1H), 7.46 (t, J = 7.6 Hz, 1H), 7.07 (d, J = 8.2 Hz, 1H), 4.21 (s, 3H). ^{13}C NMR (100 MHz, Chloroform-d) δ 155.82, 155.77, 136.71, 136.06, 135.13, 131.24, 125.94,

124.16, 123.75, 122.53, 122.01, 120.23, 119.06, 117.64, 114.31, 33.17. MS-ESI m/z: calcd for $C_{16}H_{10}Cl_2N_2$ [M + H]+: 301.0221; found: 301.1502.

3.2.5. Synthesis Method of Intermediate Phenylhydrazine

The purchased phenylhydrazine hydrochloride was dissolved in dichloromethane, and 3 M potassium hydroxide was added to carry out the reaction at room temperature, with attention to the whole process to avoid light, and the reaction lasted for about 1–3 h. The organic phase was extracted with dichlorohexane, and the solvent was removed on a rotary evaporator at low pressure. The temperature of solvent removal was not more than 40 °C. When the solvent was removed by rotary evaporation, the white solid product was phenylhydrazine.

3.2.6. Synthesis Method of Target Compounds **A1–A10**

The Intermediate IV was dissolved in N, N-dimethylformamide (DMF), and then, the corresponding alcohol hydroxyl compounds were added, and the reaction was reflux at 110 °C for 3 h. After the reaction was over, the organic phase was extracted with dichloromethane and, then, washed with salt water. After that, the organic phase was dried with anhydrous magnesium sulfate, and the solvent was removed at low pressure on the rotary evaporator. The crude product was first purified by silica gel column chromatography with the ratio of petroleum ether/ethyl acetate (2/1) eluent to remove other impurities, and then, it was purified with the ratio of dichloromethane/methanol (40/1). Finally, the target compound was obtained.

8-chloro-5-methyl-11-phenoxy-5H-indolo[2,3-b]quinoline (**A1**)

Yield, 81%; brown solid, m.p. 195–196 °C (DMSO); ^{1}H NMR (400 MHz, Chloroform-*d*) δ 8.23–8.18 (m, 1H), 7.81 (d, J = 6.3 Hz, 2H), 7.66 (s, 1H), 7.43 (d, J = 8.1 Hz, 1H), 7.32 (d, J = 2.4 Hz, 1H), 7.24–7.17 (m, 1H), 7.12–7.07 (m, 1H), 7.01 (d, J = 1.3 Hz, 1H), 7.00–6.94 (m, 2H), 6.93–6.89 (m, 1H), 6.89–6.83 (m, 1H), 4.36 (s, 3H). ^{13}C NMR (100 MHz, Chloroform-*d*) δ 161.65, 157.40, 156.01, 153.26, 150.68, 137.10, 133.47, 130.50, 129.16, 128.51, 123.61, 123.44, 122.30, 121.43, 119.47, 119.40, 118.76, 116.40, 116.25, 114.56, 114.50, 113.53, 32.46. MS-ESI m/z: calcd for $C_{22}H_{15}ClN_2O$[M + H]+: 359.0873; found: 359.1959.

8-chloro-11-(2-fluorophenoxy)-5-methyl-5H-indolo[2,3-b]quinoline (**A2**)

Yield, 73%; orange solid, m.p. 325–328 °C (DMSO); ^{1}H NMR (400 MHz, Chloroform-*d*) δ 8.23 (d, J = 8.2, 1.4 Hz, 1H), 7.95 (d, J = 8.7 Hz, 1H), 7.89 (d, J = 8.7 Hz, 1H), 7.60 (s, 1H), 7.51 (d, J = 8.1 Hz, 1H), 7.34 (d, J = 8.4 Hz, 1H), 7.31–7.25 (m, 1H), 7.11–7.04 (m, 1H), 7.00 (d, J = 8.3 Hz, 1H), 6.92–6.86 (m, 1H), 6.65 (t, J = 8.3 Hz, 1H), 4.37 (s, 3H). ^{13}C NMR (100 MHz, Chloroform-*d*) δ 158.24, 156.33, 154.27, 152.54, 151.37, 148.13, 140.16, 133.84, 132.32, 131.82, 124.99, 124.30, 121.73, 119.94, 117.85, 117.11, 116.63, 116.14, 115.10, 114.68, 113.32, 34.09. MS-ESI m/z: calcd for $C_{22}H_{14}ClFN_2O$[M + H]+: 377.0779; found: 377.1835.

8-chloro-11-(3-fluorophenoxy)-5-methyl-5H-indolo[2,3-b]quinoline (**A3**)

Yield, 82%; orange solid, m.p. 250–252 °C (DMSO); ^{1}H NMR (400 MHz, Chloroform-*d*) δ 8.18–8.10 (m, 1H), 8.01 (s, 1H), 7.88–7.77 (m, 2H), 7.66 (d, J = 1.8 Hz, 1H), 7.44 (d, J = 8.1 Hz, 1H), 7.39 (d, J = 8.2 Hz, 1H), 7.01 (d, J = 8.2 Hz, 1H), 6.85–6.80 (m, 1H), 6.80–6.68 (m, 2H), 4.37 (s, 3H). ^{13}C NMR (100 MHz, Chloroform-*d*) δ 164.92, 162.59, 158.43, 154.66, 150.84, 138.14, 134.78, 131.62, 131.09 (d, J = 9.7 Hz), 130.21 (d, J = 10.2 Hz), 124.31 (d, J = 4.4 Hz), 122.55, 120.60, 120.27, 117.51, 117.00, 114.64, 111.15, 111.12, 110.33 (d, J = 21.2 Hz), 103.70 (d, J = 25.7 Hz), 33.45. MS-ESI m/z: calcd for $C_{22}H_{14}ClFN_2O$[M + H]+: 377.0781; found:377.1899.

8-chloro-11-(4-fluorophenoxy)-5-methyl-5H-indolo[2,3-b]quinoline (**A4**)

Yield, 76%; yellow solid, m.p. 255–256 °C (DMSO); ^{1}H NMR (400 MHz, Chloroform-*d*) δ 8.21–8.15 (m, 1H), 7.86–7.77 (m, 2H), 7.66 (s, 1H), 7.44 (d, J = 8.1 Hz, 1H), 7.32 (d, J = 8.3 Hz, 1H), 7.03–6.92 (m, 5H), 4.38 (s, 3H). ^{13}C NMR (100 MHz, Chloroform-*d*) δ 158.63, 157.54,

156.22, 153.76, 152.03, 150.41, 137.15, 133.56, 130.49, 123.44, 123.33, 121.34, 119.38, 116.52, 116.13, 115.80, 115.72, 115.70, 115.62, 115.57, 115.52, 113.52, 32.34. MS-ESI m/z: calcd for $C_{22}H_{14}ClFN_2O$[M + H]+: 377.0763; found: 377.1875.

8-chloro-11-(2-methoxyphenoxy)-5-methyl-5H-indolo[2,3-b]quinoline (**A5**)

Yield, 78%; yellow solid, m.p. 244–247 °C (DMSO); ^{1}H NMR (400 MHz, Chloroform-*d*) δ 8.25 (d, J = 8.2 Hz, 1H), 7.79 (d, J = 3.5 Hz, 2H), 7.67 (s, 1H), 7.41 (d, J = 8.1 Hz, 1H), 7.36 (d, J = 8.2 Hz, 1H), 7.13 (d, J = 8.2 Hz, 1H), 7.10–7.04 (m, 1H), 6.98 (d, J = 8.2 Hz, 1H), 6.69 (t, J = 7.8 Hz, 1H), 6.58 (d, J = 8.1 Hz, 1H), 4.39 (s, 3H), 4.05 (s, 3H). ^{13}C NMR (100 MHz, Chloroform-*d*) δ 157.89, 154.14, 151.28, 148.00, 145.27, 137.12, 133.27, 130.27, 123.68, 123.37, 122.94, 121.14, 120.07, 119.84, 119.19, 116.46, 116.26, 115.49, 114.58, 113.34, 111.91, 55.27, 32.17. MS-ESI m/z: calcd for $C_{23}H_{17}ClN_2O_2$[M + H]+: 389.0979; found: 389.2214.

8-chloro-11-(3-methoxyphenoxy)-5-methyl-5H-indolo[2,3-b]quinoline (**A6**)

Yield, 83%; orange solid, m.p. 223–224 °C (DMSO); ^{1}H NMR (400 MHz, Chloroform-*d*) δ 8.21–8.16 (m, 1H), 7.80 (d, J = 6.2 Hz, 2H), 7.67 (s, 1H), 7.45–7.36 (m, 2H), 7.17 (t, J = 8.3 Hz, 1H), 7.00 (d, J = 8.2 Hz, 1H), 6.64 (d, J = 8.2 Hz, 1H), 6.60 (t, J = 2.4 Hz, 1H), 6.52 (d, J = 8.1 Hz, 1H), 4.37 (s, 3H), 3.74 (s, 4H). ^{13}C NMR (100 MHz, Chloroform-*d*) δ 161.22, 158.58, 158.11, 154.72, 151.35, 138.14, 134.47, 131.41, 130.59, 124.59, 124.48, 122.32, 120.60, 120.41, 117.42, 117.33, 116.80, 114.47, 108.52, 107.70, 102.27, 55.45, 33.35. MS-ESI m/z: calcd for $C_{23}H_{17}ClN_2O_2$[M + H]+: 389.0961; found: 389.2096.

8-chloro-11-(4-methoxyphenoxy)-5-methyl-5H-indolo[2,3-b]quinoline (**A7**)

Yield, 76%; yellow solid, m.p. 197–200 °C (DMSO); ^{1}H NMR (400 MHz, Chloroform-*d*) δ 8.22 (d, J = 8.1 Hz, 1H), 7.80 (d, J = 7.5 Hz, 2H), 7.65 (s, 1H), 7.42 (d, J = 8.2 Hz, 1H), 7.30 (d, J = 8.2 Hz, 1H), 6.94 (d, J = 9.1 Hz, 2H), 6.86–6.79 (m, 3H), 6.75 (d, J = 8.8 Hz, 1H), 4.35 (s, 3H), 3.75 (s, 3H). ^{13}C NMR (100 MHz, Chloroform-*d*) δ 158.64, 155.43, 154.49, 152.22, 151.18, 138.15, 134.31, 131.43, 124.71, 124.60, 122.31, 120.59, 120.36, 117.49, 117.30, 116.52 (2C), 116.16, 115.12 (2C), 114.78, 114.49, 58.36, 33.38. MS-ESI m/z: calcd for $C_{23}H_{17}ClN_2O_2$[M + H]+: 389.0975; found: 389.2216.

8-chloro-11-(3,4-dimethoxyphenoxy)-5-methyl-5H-indolo[2,3-b]quinoline (**A8**)

Yield, 63%; dark brown solid, m.p. 245–249 °C (DMSO); ^{1}H NMR (400 MHz, Chloroform-*d*) δ 8.23 (d, J = 8.3 Hz, 1H), 7.86–7.75 (m, 2H), 7.68 (s, 1H), 7.44 (d, J = 8.1 Hz, 1H), 7.32 (d, J = 8.2 Hz, 1H), 7.00 (d, J = 8.2 Hz, 1H), 6.80 (d, J = 2.9 Hz, 1H), 6.67 (d, J = 9.1 Hz, 1H), 6.31 (d, J = 8.8 Hz, 1H), 4.37 (s, 3H), 3.83–3.76 (m, 6H). ^{13}C NMR (100 MHz, Chloroform-*d*) δ 158.51, 154.32, 151.96, 151.31, 150.30, 145.13, 138.15, 134.42, 131.49, 124.70, 124.64, 122.37, 120.57, 120.49, 117.45, 117.32, 114.52, 112.45, 111.72, 105.91, 105.89, 101.05, 56.30, 56.16, 33.47. MS-ESI m/z: calcd for $C_{24}H_{19}ClN_2O_3$[M + H]+: 419.1084; found: 419.2344.

8-chloro-5-methyl-11-(p-tolyloxy)-5H-indolo[2,3-b]quinoline (**A9**)

Yield, 74%; brown solid, m.p. 219–220 °C (DMSO); ^{1}H NMR (400 MHz, Chloroform-*d*) δ 8.23–8.18 (m, 1H), 7.82–7.78 (m, 2H), 7.66 (s, 1H), 7.41 (d, J = 8.1 Hz, 1H), 7.33 (d, J = 8.3 Hz, 1H), 7.09 (d, J = 8.5 Hz, 2H), 6.97 (d, J = 8.2 Hz, 1H), 6.92–6.85 (m, 2H), 4.36 (s, 3H), 2.30 (s, 3H). ^{13}C NMR (100 MHz, Chloroform-*d*) δ 158.56, 155.07, 154.44, 151.97, 138.14, 134.33, 132.76, 131.44, 130.56 (2C), 129.91, 124.69, 124.54, 122.34, 120.56, 120.37, 117.49, 117.26, 116.44, 115.36 (2C), 114.51, 58.27, 18.36. MS-ESI m/z: calcd for $C_{23}H_{17}ClN_2O$[M + H]+: 373.1029; found: 373.2255.

8-chloro-11-(4-chlorophenoxy)-5-methyl-5H-indolo[2,3-b]quinoline (**A10**)

Yield, 85%; yellow solid, m.p. 258–262 °C (DMSO); ^{1}H NMR (400 MHz, Chloroform-*d*) δ 8.19–8.12 (m, 1H), 7.83 (d, J = 6.2 Hz, 2H), 7.67 (s, 1H), 7.45 (d, J = 8.1 Hz, 1H), 7.37 (d, J = 8.1 Hz, 1H), 7.28 (s, 1H), 7.02 (d, J = 8.2 Hz, 1H), 6.97–6.92 (m, 2H), 6.89–6.81 (m, 1H), 4.38 (s, 3H). ^{13}C NMR (100 MHz, Chloroform-*d*) δ 158.40, 155.54, 154.57, 151.09,

134.79, 131.63, 130.16, 129.40, 128.38, 124.39, 124.33, 122.54, 120.63, 120.26, 117.52, 117.07, 116.91, 116.78, 114.64, 33.48. MS-ESI *m*/*z*: calcd for $C_{22}H_{14}Cl_2N_2O$[M + H]+: 393.0483; found: 393.1729.

3.2.7. Synthesis Method of Target Compounds **B1–B9**

The Intermediate IV was dissolved in N, N-dimethylformamide (DMF). Then, the corresponding phenylhydrazine compounds were added and reflux at 110 °C for 3–6 h. After the reaction, dichloromethane, ethyl acetate and salt water were added to the reaction system for washing, and solids were collected to obtain the target compounds **B1–B9**.

8-chloro-5-methyl-11-(2-phenylhydrazineyl)-5H-indolo[2,3-b]quinoline (**B1**)

Yield, 70%; gray solid, m.p. > 400 °C (DMSO); ^{1}H NMR (400 MHz, DMSO-d_6) δ 13.86 (s, 1H), 10.96 (s, 1H), 9.16 (s, 1H), 8.82 (d, *J* = 8.6 Hz, 1H), 8.50 (d, *J* = 8.9 Hz, 1H), 8.16 (d, *J* = 8.7 Hz, 1H), 8.04 (t, *J* = 7.9 Hz, 1H), 7.91–7.74 (m, 1H), 7.69 (t, *J* = 7.8 Hz, 1H), 7.62 (s, 1H), 7.21 (m, 2H), 6.86 (m, 2H), 4.57 (s, 1H), 4.26 (s, 3H). ^{13}C NMR (100 MHz, DMSO-d_6) δ 152.82, 149.05, 148.47, 138.82, 137.00, 133.67, 130.70, 130.58, 129.77(2C), 124.76, 124.34, 122.34, 120.90, 120.28, 117.30, 113.87, 113.60(2C), 111.69, 97.44, 36.14. MS-ESI *m*/*z*: calcd for $C_{22}H_{17}ClN_4$[M + H]$^+$: 373.1142; found: 373.2594.

8-chloro-11-(2-(2-fluorophenyl)hydrazineyl)-5-methyl-5H-indolo[2,3-b]quinoline (**B2**)

Yield, 56%; white solid, m.p. > 400 °C (DMSO); ^{1}H NMR (400 MHz, Methanol-d_4) δ 8.87–8.71 (m, 1H), 8.51 (d, *J* = 8.9 Hz, 1H), 8.20 (d, *J* = 8.8 Hz, 1H), 8.07 (t, *J* = 8.0 Hz, 1H), 7.72 (t, *J* = 7.8 Hz, 1H), 7.59 (s, 1H), 7.29–7.18 (m, 2H), 7.00 (t, *J* = 7.7 Hz, 1H), 6.93–6.82 (m, 2H), 4.24 (s, 3H). ^{13}C NMR (100 MHz, Methanol-d_4) δ 153.54, 149.86, 139.43, 137.74, 136.47, 134.43, 131.86, 126.02, 125.55, 123.16, 121.01, 117.82, 116.68, 116.50, 116.18, 114.74, 112.40, 98.61, 57.28, 36.21. MS-ESI *m*/*z*: calcd for $C_{22}H_{16}ClFN_4$[M + H]$^+$: 391.1048; found: 391.2159.

8-chloro-11-(2-(3-fluorophenyl)hydrazineyl)-5-methyl-5H-indolo[2,3-b]quinoline (**B3**)

Yield, 73%; gray solid, m.p. > 400 °C (DMSO); ^{1}H NMR (400 MHz, DMSO-d_6) δ 8.77 (s, 1H), 8.47 (d, *J* = 8.8 Hz, 1H), 8.19 (d, *J* = 8.8 Hz, 1H), 8.06 (d, *J* = 8.5 Hz, 1H), 7.71 (t, *J* = 7.8 Hz, 1H), 7.57 (s, 1H), 7.32–7.19 (m, 2H), 6.76 (d, *J* = 8.1 Hz, 1H), 6.66 (m, 2H), 4.22 (s, 3H). ^{13}C NMR (100 MHz, DMSO-d_6) δ 152.56, 138.53, 136.91, 133.54, 131.32, 131.23, 131.09, 124.68, 122.46, 120.00, 116.89, 113.85, 111.50, 109.38, 107.29, 107.07, 100.53, 100.27, 97.70, 35.27. MS-ESI *m*/*z*: calcd for $C_{22}H_{16}ClFN_4$[M + H]$^+$: 391.1045; found: 391.2103.

8-chloro-11-(2-(4-fluorophenyl)hydrazineyl)-5-methyl-5H-indolo[2,3-b]quinoline (**B4**)

Yield, 71%; yellow solid, m.p. > 400 °C (DMSO); ^{1}H NMR (400 MHz, DMSO-d_6) δ 8.73 (s, 1H), 8.55 (d, *J* = 8.8 Hz, 1H), 8.19 (d, *J* = 8.8 Hz, 1H), 8.06 (t, *J* = 7.9 Hz, 1H), 7.70 (t, *J* = 7.8 Hz, 1H), 7.58 (s, 1H), 7.27–7.20 (m, 1H), 7.05 (t, *J* = 8.7 Hz, 2H), 6.94 (d, *J* = 9.0 Hz, 2H), 4.25 (s, 3H). ^{13}C NMR (100 MHz, DMSO) δ 153.54, 144.97, 138.62, 135.38, 134.13, 131.84, 129.43, 127.46, 125.78, 125.61, 122.51, 121.45, 117.37(2C), 116.74(2C), 116.51, 115.73, 115.64, 114.31, 111.99, 33.53. MS-ESI *m*/*z*: calcd for $C_{22}H_{16}ClFN_4$[M + H]$^+$: 391.1061; found: 391.2028.

8-chloro-11-(2-(2,4-difluorophenyl)hydrazineyl)-5-methyl-5H-indolo[2,3-b]quinoline (**B5**)

Yield, 56%; white solid, m.p. > 400 °C (DMSO); ^{1}H NMR (400 MHz, Methanol-d_4) δ 8.76 (s, 1H), 8.50 (d, *J* = 8.8 Hz, 1H), 8.20 (d, *J* = 8.7 Hz, 1H), 8.12–8.01 (m, 1H), 7.72 (t, *J* = 7.7 Hz, 1H), 7.60 (s, 1H), 7.24 (m, 2H), 6.90 (m, 2H), 4.25 (s, 3H). ^{13}C NMR (100 MHz, CD_3OD_SPE) δ 153.30, 152.37, 150.85, 149.28, 141.92, 139.78, 138.11, 134.37, 131.96, 128.69, 127.04, 125.50, 123.72, 120.55, 118.96, 116.90, 115.40, 114.75, 113.19, 107.73, 104.57, 36.00. MS-ESI *m*/*z*: calcd for $C_{22}H_{15}ClF_2N_4$[M + H]$^+$: 409.0953; found: 409.2040.

8-chloro-5-methyl-11-(2-(o-tolyl)hydrazineyl)-5H-indolo[2,3-b]quinoline (**B6**)

Yield, 74%; white solid, m.p. 255–256 °C (DMSO); ^{1}H NMR (400 MHz, DMSO-d_6) δ 8.82 (s, 1H), 8.46 (d, J = 9.3 Hz, 1H), 8.20 (d, J = 8.7 Hz, 1H), 8.07 (t, J = 8.0 Hz, 1H), 7.72 (t, J = 7.7 Hz, 1H), 7.59 (s, 1H), 7.22 (d, J = 16.6 Hz, 2H), 7.04 (t, J = 7.7 Hz, 1H), 6.83 (t, J = 7.4 Hz, 1H), 6.74 (d, J = 7.9 Hz, 1H), 4.24 (s, 3H), 3.51 (s, 3H). ^{13}C NMR (100 MHz, DMSO) δ 153.17, 148.78, 145.56, 138.03, 133.49, 133.00, 131.11, 130.93, 129.97, 127.17, 124.35, 123.54, 122.84, 122.11, 120.95, 119.56, 117.02, 114.44, 113.76, 112.53, 111.60, 33.86, 20.16. MS-ESI m/z: calcd for $C_{23}H_{19}ClN_4$[M + H]$^+$: 387.1298; found: 387.2787.

8-chloro-5-methyl-11-(2-(m-tolyl)hydrazineyl)-5H-indolo[2,3-b]quinoline (**B7**)

Yield, 80%; gray solid, m.p. > 400 °C (DMSO); ^{1}H NMR (400 MHz, DMSO-d_6) δ 8.78 (s, 1H), 8.55 (d, J = 8.8 Hz, 1H), 8.18 (d, J = 8.8 Hz, 1H), 8.09–8.02 (m, 1H), 7.70 (t, J = 7.8 Hz, 1H), 7.57 (s, 1H), 7.22 (d, J = 9.0 Hz, 1H), 7.13 (t, J = 7.8 Hz, 1H), 6.76 (d, J = 2.3 Hz, 1H), 6.72 (d, J = 7.5 Hz, 2H), 4.23 (s, 3H), 2.23 (s, 3H). ^{13}C NMR (100 MHz, DMSO-d_6) δ 152.79, 148.12, 139.19, 138.44, 136.94, 133.49, 130.94, 129.46, 124.61, 122.38, 121.90, 120.24, 116.85, 114.06, 113.85, 111.40, 110.85, 97.50, 56.51, 35.17, 18.18. MS-ESI m/z: calcd for $C_{23}H_{19}ClN_4$[M + H]$^+$: 387.1291; found: 387.2803.

8-chloro-5-methyl-11-(2-(p-tolyl)hydrazineyl)-5H-indolo[2,3-b]quinoline (**B8**)

Yield, 71%; light yellow solid, m.p. > 400 °C (DMSO); ^{1}H NMR (400 MHz, DMSO-d_6) δ 8.76 (s, 1H), 8.57 (d, J = 8.8 Hz, 1H), 8.17 (d, J = 8.7 Hz, 1H), 8.05 (d, J = 8.5 Hz, 1H), 7.70 (m, 1H), 7.57 (s, 1H), 7.21 (d, J = 8.9 Hz, 1H), 7.06 (d, J = 8.1 Hz, 2H), 6.88–6.78 (m, 2H), 4.23 (s, 3H), 2.21 (s, 3H). ^{13}C NMR (100 MHz, DMSO) δ 152.81, 148.40, 145.69, 138.41, 136.92, 134.11, 130.93, 130.85, 129.94(2C), 128.38, 124.58, 122.35, 120.18, 116.79, 113.71(2C), 111.35, 100.65, 98.74, 97.10, 33.57, 19.93. MS-ESI m/z: calcd for $C_{23}H_{19}ClN_4$[M + H]$^+$: 387.1285; found: 387.2360.

8-chloro-11-(2-(4-methoxyphenyl)hydrazineyl)-5-methyl-5H-indolo[2,3-b]quinoline (**B9**)

Yield, 70%; brownish red solid, m.p. > 400 °C (DMSO); ^{1}H NMR (400 MHz, DMSO-d_6) δ 8.77 (s, 1H), 8.59 (d, J = 8.8 Hz, 1H), 8.21 (d, J = 8.8 Hz, 1H), 8.16 (d, J = 8.9 Hz, 1H), 8.04 (t, J = 8.0 Hz, 1H), 7.68 (t, J = 7.7 Hz, 1H), 7.56 (s, 1H), 7.31 (d, J = 8.7 Hz, 0H), 7.26–7.17 (m, 1H), 6.93–6.80 (m, 4H), 4.42 (s, 1H), 4.22 (s, 3H), 3.68 (s, 3H). ^{13}C NMR (100 MHz, DMSO) δ 154.59, 151.36, 148.39, 147.17, 141.69, 139.42, 138.20, 136.66, 133.47, 130.83, 127.22, 124.56, 122.82, 120.59, 116.85, 115.21(2C), 114.96(2C), 113.84, 111.08, 54.29, 34.56. MS-ESI m/z: calcd for $C_{23}H_{19}ClN_4O$[M + H]$^+$: 403.1247; found: 403.2404.

3.2.8. Synthesis Method of the Target Compounds **C1–C10**, **D1–D6**

The Intermediate IV was dissolved in N, N-dimethylformamide (DMF). Then, the corresponding amide compound was added, and the reaction was reflux at 110 °C for 3–6 h. After the reaction, dichloromethane, ethyl acetate, and salt water were added to the reaction system to wash, and solids were collected to obtain the target compound.

N-(8-chloro-5-methyl-5H-indolo[2,3-b]quinolin-11-yl)acetamide (**C1**)

Yield, 83%; yellow solid, m.p. 324–325 °C (DMSO); ^{1}H NMR (400 MHz, DMSO-d_6) δ 8.25 (d, J = 8.3 Hz, 1H), 7.98 (d, J = 8.7 Hz, 1H), 7.86 (t, J = 7.6 Hz, 1H), 7.75 (d, J = 8.2 Hz, 1H), 7.55 (s, 1H), 7.53 (s, 1H), 7.14 (d, J = 8.1 Hz, 1H), 4.29 (s, 3H), 2.32 (s, 3H). ^{13}C NMR (100 MHz, DMSO-d_6) δ 169.34, 157.58, 155.96, 137.63, 132.79, 131.55, 126.10, 125.27, 122.69, 122.23, 120.05, 119.93, 119.20, 118.92, 116.85, 115.74, 33.40, 23.88. MS-ESI m/z: calcd for $C_{18}H_{14}ClN_3O$[M + H]$^+$: 324.0825; found: 324.1824.

N-(8-chloro-5-methyl-5H-indolo[2,3-b]quinolin-11-yl)benzamide (**C2**)

Yield, 89%; yellow solid, m.p. 275–277 °C (DMSO); ^{1}H NMR (400 MHz, DMSO-d_6) δ 11.96 (s, 1H), 8.57 (d, J = 8.5 Hz, 1H), 8.46 (d, J = 8.8 Hz, 1H), 8.30 (d, J = 7.6 Hz, 2H), 8.20 (t, J = 8.0 Hz, 1H), 7.86 (s, 1H), 7.81–7.74 (m, 4H), 7.74–7.64 (m, 2H), 7.51 (d, J = 8.5 Hz,

1H), 4.58 (s, 3H). ^{13}C NMR (100 MHz, DMSO-d_6) δ 166.35, 149.50, 143.45, 141.47, 137.27, 134.48, 134.27, 133.44, 133.12, 129.36 (2C), 129.03 (2C), 126.96, 126.22, 126.08, 123.81, 121.10, 118.86, 117.74, 116.96, 113.04, 37.82. MS-ESI *m/z*: calcd for $C_{23}H_{16}ClN_3O[M + H]^+$: 386.0982; found: 387.2003.

N-(8-chloro-5-methyl-5H-indolo[2,3-b]quinolin-11-yl)-2-fluorobenzamide (**C3**)

Yield, 64%; brownish red solid, m.p. 361–362 °C (DMSO); ^{1}H NMR (400 MHz, DMSO-d_6) δ 11.94 (s, 1H), 8.54 (d, *J* = 8.4 Hz, 1H), 8.40 (d, *J* = 8.8 Hz, 1H), 8.15 (m, 1H), 8.01 (t, *J* = 7.4, 1H), 7.90 (d, *J* = 8.4 Hz, 1H), 7.85 (t, *J* = 7.7 Hz, 1H), 7.81 (s, 1H), 7.79–7.72 (m, 1H), 7.51 (m, 3H), 4.55 (s, 3H). ^{13}C NMR (100 MHz, DMSO-d_6) δ 163.70, 161.20, 158.71, 141.87, 137.34, 134.39, 134.33, 134.25, 133.87, 130.97, 126.41, 126.14, 125.72, 125.46 (d, *J* = 3.3 Hz), 123.07, 121.71, 120.41, 119.44, 117.52, 117.17, 116.95, 113.78, 37.14. MS-ESI *m/z*: calcd for $C_{23}H_{15}ClFN_3O[M + H]^+$: 404.0888; found: 404.1265.

N-(8-chloro-5-methyl-5H-indolo[2,3-b]quinolin-11-yl)-3-fluorobenzamide (**C4**)

Yield, 77%; light yellow solid, m.p. > 400 °C; ^{1}H NMR (400 MHz, DMSO-d_6) δ 11.98 (s, 1H), 8.66–8.49 (m, 1H), 8.43 (d, *J* = 8.9 Hz, 1H), 8.28–8.00 (m, 3H), 7.92–7.68 (m, 5H), 7.56 (d, *J* = 62.1 Hz, 1H), 4.55 (s, 3H). ^{13}C NMR (100 MHz, DMSO-d_6) δ 165.07, 159.83, 155.64, 143.30, 137.30, 134.49, 134.85, 134.50, 131.56, 129.78, 126.86, 126.07, 125.89, 125.19 (d, *J* = 5.4 Hz), 123.50, 122.07, 120.84, 118.93, 117.57, 115.95, 115.71, 113.50, 37.26. MS-ESI *m/z*: calcd for $C_{23}H_{15}ClFN_3O[M + H]^+$: 404.0876; found: 404.1280.

N-(8-chloro-5-methyl-5H-indolo[2,3-b]quinolin-11-yl)-4-fluorobenzamide (**C5**)

Yield, 71%; yellow solid, m.p. > 400 °C (DMSO); ^{1}H NMR (400 MHz, DMSO-d_6) δ 11.98 (s, 1H), 8.57 (d, *J* = 8.4 Hz, 1H), 8.46 (d, *J* = 8.9 Hz, 1H), 8.39 (d, *J* = 8.6 Hz, 2H), 8.21 (t, *J* = 8.0 Hz, 1H), 7.88 (t, *J* = 7.9 Hz, 1H), 7.84 (s, 1H), 7.73 (d, *J* = 8.5 Hz, 1H), 7.59–7.45 (m, 3H), 4.57 (s, 3H). ^{13}C NMR (100 MHz, DMSO-d_6) δ 165.28, 159.56, 149.61, 143.39, 143.26, 137.27, 134.53, 134.30, 131.97 (2C, d, *J* = 9.7 Hz), 129.63, 126.97, 126.18 (d, *J* = 9.1 Hz), 123.82, 121.05, 118.85, 117.74, 116.98, 116.49 (2C), 116.27, 113.06, 37.73. MS-ESI *m/z*: calcd for $C_{23}H_{15}ClFN_3O[M + H]^+$: 404.0891; found: 404.1273.

N-(8-chloro-5-methyl-5H-indolo[2,3-b]quinolin-11-yl)-2-methoxybenzamide (**C6**)

Yield, 65%; orange solid, m.p. 250–252 °C (DMSO); ^{1}H NMR (400 MHz, DMSO-d_6) δ 11.51 (s, 1H), 8.52 (d, *J* = 8.3 Hz, 1H), 8.38 (d, *J* = 8.8 Hz, 1H), 8.15 (t, *J* = 7.9 Hz, 1H), 8.00 (d, *J* = 8.4 Hz, 1H), 7.87 (t, *J* = 7.0 Hz, 2H), 7.80 (s, 1H), 7.66 (t, *J* = 7.9 Hz, 1H), 7.53 (d, *J* = 8.4 Hz, 1H), 7.36 (d, *J* = 8.4 Hz, 1H), 7.20 (t, *J* = 7.5 Hz, 1H), 4.54 (s, 3H), 4.08 (s, 3H). ^{13}C NMR (100 MHz, DMSO-d_6) δ 165.38, 157.34, 141.73, 137.27, 134.21, 133.74, 133.53, 130.50, 129.15, 126.55, 126.44, 125.66, 124.01, 123.05, 121.30, 120.61, 119.69, 117.45, 113.64, 112.73, 104.16, 99.82, 56.61, 37.11. MS-ESI *m/z*: calcd for $C_{24}H_{18}ClN_3O_2[M + H]^+$: 416.1088; found: 416.1328.

N-(8-chloro-5-methyl-5H-indolo[2,3-b]quinolin-11-yl)-3-methoxybenzamide (**C7**)

Yield, 69%; yellow solid, m.p. 240–241 °C (DMSO); ^{1}H NMR (400 MHz, DMSO-d_6) δ 11.95 (s, 1H), 8.59–8.51 (m, 1H), 8.44 (d, *J* = 8.8 Hz, 1H), 8.19 (t, *J* = 8.7, 7.1, 1.5 Hz, 1H), 7.90–7.84 (m, 3H), 7.82 (s, 1H), 7.74 (d, *J* = 8.4 Hz, 1H), 7.61 (t, *J* = 8.0 Hz, 1H), 7.51 (d, *J* = 8.4 Hz, 1H), 7.34 (d, *J* = 8.3 Hz, 1H), 4.57 (s, 3H), 3.92 (s, 4H). ^{13}C NMR (100 MHz, DMSO-d_6) δ 166.06, 159.98, 140.92, 137.28, 134.45, 134.20, 133.12, 130.56, 128.73, 126.94, 126.07, 125.39, 124.34, 123.70, 121.23, 121.02, 119.37, 117.68, 113.97, 113.20, 105.64, 99.99, 56.04, 37.67. MS-ESI *m/z*: calcd for $C_{24}H_{18}ClN_3O_2[M + H]^+$: 416.1081; found: 416.1336.

N-(8-chloro-5-methyl-5H-indolo[2,3-b]quinolin-11-yl)-4-methoxybenzamide (**C8**)

Yield, 52%; brown solid, m.p. 310–312 °C (DMSO); ^{1}H NMR (400 MHz, DMSO-d_6) δ 11.76 (s, 1H), 8.55 (d, *J* = 8.5 Hz, 1H), 8.45 (d, *J* = 8.8 Hz, 1H), 8.28 (d, *J* = 8.4 Hz, 2H), 7.99–7.84 (m, 1H), 7.83 (s, 1H), 7.69 (d, *J* = 8.5 Hz, 1H), 7.49 (d, *J* = 9.3 Hz, 1H), 7.22

(d, J = 8.4 Hz, 3H), 4.56 (s, 3H), 3.92 (s, 3H). ^{13}C NMR (100 MHz, DMSO-d_6) δ 164.13, 159.40, 141.21, 137.57, 134.20, 134.09, 133.57, 131.17 (2C), 128.24, 126.53, 126.38, 124.10, 122.41, 121.53, 119.93, 117.15, 114.62 (2C), 113.74, 105.36, 99.87, 56.15, 37.66. MS-ESI m/z: calcd for $C_{24}H_{18}ClN_3O_2[M + H]^+$: 416.1063; found: 416.1347.

N-(8-chloro-5-methyl-5H-indolo[2,3-b]quinolin-11-yl)hexanamide (**C9**)

Yield, 73%; white solid, m.p. 284–286 °C (DMSO); ^{1}H NMR (400 MHz, DMSO-d_6) δ 11.64 (s, 1H), 8.54 (d, J = 8.4 Hz, 1H), 8.40 (d, J = 9.0 Hz, 1H), 8.16 (t, J = 8.1 Hz, 1H), 7.92–7.70 (m, 3H), 7.51 (d, J = 8.6 Hz, 1H), 4.53 (s, 3H), 2.83 (t, J = 8.0 Hz, 2H), 1.77 (m, 2H), 1.40 (m, 4H), 0.94 (t, J = 7.0 Hz, 3H). ^{13}C NMR (100 MHz, DMSO-d_6) δ 172.28, 155.32, 141.07, 137.62, 135.13, 130.64, 129.75, 127.92, 126.73, 126.48, 125.11, 123.61, 120.74, 117.65, 113.30, 102.48, 36.16, 31.52, 24.93, 22.40, 14.42. MS-ESI m/z: calcd for $C_{22}H_{22}ClN_3O[M + H]^+$: 380.1451; found: 380.1520.

N-(8-chloro-5-methyl-5H-indolo[2,3-b]quinolin-11-yl)-3-methylbutanamide (**C10**)

Yield, 81%; white solid, m.p. > 400 °C (DMSO); ^{1}H NMR (400 MHz, DMSO-d_6) δ 11.56 (s, 1H), 8.49 (d, J = 8.3 Hz, 1H), 8.41 (d, J = 8.9 Hz, 1H), 8.17 (t, J = 8.0 Hz, 1H), 7.88 (m, 2H), 7.80 (s, 1H), 7.52 (d, J = 8.4 Hz, 1H), 4.51 (s, 3H), 2.82–2.61 (m, 2H), 2.33–2.17 (m, 1H), 1.08 (d, J = 6.7 Hz, 6H). ^{13}C NMR (100 MHz, DMSO-d_6) δ 171.64, 156.39, 142.78, 137.24, 134.07, 131.54, 129.15, 128.32, 126.71, 126.48, 124.85, 123.35, 120.63, 119.24, 117.69, 100.58, 45.12, 34.61, 25.83, 22.93 (2C). MS-ESI m/z: calcd for $C_{21}H_{20}ClN_3O[M + H]^+$: 366.1295; found: 366.1364.

N-(8-chloro-5-methyl-5H-indolo[2,3-b]quinolin-11-yl)-2-fluorobenzenesulfonamide (**D1**)

Yield, 73%; yellow solid, m.p. 302–305 °C (DMSO); ^{1}H NMR (400 MHz, DMSO-d_6) δ 12.82 (s, 1H), 8.85 (d, J = 8.3 Hz, 1H), 8.12 (d, J = 8.3 Hz, 1H), 8.01 (d, J = 8.8 Hz, 1H), 7.96 (t, J = 5.2 Hz, 1H), 7.89 (t, J = 7.6 Hz, 1H), 7.59 (t, J = 7.3 Hz, 1H), 7.56–7.50 (m, 1H), 7.50 (s, 1H), 7.32 (m, 2H), 7.13 (d, J = 8.4 Hz, 1H), 4.16 (s, 3H). ^{13}C NMR (100 MHz, DMSO-d_6) δ 162.75, 159.84, 157.34, 155.04, 148.19, 138.47, 138.30, 133.46 (d, J = 8.0 Hz), 132.61, 129.91, 129.63, 128.09, 124.54 (d, J = 3.5 Hz), 123.88, 123.20, 121.82 (d, J = 5.0 Hz), 117.30, 117.09, 116.32, 111.58, 107.23, 35.20. MS-ESI m/z: calcd for $C_{22}H_{15}ClFN_3O_2S[M + H]^+$: 440.0547; found: 440.1713.

N-(8-chloro-5-methyl-5H-indolo[2,3-b]quinolin-11-yl)-3-fluorobenzenesulfonamide (**D2**)

Yield, 69%; white solid, m.p. 321–323 °C (DMSO); ^{1}H NMR (400 MHz, DMSO-d_6) δ 12.73 (s, 1H), 8.87 (d, J = 8.4 Hz, 1H), 8.04 (d, J = 8.5 Hz, 1H), 7.99 (d, J = 8.6 Hz, 1H), 7.88 (t, J = 7.9 Hz, 1H), 7.72 (d, J = 7.7 Hz, 1H), 7.63–7.56 (m, 2H), 7.53 (t, J = 7.6 Hz, 1H), 7.48 (s, 1H), 7.40 (t, J = 8.6, 2.7 Hz, 1H), 7.13 (d, J = 8.4 Hz, 1H), 4.15 (s, 3H). ^{13}C NMR (100 MHz, DMSO-d_6) δ 163.31, 160.86, 154.96, 149.91 (d, J = 6.0 Hz), 147.97, 138.32, 132.65, 131.36 (d, J = 7.9 Hz), 129.95, 129.66, 124.02, 123.27, 122.12, 121.88 (d, J = 2.6 Hz), 121.56, 117.84 (d, J = 20.9 Hz), 116.39, 112.69, 112.46, 111.51, 107.10, 35.25. MS-ESI m/z: calcd for $C_{22}H_{15}ClFN_3O_2S[M + H]^+$: 440.0558; found: 440.1708.

N-(8-chloro-5-methyl-5H-indolo[2,3-b]quinolin-11-yl)-4-fluorobenzenesulfonamide (**D3**)

Yield, 75%; white solid, m.p. > 400 °C (DMSO); ^{1}H NMR (400 MHz, DMSO-d_6) δ 12.71 (s, 1H), 8.96 (d, J = 8.4 Hz, 1H), 8.04 (d, J = 8.4 Hz, 1H), 7.99 (d, J = 8.7 Hz, 1H), 7.93 (m, 2H), 7.87 (d, J = 8.3 Hz, 1H), 7.53 (t, J = 7.7 Hz, 1H), 7.48 (s, 1H), 7.36 (t, J = 8.8 Hz, 2H), 7.15 (d, J = 8.4 Hz, 1H), 4.14 (s, 3H). ^{13}C NMR (100 MHz, DMSO-d_6) δ 164.65, 162.19, 153.50, 149.74, 147.83, 144.10, 138.42, 137.97, 132.63, 129.84 (d, J = 7.4 Hz), 128.40 (d, J = 9.0 Hz, 2C), 124.02, 123.18, 121.96, 121.37, 116.38, 116.06 (2C), 115.84, 111.45, 35.20. MS-ESI m/z: calcd for $C_{22}H_{15}ClFN_3O_2S[M + H]^+$: 440.0543; found: 440.1703.

N-(8-chloro-5-methyl-5H-indolo[2,3-b]quinolin-11-yl)-2-methylbenzenesulfonamide (**D4**)

Yield, 67%; yellow solid, m.p. > 400 °C (DMSO); ^{1}H NMR (400 MHz, DMSO-d_6) δ 12.64 (s, 1H), 9.05 (d, J = 8.4 Hz, 1H), 7.98 (m, 3H), 7.88 (t, J = 7.9 Hz, 1H), 7.54 (t, J = 7.6 Hz, 1H), 7.49 (s, 1H), 7.46 (d, J = 7.6 Hz, 1H), 7.36 (d, J = 13.3 Hz, 2H), 7.07 (d, J = 8.4 Hz, 1H), 4.14 (s, 3H). ^{13}C NMR (100 MHz, DMSO-d_6) δ 154.98, 147.81, 145.37, 138.55, 136.23, 132.58, 132.25, 131.23, 130.11, 129.55, 126.33, 126.10, 124.72, 123.57, 123.00, 122.47, 121.73, 121.33, 116.34, 111.50, 106.04, 35.09, 20.48. MS-ESI m/z: calcd for $C_{23}H_{18}ClN_3O_2S$[M + H]$^+$: 436.0808; found: 436.1984.

N-(8-chloro-5-methyl-5H-indolo[2,3-b]quinolin-11-yl)-4-methylbenzenesulfonamide (**D5**)

Yield, 84%; white solid, m.p. > 400 °C (DMSO); ^{1}H NMR (400 MHz, DMSO-d_6) δ 12.67 (s, 1H), 9.02 (d, J = 8.2 Hz, 1H), 8.10 (d, J = 8.3 Hz, 1H), 7.97 (d, J = 8.6 Hz, 1H), 7.87 (t, J = 7.8 Hz, 1H), 7.79 (d, J = 7.8 Hz, 2H), 7.52 (t, J = 7.8 Hz, 1H), 7.47 (s, 1H), 7.34 (d, J = 7.8 Hz, 2H), 7.13 (d, J = 8.3 Hz, 1H), 4.13 (s, 3H), 2.40 (s, 3H). ^{13}C NMR (100 MHz, DMSO-d_6) δ 155.02, 147.63, 144.82, 140.83, 138.48, 137.78, 132.57, 130.07, 129.59, 129.42 (2C), 125.76 (2C), 124.13, 123.06, 122.36, 121.88, 121.32, 116.33, 112.41, 111.34, 99.99, 35.14, 21.41. MS-ESI m/z: calcd for $C_{23}H_{18}ClN_3O_2S$[M + H]$^+$: 436.0804; found: 436.1940.

4-(tert-butyl)-N-(8-chloro-5-methyl-5H-indolo[2,3-b]quinolin-11-yl)benzenesulfonamide (**D6**)

Yield, 61%; white solid, m.p. > 400 °C (DMSO); ^{1}H NMR (400 MHz, DMSO-d_6) δ 12.73 (s, 1H), 9.01 (d, J = 9.9 Hz, 1H), 8.06 (d, J = 8.3 Hz, 1H), 8.02 (d, J = 8.7 Hz, 1H), 7.91 (t, J = 7.8 Hz, 1H), 7.80 (d, J = 8.1 Hz, 2H), 7.57–7.53 (m, 3H), 7.51 (s, 1H), 7.09 (d, J = 8.4 Hz, 1H), 4.16 (s, 3H), 1.33 (s, 9H). ^{13}C NMR (100 MHz, DMSO-d_6) δ 156.71, 148.30, 144.72, 141.53, 138.53, 137.83, 132.58, 130.04, 129.60, 125.74 (2C), 125.53 (2C), 124.22, 123.05, 122.44, 121.60, 118.08, 116.34, 110.53, 99.61, 35.14, 34.73, 31.46 (3C). MS-ESI m/z: calcd for $C_{26}H_{24}ClN_3O_2S$[M + H]$^+$: 478.1278; found: 478.2500.

3.3. Cell Culture

The human gastric cell lines AGS was obtained from the American Type Culture Collection (ATCC), AGS(LOT:70012225). The human gastric cancer cell lines HGC27, MKN45, SGC7901, MGC803, liver cancer cell SMMC7721, and gastric mucosa GES-1 were obtained from the genetic resource reserve of our laboratory. The AGS, HGC27, MKN45, and SMMC7721 cells were cultured in RPMI medium (Solarbio Invitrogen Corp., Beijing, China), and the SGC7901, MGC803, and GES-1 cells were cultured in a DMEM (high glucose) medium (Solarbio Invitrogen Corp., Beijing, China) containing 10% heat-inactivated fetal bovine serum and 1% penicillin/streptomycin at 37 °C in humidified atmosphere of 5% CO_2 in air.

3.4. MTT Assay

The cells were seeded in 96 well plates at the density of 8000 per well. Then, the cells were incubated in the cell incubator for about 24 h. The experiment included the treatment group, negative DMSO group, and positive group. Each group was set with 4–8 repeated wells. After the cells were incubated in the cell incubator for the corresponding time, 10 μL MTT solution of 5 mg/mL was added. The plates were incubated in the cell incubator for another 4 h. The formazan was solved in DMSO, and the absorbance value at 490 nm was measured with a microplate reader.

3.5. Colony Formation Assay

When AGS and HGC27 cells were in the logarithmic growth phase, AGS and HGC27 cells were inoculated into 24-well plates at a density of 1000 cells/well, and incubated in a cell incubator for 24 h. Cells were treated with compound **C5** or **C8** for 8–10 days. The cells were washed twice with PBS buffer, fixed in 4% paraformaldehyde solution for 40 min, and then stained with 1% crystal violet solution for 20 min. After staining, the cells were washed twice with fresh PBS buffer solution. The photos were taken, and Image J (National Institutes of Health, Bethesda, MD, USA) was used for counting analysis.

3.6. Migration Assay

A 600 μL complete medium, containing 20% fetal bovine serum, was added to the lower chamber of the transwell chamber. The cells were counted, and compounds with different concentrations were prepared using 1% complete medium. There was 150 μL cells suspension added into the upper chamber of transwell with a cell density of 50,000 cells/well. The suspension was placed in a cell incubator for further incubation for 48 h. The cells were washed twice with PBS and were fixed with 4% paraformaldehyde solution for 40 min, followed by staining with 1% crystal violet solution for 20 min. The cells in the upper transwell cells were carefully erased with cotton swabs. The number of migrating cells of the lower compartment were observed under a microscope and analyzed by Image J counting.

3.7. Cell Cycle Analysis

The AGS or HGC27 cells were seeded in six-well plates at a density of 800,000 cells/well. The plates were incubated in a cell incubator for about 24 h and treated with different concentrations of compounds. After 24 h, cells were collected and fixed with 1 mL of precooled 70% anhydrous ethanol for overnight. Additionally, 100 μL RNase A were added and incubated at 37 °C for 30 min. Then, the cells suspension was transferred to flow tube, and 400 μL PI solution was added and incubated at 4 °C for 30 min. The cells proportion of different cell cycles were detected by A BD FACSCanto II (BD LSRFortessa, USA). Modfit is used to process and analyze data.

3.8. Cell Apoptosis Analysis

AGS and HGC27 cells were seeded out in six-well plates with a cell density of 700,000 cells/well and incubated in a cell incubator for 24 h. Then, the cells were treated with different concentrations for 48 h. The supernatant was collected, the cells were washed with PBS twice, and the washing solution was collected. Then, the cells were digested and collected with trypsin without EDTA, centrifuged at 1000 r/min for 5 min, the cells were washed with PBS twice, and the cells were collected. The cell density was adjusted to $1-5 \times 10^6$ cells/mL. Then, 100 μL cell suspension was added into the flow tube, and 5 μL Annexin V/Alexa Fluor 488 solution was added. After incubation for 5 min, 10 μL PI and 400 μL PBS solution were added. A BD FACSCanto II (BD Biosciences, USA) was used for detection, and Flowjo was used for statistical analysis.

3.9. Molecular Docking Analysis

Schrödinger 10.1 software (Schrödinger, USA) was used for molecular docking correlation analysis. The crystal structure of AKT protein binding to the molecule during docking was obtained from the PDB database (PDB: 6hhf). In this experiment, we used the Prime module in the Schrödinger software to fill in the missing side chains and loops in the protein, processed the protein by protonation, dehydration, hydrogenation, etc., and then minimized and initially optimized the protein under the OPLS2005 force field. The compound was then docked with the protein AKT appropriately. During the docking process, the small molecular center bound to the protein was used as the docking site of the compound to complete the whole docking process. The crystal structures of all proteins bound to molecules in docking were obtained from the PDB database, and their PDB ID, resolution, and sources could be obtained in Supplementary Information Tables S1 and S2.

3.10. Western Blotting Assay

When AGS or HGC27 cells grew to about 80–90%, they were inoculated in six-well plates at a density of 500,000 cells/well and, then, incubated in cell incubator for 24 h. The cells were treated with a certain concentration of compounds for 48 h and DMSO was used as a negative control group. Cells were lysed with a high-potency tissue cell lysate containing 1% protease inhibitor PMSF and phosphatase inhibitor RIPA on ice for 30 min. Cell suspension was suspended every 10 min. After centrifugation, the supernatant was collected, and 5× protein denaturation buffer was added. The supernatant was placed in a constant temperature dry metal bath at 100 °C for denaturation for 10 min. The supernatant was stored at −20 °C. The protein was isolated with 10% separation gel and 5% concentrate gel. The total protein content was 25 μg per well. After electrophoresis, the protein was transferred to 0.22 μm PVDF membrane and blocked on a 5% skim milk shaker for 2 h. Then, the PVDF membrane was washed three times on the shaker with TBST buffer solution, 10 min each time, and blocked with primary antibody overnight at a ratio of 1:2000 at 4 °C. The PVDF membrane was washed with TBST buffer solution and incubated with a second antibody, at the ratio of 1:10,000, at room temperature for about 1 h. BCL luminescence system was used to record the photo, and the recorded protein bands were saved. Image J was used for statistical analysis of gray values.

3.11. Statistical Analysis

All the data were made with SPSS 22.0 (IBM, Armonk, NY, USA), GraphPad PriM 8.0 (Insightful Science, Boston, MA, USA), and AI 2020 (Adobe Systems, San Jose, CA, USA), and the error bars of all data results were represented by mean ± standard deviation. One-way ANOVA and *t*-test were used to test the differences between the analyzed data.

4. Conclusions

In summary, we designed and synthesized 36 neocryptolepine derivatives, based on 8-chloroneocryptolepine-based, and performed an in-depth structure-activity relationship study on five human gastric cancer cells, as well as evaluated toxicity on human normal gastric mucosa cells. Compounds **C5** and **C8** showed strong cytotoxicity to AGS and HGC27 cells. Moreover, compound **C8** inhibited the proliferation of AGS and HGC27 cells in a concentration-dependent and time-dependent manner. Cell colony formation and cell migration experiments showed that compound **C8** could inhibit the proliferation and migration of AGS and HGC27 cells, and compound **C5** could also inhibit the proliferation of AGS and HGC27 cells. Compound **C5** had a significant inhibitory effect on HGC cell migration. However, compound **C5** did not significantly affect the migration of AGS cells. In cell cycle and apoptosis experiments, the results showed that compounds **C5** and **C8** did not induce apoptosis of AGS and HGC27 cells but, mainly, caused cell necrosis. Compound **C5** had no significant effect on AGS and HGC27 cell cycle at low concentration. After treatment with 5 μM compound **C5** for 24 h, the AGS cell cycle could be significantly arrested in the G2/M phase. Compound **C8** had no significant effect on AGS and HGC27 cell cycles at 2.5 μM and 5 μM concentrations. The results of molecular docking and Western blot showed that compounds **C5** and **C8** might produce cytotoxic effects by the PI3K/AKT signaling pathway. Compounds **C5** and **C8** showed the best scores with AKT protein in molecular docking results. The experimental results showed that AKT might be the target of the compounds **C5** and **C8** acting on gastric cancer cells. In conclusion, by structural modification of neocryptolepine, two neocryptolepine derivatives with good activity were obtained, compounds **C5** and **C8**, which provided a lead compound for the development of drugs for the clinical treatment of gastric cancer.

Supplementary Materials: The following supporting information can be downloaded at: https://www.mdpi.com/article/10.3390/ijms231911924/s1.

Author Contributions: P.C. conceived the project and contributed to the experimental designs. Conceptualization, Y.M. and Y.T.; methodology, Z.Z.; software, Y.T., H.L. and S.C.; validation, K.D., H.Z. (Hao Zhang) and X.J.; formal analysis, J.L.; investigation, Y.N.; resources, Y.L.; data curation, L.T.; writing—original draft preparation, Y.M.; writing—review and editing, Y.M. and P.C.; visualization, J.W. and H.Z. (Hongmei Zhu); supervision, P.C. and Y.L. All authors have read and agreed to the published version of the manuscript.

Funding: This work was supported by the Key Research and Development Program of Gansu Province (Grant No. 21YF5FA112), the Technological Innovation Guidance Program of Gansu Province (Grant No. 21CX6QA127), the Key Program for International S&T Cooperation Projects of China Gansu Province (18YF1WA115), National College Students' Innovation and Entrepreneurship Training Program (Grant No. 202210730011), the College Students' Innovation and Entrepreneurship Training Program of Lanzhou University, China (Grant No. 20220260010) and Innovation and Entrepreneurship Training Program of Lanzhou University, China (Grant No. cxcy202207).

Institutional Review Board Statement: Not applicable.

Informed Consent Statement: Not applicable.

Data Availability Statement: Not applicable.

Acknowledgments: The authors are grateful to all lab members for their useful suggestions, support and encouragement.

Conflicts of Interest: The authors declare no conflict of interest.

References

1. Herszényi, L.; Tulassay, Z. Epidemiology of gastrointestinal and liver tumors. *Eur. Rev. Med. Pharmacol. Sci.* **2010**, *14*, 249–258. [PubMed]
2. Bray, F.; Ferlay, J.; Soerjomataram, I.; Siegel, R.L.; Torre, L.A.; Jemal, A. Global cancer statistics 2018: GLOBOCAN estimates of incidence and mortality worldwide for 36 cancers in 185 countries. *CA Cancer J. Clin.* **2018**, *68*, 394–424. [CrossRef] [PubMed]
3. Van Cutsem, E.; Sagaert, X.; Topal, B.; Haustermans, K.; Prenen, H. Gastric cancer. *Lancet* **2016**, *388*, 2654–2664. [CrossRef]
4. Ding, M.; Wang, H.; Qu, C.; Xu, F.; Zhu, Y.; Lv, G.; Lu, Y.; Zhou, Q.; Zhou, H.; Zeng, X.; et al. Pyrazolo[1,5-a]pyrimidine TRPC6 antagonists for the treatment of gastric cancer. *Cancer Lett.* **2018**, *432*, 47–55. [CrossRef]
5. Bukowski, K.; Kciuk, M.; Kontek, R. Mechanisms of Multidrug Resistance in Cancer Chemotherapy. *Int. J. Mol. Sci.* **2020**, *21*, 3233. [CrossRef]
6. Tao, C.; Chen, J.; Huang, X.; Chen, Z.; Li, X.; Li, Y.; Xu, Y.; Ma, M.; Wu, Z. CT1-3, a novel magnolol-sulforaphane hybrid suppresses tumorigenesis through inducing mitochondria-mediated apoptosis and inhibiting epithelial mesenchymal transition. *Eur. J. Med. Chem.* **2020**, *199*, 112441. [CrossRef]
7. Amirkia, V.; Heinrich, M. Alkaloids as drug leads–A predictive structural and biodiversity-based analysis. *Phytochem. Lett.* **2014**, *10*, xlviii–liii. [CrossRef]
8. Bracca, A.B.J.; Heredia, D.A.; Larghi, E.L.; Kaufman, T.S. Neocryptolepine (Cryprotackieine), A Unique Bioactive Natural Product: Isolation, Synthesis, and Profile of Its Biological Activity. *Eur. J. Org. Chem.* **2014**, *2014*, 7979–8003. [CrossRef]
9. Shang, X.F.; Morris-Natschke, S.L.; Yang, G.Z.; Liu, Y.Q.; Guo, X.; Xu, X.S.; Goto, M.; Li, J.C.; Zhang, J.Y.; Lee, K.H. Biologically active quinoline and quinazoline alkaloids part II. *Med. Res. Rev.* **2018**, *38*, 1614–1660. [CrossRef]
10. Yoo, E.U.N.; Choo, G.; Kim, S.; Woo, J.; Kim, H.; Park, Y.; Kim, B.; Kim, S.; Park, B.; Cho, S.; et al. Antitumor and Apoptosis-inducing Effects of Piperine on Human Melanoma Cells. *Anticancer Res.* **2019**, *39*, 1883–1892. [CrossRef]
11. Bhagya, N.; Chandrashekar, K.; Prabhu, A.; Rekha, P.D. Tetrandrine isolated from Cyclea peltata induces cytotoxicity and apoptosis through ROS and caspase pathways in breast and pancreatic cancer cells. *In Vitro Cell. Dev. Biol.-Anim.* **2019**, *55*, 331–340.
12. Zhang, Y.; Goto, M.; Oda, A.; Hsu, P.-L.; Guo, L.-L.; Fu, Y.-H.; Morris-Natschke, S.; Hamel, E.; Lee, K.-H.; Hao, X.-J. Antiproliferative Aspidosperma-Type Monoterpenoid Indole Alkaloids from Bousigonia mekongensis Inhibit Tubulin Polymerization. *Molecules* **2019**, *24*, 1256. [CrossRef] [PubMed]
13. Son, Y.; An, Y.; Jung, J.; Shin, S.; Park, I.; Gwak, J.; Ju, B.; Chung, Y.-H.; Na, M.; Oh, S. Protopine isolated from Nandina domestica induces apoptosis and autophagy in colon cancer cells by stabilizing p53. *Phytother. Res.* **2019**, *33*, 1689–1696. [CrossRef] [PubMed]
14. Sun, G.-C.; Chen, H.-H.; Liang, W.-Z.; Jan, C.-R. Exploration of the effect of the alkaloid colchicine on Ca2+ handling and its related physiology in human oral cancer cells. *Arch. Oral Biol.* **2019**, *102*, 179–185. [CrossRef] [PubMed]
15. Pawłowska, N.; Gornowicz, A.; Bielawska, A.; Surażyński, A.; Szymanowska, A.; Czarnomysy, R.; Bielawski, K. The molecular mechanism of anticancer action of novel octahydropyrazino[2,1-a:5,4-a′]diisoquinoline derivatives in human gastric cancer cells. *Investig. New Drugs* **2018**, *36*, 970–984. [CrossRef]
16. Dassonneville, L.; Lansiaux, A.; Wattelet, A.; Wattez, N.; Mahieu, C.; Van Miert, S.; Pieters, L.; Bailly, C. Cytotoxicity and cell cycle effects of the plant alkaloids cryptolepine and neocryptolepine: Relation to drug-induced apoptosis. *Eur. J. Pharmacol.* **2000**, *409*, 9–18. [CrossRef]
17. Shaban, E.; Switalska, M.; Wang, L.; Wang, N.; Xiu, F.; Hayashi, I.; Ngoc, T.A.; Nagae, S.; El-Ghlban, S.; Shimoda, S.; et al. Synthesis and In Vitro Antiproliferative Activity of 11-Substituted Neocryptolepines with a Branched omega-Aminoalkylamino Chain. *Molecules* **2017**, *22*, 1954. [CrossRef]

18. Altwaijry, N.; El-Ghlban, S.; El Sayed, I.E.; El-Bahnsawye, M.; Bayomi, A.I.; Samaka, R.M.; Shaban, E.; Elmongy, E.I.; El-Masry, T.A.; Ahmed, H.M.A.; et al. In Vitro and In Vivo Antitumor Activity of Indolo[2,3-b] Quinolines, Natural Product Analogs from Neocryptolepine Alkaloid. *Molecules* **2021**, *26*, 754. [CrossRef]
19. Zhu, J.K.; Gao, J.M.; Yang, C.J.; Shang, X.F.; Zhao, Z.M.; Lawoe, R.K.; Zhou, R.; Sun, Y.; Yin, X.D.; Liu, Y.Q. Design, Synthesis, and Antifungal Evaluation of Neocryptolepine Derivatives against Phytopathogenic Fungi. *J. Agric. Food Chem.* **2020**, *68*, 2306–2315. [CrossRef]
20. Cimanga, K.; De Bruyne, T.; Pieters, L.; Totte, J.; Tona, L.; Kambu, K.; Berghe, D.V.; Vlietinck, A.J. Antibacterial and antifungal activities of neocryptolepine, biscryptolepine and cryptoquindoline, alkaloids isolated from Cryptolepis sanguinolenta. *Phytomedicine* **1998**, *5*, 209–214. [CrossRef]
21. Sidoryk, K.; Switalska, M.; Wietrzyk, J.; Jaromin, A.; Pietka-Ottlik, M.; Cmoch, P.; Zagrodzka, J.; Szczepek, W.; Kaczmarek, L.; Peczynska-Czoch, W. Synthesis and biological evaluation of new amino acid and dipeptide derivatives of neocryptolepine as anticancer agents. *J. Med. Chem.* **2012**, *55*, 5077–5087. [CrossRef]
22. Mondal, A.; Gandhi, A.; Fimognari, C.; Atanasov, A.G.; Bishayee, A. Alkaloids for cancer prevention and therapy: Current progress and future perspectives. *Eur. J. Pharmacol.* **2019**, *858*, 172472. [CrossRef]
23. Ouyang, L.; Luo, Y.; Tian, M.; Zhang, S.Y.; Lu, R.; Wang, J.H.; Kasimu, R.; Li, X. Plant natural products: From traditional compounds to new emerging drugs in cancer therapy. *Cell Prolif.* **2014**, *47*, 506–515. [CrossRef] [PubMed]
24. Feng, Y.; Lu, Y.; Li, J.; Zhang, H.; Li, Z.; Feng, H.; Deng, X.; Liu, D.; Shi, T.; Jiang, W.; et al. Design, synthesis and biological evaluation of novel o-aminobenzamide derivatives as potential anti-gastric cancer agents in vitro and in vivo. *Eur. J. Med. Chem.* **2022**, *227*, 113888. [CrossRef] [PubMed]
25. Jokinen, E.; Koivunen, J.P. MEK and PI3K inhibition in solid tumors: Rationale and evidence to date. *Ther. Adv. Med. Oncol.* **2015**, *7*, 170–180. [CrossRef]
26. Molaei, F.; Forghanifard, M.M.; Fahim, Y.; Abbaszadegan, M.R. Molecular Signaling in Tumorigenesis of Gastric Cancer. *Iran. J. Biotechnol.* **2018**, *22*, 217–230. [CrossRef]
27. Zhang, Y.; Bao, C.; Mu, Q.; Chen, J.; Wang, J.; Mi, Y.; Sayari, A.; Chen, Y.; Guo, M. Reversal of cisplatin resistance by inhibiting PI3K/Akt signal pathway in human lung cancer cells. *Neoplasma* **2016**, *63*, 362–370. [CrossRef]
28. Zhu, Y.; Rao, Q.; Zhang, X.; Zhou, X. Galangin induced antitumor effects in human kidney tumor cells mediated via mitochondrial mediated apoptosis, inhibition of cell migration and invasion and targeting PI3K/AKT/mTOR signalling pathway. *J. BUON* **2018**, *23*, 795–799.
29. Gershtein, E.; Scherbakov, A.; Shatskaya, V.; Kushlinsky, N.; Krasil'nikov, M. Phosphatidylinositol 3-kinase/AKT signalling pathway components in human breast cancer: Clinicopathological correlations. *Anticancer Res.* **2007**, *27*, 1777–1782.
30. Kuo, P.-L.; Hsu, Y.-L.; Lin, T.-C.; Chang, J.-K.; Lin, C.-C. Induction of cell cycle arrest and apoptosis in human non-small cell lung cancer A549 cells by casuarinin from the bark of Terminalia arjuna Linn. *Anti-Cancer Drugs* **2005**, *16*, 409–415. [CrossRef]
31. Fresno, J.A.; Casado, E.; Carpeño, J.; Cejas, P.; Belda-Iniesta, C.; González-Barón, M. PI3K/AKT signalling pathway and cancer. *Cancer Treat. Rev.* **2004**, *30*, 193–204.
32. Sabbah, D.A.; Hajjo, R.; Bardaweel, S.K.; Zhong, H.A. Phosphatidylinositol 3-kinase (PI3K) inhibitors: A recent update on inhibitor design and clinical trials (2016-2020). *Expert Opin. Ther. Pat.* **2021**, *31*, 877–892. [CrossRef]
33. El-Gokha, A.A.; Boshta, N.M.; Abo Hussein, M.K.; El Sayed, I.E.-T. Synthesis and structure-activity relationships of novel neocryptolepine derivatives. *Chem. Res. Chin. Univ.* **2017**, *33*, 373–377. [CrossRef]
34. Emam, S.M.; El Sayed, I.E.T.; Ayad, M.I.; Hathout, H.M.R. Synthesis, characterization and anticancer activity of new Schiff bases bearing neocryptolepine. *J. Mol. Struct.* **2017**, *1146*, 600–619. [CrossRef]
35. Sidoryk, K.; Jaromin, A.; Edward, J.A.; Switalska, M.; Stefanska, J.; Cmoch, P.; Zagrodzka, J.; Szczepek, W.; Peczynska-Czoch, W.; Wietrzyk, J.; et al. Searching for new derivatives of neocryptolepine: Synthesis, antiproliferative, antimicrobial and antifungal activities. *Eur. J. Med. Chem.* **2014**, *78*, 304–313. [CrossRef]
36. El Sayed, I.; Van der Veken, P.; Steert, K.; Dhooghe, L.; Hostyn, S.; Van Baelen, G.; Lemière, G.; Maes, B.U.W.; Cos, P.; Maes, L.; et al. Synthesis and Antiplasmodial Activity of Aminoalkylamino-Substituted Neocryptolepine Derivatives. *J. Med. Chem.* **2009**, *52*, 2979–2988. [CrossRef]
37. Wang, L.; Switalska, M.; Mei, Z.W.; Lu, W.J.; Takahara, Y.; Feng, X.W.; El-Sayed Iel, T.; Wietrzyk, J.; Inokuchi, T. Synthesis and in vitro antiproliferative activity of new 11-aminoalkylamino-substituted 5H- and 6H-indolo[2,3-b]quinolines; structure-activity relationships of neocryptolepines and 6-methyl congeners. *Bioorg. Med. Chem.* **2012**, *20*, 4820–4829. [CrossRef]
38. Okada, M.; Mei, Z.-W.; Imran Hossain, M.; Wang, L.; Tominaga, T.; Takebayashi, T.; Murakami, M.; Yasuda, M.; Shigehiro, T.; Kasai, T.; et al. Synthesis and in vitro cancer cell growth inhibition evaluation of 11-amino-modified 5-Me-indolo[2,3-b]quinolines and their COMPARE analyses. *Med. Chem. Res.* **2016**, *25*, 879–892. [CrossRef]
39. Jia, X.; Wen, Z.; Sun, Q.; Zhao, X.; Yang, H.; Shi, X.; Xin, T. Apatinib suppresses the Proliferation and Apoptosis of Gastric Cancer Cells via the PI3K/Akt Signaling Pathway. *J. BUON* **2019**, *24*, 1985–1991.

International Journal of
Molecular Sciences

MDPI

Article

FOXO1 Is a Key Mediator of Glucocorticoid-Induced Expression of Tristetraprolin in MDA-MB-231 Breast Cancer Cells

Do Yong Jeon [1,†], So Yeon Jeong [1,†], Ju Won Lee [1], Jeonghwan Kim [2], Jee Hyun Kim [3], Hun Su Chu [3], Won Jin Jeong [3], Byung Ju Lee [1], Byungyong Ahn [4], Junil Kim [2], Seong Hee Choi [3,*] and Jeong Woo Park [1,*]

1 Department of Biological Sciences, University of Ulsan, Ulsan 44610, Korea
2 School of System Biomedical Science, Soongsil University, Seoul 06978, Korea
3 RopheLBio, B102, Seoul Forest M Tower, Seoul 04778, Korea
4 Department of Food Science and Nutrition, University of Ulsan, Ulsan 44610, Korea
* Correspondence: nacchal@ulsan.ac.kr (S.H.C.); jwpark@ulsan.ac.kr (J.W.P.)
† These authors contributed equally to this work.

Abstract: The mRNA destabilizing factor tristetraprolin (TTP) functions as a tumor suppressor by down-regulating cancer-associated genes. *TTP* expression is significantly reduced in various cancers, which contributes to cancer processes. Enforced expression of *TTP* impairs tumorigenesis and abolishes maintenance of the malignant state, emphasizing the need to identify a *TTP* inducer in cancer cells. To search for novel candidate agents for inducing TTP in cancer cells, we screened a library containing 1019 natural compounds using MCF-7 breast cancer cells transfected with a reporter vector containing the *TTP* promoter upstream of the luciferase gene. We identified one molecule, of which the enantiomers are betamethasone 21-phosphate (BTM-21-P) and dexamethasone 21-phosphate (BTM-21-P), as a potent inducer of *TTP* in cancer cells. We confirmed that BTM-21-P, DXM-21-P, and dexamethasone (DXM) induced the expression of *TTP* in MDA-MB-231 cells in a glucocorticoid receptor (GR)-dependent manner. To identify potential pathways linking BTM-21-P and DXM-21-P to *TTP* induction, we performed an RNA sequencing-based transcriptome analysis of MDA-MB-231 cells at 3 h after treatment with these compounds. A heat map analysis of FPKM expression showed a similar expression pattern between cells treated with the two compounds. The KEGG pathway analysis results revealed that the upregulated DEGs were strongly associated with several pathways, including the Hippo signaling pathway, PI3K-Akt signaling pathway, FOXO signaling pathway, NF-κB signaling pathway, and p53 signaling pathway. Inhibition of the FOXO pathway using a FOXO1 inhibitor blocked the effects of BTM-21-P and DXM-21-P on the induction of *TTP* in MDA-MB-231 cells. We found that DXM enhanced the binding of FOXO1 to the *TTP* promoter in a GR-dependent manner. In conclusion, we identified a natural compound of which the enantiomers are DXM-21-P and BTM-21-P as a potent inducer of *TTP* in breast cancer cells. We also present new insights into the role of FOXO1 in the DXM-21-P- and BTM-21-P-induced expression of *TTP* in cancer cells.

Keywords: tristetraprolin; FOXO1; dexamethasone; betamethasone; cancer cells

Citation: Jeon, D.Y.; Jeong, S.Y.; Lee, J.W.; Kim, J.; Kim, J.H.; Chu, H.S.; Jeong, W.J.; Lee, B.J.; Ahn, B.; Kim, J.; et al. FOXO1 Is a Key Mediator of Glucocorticoid-Induced Expression of Tristetraprolin in MDA-MB-231 Breast Cancer Cells. *Int. J. Mol. Sci.* **2022**, *23*, 13673. https://doi.org/10.3390/ijms232213673

Academic Editors: Barbara De Filippis, Marialuigia Fantacuzzi and Alessandra Ammazzalorso

Received: 7 October 2022
Accepted: 4 November 2022
Published: 8 November 2022

1. Introduction

Tristetraprolin (TTP, ZFP36) is an RNA binding protein that binds to AU-rich elements (AREs) within the 3′-untranslated region (3′-UTR) of mRNAs and promotes the degradation of these mRNAs [1,2]. AREs are found within the 3′-UTR of many short-lived mRNAs, such as cytokines and proto-oncogenes mRNAs [3]. TTP functions as a tumor suppressor by destabilizing the mRNA of critical genes implicated in both tumor onset and progression [4,5]. *TTP* is widely expressed, with particularly high levels in spleen, lymph nodes, and thymus [6]. However, *TTP* expression is significantly decreased in various cancers [7]; its downregulation correlates with increased expression of proto-oncogenes and may contribute to cancer processes. Re-expression of TTP in cancer cells has a growth inhibitory effect [8–10]. The expression of *TTP* in cancer cells is induced by p53 [11] and inhibited by Myc [12]. Notably, nearly all types of cancers have abnormalities in the p53 pathway [13], and c-Myc is often activated in human cancers [14]. Together, these features may lead to a widespread decrease in the expression of *TTP* in human cancers. Thus, enforced expression of *TTP* may represent a new therapeutic avenue for cancer prevention and treatment.

Previously it has been reported that glucocorticoids (GCs) induce the expression of *TTP* in cells [15–18]. However, the mechanisms underlying the GC-mediated TTP induction in cancer cells remain unclear. GCs are steroid hormones synthesized and released by the adrenal glands in response to physiological cues and stress [19]. GCs regulate fundamental body functions in mammals, including control of cell growth, development, metabolic homeostasis, cognition, mental health, immune homeostasis, and apoptosis [20–23]. Various synthetic GCs (e.g., prednisolone, aldosterone, dexamethasone, and betamethasone) have been developed by the pharmaceutical industry and serve as treatments for various diseases. Both natural and synthetic glucocorticoid hormones exert their biological effects predominantly via the glucocorticoid receptor (GR; NR3C1) [24], a ligand-activated transcription factor that is constitutively and ubiquitously expressed throughout the body [25]. GR functions by regulating the expression of GC responsive genes in a positive or negative manner. Upon ligand binding, GR shuttles into the nucleus [22] and binds to DNA sequences called glucocorticoid response elements (GREs) as a homodimeric complex [26]. The binding of GR homodimers to GRE sequences leads to an enhancement of gene expression [27]. GR also interacts with DNA as a monomer by binding to GRE half-sites and positively or negatively influences the transcription of target genes by interacting with promoter-bound STAT5, activator protein 1 (AP-1), or NF-κB transcription factors [28,29]. Independent of binding to GRE, monomeric GR can also regulate gene expression in a mechanism known as tethering, which involves physical interaction of monomeric GR with another transcription factor, such as AP-1 and NF-κB [30]. GCs also exert rapid non-genomic effects that do not require transcription processes or protein synthesis [31]. Interestingly, GCs not only increase the expression of *FOXO* [32–34] but also increase FOXO activity [35,36] in a variety cells.

The FOXO family of transcription factors comprises four closely related members—FOXO1, FOXO3, FOXO4, and FOXO6—that are direct downstream targets of AKT [37,38]. FOXOs play central roles in regulating normal hematopoiesis and are integral mediators of AKT actions in cellular growth and survival [38,39]. In the absence of active AKT, FOXOs localize to the nucleus, where they regulate the transcription of genes involved in cell-cycle arrest, apoptosis, and reactive oxygen species (ROS) detoxification. Previous studies have reported that GCs increase *FOXO1* level in a variety of cells, including hepatocytes, cardiomyocytes, and tenocytes [32–34]. A reduction in FOXO1 protein protects against beta cell death induced by the synthetic GC dexamethasone, suggesting that FOXO1 activation mediates the pro-apoptotic effects of GCs [40].

Several compounds and cytokines have been identified to induce *TTP* expression [4,5]. However, until now, there has been no report regarding the identification of compounds from library screening. The purpose of this study was to identify natural compounds that induce the expression of *TTP* in cancer cells by screening a natural compound library using a cell-based reporter assay. Among the 1019 natural compounds in the library, we identified one molecule, of which the enantiomers are betamethasone 21-phosphate (BTM-21-P) and dexamethasone 21-phosphate (DXM-21-P), as the best inducer of *TTP* in the cell-based reporter assay. We show here, for the first time, that GCs such as BTM-21-P, DXM-21-P, and DXM induce the expression of *TTP* in a FOXO1-dependent manner, even in p53 mutant breast cancer cells. The inhibition of GR or FOXO1 by inhibitors abrogated the effects of GCs with respect to *TTP* induction. We also found that GC-induced *TTP* is required for the growth inhibitory effect of GC on breast cancer cells. Together, these studies identify a novel signaling pathway by which GCs induce *TTP* expression in a FOXO1-dependent manner, representing a possible novel pharmacological approach to treat p53 mutant breast cancer cells.

2. Results

2.1. Screening of a Natural Compound Library Identified an Enantiomer of Betamethasone 21-Phosphate and Dexamethasone 21-Phosphate as a Potent Inducer of TTP in Cancer Cells

To perform cell-based screening for compounds that induce *TTP* expression in breast cancer cells, we used a library containing 1019 natural compounds and MCF-7 cells transiently transfected with the pGL3/TTPp-1343 construct containing the *TTP* promoter upstream of a luciferase reporter gene. Each natural compound was added to the transfected cells, and the effect of the compound on *TTP* induction was measured at 24 h post-treatment by luciferase assay. After three rounds of screening, we identified five compounds that induced a greater than two-fold increase in luciferase activity (Tables S1 and S2). To determine whether the selected compounds enhanced *TTP* promoter activity in p53 mutant breast cancer cells, we conducted luciferase reporter assays with the reporter vector in MDA-MB-231 cells that express mutant p53. Among the five identified compounds, three increased the luciferase activity in a dose-dependent manner (Table S2 and Figure 1A). We next tested these three compounds for their effect on the expression of endogenous *TTP* in MDA-MB-231 cells. Among the three compounds, compound 05-A06 was the most potent inducer of endogenous *TTP* at low volume (5 μL) in MDA-MB-231 cells (Figure 1B–D). At 50 μL, compounds 01-G05 and 05-A06 were toxic to MDA-MB-231 cells, which might lead to a decrease in *TTP* expression (Figure 1C,D). Compound 05-A06 is an enantiomer of betamethasone 21-phosphate (BTM-21-P) and dexamethasone 21-phosphate (DXM-21-P) (Figure 1E).

2.2. Betamethasone 21-Phosphate, Dexamethasone 21-Phosphate, and Dexamethasone Induce the Expression of TTP in MDA-MB-231 Cells

We next tested whether BTM-21-P and DXM-21-P, enantiomers of the identified compound, induced the expression of endogenous *TTP* in MDA-MB-231 TNBC cells. DXM-21-P is a prodrug that is converted to DXM. We also used dexamethasone (DXM) to compare its *TTP*-inducing ability with those of BTM-21-P and DXM-21-P. All three compounds induced the expression of endogenous *TTP* in MDA-MB-231 cells at 24 h post-treatment (Figure 2A). To determine the optimal concentration for *TTP* induction, MDA-MB-231 cells were treated with various concentrations of BTM-21-P for 48 h, and *TTP* mRNA expression was examined by by qRT-PCR. *TTP* mRNA expression was highest in response to 500 nM of BTM-21-P in MDA-MB-231 cells (Figure 2B). TTP protein level in MDA-MB-231 cells also was increased by treatment with 500 nM of BTM-21-P for 48 h (Figure 2C). We next treated MDA-MB-231 cells with 500 nM BTM-21-P and collected cells from 3 h to 30 h post-treatment at 3-h intervals and at 48 h post-treatment. *TTP* expression level fluctuated with time after BTN-21-P treatment and peaked at 3 h and 48 h post-treatment (Figure 2D). These data suggest that BTM-21-P may induce *TTP* expression earlier than 3 h post-treatment. We thus analyzed *TTP* expression at 30-min intervals after BTM-21-P treatment. As shown in Figure 2E, *TTP* expression level reached a peak at 1 h after BTM-21-P treatment (Figure 2E). We further analyzed the effect of BTM-21-P on *TTP* expression in other breast cancer cell lines such as HCC-1143, BT20, HCC-1187, MCF-7, BT-474, and T47D. BTM-21-P induced *TTP* expression in all breast cancer cell lines except the T47D cell line (Figure 2F). MDA-MB-231 cells treated with 500 nM DXM expressed a similar level of *TTP* as cells treated with 500 nM BTM-21-P at 3 h and 48 h post-treatment (Figure 2G).

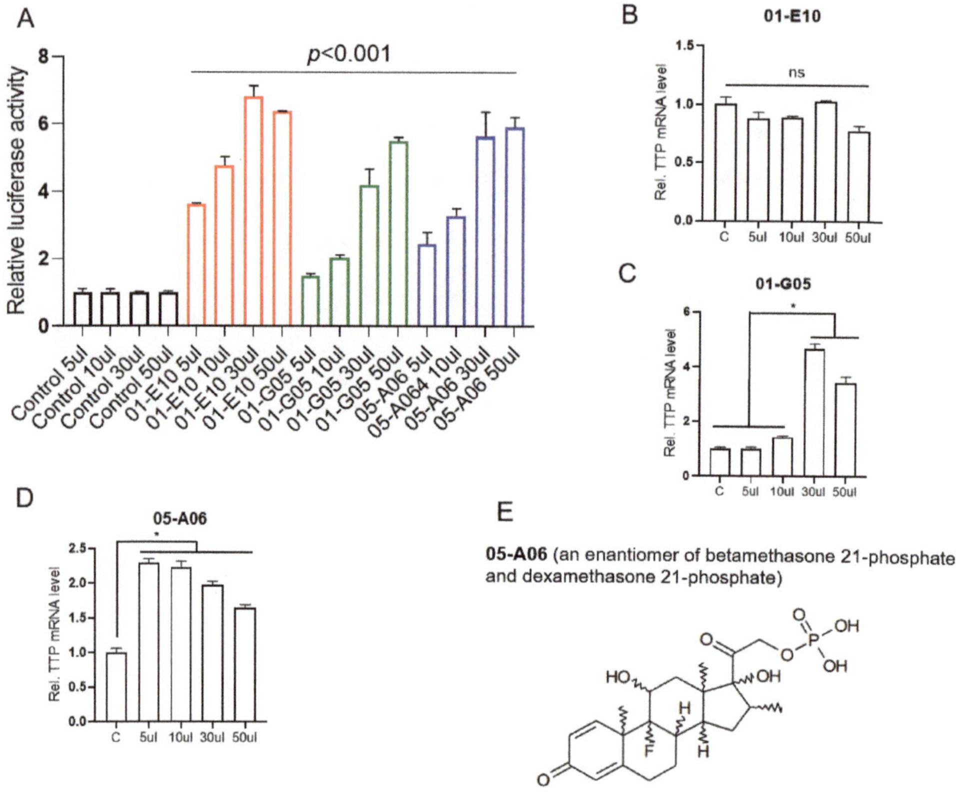

Figure 1. Dose-dependent induction of *TTP* in MDA-MB-231 cells by three compounds selected from the fourth screening of the natural compound library. (**A**) Dose-dependent changes in luciferase activity. MDA-MB-231 cells were transfected with pGL3/TTPp-1343 luciferase reporter vector containing the human *TTP* promoter, followed by stimulation with different concentrations of three selected compounds solubilized in DMSO for 48 h. The same volume of DMSO was added to the cells as controls. For each compound, the fold change in luciferase activity of stimulated cells was calculated relative to that of the DMSO control. The graphs are mean ± SD of three independent experiments (Two-way ANOVA). Black bars, control; red bars, 01-E10; green bars, 01-G05; violet bars, 05-A06. (**B–D**) Dose-dependent changes in endogenous *TTP* level. MDA-MB-231 cells were stimulated with different concentrations of compounds (**B**) 01-E10, (**C**) 01-G05, and (**D**) 05-A06 for 48 h. The expression level of *TTP* mRNA was analyzed by qRT-PCR. For each compound, the fold change in expression level was calculated relative to that of the DMSO control. The graphs are mean ± SD of three independent experiments (one-way ANOVA, * $p < 0.01$). (**E**) Structure of compound 05-A06, an enantiomer of BTM-21-P and DXM-21-P.

GCs exert their biological effects predominantly via GR [24]. Mifepristone is a potent antagonist of progesterone receptors and GR and has been used as an abortifacient. To determine whether BTM-21-P and DXM induce *TTP* expression via GR, we pretreated MDA-MB-231 cells with the GR inhibitor mifepristone and tested the effects of BTM-21-P and DXM on *TTP* expression. The inhibition of GR using mifepristone blocked the BTM-21-P- and DXM-induced expression of *TTP* in a dose-dependent manner in MDA-MB-231 cells (Figure 2H).

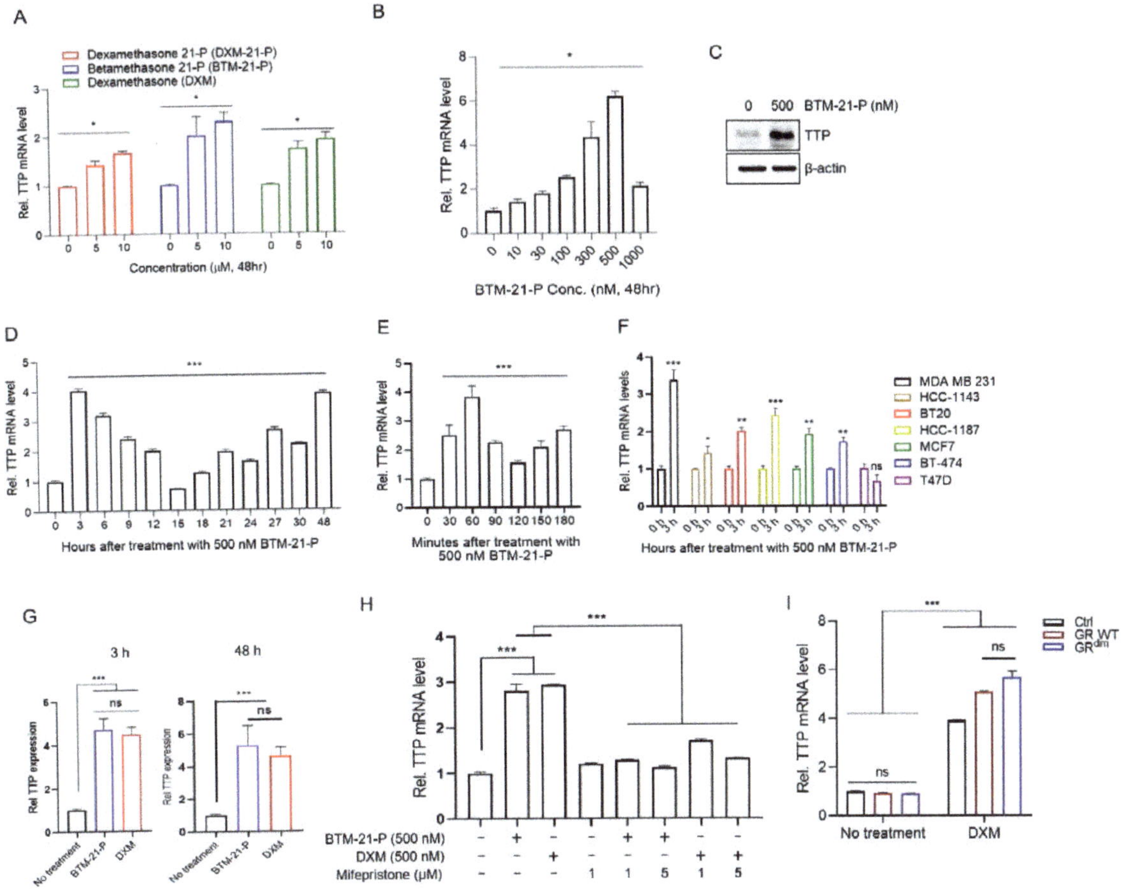

Figure 2. Induction of *TTP* expression by BTM-21-P, DXM-21-P, and DXM in breast cancer cells in a glucocorticoid receptor (GR)-dependent manner. (**A**,**B**) Dose-dependent changes in *TTP* expression level in MDA-MB-231 cells. MDA-MB-231 cells were stimulated with the indicated concentration of BTM-21-P, DXM-21-P, or DXM for 48 h. The expression level of *TTP* was analyzed by qRT-PCR. For each compound, the fold change in expression level was calculated relative to that of the DMSO control. The graphs are mean ± SD of three independent experiments (one-way ANOVA, * $p < 0.01$). (**C**) Western blotting analysis for TTP in MDA-MB-231 cells stimulated by 500 nM BTM-21-P for 48 h. (**D**,**E**) Time-dependent changes in *TTP* expression level in MDA-MB-231 cells. MDA-MB-231 cells were stimulated with 500 nM BTM-21-P for the indicated times. The expression level of *TTP* mRNA was analyzed by qRT-PCR. Fold change in expression level was calculated relative to that of the DMSO control. The graphs are mean ± SD of three independent experiments (one-way ANOVA, *** $p < 0.001$). (**F**) Effects of BTM-21-P on *TTP* expression in several breast cancer cell lines (MDA-MB-231, HCC-1143, BT20, HCC-1187, MCF-7, BT-474, and T47D) stimulated with 500 nM BTM-21-P for 3 h. The expression level of *TTP* was analyzed by qRT-PCR. Fold change in expression level was calculated relative to that of the DMSO control. The graphs are mean ± SD of three independent experiments (Student's *t* test, * $p < 0.01$; ** $p < 0.005$; *** $p < 0.001$). ns, not significant. (**G**) Comparison of the effects of BTM-21-P and DXM on *TTP* expression in MDA-MB-231 cells. MDA-MB-231 cells were stimulated with 500 nM BTM-21-P or 500 nM DXM for 3 h or 48 h. The expression level of *TTP* mRNA was analyzed by qRT-PCR. Fold change in expression level was calculated relative to that of the DMSO control. The graphs are mean ± SD of three independent experiments (Student's *t* test,

*** $p < 0.001$). ns, not significant. Blue bars, BTM-21-P; red bars, DXM. (**H**) The effect of the GR inhibitor on the BTM-21-P- and DXM-mediated induction of *TTP* expression in MDA-MB-231 cells. MDA-MB-231 cells were treated with indicated concentrations of the GR inhibitor mifepristone for 30 min, followed by stimulation with 500 nM BTM-21-P or 500 nM DXM for 3 h. The expression level of *TTP* mRNA was analyzed by qRT-PCR. Fold change in expression level was calculated relative to that of the DMSO control. The graphs are mean ± SD of three independent experiment (one-way ANOVA, *** $p < 0.001$). (**I**) The effect of dimerization-defective GR (GR^{dim}) on the DXM-mediated induction of *TTP* expression in MDA-MB-231 cells. MDA-MB-231 cells were transfected with empty vector, pGR, or pGRdim, followed by 500 nM DXM for 3 h. The expression level of *TTP* mRNA was analyzed by qRT-PCR. Fold change in expression level was calculated relative to that of the DMSO control. The graphs are mean ± SD of three independent experiments (two-way ANOVA, *** $p < 0.001$). ns, not significant.

GR regulates gene expression as either a homodimer or monomer [27–29]. To determine whether GR dimerization is required for TTP induction, we transfected MDA-MB-231 cells with plasmid expressing wild-type GR or dimerization-defective GR (GR^{dim}) and analyzed the expression of *TTP* after DXM treatment. In the absence of DXM treatment, ectopic expression of either wild-type GR or GR^{dim} did not induce the expression of *TTP* (Figure 2I). DXM treatment significantly increased *TTP* expression in both wild-type GR– and GR^{dim}-transfected cells, and there was no significant difference in *TTP* expression levels (Figure 2I). This result indicates that GR dimerization is not required for *TTP* induction by DXM.

2.3. *RNA-Seq Transcriptome Analysis of Betamethasone 21-Phosphate and Dexamethasone-Treated MDA-MB-231 Cells*

To gain insights into the molecular mechanism underlying the DXM-mediated induction of *TTP* in MDA-MB-231 cells, we performed RNA-seq analysis of DXM-treated MDA-MB-231 cells. To determine whether the gene expression profiles of DXM-treated cells were similar to those of BTM-21-P-treated cells, we also performed an RNA-seq analysis of BTM-21-P-treated MDA-MB-231 cells. We collected cells at 3 h post-treatment, as both DXM and BTM-21-P induced TTP expression in MDA-MB-231 cells at this time point. Non-treated cells were used as controls. We determined differential gene expression between non-treated and BTM-21-P- or DXM-treated cells by comparing the three groups using EdgeR [41]. A total of 1260 differentially expressed genes (DEGs) (FDR < 0.01) with an absolute log2fold change of 0.3 or greater was detected in BTM-21-P-treated cells and DXM-treated cells compared with non-treated cells (Table S3). In the comparison of BTM-21-P-treated cells with non-treated cells, 927 DEGs were identified, with 544 up-regulated and 383 down-regulated DEGs, as shown in the volcano plot (Figure 3A). Similarly, in the comparison of DXM-treated cells with non-treated cells, 1107 DEGs were identified, with 655 up-regulated and 452 down-regulated DEGs (Figure 3B). Two-way unsupervised hierarchical clustering of the union of the DEGs showed a clear separation of BTM-21-P-treated cells (B1–B4) and DXM-treated cells (D1–D4) from non-treated cells (N1–N4) (Figure 3C). However, no recognizable clustering pattern from BTM-21-P-treated cells (B1–B4) and DXM-treated cells (D1–D4) was detected in unsupervised hierarchical clustering (Figure 3C), suggesting a high degree of similarity among them. The DEGs were separated into two clusters of 729 up-regulated and 531 down-regulated DEGs, both in BTM-21-P- and DXM-treated cells (Figure 3D). DEGs identified in biological replicates clustered together, indicating good reproducibility of the treatments (Figure 3D). DEGs identified in BTM-21-P-treated cells and DXM-treated cells showed no significant intergroup differences (Figure 3D), suggesting that BTM-21-P and DXM affect similar signaling pathways in MDA-MB-231 cells.

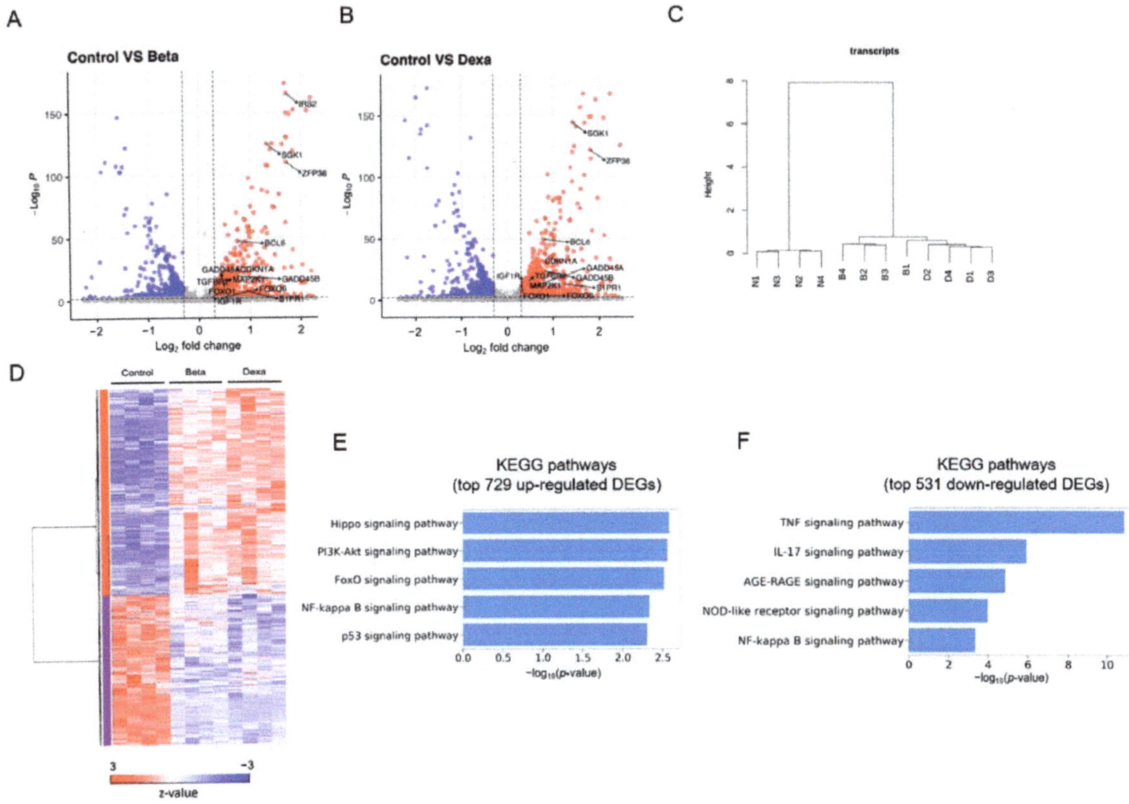

Figure 3. RNA-Seq data analysis and KEGG pathways. (**A**,**B**) Volcano plots for the differentially expressed genes (DEGs) in BTM-21-P-treated and DXM-21-P-treated cells compared with untreated cells. The *y*-axis corresponds to the significance level represented with $-\log_{10}p$ value, and the *x*-axis displays the $\log_2$ (FC) value. The red dots represent the significant ($p \leq 0.01$ and $|FC| \geq 0.3$) DEGs in (**A**) BTM-21-P-treated cells and (**B**) DXM-21-P-treated cells. The dotted horizontal line means $p = 0.01$, and the dotted vertical lines mean $|FC| = 0.3$. (**C**) Unsupervised hierarchical clustering of RNA-Seq data from untreated (N1–N4), BTM-21-P-treated (B1–B4), and DXM-21-P-treated (D1–D4) MDA-MB-231 cells. The similarities were calculated by Ward's criterion for 1-(Pearson's correlation coefficient). (**D**) Unsupervised hierarchical clustering and heatmap of DEGs clustered into up-regulated and down-regulated DEGs. (**E**,**F**) The *p* values and names of the 5 most over-represented KEGG pathways, calculated on the basis of (**E**) the top 729 up-regulated DEGs and (**F**) the top 531 down-regulated DEGs after treatment with BTM-21-P and DXM-21-P.

To identify pathways modulated by BTM-21-P and DXM, we analyzed the Kyoto Encyclopedia of Genes and Genomes (KEGG) pathways of 729 upregulated and 531 down-regulated DEGs in BTM-21-P- and DXM-21-P-treated cells. The KEGG pathway analysis results showed that the upregulated DEGs were associated with several signaling pathways, including the Hippo signaling pathway, PI3K-AKT signaling pathway, FOXO signaling pathway, NF-κB signaling pathway, and p53 signaling pathway (Figure 3E). The down-regulated DEGs were associated with the TNF signaling pathway, IL-17 signaling pathway, AGE-RAGE signaling pathway, NOD-like receptor signaling pathway, and NF-κB signaling pathway (Figure 3F).

2.4. FOXO1 Mediates Dexamethasone- and Betamethasone 21-Phosphate-Induced TTP Expression in MDA-MB-231 Cells

To further uncover the signal pathways involved in DXM- and BTM-21-P-induced expression of *TTP* in MDA-MB-231 cells, and to determine whether any of the up-regulated KEGG pathways mediated the DXM- and BTM-21-P-induced expression of TTP in MDA-MB-231 cells, we analyzed the effects of inhibitors against PI3K (Wortmannin) (Figures 4A and S1A), NF-κB (QNZ) (Figures 4B and S1B), AKT (MK2206) (Figures 4C and S1C), and FOXO1 (AS1842856) (Figures 4D and S1D) on the DXM- and BTM-21-P-induced expression of *TTP* in cancer cells. Only the FOXO1 inhibitor blocked the effects of both DXM and BTM-21-P on the induction of *TTP* in MDA-MB-231 cells (Figures 4D and S1D).

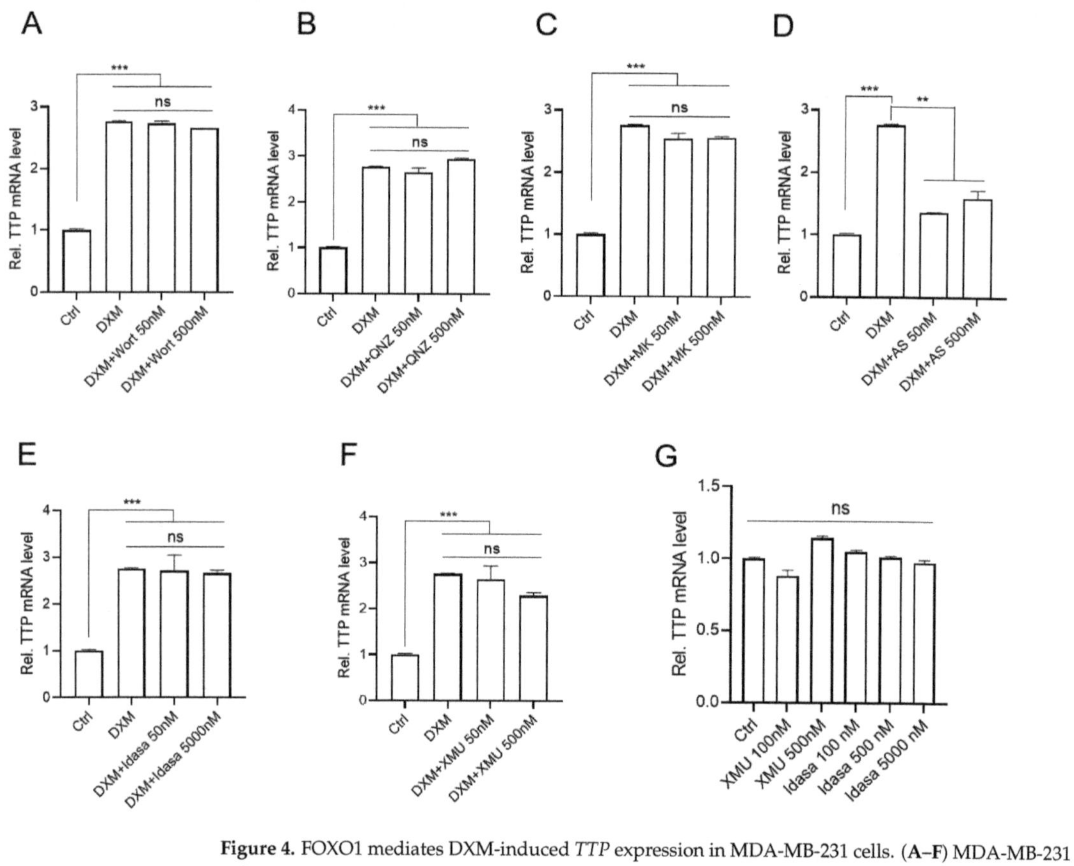

Figure 4. FOXO1 mediates DXM-induced *TTP* expression in MDA-MB-231 cells. (**A**–**F**) MDA-MB-231 cells were incubated with the indicated concentrations of inhibitors against (**A**) PI3K (Wortmannin) (**B**) NF-κB (QNZ), (**C**) AKT (MK2206), (**D**) FOXO1 (AS1842856), (**E**) MDM2 (Idasanutlin), and (**F**) MST1/2 (XMU-MP-1) for 12 h, followed by stimulation with 500 nM DXM for 3 h. The expression level of *TTP* mRNA was analyzed by qRT-PCR. Fold change in expression level was calculated relative to that of the DMSO control. The graphs are mean± SD of three independent experiment (one-way ANOVA, ** $p < 0.005$; *** $p < 0.001$). ns, not significant. (**G**) MDA-MB-231 cells were incubated in the presence of the indicated concentration of inhibitors against MST1/2 (XMU-MP-1) and MDM2 (Idasanutlin) for 12 h. The expression level of *TTP* mRNA was analyzed by qRT-PCR. Fold change in expression level was calculated relative to that of the DMSO control. The graphs are mean ± SD of three independent experiments (one-way ANOVA). ns, not significant.

To determine the involvement of the p53 and Hippo pathways in the induction of *TTP* expression in MDA-MB-231 cells, we treated MDA-MB-231 cells with inhibitors against MDM2 (Idasanutlin) and MST1/2 (XMU-MP-1) to activate the p53 and the Hippo pathways, respectively. Neither inhibitor enhanced the expression of *TTP* in MDA-MB-231 cells, either in the presence of DXM (Figure 4E,F) or BTM-21-P (Figure S1E,F) or in the absence of DXM (Figure 4G). These results, combined with the inhibitor results, suggest that the FOXO1 pathway may mediate the DXM- and BTM-21-phosphate-induced expression of *TTP* in MDA-MB-231 cells. Since both BTM-21-P and DXM induced *TTP* expression in MDA-MB-231 cells through the FOXO1 pathway, we used DXM to induce *TTP* expression in further experiments. qRT-PCR was performed to examine the expression of six genes involved in the FOXO signaling pathway in KEGG analysis: *CDKN1A*, *GADD45A*, *BCL6*, *IRS2*, *SGK1* and *S1PR1*. Consistent with the RNA-seq results, all six genes were significantly increased by DXM treatment in MDA-MB-231 cells (Figure 5A).

The mammalian FOXOs have four members: FOXO1, FOXO3, FOXO4, and FOXO6 [42]. Interestingly, none of the four FOXO members was involved in the upregulated FOXO signaling pathway, and we could not detect them from upregulated DEGs in BTM-21-P and DXM-treated cells (Table S3). qRT-PCR and western blot analyses also confirmed that DXM did not increase the expression of FOXO1 in MDA-MB-231 cells (Figure 5B). However, DXM increased the phosphorylation of GR (Figure 5B). We also found that overexpression of *FOXO1* did not induce the expression of *TTP* in the absence of DXM and did not affect the DXM-induced expression of *TTP* in MDA-MB-231 cells (Figure 5C). In addition, the treatment of cells with a GR inhibitor, mifepristone, blocked the DXM-induced expression of *TTP*, even in *FOXO1*-overexpressing cells (Figure 5C). Collectively, our results suggest that even though DXM induces the expression of *TTP* in a monomeric GR-FOXO1 pathway-dependent manner, the induction of *FOXO1* expression is not required for DXM-induced expression of *TTP*.

The mammalian FOXO family has four members: FOXO1, FOXO3, FOXO4, and FOXO6 [35]. Notably, none of the FOXO members was involved in the upregulated FOXO signaling pathway, and none was not detected from upregulated DEGs in BTM-21-P- and DXM-treated cells (Table S3). qRT-PCR analyses also confirmed that DXM did not increase the expression of *FOXO1* in MDA-MB-231 cells (Figure 5B). We also found that overexpression of *FOXO1* did not induce the expression of *TTP* in the absence of DXM and did not affect the DXM-induced expression of *TTP* in MDA-MB-231 cells (Figure 5C). In addition, the treatment of cells with the GR inhibitor mifepristone blocked the DXM-induced expression of *TTP*, even in *FOXO1*-overexpressing cells (Figure 5C). Collectively, our results suggest that while DXM induced the expression of *TTP* in a monomeric GR-FOXO1 pathway–dependent manner, the induction of *FOXO1* expression is not required for DXM-induced expression of *TTP*.

Inhibition of GR (Figure 2H) or FOXO1 (Figure 4D) abrogated the DXM-induced expression of *TTP*, indicating the requirement for GR and FOXO1 in DXM-induced expression of *TTP* in MDA-MB-231 cells. A search for transcription factor binding sites using online software (JASPAR) revealed the presence of putative FOXO1 binding sites within the *TTP* promoter, but no putative binding sites for FOXO3, FOXO4, FOXO6, and GR were found (Figure S2), indicating that DXM may enhance FOXO1 binding to the *TTP* promoter in a GR-dependent manner in MDA-MB-231 cells.

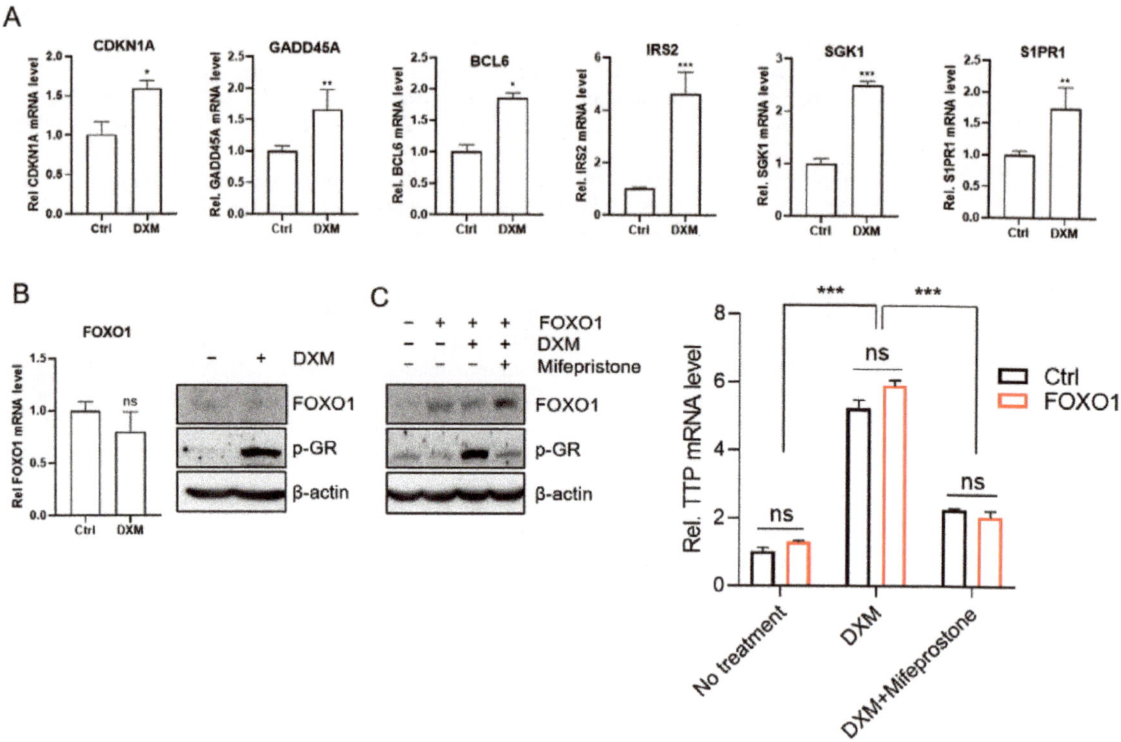

Figure 5. DXM induces *TTP* expression without induction of FOXO1 expression. (**A**) Validation of the DEGs in the FOXO signaling pathway in KEGG analysis by qRT-PCR analysis. MDA-MB-231 cells were stimulated with 500 nM DXM for 3 h. The mRNA expression levels of *CDKN1A*, *BCL6*, *GADD45A*, *S1PR1*, *IRS2*, and *SGK1* were analyzed by qRT-PCR. Fold change in expression level was calculated relative to that of the DMSO control. The graphs are mean ± SD of three independent experiments (Student's *t* test, * $p < 0.05$; ** $p < 0.005$; *** $p < 0.001$). (**B**) Effect of DXM on the expression of the *FOXO1* in MDA-MB-231 cells. MDA-MB-231 cells were stimulated with 500 nM DXM for 3 h. The expression level of FOXO1 was analyzed by qRT-PCR and western blot analysis. In addition, phosphorylation of GR was determined by western blot. Fold change in expression level was calculated relative to that of the DMSO control. The graphs are mean ± SD of three independent experiments (Student's *t* test). (**C**) Effect of ectopic expression of *FOXO1* on the DXM-induced expression of TTP in MDA-MB-231 cells. MDA-MB-231 cells were transfected with pFOXO1 plasmid. After 24 h incubation, cells were stimulated with 500 nM DXM in the presence or absence of mifepristone for 3 h. Expression of FOXO1 and phosphorylation of GR were determined by western blot analysis. The expression level of *TTP* mRNA was analyzed by qRT-PCR. Fold change in expression level was calculated relative to that of the DMSO control. The graphs are mean ± SD of three independent experiments (Student's *t* test and one-way ANOVA, *** $p < 0.001$). ns, not significant.

2.5. Dexamethasone-Induced TTP Down-Regulates ARE-Containing Genes in Cancer Cells and Mediates the Anti-Viability Effect of Dexamethasone

TTP contributes to the down-regulation of ARE-containing genes [1,2]. We next determined whether dexamethasone-induced TTP down-regulated the expression of ARE-containing genes. After treatment with DXM, cells were analyzed for the expression level of TTP-target genes, including *VEGF*, *COX2*, and *Myc* [9,10,12]. DXM treatment led to a decrease in ARE-containing genes in MDA-MB-231 cells (Figure 6A–C).

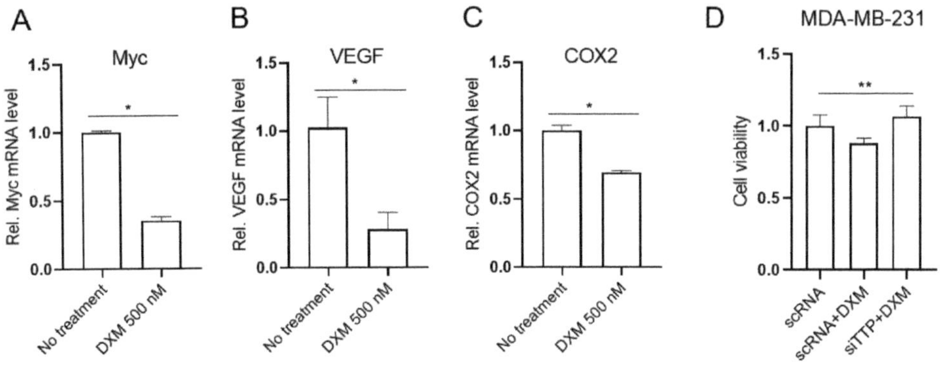

Figure 6. DXM-induced TTP mediates the anti-viability function of DXM in MDA-MB-231 cells. (**A–C**) DXM treatment decreases expression of ARE-containing genes in MDA-MB-231 cells. MDA-MB-231 cells were stimulated with 500 nM DXM, and the expression of ARE-containing genes such as (**A**) *Myc*, (**B**) *VEGF*, and (**C**) *COX2* was analyzed by qRT-PCR. Fold change in expression level was calculated relative to that of the DMSO control. The graphs are mean ± SD of three independent experiments (Student's t test, * $p < 0.05$). (**D**) TTP mediates the anti-viability function of DXM in MDA-MB-231 cells. MDA-MB-231 cells were transfected with *TTP*-specific siRNA (siTTP) or control scrambled siRNA (scRNA) and stimulated with 500 nM DXM. Viability of MDA-MB-231 cells was assessed using MTS assays. Graphs show relative cell viability. Data are mean ± SD of three independent experiments (one-way ANOVA, ** $p < 0.01$).

GCs have been reported to exert anti-tumorigenic effects [43]. To determine whether DXM exhibited anti-viability effects in MDA-MB-231 cells, we incubated cells with 500 nM DXM and analyzed viability using MTS assays. Consistent with previous reports [44,45], DXM (500 nM) significantly inhibited the viability of MDA-MB-231 cells (Figure 6D). TTP exerts anti-viability functions by destabilizing the mRNAs of genes involved in cell viability [4,5]. Thus, we speculated that TTP induced by DXM may mediate the anti-viability effects of DXM in cancer cells. We next tested whether TTP was required for the anti-viability activity of the combined treatment with these compounds. The inhibition of *TTP* using siRNA against *TTP* (TTP-siRNA) attenuated the inhibitory effects of DXM on the viability of MDA-MB-231 cells (Figure 6D). These results suggest that TTP mediates the anti-viability functions of DXM in breast cancer cells.

3. Discussion

Approximately 16% of human genes have ARE motifs within their mRNA 3′UTR [46], and many of them are implicated in immune response and tumorigenesis [47,48]. TTP can bind to ARE and enhance the degradation of ARE-containing mRNA by recruiting protein components of P-body to the TTP-mRNA complexes [49,50]. By post-transcriptional down-regulation of the genes involved in tumor onset and progression (4, 5), TTP functions as a tumor suppressor. However, the expression of the TTP tumor suppressor is significantly decreased in various cancers [7]. Thus, inducers of *TTP* in cancer cells with low *TTP* expression may be good candidates for new therapeutic drugs for cancer treatment.

Compounds derived from natural products can demonstrate structural diversity and have the potential to act via diverse mechanisms. Until now, there has been no report of the identification of compounds from a natural compound library that induce TTP expression in cancer cells. The natural compound library provided by the Korea Chemical Bank (http://www.chembank.org/. accessed on 26 January 2017) contains 1019 pure natural compounds from medicinal plants. In this study, we used this library in conjunction with a cell-based reporter assay to discover novel compounds to induce *TTP* expression in cancer cells. By screening the library, we identified one molecule of which the enantiomers are the GCs BTM-21-P and DXM-21-P as a potent inducer of *TTP* in cancer cells. Further characterization revealed that BTM-21-P and DXM-21-P induce *TTP* expression in breast cancer cells in a GR-dependent manner.

Both natural and synthetic GC hormones exert their biological effects predominantly via the GR, a ligand-activated transcription factor that is expressed in nearly all cells [24,25]. DXM, DXM-21-P, and BTM-21-P induced *TTP* expression in a GR-dependent manner in MDA-MB-231 cells. Both monomeric and homodimeric GRs regulate gene expression [27–29]. In our study, MDA-MB-231 cells transfected with either wild-type or dimerization-defective GR (GR^{dim}) induced similar levels of *TTP* after DXM treatment, indicating that monomeric GR is involved in the DXM-induced expression of *TTP* in MDA-MB-231 cells.

Upon ligand binding, the GR becomes localized in the cell nucleus and binds to DNA sequences called glucocorticoid response elements (GREs) to either inhibit [51,52] or enhance [27,53,54] the expression of numerous genes. However, when predicting transcription factor binding sites, we did not identify GREs within the promoter region of the TTP gene, suggesting that GR may induce the expression of *TTP* in a GRE-independent manner. GR can regulate gene expression without direct binding to GRE by interacting with promoter-bound transcription factors, such as NF-κB, STAT5, and AP-1 [29,30], in a mechanism known as tethering. To better understand the signaling pathways involved in the *TTP* induction in DXM- and BTM-21-P-treated cells, we performed whole genome transcriptome analysis of MDA-MB-231 cells treated with DXM or BTM-21-P for 3 h using RNA-Seq. Both unsupervised hierarchical clustering and DEG clustering in a heat map showed no significant difference between DXM- and BTM-21-P-treated cells, suggesting that they affect similar signaling pathways in MDA-MB-231 cells. A KEGG pathway analysis of up-regulated DEGs in DXM- and BTM-21-P-treated cells revealed upregulation of the FOXO signaling pathway, and inhibition of FOXO1 blocked the DXM- and BTM-21-P-mediated induction of *TTP* expression in MDA-MB-231 cells. In addition, the JASPAR prediction revealed the presence of putative FOXO1 binding sites within the *TTP* promoter. These results suggest that FOXO1 may mediate the effect of GCs on TTP expression in cancer cells. In this study, DXM treatment induced *TTP* expression without increasing FOXO1 level. The over-expression of FOXO1 without DXM stimulation did not enhance TTP expression in MDA-MB-231 cells. Collectively, these results suggest that the GC/GR signal pathway does not increase *FOXO1* expression but may increase FOXO1 binding to the *TTP* promoter, which leads to induction of *TTP* expression in MDA-MB-231 cells.

GCs have been reported to inhibit the growth of cells [43–45], and TTP also inhibits the growth of cancer cells by down-regulation of ARE-containing genes involved in cell proliferation [9,10,12]. In our study, *TTP* expression was induced in MDA-MB-231 cells. This suggests that GC-induced *TTP* may inhibit the growth of cancer cells through down-regulation of ARE-containing genes. Indeed, GC treatment down-regulated the expression of ARE-containing TTP target genes such as *Myc*, *VEGF*, and *COX-2* and inhibited the viability of MDA-MB-231 cells. Inhibition of *TTP* by siRNA against *TTP* attenuated DXM-induced inhibition of cell viability, indicating that DXM-induced TTP plays a role in the anti-viability effect of DXM. Even though we found that GCs increased the TTP expression and inhibited viability of MDA-MB-231 cells, it is not likely that all kinds of breast cancer cells will show a similar response to GCs. GCs can promote metastasis of certain type of breast cancer cells [55,56], and TTP inhibits the migration of cancer cells by suppressing the expression of *Twist1* and *Snail1* [57]. Further study is required to determine whether GCs induces TTP expression in breast cancer cells in which metastasis is promoted by GCs.

4. Materials and Methods

4.1. Cells and Chemicals

The human MCF-7, MDA-MB-231, HCC-1143, HCC-1187, BT20, BT-474, and T47D breast cancer cell lines were purchased from the Korean Cell Line Bank (Seoul, Korea). Cells were cultured in RPMI 1640 media supplemented with 10% heat-inactivated fetal bovine serum (FBS) (Welgene, Korea) and were maintained at 37 °C in a humidified 5%

CO_2 atmosphere. Dexamethasone (DXM), dexamethasone 21-phosphate (DXM-21-P), betamethasone 21-phosphate (BTM-21-P), mifepristone (Sigma Aldrich, St. Louis, MO, USA), Wortmannin, QNZ, MK2206, idasanutlin, AS1842856, XMU-MP-1 and p38 MAPK inhibitor (Selleckchem, Houston, TX, USA) were used in this study.

4.2. Cell Viability

For the MTS assay, cells were plated in triplicate at 1.0×10^4 cells/well in 96-well culture plates in culture media. At 24 h after plating, CellTiter 96 AQueous One Solution reagent (Promega, Madison, WI, USA) was added to each well according to the manufacturer's instructions, and absorbance at 490 nm was determined for each well using a Victor 1420 Multilabel Counter (EG&G Wallac, Turku, Finland).

4.3. Plasmids, Small Interfering RNAs, Transfections, and Dual-Luciferase Assay

The pGL3/TTPp-1343 plasmid containing the human *TTP* promoter was described previously [11]. The pGR-wt, pGR^{dim}, and pFOXO1-Flag plasmids were purchased from Addgene (Watertown, MA, USA).

Small interfering RNAs (siRNAs) against human *TTP* (TTP-siRNA, sc-36761) and control siRNA [scrambled siRNA (scRNA), sc-37007] were purchased from Santa Cruz Biotechnology (Santa Cruz, Santa Cruz, CA, USA). Cells were transfected 24 h after plating using LipofectamineTM RNAiMAX (Invitrogen, Carlsbad, CA, USA) and harvested at 48 h after transfection. The expression levels of *TTP* mRNA were analyzed by qRT-PCR.

4.4. Screening of the Natural Product Library and Luciferase Assay

Natural compounds have been used to develop drugs for cancer and infectious diseases, since they are structurally optimized by evolution to serve particular biological functions, and their use in traditional medicine provides insights regarding efficacy and safety [58]. Thus, in this study, we used a natural product library to select natural compounds which can induce TTP expression in cancer cells. A library containing 1019 natural products was provided by the Korea Chemical Bank (http://www.chembank.org/. accessed on 26 January 2017) of the Korea Research Institute of Chemical Technology. MCF-7 cells in culture dishes (100 mm diameter) were co-transfected with the pGL3/TTPp-1343-luciferase reporter construct and pRL-SV40 Renilla luciferase construct using TurboFectTM in vitro transfection reagent (Fermentas, Waltham, MA, USA). After incubation for 24 h, cells were harvested and seeded in 96-well plates at a density of 4×10^3 cells per well in 100 μL and cultured with 30 μL of natural compounds diluted in fresh culture media. After further incubation for 24 h, cells were lysed with lysis buffer and mixed with luciferase assay reagent (Promega, Madison, WI, USA). Cells were also treated with the same volume of DMSO to detect luciferase activity induced by the native signal pathway. The chemiluminescent signal was measured using a SpectraMax L Microplate (Molecular Devices, Sunnyvale, CA, USA). Firefly luciferase was normalized to Renilla luciferase in each sample. All luciferase assays reported in this study represent at least three independent experiments, each consisting of three wells per transfection. We selected compounds that induced a greater than two-fold increase in luciferase activity.

4.5. Quantitative Real-Time PCR and Semi-qRT-PCR

DNase I–treated total RNA (3 μg) was reverse transcribed using oligo-dT and Superscript II reverse transcriptase (Invitrogen, Carlsbad, CA, USA) according to the manufacturer's instructions. Quantitative real-time PCR (qRT-PCR) was performed by monitoring in real-time the increase in fluorescence of SYBR Green dye (QIAGEN, Hilden, Germany) using the $StepOnePlus^{TM}$ real-time PCR system (Applied Biosystems, Waltham, MA, USA). Semi-qRT-PCR was performed using Taq polymerase (Solgent, Daejeon, Korea) and the PCR primer pairs (Table 1).

Table 1. PCR primers used in this study.

	Genes		Primer Sequences (5′-3′)
Gene expression analysis	*β-actin*	F	ATCGTGCGTGACATTAAGGAGAAG
		R	AGGAAGGAAGGCTGCAAG
	BCL6	F	CATGCAGAGATGTGCCTCCACA
		R	TCAGAGAAGCGGCAGTCACACT
	CDKN1A	F	AGGTGGACCTGGAGACTCTCAG
		R	TCCTCTTGGAGAAGATCAGCCG
	FOXO1	F	CTACGAGTGGATGGTCAAGAGC
		R	CCAGTTCCTTCATTCTGCACACG
	GADD45A	F	CTGGAGGAAGTGCTCAGCAAAG
		R	AGAGCCACATCTCTGTCGTCGT
	GAPDH	F	AATCCCATCACCATCTTCCAG
		R	AAATGAGCCCCAGCCTTC
	IRS2	F	CCTGCCCCCTGCCAACACCT
		R	TGTGACATCCTGGTGATAAAGCC
	S1PR1	F	CCTGTGACATCCTCTTCAGAGC
		R	CACTTGCAGCAGGACATGATCC
	SGK1	F	GCTGAAATAGCCAGTGCCTTGG
		R	GTTCTCCTTGCAGAGTCCGAAG
	TTP	F	TCTTCGAGGCGGGAGTTTTT
		R	TGCGATTGAAGATGGGGAGTC

4.6. SDS-PAGE and Immunoblotting

Proteins were resolved by SDS-PAGE and transferred onto Hybond-P membranes (Amersham Biosciences Inc., Amersham, UK). The membranes were blocked and then probed with appropriate dilutions of the following antibodies: rabbit anti-human TTP (T5327, Sigma, St. Louis, MO, USA) and anti-β-actin (A2228, Sigma, St. Louis, MO, USA). Immunoreactivity was detected using an ECL detection system (Amersham Biosciences Inc., Amersham, UK). Films were exposed at multiple time points to ensure that the images were not saturated.

4.7. RNA Preparation and RNA-Seq

We performed RNA-Seq on total RNA samples (RIN above 8.5) collected from MDA-MB-231 cells at 4 h after treatment with growth media control, 500 nM DXM-21-P or 500 nM BTM-21-P. Residual DNA from each sample was removed using the RNeasyMinElute-Cleanup Kit (Qiagen, Hilden, Germany). The cDNA library was prepared with 1.0 μg of total RNA using the TrueSeq RNA library Preparation Kit (Illumina, San Diego, CA, USA) following manufacturer's recommendations, followed by paired-end sequencing (2 × 100 bp) using the HiSeq1500 platform (Illumina, San Diego, CA, USA). cDNAs were amplified according to the RNAseq protocol provided by Illumina and sequenced using an Illumina HiSeq 2500 system to obtain 150-bp paired-end reads. The sequencing depth for each sample was >20 million reads. RNA-seq reads were mapped using STAR 2.7.9a [59] to the human genome GRCh38. Gene expression counts were measured using multicov implemented in bedtools [60]. Differentially expressed genes (DEGs) were obtained by comparing groups (Control, Beta, and Dexa) using EdgeR [41]. Genes with false discovery rate (FDR) <0.01 and log2fold change >0.3 were selected as DEGs. The DEGs were clustered using hierarchical clustering implemented in R. Ward's criterion. Pearson's correlation coefficient was used as a distance measure. A clustering heatmap was drawn using a z-score scaled across samples for each gene. The enriched KEGG pathway terms were obtained from Enrichr software [61].

4.8. Statistical Analysis

Differences in the expression of genes were evaluated by Student's t-test or one-way ANOVA. A p value less than 0.05 was considered statistically significant.

5. Conclusions

Herein, we have reported that GC compound, an enantiomer of BTM-21-P and DXM-21-P, identified from a natural compound library, induces *TTP* expression in a GR-dependent manner in breast cancer cells. Furthermore, we found that GR does not induce *FOXO1* expression but may stimulate FOXO1 to bind to the TTP promoter and thus to induce TTP expression. Importantly, GC-induced TTP down-regulated ARE-containing TTP target genes and mediated the anti-viability function of GCs. The inhibition of *TTP* by siRNA attenuated the anti-viability effect of GCs. Thus, our data indicate that GCs induce *TTP* expression in a FOXO1-dependent manner, and that GC-induced TTP mediates the anti-viability activity of GCs in breast cancer cells.

Supplementary Materials: The following supporting information can be downloaded at: https://www.mdpi.com/article/10.3390/ijms232213673/s1.

Author Contributions: J.W.P. designed experiments and wrote the manuscript. D.Y.J., S.Y.J. and J.W.L. performed most of the experiments and wrote the manuscript. J.K. (Jeonghwan Kim), B.A. and J.K. (Junil Lim) performed RNA-Seq analysis. J.H.K., H.S.C., W.J.J. and B.J.L. analyzed the results. S.H.C. designed experiments. All authors have read and agreed to the published version of the manuscript.

Funding: This work was supported by the National Research Foundation of Korea (NRF- 2014R1A6A 1030318).

Institutional Review Board Statement: Not applicable.

Informed Consent Statement: Not applicable.

Acknowledgments: The chemical library used in this study was kindly provided by Korea Chemical Bank (http://www.chembank.org/. accessed on 26 January 2017) of Korea Research Institute of Chemical Technology.)

Conflicts of Interest: The authors declare no conflict of interest.

References

1. Brooks, S.A.; Blackshear, P.J. Tristetraprolin (TTP): Interactions with mRNA and proteins, and current thoughts on mechanisms of action. *Biochim. Biophys. Acta* **2013**, *1829*, 666–679. [CrossRef] [PubMed]
2. Carballo, E.; Lai, W.S.; Blackshear, P.J. Feedback inhibition of macrophage tumor necrosis factor-alpha production by tristetraprolin. *Science* **1998**, *281*, 1001–1005. [CrossRef] [PubMed]
3. Shaw, G.; Kamen, R. A conserved AU sequence from the 3′ untranslated region of GM-CSF mRNA mediates selective mRNA degradation. *Cell* **1986**, *46*, 659–667. [CrossRef]
4. Park, J.M.; Lee, T.H.; Kang, T.H. Roles of Tristetraprolin in Tumorigenesis. *Int. J. Mol. Sci.* **2018**, *19*, 3384. [CrossRef]
5. Zhang, D.; Zhou, Z.; Yang, R.; Zhang, S.; Zhang, B.; Tan, Y.; Chen, L.; Li, T.; Tu, J. Tristetraprolin, a Potential Safeguard Against Carcinoma: Role in the Tumor Microenvironment. *Front. Oncol.* **2021**, *11*, 632189. [CrossRef] [PubMed]
6. Lai, W.S.; Stumpo, D.J.; Blackshear, P.J. Rapid insulin-stimulated accumulation of an mRNA encoding a proline-rich protein. *J. Biol. Chem.* **1990**, *265*, 16556–16563. [CrossRef]
7. Brennan, S.E.; Kuwano, Y.; Alkharouf, N.; Blackshear, P.J.; Gorospe, M.; Wilson, G.M. The mRNA-destabilizing protein tristetraprolin is suppressed in many cancers, altering tumorigenic phenotypes and patient prognosis. *Cancer Res.* **2009**, *69*, 5168–5176. [CrossRef]
8. Marderosian, M.; Sharma, A.; Funk, A.P.; Vartanian, R.; Masri, J.; Jo, O.D.; Gera, J.F. Tristetraprolin regulates Cyclin D1 and c-Myc mRNA stability in response to rapamycin in an Akt-dependent manner via p38 MAPK signaling. *Oncogene* **2006**, *25*, 6277–6290. [CrossRef]
9. Young, L.E.; Sanduja, S.; Bemis-Standoli, K.; Pena, E.A.; Price, R.L.; Dixon, D.A. The mRNA binding proteins HuR and tristetraprolin regulate cyclooxygenase 2 expression during colon carcinogenesis. *Gastroenterology* **2009**, *136*, 1669–1679. [CrossRef]

10. Lee, H.H.; Son, Y.J.; Lee, W.H.; Park, Y.W.; Chae, S.W.; Cho, W.J.; Kim, Y.M.; Choi, H.J.; Choi, D.H.; Jung, S.W.; et al. Tristetraprolin regulates expression of VEGF and tumorigenesis in human colon cancer. *Int. J. Cancer* **2010**, *126*, 1817–1827. [CrossRef]
11. Lee, J.Y.; Kim, H.J.; Yoon, N.A.; Lee, W.H.; Min, Y.J.; Ko, B.K.; Lee, B.J.; Lee, A.; Cha, H.J.; Cho, W.J.; et al. Tumor suppressor p53 plays a key role in induction of both tristetraprolin and let-7 in human cancer cells. *Nucleic Acids Res.* **2013**, *41*, 5614–5625. [CrossRef]
12. Rounbehler, R.J.; Fallahi, M.; Yang, C.; Steeves, M.A.; Li, W.; Doherty, J.R.; Schaub, F.X.; Sanduja, S.; Dixon, D.A.; Blackshear, P.J.; et al. Tristetraprolin impairs myc-induced lymphoma and abolishes the malignant state. *Cell* **2012**, *150*, 563–574. [CrossRef]
13. Soussi, T.; Beroud, C. Assessing TP53 status in human tumours to evaluate clinical outcome. *Nat. Rev. Cancer* **2001**, *1*, 233–240. [CrossRef]
14. Cole, M.D. The myc oncogene: Its role in transformation and differentiation. *Ann. Rev. Genet.* **1986**, *20*, 361–384. [CrossRef] [PubMed]
15. Smoak, K.; Cidlowski, J.A. Glucocorticoids regulate tristetraprolin synthesis and posttranscriptionally regulate tumor necrosis factor alpha inflammatory signaling. *Mol. Cell Biol.* **2006**, *26*, 9126–9135. [CrossRef]
16. Ishmael, F.T.; Fang, X.; Galdiero, M.R.; Atasoy, U.; Rigby, W.F.; Gorospe, M.; Cheadle, C.; Stellato, C. Role of the RNA-binding protein tristetraprolin in glucocorticoid-mediated gene regulation. *J. Immunol.* **2008**, *180*, 8342–8353. [CrossRef] [PubMed]
17. Kaur, M.; Chivers, J.E.; Giembycz, M.A.; Newton, R. Long-acting beta2-adrenoceptor agonists synergistically enhance glucocorticoid-dependent transcription in human airway epithelial and smooth muscle cells. *Mol. Pharmacol.* **2008**, *73*, 203–214. [CrossRef] [PubMed]
18. King, E.M.; Kaur, M.; Gong, W.; Rider, C.F.; Holden, N.S.; Newton, R. Regulation of tristetraprolin expression by interleukin-1 beta and dexamethasone in human pulmonary epithelial cells: Roles for nuclear factor-kappa B and p38 mitogen-activated protein kinase. *J. Pharmacol. Exp. Ther.* **2009**, *330*, 575–585. [CrossRef]
19. Miller, W.L.; Auchus, R.J. The molecular biology, biochemistry, and physiology of human steroidogenesis and its disorders. *Endocr. Rev.* **2011**, *32*, 81–151. [CrossRef]
20. Sapolsky, R.M.; Romero, L.M.; Munck, A.U. How do glucocorticoids influence stress responses? Integrating permissive, suppressive, stimulatory, and preparative actions. *Endocr. Rev.* **2000**, *21*, 55–89.
21. Rhen, T.; Cidlowski, J.A. Antiinflammatory action of glucocorticoids–new mechanisms for old drugs. *N. Engl. J. Med.* **2005**, *353*, 1711–1723. [CrossRef] [PubMed]
22. Oakley, R.H.; Cidlowski, J.A. The biology of the glucocorticoid receptor: New signaling mechanisms in health and disease. *J. Allergy Clin. Immunol.* **2013**, *132*, 1033–1044. [CrossRef] [PubMed]
23. Vandewalle, J.; Luypaert, A.; De Bosscher, K.; Libert, C. Therapeutic Mechanisms of Glucocorticoids. *Trends Endocrinol. Metab.* **2018**, *29*, 42–54. [CrossRef] [PubMed]
24. Wright, A.P.; Zilliacus, J.; McEwan, I.J.; Dahlman-Wright, K.; Almlof, T.; Carlstedt-Duke, J.; Gustafsson, J.A. Structure and function of the glucocorticoid receptor. *J. Steroid Biochem. Mol. Biol.* **1993**, *47*, 11–19. [CrossRef]
25. Kadmiel, M.; Cidlowski, J.A. Glucocorticoid receptor signaling in health and disease. *Trends Pharmacol. Sci.* **2013**, *34*, 518–530. [CrossRef] [PubMed]
26. Beato, M.; Chalepakis, G.; Schauer, M.; Slater, E.P. DNA regulatory elements for steroid hormones. *J. Steroid Biochem.* **1989**, *32*, 737–747. [CrossRef]
27. Lim, H.W.; Uhlenhaut, N.H.; Rauch, A.; Weiner, J.; Hubner, S.; Hubner, N.; Won, K.J.; Lazar, M.A.; Tuckermann, J.; Steger, D.J. Genomic redistribution of GR monomers and dimers mediates transcriptional response to exogenous glucocorticoid in vivo. *Genome Res.* **2015**, *25*, 836–844. [CrossRef]
28. Diamond, M.I.; Miner, J.N.; Yoshinaga, S.K.; Yamamoto, K.R. Transcription factor interactions: Selectors of positive or negative regulation from a single DNA element. *Science* **1990**, *249*, 1266–1272. [CrossRef]
29. Tuckermann, J.P.; Kleiman, A.; McPherson, K.G.; Reichardt, H.M. Molecular mechanisms of glucocorticoids in the control of inflammation and lymphocyte apoptosis. *Crit. Rev. Clin. Lab. Sci.* **2005**, *42*, 71–104. [CrossRef]
30. Ratman, D.; Vanden Berghe, W.; Dejager, L.; Libert, C.; Tavernier, J.; Beck, I.M.; De Bosscher, K. How glucocorticoid receptors modulate the activity of other transcription factors: A scope beyond tethering. *Mol. Cell Endocrinol.* **2013**, *380*, 41–54. [CrossRef]
31. Song, I.H.; Buttgereit, F. Non-genomic glucocorticoid effects to provide the basis for new drug developments. *Mol. Cell Endocrinol.* **2006**, *246*, 142–146. [CrossRef] [PubMed]
32. Puthanveetil, P.; Wang, Y.; Wang, F.; Kim, M.S.; Abrahani, A.; Rodrigues, B. The increase in cardiac pyruvate dehydrogenase kinase-4 after short-term dexamethasone is controlled by an Akt-p38-forkhead box other factor-1 signaling axis. *Endocrinology* **2010**, *151*, 2306–2318. [CrossRef] [PubMed]
33. Poulsen, R.C.; Carr, A.J.; Hulley, P.A. Protection against glucocorticoid-induced damage in human tenocytes by modulation of ERK, Akt, and forkhead signaling. *Endocrinology* **2011**, *152*, 503–514. [CrossRef]
34. Kaiser, G.; Gerst, F.; Michael, D.; Berchtold, S.; Friedrich, B.; Strutz-Seebohm, N.; Lang, F.; Haring, H.U.; Ullrich, S. Regulation of forkhead box O1 (FOXO1) by protein kinase B and glucocorticoids: Different mechanisms of induction of beta cell death in vitro. *Diabetologia* **2013**, *56*, 1587–1595. [CrossRef] [PubMed]
35. Wang, X.J.; Xiao, J.J.; Liu, L.; Jiao, H.C.; Lin, H. Excessive glucocorticoid-induced muscle MuRF1 overexpression is independent of Akt/FoXO1 pathway. *Biosci. Rep.* **2017**, *37*, BSR20171056. [CrossRef]

36. Felice, F.; Cesare, M.M.; Fredianelli, L.; De Leo, M.; Conti, V.; Braca, A.; Di Stefano, R. Effect of Tomato Peel Extract Grown under Drought Stress Condition in a Sarcopenia Model. *Molecules* **2022**, *27*, 2563. [CrossRef]
37. Arden, K.C. Multiple roles of FOXO transcription factors in mammalian cells point to multiple roles in cancer. *Exp. Gerontol.* **2006**, *41*, 709–717. [CrossRef]
38. Fu, Z.; Tindall, D.J. FOXOs, cancer and regulation of apoptosis. *Oncogene* **2008**, *27*, 2312–2319. [CrossRef]
39. Miyamoto, K.; Araki, K.Y.; Naka, K.; Arai, F.; Takubo, K.; Yamazaki, S.; Matsuoka, S.; Miyamoto, T.; Ito, K.; Ohmura, M.; et al. Foxo3a is essential for maintenance of the hematopoietic stem cell pool. *Cell Stem. Cell* **2007**, *1*, 101–112. [CrossRef]
40. Zhang, X.; Yong, W.; Lv, J.; Zhu, Y.; Zhang, J.; Chen, F.; Zhang, R.; Yang, T.; Sun, Y.; Han, X. Inhibition of forkhead box O1 protects pancreatic beta-cells against dexamethasone-induced dysfunction. *Endocrinology* **2009**, *150*, 4065–4073. [CrossRef]
41. Robinson, M.D.; McCarthy, D.J.; Smyth, G.K. edgeR: A Bioconductor package for differential expression analysis of digital gene expression data. *Bioinformatics* **2010**, *26*, 139–140. [CrossRef] [PubMed]
42. Ma, J.; Matkar, S.; He, X.; Hua, X. FOXO family in regulating cancer and metabolism. *Semin. Cancer Biol.* **2018**, *50*, 32–41. [CrossRef] [PubMed]
43. Kalfeist, L.; Galland, L.; Ledys, F.; Ghiringhelli, F.; Limagne, E.; Ladoire, S. Impact of Glucocorticoid Use in Oncology in the Immunotherapy Era. *Cells* **2022**, *11*, 770. [CrossRef]
44. Almawi, W.Y.; Saouda, M.S.; Stevens, A.C.; Lipman, M.L.; Barth, C.M.; Strom, T.B. Partial mediation of glucocorticoid antiproliferative effects by lipocortins. *J. Immunol.* **1996**, *157*, 5231–5239.
45. Almawi, W.Y.; Tamim, H. Posttranscriptional mechanisms of glucocorticoid antiproliferative effects: Glucocorticoids inhibit IL-6-induced proliferation of B9 hybridoma cells. *Cell Transpl.* **2001**, *10*, 161–164. [CrossRef]
46. Gruber, A.R.; Fallmann, J.; Kratochvill, F.; Kovarik, P.; Hofacker, I.L. Aresite: A database for the comprehensive investigation of au-rich elements. *Nucleic Acids Res.* **2011**, *39*, D66–D69. [CrossRef]
47. Khabar, K.S.A. Hallmarks of cancer and AU-rich elements. *Wiley Interdiscip. Rev. RNA* **2017**, *8*, 1368. [CrossRef]
48. Bisogno, L.S.; Keene, J.D. RNA regulons in cancer and inflammation. *Curr. Opin. Genet. Dev.* **2018**, *48*, 97–103. [CrossRef] [PubMed]
49. Lykke-Andersen, J.; Wagner, E. Recruitment and activation of mRNA decay enzymes by two ARE-mediated decay activation domains in the proteins TTP and BRF-1. *Genes Dev.* **2005**, *19*, 351–361. [CrossRef]
50. Jing, Q.; Huang, S.; Guth, S.; Zarubin, T.; Motoyama, A.; Chen, J.; Padova, F.D.; Lin, S.; Gram, H.; Han, J. Involvement of microRNA in AU-rich element-mediated mRNA instability. *Cell* **2005**, *120*, 623–634. [CrossRef]
51. Surjit, M.; Ganti, K.P.; Mukherji, A.; Ye, T.; Hua, G.; Metzger, D.; Li, M.; Chambon, P. Widespread negative response elements mediate direct repression by agonist-liganded glucocorticoid receptor. *Cell* **2011**, *145*, 224–241. [CrossRef] [PubMed]
52. Hua, G.; Ganti, K.P.; Chambon, P. Glucocorticoid-induced tethered transrepression requires SUMOylation of GR and formation of a SUMO-SMRT/NCoR1-HDAC3 repressing complex. *Proc. Natl. Acad. Sci. USA* **2016**, *113*, E635–E643. [CrossRef] [PubMed]
53. Chandler, V.L.; Maler, B.A.; Yamamoto, K.R. DNA sequences bound specifically by glucocorticoid receptor in vitro render a heterologous promoter hormone responsive in vivo. *Cell* **1983**, *33*, 489–499. [CrossRef]
54. Schiller, B.J.; Chodankar, R.; Watson, L.C.; Stallcup, M.R.; Yamamoto, K.R. Glucocorticoid receptor binds half sites as a monomer and regulates specific target genes. *Genome Biol.* **2014**, *15*, 418. [CrossRef]
55. Obradović, M.M.S.; Hamelin, B.; Manevski, N.; Couto, J.P.; Sethi, A.; Coissieux, M.M.; Münst, S.; Okamoto, R.; Kohler, H.; Schmidt, A.; et al. Glucocorticoids promote breast cancer metastasis. *Nature* **2019**, *567*, 540–544. [CrossRef]
56. Crozier, M.; Tubman, J.; Fifield, B.; Ferraiuolo, R.; Ritchie, J.; Zuccato, K.; Mailloux, E.; Sinha, I.; Hamm, C.; Porter, L.A. Frequently used antiemetic agent dexamethasone enhances the metastatic behaviour of select breast cancer cells. *PLoS ONE* **2022**, *17*, e0274675. [CrossRef]
57. Yoon, N.A.; Jo, H.G.; Lee, U.H.; Park, J.H.; Yoon, J.E.; Ryu, J.; Kang, S.S.; Min, Y.J.; Ju, S.A.; Seo, E.H.; et al. Tristetraprolin suppresses the EMT through the down-regulation of Twist1 and Snail1 in cancer cells. *Oncotarget* **2016**, *7*, 8931–8943. [CrossRef]
58. Atanasov, A.G.; Zotchev, S.B.; Dirsch, V.M.; The International Natural Product Sciences Taskforce; Claudiu, T.; Supuran, C.T. Natural products in drug discovery: Advances and opportunities. *Nat. Rev. Drug Dis.* **2021**, *20*, 200–216. [CrossRef]
59. Dobin, A.; Davis, C.A.; Schlesinger, F.; Drenkow, J.; Zaleski, C.; Jha, S.; Batut, P.; Chaisson, M.; Gingeras, T.R. STAR: Ultrafast universal RNA-seq aligner. *Bioinformatics* **2013**, *29*, 15–21. [CrossRef]
60. Quinlan, A.R.; Hall, I.M. BEDTools: A flexible suite of utilities for comparing genomic features. *Bioinformatics* **2010**, *26*, 841–842. [CrossRef]
61. Kuleshov, M.V.; Jones, M.R.; Rouillard, A.D.; Fernandez, N.F.; Duan, Q.; Wang, Z.; Koplev, S.; Jenkins, S.L.; Jagodnik, K.M.; Lachmann, A.; et al. Enrichr: A comprehensive gene set enrichment analysis web server 2016 update. *Nucleic Acids Res.* **2016**, *44*, W90–W97. [CrossRef] [PubMed]

International Journal of
Molecular Sciences

MDPI

Article

New Angucycline Glycosides from a Marine-Derived Bacterium *Streptomyces ardesiacus*

Cao Van Anh [1,2], Joo-Hee Kwon [3], Jong Soon Kang [3], Hwa-Sun Lee [1], Chang-Su Heo [1,2] and Hee Jae Shin [1,2,*]

1 Marine Natural Products Chemistry Laboratory, Korea Institute of Ocean Science and Technology, 385 Haeyang-ro, Yeongdo-gu, Busan 49111, Korea
2 Department of Marine Biotechnology, University of Science and Technology (UST), 217 Gajungro, Yuseong-gu, Daejeon 34113, Korea
3 Laboratory Animal Resource Center, Korea Research Institute of Bioscience and Biotechnology, 30 Yeongudanjiro, Cheongju 28116, Korea
* Correspondence: shinhj@kiost.ac.kr; Tel.: +82-51-664-3341; Fax: +82-51-664-3340

Abstract: Chemical investigation of the ethyl acetate extract from the culture broth of the marine-derived actinobacterium *Streptomyces ardesiacus* 156VN-095 led to the isolation of three hitherto undescribed angucycline glycosides, including urdamycins W and X (**1** and **2**) and grincamycin U (**9**), as well as their seven known congeners. The structures of the new compounds were elucidated by means of spectroscopic methods (HRESIMS, 1D and 2 D NMR) and comparison of their experimental data with literature values. Compounds **1–3** and **9** were evaluated for their anti-Gram-positive bacterial effect and cytotoxicity against six cancer cell lines. Compound **1** displayed significant cytotoxicity against all the tested cell lines with GI_{50} values of 0.019–0.104 μM. Collectively, these findings highlight the potential of angucycline glycosides as leading structures for the development of new anti-cancer drugs.

Keywords: *Streptomyces ardesiacus*; urdamycin; grincamycin; anti-bacterial; cytotoxicity

Citation: Anh, C.V.; Kwon, J.-H.; Kang, J.S.; Lee, H.-S.; Heo, C.-S.; Shin, H.J. New Angucycline Glycosides from a Marine-Derived Bacterium *Streptomyces ardesiacus*. *Int. J. Mol. Sci.* **2022**, 23, 13779. https://doi.org/10.3390/ijms232213779

Academic Editors: Barbara De Filippis, Marialuigia Fantacuzzi and Alessandra Ammazzalorso

Received: 17 October 2022
Accepted: 3 November 2022
Published: 9 November 2022

1. Introduction

The genus *Streptomyces* are renowned as the largest contributor of currently used antibiotics [1]. Over the past decades, the most important classes of antimicrobial drugs have been isolated from this genus, such as tetracyclines, aminoglycosides, macrolides, and lypopeptides [2]. However, bioassay-guided screening of common actinomycetes, particularly the genus *Streptomyces*, often led to the rediscovery of known compounds and it is not an efficient approach to identifying new natural scaffolds [3]. Over the last decades, several dereplication strategies in natural product research were conducted to search for novel chemical structures from natural resources, such as bioactivity-guided fractionation, chemical profiles of crude extract collections and target compounds, and taxonomic identification of microbial strains [4]. Since terrestrial microbes have been well studied, several different approaches, including the investigation of unexploited habitats such as marine and extreme environments, have been employed to yield novel chemistry [5].

Polyketides are one of the largest classes of natural products isolated from the genus *Streptomyces* [6,7]. Among them, polycyclic aromatic polyketides, which are called "cytotoxic antibiotics", are one of the chemically richest classes of secondary metabolites and possess various biological activities, predominantly anticancer and antibacterial, and some of them are currently used as anti-cancer or anti-bacterial drugs, such as doxorubicin, epirubicin, and tetracycline [8–10]. The angucycline group is the largest group of type II PKS-engineered natural products, and is abundant in biological activities and chemical scaffolds [8], and the majority of angucycline producers were classified to be *Streptomycetes* of various species [11]. Besides possessing an interesting cytotoxicity, some of the angucyclines act as hydroxylase and/or mono-oxygenase inhibitors, some potentially inhibit blood platelet aggregation and others demonstrate antibacterial or antiviral activity [11]. Therefore, angucyclines may serve as leading structures for new drug discovery.

As part of our ongoing studies on bioactive secondary metabolites isolated from marine-derived microorganisms, an actinomycetal strain was isolated near Nha Trang Bay, Vietnam, and identified as *Streptomyces ardesiacus* 156VN-095 by 16S rRNA gene sequence analysis. NMR and HPLC profiling of the ethyl acetate (EtOAc) extract from the culture broth of the strain showed characteristic signals of polycyclic aromatic polyketides. Chemical investigations of a large-scale culture of the strain were carried out and resulted in the isolation of three previously undescribed angucycline polyketides (**1**, **2**, and **9**) and their seven known congeners. Herein, we describe the isolation, structure elucidation, and their anti-Gram-positive bacterial and cytotoxic activities.

2. Results and Discussion

The strain *Streptomyces ardesiacus* 156VN-095 cultured on Bennett's agar medium produced dark purple pigments. A small-culture test in Bennett's modified broth led to the isolation of urdamycins A and B as major metabolites (Figure S1). To further discover other unknown chemical constituents, a large-scale culture was conducted, and consequently, three unreported congeners were isolated. The structures and biological activities of these compounds are described below.

Compound **1** was isolated as a dark red powder, and the molecular formula of **1** was determined as $C_{38}H_{48}O_{15}S$ based on its HRESIMS peak at m/z 799.2612, $[M + Na]^+$ (calcd. for $C_{38}H_{48}O_{15}SNa$, 799.2612, Figure S8). The ^{1}H NMR spectrum of **1** showed signals of three aromatic protons at δ_H 7.73 (d, J = 7.6 Hz, H-10), 7.42 (d, J = 6.8 Hz, H-11), and 6.42 (s, H-6); two anomeric protons at δ_H 4.96 (s, H-1″) and 4.57 (d, J = 9.6 Hz, H-1‴); nine oxygenated methines at δ_H 2.91–4.75; twelve methylene protons at δ_H 1.22–2.85; and signals of five methyl groups at δ_H 1.17–2.49 (Figure S2). The ^{13}C NMR data, in combination with HSQC spectrum, demonstrated signals of 13 sp^2 carbons including three ketones at δ_C 206.6 (C-1), 190.1 (C-7), and 183.1 (C-12); three protonated aromatic carbons at δ_C 134.4 (C-10), 119.7 (C-11), and 106.5 (C-6); and seven non-protonated sp^2 carbons at δ_C 115.3–165.8 (Figures S3 and S4). In addition, the ^{13}C NMR spectrum also revealed signals of two anomeric carbons at δ_C 102.8 (C-1‴) and 95.2 (C-1″); nine protonated oxygenated methines at δ_C 67.8–78.4; three tertiary alcohols at δ_C 84.2 (C-4a), 79.5 (C-12b), and 77.3 (C-3); six methylenes at δ_C 25.4–53.3; and five methyl groups at δ_C 14.6–30.3. The ^{1}H NMR spectrum of **1** was quite similar to that of urdamycin E (**3**), except for the obvious missing signals for a sugar moiety attached to C-12b, indicating **1** was a new derivative of **3** with one less sugar unit [12] as shown in Figure 1. Further detailed analysis of HMBC and COSY data (Figure 2 and Figures S5 and S6) confirmed the planar structure of **1**. The relative configuration of trisaccharide moiety was deduced by analysis of $^3J_{H,H}$ coupling constants and NOESY data. The strong NOESY correlations from H-1′ to H-3′ and H-5′ indicated H-1′, H-3′, and H-5′ had a co-facial relationship, and H-4′ was observed at δ_H 3.12 (t), with a large coupling constant (J = 8.9 Hz), indicating H-4′ had a diaxial relationship with H-3′ and H-5′ (Figure 3 and Figure S7). Thus, the first sugar was determined as *D*-olivose and, similarly, the third sugar was also determined as *D*-olivose. The strong NOESY correlation between H-4″ and H_3-5″ and the lack of NOESY correlation from H-1″ to H-5″ identified the second sugar as *L*-rhodinose. Urdamycins are a group of angucycline glycosides firstly isolated from *Streptomyces fradiae* and the absolute stereochemistry of urdamycin A (**5**) was unambiguously determined by an X-ray analysis [13]. Urdamycin E (**3**) with an additional thiomethyl group (CH_3S-) at C-5 position of urdamycin A (**5**) was also isolated from the same strain, and **3** was transformed into **5** by treatment with Raney nickel reagent [14]. Hydrolysis of **3** yielded urdamycinone E (**4**) [14]. These studies revealed that urdamycin A (**5**) and its congeners (**3** and **4**) have the same absolute stereochemistry. Therefore, the absolute stereochemistry of **1** was determined by comparison experimental ECD between

1 and **4** (Figure 4 and Figure S28), and by considering the similarity of ^{1}H and ^{13}C NMR data and biosynthetic correlation of **1** and **4**. Thus, the structure of **1** was determined as 12b-desrhodinosyl urdamycin E and named urdamycin W.

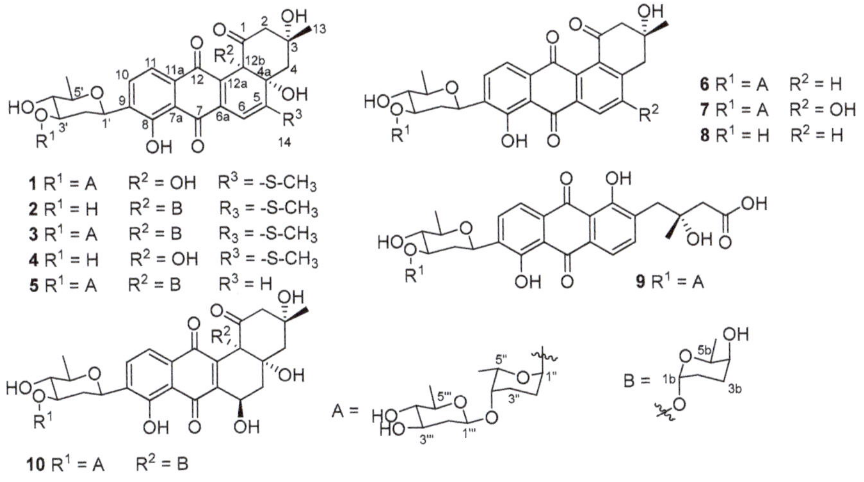

Figure 1. Structures of **1–10** isolated from *Streptomyces ardesiacus* 156VN-095.

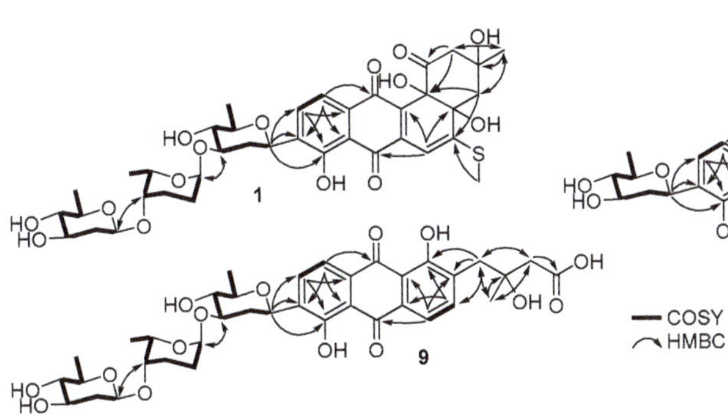

Figure 2. Key COSY and HMBC correlations for **1**, **2**, and **9**.

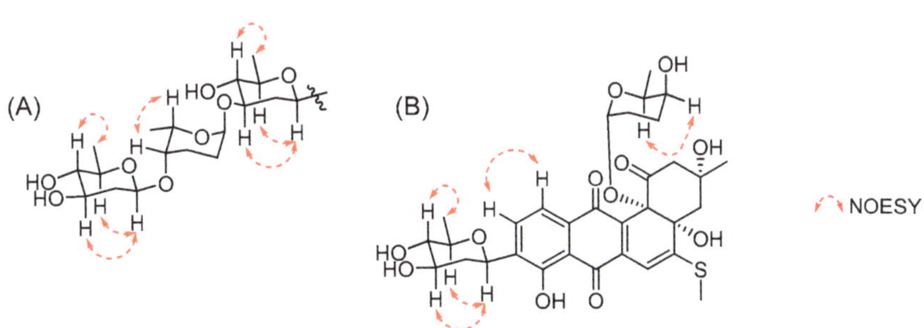

Figure 3. (**A**). Key NOESY correlations for trisaccharide moiety of **1** and **9**. (**B**). Key NOESY correlations for **2**.

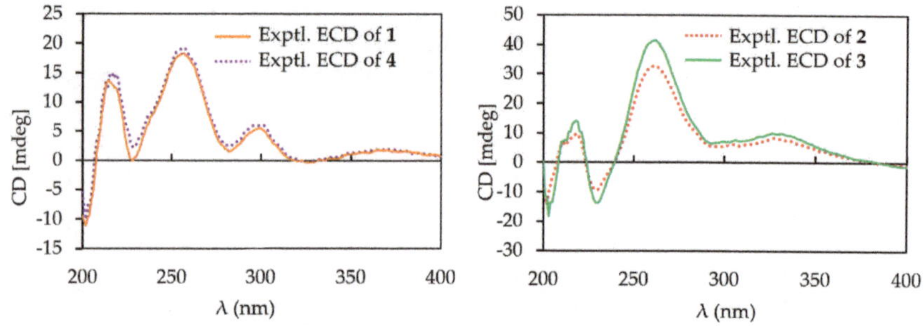

Figure 4. Experimental ECD spectra of **1–4**.

Compound **2** was also isolated as a dark red powder, the molecular formula of **2** was determined as $C_{32}H_{38}O_{12}S$ based on its HRESIMS peak at m/z 669.1984, $[M + Na]^+$ (calcd. for $C_{32}H_{38}O_{12}SNa$, 669.1982, Figure S15). The ^1H NMR spectrum of **2** revealed signals of three aromatic protons at δ_H 7.84 (d, J = 7.8 Hz, H-10), 7.57 (d, J = 7.8 Hz, H-11), and 6.49 (s, H-6); an anomeric proton at δ_H 5.28 (s, H-1b); six oxygenated methines at δ_H 3.03–4.89; ten methylene protons at δ_H 1.38–2.78; and signals of four methyl groups at δ_H 0.55–2.48 (Figure S9). The ^{13}C NMR data, in collaboration with HSQC spectrum, showed signals of 13 sp^2 carbons including three ketocarbonyls at δ_C 204.7 (C-1), 190.3 (C-7), and 183.9 (C-12); three protonated aromatic carbons δ_C 134.4 (C-10), 120.1 (C-11), and 106.0 (C-6); and seven non-protonated sp^2 carbons at δ_C 115.5–165.8 (Figures S10 and S11). Additionally, the ^{13}C NMR spectrum also showed signals of an anomeric carbon at δ_C 95.7 (C-1b), six protonated oxygenated methines at δ_C 67.8–78.8, three tertiary alcohols at δ_C 84.7 (C-4a), 83.5 (C-12b), and 76.8 (C-3), five methylenes at δ_C 24.2–55.0, and four methyl groups at δ_C 14.6–30.0 (Figure S10). The ^1H NMR spectrum of **2** was similar to that of urdamycin V, except for the obvious missing signals of a doublet anomeric proton at δ_H 4.98 and a doublet methyl group at δ_H 1.14 in urdamycin V, indicating **2** was a new derivative of urdamycin V with a missing sugar moiety attached to C-3′ position [12]. Further detailed analysis of HMBC and COSY data confirmed the planar structure of **2** as depicted in Figure 1 (Figures S12 and S13). Two sugar units were determined as *D*-olivose and *L*-rhodinose by a similar procedure for **1** (Figure S14). The absolute stereochemistry of **2** was determined by comparison of its experimental ECD spectrum with that of **3** (Figure 4 and Figure S29). Thus, the structure of **2** was determined as 3′-desrhodinosyl urdamycin V and named urdamycin X.

Compound **9** was isolated as an orange powder. The molecular formula of **9** was determined as $C_{37}H_{46}O_{15}$ based on its HRESIMS peak at m/z 753.2734, $[M + Na]^+$ (calcd. for $C_{37}H_{46}O_{15}Na$, 753.2734, Figure S27), with two hydroxy groups (-OH) more than that of **6** (urdamycin B). The ^1H NMR spectrum of **9** showed a similar pattern to that of **6**, and the obvious differences were the upfield-shifted chemical shift values of H-5 and H_3-13 (Figures S16 and S22)). The ^{13}C NMR spectrum of **9** showed an additional carbonyl signal at δ_C 175.7 and a missed ketone signal at δ_C 196.7 [14], indicating **9** was a new derivative of **6** with a ring-opening type of ring A and the ketone was hydrolyzed to a carboxylic acid (grincamycin type, Figures S17 and S23) [15]. The planar structure of **9** was further confirmed by detailed analysis of HSQC, ^1H-^1H COSY, and HMBC data (Figures S18–S20 and S24–S26). The relative configuration of the trisaccharide moiety was determined to be the same as that of **1** by analysis of NOESY data and $^3J_{H,H}$ coupling constants (Figures S21). The absolute configuration of **9** was the same as that of other gricamycin derivatives by considering the biosynthetic correlation and comparison of experimental ECD spectra of **9** with grincamycin L (Figure S30) [15]. Thus, the structure of **9** was determined as depicted in Figure 1 and named grincamycin U [16].

The structures of known compounds were identified as urdamycin E (**3**) [12], urdamycinone E (**4**) [14], urdamycin A (**5**) [13], urdamycin B (**6**) [14], 5-hydroxyurdamycin B (**7**) [17], urdamycinone B (**8**) [14], and urdamycin F (**10**) [14] by comparison of their spectroscopic data with those reported in the literature (Figures S31–S37).

Since previously described angucyline glycosides showed anti-Gram-positive bacterial or cytotoxic activities [9], the new compounds (**1**, **2**, and **9**) were primarily evaluated for their anti-bacterial activity against three Gram-positive bacterial strains (Table 1). The tested compounds showed selective anti-microbial activity, and of them, **1** showed the strongest activity against *Bacillus substilis* (KCTC 1021) with a MIC value of 8.0 μg/mL.

Table 1. Antibacterial activity of **1**, **2**, and **9**.

	MIC (μg/mL)		
	B. subtilis KCTC 1021	*Micrococcus luteus* KCTC 1915	*Staphylococcus aureus* KCTC 1927
1	8.0	64.0	32.0
2	>128	64.0	64.0
9	32.0	>128	>128
Kanamycin	0.25	1.0	0.5

Compounds **1–3** and **9** were also tested for their cytotoxicity against six cancer cell lines (PC-3 (prostate), NCI-H23 (lung), HCT-15 (colon), NUGC-3 (stomach), ACHN (renal), and MDA-MB-231 (breast)). All compounds showed cytotoxic effect with a different tendency (Table 2 and Figure S38). Compound **1** showed the strongest cytoxicity against all tested cell lines, which was more potent than the positive control (adriamycin). The cytotoxic and anti-bacterial results indicated that a longer saccharide chain at C-3′ could enhance the activities (**1** and **2**) and ring-opening type (**9**) led to a significant reduction in their biological effects.

Table 2. Growth inhibition (GI_{50}, μM) of **1–3**, and **9** against human cancer cell lines.

Compounds	1	2	3	9	Adr.
ACHN	0.104 ± 0.012	0.093 ± 0.004	0.060 ± 0.001	3.422 ± 0.357	0.140 ± 0.009
HCT-15	0.075 ± 0.012	0.150 ± 0.015	0.095 ± 0.037	3.886 ± 0.351	0.162 ± 0.012
MDA-MB-231	0.033 ± 0.008	0.077 ± 0.017	0.093 ± 0.005	3.500 ± 0.472	0.162 ± 0.000
NCI-H23	0.031 ± 0.002	0.050 ± 0.004	0.036 ± 0.002	3.245 ± 0.179	0.145 ± 0.003
NUGC-3	0.019 ± 0.003	0.028 ± 0.006	0.030 ± 0.006	3.037 ± 0.045	0.151 ± 0.014
PC-3	0.022 ± 0.006	0.103 ± 0.002	0.062 ± 0.012	2.750 ± 0.344	0.148 ± 0.005

Adr., Adriamycin as a positive control. GI_{50} values are the concentration corresponding to 50% growth inhibition.

3. Materials and Methods

3.1. General Experimental Procedures

The 1D and 2D NMR spectra were recorded using a Bruker AVANCE III 600 spectrometer with a 3 mm probe operating at 600 MHz (^{1}H) and 150 MHz (^{13}C). HRESIMS data were acquired by a Waters SYNPT G2 Q-TOF mass spectrometer at the Korea Basic Science Institute (KBSI) in Cheongju, Korea. UV spectra were measured by a Shimadzu UV-1650PC spectrophotometer. ECD spectra were obtained on a JASCO J-1500 polarimeter at the Center for Research Facilities, Changwon National University, Changwon, Korea. IR spectra were recorded on a JASCO FT/IR-4100 spectrophotometer. HPLC was carried out using a PrimeLine binary pump coupled with a Shodex RI-101 refractive index detector and S3210 variable UV detector. Columns used for HPLC were YMC-Triart C_{18} (250 mm × 10 mm, 5 μm and 250 mm × 4.6 mm, 5 μm). Reversed-phase silica gel (YMC-Gel ODS-A, 12 nm, S-75 μm) was used for open-column chromatography. Mass culture was conducted using a Fermentec 100 L fermenter. All solvents were either HPLC grade or distilled prior to use.

3.2. Bacterial Strain, Fermentation, and Isolation of 1–10 from Streptomyces ardesiacus 156VN-095

The strain 156VN-095 was isolated from an unidentified sponge collected near Nha Trang Bay, Vietnam, in June 2015. The strain was identified as *Streptomyces ardesiacus* based on 16S rRNA gene sequence analysis (GenBank accession number OP604346) by Macrogen Inc. (Seoul, Korea). The seed and mass cultures of the strain were conducted in Bennett's modified medium (BN broth, 0.5% glucose, 0.05% yeast extract, 0.1% tryptone, 0.05% beef extract, 0.25% glycerol, and 3.2% sea salt). The strain was grown on BN agar plates at 28 °C for 7 days. The bacterial spores were then inoculated into BN broth medium (50 mL) in a 100 mL flask and incubated in a rotation shaker (140 rpm) at 28 °C for 4 days. An aliquot (10 mL) of the seed culture was then transferred into the BN broth medium (1.0 L) in a 2.0 L flask and grown under the same afore-mentioned conditions. The culture was then inoculated into a 100 L fermenter filled with 70 L of BN medium and cultured for 11 days and then harvested. The culture broth and the cells were separated by centrifugation and the broth was extracted with an equal volume of EtOAc, twice. The organic layer was evaporated under reduced pressure to yield a crude extract (6.0 g). The extract was fractionated into 10 fractions (F1 to F10) by liquid vacuum chromatography on an OSD column using a stepwise elution of 10 to 100% MeOH in H_2O. The F6 fraction was subjected to a semi-preparative HPLC (YMC-PackODS-A, 250 × 10 mm i.d., 5 μm, flow rate 2.0 mL/min) with an isocratic elution of 53% MeOH in H_2O to obtain compounds **1** (3.0 mg, t_R = 48.5 min), **3** (4.0 mg, t_R = 54.0 min), **5** (4.2 mg, t_R = 33.2 min), **6** (5.0 mg, t_R = 75.0 min), and **7** (1.0 mg, t_R = 80.3 min) and subfraction F6-1. The subfraction F6-1 was repurified by a semi-preparative HPLC (YMC-PackODS-A, 250 × 10 mm i.d., 5 μm, flow rate 2.0 mL/min) with an isocratic elution of 23% MeCN in H_2O to obtain compounds **10** (1.3 mg, t_R = 26.5 min), **8** (7.0 mg, t_R = 37.0 min), **4** (1.0 mg, t_R = 40.2 min), and **2** (3.0 mg, t_R = 50.6 min). Compound **9** (3.2 mg, t_R = 30.1 min) was isolated from the F8 fraction by a semi-preparative HPLC (YMC-PackODS-A, 250 × 10 mm i.d., 5 μm, flow rate 2.0 mL/min) with an isocratic elution of 75% MeOH in H_2O.

Urdamycin W (**1**): dark red powder; IR ν_{max} 3398, 2929, 1632, 1515, 1430, 1367, 1293, 1063 cm^{-1}; UV (MeOH) λ_{max} (log ε) 291 (4.7), 475 (4.2) nm; HRESIMS *m/z* 799.2612, $[M + Na]^+$ (calcd. for $C_{38}H_{48}O_{15}SNa$, 799.2612), ^{1}H NMR (CD_3OD, 600 MHz) and ^{13}C NMR (CD_3OD, 150 MHz) see Table 3.

Table 3. ^{1}H and ^{13}C NMR spectroscopic data of **1**, **2**, and **9** (600 MHz for ^{1}H and 150 MHz for ^{13}C).

	1 [a]			**2** [a]			**9** [b]	
Pos.	**δ_H, Mult (*J* in Hz)**	**δ_C**	**Pos.**	**δ_H, Mult (*J* in Hz)**	**δ_C**	**Pos.**	**δ_H, Mult (*J* in Hz)**	**δ_C**
1		206.6	1		204.7	1		175.7
2	2.85, d (13.0) 2.66, d (13.3)	53.3	2	2.78, d (13.1) 2.56, dd (13.1, 2.6)	55.0	2	3.00, m	47.0
3		77.3	3		76.8	3		72.4
4	2.13, s	46.6	4	2.21, d (14.9) 2.06, dd (15.0, 2.6)	46.1	4	3.44, m	41.4
4a		84.2	4a		84.7	4a		136.6
5		165.8	5		165.8	5	8.03, d (7.6)	140.6
6	6.42, s	106.5	6	6.49, s	106.0	6	7.88, d (7.6)	119.3
6a		139.6	6a		138.7	6a		132.3
7		190.1	7		190.3	7		188.9
7a		115.3	7a		115.5	7a		116.3
8		158.7	8		158.7	8		159.5
9		138.5	9		138.6	9		139.4
10	7.73, d (7.6)	134.4	10	7.84, d (7.8)	134.4	10	8.09, d (7.8)	134.1
11	7.42, d (6.8)	119.7	11	7.57, d (7.8)	120.1	11	7.98, d (7.8)	119.7

Table 3. *Cont.*

	1 [a]			2 [a]			9 [b]	
Pos.	**δ_H, Mult (*J* in Hz)**	**δ_C**	**Pos.**	**δ_H, Mult (*J* in Hz)**	**δ_C**	**Pos.**	**δ_H, Mult (*J* in Hz)**	**δ_C**
11a		132.3	11a		132.6	11a		132.7
12		183.1	12		183.9	12		188.8
12a		134.7	12a		135.4	12a		116.3
12b		79.5	12b		83.5	12b		162.3
13	1.24, s	30.3	13	1.21, s	30.0	13	1.69, s	28.1
14	2.49, s	14.6	14	2.48, s	14.6	14		
1′	4.75, d (11.1)	72.3	1′	4.89, d (11.0)	72.4	1′	5.11, d (11.2)	72.1
2′	2.45, m 1.22, m	37.6	2′	2.40, dd (12.7, 4.7) 1.38, m	41.1	2′	2.81, dd (12.0, 3.1) 1.61, m	37.7
3′	3.73, m	77.8	3′	3.69, m	73.6	3′	4.21, m	78.2
4′	3.12, t (8.9)	76.8	4′	3.03, t (8.9)	78.8	4′	3.64, m	76.4
5′	3.45, m	77.7	5′	3.44, dq (12.2, 6.1)	77.8	5′	3.81, m	77.8
6′	1.38, d (5.9)	18.9	6′	1.37, d (6.2)	18.6	6′	1.69, d (6.3)	19.4
1″	4.96, s	95.2	1b	5.28, s	95.7	1″	5.27, s	95.1
2″	2.05, m 1.44, m	25.6	2b	1.86, m	24.2	2″	2.38, m 2.25, m	25.7
3″	2.05, m 1.94, m	25.4	3b	2.01, m 1.58, dd (2.5, 13.2)	26.5	3″	2.25, m 1.62, m	25.7
4″	3.55, s	77.7	4b	3.35, s	67.8	4″	3.67, s	76.9
5″	4.24, q (6.4)	67.8	5b	3.64, q (6.5)	68.3	5″	4.67, q (6.0)	67.3
6″	1.17, d (6.4)	17.4	6b	0.55, d (6.6)	17.0	6″	1.38, d (6.4)	17.9
1‴	4.57, d (9.6)	102.8				1‴	4.80, d (9.6)	102.9
2‴	2.20, dd (12.3, 4.9) 1.55, m	40.6				2‴	2.66, dd (12.1, 4.3) 2.17, m	41.4
3‴	3.50, m	72.3				3‴	4.08, m	72.5
4‴	2.91, t (9.0)	78.4				4‴	3.56, t (8.7)	78.9
5‴	3.23, dq (12.5, 6.1)	73.2				5‴	3.64, m	73.4
6‴	1.26, d (6.0)	18.4				6‴	1.61, d (6.1)	19.2

[a] measured in methanol-d_4; [b] measured in pyridine-d_5.

Urdamycin X (**2**): dark red powder; IR ν_{max} 3417, 2929, 1632, 1515, 1430, 1299, 1088 cm^{-1}; UV (MeOH) λ_{max} (log ε) 298 (4.9), 470 (4.3) nm; HRESIMS *m*/*z* 669.1984, [M + Na]$^+$ (calcd. for $C_{32}H_{38}O_{12}SNa$, 669.1982), ^{1}H NMR (CD_3OD, 600 MHz) and ^{13}C NMR (CD_3OD, 150 MHz) see Table 3.

Grincamycin U (**9**): orange powder; IR ν_{max} 3396, 2929, 1628, 1430, 1371, 1257, 1070 cm^{-1}; UV (MeOH) λ_{max} (log ε) 230 (4.8), 255 (3.9), 442 (3.2) nm; HRESIMS *m*/*z* 753.2734, [M + Na]$^+$ (calcd. for $C_{37}H_{46}O_{15}Na$, 753.2734), ^{1}H NMR (pyridine-d_5, 600 MHz) and ^{13}C NMR (pyridine-d_5, 150 MHz) see Table 3.

3.3. Antibacterial Assay

The antimicrobial assay of **1**, **2**, and **9** was conducted using a standard broth dilution assay. Difco™ Mueller–Hinton broth (BD, 275730) was used for determination of MIC values. Compounds **1**, **2**, and **9** were tested against three Gram-positive bacteria including, *Staphylococcus aureus* (KCTC 1927), *Micrococcus luteus* (KCTC 1915), and *Bacillus subtilis* (KCTC 1021). The tested compounds were prepared in the range of 0.5–256 µg/mL in 96-microtiter plates by a serial double dilution. An overnight culture broth of each strain was dispensed in sterilized 0.9% saline to an inoculum density of 5×10^5 cfu by comparison with a McFarland standard [18]. The diluted culture broth (100 μL) was added to each dilution of the tested compounds (**1**, **2**, and **9**, 100 μL), in the plate to yield final concentrations from 0.25 to 128 μg/mL. The plates were maintained for 24 h at 37 °C. The MIC value is the lowest concentration at which the microorganism did not demonstrate visible growth, as indicated by the presence of turbidity. Kanamycin was used as a positive control. All experiments were conducted twice to check reproducibility.

3.4. Cytotoxicity Test by SRB Assay

The SRB cytotoxicity test for **1–3**, and **9** was performed as previously described [19]. Cancer cell lines were obtained from Japanese Cancer Research Resources Bank (JCRB) (NUGC-3, JCRB Cell Bank/Cat. #JCRB0822) and American Type Culture Collection (ATCC) (PC-3, ATCC/Cat. #CRL-1435; MDA-MB-231, ATCC/Cat. #HTB-26; ACHN, ATCC/Cat. #CRL-1611; NCI-H23, ATCC/Cat. #CRL-5800; HCT-15, ATCC/Cat. #CCL-225).

3.5. Statistical Analysis

Statistical analysis was evaluated by one-way ANOVA followed by Dunnett's t-test and the GI_{50} values were determined by the software of GraphPad Prism 8 (GraphPad Software Inc., San Diego, CA, USA).

4. Conclusions

In conclusion, we have isolated 10 angucycline glycosides from the culture broth of *Streptomyces ardesiacus* 156VN-095 and three of them were new compounds (**1**, **2**, and **9**). The structures of the new metabolites were elucidated by spectroscopic analysis and comparison of their experimental data with those reported in the literature. The new compounds showed selective anti-bacterial effects against three Gram-positive bacterial strains and significant cytotoxicity against a panel of cancer cell lines with a different potency. Among them, **1** showed the strongest activities against all the tested cell lines with GI_{50} values of 0.019–0.104 μM. These results expanded biochemical diversities of naturally occurring angucycline glycosides.

Supplementary Materials: The following supporting information can be downloaded at: https://www.mdpi.com/article/10.3390/ijms232213779/s1.

Author Contributions: Conceptualization, H.J.S.; investigation, C.V.A. and J.-H.K.; resources, H.-S.L. and C.-S.H.; writing—original draft preparation, C.V.A.; writing—review and editing, H.J.S.; visualization, J.S.K.; project administration, H.J.S.; funding acquisition, H.J.S. All authors have read and agreed to the published version of the manuscript.

Funding: This research was supported by the project titled "Development of potential antibiotic compounds using polar organism resources (No. 20200610, KIOST Grant PM62930)" and PM58482, funded by the Ministry of Oceans and Fisheries, Korea.

Institutional Review Board Statement: Not applicable.

Informed Consent Statement: Not applicable.

Data Availability Statement: The data presented in the article are available in the Supplementary Mater

Acknowledgments: The authors express gratitude to Jung Hoon Choi, Korea Basic Science Institute, Ochang, Korea, for providing mass data. Authors would like to thank the Vietnam Government for allowing us to do marine microbial research.

Conflicts of Interest: The authors declare no conflict of interest.

References

1. Quinn, G.A.; Banat, A.M.; Abdelhameed, A.M.; Banat, I.M. *Streptomyces* from traditional medicine: Sources of new innovations in antibiotic discovery. *J. Med. Microbiol.* **2020**, *69*, 1040–1048. [CrossRef] [PubMed]
2. Mast, Y.; Stegmann, E. Actinomycetes: The Antibiotics Producers. *Antibiotics* **2019**, *8*, 105. [CrossRef] [PubMed]

3. Saito, S.; Xiaohanyao, Y.; Zhou, T.; Nakajima-Shimada, J.; Tashiro, E.; Triningsih, D.W.; Harunari, E.; Oku, N.; Igarashi, Y. Phytohabitols A–C, δ-Lactone-Terminated Polyketides from an Actinomycete of the Genus *Phytohabitans*. *J. Nat. Prod.* **2022**, *85*, 1697–1703. [CrossRef] [PubMed]
4. Hubert, J.; Nuzillard, J.-M.; Renault, J.-H. Dereplication strategies in natural product research: How many tools and methodologies behind the same concept? *Phytochem. Rev.* **2017**, *16*, 55–95. [CrossRef]
5. Voser, T.M.; Campbell, M.D.; Carroll, A.R. How different are marine microbial natural products compared to their terrestrial counterparts? *Nat. Prod. Rep.* **2021**, *39*, 7–19. [CrossRef] [PubMed]
6. Risdian, C.; Mozef, T.; Wink, J. Biosynthesis of Polyketides in *Streptomyces*. *Microorganisms* **2019**, *7*, 124. [CrossRef] [PubMed]
7. Lacey, H.J.; Rutledge, P.J. Recently Discovered Secondary Metabolites from *Streptomyces* Species. *Molecules* **2022**, *27*, 887. [CrossRef] [PubMed]
8. Kharel, M.K.; Pahari, P.; Shepherd, M.D.; Tibrewal, N.; Nybo, S.E.; Shaaban, K.A.; Rohr, J. Angucyclines: Biosynthesis, mode-of-action, new natural products, and synthesis. *Nat. Prod. Rep.* **2012**, *29*, 264–325. [CrossRef] [PubMed]
9. Hulst, M.B.; Grocholski, T.; Neefjes, J.J.C.; van Wezel, G.P.; Metsä-Ketelä, M. Anthracyclines: Biosynthesis, engineering and clinical applications. *Nat. Prod. Rep.* **2022**, *39*, 814–841. [CrossRef] [PubMed]
10. Hu, Y.; Nie, Q.-Y.; Pan, H.-X.; Tang, G.-L. 1.07-Bacterial Type II Polyketide Synthases. In *Comprehensive Natural Products III*; Liu, H.-W., Begley, T.P., Eds.; Elsevier: Oxford, UK, 2020; Volume 1, pp. 198–249. [CrossRef]
11. Rohr, J.; Thiericke, R. Angucycline group antibiotics. *Nat. Prod. Rep.* **1992**, *9*, 103–137. [CrossRef] [PubMed]
12. Dan, V.M.; Vinodh, J.S.; Sandesh, C.J.; Sanawar, R.; Lekshmi, A.; Kumar, R.A.; Santhosh Kumar, T.R.; Marelli, U.K.; Dastager, S.G.; Pillai, M.R. Molecular networking and whole-genome analysis aid discovery of an angucycline that inactivates mTORC1/C2 and induces programmed cell death. *ACS Chem. Biol.* **2020**, *15*, 780–788. [CrossRef] [PubMed]
13. Drautz, H.; Zähner, H.; Rohr, J.; Zeeck, A. Metabolic products of microorganisms. 234. Urdamycins, new angucycline antibiotics from *Streptomyces fradiae*. I. Isolation, characterization and biological properties. *J. Antibiot.* **1986**, *39*, 1657–1669. [CrossRef] [PubMed]
14. Rohr, J.; Zeeck, A. Metabolic products of microorganisms. 240 Urdamycins, new angucycline antibiotics from *Streptomyces fradiae*. II Structural studies of urdamycins B to F. *J. Antibiot.* **1987**, *40*, 459–467. [CrossRef] [PubMed]
15. Yang, L.; Hou, L.K.; Li, H.Y.; Li, W.L. Antibiotic angucycline derivatives from the deepsea-derived *Streptomyces lusitanus*. *Nat. Prod. Res.* **2020**, *34*, 3444–3450. [CrossRef] [PubMed]
16. Shang, Z.; Ferris, Z.E.; Sweeney, D.; Chase, A.B.; Yuan, C.; Hui, Y.; Hou, L.; Older, E.A.; Xue, D.; Tang, X.; et al. Grincamycins P–T: Rearranged Angucyclines from the Marine Sediment-Derived *Streptomyces* sp. CNZ-748 Inhibit Cell Lines of the Rare Cancer Pseudomyxoma Peritonei. *J. Nat. Prod.* **2021**, *84*, 1638–1648. [CrossRef] [PubMed]
17. Rohr, J.; Schoenewolf, M.; Udvarnoki, G.; Eckardt, K.; Schumann, G.; Wagner, C.; Beale, J.M.; Sorey, S.D. Investigations on the biosynthesis of the angucycline group antibiotics aquayamycin and the urdamycins A and B. Results from the structural analysis of novel blocked mutant products. *J. Org. Chem.* **1993**, *58*, 2547–2551. [CrossRef]
18. Appendino, G.; Gibbons, S.; Giana, A.; Pagani, A.; Grassi, G.; Stavri, M.; Smith, E.; Rahman, M.M. Antibacterial cannabinoids from *Cannabis sativa*: A structure-activity study. *J. Nat. Prod.* **2008**, *71*, 1427–1430. [CrossRef] [PubMed]
19. Choi, B.-K.; Trinh, P.T.H.; Lee, H.-S.; Choi, B.-W.; Kang, J.S.; Ngoc, N.T.D.; Van, T.T.T.; Shin, H.J. New Ophiobolin Derivatives from the Marine Fungus *Aspergillus flocculosus* and Their Cytotoxicities against Cancer Cells. *Mar. Drugs* **2019**, *17*, 346. [CrossRef] [PubMed]

International Journal of
Molecular Sciences

MDPI

Article

Flavones, Flavonols, Lignans, and Caffeic Acid Derivatives from *Dracocephalum moldavica* and Their In Vitro Effects on Multiple Myeloma and Acute Myeloid Leukemia

Karin Jöhrer [1], Mayra Galarza Pérez [2], Brigitte Kircher [1,3] and Serhat Sezai Çiçek [2,*]

1 Tyrolean Cancer Research Institute, Innrain 66, 6020 Innsbruck, Austria
2 Department of Pharmaceutical Biology, Kiel University, Gutenbergstraße 76, 24118 Kiel, Germany
3 Department of Internal Medicine V (Hematology and Oncology), Medical University Innsbruck, Anichstraße 35, 6020 Innsbruck, Austria
* Correspondence: scicek@pharmazie.uni-kiel.de; Tel.: +49-431-880-1077

Abstract: Phenolic plant constituents are well known for their health-promoting and cancer chemopreventive properties, and products containing such constituents are therefore readily consumed. In the present work, we isolated 13 phenolic constituents of four different compound classes from the aerial parts of the Moldavian dragonhead, an aromatic and medicinal plant with a high diversity on secondary metabolites. All compounds were tested for their apoptotic effect on myeloma (KMS-12-PE) and AML (Molm-13) cells, with the highest activity observed for the flavone and flavonol derivatives. While diosmetin (**6**) exhibited the most pronounced effects on the myeloma cell line, two polymethylated flavones, namely cirsimaritin (**1**) and xanthomicrol (**3**), were particularly active against AML cells and therefore subsequently investigated for their antiproliferative effects at lower concentrations. At a concentration of 2.5 μM, cirsimaritin (**1**) reduced proliferation of Molm-13 cells by 72% while xanthomicrol (**3**) even inhibited proliferation to the extent of 84% of control. In addition, both compounds were identified as potent FLT3 inhibitors and thus display promising lead structures for further drug development. Moreover, our results confirmed the chemopreventive properties of flavonoids in general, and in particular of polymethylated flavones, which have been intensively investigated especially over the last decade.

Keywords: hematologic cancer; FLT3 inhibitor; natural product; cytotoxicity; apoptosis; structure-activity relationship; apigenin; luteolin; quercetin; kaempferol

Citation: Jöhrer, K.; Galarza Pérez, M.; Kircher, B.; Çiçek, S.S. Flavones, Flavonols, Lignans, and Caffeic Acid Derivatives from *Dracocephalum moldavica* and Their In Vitro Effects on Multiple Myeloma and Acute Myeloid Leukemia. *Int. J. Mol. Sci.* **2022**, 23, 14219. https://doi.org/10.3390/ijms232214219

Academic Editors: Barbara De Filippis, Marialuigia Fantacuzzi, Alessandra Ammazzalorso and Haifa Kathrin Al-Ali

Received: 30 August 2022
Accepted: 15 November 2022
Published: 17 November 2022

1. Introduction

Multiple myeloma (MM) is a hematologic malignancy where mature B-cells, i.e., plasma cells, proliferate extensively within the bone marrow [1]. Myeloma cells display a variety of genetic aberrations and, especially upon treatment, resistant clones are selected which finally leads to disease relapse in most patients. Likewise, acute myeloid leukemia (AML) is a heterogenous hematologic disorder caused by multiple genetic abnormalities that occur in the myeloid precursor cells within the bone marrow [2]. Both diseases predominantly affect the bone marrow of patients. Although several treatment lines are available for myeloma and AML, relapses are usual and most patients finally succumb to their disease. Thus, novel therapies are urgently needed.

In our ongoing search for new lead compounds in the treatment of hematologic cancers [3–5], we investigated the aerial parts of *Dracocephalum moldavica* L. (Lamiaceae), one of 74 accepted species of the dragonhead genus [6]. *D. moldavica* can be found on mountains and in semiarid areas of Europe and Asia, where it has been used as a folk medicine for treating various chronic diseases, such as cardiac disease, hypertension, atherosclerosis, asthma, and other oxidative-stress related disorders [7–10]. Extensive phytochemical studies on its metabolome revealed a plethora of chemical constituents from different compound classes, including alkaloids, coumarins, cyanogenic glucosides, flavonoids, phenylpropanoids, polysaccharides, and terpenoids, which showed anti-inflammatory, antioxidant, and antitumor activities [10–15]. The variety of potential drug candidates and the activity of a crude acetone extract against Molm-13 and KMS-12-PE cells prompted us to further investigate this interesting plant species. In the present work, 13 constituents from four different compound classes were isolated and subsequently evaluated for their effects on the above-mentioned myeloma and AML cell lines.

2. Results and Discussion

2.1. Isolation and Identification

Exhaustive extraction followed by liquid–liquid partitioning and repeated chromatographic separation led to the isolation of six flavones (**1–6**), two flavonols (**7** and **8**), two lignans (**9** and **10**), and three caffeic acid derivatives (**11–13**) (Figures 1 and S1). After comparison of MS and NMR data and optical rotation values (see Supporting Information) with the values reported in the literature, the compounds were identified as cirsimaritin (**1**) [16], 5-desmethylsinensetin (**2**) [17], xanthomicrol (**3**) [18], apigenin (**4**) [19], luteolin (**5**) [20], diosmetin (**6**) [21], kaempferol (**7**) [19], quercetin (**8**) [22], (+)-piperitol (**9**) [23], (+)-9α-hydroxysesamin (**10**) [24], caffeic acid (**11**) [25], (R)-(+)-rosmarinic acid (**12**) [26], and (R)-(+)-3′-O-methylrosmarinic acid (**13**) [27].

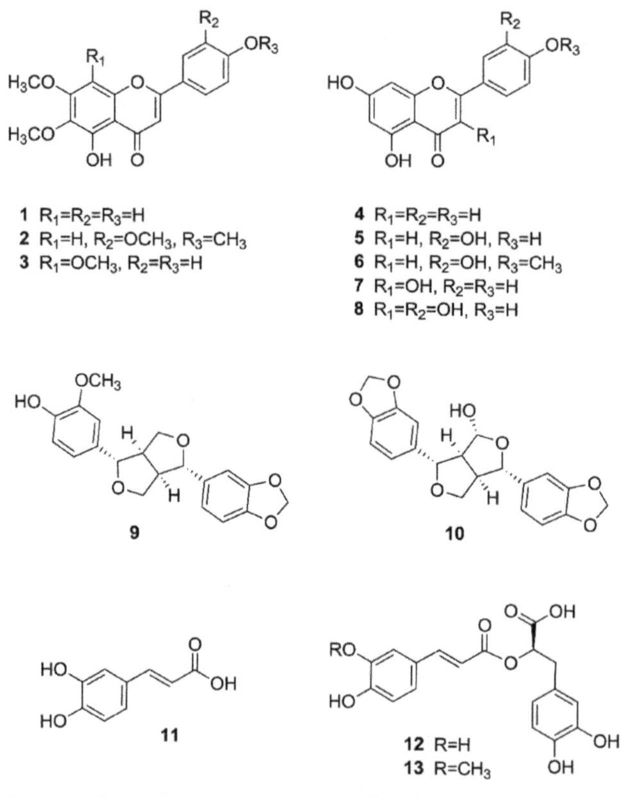

Figure 1. Chemical structures of compounds isolated from *D. moldavica*.

2.2. Biological Activity

All isolated substances were tested at different concentrations for their potential to induce programmed cell death (apoptosis) in myeloma cells and AML cells (Figure 2, Table 1).

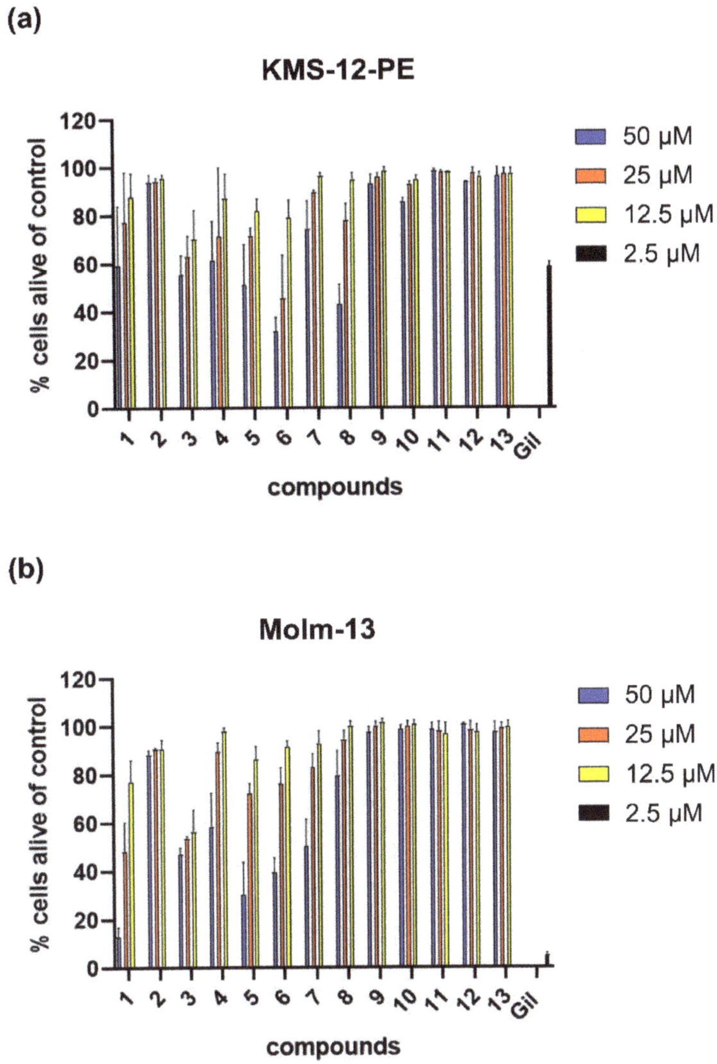

Figure 2. Apoptosis of cancer cells after treatment with isolated compounds. Percentage of cells alive after treatment with compounds **1** to **13**: (**a**) KMS-12-PE and (**b**) Molm-13 cells were treated with indicated concentrations (50 µM/25 µM/12.5 µM) of compounds for 48 h. Gilteritinib (2.5 µM) was used as positive control. Cell survival was measured by calculating cells which did not stain with AnnexinV/PI in comparison to untreated controls. Mean +/− SD of 2–4 independent experiments in duplicates are shown.

While no cytotoxic effect was found for lignans and caffeic acid derivatives, five out of six flavones (**1** and **3–6**) and both flavonols (**7** and **8**) induced apoptosis in both cancer cell types in a dose-dependent and time-dependent manner. In the KMS-12-PE cell line, the effects were more pronounced for the flavone compounds (except **2**) generally being more apoptotic than the flavonols, which were not active at the lowest concentration. With an EC_{50} value of 26 µM, diosmetin (**6**) was the most potent compound on the KMS-12-PE cell line.

Table 1. Results of apoptosis measurements on KMS-12-PE and Molm-13 cells after treatment with different compounds and concentrations for 48 h. Results are given in percentage of cells alive of control. Number of independent experiments is given in parentheses. EC_{50} values were calculated using the "best-fit" model and are given in µM.

		KMS-12-PE		Molm-13	
Compound	**Concentration**	**% Alive**	**EC_{50}**	**% Alive**	**EC_{50}**
1	50 µM 25 µM 12.5 µM	58.9 ± 28.6 (4) 76.6 ± 25.6 (4) 86.8 ± 14.5 (4)	>50	12.9 ± 4.1 (4) 48.4 ± 12.0 (4) 77.3 ± 9.0 (4)	21.74
2	50 µM 25 µM 12.5 µM	93.1 ± 10.2 (3) 93.4 ± 9.3 (3) 94.6 ± 10.2 (3)	>50	88.6 ± 1.8 (2) 90.9 ± 0.4 (2) 91.1 ± 3.4 (2)	>50
3	50 µM 25 µM 12.5 µM	55.4 ± 13.1 (4) 62.6 ± 13.1 (4) 69.5 ± 16.0 (4)	45.39	47.0 ± 2.7 (4) 53.5 ± 1.0 (4) 56.4 ± 9.1 (4)	27.98
4	50 µM 25 µM 12.5 µM	59.6 ± 16.1 (4) 69.4 ± 31.3 (4) 85.5 ± 10.6 (4)	>50	58.4 ± 14.2 (4) 89.5 ± 3.9 (4) 98.0 ± 1.6 (4)	>50
5	50 µM 25 µM 12.5 µM	50.3 ± 18.4 (4) 70.5 ± 5.6 (4) 80.3 ± 5.4 (4)	>50	30.2 ± 13.7 (4) 72.4 ± 4.0 (4) 86.5 ± 5.2 (4)	42.31
6	50 µM 25 µM 12.5 µM	31.1 ± 5.3 (4) 44.2 ± 19.0 (4) 77.3 ± 6.9 (4)	25.65	39.8 ± 5.8 (4) 76.2 ± 6.7 (4) 91.5 ± 2.8 (4)	>50
7	50 µM 25 µM 12.5 µM	76.3 ± 17.3 (3) 91.2 ± 15.0 (3) 98.0 ± 2.7 (3)	>50	50.2 ± 11.4 (4) 83.1 ± 5.7 (4) 93.1 ± 5.1 (4)	>50
8	50 µM 25 µM 12.5 µM	43.7 ± 8.3 (3) 79.0 ± 4.8 (3) 96.6 ± 2.7 (3)	>50	79.8 ± 10.2 (4) 94.4 ± 3.9 (4) 100.1 ± 2.2 (4)	>50
9	50 µM 25 µM 12.5 µM	97.1 ± 4.1 (2) 100.1 ± 0.8 (2) 102.8 ± 0.8 (2)	>50	97.5 ± 2.4 (2) 100.0 ± 2.1 (2) 101.8 ± 1.3 (2)	>50
10	50 µM 25 µM 12.5 µM	89.4 ± 0.8 (2) 96.7 ± 0.5 (2) 99.0 ± 0.6 (2)	>50	98.7 ± 1.7 (2) 100.2 ± 2.0 (2) 101.1 ± 1.4 (2)	>50
11	50 µM 25 µM 12.5 µM	102.6 ± 0.5 (2) 102.5 ± 0.9 (2) 102.3 ± 1.8 (2)	>50	98.8 ± 2.8 (2) 98.1 ± 3.8 (2) 96.9 ± 4.6 (2)	>50
12	50 µM 25 µM 12.5 µM	98.2 ± 1.5 (2) 101.6 ± 1.5 (2) 100.2 ± 0.9 (2)	>50	100.8 ± 0.6 (2) 98.5 ± 3.6 (2) 97.6 ± 3.2 (2)	>50
13	50 µM 25 µM 12.5 µM	100.7 ± 3.4 (2) 101.3 ± 1.8 (2) 101.5 ± 1.6 (2)	>50	97.8 ± 4.0 (2) 99.4 ± 1.9 (2) 99.6 ± 2.6 (2)	>50

For the AML cell line Molm-13, the overall picture was similar, also showing stronger apoptotic effects for the flavone components. However, even more evident was the higher activity of the two polymethylated derivatives, cirsimaritin (**1**) and xanthomicrol (**3**), compared to the other flavone (and flavonol) derivatives, with EC_{50} values of around 22 µM (**1**) and 28 µM (**3**). The latter two compounds were further investigated at lower concentrations in proliferation assays (Figure 3).

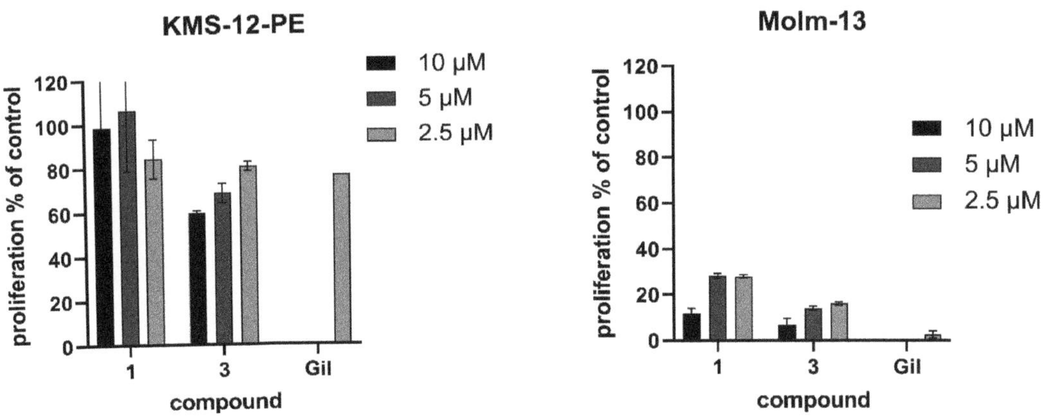

(a) (b)

Figure 3. Proliferation of cancer cells after treatment with selected compounds. Percentage of proliferation after treatment with different compounds for 48 h was measured with a modified MTT assay. (**a**) KMS-12-PE and (**b**) Molm-13 cells were treated with indicated concentrations (10 µM/5 µM/2.5 µM) of compounds **1** and **3** and gilteritinib (2.5 µM) as positive control. Percentage of proliferation was calculated compared to untreated (set at 100%). Mean +/− SD of 3 (AML)—2 (MM) independent experiments are shown.

At concentrations ranging from 10 to 2.5 µM, cirsimaritin (**1**) and xanthomicrol (**3**) induced an inhibition of proliferation, which was marginally in the myeloma cell line but clearly induced in AML cells. Here, cirsimaritin (**1**) was inhibiting proliferation to an extent of 88 to 72% compared to untreated cells, while xanthomicrol (**3**) showed an inhibition of up to 93% (and of still 84% at a concentration of 2.5 µM). The FLT3 inhibitor gilteritinib was added as a positive control and showed high effect on AML cells but not on myeloma cells. These clear anticancer effects on AML cells at reasonably low and certainly further titratable concentrations are promising and warrant further testing.

Polymethylated flavones were previously found to inhibit the FLT3 pathway in a study on 45 natural and synthetic flavonoids using AML cell lines Molm-13 and MV-4-11 [27]. This specific potential to inhibit FLT3 is of major interest for AML. Cells harboring an activating mutation in FLT3 represent approximately one third of the AML cases, and activation of FLT3 is a risk factor for high relapse and bad prognosis [28,29]. Gilteritinib, a second-generation FLT3 inhibitor, is approved for relapsed/refractory FLT3 + AML. However, the FLT3 pathway can also play an important role in multiple myeloma.

In our previous work [30], we found that MM patients with advanced disease showed high levels of FLT3 ligand in the blood and bone marrow. In addition, we could show that the FLT3-receptor is overexpressed in a subgroup of MM patients and this overexpression correlated with inferior prognosis [31]. Inhibitors of FLT3 (midostaurin, gilteritinib) demonstrated anti-myeloma activity in vitro. Therefore, we are especially interested in novel inhibitors of FLT3 and further testing of xanthomicrol (**3**) and cirsimaritin (**1**) on primary myeloma cells is guaranteed. The lack of significant effects of compound **1** and the smaller effect of compound **3** on the tested MM cell line (KMS-12-PE) compared to AML cells might be explained by its lower dependence on the FLT3 pathway. This is corroborated by the fact that also second generation FLT3 inhibitor, gilteritinib, had a lower effect on this myeloma cell proliferation.

Regarding the structural requirements for FLT3 inhibition, Yen et al. investigated five subclasses of flavonoids [27]. Thereby, the average inhibitions were highest for flavonols, flavones, and chalcones, all of which show a planar chromone substructure. In contrast, the tested flavanones and prenylflavanones were not effective. Apart from the planar structure, several other necessary structural features for FLT3 inhibition were identified by molecular docking studies, such as a carbonyl group in position 4, a hydroxy group in position 3 or 5, a hydroxy or methoxy group in position 4′, as well as a hydroxy group in position 7. Except for the last point, all of these structural features are fulfilled by cirsimaritin (**1**) and xanthomicrol (**3**). Therefore, we investigated both compounds on their potential to reduce FLT3 kinase activity. Cirsimaritin (**1**) and xanthomicrol (**3**) effectively inhibited FLT3 kinase at concentrations of 25 to 6.25 nM, with inhibition rates of 81% (**1**) and 88% (**3**) of 20 ng protein at the lowest concentration.

With the results of our study, we could identify two novel FLT3 inhibitors of flavonoid origin. Moreover, additional findings can now be added to the structural requirements for FLT3 binding. One such finding becomes evident while looking at the structure of compound **2**, which differs from salvigenin, the second most active compound in the study of Yen et al. [27], by only one methoxy group in position 3 and which showed no effects in any of the tested cell lines. The negative effect of this additional methoxy group is corroborated by the results of the other flavonoids with this feature in the study of Yen et al., which also showed much lower activities.

An even more interesting structural feature is indicated by xanthomicrol (**3**), which possesses an additional methoxy group in position 8. This specific feature did not seem to reduce the cytotoxic effects and therefore the structure of xanthomicrol (**3**) might as well be proposed as a valuable lead compound for further optimization. Not only because this specific structural feature was missing in the study by Yen et al., but because methoxylated flavonoids are not as common as their unmethoxylated counterparts, and those bearing several methoxy groups are even more rare [32].

This particular subgroup of flavonoids, which is also referred to as polymethylated or polymethoxylated flavonoids (PMFs), became of increased interest over the last decade [32,33]; firstly, because many PMFs exhibit pronounced cancer chemopreventive properties and secondly, because they show a dramatically increased bioavailability compared to unmethylated flavonoids [34,35]. The higher bioavailability of PMFs results from a lower polarity and thus an elevated membrane penetration, as well as an increased metabolic stability caused by hindered glucuronidation and sulfation processes [35].

Nevertheless, unmethylated or monomethylated flavonoids, such as diosmetin (**6**), also contribute towards cancer chemoprevention. Even though they may show lower effects in vitro and decreased bioavailability, they are much more abundant in the plant kingdom and in our daily nutrition and are therefore consumed in significantly higher amounts. Thus, not only the discovery of a new potent lead structure for AML treatment (**3**), but also the results obtained for the more common flavonoids (**4** to **8**) are of interest. Following our report on the activity of apigenin (**4**) and luteolin (**5**) and some of their glycosides against myeloma cell lines NCI-H929, U266, and OPM2 [5], our present study demonstrates their activity against KMS-12-PE cells and the AML cell line Molm-13. In addition, cytotoxic effects of the highly abundant flavonols kaempferol (**7**) and quercetin (**8**) are presented in our study.

Due to their high abundance and availability, these compounds have been the target of repeated investigations for their cytotoxic and anticancer effects [36]. Apart from their antioxidant properties, apigenin (**4**) and quercetin (**8**) were found to modulate a number of signaling pathways involved in carcinogenesis, with apigenin also being suggested as a general cancer medication [37–39]. In addition, for luteolin (**5**), interesting antitumor effects have been discovered, which showed the compound to suppress metastasis in breast and colorectal cancer cells [40,41].

Summarizing, our study reveals new data for the chemopreventive effects of several prominent and some more particular flavonoids against multiple myeloma and acute myeloid leukemia. While diosmetin (**6**) was effective against myeloma cell line KMS-12-PE, two compounds (**1** and **3**) showed pronounced effects on AML cell line Molm-13, also at lower concentrations. Thereby, the latter two compounds, namely cirsimaritin (**1**) and xanthomicrol (**3**), were identified as novel FLT3 inhibitors.

3. Materials and Methods

3.1. Plant Material, Reagents and Experimental Procedures

Dried aerial parts (leaves and flowers) of *D. moldavica* were obtained from Dr. Vasilica Onofrei of the University of Agricultural Sciences and Veterinary Medicine, Faculty of Agriculture, in Iaşi, Romania. LC–MS grade acetonitrile and water and other (analytical grade) solvents and reagents were purchased from VWR International GmbH (Darmstadt, Germany). LC–MS grade formic acid was obtained from Sigma Aldrich Co. (St. Louis, MO, USA). Water used for isolation was twice distilled in-house. DMSO-d_6 (99.80%, Lot S1051, Batch 0119E) and MeOH-d_4 (99.80%, Lot P3021, Batch 1016B) for NMR spectroscopy were purchased from Euriso-top GmbH, Saarbrücken, Germany. TLC was performed on silica gel 60 F254 plates (VWR International, Darmstadt, Germany) using toluene-ethyl acetate-formic acid (5.5:3.5:1) as the mobile phase and vanillin-sulphuric acid for detection. Flash chromatography was carried out with a Büchi PrepChrom C-700 chromatograph using a FlashPure EcoFlex Silica Gel SL cartridge (100 g/135 mL, irregular 40–63 µm particle size, Büchi Labortechnik GmbH, Essen, Germany). Column chromatography was performed with Sephadex LH-20 (GE Healthcare AB, Uppsala, Sweden). Semi-preparative HPLC was carried out on a Waters Alliance e2695 Separations Module coupled to a 2998 Photodiode Array detector and a WFC III fraction collector using a Phenomenex Aqua column (5 µm. 250 × 10.0 mm). Extracts, fractions, and pure compounds were analyzed on a Shimadzu Nexera 2 liquid chromatograph connected to an LC–MS triple quadrupole mass spectrometer with electrospray ionization (Shimadzu, Kyoto, Japan). A Phenomenex Luna Omega C18 column (100 × 2.1 mm, 1.6 µm particle size, Phenomenex, Aschaffenburg, Germany) was used for separation. 1D (^{1}H, ^{13}C) and 2D (HSQC, HMBC, COSY) NMR spectra were recorded on a Bruker Avance III 400 NMR spectrometer operating at 400 MHz for the proton channel and 100 MHz for the ^{13}C channel with a 5 mm PABBO broad band probe with a z gradient unit at 298 K (Bruker BioSpin GmbH, Rheinstetten, Germany). Reference values were 2.50 (^{1}H) and 39.51 ppm (^{13}C) for dimethyl sulfoxide as well as 3.31 (^{1}H) and 49.15 ppm (^{13}C) for MeOH, respectively. Structure elucidation and spectra simulations were performed using the Topspin 3.6 software (Bruker Biospin GmbH, Rheinstetten, Germany). 5 mm NMR sample tubes were obtained from Rototec-Spintec GmbH, Griesheim, Germany. The specific rotation of compounds was measured on a Jasco P-2000 polarimeter (Jasco, Pfungstadt, Germany).

3.2. Extraction and Isolation

1140 g of dried plant material were ground and extracted five times with 6 L of an 85% aqueous acetone solution using ultrasonication followed by 24 h of maceration. The acetone was evaporated under reduced pressure and the remaining aqueous solution (2224 mL) was extracted five times with 500 mL of dichloromethane to afford 9.021 g of extract. The extract was subjected to flash chromatography using silica gel as the stationary phase and a mixture of *n*-hexane (A) and acetone (B) as the mobile phase with the following gradient: 1%B to 2%B in 10 min, to 5%B in 10 min, to 10%B in 10 min, to 20%B in 10 min, to 33%B in 10 min and to 50%B in 40 min. Of the resulting ten fractions (A–J), fractions H (1389 mg) and J (1097 mg) were further processed. Fraction H was subjected to Sephadex LH-20 chromatography (100 × 3 cm) and methanol as the solvent to give eleven fractions (H1–H11). Fraction H9 (30.74 mg) was subjected to semi-preparative chromatography using a mixture of 0.025% formic acid and acetonitrile (55:45) to give 3.30 mg of 5-desmethylsinensetin (**2**), 11.99 mg of xanthomicrol (**3**), and 3.69 mg of (+)-piperitol (**9**). Fraction H10 (16.58 mg) was chromatographed in the same manner to yield 3.46 mg of cirsimaritin (**1**), 8.6 mg of 9α-hydroxysesamin (**10**), and another 2.93 mg of xanthomicrol (**3**). Fraction J was also subjected to Sephadex LH-20 chromatography (100 × 3 cm) and methanol as the solvent to give 16 fractions (J1–J16). Fraction J12 (30.80 mg) was subjected to semi-preparative chromatography using a mixture of 0.025% formic acid and acetonitrile (70:30) to give 4.06 mg of caffeic acid (**11**), 3.31 mg of rosmarinic acid (**12**), and 5.44 mg of 3-methylrosmarinic acid (**13**). Fraction J14 (25.19 mg) was subjected to semi-preparative chromatography using a mixture of 0.025% formic acid and acetonitrile (65:35) to yield 3.02 mg of apigenin (**4**), 2.86 mg of luteolin (**5**), and 4.85 mg of diosmetin (**6**). Fraction J15 (12.74 mg) was subjected to semi-preparative chromatography using a mixture of 0.025% formic acid and acetonitrile (55:45) to give 3.25 mg of kaempferol (**7**) and another 4.38 mg of luteolin (**5**). Fraction J16 (16.29 mg) was subjected to Sephadex LH-20 chromatography (100 × 1 cm) using methanol as the solvent yielding 11.47 mg of quercetin (**8**).

3.3. *Cytotoxicity Assays, Proliferation Assays, and FLT3 Kinase Assay*

Cytotoxicity was measured as induction of apoptosis in myeloma cell line KMS-12-PE and AML cell line Molm-13, staining the cells with AnnexinV-fluorescein isothiocyanate (AnnexinV-FITC) and propidium iodide (PI). Cell lines were purchased from DSMZ (Braunschweig, Germany) and routinely fingerprinted and tested for mycoplasma negativity. All cell lines were grown in RPMI-1640 medium (Life Technologies, Paisley, UK), and supplemented with 10% fetal calf serum (FCS; PAA, Linz, Austria), L-glutamine 100 μg/mL, and penicillin-streptomycin 100 U/mL. Compounds were dissolved in DMSO at a stock concentration of 50 mM and stored at −20 °C. Briefly, 0.5 × 10^6 cancer cells/mL were incubated for 24 h and 48 h with or without the tested compounds at indicated concentrations. Analyses were performed in duplicates and a solvent control was included. The extent of non-apoptotic cells (AnnexinV/propidium iodide negativity) was calculated as the percentage of viable cells in respect to the untreated control. Data are shown as the mean percentage of viable cells +/− standard deviation (SD) (error bars).

Proliferation was measured using a modified MTT assay (EZ4U kit, Biomedica, Vienna, Austria) according to the manufacturer's instructions. In brief, 2.5 × 10^4 (Molm-13)—5.0 × 10^4 cells (KMS-12-PE cells) were seeded in 96-well plates and substances were added as indicated. Different concentrations are due to the different doubling time of the cells (24 h vs. 48 h). Cells were incubated for 48 h and during the last 7 h of incubation, 3-(4,5-dimethylthiazol-2-yl)-2,5-diphenyltetrazolium bromide was added as a substrate. Reduction of the tetrazolium salt to formazan by the mitochondrial activity of the growing cells was measured as optical density at 492 nm (with 620 nm as reference) on a plate reader. Proliferation (mean +/− SD) was calculated as the percentage of control (without substances). Concentrations used were 10 μM/5 μM/2.5 μM for all substances. Gilteritinib was used as a positive control at 2.5 μM.

FLT3 inhibitory activity of compounds **1** and **3** was determined using the Z′-LYTE screening protocol. Z′-LYTE Kinase Assay—Tyrosine 2 Peptide Kit and FLT3 were purchased from Thermo Fisher Scientific Inc. (Waltham, MA, USA). The assay was performed according to the manufacturer's instructions using a kinase buffer (50 mM HEPES pH 7.5, 0.01% BRIJ-35, 10 mM $MgCl_2$, 1 mM EGTA) containing 0.01 to 20 ng of FLT3. Compounds were measured at concentrations of 50 nM/25 nM/12.5 nM/6.25 nM using gilteritinib as a positive control.

4. Conclusions

In the present study, a series of phenolic compounds was studied for their activity against myeloma cell line KMS-12-PE and AML cell line Molm-13. Of the 13 tested compounds, five out of six flavones (**1**, **3–6**), and the two investigated flavonols, kaempferol (**7**) and quercetin (**8**), induced apoptosis in a dose-dependent manner, confirming once more the broad chemoprotective potential of flavonoids in carcinogenesis. The two polymethylated flavones, cirsimaritin (**1**) and xanthomicrol (**3**), were further examined for their antiproliferative effects at lower concentrations and showed clear impact on the AML cell line. Subsequent experiments revealed both compounds to effectively inhibit FLT3 kinase activity, which will be further examined in future studies.

Supplementary Materials: The following supporting information can be downloaded at: https://www.mdpi.com/article/10.3390/ijms232214219/s1.

Author Contributions: Conceptualization, S.S.Ç. and K.J.; investigation, S.S.Ç., M.G.P., B.K., and K.J.; writing—original draft preparation, S.S.Ç. and K.J.; writing—review and editing, K.J. and S.S.Ç. All authors have read and agreed to the published version of the manuscript.

Funding: The authors acknowledge financial support by the DFG within the funding program "Open Access-Publikationskosten".

Institutional Review Board Statement: Not applicable.

Informed Consent Statement: Not applicable.

Data Availability Statement: Not applicable.

Acknowledgments: The authors thank Claudia Ramisch for the extraction and fractionation of the compounds.

Conflicts of Interest: The authors declare no conflict of interest.

References

1. Abdallah, N.; Rajkumar, S.V.; Greipp, P.; Kapoor, P.; Gertz, M.A.; Dispenzieri, A.; Baughn, L.B.; Lacy, M.Q.; Hayman, S.R.; Buadi, F.K.; et al. Cytogenetic Abnormalities in Multiple Myeloma: Association with Disease Characteristics and Treatment Response. *Blood Cancer J.* **2020**, *10*, 82. [CrossRef]
2. Döhner, H.; Estey, E.; Grimwade, D.; Amadori, S.; Appelbaum, F.R.; Büchner, T.; Dombret, H.; Ebert, B.L.; Fenaux, P.; Larson, R.A.; et al. Diagnosis and Management of AML in Adults: 2017 ELN Recommendations from an International Expert Panel. *Blood* **2017**, *129*, 424–447. [CrossRef] [PubMed]
3. Willer, J.; Jöhrer, K.; Greil, R.; Zidorn, C.; Çiçek, S.S. Cytotoxic Properties of Damiana (*Turnera diffusa*) Extracts and Constituents and A Validated Quantitative UHPLC-DAD Assay. *Molecules* **2019**, *24*, 855. [CrossRef] [PubMed]
4. Jöhrer, K.; Stuppner, H.; Greil, R.; Çiçek, S.S. Structure-Guided Identification of Black Cohosh (*Actaea racemosa*) Triterpenoids with In Vitro Activity against Multiple Myeloma. *Molecules* **2020**, *25*, 766. [CrossRef] [PubMed]
5. Çiçek, S.S.; Willer, J.; Preziuso, F.; Sönnichsen, F.; Greil, R.; Girreser, U.; Zidorn, C.; Jöhrer, K. Cytotoxic Constituents and a New Hydroxycinnamic Acid Derivative from *Leontodon saxatilis* (Asteraceae, Cichorieae). *RSC Adv.* **2021**, *11*, 10489–10496. [CrossRef]
6. The Plant List. Version 1.1. Available online: http://www.theplantlist.org/ (accessed on 15 August 2022).
7. Cao, W.; Hu, N.; Yuan, Y.; Cheng, J.; Guo, X.; Wang, Y.; Wang, X.; Hu, P. Effects of Tilianin on Proliferation, Migration and TGF-β/Smad Signaling in Rat Vascular Smooth Muscle Cells Induced with Angiotensin II. *Phytother. Res.* **2017**, *31*, 1240–1248. [CrossRef]
8. Wang, J.; Sun, J.; Wang, M.; Cui, H.; Zhou, W.; Li, G. Chemical Constituents from *Dracocephalum moldavica* L. and Their Chemotaxonomic Significance. *Biochem. Syst. Ecol.* **2022**, *102*, 104422. [CrossRef]
9. Zhang, H.; Xu, L.; Liu, X.; Fan, J.; Wang, X.; Shen, T.; Wang, S.; Ren, D. Dracomolphesin A–E, Five 3,4-Seco-Phenylpropanoids with Nrf2 Inducing Activity from *Dracocephalum moldavica*. *Chin. Chem. Lett.* **2020**, *31*, 1259–1262. [CrossRef]
10. Zeng, Q.; Jin, H.-Z.; Qin, J.-J.; Fu, J.-J.; Hu, X.-J.; Liu, J.-H.; Yan, L.; Chen, M.; Zhang, W.-D. Chemical Constituents of Plants from the Genus *Dracocephalum*. *Chem. Biodivers.* **2010**, *7*, 1911–1929. [CrossRef]
11. Yang, L.-N.; Xing, J.-G.; He, C.-H.; Wu, T. The Phenolic Compounds from *Dracocephalum moldavica* L. *Biochem. Syst. Ecol.* **2014**, *54*, 19–22. [CrossRef]
12. Zhang, J.-L.; Yan, R.-J.; Yu, N.; Zhang, X.; Chen, D.-J.; Wu, T.; Xin, J.-G. A New Caffeic Acid Tetramer from the *Dracocephalum moldavica* L. *Nat. Prod. Res.* **2018**, *32*, 370–373. [CrossRef] [PubMed]
13. Tan, M.; He, C.; Jiang, W.; Zeng, C.; Yu, N.; Huang, W.; Gao, Z.; Xing, J. Development of Solid Lipid Nanoparticles Containing Total Flavonoid Extract from *Dracocephalum moldavica* L. and Their Therapeutic Effect against Myocardial Ischemia-Reperfusion Injury in Rats. *Int. J. Nanomed.* **2017**, *12*, 3253–3265. [CrossRef] [PubMed]
14. Hu, Z.; Wang, J.; Jin, L.; Duan, Y.; Zhang, X.; Sun, J.; Zhou, W.; Li, G. Isolation and Structural Characterization of Two Polysaccharides from *Dracocephalum moldavica* and Their Anti-Complementary Activity. *Chem. Biodivers.* **2022**, *19*, e202200294. [CrossRef]
15. Nie, L.; Li, R.; Huang, J.; Wang, L.; Ma, M.; Huang, C.; Wu, T.; Yan, R.; Hu, X. Abietane Diterpenoids from *Dracocephalum moldavica* L. and Their Anti-Inflammatory Activities in Vitro. *Phytochemistry* **2021**, *184*, 112680. [CrossRef] [PubMed]
16. Bai, N.; He, K.; Roller, M.; Lai, C.-S.; Shao, X.; Pan, M.-H.; Bily, A.; Ho, C.-T. Flavonoid Glycosides from Microtea Debilis and Their Cytotoxic and Anti-Inflammatory Effects. *Fitoterapia* **2011**, *82*, 168–172. [CrossRef]
17. Zhao, H.-Y.; Yang, L.; Wei, J.; Huang, M.; Jiang, J.-G. Bioactivity Evaluations of Ingredients Extracted from the Flowers of *Citrus aurantium* L. Var. *Amara Engl. Food Chem.* **2012**, *135*, 2175–2181. [CrossRef]
18. El-Ansari, M.A.; Abdalla, M.F.; Saleh, N.A.M.; Barron, D.; Le Quéré, J.L. Flavonoid Constituents of *Stachys aegyptiaca*. *Phytochemistry* **1991**, *30*, 1169–1173. [CrossRef]
19. Xu, Y.; Tao, Z.; Jin, Y.; Yuan, Y.; Dong, T.T.X.; Tsim, K.W.K.; Zhou, Z. Flavonoids, a Potential New Insight of *Leucaena leucocephala* Foliage in Ruminant Health. *J. Agric. Food Chem.* **2018**, *66*, 7616–7626. [CrossRef]

20. Lin, L.-C.; Pai, Y.-F.; Tsai, T.-H. Isolation of Luteolin and Luteolin-7-O-Glucoside from *Dendranthema Morifolium* Ramat Tzvel and Their Pharmacokinetics in Rats. *J. Agric. Food Chem.* **2015**, *63*, 7700–7706. [CrossRef]
21. Kipchakbaeva, A.K.; Eskalieva, B.K.; Burasheva, G.S.; Aisa, H.A. Polyphenols from the Plant Climacoptera Korshinskyi. *Chem. Nat. Compd.* **2019**, *55*, 131–132. [CrossRef]
22. Yang, Z.; Wang, Y.; Wang, Y.; Zhang, Y. Bioassay-Guided Screening and Isolation of α-Glucosidase and Tyrosinase Inhibitors from Leaves of *Morus alba*. *Food Chem.* **2012**, *131*, 617–625. [CrossRef]
23. Iida, T.; Noro, Y.; Ito, K. Magnostellin A and B, Novel Lignans from Magnolia Stellata. *Phytochemistry* **1983**, *22*, 211–213. [CrossRef]
24. Wang, Y.; Zhang, L.-T.; Zhang, D.; Guo, S.-S.; Xi, C.; Du, S.-S. Repellent and Feeding Deterrent Activities of Butanolides and Lignans Isolated from *Cinnamomum camphora* against *Tribolium castaneum*. *J. Chem.* **2020**, *2020*, 5685294. [CrossRef]
25. Anh, L.T.T.; Son, N.T.; Van Tuyen, N.; Thuy, P.T.; Quan, P.M.; Ha, N.T.T.; Tra, N.T. Antioxidative and α-Glucosidase Inhibitory Constituents of *Polyscias guilfoylei*: Experimental and Computational Assessments. *Mol. Divers.* **2022**, *26*, 229–243. [CrossRef] [PubMed]
26. Khan, S.; Taning, C.N.T.; Bonneure, E.; Mangelinckx, S.; Smagghe, G.; Ahmad, R.; Fatima, N.; Asif, M.; Shah, M.M. Bioactivity-Guided Isolation of Rosmarinic Acid as the Principle Bioactive Compound from the Butanol Extract of *Isodon rugosus* against the Pea Aphid, *Acyrthosiphon pisum*. *PLoS ONE* **2019**, *14*, e0215048. [CrossRef]
27. Baba, S.; Osakabe, N.; Natsume, M.; Terao, J. Orally Administered Rosmarinic Acid Is Present as the Conjugated and/or Methylated Forms in Plasma, and Is Degraded and Metabolized to Conjugated Forms of Caffeic Acid, Ferulic Acid and m-Coumaric Acid. *Life Sci.* **2004**, *75*, 165–178. [CrossRef]
28. Yen, S.-C.; Chen, L.-C.; Huang, H.-L.; Ngo, S.-T.; Wu, Y.-W.; Lin, T.E.; Sung, T.-Y.; Lien, S.-T.; Tseng, H.-J.; Pan, S.-L.; et al. Investigation of Selected Flavonoid Derivatives as Potent FLT3 Inhibitors for the Potential Treatment of Acute Myeloid Leukemia. *J. Nat. Prod.* **2021**, *84*, 1–10. [CrossRef]
29. Arai, Y.; Chi, S.; Minami, Y.; Yanada, M. FLT3-Targeted Treatment for Acute Myeloid Leukemia. *Int. J. Hematol.* **2022**, *116*, 351–363. [CrossRef]
30. Acharya, B.; Saha, D.; Armstrong, D.; Lakkaniga, N.R.; Frett, B. FLT3 Inhibitors for Acute Myeloid Leukemia: Successes, Defeats, and Emerging Paradigms. *RSC Med. Chem.* **2022**, *13*, 798–816. [CrossRef]
31. Steiner, N.; Hajek, R.; Sevcikova, S.; Borjan, B.; Jöhrer, K.; Göbel, G.; Untergasser, G.; Gunsilius, E. High Levels of FLT3-Ligand in Bone Marrow and Peripheral Blood of Patients with Advanced Multiple Myeloma. *PLoS ONE* **2017**, *12*, e0181487. [CrossRef]
32. Steiner, N.; Jöhrer, K.; Plewan, S.; Brunner-Véber, A.; Göbel, G.; Nachbaur, D.; Wolf, D.; Gunsilius, E.; Untergasser, G. The FMS like Tyrosine Kinase 3 (FLT3) Is Overexpressed in a Subgroup of Multiple Myeloma Patients with Inferior Prognosis. *Cancers* **2020**, *12*, 2341. [CrossRef] [PubMed]
33. Murakami, A.; Ohigashi, H. Polymethylated Flavonoids: Cancer Preventive and Therapeutic Potentials Derived from Anti-Inflammatory and Drug Metabolism-Modifying Properties. In *Phytochemicals in Health and Disease*, 1st ed.; Bao, Y., Fenwick, R., Eds.; CRC Press: Boca Raton, FL, USA, 2004; pp. 169–192.
34. Guo, L.; Li, Y.; Mao, X.; Tao, R.; Tao, B.; Zhou, Z. Antifungal Activity of Polymethoxylated Flavonoids (PMFs)-Loaded Citral Nanoemulsion against *Penicillium italicum* by Causing Cell Membrane Damage. *J. Fungi* **2022**, *8*, 388. [CrossRef]
35. Park, E.-J.; Pezzuto, J.M. Flavonoids in Cancer Prevention. *Anti-Cancer Agents Med. Chem.* **2012**, *12*, 836–851. [CrossRef] [PubMed]
36. Walle, T. Methoxylated Flavones, a Superior Cancer Chemopreventive Flavonoid Subclass? *Semin. Cancer Biol.* **2007**, *17*, 354–362. [CrossRef] [PubMed]
37. Jöhrer, K.; Çiçek, S.S. Multiple Myeloma Inhibitory Activity of Plant Natural Products. *Cancers* **2021**, *13*, 2678. [CrossRef]
38. Almatroodi, S.A.; Alsahli, M.A.; Almatroudi, A.; Verma, A.K.; Aloliqi, A.; Allemailem, K.S.; Khan, A.A.; Rahmani, A.H. Potential Therapeutic Targets of Quercetin, a Plant Flavonol, and Its Role in the Therapy of Various Types of Cancer through the Modulation of Various Cell Signaling Pathways. *Molecules* **2021**, *26*, 1315. [CrossRef]
39. Ahmed, S.A.; Parama, D.; Daimari, E.; Girisa, S.; Banik, K.; Harsha, C.; Dutta, U.; Kunnumakkara, A.B. Rationalizing the Therapeutic Potential of Apigenin against Cancer. *Life Sci.* **2021**, *267*, 118814. [CrossRef]
40. Feng, J.; Zheng, T.; Hou, Z.; Lv, C.; Xue, A.; Han, T.; Han, B.; Sun, X.; Wei, Y. Luteolin, an Aryl Hydrocarbon Receptor Ligand, Suppresses Tumor Metastasis in Vitro and in Vivo. *Oncol. Rep.* **2020**, *44*, 2231–2240. [CrossRef]
41. Yao, Y.; Rao, C.; Zheng, G.; Wang, S. Luteolin Suppresses Colorectal Cancer Cell Metastasis via Regulation of the MiR-384/Pleiotrophin Axis. *Oncol. Rep.* **2019**, *42*, 131–141. [CrossRef]

International Journal of
Molecular Sciences

MDPI

Article

Anti-Cancer Effects of a New Herbal Medicine PSY by Inhibiting the STAT3 Signaling Pathway in Colorectal Cancer Cells and Its Phytochemical Analysis

Sanghee Han [1], Hail Kim [1], Min Young Lee [2], Junhee Lee [1,2], Kwang Seok Ahn [1], In Jin Ha [1,2,*] and Seok-Geun Lee [1,2,3,*]

1 Graduate School, Kyung Hee University, Seoul 02447, Republic of Korea
2 Korean Medicine Clinical Trial Center, Kyung Hee University Korean Medicine Hospital, Seoul 02454, Republic of Korea
3 BioNanocomposite Research Center, Kyung Hee University, Seoul 02447, Republic of Korea
* Correspondence: ijha@khu.ac.kr (I.J.H.); seokgeun@khu.ac.kr (S.-G.L.); Tel.: +82-958-9493 (I.J.H.); +82-2-961-2355 (S.-G.L.)

Abstract: Colorectal cancer (CRC) is an inflammation-associated common cancer worldwide. Paejangsan and Mori Cortex Radicis have been traditionally used for treating intestinal inflammatory diseases in Korea and China. In the present study, we developed a new herbal formula as an alternative to CRC treatments, which is composed of two main components of Paejangsan (Patriniae Radix (Paejang in Korean) and Coix Seed (Yiyiin in Korean)), and Mori Cortex Radicis (Sangbekpi in Korean) based on the addition and subtraction theory in traditional medicine, hence the name PSY, and explored the potential therapeutic effects of the new formula PSY in human CRC cells by analyzing viability, cell cycle and apoptosis. We found that PSY ethanol extract (EtOH-Ex), but not water extract, significantly suppressed the viability of human CRC cells, and synergistically decreased the cell proliferation compared to each treatment of Patriniae Radix and Coix Seed extract (PY) or Mori Cortex Radicis extract (S), suggesting the combination of PY and S in a 10-to-3 ratio for the formula PSY. PSY EtOH-Ex in the combination ratio reduced cell viability but induced cell cycle arrest at the G_2/M and sub-G_1 phases as well as apoptosis in CRC cells. In addition, the experimental results of Western blotting, immunofluorescence staining and reporter assays showed that PSY also inhibited STAT3 by reducing its phosphorylation and nuclear localization, which resulted in lowering STAT3-mediated transcriptional activation. In addition, PSY regulated upstream signaling molecules of STAT3 by inactivating JAK2 and Src and increasing SHP1. Moreover, the chemical profiles of PSY from UPLC-ESI-QTOF MS/MS analysis revealed 38 phytochemicals, including seven organic acids, eight iridoids, two lignans, twelve prenylflavonoids, eight fatty acids, and one carbohydrate. Furthermore, 21 potentially bioactive compounds were highly enriched in the PSY EtOH-Ex compared to the water extract. Together, these results indicate that PSY suppresses the proliferation of CRC cells by inhibiting the STAT3 signaling pathway, suggesting PSY as a potential therapeutic agent for treating CRC and 21 EtOH-Ex-enriched phytochemicals as anti-cancer drug candidates which may act by inhibiting STAT3.

Keywords: Patriniae Radix; Mori Cortex Radicis; Coix Seed; PSY; colorectal cancer; STAT3

Citation: Han, S.; Kim, H.; Lee, M.Y.; Lee, J.; Ahn, K.S.; Ha, I.J.; Lee, S.-G. Anti-Cancer Effects of a New Herbal Medicine PSY by Inhibiting the STAT3 Signaling Pathway in Colorectal Cancer Cells and Its Phytochemical Analysis. *Int. J. Mol. Sci.* **2022**, *23*, 14826. https://doi.org/10.3390/ijms232314826

Academic Editors: Barbara De Filippis, Alessandra Ammazzalorso and Marialuigia Fantacuzzi

Received: 12 October 2022
Accepted: 22 November 2022
Published: 27 November 2022

1. Introduction

Colorectal cancer (CRC) is the third most common cancer in the world, the third most diagnosed cancer among men, and the second most common among women. Overall, CRC ranks third in terms of incidence but second in terms of mortality [1]. Incidence rates have steadily risen in many countries in eastern Europe, southeastern and south-central Asia, and South America. Risk factors include the consumption of red or processed meat and heavy alcohol consumption, whereas adequate consumption of whole grains, fiber, and dairy products decreases the risk [2]. Primary prevention remains a key strategy for reducing the increasing global burden of CRC. The largest proportion of CRC cases has been linked to environmental mutations rather than heritable genetics [2]. Inflammatory bowel disease (IBD) is an important risk factor for colon cancer. In this regard, colitis-associated cancer is a CRC subtype associated with IBD, is challenging to treat, and has high mortality [3]. Moreover, CRC exhibits constitutive activation of NF-κB and STAT3, transcription factors that influence interactions between tumor cells and tumor microenvironment and play integrated roles in cancer-promoting inflammation [4]. Further, inflammation is associated with tumor cell proliferation, survival, metastasis, angiogenesis, and chemoresistance and may also affect the efficacy of CRC therapies, including STAT3 inhibitors [4,5]. However, NF-κB is also involved in anti-tumor immune responses, and in contrast, STAT3 restrains the NF-κB-mediated anti-tumor immunity [4]. Thus, STAT3 has been suggested as a more promising target for cancer therapy by redirecting inflammation [4,5]. Recent studies have also indicated that CRC progression occurs by activating tumorigenic JAK/STAT3 signaling [5,6].

Although many cancer medications such as oxaliplatin for treating CRC are available, better options have been requested for cancer patients because of the low efficacy and severe side effects of conventional chemotherapies [7,8]. Thus, medicinal plants and dietary phytochemicals have attracted great attention due to strong beliefs that as these substances are edible they have minimal toxicity [9].

Roots of *Patrinia scabiosaefolia* Fisch. (Patriniae Radix (PR)) and seeds of *Coix lacryma-jobi* L. var. *ma-yuen* Stapf (Coix Seed (CS)) are the main components of Paejangsan which has been traditionally used to treat intestinal inflammatory diseases in Korea and China [10]. The root bark of *Morus alba* L. (Mori Cortex Radicis (MCR)) has been used for inflammation-related diseases in the intestine and lungs in traditional Korean and Chinese medicine [10]. Recent studies have also shown that the extract of each medicinal plant inhibits the proliferation of CRC cells [11–16]. Moreover, a basic theory of herbal combination in traditional medicine is the addition and subtraction theory that adds or/and removes one or more herbal medicines or dosages from an original foundational formula, thus generating another new formula for personalized medicine or better therapeutic effects [17]. Based on the information, we hypothesized that the addition of MCR to the main components of Paejangsan generating a new herbal formula might have anti-cancer properties for CRC. Therefore, we have in the present study developed a new herbal formula as an alternative to CRC treatments, which is comprised of PR (Paejang in Korean), MCR (Sangbekpi in Korean), and CS (Yiyiin in Korean), hence the name PSY, and have investigated whether this formula could be a potential therapeutic intervention for treating CRC.

2. Results and Discussion

2.1. PSY Synergistically Suppresses Cell Viability in Human CRC Cells

Since we aimed to develop PSY as a potential therapeutic intervention for CRC based on the addition and subtraction theory, we first examined whether PSY ethanol extract (EtOH-Ex) would synergistically affect the viability of human CRC cells compared to two main components of Paejangsan (PR and CS combination: PY) and MCR (S). Human CRC cells were treated with PY EtOH-Ex for 72 h, and cell viability was determined. As shown in Figure 1a, PY decreased cell viability in a dose-dependent manner in all CRC cell lines, but IC_{50} values in each cell line were quite high. In addition, the results indicated that HT-29 cells are quite resistant to PY (Figure 1a). We then performed the combination of IC_{30} (125 μg/mL) and IC_{50} (200 μg/mL) concentrations of PY in HCT116 with various concentrations of S EtOH-Ex to evaluate the potential effect of the combination and determine the best combination ratio. As shown in Figure 1b, an increase of S together with 125 μg/mL or 200 μg/mL of PY reduced cell viability in a dose-dependent manner in all CRC cell lines including HCT116. In addition, combinations of 37.5 μg/mL of S with 125 μg/mL of PY and 60 μg/mL of S with 200 μg/mL of PY were the lowest concentrations showing significant effects in all CRC cells including HT-29 (Figure 1b). These results suggested the combination of PY and S in a 10-to-3 ratio for the formula PSY. Additionally, the increase of PSY in the combination ratio (PY:S = 10:3) dramatically and synergistically suppressed the cell viability of all CRC cell lines tested compared to PY or S treatment (Figure 1c). However, PSY water extract (Water-Ex) did not show any significant effect (Figure 1d). These results indicated that PSY is potent to suppress the viability of CRC cells, and we further evaluated PSY EtOH-Ex in the combination ratio (PY:S = 10:3) as a potential anti-CRC agent.

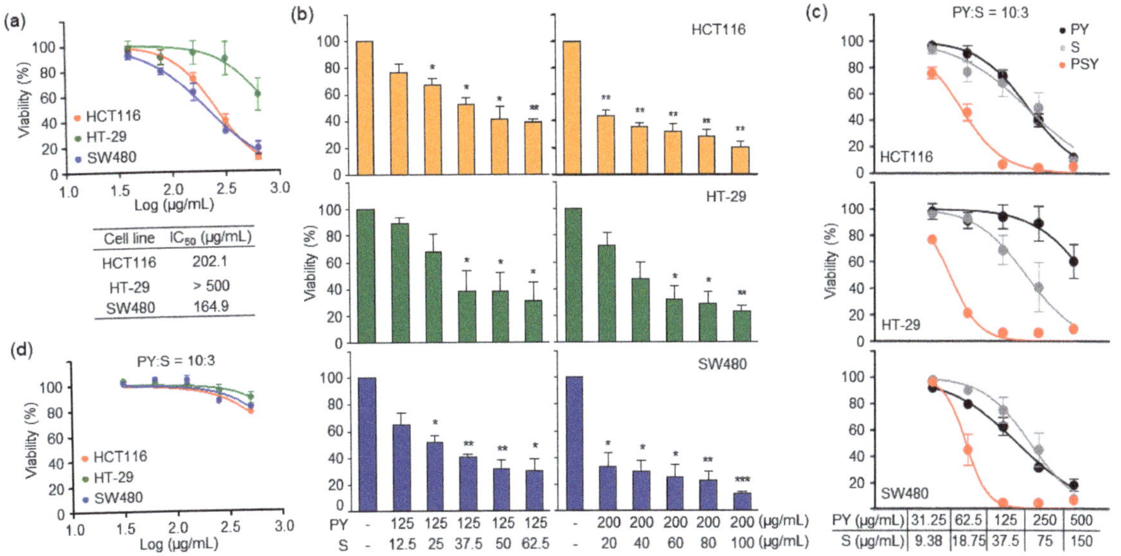

Figure 1. Effects of PSY extracts on the viability of human CRC cells. (**a**) Human CRC cells were treated with ethanol extract (EtOH-Ex) of Patriniae Radix and Coix Seed (PY) for 72 h as indicated. Cell viability was determined by MTT assays. IC_{50} values of PY EtOH-Ex in CRC cell lines were determined. (**b**) CRC cells were treated with five concentrations of Mori Cortex Radicis (S) EtOH-Ex in combination with PY EtOH-Ex (125 and 200 μg/mL) for 72 h. The ratio of PY and S was from 10-to-1 to 10-to-5. (**c**) CRC cells were treated with PSY EtOH-Ex in a 10-to-3 combination ratio and compared to each treatment of PY or S EtOH-Ex. (**d**) CRC cells were treated with PSY water extract (Water-Ex) in the combined ratio as indicated. Data are presented as the mean ± standard error of the mean (SEM) of results from at least three independent experiments performed in triplicates. *, $p < 0.05$, **, $p < 0.01$, ***, $p < 0.001$.

2.2. PSY Induces Cell Cycle Arrest in the G_2/M Phase and Apoptosis in Human CRC Cells

As cell viability is regulated by cell proliferation and death, we investigated the effect of PSY on the cell cycle. As shown in Figure 2a, PSY increased the number of human CRC cells in the G_2/M phase while gradually decreasing the number of cells in the G_0/G_1 phase. Accordingly, PSY decreased the expression levels of CDK1 and cyclin B1 in HCT116 cells and increased the phosphorylation of CDK1 in SW480 cells (Figure 2b), indicating that the inactivation of CDK1 leads to G_2/M arrest. At the same time, PSY increased the CRC cell population in the sub-G_1 phase (Figure 2a), suggesting the induction of apoptotic cell death. To further confirm whether PSY induces apoptosis, we stained PSY-treated CRC cells with annexin V-FITC and PI, and the proportion of apoptotic cells was determined. As shown in Figure 3a, PSY increased the number of annexin V-positive cells, indicating apoptosis. These results were also confirmed by terminal deoxynucleotidyl transferase dUTP nick end labeling (TUNEL) assays and examination of increased cleaved PARP, another apoptosis marker (Figure 3b,c). These results indicate that PSY decreases the viability of human CRC cells by inducing cell cycle arrest at the G_2/M phase and apoptosis.

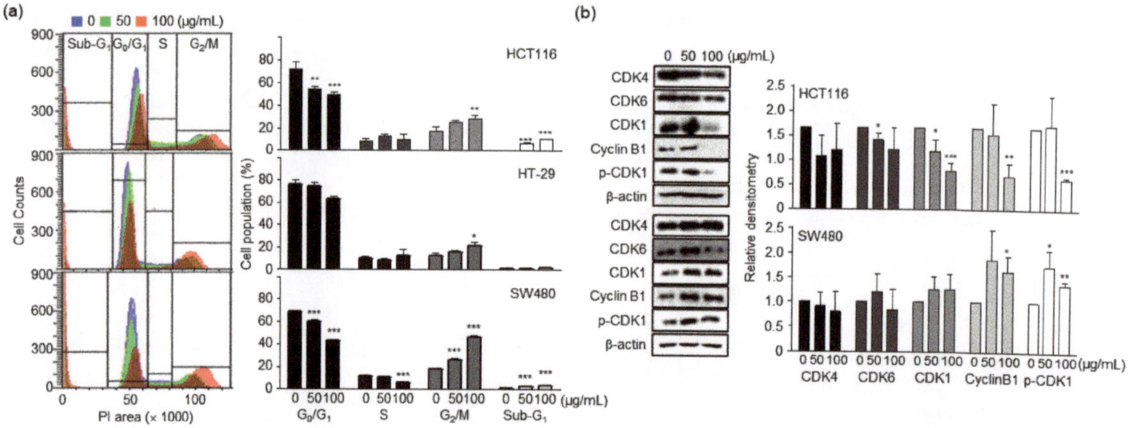

Figure 2. Effects of PSY on cell cycle in human CRC cells. CRC cells were treated with PSY EtOH-Ex for 48 h. (**a**) The treated cells were stained with PI, and the staining was analyzed using flow cytometry. The representative analysis is shown in the left panel. Every PI staining and analysis was performed at least three times in duplicate or triplicate. Cells were quantitated as a percentage of cells in each phase. Data in the right panel represent the mean ± SEM (*, $p < 0.05$; **, $p < 0.01$ and ***, $p < 0.001$ versus control). (**b**) Whole lysates of the treated cells were prepared, and Western blot analysis for CDK1, CDK4, CDK6, Cyclin B1, and phospho (p)-CDK1 was performed, and β-actin was used as an internal control. Data represent the mean ± standard deviation (SD) of three independent experiments (*, $p < 0.05$; **, $p < 0.01$ and ***, $p < 0.001$ versus control).

2.3. PSY Inhibits the STAT3 Pathway in Human CRC Cells

In the next step of the study, we attempted to determine the mechanism by which PSY induced cell cycle arrest and apoptosis in human CRC cells. The CRC development and progression are closely related to inflammation and the key molecule STAT3 [4]. Therefore, we prepared PSY with PR, MCR, and CS, each of which was traditionally used for treating inflammatory diseases. In this regard, we explored the effect of PSY on STAT3 expression. As shown in Figure 4a, PSY effectively reduced the phosphorylation of STAT3 in human CRC cells. PSY also inhibited the nuclear translocation of STAT3 (Figure 4b). Furthermore, PSY significantly decreased luciferase expression of the heterologous promoter system, which is regulated by STAT3 transcriptional activation in HCT116 cells (Figure 4c). STAT3 is constitutively activated in various types of human cancers and is associated with adverse clinical outcomes and poor prognosis in human CRC [18,19]. Recent studies have shown that PR and MCR induce apoptosis by inhibiting STAT3 in human multiple myeloma and CRC cells, respectively [15,16,20]. These results suggested that PSY induces apoptosis by inhibiting STAT3 in human CRC cells. Considering that JAK2, Src, and protein tyrosine phosphatases (PTPs), including SHP1 and SHP2, have been associated with STAT3 activation [6], we further examined the upstream signaling molecules of STAT3. As shown in Figure 5a, PSY decreased the phosphorylation of JAK2 and Src in HCT116 cells, while it only reduced the phosphorylation of JAK2 in SW480 cells. PSY also increased the expression of SHP1, a negative regulator of the JAK-STAT pathway, but not SHP2 in CRC cells (Figure 5b). In addition, pervanadate reversed PSY-mediated inhibition of STAT3 in HCT116 cells (Figure 5c), indicating a crucial role of SHP1 in the PSY mechanism of action. Accordingly, these results suggest that PSY suppresses human CRC cell proliferation by inducing cell cycle arrest and apoptosis via inhibiting the STAT3 signaling pathway.

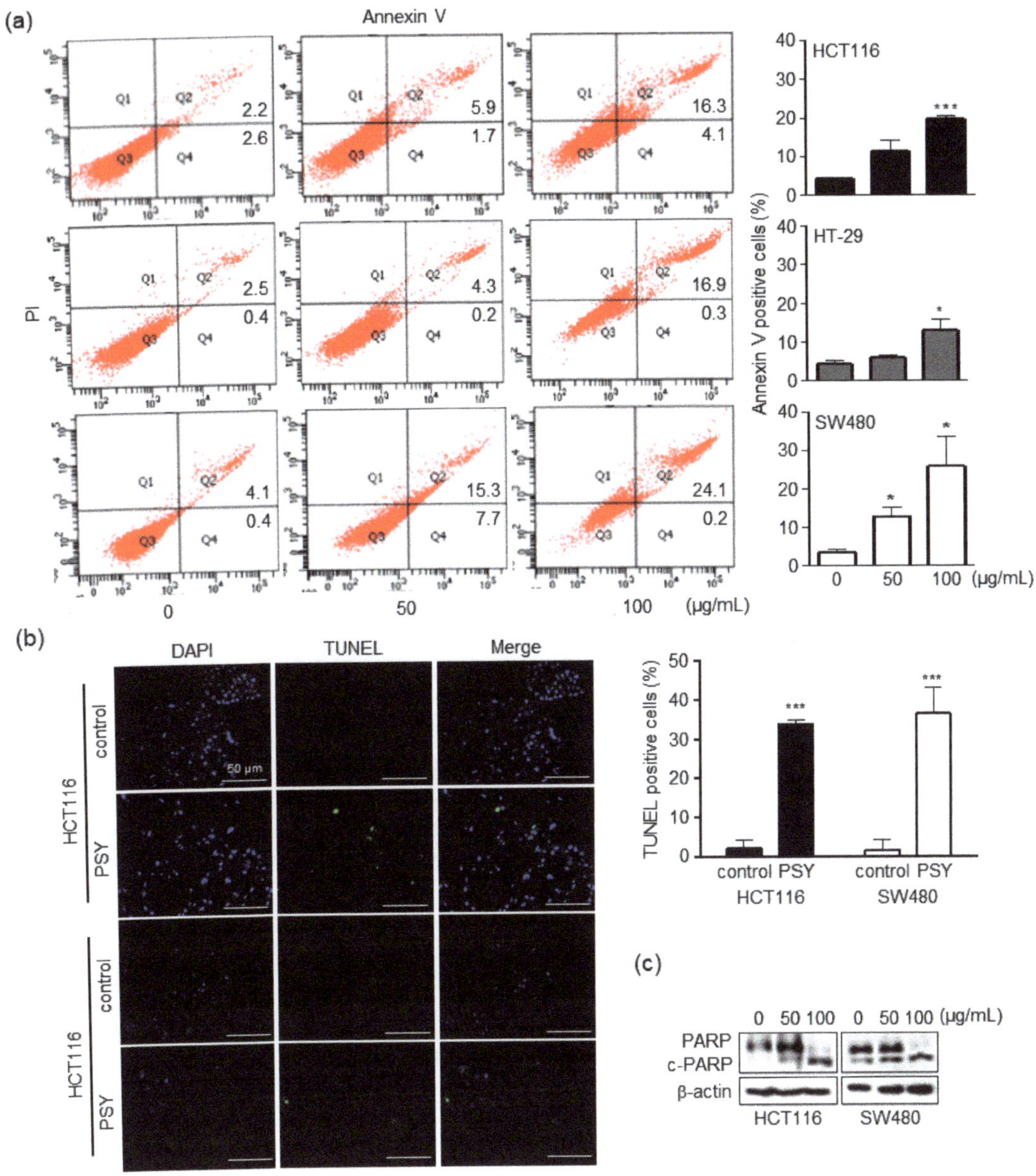

Figure 3. Effects of PSY on apoptosis in human CRC cells. CRC cells were treated with PSY EtOH-Ex for 48 h. (**a**) The cells were double-stained with FITC-Annexin V and PI and analyzed using flow cytometry (left panel). (**b**) The TUNEL and DAPI staining of the PSY (50 μg/mL)-treated cells were analyzed by confocal microscopy (left panel). Scale bar, 50 μm. Apoptotic cells were quantified as a percentage of Annexin V-positive and TUNEL-positive cells (right panel in **a**,**b**, respectively). Data present the mean ± SEM of three independent experiments (*, $p < 0.05$ and ***, $p < 0.001$ versus control). (**c**) Whole lysates of the treated cells were subjected to Western blotting for PARP and cleaved PARP (c-PARP). β-actin was used as an internal control.

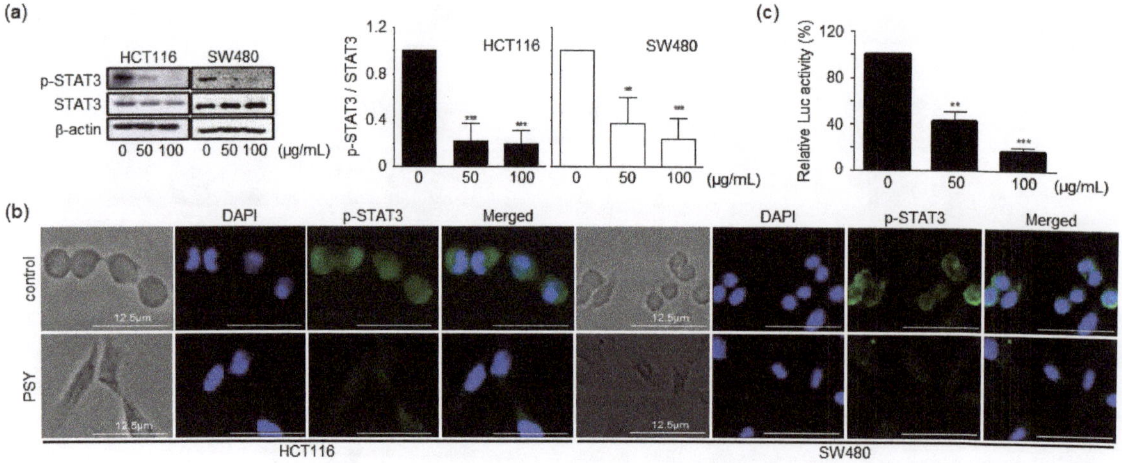

Figure 4. Effects of PSY on STAT3 in human CRC cells. (**a**) CRC cells were treated with PSY EtOH-Ex for 24 h, and cell lysates were subjected to Western blot analysis for STAT3 and p-STAT3. β-actin was used as an internal control. Data in the graphs represent the mean ± SD to that of the mock-treated cells taken as 1 (**, $p < 0.01$ and ***, $p < 0.001$ versus control). (**b**) Immunofluorescence staining of p-STAT3 and DAPI in the PSY (50 μg/mL)-treated CRC cells were analyzed by confocal microscopy. Scale bar, 12.5 μm. (**c**) HCT116 cells transfected with pSTAT3-Luc plasmid were treated with PSY for 24 h to analyze the transcriptional activity of STAT3. Data in the graphs are presented as the mean of fold-normalized luciferase (Luc) activities ± SEM to that of the untreated cells taken as 100% (**, $p < 0.01$ and ***, $p < 0.001$ versus control).

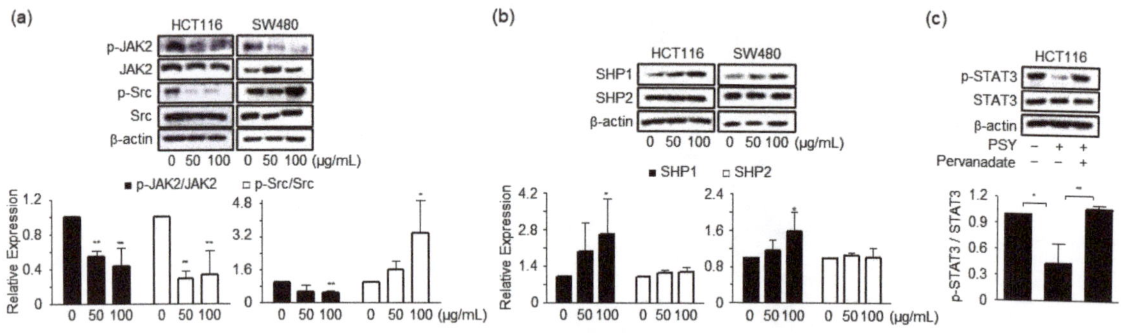

Figure 5. Effects of PSY on the STAT3 signaling pathway in human CRC cells. Whole lysates of CRC cells treated with PSY EtOH-Ex for 24 h were subjected to Western blot analysis for JAK2, p-JAK2, Src, and p-Src (**a**), and SHP1 and SHP2 (**b**). In addition, lysates of HCT116 cells treated with pervanadate (5 μM) and PSY (50 μg/mL) for 24 h were subjected to Western blot analysis for STAT3 and p-STAT3 (**c**). β-actin was used as an internal control. Data in graphs present the mean ± SD to that of the untreated cells taken as 1 (*, $p < 0.05$ and **, $p < 0.01$ versus control).

2.4. Chemical Identification in PSY Extracts

The chemical compositions of PSY EtOH-Ex and Water-Ex were characterized using UPLC-ESI-QTOF MS/MS in positive and negative ion modes. Representative base peak chromatograms (BPCs) of PSY Water-Ex and EtOH-Ex are shown in Figure 6a,b, and the identified minor or overlapping peaks on the BPCs are divided in the extracted-ion chromatograms (XICs) (Figure 6c,d). Detailed chemical and chromatographic information on the identified peaks (Figure 6) are summarized in Table 1, and their chemical profiles revealed 38 compounds of PSY, 7 organic acids, 8 iridoids, 2 lignans, 12 prenylflavonoids, 8 fatty acids, and 1 carbohydrate.

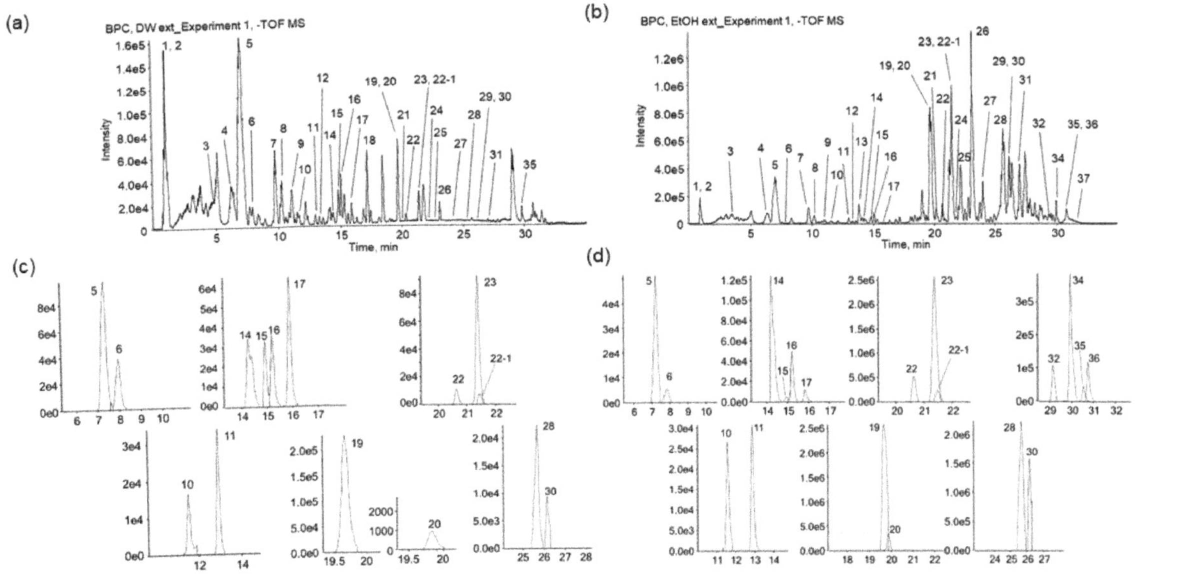

Figure 6. Chemical identification in PSY extracts. Representative BPCs of the Water-Ex (**a**) and EtOH-Ex (**b**) and expanded XICs from the Water-Ex (**c**) and EtOH-Ex (**d**) are presented. The scale of Y axis for intensity (CPS) on the chromatograms indicate that 1.6e5 equals 1.6×10^5.

Quinic acid (peak **2**) was identified using molecular networking (MN) analysis through Global Natural Products Social Molecular Networking (GNPS), and its derivatives, neochlorogenic acid (**3**), chlorogenic acid (**5**), cryptochlorogenic acid (**6**), 1,4-dicaffeoylquinic acid (**15**), 1,3-dicaffeoylquinic acid (**16**), and 4,5-dicaffeoylquinic acid (**17**), were identified by comparison with the retention time and fragmentation patterns of the reference standard in both positive and negative ion modes. Peaks **2**, **5**, **15**, **16**, and **17** have been reported as constituents of *P. scabiosaefolia* and *Partinia* [21,22].

Eight iridoids were identified in the PSY extracts. Loganic acid (**4**) and loganin (**8**) were identified using the reference standard and MN analysis on the GNPS. The loganic acid yielded its quasi-molecular ion $[M-H]^-$ at m/z 375.1287 (mass error = −1.72), and its fragment ions were m/z 213.0762 $[M-H-Glc]^-$, 169.0864 $[M-H-Glc-CO_2]$, 151.0757 $[M-H-Glc-CO_2-H_2O]$, 113.0243 $[M-H-Glc-C_3O_4]$, and 69.0369 (C_5H_9, isoprenyl moiety). The precursor ion at m/z 359.1344 was putatively identified as a deoxyloganic acid isomer (**9** and **11**) in MN analysis (Figure 7a). The mass difference (15.9943 Da, oxygen) of the precursor ion between loganic acid and deoxyloganic acid was found at m/z 197.0823, 135.0823, and 153.0915 from the fragment ions of **9** and **11**, respectively. The precursor ions of deoxyloganic acid were detected at peaks **9** (RT 11.1 min) and **11** (RT 12.9 min) on BPC and XIC (Figure 6). Although compounds **9** and **11** were identified as deoxyloganic acid isomers, they could not be clearly classified as 7-deoxyloganic acid or 8-epideoxyloganic acid. Geniposide (**7**) was putatively identified through MN analysis on the GNPS (Figure 7b). Patrinalloside (**10**) and patrinoside isomers (**13** and **14**) have been identified in the literature [23–26]. Some iridoids (**4**, **8**, **9**, **10**, and **11**) are representative components of *P. scabiosaefolia* [21,22].

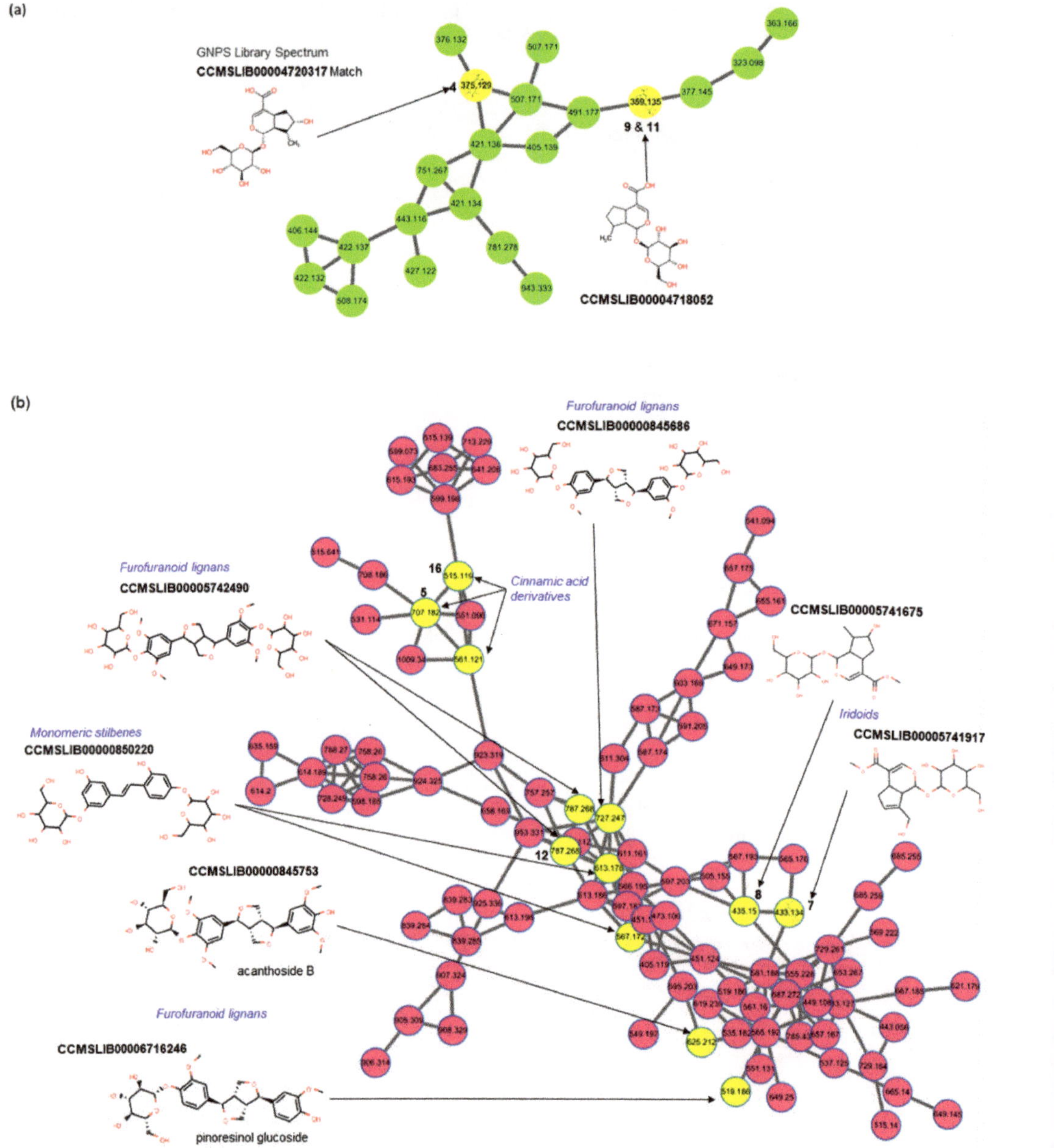

Figure 7. *Cont.*

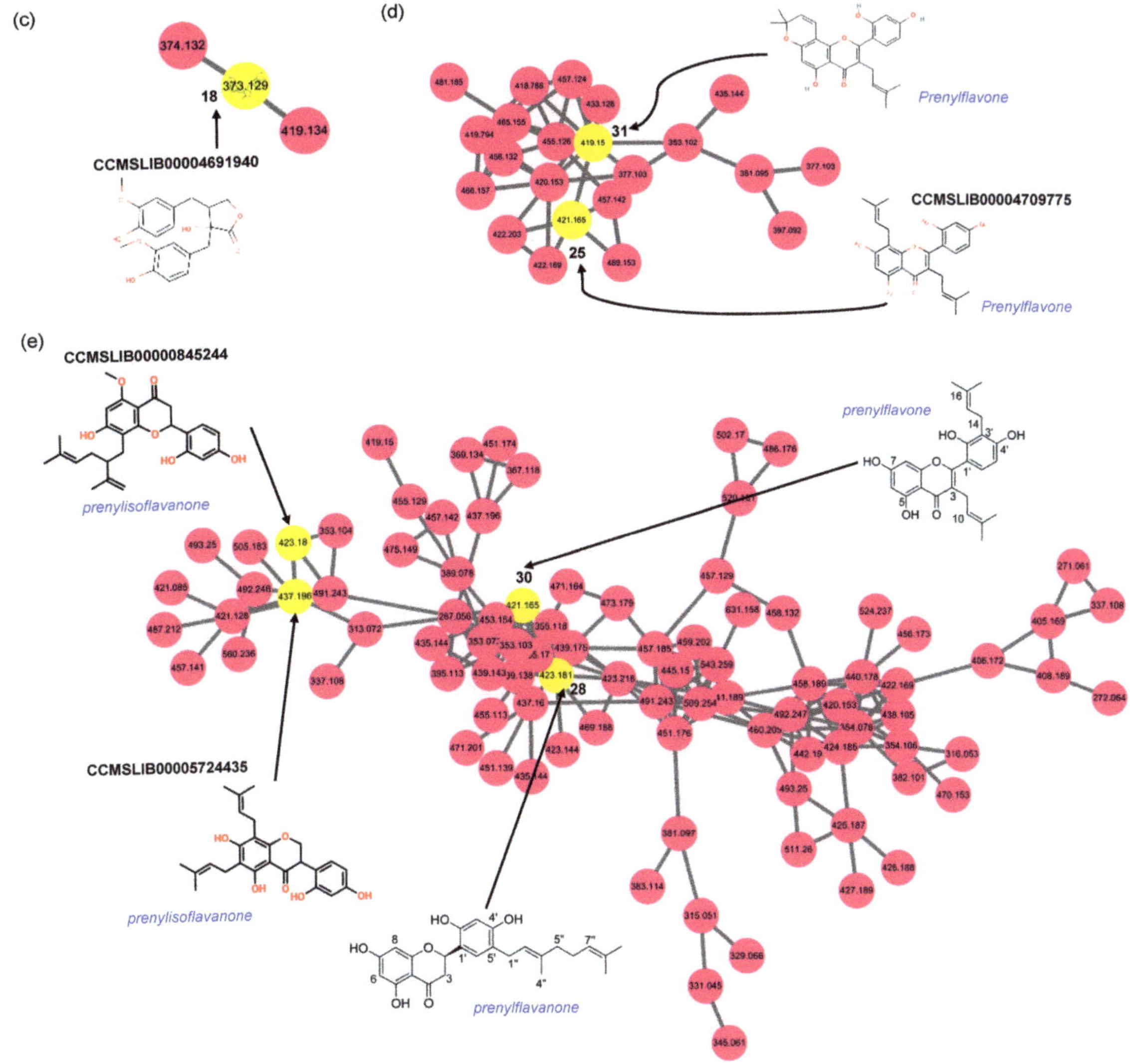

Figure 7. The representative MS/MS spectral network of identified phytochemical compounds in PSY extracts. Spectral nodes indicating identified compounds are noted with numbers (yellow nodes with peak numbers in Table 1). Annotated candidates for selected spectral nodes (yellow nodes without numbers) show compound name, GNPS library spectrum matching (in bold), and chemical class and subclass (in italic with blue). Molecular networks of representative chemical classes or biosynthetic pathways of natural products in PSY extracts. (**a**) iridoid class, (**b**) shikimate pathway including cinnamic (or quinic) acid derivatives, iridoid, furofuranoid lignan subclass in lignan, and stilbene class, (**c**) lignan class, (**d**) prenylflavone subclass in prenylflavonoid class, and (**e**) prenylisoflavanone, prenylflavanone, and prenylflavone subclasses in prenylflanoid class. Further information can be found at the GNPS job link (https://gnps.ucsd.edu/ProteoSAFe/status.jsp?task=e4406e69e619467b9a347a905d6c383a accessed on 31 March 2022).

Eleutheroside E (**12**) and nortrachelogenin (**18**) were detected and putatively identified as lignans by matching the MS/MS fragment ions with the MN analysis on the GNPS (Figure 7b,c). Nortrachelogenin has been previously isolated from PR [27].

Twelve prenylflavonoids originating from MCR were detected, and **23** and **31** were identified as kuwanon G and morusin [28,29], representative components in MCR with each reference standard, respectively. Peak **23** is the Diels-Alder (DA)-type adduct of a chalcone and prenylflavone and exhibited an $[M-H]^-$ ion at m/z 691.2182. In negative ion mode, fragment ions were observed at m/z 581.1820 [M−H−resorcinol ($C_6H_6O_2$, 110 Da)]$^-$, 353.1029 [M−H−resorcinol−$C_{14}H12O_3$]$^-$, 419.1501, 379.1189 [M-H-2resorcinol−C_4H_8O−H_2O]$^-$, and 539.1719 [M−H−resorcinol−C_3H_6]$^-$. Morusin exhibited characteristic fragment ions at m/z 297.1134, 191.0716, 309.1139 [M−H−resorcinol]$^-$, and 350.04804 [M−H−isoprenyl]$^-$. The fragment ion at m/z 191.0716 lost one CO and received two hydrogens at C-10 from m/z 217.0507, produced by retro-DA cleavage [30]. Peak **25** was detected and putatively identified as Kuwanon C through MN analysis and clustered with **31** as prenylflavones (Figure 7d). The mass difference (2 Da, two hydrogens) between the precursor ions of peaks **31** and **25** was found in the characteristic fragmentation patterns (Table 1). Peaks **28** and **30** were putatively identified as Kuwanon E and Kuwanon T using PeakView 2.2, using exact mass and isotope patterns. Kuwanon E was further identified by fragmentation patterns in FooDB. Additionally, **28** and **30** (prenylflavones) were clustered by MN analysis, with two isoflavanones (not shown in Table 1) identified by library matching (Figure 7e). Mulberrofuran G, kuwanon G, kuwanon T, sanggenon F, and morusin, found in MCR, are known to exert anti-inflammatory and anti-cancer activities [15,31]. Kuwanon G also ameliorates lipopolysaccharide-induced disruption of the gut epithelial barrier [32,33]. In addition, morusin induces autophagy and apoptosis by regulating various signaling molecules, including STAT3, in several types of cancer cells [31,32].

Peaks **27**, **29**, and **32–37** were identified as fatty acids (Table 1), and linoleic (**34**) and oleic (**37**) acids are known to be present in CS [34]. Moreover, Linolenic, linoleic, and oleic acids are known to have various pharmacological activities, including anti-inflammatory, anti-cancer, and anti-microbial activities [35,36].

2.5. Identification of Potential Bioactive Phytochemicals in PSY EtOH-Ex

To investigate the potential bioactive candidates in EtOH-Ex, due to its potent anti-cancer activity compared to that of Water-Ex, the fold change in the peak area of every compound in EtOH-Ex versus Water-Ex was calculated and compared because the fold change reflects the degree of differences in chemical concentration. As shown in Figure 8, the comparison of ploidy area variation was significant for 21 phytochemicals (fold change > 2), including 12 prenylflavonoids, two iridoids, and seven fatty acids. All prenylflavonoids were significantly enriched in EtOH-Ex. Intriguingly, four fatty acids (**32**, **35**, **36**, and **37**) and one iridoid (**13**) were found only in the EtOH-Ex. These results suggest that the EtOH-Ex-enriched compounds could be potential bioactive molecules, indicating the PSY effect to suppress CRC cell proliferation, and could be a useful source for developing anti-cancer drugs. Additionally, other phytochemicals remain unknown. Since these candidates may also contribute to anti-cancer effects, further identification of novel compounds, evaluation of their anti-cancer effects, and further investigation of their mechanisms of action seem to be necessary.

Table 1. Identification of chemical components in PSY using LC-ESI-QTOF MS/MS.

Peak No.	Name	Formula	Mass (Da)	Expected RT (min)	Adduct	Detected at Mass (Da)	Error (ppm)	Fragment Ions (MS/MS Product Ions)	Identified with	Chemical Class
1	Sucrose	$C_{12}H_{22}O_{11}$	342.1162	0.9	[M−H]⁻	341.1091	0.3	89.0258, 179.0565, 119.0359, 59.0166, 71.0166, 113.0253	# GNP	*Carbohydrate*
2	Quinic acid	$C_7H_{12}O_6$	192.0634	0.9	[M−H]⁻	191.0567	0.8	85.0315, 93.0362	# in-house & GNP	*Quinic acid derivatives*
3	Neochlorogenic acid (3-O-caffeoylquinic acid, 3-CQA)	$C_{16}H_{18}O_9$	354.0951	4.5	[M+H]⁺ [M−H]⁻	355.1021 353.0877	−0.6 −0.3	163.0373, 145.0284, 135.0438, 117.0326 191.0564, 179.0345, 135.0462, 134.0372	†	*Quinic acid derivatives* *Quinic acid derivatives*
4	Loganic acid	$C_{16}H_{24}O_{10}$	376.1370	6.6	[M−H]⁻	375.1287	−1.7	213.0762, 169.0864, 151. 0757, 113.0243, 69.0369	†	*Iridoids*
5	Chlorogenic acid (5-O-caffeoylquinic acid, 5-CQA)	$C_{16}H_{18}O_9$	354.0951	7.3	[M+H]⁺ [M−H]⁻	355.1025 353.0871	0.3 −2.1	163.0388, 145.0283, 135.0439, 117.0333 191.0566, 161.0252, 173.0464	†	*Quinic acid derivatives* *Quinic acid derivatives*
6	Cryptochlorogenic acid (4-O-caffeoylquinic acid, 4-CQA)	$C_{16}H_{18}O_9$	354.0951	7.9	[M+H]⁺ [M−H]⁻	355.1024 353.0874	0.2 −1.1	163.0390, 145.0284, 135.0442, 117.0343 191.0557, 173.0449, 135.0451, 179.0350	†	*Quinic acid derivatives* *Quinic acid derivatives*
7	Geniposide	$C_{17}H_{24}O_{10}$	388.1370	9.7	[M−H+FA]⁻	433.1341	0.2	225.0772, 387.1270, 101.0255, 123.0455	# GNP	*Iridoids*
8	Loganin	$C_{17}H_{26}O_{10}$	390.1526	10.2	[M−H+FA]⁻	435.1498	0.3	227.0929, 127.0414, 101.0264, 389.1474	†	*Iridoids*
9	Deoxyloganic acid (7- or 8-epi)	$C_{16}H_{24}O_9$	360.1420	11.1	[M−H]⁻	359.1344	−2.0	197.0823, 135.0823, 153.0915	# FooDB, GNP & Ref. [21]	*Iridoids*
10	Patrinalloside	$C_{21}H_{34}O_{11}$	462.2101	11.6	[M−H+FA]⁻	507.2070	−0.9	361.1498, 403.1605, 343.1391, 161.0449	Refs. [25,26]	*Iridoids*
11	Deoxyloganic acid (7- or 8-epi)	$C_{16}H_{24}O_9$	360.1420	12.9	[M−H]⁻	359.1344	−1.1	197.0818, 135.0817, 153.0916,59.0167	# FooDB, GNP & Ref. [21]	*Iridoids*
12	Eleutheroside E	$C_{34}H_{46}O_{18}$	742.2684	13.4	[M−H+FA]⁻	787.2670	1.8	579.2089, 417.1554, 181.0506	# GNP	*lignans*
13	Patrinoside/isomers	$C_{21}H_{34}O_{11}$	462.2101	13.8	[M−H+FA]⁻	507.2070	−0.4	179.0564, 89.0260, 119.0356, 161.0459, 377.1444	Refs. [23,24]	*Iridoids*
14	Patrinoside/isomers	$C_{21}H_{34}O_{11}$	462.2101	14.3	[M−H+FA]⁻	507.2070	−0.1	179.0559, 461.2007, 89.0262, 377.1447, 119.0358, 161.0457	Refs. [23,24]	*Iridoids*
15	1,4-Dicaffeoylquinic acid	$C_{25}H_{24}O_{12}$	516.1268	14.9	[M+H]⁺ [M−H]⁻	517.1316 515.1183	−2.4 −2.3	163.0377, 145.0273, 499.1216, 319.0789 353.0869, 179.0340, 173.0452, 191.0553	†	*Quinic acid derivatives*
16	1,3-Dicaffeoylquinic acid	$C_{25}H_{24}O_{12}$	516.1268	15.2	[M+H]⁺ [M−H]⁻	517.1332 515.1188	−1.7 −1.4	163.0391, 145.0294, 135.0431, 117.0331 353.0866, 191.0556, 179.0338, 135.0455	†	*Quinic acid derivatives*
17	4,5-Dicaffeoyl quinic acid	$C_{25}H_{24}O_{12}$	516.1268	15.9	[M+H]⁺ [M−H]⁻	517.1338 515.1191	−0.6 −0.8	163.0382, 145.0260, 135.0421,337.0906 353.0874, 173.0454, 179.0346, 191.0556	†	*Quinic acid derivatives*
18	Nortrachelogenin	$C_{20}H_{22}O_7$	374.1366	17.1	[M−H]⁻	373.1291	−0.5	179.0714, 164.0476, 99.0099, 327.1238, 163.0476	# GNP	*lignans*
19	Kuwanon L	$C_{35}H_{30}O_{11}$	626.1788	19.7	[M+H]⁺ [M−H]⁻	627.1853 625.1716	−1.2 0.1	309.1740, 153.0181, 137.0233, 433.0908, 499.1374 499.1406, 389.1025, 125.0253, 109.0306	*	*Diels-Alder (DA)-type flavonoids*
20	Kuwanon Y	$C_{34}H_{30}O_9$	582.1890	19.8	[M+H]⁺ [M−H]⁻	583.1947 581.1813	−2.6 −0.6	203.0706, 137.0237, 339.1218, 473.1585 361.1089, 471.1463, 227.0716, 243.0666, 563.1738	# FooDB	*Diels-Alder (DA)-type flavonoids*
21	Mulberrofuran G	$C_{34}H_{26}O_8$	562.1628	20.2	[M+H]⁺ [M−H]⁻	563.1695 561.1540	−0.9 −1.1	441.1345, 255.0661, 123.0449, 387.0873 451.12190, 439.1187, 433.1072, 241.0508	* *	*Diels-Alder (DA)-type flavonoids*

Table 1. *Cont.*

Peak No.	Name	Formula	Mass (Da)	Expected RT (min)	Adduct	Detected at Mass (Da)	Error (ppm)	Fragment Ions (MS/MS Product Ions)	Identified with	Chemical Class
22	Sangenon F/isomers	$C_{20}H_{18}O_6$	354.1103	20.6	[M+H] + [M−H] −	355.1178 353.1027	0.4 −1.0	153.0189 227.0712, 125.0251, 201.0920	*	*Prenylflavonoids*
23	Kuwanon G	$C_{40}H_{36}O_{11}$	692.2258	21.4	[M+H] + [M−H] −	693.2321 691.2182	−1.4 −1.0	137.0235, 203.0708, 365.1026, 299.0556, 421.1654 581.1820, 353.1029, 419.1501, 379.1189, 539.1719	†	*Diels-Alder (DA)-type flavonoids*
22-1	Sangenon F/ isomers	$C_{20}H_{18}O_6$	354.1103	21.5	[M+H] + [M−H] −	355.1178 353.1027	0.7 −0.8	153.0184 125.0257, 201.0927, 227.0712	*	*Prenylflavonoids*
24	Kuwanon O or Sanggenon G/isomers	$C_{40}H_{38}O_{11}$	694.2374 694.2433	22.1 22.1	[M+H] + [M−H] −	695.2452 693.2350	−2.2 −0.7	205.0858, 341.1381, 267.0650, 677.2367 567.2098, 389.1034, 177.0919, 125.0243	Ref. [29]	*Diels-Alder (DA)-type flavonoids*
25	Kuwanon C	$C_{25}H_{26}O_6$	422.1729	22.8	[M+H] + [M−H] −	423.1802 421.1654	−1.8 −0.7	311.0549, 241.0494, 283.0599, 367.1179 299.1292, 309.0411, 193.0870, 219.0667, 297.0408	# GNP	*Prenylflavonoids*
26	Kuwanon O/isomer	$C_{40}H_{38}O_{11}$	694.2374 694.2433	23.1 23.1	[M+H] + [M−H] −	695.2452 693.2350	0.7 −1.5	271.1323, 137.0234, 407.1849, 297.1482 531.2031, 287.0563, 259.1341, 125.0253, 583.1993	* *	*Diels-Alder (DA)-type flavonoids*
27	13-keto-9Z,11E-octadecadienoic acid	$C_{18}H_{30}O_3$	294.2195	24.1	[M−H] −	293.2120	−0.6	275.2007, 235.1692, 183.1383, 171.1018	*	*Fatty acids*
28	Kuwanon E	$C_{25}H_{28}O_6$	424.1886	25.7	[M+H] + [M−H] −	425.1955 423.1806	−0.8 −1.7	153.0183, 175.3939 297.1492, 125.0250, 271.1705, 177.0195, 245.1545, 405.1703	# FooDB	*Prenylflavonoids*
29	13-Hydroxyoctadecadienoic acid	$C_{18}H_{32}O_3$	296.2352	26.0	[M−H] −	295.2272	0.0	277.2181, 195.1392, 171.1033	*	*Fatty acids*
30	Kuwanon T	$C_{25}H_{26}O_6$	422.1729	26.2	[M+H] + [M−H] −	423.1796 421.1657	−1.5 0.1	153.0178, 175.0385 295.1341, 125.0252, 269.1550, 174.0329, 151.0040	*	*Prenylflavonoids*
31	Morusin	$C_{25}H_{24}O_6$	420.1573	27.0 27.0	[M+H] + [M−H] −	421.1645 419.1501	−0.3 0.2	365.1012, 347.0913, 332.0682, 295.0953 297.1134, 191.0716, 309.1139, 350.04804, 217.0507	†	*Prenylflavonoids*
32	Linolenic acid	$C_{18}H_{30}O_2$	278.2246	29.2	[M−H] −	277.2175	0.8	277.2175	# GNP	*Fatty acids*
33	Oleamide	$C_{18}H_{35}NO$	281.2719	29.8	[M+H] +	282.2794	0.9	247.2419, 265.2525, 97.1019, 135.1168, 121.1013,149.1321	# GNP	*Fatty acid amide*
34	Linoleic acid	$C_{18}H_{32}O_2$	280.2402	29.9	[M−H] −	279.2335	1.9	279.2335	†	*Fatty acids*
35	3-Oxo-olean-12-en-28-oic acid	$C_{30}H_{46}O_3$	454.3447	30.4	[M−H] −	453.3365	−2.1	453.3365	†	*Fatty acids*
36	Palmitic acid	$C_{16}H_{32}O_2$	256.2402	30.5	[M−H] −	255.2329	−0.4	255.2329	†	*Fatty acids*
37	Oleic acid	$C_{18}H_{34}O_2$	282.2559	31.7	[M−H] −	281.2485	−0.6	283.2643	†	*Fatty acids*

In-house ms/ms library and online database; such as GNPS, MASS bank or Metlin; † Reference standard; and * Extract MS with isotope mass.

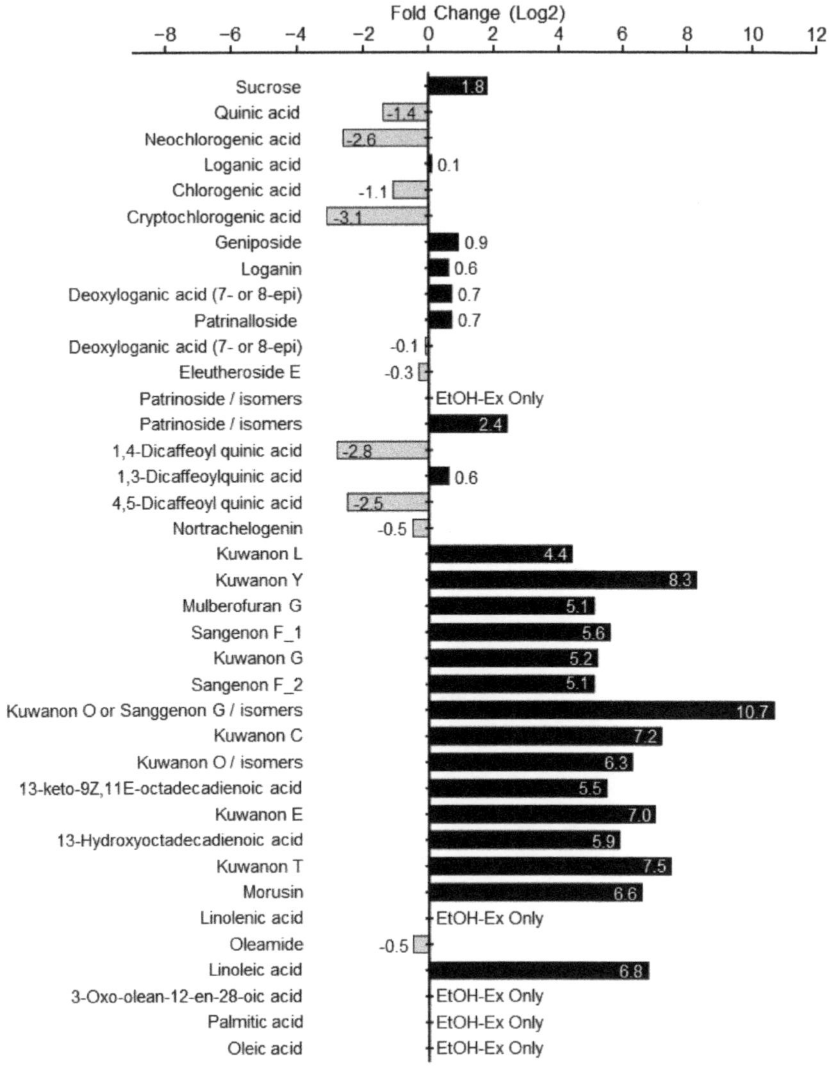

Figure 8. Identification of PSY EtOH-Ex-enriched phytochemicals. Peak area fold change of 38 compounds from PSY EtOH-Ex and Water-Ex. Fold change > 0 means that the relative content of chemical compounds in EtOH-Ex is higher than Water-Ex. The fold changes in peak area were calculated using the formula log2 for the ratio of peak area values of the phytochemicals extracted by different solvents.

Although many early stage CRC patients undergo surgery such as colectomy or proctectomy without chemotherapy, most patients, especially those suffering from metastatic CRC require chemotherapy with or without surgery and radiotherapy [37]. Conventional combinatorial strategies, FOLFOX (folinic acid, 5-fluorouracil (5-FU), and oxaliplatin) or FOLFIRI (folinic acid, 5-FU, and irinotecan) have been the most appropriate first-line chemotherapy options for CRC patients since their development in the early 2000s [38,39]. The recent addition of molecular-targeted drugs such as cetuximab and encorafenib has been a major improvement with more effective therapeutic options [39]. These therapeutic advances have resulted in clinically relevant survival improvements, but the five-year survival rate is still less than 15% for stage IV disease and most survivors suffer from severe side effects including neuropathy, bowel and bladder dysfunction, and sexual dysfunction [1,38,39]. Therefore, novel therapeutic strategies are still required for this fatal disease. We, thus, have focused on medicinal plants which have been traditionally used for thousands of years and are edible, expecting at least fewer adverse effects, and found the combination of PSY in the present study.

Altogether, these results demonstrate that PSY likely suppresses CRC cell proliferation by inducing cell cycle arrest and apoptosis via inhibiting oncogenic STAT3 signals. Further, we found 21 EtOH-Ex-enriched PSY phytochemicals, suggesting further studies investigating the potential anti-cancer activities of these compounds and their mechanisms of action involved in STAT3 (Figure 9). In conclusion, these results suggest that PSY could be a potentially effective therapeutic for patients with CRC. More research about the potential combination of PSY or an EtOH-Ex-enriched PSY phytochemical with any conventional drug including 5-FU, oxaliplatin, and irinotecan would be also interesting and facilitate the development of a more effective and therapeutic strategy with less adverse effects for CRC patients.

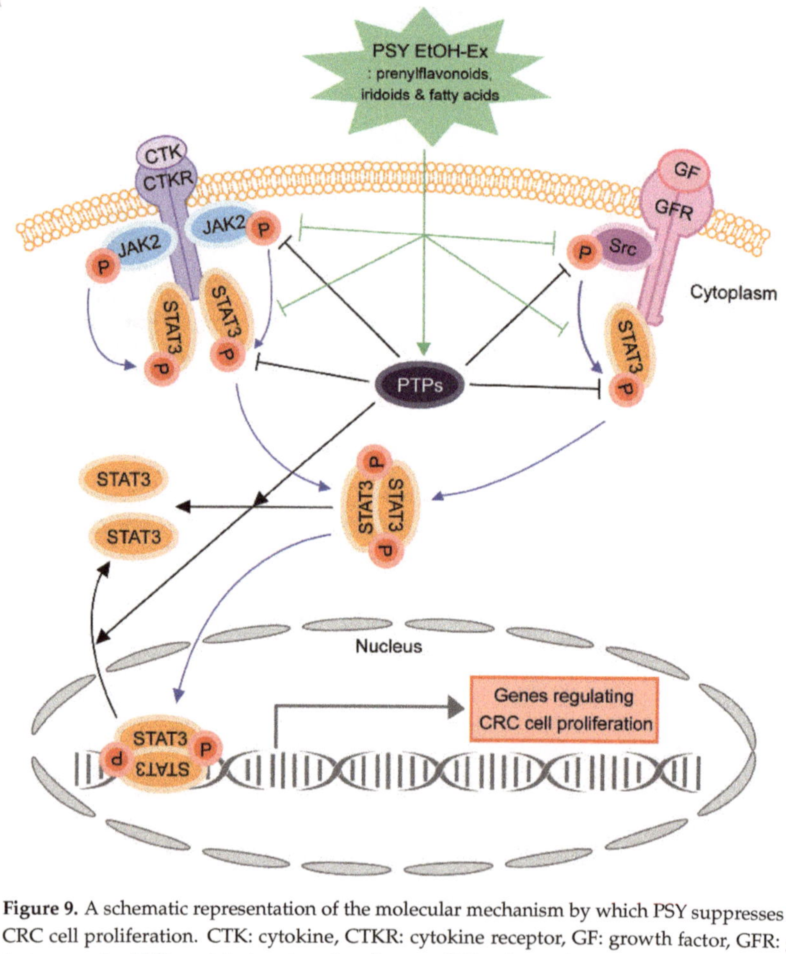

Figure 9. A schematic representation of the molecular mechanism by which PSY suppresses human CRC cell proliferation. CTK: cytokine, CTKR: cytokine receptor, GF: growth factor, GFR: growth factor receptor, PTP: protein tyrosine phosphatase, CRC: colorectal cancer.

3. Materials and Methods

3.1. PSY Preparation

Dried PR, MCR, and CS were purchased from Omniherb (Daegu, Republic of Korea), regulated in herbal Good Manufacturing Practices (hGMP), and each voucher specimen was deposited in the herbarium of the Korean Medicine Clinical Trial Center, Kyung Hee University Korean Medicine Hospital (Seoul, Republic of Korea). For EtOH-Ex preparation, 37.5 g of PR, 22.5 g of MCR, and 37.5 g of CS were extracted with 877.5 mL of ethanol by refluxing at room temperature sonication. Similarly, for the preparation of PSY Water-Ex, the amount of PR, MCR, and CS was extracted with 877.5 mL of distilled water by refluxing at 100 °C for 1.5 h. Each extract was filtered through vacuum filter paper and concentrated in a rotary evaporator (Eyela N-1200 system, Tokyo, Japan) at 40 °C under lower pressure. The extracts were lyophilized, and the yields of dried EtOH-Ex and Water-Ex were 3.21% and 10.13%, respectively. Each extract was dissolved in dimethyl sulfoxide (DMSO) to obtain a 500 mg/mL stock solution.

3.2. Chemicals and Reagents

Standard references, including neochlorogenic acid, loganic acid, cryptochlorogenic acid, loganin, kuwanon G, and 3-Oxo-olean-12-en-28-oic acid, were purchased from ChemFaces (Wuhan, China). Linoleic and palmitic acids were obtained from Sigma-Aldrich (St. Louis, MO, USA). Morusin and chlorogenic acid were obtained from Biopurity Phytochemicals, Ltd. (Chengdu, China). Further, mixed references were prepared by dissolving the references in a 50% methanol in water (v/v) solution for qualitative analysis using UPLC-ESI-QTOF MS/MS.

3.3. Cell Lines and Culture Condition

HCT116, HT-29, and SW480 human CRC cell lines were acquired from the Korean Cell Line Bank (Seoul, Republic of Korea) and were cultured according to the manufacturer's instructions.

3.4. Cell Viability Assays

CRC cells (3–5 $\times$ 10^3 cells/well) were seeded in 96-well plates and incubated overnight. Then, the cells were treated with PSY for 72 h. After the treatment, cell viability was measured by 3-(4,5-dimethylthiazol-2-yl)-2,5-diphenyl-tetrazolium bromide (MTT) assays as previously described [40]. After dissolving formazan crystals with DMSO, the absorbance was monitored at 570 nm using a microplate reader (Molecular Devices, CA, USA Data are presented as standard error of means (SEM) from at least three independent experiments in triplicate.

3.5. Cell Cycle Analysis

CRC cells (2–3 $\times$ 10^5 cells/well) in 6-well plates were treated with PSY for 48 h. Then, the cells were harvested by trypsinization, rinsed twice with cold PBS, and pelleted by centrifugation at 1200 rpm for 3 min. Pellets were re-suspended in 70% ice-cold EtOH for 30 min at 4 °C to perform cell fixation. Then, samples were rinsed twice with PBS and stained using a solution containing 100 µg/mL of RNase A, 50 µg/mL propidium iodide (PI) in PBS for 30 min in the dark ([31]). Then, the cell cycle of the treated cells was analyzed using a BD FACS Canto™ II (Franklin Lakes, NJ, USA).

3.6. Apoptosis Analysis

Apoptosis of CRC cells was analyzed using a fluorescein isothiocyanate (FITC) Annexin V apoptosis detection kit (Biovision, Inc. K101-100, Waltham, MA, USA). Cells (2–3 $\times$ 10^5 cells/well) in 6-well plates were treated with PSY for 48 h. After the treatment, both adherent and floating cells were harvested by centrifugation, washed with PBS, and resuspended in 1$\times$ binding buffer at 1 $\times$ 10^6 cells/mL. Then, 100 µL of the cell suspension was transferred to a 5 mL culture tube and incubated with 5 µL FITC Annexin V and 5 µL PI for 15 min at room temperature in the dark. Then, 400 µL of 1$\times$ binding buffer was added in the 5 mL culture tube. Fluorescence intensity was analyzed using a BD FACS canto II (Franklin Lakes, NJ, USA). In addition, TUNEL assays were performed using a DeadEnd™ Fluorometric TUNEL assay kit (Promega, Madison, WI, USA) according to the manufacturer's protocol.

3.7. Immunofluorescence Staining

Cells were seeded in 8-well chamber slides and treated with PSY for 24 h. After the cells were fixed and permeabilized, the cells were stained with rabbit polyclonal anti-phospho (p)-STAT3 (1:100), Alexa Flour 488 goat anti-rabbit antibody (1:1000) (Invitrogen, Carlsbad, CA, USA) and 4′,6-diamidino-2-phenylindole (DAPI) (Sigma-Aldrich) as described ([31]. Images were obtained using an iRiSTM Digital Cell Imaging System (Logos Biosystems, Anyang, Republic of Korea).

3.8. Transient Transfection and Luciferase (Luc) Assays

Transient transfection and Luc assays were performed to measure STAT3 activity in PSY-treated cells as previously described ([31]). Cells were transfected with pSTAT3-Luc reporter containing STAT3 binding sites to measure STAT3 activity (Clontech, Palo Alto, CA, USA) in a 60 mm plate using Lipofectamine 2000 (Invitrogen). One day after transfection, cells were re-plated into a 48-well plate. Then, the cells were treated with PSY for 24 h. Luc assays were performed using a Luc assay system (Promega, Madison, WI, USA) according to the manufacturer's instructions. Luc activity was normalized by protein concentration.

3.9. Western Blotting Analysis

Whole-cell lysates were prepared, and Western blotting was performed as previously described ([31]). Primary antibodies against STAT3, p-STAT3 (Tyr705), JAK2, Src, p-Src (Tyr416), CDK4, CDK6, and p-CDK1 (Tyr15) were purchased from Cell Signaling Technology (Danvers, MA, USA). Additionally, p-JAK2 (Tyr1007/1008), CDK1, cyclin B1, PARP, SHP1, SHP2, and β-actin were purchased from Santa Cruz Biotechnology (Santa Cruz, CA, USA), and HRP-conjugated anti-mouse IgG and anti-rabbit (Cell Signaling Biotechnology) were used. Densitometric analysis of each band was performed using the ImageJ software (https://imagej.nih.gov/ij accessed and downloaded the updated software on 27 September 2021). Data are presented as the mean ± standard deviation (SD) from at least three independent experiments.

3.10. Ultra-Performance Liquid Chromatography Quadrupole Time of Flight Mass Spectrophotometry (UPLC-ESI-QTOF MS/MS) Analysis

Chromatographic analysis of the extract was performed to identify and assess the quality of the chemical components of the EtOH-Ex and Water-Ex. The LC-MS/MS system consisted of a Thermo Scientific Vanquish UHPLC system (Sunnyvale, CA, USA) with an ACQUITY UPLC HSS T3 column (2.1 mm × 100 mm, 1.8 μm; Waters™, Milford, MA, USA) and a Triple TOF 5600+ MS system (QTOF MS/MS, SCIEX, Foster City, CA, USA). The QTOF MS was equipped with an ESI source and used to complete the high-resolution experiment.

3.11. Phytochemical Identification in PSY

Raw data detected by UPLC-QTOF MS/MS were analyzed using PeakView 2.2, including MasterView software (SCIEX) for peak identification and matching with the reference standard and in-house MS/MS library, and the chemical structural information was analyzed using the GNPS website (http://gnps.ucsd.edu, accessed on 31 March 2022). Subsequently, accurate MS/MS fragmentation information was queried in MassBank (https://massbank.eu/MassBank), FooDB (https://foodb.ca), and Metlin databases (http://metlin.scripps.edu/website) to screen and identify potential compound information.

3.12. Statistical Analysis

All experiments were performed at least thrice. Data were analyzed using GraphPad Prism software (version 5.03; GraphPad Software, Inc., La Jolla, CA, USA) and expressed as mean ± SEM or SD. Differences between groups were assessed using analysis of variance, followed by ANOVA-Tukey's post hoc test, and $p < 0.05$ was considered to indicate a statistically significant difference.

Author Contributions: Conceptualization, S.H., J.L., K.S.A., I.J.H. and S.-G.L.; methodology, S.H., I.J.H. and S.-G.L.; validation, H.K., M.Y.L. and K.S.A.; formal analysis, S.H., H.K., K.S.A., I.J.H. and S.-G.L.; investigation, S.H., H.K., M.Y.L., K.S.A., I.J.H. and S.-G.L.; resources, J.L., K.S.A., I.J.H. and S.-G.L.; data curation, S.H., M.Y.L., I.J.H. and S.-G.L.; writing—original draft preparation, S.H., I.J.H. and S.-G.L.; writing—review and editing, I.J.H. and S.-G.L.; supervision, I.J.H. and S.-G.L.; project administration, I.J.H. and S.-G.L.; funding acquisition, I.J.H. and S.-G.L. All authors have read and agreed to the published version of the manuscript.

Funding: This study was supported by grants from the National Research Foundation of Korea: NRF-2021R1I1A2054560 (S.-G.L) and NRF-2021R1F1A1049427 (I.J.H.).

Institutional Review Board Statement: Not applicable.

Informed Consent Statement: Not applicable.

Data Availability Statement: Not applicable.

Conflicts of Interest: The authors declare no conflict of interest.

References

1. Sung, H.; Ferlay, J.; Siegel, R.L.; Laversanne, M.; Soerjomataram, I.; Jemal, A.; Bray, F. Global Cancer Statistics 2020: GLOBOCAN Estimates of Incidence and Mortality Worldwide for 36 Cancers in 185 Countries. *CA Cancer J. Clin.* **2021**, *71*, 209–249. [CrossRef] [PubMed]
2. Clinton, S.K.; Giovannucci, E.L.; Hursting, S.D. The World Cancer Research Fund/American Institute for Cancer Research Third Expert Report on Diet, Nutrition, Physical Activity, and Cancer: Impact and Future Directions. *J. Nutr.* **2020**, *150*, 663–671. [CrossRef] [PubMed]
3. Terzic, J.; Grivennikov, S.; Karin, E.; Karin, M. Inflammation and colon cancer. *Gastroenterology* **2010**, *138*, 2101–2114.e5. [CrossRef] [PubMed]
4. Yu, H.; Pardoll, D.; Jove, R. STATs in cancer inflammation and immunity: A leading role for STAT3. *Nat. Rev. Cancer* **2009**, *9*, 798–809. [CrossRef]
5. Chalikonda, G.; Lee, H.; Sheik, A.; Huh, Y.S. Targeting key transcriptional factor STAT3 in colorectal cancer. *Mol. Cell. Biochem.* **2021**, *476*, 3219–3228. [CrossRef]
6. Zhang, Z.H.; Li, M.Y.; Wang, Z.; Zuo, H.X.; Wang, J.Y.; Xing, Y.; Jin, C.; Xu, G.; Piao, L.; Piao, H.; et al. Convallatoxin promotes apoptosis and inhibits proliferation and angiogenesis through crosstalk between JAK2/STAT3 (T705) and mTOR/STAT3 (S727) signaling pathways in colorectal cancer. *Phytomedicine* **2020**, *68*, 153172. [CrossRef]
7. Huehnchen, P.; van Kampen, A.; Boehmerle, W.; Endres, M. Cognitive impairment after cytotoxic chemotherapy. *Neurooncol. Pract.* **2020**, *7*, 11–21. [CrossRef]
8. Tofthagen, C. Surviving chemotherapy for colon cancer and living with the consequences. *J. Palliat. Med.* **2010**, *13*, 1389–1391. [CrossRef]
9. Guldiken, B.; Ozkan, G.; Catalkaya, G.; Ceylan, F.D.; Ekin Yalcinkaya, I.; Capanoglu, E. Phytochemicals of herbs and spices: Health versus toxicological effects. *Food Chem. Toxicol.* **2018**, *119*, 37–49. [CrossRef]
10. Heo, J. *DONGUIBOGAM Treasured Mirror of Eastern Medicine*; Bubin Publishers Co.: Seoul, Republic of Korea, 2005.
11. Huang, S.Z.; Liu, W.Y.; Huang, Y.; Shen, A.L.; Liu, L.Y.; Peng, J. Patrinia scabiosaefolia Inhibits Growth of 5-FU-Resistant Colorectal Carcinoma Cells via Induction of Apoptosis and Suppression of AKT Pathway. *Chin. J. Integr. Med.* **2019**, *25*, 116–121. [CrossRef]
12. Liu, L.; Shen, A.; Chen, Y.; Wei, L.; Lin, J.; Sferra, T.J.; Hong, Z.; Peng, J. Patrinia scabiosaefolia induces mitochondrial-dependent apoptosis in a mouse model of colorectal cancer. *Oncol. Rep.* **2013**, *30*, 897–903. [CrossRef] [PubMed]
13. Lee, M.Y.; Lin, H.Y.; Cheng, F.; Chiang, W.; Kuo, Y.H. Isolation and characterization of new lactam compounds that inhibit lung and colon cancer cells from adlay (*Coix lachryma-jobi* L. var. *ma-yuen* Stapf) bran. *Food Chem. Toxicol.* **2008**, *46*, 1933–1939. [CrossRef]
14. Son, E.S.; Kim, Y.O.; Park, C.G.; Park, K.H.; Jeong, S.H.; Park, J.W.; Kim, S.H. Coix lacryma-jobi var. ma-yuen Stapf sprout extract has anti-metastatic activity in colon cancer cells in vitro. *BMC Complement. Altern. Med.* **2017**, *17*, 486. [CrossRef] [PubMed]

15. Eo, H.J.; Park, J.H.; Park, G.H.; Lee, M.H.; Lee, J.R.; Koo, J.S.; Jeong, J.B. Anti-inflammatory and anti-cancer activity of mulberry (*Morus alba* L.) root bark. *BMC Complement. Altern. Med.* **2014**, *14*, 200. [CrossRef] [PubMed]
16. Park, H.J.; Park, S.H. Root Bark of Morus Alba L. Induced p53-Independent Apoptosis in Human Colorectal Cancer Cells by Suppression of STAT3 Activity. *Nutr. Cancer* **2022**, *74*, 1837–1848. [CrossRef]
17. Li, B.; Tao, W.; Zheng, C.; Shar, P.A.; Huang, C.; Fu, Y.; Wang, Y. Systems pharmacology-based approach for dissecting the addition and subtraction theory of traditional Chinese medicine: An example using Xiao-Chaihu-Decoction and Da-Chaihu-Decoction. *Comput. Biol. Med.* **2014**, *53*, 19–29. [CrossRef]
18. Huynh, J.; Chand, A.; Gough, D.; Ernst, M. Therapeutically exploiting STAT3 activity in cancer—Using tissue repair as a road map. *Nat. Rev. Cancer* **2019**, *19*, 82–96. [CrossRef]
19. Morikawa, T.; Baba, Y.; Yamauchi, M.; Kuchiba, A.; Nosho, K.; Shima, K.; Tanaka, N.; Huttenhower, C.; Frank, D.A.; Fuchs, C.S.; et al. STAT3 expression, molecular features, inflammation patterns, and prognosis in a database of 724 colorectal cancers. *Clin. Cancer Res.* **2011**, *17*, 1452–1462. [CrossRef]
20. Peng, J.; Chen, Y.; Lin, J.; Zhuang, Q.; Xu, W.; Hong, Z.; Sferra, T.J. Patrinia scabiosaefolia extract suppresses proliferation and promotes apoptosis by inhibiting the STAT3 pathway in human multiple myeloma cells. *Mol. Med. Rep.* **2011**, *4*, 313–318.
21. Zhong, Y.-M.; Zhong, X.-L.; Wang, J.-H.; Han, L. Rapid analysis and identification of the main constituents in *Patrinia scabiosaefolia* Fisch. by UPLC/Q-TOF-MS/MS. *Acta Chromatogr.* **2017**, *29*, 267–277. [CrossRef]
22. Gong, L.; Zou, W.; Zheng, K.; Shi, B.; Liu, M. The *Herba Patriniae* (Caprifoliaceae): A review on traditional uses, phytochemistry, pharmacology and quality control. *J. Ethnopharmacol.* **2021**, *265*, 113264. [CrossRef]
23. Taguchi, H.; Endo, T. Letter: Patrinoside, a new iridoid glycoside from Patrinia scabiosaefolia. *Chem. Pharm. Bull.* **1974**, *22*, 1935–1937. [CrossRef] [PubMed]
24. Taguchi, H.; Endo, T.; Yosioka, I.; Iitaka, Y. The revised stereostructure of patrinoside X-ray crystallographic analysis. *Chem. Pharm. Bull.* **1979**, *27*, 1275–1276. [CrossRef]
25. Kim, J.S.; Kang, S.S. Chemical constituents of plants from the genus Patrinia. *Nat. Prod. Sci.* **2013**, *19*, 77–119.
26. Huang, L.; Zhang, R.S.; Wang, C.F.; Zhang, S.F. Studies on chemical constituents of Patrinia villosa. *Zhong Yao Cai* **2007**, *30*, 415–417.
27. Choi, E.J.; Shin, J.E.; Kim, H.G.; Kim, J.J.; Woo, E.-R. Lignans Isolated from the Roots of *Patrinia scabiosaefolia* F. and their IL(Interleukin)-6 Inhibitory Activity. *Yakhak Hoeji* **2009**, *53*, 201–205.
28. Park, D.; Ha, I.J.; Park, S.Y.; Choi, M.; Lim, S.L.; Kim, S.H.; Lee, J.H.; Ahn, K.S.; Yun, M.; Lee, S.G. Morusin Induces TRAIL Sensitization by Regulating EGFR and DR5 in Human Glioblastoma Cells. *J. Nat. Prod.* **2016**, *79*, 317–323. [CrossRef]
29. Jing, W.; Yan, R.; Wang, Y. A practical strategy for chemical profiling of herbal medicines using ultra-high performance liquid chromatography coupled with hybrid triple quadrupole-linear ion trap mass spectrometry: A case study of Mori Cortex. *Anal. Methods* **2015**, *7*, 443–457. [CrossRef]
30. Shi, X.; Mackie, B.; Zhang, G.; Yang, S.; Song, Y.; Su, D.; Liu, Y.; Shan, L. Identification of the Metabolic Enzyme Involved Morusin Metabolism and Characterization of Its Metabolites by Ultraperformance Liquid Chromatography Quadrupole Time-of-Flight Mass Spectrometry (UPLC/Q-TOF-MS/MS). *Evid. Based Complement. Altern. Med.* **2016**, *2016*, 9240103. [CrossRef]
31. Lim, S.-L.; Park, S.-Y.; Kang, S.; Park, D.; Kim, S.-H.; Um, J.-Y.; Jang, H.-J.; Lee, J.-H.; Jeong, C.-H.; Jang, J.-H.; et al. Morusin induces cell death through inactivating STAT3 signaling in prostate cancer cells. *Am. J. Cancer Res.* **2015**, *5*, 289–299.
32. Choi, D.W.; Cho, S.W.; Lee, S.G.; Choi, C.Y. The Beneficial Effects of Morusin, an Isoprene Flavonoid Isolated from the Root Bark of Morus. *Int. J. Mol. Sci* **2020**, *21*, 6541. [CrossRef]
33. Guo, H.; Xu, Y.; Huang, W.; Zhou, H.; Zheng, Z.; Zhao, Y.; He, B.; Zhu, T.; Tang, S.; Zhu, Q. Kuwanon G Preserves LPS-Induced Disruption of Gut Epithelial Barrier In Vitro. *Molecules* **2016**, *21*, 1597. [CrossRef]
34. Numata, M.; Yamamoto, A.; Moribayashi, A.; Yamada, H. Antitumor components isolated from the Chinese herbal medicine Coix lachryma-jobi. *Planta Med.* **1994**, *60*, 356–359. [CrossRef] [PubMed]
35. Jozwiak, M.; Filipowska, A.; Fiorino, F.; Struga, M. Anticancer activities of fatty acids and their heterocyclic derivatives. *Eur. J. Pharm.* **2020**, *871*, 172937. [CrossRef] [PubMed]
36. Liu, S.; Shen, H.; Li, J.; Gong, Y.; Bao, H.; Zhang, J.; Hu, L.; Wang, Z.; Gong, J. Loganin inhibits macrophage M1 polarization and modulates sirt1/NF-kappaB signaling pathway to attenuate ulcerative colitis. *Bioengineered* **2020**, *11*, 628–639. [CrossRef] [PubMed]
37. Miller, K.D.; Nogueira, L.; Devasia, T.; Mariotto, A.B.; Yabroff, K.R.; Jemal, A.; Kramer, J.; Siegel, R.L. Cancer treatment and survivorship statistics, 2022. *CA Cancer J. Clin.* **2022**, *72*, 409–436. [CrossRef]
38. Hofmann, C.; Buttenschoen, K.; Straeter, J.; Henne-Bruns, D.; Kornmann, M. Pre-clinical evaluation of the activity of irinotecan as a basis for regional chemotherapy. *Anticancer Res.* **2005**, *25*, 795–804.
39. Ciardiello, F.; Ciardiello, D.; Martini, G.; Napolitano, S.; Tabernero, J.; Cervantes, A. Clinical management of metastatic colorectal cancer in the era of precision medicine. *CA Cancer J. Clin.* **2022**, *72*, 372–401. [CrossRef]
40. Lee, S.G.; Jeon, H.Y.; Su, Z.Z.; Richards, J.E.; Vozhilla, N.; Sarkar, D.; Van Maerken, T.; Fisher, P.B. Astrocyte elevated gene-1 contributes to the pathogenesis of neuroblastoma. *Oncogene* **2009**, *28*, 2476–2484. [CrossRef]

biomolecules

MDPI

Article

Combination Therapy of Curcumin and Disulfiram Synergistically Inhibits the Growth of B16-F10 Melanoma Cells by Inducing Oxidative Stress

Sheila S. Fontes [1], Mateus L. Nogueira [1], Rosane B. Dias [1,2], Clarissa A. Gurgel Rocha [1,2], Milena B. P. Soares [1,3], Marcos A. Vannier-Santos [4,*] and Daniel P. Bezerra [1,*]

1 Gonçalo Moniz Institute, Oswaldo Cruz Foundation (IGM-FIOCRUZ/BA), Salvador 40296-710, BA, Brazil
2 Department of Propedeutics, School of Dentistry of the Federal University of Bahia, Salvador 40110-909, BA, Brazil
3 SENAI Institute for Innovation in Advanced Health Systems, SENAI CIMATEC, Salvador 41650-010, BA, Brazil
4 Oswaldo Cruz Institute, LITEB, Oswaldo Cruz Foundation, Rio de Janeiro 21040-360, RJ, Brazil
* Correspondence: marcos.vannier@ioc.fiocruz.br (M.A.V.-S.); daniel.bezerra@fiocruz.br (D.P.B.); Tel./Fax: +55-71-3176-2272 (D.P.B.)

Abstract: Oxidative stress plays a central role in the pathophysiology of melanoma. Curcumin (CUR) is a polyphenolic phytochemical that stimulates reactive oxygen species (ROS) production, while disulfiram (DSS) is a US FDA-approved drug for the treatment of alcoholism that can act by inhibiting the intracellular antioxidant system. Therefore, we hypothesized that they act synergistically against melanoma cells. Herein, we aimed to study the antitumor potential of the combination of CUR with DSS in B16-F10 melanoma cells using in vitro and in vivo models. The cytotoxic effects of different combination ratios of CUR and DSS were evaluated using the Alamar Blue method, allowing the production of isobolograms. Apoptosis detection, DNA fragmentation, cell cycle distribution, and mitochondrial superoxide levels were quantified by flow cytometry. Tumor development in vivo was evaluated using C57BL/6 mice bearing B16-F10 cells. The combinations ratios of 1:2, 1:3, and 2:3 showed synergic effects. B16-F10 cells treated with these combinations showed improved apoptotic cell death and DNA fragmentation. Enhanced mitochondrial superoxide levels were observed at combination ratios of 1:2 and 1:3, indicating increased oxidative stress. In vivo tumor growth inhibition for CUR (20 mg/kg), DSS (60 mg/kg), and their combination were 17.0%, 19.8%, and 28.8%, respectively. This study provided data on the potential cytotoxic activity of the combination of CUR with DSS and may provide a useful tool for the development of a therapeutic combination against melanoma.

Keywords: curcumin; disulfiram; melanoma; apoptosis; oxidative stress

Citation: Fontes, S.S.; Nogueira, M.L.; Dias, R.B.; Rocha, C.A.G.; Soares, M.B.P.; Vannier-Santos, M.A.; Bezerra, D.P. Combination Therapy of Curcumin and Disulfiram Synergistically Inhibits the Growth of B16-F10 Melanoma Cells by Inducing Oxidative Stress. *Biomolecules* **2022**, *12*, 1600. https://doi.org/10.3390/biom12111600

Academic Editor: Vladimir N. Uversky

Received: 27 September 2022
Accepted: 16 October 2022
Published: 31 October 2022

1. Introduction

Melanoma is one of the most aggressive forms of malignant skin neoplasms and one of the main causes of cancer mortality. Although it represents only 4% of dermatological cancers, it is responsible for 80% of skin cancer deaths due to its high metastatic capacity and high refractoriness to chemotherapy [1–4]. The 5-year survival rate of patients with metastatic melanoma is less than 20% [5]. Dacarbazine, an alkylating agent, is the main treatment for advanced melanoma. However, serious side effects have been observed, and the therapeutic response rate is approximately 10% [5,6]. These results indicate that new therapies for melanoma are urgently required.

Oxidative stress plays a central role in the pathophysiology of melanoma since the generation of melanin leads to the generation of hydrogen peroxide and consumption of reduced glutathione (GSH) [7,8]. Consequently, melanoma maintains high baseline

ROS levels compared to normal cells, which makes melanoma cells more susceptible to oxidative stress [7,9].

Curcumin (CUR) is a polyphenolic phytochemical isolated from turmeric, a food spice made from the rhizome of *Curcuma longa* L. [10]. Turmeric is traditionally used in many South Asian countries, both in traditional medicine and cooking, and has been used for over 2000 years as a medicine in China and India [11]. Curiously, many studies have reported that CUR causes cell death by stimulating reactive oxygen species (ROS) production in fibroblasts [12], leukemia [13], lymphoma [14], melanoma [15], and colon cancer [16].

Disulfiram (DSS) is a thiocarbamate drug approved by the United States Food and Drug Administration (US-FDA) for the clinical treatment of alcoholism and has been used for over 60 years [17]. DSS is an irreversible inhibitor of aldehyde dehydrogenase (ALDH). Interestingly, ALDH can decrease intracellular oxidative stress due to its ROS scavenger action. Consequently, DSS can act by inhibiting the intracellular antioxidant system [18,19].

Importantly, both DSS and CUR not only have antitumor activities but can also potentiate the action of anticancer chemotherapy drugs by blocking drug efflux pumps [20–26]. Furthermore, these compounds have been reported as agents capable of reducing the adverse reactions of highly toxic chemotherapeutic agents [27,28].

Therefore, we hypothesized that CUR, an oxidative stress inducer [29], combined with DSS, which acts as an antagonist of the intracellular antioxidant system [22], will have a synergistic effect, providing greater sensitization of cancer cells and resulting in cell death. Herein, we aimed to study the antitumor potential of the combination of CUR with DSS in B16-F10 melanoma cells using in vitro and in vivo models.

2. Material and Methods

2.1. CUR and DSS Obtaining

CUR and DSS were purchased from Sigma-Aldrich (Sigma-Aldrich Co., Saint Louis, MO, USA).

2.2. In Vitro Assays

2.2.1. Cells

The mouse melanoma B16-F10 cell line and human lung fibroblast MRC-5 cell line were obtained from the American Type Culture Collection (ATCC, Manassas, VA, USA) and were cultured as recommended by the ATCC animal cell culture guide. All cell lines were tested for mycoplasma using a mycoplasma staining kit (Sigma-Aldrich Co.) and were free from contamination. Cell viability was examined using the trypan blue exclusion method for all experiments. Over 90% of the cells were viable at the beginning of culture.

2.2.2. Alamar Blue Method

The quantification of cell viability was carried out by the Alamar Blue method, as previously described in refs. [30–32]. Briefly, the cells were seeded in 96-well plates and incubated for 72 h. CUR and DSS were tested on a concentration-response curve obtained by serial dilution of a stock dissolved in dimethyl sulfoxide (DMSO; Vetec Química Fina Ltd.a, Duque de Caxias, RJ, Brazil), with concentrations based on previous studies [33–35]. Doxorubicin (DOX, doxorubicin hydrochloride, purity $\geq$ 95%, Laboratory IMA S.A.I.C., Buenos Aires, Argentina) was used as a positive control. At the end of the treatment, 20 μL of a stock solution (0.312 mg/mL) of resazurin (Sigma-Aldrich Co.) were added to each well. Absorbances at 570 and 600 nm were measured using a SpectraMax 190 Microplate Reader (Molecular Devices, Sunnyvale, CA, USA).

2.2.3. Flow Cytometry Assays

To quantify cell death, the FITC Annexin V Apoptosis Detection Kit I (BD Biosciences, San Jose, CA, USA) was used, and the analysis was performed according to the manufacturer's instructions. Cell fluorescence was determined by flow cytometry.

DNA fragmentation and cell cycle distribution were determined using 2 μg/mL propidium iodide (PI) in cells permeabilized with 0.1% Triton X-100, 0.1% sodium citrate and 100 μg/mL RNAse (all from Sigma-Aldrich Co.), as previously described in ref. [36], and cell fluorescence was assessed by flow cytometry.

Detection of superoxide levels was performed using MitoSOX™ Red reagent, a fluorogenic dye specifically targeted to mitochondria in living cells (Thermo Fisher Scientific, Waltham, MA, USA), and the analysis was performed according to the manufacturer's instructions. Cell fluorescence was determined by flow cytometry.

For all analyses using flow cytometry, 10,000 events were recorded per sample with a BD LSRFortessa cytometer and analyzed with BD FACSDiva Software (BD Biosciences, San Jose, CA, USA) and FlowJo Software 10 (Flowjo LCC, Ashland, OR, USA), and cellular debris was omitted from the analysis.

2.3. *In Vivo Assay*

2.3.1. Animals

A total of 50 specific pathogen-free C57BL/6 mice (males, 25–30 g) were obtained and maintained at the animal facilities of the Gonçalo Moniz Institute-FIOCRUZ (Salvador, BA, Brazil). Animals were housed in cages with free access to food and water. All animals were kept under a 12:12 h light–dark cycle (lights on at 6:00 a.m.). The animals were treated according to the ethical principles for animal experimentation of SBCAL (Brazilian Association of Laboratory Animal Science), Brazil. The Animal Ethics Committee of the Oswaldo Cruz Foundation (Salvador, BA, Brazil) approved the experimental protocol (number 01/2013).

2.3.2. In Vivo B16-F10 Melanoma Model

The in vivo antitumor effect was evaluated in C57BL/6 mice inoculated with B16-F10 melanoma cells, as previously described in ref. [37]. Tumor cells (2×10^6 cells per 500 μL) were implanted subcutaneously into the left hind groin of mice. The compounds were dissolved in 5% DMSO and provided to the mice intraperitoneally once a day for 15 consecutive days. Mice were divided into five groups at the beginning of the experiment: Group 1 (negative control, $n = 10$): animals treated with vehicle (5% DMSO); Group 2 (positive control, $n = 10$): animals treated with DOX (1 mg/kg/day); Group 3: animals treated with CUR (20 mg/kg/day, $n = 10$); Group 4: animals treated with DSS (60 mg/kg/day, $n = 10$); Group 5: animals treated with CUR (20 mg/kg/day) plus DSS (60 mg/kg/day) ($n = 10$). The treatments were initiated one day after tumor injection. On day 16, the animals were anesthetized (thiopental, 50 mg/kg), and samples of peripheral blood were collected from the brachial artery for hematological analyses, as described below. The animals were euthanized by anesthetic overdose (thiopental, 100 mg/kg), and the tumors were excised and weighed. Drug effects are expressed as the percentage inhibition in relation to the control.

2.3.3. Systemic Toxicological Evaluation

Systemic toxicological effects were also investigated, as previously described in ref. [37]. The mice were weighed at the beginning and end of the experiment. The animals were observed for signs of abnormalities throughout the study. Hematological analyses were performed using an Advia 60 hematology system (Bayer, Leverkusen, Germany). Their livers, kidneys, lungs, and hearts were removed, weighed, and examined for any signs of gross lesions or color changes and hemorrhage. Following macroscopic analysis, representative tissue sections of the tumors, livers, kidneys, lungs, and hearts were fixed in 4% buffered formalin and embedded in paraffin. Tissue sections with a thickness of 4 μm were stained with hematoxylin and eosin, and the analyses were performed under light microscopy.

2.4. *Statistical Analysis*

Inhibitory concentrations of 50% (IC_{50}) values and their 95% confidence intervals (CI 95%) were obtained via nonlinear regression. The fractional inhibitory concentration

(FIC) was calculated following the formula FIC(a) = effect (a) of the compound in combination/effect (a) of the compound alone where (a) are the effects of 25%, 50%, and 75% inhibition resulting in FIC25, FIC50, and FIC75. Isobolograms were constructed using the coordinates formed by the FIC (CUR + DSS) of the 25%, 50%, and 75% effects. The line linking the number 1 in both axes was used. Points below this line indicate synergistic results of combination, and points above the line indicate antagonism. Points upon the line indicate an addictive effect [38].

Data are presented as the means ± SEMs or IC_{50} values. Differences between experimental groups were compared using ANOVA (analysis of variance) followed by the Student Newman-Keuls test ($p < 0.05$). Statistical analyses were performed using GraphPad software (GraphPad Software, Inc., San Diego, CA, USA).

3. Results

3.1. Combination Therapy of CUR and DSS Synergistically Inhibits the Growth of B16-F10 Melanoma Cells

CUR and DSS showed cytotoxic effects on B16-F10 and MRC-5 cells in a concentration-dependent manner after 72 h of incubation, as evaluated using the Alamar Blue method (Figure 1). The IC_{50} values found in B16-F10 cells were 9.69, 16.49, and 0.19 µg/mL for CUR, DSS, and DOX, respectively, while those in MRC-5 cells were 3.60, 13.63, and 1.60 µg/mL, respectively.

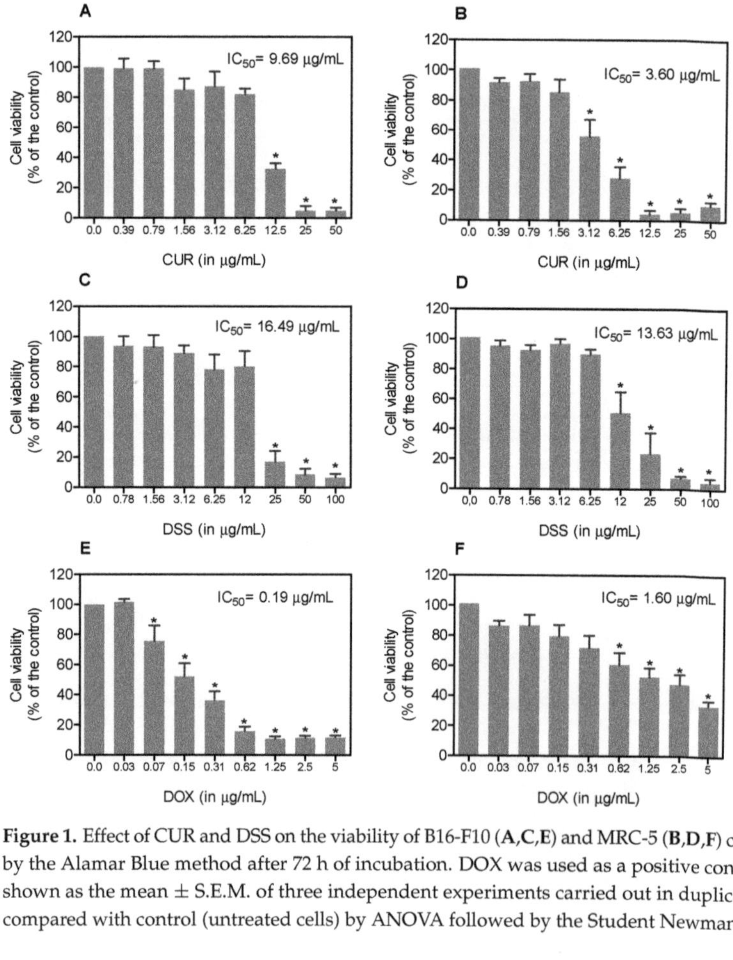

Figure 1. Effect of CUR and DSS on the viability of B16-F10 (**A**,**C**,**E**) and MRC-5 (**B**,**D**,**F**) cells measured by the Alamar Blue method after 72 h of incubation. DOX was used as a positive control. Data are shown as the mean ± S.E.M. of three independent experiments carried out in duplicate. * $p < 0.05$ compared with control (untreated cells) by ANOVA followed by the Student Newman-Keuls test.

Next, we tested the combination of CUR with DSS in five different ratios: 1:2, 1:3, 1:4, 2:3. and 1:10 (Figures S1–S5). Although these combinations were also toxic to noncancerous MRC-5 cells, enhanced cytotoxicity was observed in B16-F10 cells. The effect on B16-F10 cells was evaluated using FIC25, FIC50, and FIC75, revealing the magnitude of the concentration of each compound in relation to the same compound alone (Table S1). These data were also observed in isobolograms (Figure 2), where we found synergic effects for the combinations 1:2, 1:3, and 2:3 in FIC50. Therefore, these combinations were selected for further studies.

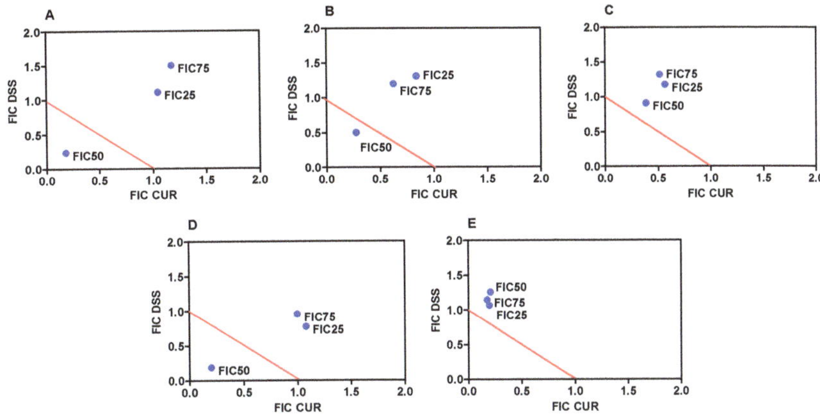

Figure 2. Isobolograms of the effects of the combination of CUR with DSS at ratios of 1:2 (**A**), 1:3 (**B**), 1:4 (**C**), 2:3 (**D**), and 1:10 (**E**) on the viability of B16-F10 cells. The fractional inhibitory concentration (FIC) values were calculated following the formula FIC(a) = effect (a) of the compound in combination/effect (a) of the compound alone, where (a) are the effects of 25%, 50%, and 75% inhibition resulting in FIC25, FIC50, and FIC75, respectively. Isobolograms were constructed using the coordinates formed by the FIC (CUR + DSS) of the 25%, 50%, and 75% effects. The line linking the number 1 in both axes was used. Points below this line indicate synergistic results of combination, and points above the line indicate antagonism. Points upon the line indicate an addictive effect.

3.2. Combination Therapy with CUR and DSS Causes Apoptotic Cell Death in B16-F10 Melanoma Cells

In a new set of experiments, apoptosis quantification was evaluated in B16-F10 cells by annexin-V/PI double staining using flow cytometry after 48 and 72 h incubation. The numbers of viable (annexin-V/PI double-negative cells), apoptotic (all annexin-V-positive cells), and necrotic cells (annexin-V-negative/PI-positive cells) were quantified. The IC_{50} values of each compound were used (CUR 10 μg/mL and DSS 18 μg/mL). The ratios of 1:2 (CUR 2 μg/mL and DSS 4 μg/mL), 1:3 (CUR 2 μg/mL and DSS 6 μg/mL), and 2:3 (CUR 2 μg/mL and DSS 3 μg/mL) were also tested.

In B16-F10, CUR treatment led to 56.6% and 71.5% apoptosis after 48 and 72 h incubation, respectively, whereas DSS caused 39.7% and 36.3% apoptosis (Figures 3 and S6). The combinations tested significantly increased apoptosis after 72 h of incubation. Combination 1:2 led to 32.0% apoptosis in B16-F10 cells (Figures 4 and S7), while combination 1:3 caused 22.7% apoptosis (Figures 5 and S8), and combination 2:3 caused 31.6% apoptosis (Figures 6 and S9) after 72 h of incubation. A statistically significant proportional reduction in the viable cells was also observed.

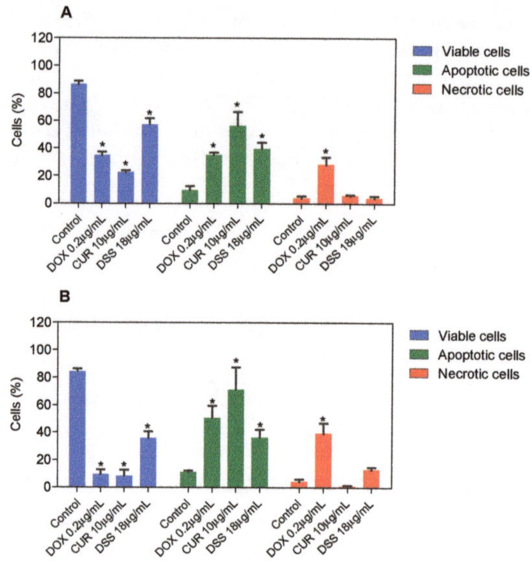

Figure 3. Effect of CUR and DSS on the viability of B16-F10 cells measured by annexin V-FITC/PI staining after 48 (**A**) and 72 (**B**) h of incubation. DOX was used as a positive control. Data are shown as the mean ± S.E.M. of three independent experiments carried out in duplicate. * $p < 0.05$ compared with control (0.5% DMSO) by ANOVA followed by Student Newman-Keuls test.

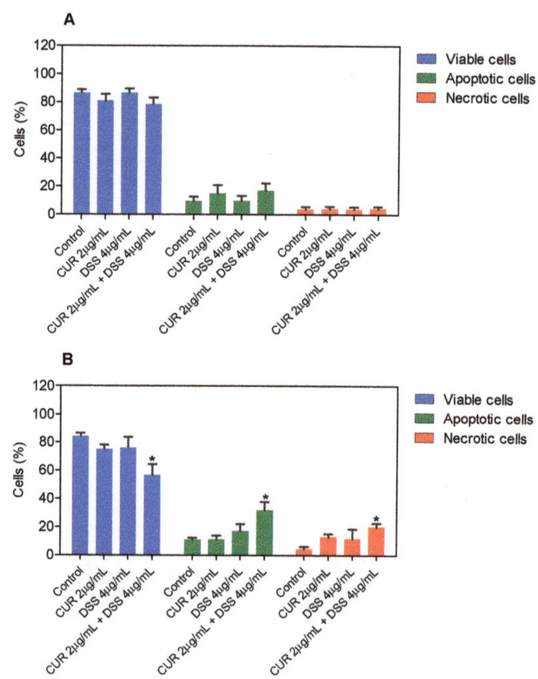

Figure 4. Effect of the combination of CUR with DSS at a ratio of 1:2 on the viability of B16-F10 cells measured by annexin V-FITC/PI staining after 48 (**A**) and 72 (**B**) h of incubation. Data are shown as the mean ± S.E.M. of three independent experiments carried out in duplicate. * $p < 0.05$ compared with control (0.5% DMSO) by ANOVA followed by Student Newman-Keuls test.

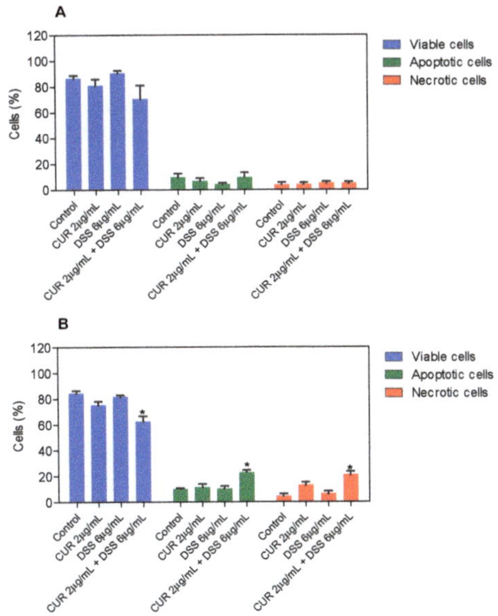

Figure 5. Effect of the combination of CUR with DSS at a ratio of 1:3 on the viability of B16-F10 cells measured by annexin V-FITC/PI staining after 48 (**A**) and 72 (**B**) h of incubation. Data are shown as the mean ± S.E.M. of three independent experiments carried out in duplicate. * $p < 0.05$ compared with control (0.5% DMSO) by ANOVA followed by Student Newman-Keuls test.

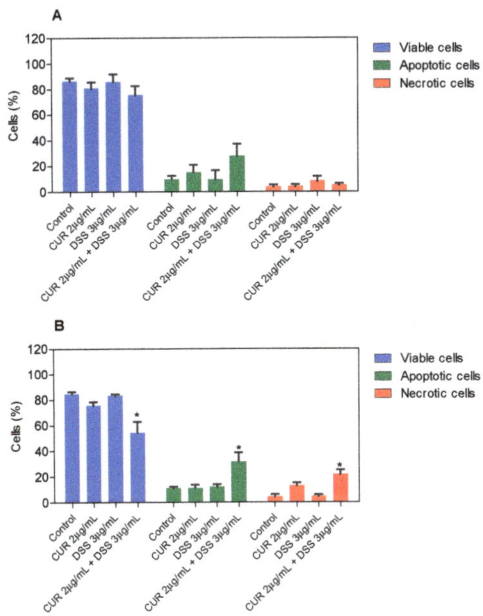

Figure 6. Effect of the combination of CUR with DSS at a ratio of 2:3 on the viability of B16-F10 cells measured by annexin V-FITC/PI staining after 48 (**A**) and 72 (**B**) h of incubation. Data are shown as the mean ± S.E.M. of three independent experiments carried out in duplicate. * $p < 0.05$ compared with control (0.5% DMSO) by ANOVA followed by Student Newman-Keuls test.

Next, the DNA content was measured by flow cytometry to quantify the internucleosomal DNA fragmentation and cell cycle distribution in B16-F10 cells treated with CUR and DSS alone or in combination after 48 and 72 h incubation. All DNA that was subdiploid (sub-G_0/G_1) was considered fragmented. CUR induced 33.5% and 34.4% DNA fragmentation in B16-F10 cells, while DSS caused 34.0% and 32.7% DNA fragmentation after 48 and 72 h of incubation, respectively (Figures 7 and S10). After 72 h of incubation, the 1:2 combination induced 24.9% DNA fragmentation in B16-F10 cells (Figures 8 and S11), while the 1:3 (Figures 9 and S12) and 2:3 (Figures 10 and S13) combinations caused 23.4% DNA fragmentation. No significant changes were observed after 48 h of incubation. A proportional reduction in the cell cycle phase was also observed. An increase in the cell cycle phase G_2/M was found after 48 h of incubation with CUR, as well as in the combination 1:2 after 72 h of incubation. DOX caused cell cycle arrest at the G_2/M phase, which was followed by DNA fragmentation in B16-F10 cells.

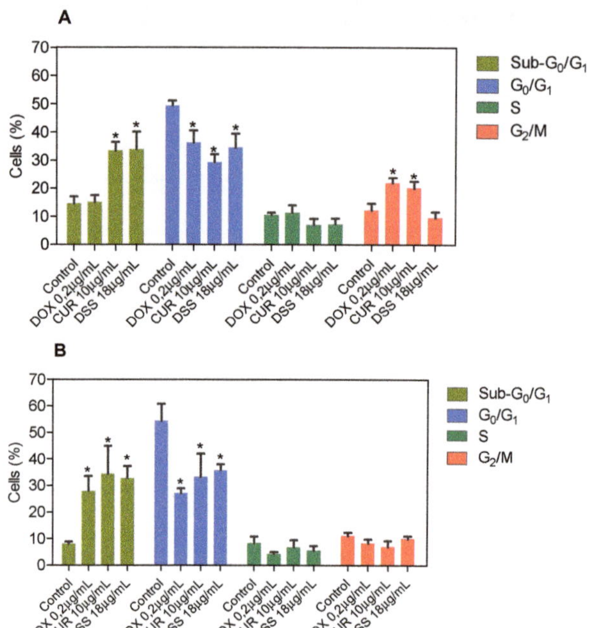

Figure 7. Effect of CUR and DSS on DNA fragmentation and cell cycle distribution of B16-F10 cells after 48 (**A**) and 72 (**B**) h of incubation. DOX was used as a positive control. Data are shown as the mean ± S.E.M. of three independent experiments carried out in duplicate. * $p < 0.05$ compared with control (0.5% DMSO) by ANOVA followed by Student Newman-Keuls test.

3.3. Combination Therapy with CUR and DSS Induces Oxidative Stress in B16-F10 Melanoma Cells

MitoSOX™ Red was used to quantify mitochondrial superoxide levels in B16-F10 cells treated with CUR and DSS alone or in combination after 24 h of incubation (Figure 11). CUR or DSS significantly increased MitoSOX™ Red staining in B16-F10 cells, showing an MFI of 3313 ± 204.3 for CUR and 3532 ± 661.9 for DSS, against 1641 ± 292.6 found for the negative control, indicating increased oxidative stress. A significant increase in oxidative stress was also observed in B16-F10 cells treated with the combinations 1:2 (MFI of 3168 ± 156.7) and 1:3 (MFI of 3571 ± 360.1).

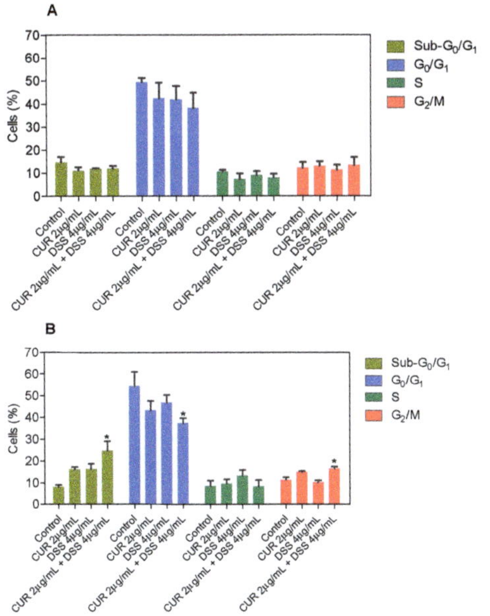

Figure 8. Effect of the combination of CUR with DSS at a ratio of 1:2 on DNA fragmentation and cell cycle distribution of B16-F10 cells after 48 (**A**) and 72 (**B**) h of incubation. Data are shown as the mean ± S.E.M. of three independent experiments carried out in duplicate. * $p < 0.05$ compared with control (0.5% DMSO) by ANOVA followed by Student Newman-Keuls test.

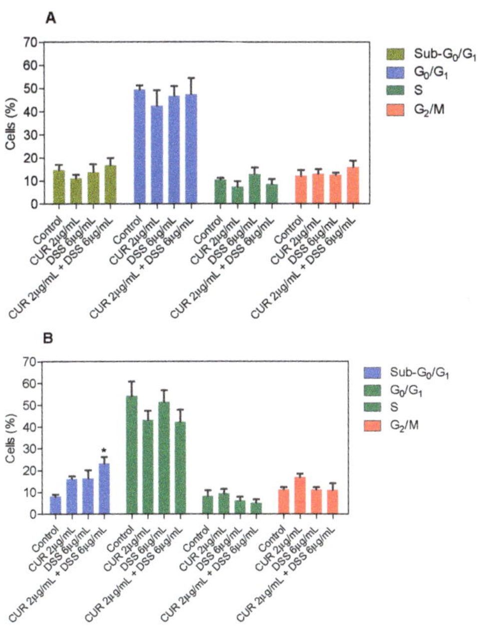

Figure 9. Effect of the combination of CUR with DSS at a ratio of 1:3 on DNA fragmentation and cell cycle distribution of B16-F10 cells after 48 (**A**) and 72 (**B**) h of incubation. Data are shown as the mean ± S.E.M. of three independent experiments carried out in duplicate. * $p < 0.05$ compared with control (0.5% DMSO) by ANOVA followed by Student Newman-Keuls test.

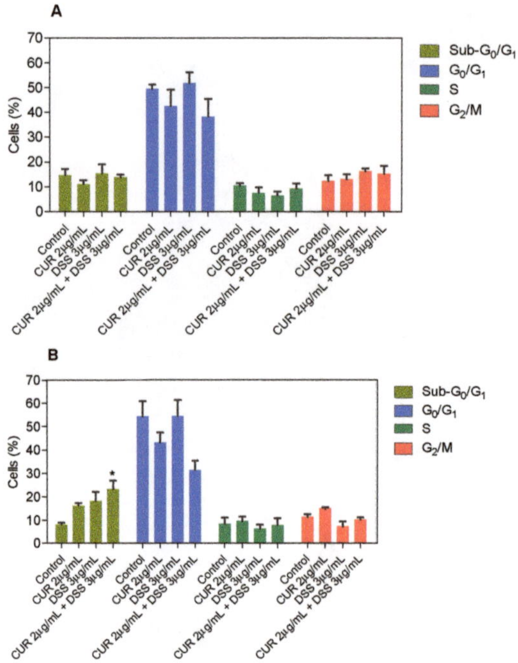

Figure 10. Effect of the combination of CUR with DSS at a ratio of 2:3 on DNA fragmentation and cell cycle distribution of B16-F10 cells after 48 (**A**) and 72 (**B**) h of incubation. Data are shown as the mean ± S.E.M. of three independent experiments carried out in duplicate. * $p < 0.05$ compared with control (0.5% DMSO) by ANOVA followed by Student Newman-Keuls test.

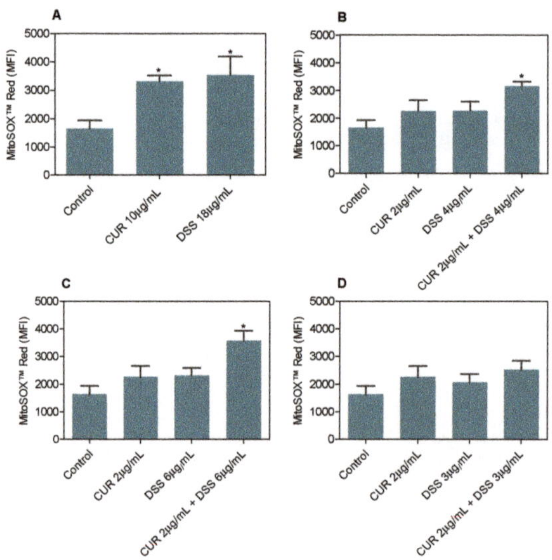

Figure 11. Effect of CUR and DSS (**A**) and their combinations at ratios of 1:2 (**B**), 1:3 (**C**), and 2:3 (**D**) on the mitochondrial superoxide level of B16-F10 cells measured by MitoSOX™ Red staining after 24 h of incubation. Data are shown as the mean ± S.E.M. of three independent experiments carried out in duplicate. * $p < 0.05$ compared with control (0.5% DMSO) by ANOVA followed by Student Newman-Keuls test. MFI = Mean Fluorescence Intensity.

3.4. Combination Therapy with CUR and DSS Inhibits B16-F10 Melanoma Cells Grown In Vivo

The antitumor activities of CUR and DSS alone and in combination were evaluated in C57BL/6 mice bearing B16-F10 cells (Figure 12). The treatment was performed by intraperitoneal injection of 20 mg/kg CUR, 60 mg/kg DSS and their combination at a ratio of 1:3 (20 mg/kg CUR + 60 mg/kg DSS) for 15 days. DOX was used as a positive control at 1 mg/kg. At the end of treatment, the mean tumor mass weight of the control group was 6.9 ± 0.3 g. CUR and DSS showed mean tumor mass weights of 5.7 ± 0.5 and 5.6 ± 0.3 g, respectively, while an average tumor mass of 4.9 ± 0.6 g was found for the combination of CUR with DSS. Tumor mass inhibition rates were 17.0%, 19.8%, and 28.8% for CUR, DSS, and the combination, respectively. DOX (1 mg/kg) reduced tumor weight by 43.9%.

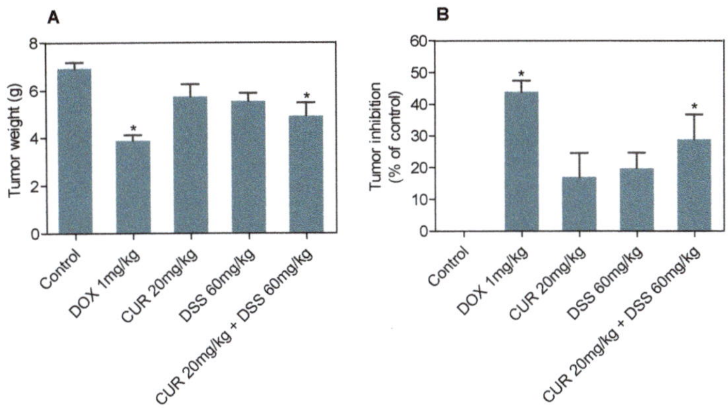

Figure 12. Effect of CUR and DSS and their combination at a ratio of 1:3 on the in vivo development of B16-F10 cells measured by tumor weight (**A**) and tumor inhibition (**B**). DOX was used as a positive control. Data are shown as the mean ± S.E.M. of 7–10 animals. * $p < 0.05$ compared with control (5% DMSO) by ANOVA followed by Student Newman-Keuls test.

In the histological analysis of tumors (Figure 13), a highly proliferative tumor exhibiting rounded and disrupted cells was observed. Atypical mitosis, apoptosis, and necrosis were frequent features. In CUR-treated animals, we observed more delimitated and less vascularized tumors.

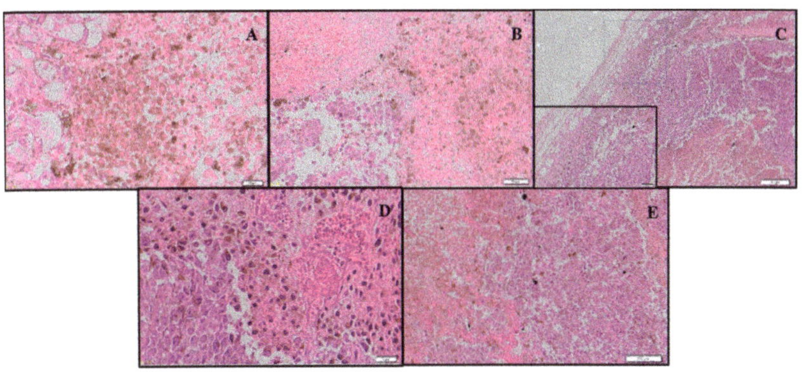

Figure 13. Representative histological analysis of B16-F10 tumor tissues stained with hematoxylin and eosin and analyzed by light microscopy. The animals were treated with 5% DMSO (**A**), 1 mg/kg DOX (**B**), 20 mg/kg CUR (**C**), 60 mg/kg DSS (**D**), or 20 mg/kg CUR + 60 mg/kg DSS (**E**). Bars = 20 µm (**A**,**D**), 50 µm (**B**), 200 µm (**C**), or 100 µm (**E**).

The systemic toxic effect of the CUR and DSS treatments or their combination was also evaluated. Three animals died in the combination group, and one animal died in each group, with the exception of the control group. No significant changes were found in the relative mass of the organs or body weights (Table S2). In the hematological parameter analyses, an increase in erythrocytes, hemoglobin, MCV, and platelets was found in the groups treated with DOX and DSS compared to the control (Table S3).

The histopathological examinations of hearts and kidneys showed well-preserved structures in all experimental groups (Figures S14 and S15). In the liver, areas of hydropic degeneration, vascular hyperemia and inflammation were frequent in the control groups, although swelling of hepatocytes was seen in the CUR and DSS groups (Figure S16). Single treatment with CUR or DSS resulted in mild inflammation and areas of fibrosis in the kidney and liver. In the combination treatment group, mild edema was identified. Focal areas of microgoticular steatosis were observed in some animals of the control and groups treated with DOX, CUR, and the combination treatment. In the lungs, areas of inflammation, vascular hyperemia, and alveolar septal thickening were observed in all groups (Figure S17).

4. Discussion

The treatment for patients with melanoma usually shows low response rates associated with the development of resistance and side effects with low overall survival [1–6]. In this work, we demonstrated for the first time that CUR and DSS inhibit the in vitro and in vivo development of melanoma B16-F10 cells and, when combined, presented synergistic action. Induction of apoptosis and oxidative stress was also found.

Repositioning clinically approved drugs has been considered a viable approach to building new anti-cancer drugs. The repositioning allows prior knowledge of safety factors, bioavailability, and formulations, offering advantages such as shorter development time and lower research costs, providing agility in accessing new therapeutic options for cancer patients [39,40]. The time between new drug development and clinical trials averages 9 years, with a success rate of less than 10% and an average patient cost per drug of several hundred million dollars. In contrast, drug repositioning can take 3 to 4 years for clinical trials and costs only a fraction of the amounts needed to test a new class of drug in patients [41].

CUR is a nutraceutical drug, and DSS is an FDA-approved drug, both of which are used long-term by humans. This indicates that their combination can be safe, even if it has an effect on noncancerous MRC-5 cells. Nevertheless, drug repositioning may be accompanied by side effects that have not been previously identified and described [42]. Therefore, more experiments are required to validate the safety of the CUR and DSS combination.

Apoptosis has been reported as a mechanism of programmed cell death in the presence of cytotoxic agents with chemotherapeutic potential. Treatment with high concentrations of CUR has been described as capable of inducing apoptosis, depending on the cell and tissue type, by both extrinsic and intrinsic pathways, as well as by increased endoplasmic reticulum stress [43]. The intrinsic induction of apoptosis by CUR is activated in response to cellular signals, including stress or DNA damage [34,44]. DSS is responsible for activating the extrinsic pathway of apoptosis [35]. In this work, we showed that B16-F10 cells treated with the combination of CUR with DSS for a period of 72 h showed increased externalization of phosphatidylserine, suggesting cell death by apoptosis.

Considering that the redox mechanism of melanocytes is extremely important for tumor progression, our result here was obtained by the combination of the pro-oxidant profile, favored by the use of CUR, and by the antagonistic action of the antioxidant system performed by DSS, resulting in increased oxidative stress in tumor cells, which was confirmed by the presence of superoxide radicals in B16-F10 cells. In addition, other targets, including the inhibition of the ubiquitin-proteasome system, were reported for these compounds and may contribute to their cytotoxicity [45,46].

The antitumor activities of CUR have been demonstrated in melanoma cells [15] and animal models [47]. DSS has been shown to exert protective effects on organs in experimental studies, preventing myocardial damage [48], in addition to sensitizing tumor cells to radiotherapy and increasing the cytotoxicity of antineoplastic drugs, which can be used as adjuvant therapy [49]. In our in vivo experiment, we also observed that lower doses of the combined drugs led to a significant reduction in the progression of B16F10 cells in mice.

This study provided data on the potential cytotoxic activity of the combination of CUR with DSS and may provide a useful tool for the development of novel therapeutic combinations against melanoma.

Supplementary Materials: The following supporting information can be downloaded at: https://www.mdpi.com/article/10.3390/biom12111600/s1, Figure S1. Effect of the combination of CUR and DSS at a ratio of 1:2 on the viability of B16-F10 (A) and MRC-5 (B) cells measured by the alamar blue method after 72 h of incubation. Figure S2. Effect of the combination of CUR and DSS at a ratio of 1:3 on the viability of B16-F10 (A) and MRC-5 (B) cells measured by the alamar blue method after 72 h of incubation. Figure S3. Effect of the combination of CUR and DSS at a ratio of 1:4 on the viability of B16-F10 (A) and MRC-5 (B) cells measured by the alamar blue method after 72 h of incubation. Figure S4. Effect of the combination of CUR and DSS at a ratio of 2:3 on the viability of B16-F10 (A) and MRC-5 (B) cells measured by the alamar blue method after 72 h of incubation. Figure S5. Effect of the combination of CUR and DSS at a ratio of 1:10 on the viability of B16-F10 (A) and MRC-5 (B) cells measured by the alamar blue method after 72 h of incubation. Figure S6. Representative dotplots of the effect of CUR and DSS on the viability of B16-F10 cells measured by annexin V-FITC/PI staining. Figure S7. Representative dotplots of the effect of the combination of CUR with DSS at a ratio of 1:2 on the viability of B16-F10 cells measured by annexin V-FITC/PI staining. Figure S8. Representative dotplots of the effect of the combination of CUR with DSS at a ratio of 1:3 on the viability of B16-F10 cells measured by annexin V-FITC/PI staining. Figure S9. Representative dotplots of the effect of the combination of CUR with DSS at a ratio of 2:3 on the viability of B16-F10 cells measured by annexin V-FITC/PI staining. Figure S10. Representative histograms of the effect of CUR and DSS on DNA fragmentation and cell cycle distribution of B16-F10 cells. Figure S11. Representative histograms of the effect of the combination of CUR with DSS at a ratio of 1:2 on DNA fragmentation and cell cycle distribution of B16-F10 cells. Figure S12. Representative histograms of the effect of the combination of CUR with DSS at a ratio of 1:3 on DNA fragmentation and cell cycle distribution of B16-F10 cells. Figure S13. Representative histograms of the effect of the combination of CUR with DSS at a ratio of 2:3 on DNA fragmentation and cell cycle distribution of B16-F10 cells. Figure S14. Representative histological analysis of hearts stained with hematoxylin and eosin and analyzed by light microscopy. Figure S15. Representative histological analysis of kidneys stained with hematoxylin and eosin and analyzed by light microscopy. Figure S16. Representative histological analysis of livers stained with hematoxylin and eosin and analyzed by light microscopy. Figure S17. Representative histological analysis of lungs stained with hematoxylin and eosin and analyzed by light microscopy. Table S1. Inhibitory concentrations of CUR and DSS alone and in combination. Table S2. Effect of CUR and DSS and their combination on body and relative organ weight from C57BL/6 mice bearing B16-F10 cells. Table S3. Effect of CUR and DSS and their combination on hematological parameters of peripheral blood from C57BL/6 mice bearing B16-F10 cells.

Author Contributions: S.S.F.: conceptualization, formal analysis, investigation, visualization; M.L.N.: formal analysis, investigation, visualization; R.B.D.: formal analysis, investigation, visualization; C.A.G.R.: formal analysis, writing—review and editing, funding acquisition; M.B.P.S.: writing—review and editing, supervision, funding acquisition; M.A.V.-S.: conceptualization, writing—review and editing, supervision, project administration, funding acquisition; D.P.B.: conceptualization, writing—original draft, supervision, project administration, funding acquisition. All authors have read and agreed to the published version of the manuscript.

Funding: This work was financially supported by Brazilian agencies Coordenação de Aperfeiçoamento de Pessoal de Nível Superior (CAPES), Conselho Nacional de Desenvolvimento Científico e Tecnológico (CNPq), and Fundação de Amparo à Pesquisa do Estado da Bahia (FAPESB). The design of the study, collection, analysis, and interpretation of data, and the writing of the manuscript were not influenced by funding agencies.

Institutional Review Board Statement: The Animal Ethics Committee of the Oswaldo Cruz Foundation (Salvador, Bahia, Brazil) approved the experimental protocol (number 01/2013).

Informed Consent Statement: Not applicable.

Data Availability Statement: Data will be made available upon reasonable request.

Acknowledgments: The authors are grateful to the flow cytometry and histotechnology cores of FIOCRUZ-Bahia for collecting flow cytometry data and performing histological techniques, respectively.

Conflicts of Interest: The authors declare no conflict of interest.

References

1. Miller, A.J.; Mihm, M.C., Jr. Melanoma. *N. Engl. J. Med.* **2006**, *355*, 51–65. [CrossRef] [PubMed]
2. Wagstaff, W.; Mwamba, R.N.; Grullon, K.; Armstrong, M.; Zhao, P.; Hendren-Santiago, B.; Qin, K.H.; Li, A.J.; Hu, D.A.; Youssef, A.; et al. Melanoma: Molecular genetics, metastasis, targeted therapies, immunotherapies, and therapeutic resistance. *Genes Dis.* **2022**, *9*, 1608–1623. [CrossRef] [PubMed]
3. Davis, L.E.; Shalin, S.C.; Tackett, A.J. Current state of melanoma diagnosis and treatment. *Cancer Biol. Ther.* **2019**, *20*, 1366–1379. [CrossRef] [PubMed]
4. Sung, H.; Ferlay, J.; Siegel, R.L.; Laversanne, M.; Soerjomataram, I.; Jemal, A.; Bray, F. Global Cancer Statistics 2020: GLOBOCAN Estimates of Incidence and Mortality Worldwide for 36 Cancers in 185 Countries. *CA Cancer J. Clin.* **2021**, *71*, 209–249. [CrossRef] [PubMed]
5. Maio, M.; Grob, J.J.; Aamdal, S.; Bondarenko, I.; Robert, C.; Thomas, L.; Garbe, C.; Chiarion-Sileni, V.; Testori, A.; Chen, T.T.; et al. Five-year survival rates for treatment-naive patients with advanced melanoma who received ipilimumab plus dacarbazine in a phase III trial. *J. Clin. Oncol.* **2015**, *33*, 1191–1196. [CrossRef]
6. Hao, M.; Song, F.; Du, X.; Wang, G.; Yang, Y.; Chen, K.; Yang, J. Advances in targeted therapy for unresectable melanoma: New drugs and combinations. *Cancer Lett.* **2015**, *359*, 1–8. [CrossRef]
7. Obrador, E.; Liu-Smith, F.; Dellinger, R.W.; Salvador, R.; Meyskens, F.L.; Estrela, J.M. Oxidative stress and antioxidants in the pathophysiology of malignant melanoma. *Biol. Chem.* **2019**, *400*, 589–612. [CrossRef]
8. Kim, E.; Panzella, L.; Napolitano, A.; Payne, G.F. Redox Activities of melanins investigated by electrochemical reverse engineering: Implications for their roles in oxidative stress. *J. Investig. Dermatol.* **2020**, *140*, 537–543. [CrossRef]
9. Liu-Smith, F.; Dellinger, R.; Meyskens, F.L., Jr. Updates of reactive oxygen species in melanoma etiology and progression. *Arch. Biochem. Biophys.* **2014**, *563*, 51–55. [CrossRef]
10. Ghasemi, F.; Shafiee, M.; Banikazemi, Z.; Pourhanifeh, M.H.; Khanbabaei, H.; Shamshirian, A.; Amiri Moghadam, S.; ArefNezhad, R.; Sahebkar, A.; Avan, A.; et al. Curcumin inhibits NF-kB and Wnt/β-catenin pathways in cervical cancer cells. *Pathol. Res. Pract.* **2019**, *215*, 152556. [CrossRef]
11. Sarkar, F.H.; Li, Y.; Wang, Z.; Padhye, S. Lesson learned from nature for the development of novel anti-cancer agents: Implication of isoflavone, curcumin, and their synthetic analogs. *Curr. Pharm. Des.* **2010**, *16*, 1801–1812. [CrossRef]
12. Thayyullathil, F.; Chathoth, S.; Hago, A.; Patel, M.; Galadari, S. Rapid reactive oxygen species (ROS) generation induced by curcumin leads to caspase-dependent and -independent apoptosis in L929 cells. *Free Radic. Biol. Med.* **2008**, *45*, 1403–1412. [CrossRef]
13. Sánchez, Y.; Simón, G.P.; Calviño, E.; de Blas, E.; Aller, P. Curcumin stimulates reactive oxygen species production and potentiates apoptosis induction by the antitumor drugs arsenic trioxide and lonidamine in human myeloid leukemia cell lines. *J. Pharmacol. Exp. Ther.* **2010**, *335*, 114–123. [CrossRef]
14. Khan, M.A.; Gahlot, S.; Majumdar, S. Oxidative stress induced by curcumin promotes the death of cutaneous T-cell lymphoma (HuT-78) by disrupting the function of several molecular targets. *Mol. Cancer Ther.* **2012**, *11*, 1873–1883. [CrossRef]
15. Liao, W.; Xiang, W.; Wang, F.F.; Wang, R.; Ding, Y. Curcumin inhibited growth of human melanoma A375 cells via inciting oxidative stress. *Biomed. Pharmacother.* **2017**, *95*, 1177–1186. [CrossRef]
16. Watson, J.L.; Hill, R.; Yaffe, P.B.; Greenshields, A.; Walsh, M.; Lee, P.W.; Giacomantonio, C.A.; Hoskin, D.W. Curcumin causes superoxide anion production and p53-independent apoptosis in human colon cancer cells. *Cancer Lett.* **2010**, *297*, 1–8. [CrossRef]
17. Gessner, P.K.; Gessner, T. *Disulfiram and Its Metabolite, Diethyldithiocarbamate: Pharmacology and Status in the Treatment of Alcoholism, Hiv Infections, Aids and Heavy Metal Toxicity*; Springer Science & Business Media: Berlin/Heidelberg, Germany, 2012.
18. Wang, N.N.; Wang, L.H.; Li, Y.; Fu, S.Y.; Xue, X.; Jia, L.N.; Yuan, X.Z.; Wang, Y.T.; Tang, X.; Yang, J.Y.; et al. Targeting ALDH2 with disulfiram/copper reverses the resistance of cancer cells to microtubule inhibitors. *Exp. Cell Res.* **2018**, *362*, 72–82. [CrossRef]

19. Guo, F.; Yang, Z.; Kulbe, H.; Albers, A.E.; Sehouli, J.; Kaufmann, A.M. Inhibitory effect on ovarian cancer ALDH+ stem-like cells by Disulfiram and Copper treatment through ALDH and ROS modulation. *Biomed. Pharmacother.* **2019**, *118*, 109371. [CrossRef]
20. Fruehauf, J.P.; Trapp, V. Reactive oxygen species: An Achilles' heel of melanoma? *Expert Rev. Anticancer Ther.* **2008**, *8*, 1751–1757. [CrossRef]
21. Lopes-Rodrigues, V.; Sousa, E.; Vasconcelos, M.H. Curcumin as a modulator of P-glycoprotein in cancer: Challenges and perspectives. *Pharmaceuticals* **2016**, *9*, 71. [CrossRef]
22. Ekinci, E.; Rohondia, S.; Khan, R.; Dou, Q.P. Repurposing disulfiram as an anti-cancer agent: Updated review on literature and patents. *Recent Pat. Anticancer Drug Discov.* **2019**, *14*, 113–132. [CrossRef] [PubMed]
23. Jangra, A.; Choi, S.A.; Yang, J.; Koh, E.J.; Phi, J.H.; Lee, J.Y.; Wang, K.C.; Kim, S.K. Disulfiram potentiates the anticancer effect of cisplatin in atypical teratoid/rhabdoid tumors (AT/RT). *Cancer Lett.* **2020**, *486*, 38–45. [CrossRef] [PubMed]
24. Wang, L.; Yu, Y.; Zhou, C.; Wan, R.; Li, Y. Anticancer effects of disulfiram: A systematic review of in vitro, animal, and human studies. *Syst. Rev.* **2022**, *11*, 109. [CrossRef] [PubMed]
25. Sukprasansap, M.; Chanvorachote, P. Evidence of potential plant-derived compounds with anticancer effects on lung cancer: Clinical and molecular pharmacology approaches. *Anticancer Res.* **2022**, *42*, 4247–4258. [CrossRef] [PubMed]
26. Ng, C.X.; Affendi, M.M.; Chong, P.P.; Lee, S.H. The potential of plant-derived extracts and compounds to augment anticancer effects of chemotherapeutic drugs. *Nutr. Cancer* **2022**, *74*, 3058–3076. [CrossRef]
27. Hussain, Y.; Islam, L.; Khan, H.; Filosa, R.; Aschner, M.; Javed, S. Curcumin-cisplatin chemotherapy: A novel strategy in promoting chemotherapy efficacy and reducing side effects. *Phytother Res.* **2021**, *35*, 6514–6529. [CrossRef]
28. Almeida-Silva, J.; Menezes, D.S.; Fernandes, J.M.P.; Almeida, M.C.; Vasco-Dos-Santos, D.R.; Saraiva, R.M.; Viçosa, A.L.; Perez, S.A.C.; Andrade, S.G.; Suarez-Fontes, A.M.; et al. The repositioned drugs disulfiram/diethyldithiocarbamate combined to benznidazole: Searching for Chagas disease selective therapy, preventing toxicity and drug resistance. *Front. Cell Infect. Microbiol.* **2022**, *12*, 926699. [CrossRef]
29. López-Lázaro, M. Anticancer and carcinogenic properties of curcumin: Considerations for its clinical development as a cancer chemopreventive and chemotherapeutic agent. *Mol. Nutr. Food Res.* **2008**, *52*, S103–S127. [CrossRef]
30. Ahmed, S.A.; Gogal, R.M., Jr.; Walsh, J.E. A new rapid and simple non-radioactive assay to monitor and determine the proliferation of lymphocytes: An alternative to [3H]-thymidine incorporation assay. *J. Immunol. Methods* **1994**, *170*, 211–224. [CrossRef]
31. Santos, L.S.; Silva, V.R.; Menezes, L.R.A.; Soares, M.B.P.; Costa, E.V.; Bezerra, D.P. Xylopine induces oxidative stress and causes G2/M phase arrest, triggering caspase-mediated apoptosis by p53-independent pathway in HCT116 cells. *Oxid. Med. Cell Longev.* **2017**, *2017*, 7126872. [CrossRef]
32. Silva, V.R.; Correa, R.S.; Santos, L.S.; Soares, M.B.P.; Batista, A.A.; Bezerra, D.P. A ruthenium-based 5-fluorouracil complex with enhanced cytotoxicity and apoptosis induction action in HCT116 cells. *Sci. Rep.* **2018**, *8*, 288. [CrossRef]
33. Bill, M.A.; Bakan, C.; Benson, D.M., Jr.; Fuchs, J.; Young, G.; Lesinski, G.B. Curcumin induces proapoptotic effects against human melanoma cells and modulates the cellular response to immunotherapeutic cytokines. *Mol. Cancer Ther.* **2009**, *8*, 2726–2735. [CrossRef]
34. Kocyigit, A.; Guler, E.M. Curcumin induce DNA damage and apoptosis through generation of reactive oxygen species and reducing mitochondrial membrane potential in melanoma cancer cells. *Cell Mol. Biol.* **2017**, *63*, 97–105. [CrossRef]
35. Morrison, B.W.; Doudican, N.A.; Patel, K.R.; Orlow, S.J. Disulfiram induces copper-dependent stimulation of reactive oxygen species and activation of the extrinsic apoptotic pathway in melanoma. *Melanoma Res.* **2010**, *20*, 11–20. [CrossRef]
36. Nicoletti, I.; Migliorati, G.; Pagliaccim, M.C.; Grignanim, F.; Riccardi, C. A rapid and simple method for measuring thymocyte apoptosis by propidium iodide staining and flow cytometry. *J. Immunol. Methods* **1991**, *139*, 271–279. [CrossRef]
37. Rodrigues, A.C.; Bomfim, L.M.; Neves, S.P.; Menezes, L.R.; Dias, R.B.; Soares, M.B.; Prata, A.P.; Rocha, C.A.; Costa, E.V.; Bezerra, D.P. Antitumor properties of the essential oil from the leaves of *Duguetia gardneriana*. *Planta Med.* **2015**, *81*, 798–803. [CrossRef]
38. Chou, T.C. Theoretical basis, experimental design, and computerized simulation of synergism and antagonism in drug combination studies. *Pharmacol. Rev.* **2006**, *58*, 621–681. [CrossRef]
39. Grammer, A.C.; Lipsky, P.E. Drug repositioning strategies for the identification of novel therapies for rheumatic autoimmune inflammatory diseases. *Rheum. Dis. Clin. N. Am.* **2017**, *43*, 467–480. [CrossRef]
40. Yang, B.; Shi, J. Developing new cancer nanomedicines by repurposing old drugs. *Angew. Chem. Int. Ed. Engl.* **2020**, *59*, 21829–21838. [CrossRef]
41. Nowak-Sliwinska, P.; Scapozza, L.; Ruiz, I.A.A. Drug repurposing in oncology: Compounds, pathways, phenotypes and computational approaches for colorectal cancer. *Biochim. Biophys. Acta Rev. Cancer* **2019**, *1871*, 434–454. [CrossRef]
42. Antoszczak, M.; Markowska, A.; Markowska, J.; Huczyński, A. Old wine in new bottles: Drug repurposing in oncology. *Eur. J. Pharmacol.* **2020**, *866*, 172784. [CrossRef]
43. Laubach, V.; Kaufmann, R.; Bernd, A. Extrinsic or intrinsic apoptosis by curcumin and light: Still a mystery. *Int. J. Mol. Sci.* **2019**, *20*, 905. [CrossRef]
44. Mortezaee, K.; Salehi, E.; Mirtavoos-Mahyari, H.; Motevaseli, E.; Najafi, M.; Farhood, B.; Rosengren, R.J.; Sahebkar, A. Mechanisms of apoptosis modulation by curcumin: Implications for cancer therapy. *J. Cell Physiol.* **2019**, *234*, 12537–12550. [CrossRef]

45. Meraz-Torres, F.; Plöger, S.; Garbe, C.; Niessner, H.; Sinnberg, T. Disulfiram as a therapeutic agent for metastatic malignant melanoma-old myth or new logos? *Cancers* **2020**, *12*, 3538. [CrossRef]
46. Banerjee, S.; Ji, C.; Mayfield, J.E.; Goel, A.; Xiao, J.; Dixon, J.E.; Guo, X. Ancient drug curcumin impedes 26S proteasome activity by direct inhibition of dual-specificity tyrosine-regulated kinase 2. *Proc. Natl. Acad. Sci. USA* **2018**, *115*, 8155–8160. [CrossRef]
47. Odot, J.; Albert, P.; Carlier, A.; Tarpin, M.; Devy, J.; Madoulet, C. In vitro and in vivo anti-tumoral effect of curcumin against melanoma cells. *Int. J. Cancer* **2004**, *111*, 381–387. [CrossRef]
48. Sonawane, V.K.; Mahajan, U.B.; Shinde, S.D.; Chatterjee, S.; Chaudhari, S.S.; Bhangale, H.A.; Ojha, S.; Goyal, S.N.; Kundu, C.N.; Patil, C.R. A chemosensitizer drug: Disulfiram prevents doxorubicin-induced cardiac dysfunction and oxidative stress in rats. *Cardiovasc. Toxicol.* **2018**, *18*, 459–470. [CrossRef] [PubMed]
49. Jiao, Y.; Hannafon, B.N.; Ding, W.Q. Disulfiram's anticancer activity: Evidence and mechanisms. *Anticancer Agents Med. Chem.* **2016**, *16*, 1378–1384. [CrossRef] [PubMed]

biomolecules

MDPI

Article

Efficient Synthesis for Altering Side Chain Length on Cannabinoid Molecules and Their Effects in Chemotherapy and Chemotherapeutic Induced Neuropathic Pain

Wesley M. Raup-Konsavage [1,†], Diana E. Sepulveda [1,2,†], Daniel P. Morris [1], Shantu Amin [1], Kent E. Vrana [1], Nicholas M. Graziane [1,2,*] and Dhimant Desai [1,*]

1 Department of Pharmacology, Penn State College of Medicine, Hershey, PA 17033, USA
2 Department of Anesthesiology & Perioperative Medicine, Penn State College of Medicine, Hershey, PA 17033, USA
* Correspondence: ngraziane@pennstatehealth.psu.edu (N.M.G.); ddesai@pennstatehealth.psu.edu (D.D.)
† These authors contributed equally to this work.

Abstract: (1) Background: Recently, a number of side chain length variants for tetrahydrocannabinol and cannabidiol have been identified in cannabis; however, the precursor to these molecules would be based upon cannabigerol (CBG). Because CBG, and its side chain variants, are rapidly converted to other cannabinoids in the plant, there are typically only small amounts in plant extracts, thus prohibiting investigations related to CBG and CBG variant therapeutic effects. (2) Methods: To overcome this, we developed an efficient synthesis of corresponding resorcinol fragments using the Wittig reaction which, under acid catalyzed coupling with geraniol, produced the desired side chain variants of CBG. These compounds were then tested in an animal model of chemotherapeutic-induced neuropathic pain and to reduce colorectal cancer cell viability. (3) Results: We found that all side-chain variants were similarly capable of reducing neuropathic pain in mice at a dose of 10 mg/kg. However, the molecules with shorter side chains (i.e., CBGV and CBGB) were better at reducing colorectal cancer cell viability. (4) Conclusions: The novel synthesis method developed here will be of utility for studying other side chain derivatives of minor cannabinoids such as cannabichromene, cannabinol, and cannabielsoin.

Keywords: cannabigerol; neuropathic pain; colorectal cancer; cannabinoid synthesis

Citation: Raup-Konsavage, W.M.; Sepulveda, D.E.; Morris, D.P.; Amin, S.; Vrana, K.E.; Graziane, N.M.; Desai, D. Efficient Synthesis for Altering Side Chain Length on Cannabinoid Molecules and Their Effects in Chemotherapy and Chemotherapeutic Induced Neuropathic Pain. *Biomolecules* **2022**, *12*, 1869. https://doi.org/10.3390/biom12121869

Academic Editors: Marialuigia Fantacuzzi, Barbara De Filippis and Alessandra Ammazzalorso

Received: 3 October 2022
Accepted: 9 December 2022
Published: 13 December 2022

Publisher's Note: MDPI stays neutral with regard to jurisdictional claims in published maps and institutional affiliations.

1. Introduction

In the United States, 150,000 new cases of colorectal cancer will be diagnosed in 2022 with an estimated 55,000 deaths caused by the disease [1]. Cisplatin, a commonly used chemotherapeutic agent, is used to treat colorectal cancer, albeit with negative side effects, including chemotherapeutic-induced peripheral neuropathy (CIPN), for which there is a lack of treatment options [2–4]. The prevalence of CIPN is agent-dependent, with reported rates varying from 19% to more than 85% [5] and is the highest in the case of platinum-based drugs (70–100%), including cisplatin [6]. This outcome results in an impaired quality of life for affected patients. Therefore, there is a need to identify alternative treatments for colorectal cancer, as well as identify anti-nociceptive agents capable of treating CIPN in patients undergoing cisplatin-based chemotherapy for colorectal cancer.

A number of cannabinoids have been found to reduce cancer cell growth with Δ^9-tetrahydrocannabinol (THC) and cannabidiol (CBD)—the two most often studied cannabinoids for anti-cancer activity [7–12]. In addition to anti-cancer effects, evidence suggests that cannabinoids (e.g., cannabigerol (CBG), THC, and CBD) have anti-nociceptive properties, resulting in ongoing clinical investigations related to cannabinoid effects on pain [13–18]. The mechanisms by which cannabinoids reduce cancer cell growth as well as mitigate pain are currently under investigation. However, it is known that cannabinoids are promiscuous molecules with the ability to bind to a number of receptors involved in pain processing and inflammation (e.g., CB1, CB2, 5-HT$_{1A}$, α2-adrenergic receptor) as well as induce immunogenic cell death [15,18–20].

Cannabis produces a number of bioactive compounds that are of pharmaceutical interest. Broadly, these molecules fall into one of three classes: terpenes, flavonoids, and cannabinoids (which are unique to the genus *Cannabis*). Over 100 different types of cannabinoids are produced by cannabis, with CBD and THC being the two most abundant and most well studied. The predominant cannabinoids in *Cannabis* cultivars have a 5-carbon side chain off of the aromatic ring; however, shortly after the discovery of the major 5-carbon phytocannabinoids, CBD and THC, two additional variations of these molecules were described with a shorter, 3-carbon, side chain, cannabidivarin (CBDV) and tetrahydrocannabivarin (THCV) [21]. More recently, CBD and THC variants with carbon side chains of 4, 6, and 7 carbons have been isolated from cannabis, albeit in much lower concentrations [22–24].

The biosynthesis of all cannabinoids begins with geranyl pyrophosphate and a benzoic acid, olivetolic acid in the case of the 5-carbon cannabinoids, by the enzyme geranylpyrophosphate-olivetolic acid geranyltransferase (GOT) [25]. This reaction produces CBG, and the respective variations, which serve as the precursor molecules to all other cannabinoids produced in the plant. However, in most cultivars, CBG is found at low levels because this precursor is efficiently converted to downstream products, which means that the variant molecules will therefore be present in trace amounts. Novel and trace side chain length variants of CBD and THC have previously been isolated from plant material [22]. Here, we set out to develop a novel synthetic mechanism to produce side-chain variants of CBG. Additionally, we tested CBG and CBG variants for potential anti-cancer activity in colorectal cancer cell lines, as well as anti-nociceptive properties in a model of chemotherapy-induced neuropathic pain (CIPN).

2. Materials and Methods

Thin-layer chromatography (TLC) was performed on aluminum-supported, precoated silica gel plates (EM Industries, Gibbstown, NJ, USA). Flash column chromatography was performed using silica gel SI 60. ^{1}H NMR spectra were recorded on a 500 MHz Bruker mass spectrometer (Billerica, MA, USA). Proton chemical shifts are reported in parts per million (δ). The following abbreviations were used to designate chemical shift multiplicities: s = singlet, d = doublet, dd = double doublet, t = triplet, dt = doublet of triplet, m = multiplet. Mass spectrometry analysis was performed on a 4000 Q-trap hybrid triple quadrupole/linear ion trap instrument (Applied Biosystems/MDS Sciex, Waltham, MA, USA) at the proteomic facility of the Penn State College of Medicine, Hershey, PA. High Resolution Mass Spectrometry (HRMS) was performed on AB Sciex TripleTOF 5600 mass spectrometer (Farmington, MA, USA) with electrospray ionization (ESI) in positive-ion mode at the metabolomics core at Penn State University, University Park, PA. The sample was analyzed by flow infusion with a Prominence UFLC system (Shimadzu, Kyoto, Japan) at flow 300 μL/min rates of 0.1% formic acid in a mixture of methanol and water 60:40. MS1 and MS2 data were acquired using a declustering potential (DP) of 80 V. MS2 data were collected in IDA mode with collision energy (CE) of 40 V and collision energy spread (CES) 20 V. During the analysis, an ion spray voltage (IS) of 5500 V, curtain gas (CUR) of 35 psi, nebulizer gas (GS1) of 50 psi, heater gas 2 (GS2) of 55, and heater temperature of 550 C were applied. CBG was purchased from a commercial source (Cayman Chemical, Ann Arbor, MI, USA). 3,5-dimethoxybenzyltriphenylphosphonium bromide (**1**) was prepared as reported in the literature [26]. Briefly, 3,5-dimethoxybenzylbromide (10 g, 43.2 mmol) was heated under reflux with triphenyl phosphine (12.6 g, 47.6 mmol) in toluene (60 mL) for 6 h to give a quantitative yield of compound **1**. All starting materials were obtained from Aldrich Chemical Co. (Milwaukee, WI) and used without further purification. Synthesis of 5-alkyl substituted-1,3-dihydroxybenzene precursors was conducted as described below (and illustrated in Scheme 1).

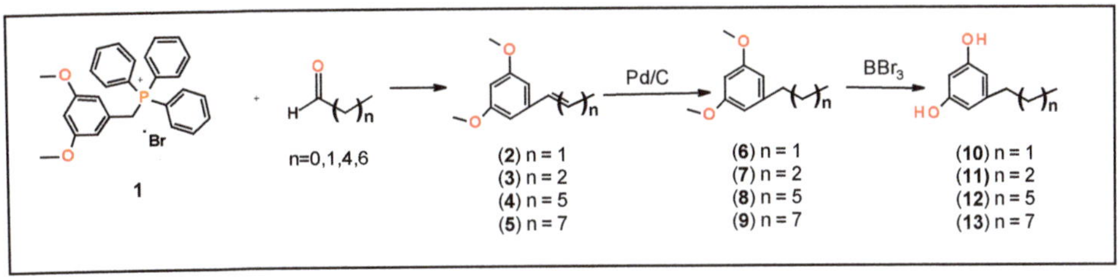

Scheme 1. Synthesis of 5-alkyl substitute-1,3-dihydroxybenezene.

(E/Z) 1,3-Dimethoxy-5-(Prop-1-en-1-yl) benzene (2)

3,5-dimethoxylbenzyltriphenylphosphonium bromide (**1**) (2 g, 4 mmol) in aqueous K_2CO_3 solution (0.1 M, 50 mL) and acetaldehyde (0.264 g, 0.337 mL, 6 mmol) were refluxed for 24 h, cooled to room temperature and cyclohexane (50 mL) was added and vigorously shaken for 30 min. The mixture was filtered, and the aqueous layer was extracted with cyclohexane (2 × 50 mL). Combined organic layers were dried over $MgSO_4$, filtered, and evaporated. The crude olefin, **2** was purified on a silica gel column using Hexane: EtOAc (95:0.5) as an eluent to give mixture of olefins, **2** in 50% yield. ^{1}H NMR (500 MHz, $CDCl_3$): δ 6.50 (d, 2H, aromatic, J = 2.0 Hz), 6.39–6.30 (m, 1H), 6.28–6.11 (m, 2H), 3.80 (s, 6H, OCH_3), and 1.87 (dd, 3H, CH_3, J = 6.5 Hz).

(E/Z) 1,3-Dimethoxy-5-(Butyl-1-en-1-yl) benzene (3)

A mixture of olefins (E/Z)—**3** was prepared as described for olefin **2** using 3,5-dimethoxybenzyltriphenylphosphonium bromide (**1**) (4.0 g, 8 mmol) and propionaldehyde (0.69 g, 0.86 mL, 12 mmol) to give **3** in 91% yield. ^{1}H NMR (500 MHz, $CDCl_3$): δ 6.51 (d, 2H, aromatic, J = 2.5 Hz), 6.33 (d, 1H, aromatic, J = 2.5 Hz), 5.95–5.75 (m, 2H, CH), 3.80 (s, 6H, OCH_3), 2.70–2.50 (m, 2H, CH_2), 1.57–1.12 (m, 4H, CH_2) and 1.12–1.00 (m, 3H, CH_3).

(E/Z) 1,3-Dimethoxy-5-(Heptyl-1-en-1-yl) benzene (4)

Olefins (E/Z)—**4** was prepared as described for **2** using 3,5-dimethoxybenzyltriphenylphosphonium bromide (**1**) (4.0 g, 8 mmol) and hexanaldehyde (1.2 g, 1.48 mL, 12 mmol) to give **4** in 56% yield. ^{1}H NMR (500 MHz, $CDCl_3$): δ 6.41–6.20 (m, 2H, aromatic), 5.95–5.75 (m, 2H, CH), 3.97 (s, 6H, OCH_3), 3.97 (s, 6H, OCH_3), 2.32 (m, 2H, CH_2), 1.46 (q, 2H, CH_2, J = 7.5 Hz), 1.41–1.20 (m, 4H, CH_2), and 0.96–0.88 (m, 3H, CH_3).

(E/Z)-1,3-Dimethoxy-5-(nonyl-1-en-1-yl) benzene (5)

A mixture of olefins (E/Z)—**5** was prepared as described for **2** using 3,5-dimethoxybenzyltriphenylphosphonium bromide (**1**) (2.0 g, 4 mmol), and octanaldehyde (0.77 g, 0.94 mL, 6 mmol) to give olefin **5** in 95% yield. ^{1}H NMR (500 MHz, $CDCl_3$): δ 6.54 (d, 1H, J = 2.0 Hz) 6.47 (d, 1H, J = 2.0 Hz), 6.39–6.30 (m, 2H), 6.28–6.20 (m, 1H), 3.82 (s, 6H, OCH_3), 2.40–2.32 (m, 1H), 2.25–2.20 (m, 1H),1.55–1.25 (m, 10H, CH_2), and 0.92 (dd, 3H, CH_3, J = 13.5 Hz and 6.5 Hz).

1,3-Dimethoxy-5-propylbenzene (6)

A mixture of **2** (1.00 g, 5.62 mmol) in EtOH (60 mL) and 10% Pd/C (100 mg) under 40psi of H_2 atmosphere were shaken in Parr Hydrogenation apparatus for 24 h. The catalyst was removed by filtration over Celite and the solvent was evaporated under reduced pressure to give compound **6** in 88% yield; ^{1}H NMR (500 MHz, $CDCl_3$): δ 6.38 (d, 2H, aromatic, J= 2.0 Hz), 6.34 (t, aromatic, J = 2.0 Hz), 3.81 (s, 6H, OCH_3), 2.57 (q, 2H, CH_2, *J* = 7.5 Hz), 1.69–1.62 (m, 2H, CH_2), and 0.97 (t, 3H, CH_3,*J*, = 7.5 Hz).

1,3-Dimethoxy-5-butylbenzene (7)

Compound **7** was prepared as described for compound **6** using a solution of **3** (576 mg, 3.0 mmol) in EtOH (30 mL) and 10% Pd/C (58 mg) to give **7** in 86% yield. ^{1}H NMR (500 MHz, $CDCl_3$): δ 6.39–6.38 (m, 2H, aromatic), 6.34 (bs,1H, aromatic), 3.81 (s, 6H, OCH_3), 2.7–2.53 (m, 2H, Ph-CH_2), 1.70–1.11 (m, 4H, CH2), and 0.97 (m, 3H, CH_3).

1,3-Dimethoxy-5-heptylbenzene (8)

Compound **8** was prepared as described for compound **6** using a solution of **4** (702 mg, 3 mmol) in EtOH (50 mL) and 10% Pd/C (70 mg) to give **8** in 86% yield: ^{1}H NMR (500 MHz,

$CDCl_3$): δ 6.38 (d, 2H, aromatic, J = 2.0 Hz), 6.34 (d, 1H, aromatic, J = 2.5 Hz), 3.81 (s, 6H, OCH_3), 2.58 (t, 2H, CH2, *J* = 7.5 Hz), 1.64 (t, 2H, CH2, J = 7.5 Hz), 1.36–1.31 (m, 8H, CH2), and 0.92 (t, 3H, CH3, J = 7.5 Hz).

1,3-Dimethoxy-5-nonylbenzene (9)

Compound **9** was prepared as described for compound **6** using a solution of **5** (792 mg, 3.00 mmol) in EtOH (30 mL) and 10% Pd/C (83 mg) to give **9** in 93% yield. ^{1}H NMR (500 MHz, $CDCl_3$): δ 6.38 (d, 2H, aromatic, J = 2.0 Hz), 6.33 (t, 1H, aromatic, J = 2.0 Hz), 3.81 (s, 6H, OCH_3), 2.58 (t, 2H, CH_2, *J* = 8.0 Hz), 1.64 (m, 2H, CH_2), 1.35–1.30 (m, 12H, CH_2), and 0.92 (t, 3H, CH_3, J = 7.0 Hz).

1,3-Dihydroxy-5-propylbenzene (10)

A stirring solution of **6** (200 mg, 1.11 mmol) in CH_2Cl_2 was cooled to −10 °C for 30 min. To this cold reaction solution, BBr_3 (1 M solution in CH_2Cl_2, 2.78 mL, 2.78 mmol) was added dropwise. After the addition, the mixture was allowed to warm up to room temperature and stirred for an additional 24 h. The mixture was cooled to 0 °C and quenched with saturated $NaHCO_3$ and stirred for an additional 30 min at room temperature. The aqueous layer was extracted with CH_2Cl_2 (2 × 25 mL), combined organic layers were dried over $MgSO_4$, filtered, and evaporated. Purification on a silica gel column by using CH_2Cl_2:MeOH (98:2) as an eluent gave 79% yield of **10 [27]**. ^{1}H NMR (500 MHz, $CDCl_3$): δ 6.28 (d, *J* = 2.0 Hz, 2H, aromatic), 6.21 (S, 1H, aromatic), 2.47 (q, 2H, CH_2, *J* = 9.0 Hz), 1.59 (q, 2H, CH_2, J = 8.0 Hz), and 0.93 (t, 3H, CH_3, J = 7.5 Hz).

1,3-Dihydroxy-5-butylbenzene (11)

Compound **11** was prepared as described for **10** using compound **7** (0.5 g, 2.58 mmol) and BBr_3 (1 M solution in CH_2Cl_2, 5.16 mL, 5.16 mmol) to give compound **11** in 68% yield [28,29]. ^{1}H NMR (500 MHz, $CDCl_3$): δ 6.28 (s, 2H, aromatic), 6.20 (d, 1H, aromatic, J = 2.0 Hz), 4.89 (bs, 2H, OH), 2.60–2.40 (m, 2H, CH_2), 1.63–1.10 (m, 4H, CH_2), and 0.92 (t, 3H, CH_3, J = 7.0 Hz).

1,3-Dihydroxy-5-heptylbenzene (12)

Compound **12** was prepared as described for **10** using compound **8** (0.98 g, 4.15 mmol) and BBr_3 (1 M solution in CH_2Cl_2, 9.5 mL, 9.5 mmol) to give compound **12** in 91% yield [30]. ^{1}H NMR (500 MHz, $CDCl_3$): δ 6.27 (d, 2H, aromatic, J = 2.0 Hz), 6.20 (d, 1H, aromatic, J = 2.0 Hz), 2.51 (t, 2H, CH, *J* = 7.5 Hz), 1.59 (q, 2H, CH_2, J = 7.5 Hz), 1.39–1.22 (m, 14H, CH_2), and 0.91 (t, 3H, CH_3, J = 6.5 Hz).

1,3-Dihydroxy-5-nonylbenzene (13)

Compound **13** was prepared as described for **10** using compound **9** (0.76 g, 2.88 mmol), and BBr_3 (1 M solution in CH_2Cl_2, 5.8 mL, 5.8 mmol) to give compound **13** in 84% yield [31]. ^{1}H NMR (500 MHz, $CDCl_3$): δ 6.27 (d, 2H, aromatic, J = 2.0 Hz), 6.20 (bs, 1H, aromatic), 4.72 (bs, OH), 2.51 (t, 2H, CH_2, *J* = 7.5 Hz), 1.61–1.58 (m, 2H, CH_2), 1.33–1.28 (m, 12H, CH_2), and 0.91 (t, 3H, CH_3, J = 7.0 Hz).

Syntheses of the CBG analogs of varying side chain lengths were conducted as described below and illustrated in Scheme 2.

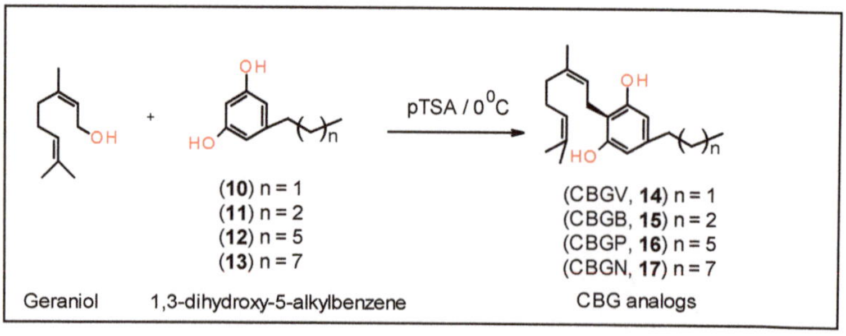

Scheme 2. Synthesis of CBG analogs, **14–17**.

Cannabigerovarin (CBGV, 14):

To a stirred cold solution of geraniol (203 mg,1.32 mmol) in anhydrous chloroform (20 mL) was added (over a period of 20 min) a solution of 1,3-dihydroxy-5-ethylbenzene (**10**) (131 mg, 0.73 mmol) and p-toluenesulfonic acid (14 mg) in anhydrous chloroform (15 mL) at 0 °C and under a positive pressure of nitrogen. After stirring in the same conditions for 14 h, the reaction was quenched with saturated of $NaHCO_3$ (5 mL). The reaction mixture was extracted with EtOAc (3 × 15 mL) and the combined organic layers were washed with water, dried ($MgSO_4$) and evaporated. The residue was purified on silica gel column by eluting with hexane:CH_2Cl_2 (1:1) to give 21% yield of CBGV (**14**) [32]. ^{1}H NMR (500 MHz, $CDCl_3$): δ 6.26 (s, 2H, aromatic), 5.33–5.28 (m, 1H, CH), 5.14 (bs, 2H, OH), 5.08 (t, 1H, CH, J = 7.0 Hz), 3.42 (d, 2H, Ph-CH_2, J = 7.0 Hz), 2.56 (t, 2H, Ph-CH_2, J = 7.5 Hz), 2.18–2.0 (m, 6H), 1.84 (s, 3H, CH_3), 1.70 (S, 3H, CH_3), 1.63 (s, 3H, CH_3), 0.95 (t, 3H, CH_3, J = 7.5 Hz); HRMS calculated for $C_{19}H_{28}O_2$ + H: 289.2169; the observed value was 289.2091.

Cannabigerobutol (CBGB, 15):

Compound **15** was prepared as described for **14** using compound **11** (250 mg, 1.50 mmol) and geraniol (416 mg, 2.7 mmol) to give compound **15** in 18% yield. ^{1}H NMR (500 MHz, CD_3OD): δ 6.16 (d, 2H, aromatic), 5.26 (t, 1H, CH, J = 7.0 Hz), 5.09 (t, 1H, CH, J = 7.0 Hz), 3.27 (d, 2H, J = 7.5 Hz, Ph-CH_2), 2.50–2.35 (m, 2H, Ph-CH_2), 2.10–1.90 (m, 4H), 1.77 (s, 3H, CH_3), 1.67 (S, 3H, CH_3), 1.58 (s, 3H, CH_3), 1.40–1.30 (m, 4H), 0.92 (t, 3H, CH_3, J = 6.5 Hz); HRMS calculated for $C_{20}H_{30}O_2$ + H: 303.2326; the observed value was 303.1941.

Cannabigerophorbol (CBGP, 16):

Compound **16** was prepared as described for **14** using compound **12** (208 mg, 1.0 mmol) and geraniol (278 mg, 1.8 mmol) to give compound **16** in 26% yield [33]. ^{1}H NMR (500 MHz, $CDCl_3$): δ 6.27 (S, 2H, aromatic), 5.30 (t, 1H, CH, J = 7.0 Hz), 5.08 (t, 1H, CH, J = 6.0 Hz), 5.02 (bs, 2H, OH), 3.42 (d, 2H, Ph-CH_2, J = 7.0 Hz), 2.48 (t, 2H, Ph-CH_2, J = 8.0 Hz), 2.19–2.10 (m, 4H), 1.84 (s, 3H, CH_3), 1.70 (S, 3H, CH_3), 1.62–1.57 (m and S, 5H, CH_2 and CH_3), 1.33–1.24 (m, 10H), 0.91 (t, 3H, CH_3, J = 7.0 Hz); HRMS calculated for $C_{23}H_{36}O_2$ + H: 344.2715; the observed value was 344.2657.

Cannabigerononol (CBGN, 17):

Compound **17** was prepared as described for **14** using compound **13** (307 mg, 1.5 mmol) and geraniol (417 mg, 2.7 mmol) to give compound **17** in 29% yield. ^{1}H NMR (500 MHz, $CDCl_3$): δ 6.27 (S, 2H, aromatic), 5.30 (t, 1H, CH, J = 7.0 Hz), 5.08 (t, 1H, CH, J = 6.5 Hz), 5.00 (bs, 2H, OH), 3.42 (d, 2H, Ph-CH_2, J = 7.0 Hz), 2.48 (t, 2H, Ph-CH_2, J = 7.5 Hz), 2.15–2.10 (m, 4H), 1.84 (s, 3H, CH_3), 1.70 (S, 3H, CH_3), 1.62 (s, 3H, CH_3), 1.62–1.57 (m, 2H), 1.33–1.24 (m, 12H), 0.91 (t, 3H, CH_3, J = 7.0 Hz); HRMS calculated for $C_{25}H_{40}O_2$ + H: 373.3108; the observed value was 373.3089.

Animals

All experiments were performed in accordance with procedures approved by the Pennsylvania State University College of Medicine Institutional Animal Care and Use Committee (protocol 202001327). Wild-type C57BL/6 (The Jackson Laboratory, Bar Harbor, ME, USA) male mice (n = 35) were used for all experiments. Animals were grouped housed with a 12-h light/dark cycle with *ad libitum* food and water.

Cisplatin-induced peripheral neuropathy was induced as previously described [13,15,34]. Mice were injected with 4% sodium bicarbonate solution (1 mL, s.c.) administered just prior to cisplatin (5 mg/kg, i.p.) to prevent neurotoxicity and to minimize damage to renal function. Cisplatin was administered once a week for four weeks [15,35]. Mechanical allodynia was assessed before and after cisplatin treatment to confirm neuropathic pain state as described below.

Mechanical hypersensitivity was assessed using an electronic von Frey anesthesiometer (IITC Life Sciences Inc., Woodland Hills, CA, USA) with a semi-flex tip (IITC Life Sciences Inc., Woodland Hills, CA, USA), which was applied to the plantar surface of the right hind-paw with increasing force to prompt a paw withdrawal response. Mice were placed in one of eight small acrylic chambers placed on a wire mesh table (IITC Life Sciences

Inc., Woodland, CA, USA), and acclimated to the chamber for 20 min before testing. The average of three tests were calculated with each test separated by at least 3 min.

To measure the effects of test compounds, 35 neuropathic male mice were randomly assigned to 7 groups (5 mice/group). During week 1, mice were injected with vehicle (DMSO, Tween 80, saline (1:1:18), i.p.), CBGV, CBGB, CBG, CBGP, CBGN, or the non-steroidal anti-inflammatory drug indomethacin (10 mg/kg, i.p., based upon our previous work with CBG [15]). Mice were then given a one-week washout period, and during week 2 were again randomly assigned to one of the 7 groups and injected with the test compounds. All von Frey experiments were performed by experimenters blinded to treatments.

Cell lines

The human CRC cell lines SW480, SW620, HT29, DLD-1, HCT115, LS174, and RKO were obtained from the American Type Culture Collection (ATCC, Manassas, VA) and cultured as previously described [7]. Briefly, cells were grown in Dulbecco's Modified Eagle's Media supplemented with 10% fetal bovine serum, 2 mM Glutamax, 10 U/mL penicillin, 10 µg/mL streptomycin, and 0.25 µg/mL Amphotericin B at 37 °C in 5% CO_2. RKO cells were grown under the same conditions except that RPMI was used in place of Dulbecco's Modified Eagle's Media.

CRC cell lines were treated as previously described, except cells were seeded at a density of 10,000 cells/well [7] and 16 h later treated with vehicle (DMSO), CBGV, CBGB, CBG, CBGP, CBGN at 10 µM for 48 h. In all treatments, the DMSO was maintained at a constant 1%. Results in two cell lines (HCT116 and SW480) were confirmed by trypan blue staining. Cells were plated and treated as described above and after 48 h adherent and nonadherent cells were collected and stained with 0.2% trypan blue; cells were counted on a Countess 3 automated cell counter (ThermoFisher, Pittsburgh, PA, USA). For dose effect curves, cells were seeded as described above and then treated with Vehicle (DMSO, CBGV, CBGB, CBG, CBGP, or CBGN at concentrations of 333 nM, 1 µM, 3.3 µM, 10 µM, 18.56 µM, 33 µM, and 56µM. Cell viability for all experiments was measured using the MTT ((3-(4,5-dimethylthiazol-2-yl)-5-(3-carboxymethoxyphenyl)-2-(4-sulfophenyl)-2H-tetrazolium), Biovision; Milpitas, CA). MTT (0.5 mg/mL, 15µL) was added to each well and incubated for 2 h at 37 °C in 5% CO_2. Formazan crystals were solubilized by adding stop solution (10% Triton X-100, 0.05% HCl in isopropanol) and vigorously pipetting the mixture. Absorbance was measured at 570 nm on a FlexStation 3 (Molecular Devices, San Jose, CA, USA). For each experiment, the cell line/treatment was measured from triplicate wells and the average was determined. Data are presented as the signal normalized to vehicle control.

Statistics

All results are shown as mean ± standard deviation. Statistical significance was determined using GraphPad Prism Software (9.3.1, San Diego, CA, USA) using a one-way ANOVA with Dunnett's multiple comparison post hoc tests.

3. Results

First, to generate CBG and CBG variants, we synthesized corresponding resorcinol fragments. Several approaches have been reported in the literature for the synthesis of resorcinol derivatives [33,35]. We have developed an efficient method to generate the resorcinol fragments as shown in Scheme 1. This was accomplished in three steps involving: (1) preparation of corresponding olefins, **2–5** using 3,5-dimethoxybenzyl triphenylphosphonium bromide (**1**) and the corresponding aldehyde (Wittig reaction); (2) hydrogenation of the resultant E/Z-olefin mixture in Parr-hydrogenation apparatus to give compounds, **6–9**; and (3) deprotection of methoxy group of compounds, **6–9** by using BBr_3 gave corresponding substituted resorcinol derivatives, **10–13**. All of these operations overall gave moderate yields (40–80%).

Each of these corresponding substituted resorcinol derivatives, **10–13**, were coupled with geraniol in the presence of catalytic amounts of *p*-toluenesulfonic acid monohydrate as shown in Scheme 2 to give the corresponding CBG analogs, **14–17**, in 20–30% yields [36].

The solubility of CBGV and CBG is between 25–50 mg/mL or around 80–180 mM in pure DMSO; the solubility drops by 100-fold or more when the compounds are in 25% DMSO [37].

Given the potential of cannabinoids to evoke cancer cell death, we next investigated the effects of the CBG side-chain variants on cancer cell viability at 10 μM for 48 h. Following the 48-h timepoint, cell viability was assessed using the MTT assay. Our results show that CBGV, across all cell lines, demonstrated the greatest reduction in cell growth (Figure 1A–G). Additionally, we found that the 4-carbon variant, CBGB, decreased cancer cell viability, although not to the same extent as CBGV. Moreover, we found that the effects of CBG were dependent upon the cell lines tested, as CBG only reduced colorectal cancer cell viability in 4 of the cell lines tested (HT-29, DLD-1, LS174, and RKO, Figure 1C,D,F,G). Even in cell lines sensitive to CBG, CBGV remained more efficacious, except in DLD-1 cells where the CBG and CBGV had a similar effect on cell viability (Figure 1D). The longer 7 and 9 carbon variants (CBGP and CBGN) did not significantly influence cell viability in any of the cell lines tested. The results of the MTT assay were confirmed in HCT116 and SW480 cell lines by trypan blue staining (data not shown).

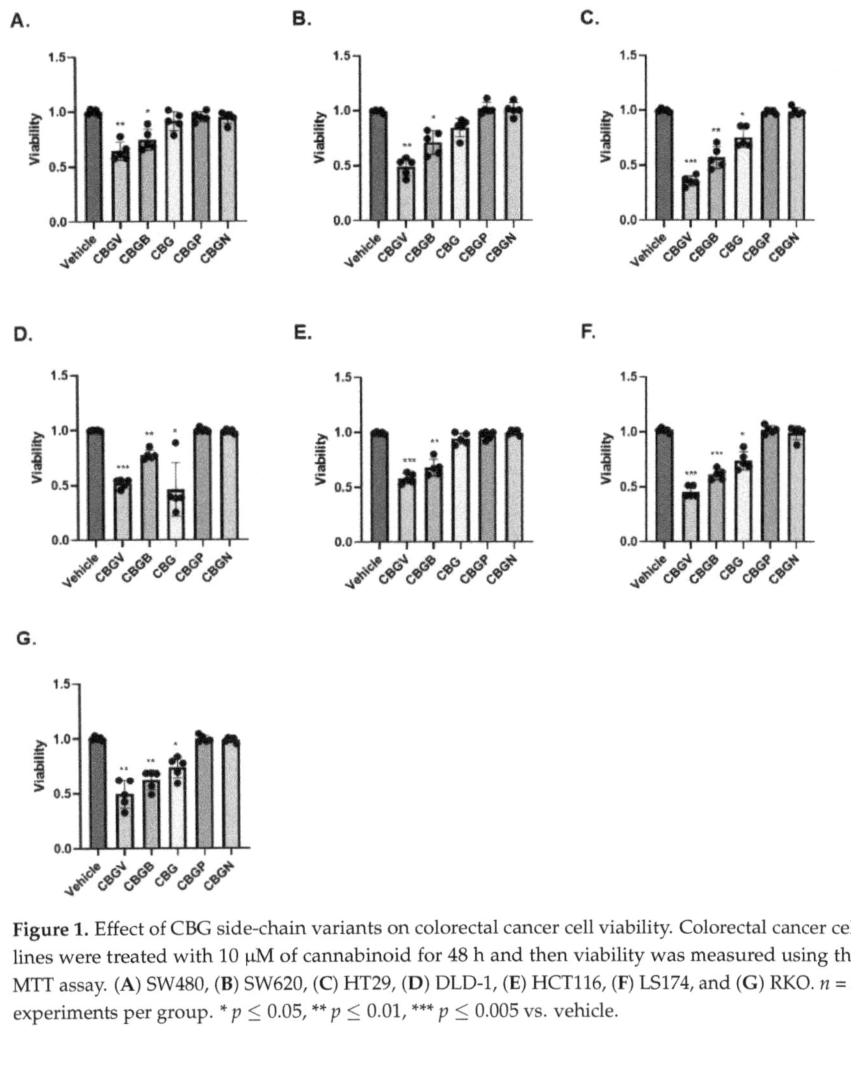

Figure 1. Effect of CBG side-chain variants on colorectal cancer cell viability. Colorectal cancer cell lines were treated with 10 μM of cannabinoid for 48 h and then viability was measured using the MTT assay. (**A**) SW480, (**B**) SW620, (**C**) HT29, (**D**) DLD-1, (**E**) HCT116, (**F**) LS174, and (**G**) RKO. $n = 5$ experiments per group. * $p \leq 0.05$, ** $p \leq 0.01$, *** $p \leq 0.005$ vs. vehicle.

To better examine the impact of these compounds on colorectal cancer cell growth, we performed dose effect curves. Consistent with our data at 10 µM, we found that CBGV had the lowest IC_{50} value across all cell lines, except DLD-1 cells (Figure 2A–G, Table 1). We also found that only in DLD-1 cells was the IC_{50} value of CBG similar to that found with CBGV (Figure 2D, Table 1). The highest IC_{50} values were found for the molecules with the longer side chains (Figure 2, Table 1). In general, the IC_{50} values for CBGB and CBG were found to be between those observed for CBGV and the larger chain molecules (CBGP and CBGN) (Figure 2, Table 1).

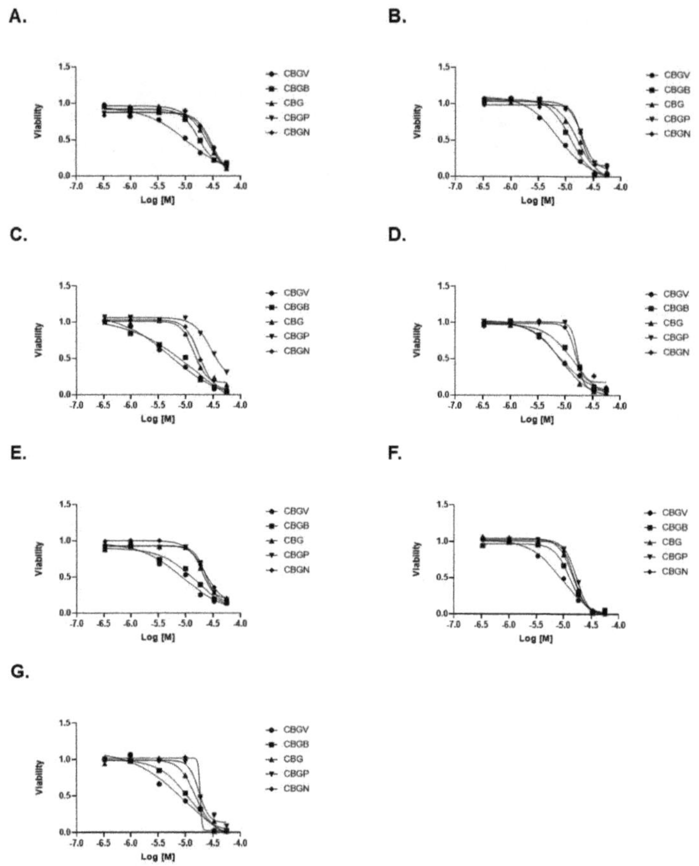

Figure 2. Dose response curves of CBG side-chain variants on colorectal cancer cell viability. Colorectal cancer cell lines were treated with varying doses of cannabinoid for 48 h and then viability was measured using the MTT assay. Representative dose response curves are shown for (**A**) SW480, (**B**) SW620, (**C**) HT29, (**D**) DLD-1, (**E**) HCT116, (**F**) LS174, and (**G**) RKO cell lines.

Next, we investigated the anti-nociceptive properties of CBG variants in a model of CIPN. Previously, we have demonstrated, using the von Frey test, that CBG (10 mg/kg i.p.) was effective at significantly reducing mechanical hypersensitivity in a preclinical model of CIPN [15]. Using this model, we investigated and compared the anti-nociceptive properties of the CBG side chain variants, CBGV, CBGB, CBG, CBGP, and CBGN. Neuropathic male mice were treated with vehicle control, a CBG variant, or the positive control indomethacin each at 10 mg/kg i.p. Mice then underwent von Frey testing of the hind-paw, 1 h following injections, to measure the force required to elicit a paw withdrawal response.

Our results show that all variants were equally as effective as CBG and the positive control, indomethacin, in reversing CIPN ($F_{(6,63)} = 9.56$, $p < 0.0001$; one-way ANOVA with Tukey's post-test). (Figure 3).

Table 1. IC_{50} values for CBG variants in Colorectal Cancer Cell Lines.

Cell Line	CBGV	CBGB	CBG	CBGP	CBGN
SW480	12.3 ± 2.5 **	15.5 ± 2.1 *	22.8 ± 3.4	23.9 ± 5.0	24.5 ± 6.0
SW620	8.1 ± 0.6 *	13.6 ± 1.7	16.2 ± 1.3	20.6 ± 3.6	23.4 ± 7.8
HT29	5.6 ± 3.3 **	12.5 ± 4.7	16.6 ± 3.3	25.2 ± 4.1 *	20.8 ± 3.6
DLD-1	8.3 ± 1.6	15.4 ± 1.4 **	7.9 ± 1.2	20.2 ± 3.9 ***	19.4 ± 3.7 ***
HCT116	9.3 ± 1.6 ****	15.8 ± 1.6 ***	21.6 ± 1.4	22.9 ± 0.1	22.3 ± 1.0
LS174	9.4 ± 1.1 ***	14.0 ± 3.1	16.7 ± 2.3	18.2 ± 1.1	17.3 ± 1.9
RKO	9.1 ± 2.9 **	13.1 ± 0.7	14.7 ± 0.5	17.5 ± 1.6	19.0 ± 1.6 *

IC_{50} values are from 3–4 independent dose effect curves and are presented as mean ± standard deviation, concentrations are in μM. * $p \leq 0.05$, ** $p \leq 0.01$, *** $p \leq 0.005$, **** $p \leq 0.001$ vs. CBG.

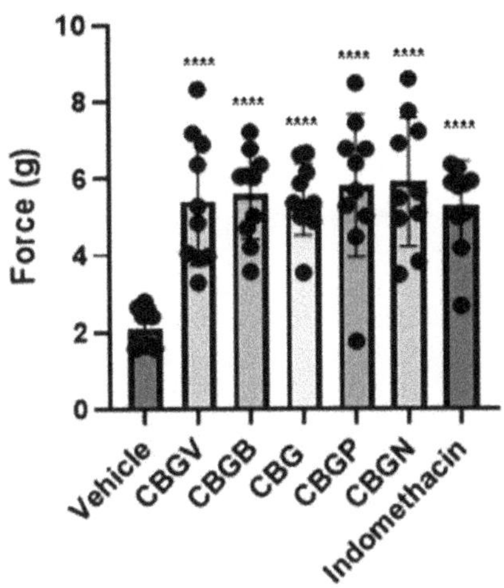

Figure 3. Effect of CBG side-chain variants on mechanical sensitivity. Neuropathic male mice were treated with 10 mg/kg of vehicle, side-chain variant of CBG, or indomethacin as a positive control and mechanical sensitivity was assessed using von Frey filaments. $n = 10$ mice per group, **** $p \leq 0.0001$.

4. Discussion

Recently, a variant of CBD and THC has been identified in which the 5-carbon side chain is two carbons longer, these molecules were termed CBDP and THCP [22]. The authors went on to show that THCP binds to cannabinoid receptors with a higher affinity and was more effective at reducing pain than THC. In contrast, we did not see any impact of side-chain length on the ability of CBG to reduce pain in a mouse model of CIPN. However, we did find a significant anti-nociceptive effect of CBG and all CBG variants in a model of CIPN.

Our data indicate that side-chain length plays a role in the ability of CBG to reduce colorectal cancer cell growth in vitro. We found that, molecules with shorter side chains are more efficacious at reducing cell growth compared to longer side chains. Our findings with CBG are in contrast with previous work on CBDV and THCV which did not find a significant difference between these compounds and the more common 5-carbon variant (CBD and THC) [38–40]. Furthermore, neither the 4 or 7 carbon variants of CBD was found to have any greater impact on breast cancer cell growth than the 5-carbon molecule [41].

This could be due to the unique nature of CBG, which has been found to be an agonist of α2-adrenogeric receptors [42] and peroxisome proliferator-activated receptors (PPAR) α and γ [43–46], and the activation of these receptors has previously been reported to inhibit colorectal cancer cell growth.

It has been shown that side chain length can influence receptor binding for cannabinoids. For example, THCP has been shown to bind to CB1 receptors with a higher affinity than THC [22]. In contrast, THCV acts as an antagonist of the CB1 receptor, the opposite activity of THC, THCB, and THCP [24,47]. It is known that CBG binds with differing affinities and activities to a variety of receptors compared to THC and CBD [25]. One possible explanation for the differences we observe between the pain assay and cytotoxicity effects of these molecules is that different receptors mediate the analgesic and cytotoxic effects of CBG. Alternatively, the varying side chain lengths may create differing pharmacokinetics in vivo, thus normalizing their effects. Further studies on the binding of these novel molecules at known CBG receptors and additional studies on the mechanism that leads to cytotoxicity may provide useful insights into the mechanism by which CBGV and CBGB are slightly more cytotoxic but not more analgesic. These studies would also provide novel insights into how CBG interacts with known receptors.

5. Conclusions

We have developed a unique and adaptable process for generating cannabinoids with varying side chain lengths. Several recent reports have identified variants of CBD and THC with 3, 4, 6, and 7 carbon side chains; however, such side chain variants also likely exist for other cannabinoids such as cannabichromene (CBC) and must exist for CBG since this is the precursor molecule for the other cannabinoids. Surprisingly, we did not observe any effect of side-chain length regarding the ability to reduce neuropathic pain, which is in contrast to the data regarding THCP. However, we did find that CBG variants, such as CBG, produced significant anti-nociceptive effects in a murine model of CIPN. Importantly, we found that shorter side-chain variants of CBG were better able to reduce colorectal-cancer cell viability compared to longer-side chains.

Author Contributions: Conceptualization, D.D., K.E.V., N.M.G., S.A. and W.M.R.-K.; formal analysis, D.E.S., N.M.G., W.M.R.-K. and D.D.; investigation, D.E.S., W.M.R.-K., D.P.M. and D.D.; resources, K.E.V.; data curation, D.D. and W.M.R.-K.; writing—original draft preparation, D.E.S., D.D. and W.M.R.-K.; writing—review and editing, D.D., K.E.V., N.M.G. and W.M.R.-K.; visualization, W.M.R.-K.; project administration, W.M.R.-K.; funding acquisition, K.E.V. and N.M.G. All authors have read and agreed to the published version of the manuscript.

Funding: This project was supported by a NARSAD Young Investigator Award (27364; NMG) and by the Pennsylvania Department of Health using Tobacco CURE Funds (NMG). KEV (and the Penn State College of Medicine) is the recipient of research support from PA Options for Wellness (a state-approved medical marijuana clinical registrant). The funding sources were not involved in: study design, providing any experimental materials, data collection, analysis and interpretation; writing of the report; or the decision to submit the article for publication.

Data Availability Statement: Not applicable.

Acknowledgments: The authors would like to acknowledge members of the state-approved medical marijuana academic clinical research center at Penn State for insights and comments on the data and study design, along with the Drug Discovery, Development, and Delivery (D4) core and Organic Synthesis core for assistance with the preparation of the compounds and viability testing.

Conflicts of Interest: The authors declare no conflict of interest.

References

1. Society, A.C. Key Statistics for Colorectal Cancer. Available online: https://www.cancer.org/cancer/colon-rectal-cancer/about/keystatistics.html#:~{}:text=Excluding%20skin%20cancers%2C%20colorectal%20cancer,new%20cases%20of%20rectal%20cancer (accessed on 3 October 2022).
2. Ranasinghe, R.; Mathai, M.L.; Zulli, A. Cisplatin for cancer therapy and overcoming chemoresistance. *Heliyon* **2022**, *8*, e10608. [CrossRef]
3. Buyana, B.; Naki, T.; Alven, S.; Aderibigbe, B.A. Nanoparticles Loaded with Platinum Drugs for Colorectal Cancer Therapy. *Int. J. Mol. Sci.* **2022**, *23*, 11261. [CrossRef]
4. Avallone, A.; Bimonte, S.; Cardone, C.; Cascella, M.; Cuomo, A. Pathophysiology and Therapeutic Perspectives for Chemotherapy-induced Peripheral Neuropathy. *Anticancer Res.* **2022**, *42*, 4667–4678. [CrossRef]
5. Fallon, M.T. Neuropathic pain in cancer. *Br. J. Anaesth.* **2013**, *111*, 105–111. [CrossRef]
6. Banach, M.; Juranek, J.K.; Zygulska, A.L. Chemotherapy-induced neuropathies-a growing problem for patients and health care providers. *Brain Behav.* **2017**, *7*, e00558. [CrossRef]
7. Raup-Konsavage, W.M.; Johnson, M.; Legare, C.A.; Yochum, G.S.; Morgan, D.J.; Vrana, K.E. Synthetic Cannabinoid Activity Against Colorectal Cancer Cells. *Cannabis Cannabinoid Res.* **2018**, *3*, 272–281. [CrossRef]
8. Raup-Konsavage, W.; Carkaci-Salli, N.; Greenland, K.; Gearhart, R.J.; Vrana, K. Cannabidiol (CBD) Oil Does Not Display an Entourage Effect in Reducing Cancer Cell Viability in Vitro. *Med. Cannabis Cannabinoids* **2020**, *3*, 95–102. [CrossRef]
9. Caffarel, M.M.; Sarrió, D.; Palacios, J.; Guzmán, M.; Sánchez, C. Delta9-tetrahydrocannabinol inhibits cell cycle progression in human breast cancer cells through Cdc2 regulation. *Cancer Res.* **2006**, *66*, 6615–6621. [CrossRef]
10. Ligresti, A.; Moriello, A.S.; Starowicz, K.; Matias, I.; Pisanti, S.; De Petrocellis, L.; Laezza, C.; Portella, G.; Bifulco, M.; Di Marzo, V. Antitumor activity of plant cannabinoids with emphasis on the effect of cannabidiol on human breast carcinoma. *J. Pharmacol. Exp. Ther.* **2006**, *318*, 1375–1387. [CrossRef]
11. Scott, K.A.; Dalgleish, A.G.; Liu, W.M. The combination of cannabidiol and Δ9-tetrahydrocannabinol enhances the anticancer effects of radiation in an orthotopic murine glioma model. *Mol. Cancer Ther.* **2014**, *13*, 2955–2967. [CrossRef]
12. Jeong, S.; Yun, H.K.; Jeong, Y.A.; Jo, M.J.; Kang, S.H.; Kim, J.L.; Kim, D.Y.; Park, S.H.; Kim, B.R.; Na, Y.J.; et al. Cannabidiol-induced apoptosis is mediated by activation of Noxa in human colorectal cancer cells. *Cancer Lett.* **2019**, *447*, 12–23. [CrossRef]
13. Henderson-Redmond, A.N.; Crawford, L.C.; Sepulveda, D.E.; Hale, D.E.; Lesperance, J.J.; Morgan, D.J. Sex Differences in Tolerance to Delta-9-Tetrahydrocannabinol in Mice With Cisplatin-Evoked Chronic Neuropathic Pain. *Front. Mol. Biosci.* **2021**, *8*, 684115. [CrossRef]
14. Sepulveda, D.E.; Morris, D.P.; Raup-Konsavage, W.M.; Sun, D.; Vrana, K.E.; Graziane, N.M. Evaluating the Antinociceptive Efficacy of Cannabidiol Alone or in Combination with Morphine Using the Formalin Test in Male and Female Mice. *Cannabis Cannabinoid Res.* **2021**, *7*, 648–657. [CrossRef]
15. Sepulveda, D.E.; Morris, D.P.; Raup-Konsavage, W.M.; Sun, D.; Vrana, K.E.; Graziane, N.M. Cannabigerol (CBG) attenuates mechanical hypersensitivity elicited by chemotherapy-induced peripheral neuropathy. *Eur. J. Pain* **2022**, *26*, 1950–1966. [CrossRef]
16. King, K.M.; Myers, A.M.; Soroka-Monzo, A.J.; Tuma, R.F.; Tallarida, R.J.; Walker, E.A.; Ward, S.J. Single and combined effects of Δ9-tetrahydrocannabinol and cannabidiol in a mouse model of chemotherapy-induced neuropathic pain. *Br. J. Pharmacol.* **2017**, *174*, 2832–2841. [CrossRef]
17. Ward, S.J.; Ramirez, M.D.; Neelakantan, H.; Walker, E.A. Cannabidiol prevents the development of cold and mechanical allodynia in paclitaxel-treated female C57Bl6 mice. *Anesth. Analg.* **2011**, *113*, 947–950. [CrossRef]
18. Ward, S.J.; McAllister, S.D.; Kawamura, R.; Murase, R.; Neelakantan, H.; Walker, E.A. Cannabidiol inhibits paclitaxel-induced neuropathic pain through 5-HT(1A) receptors without diminishing nervous system function or chemotherapy efficacy. *Br. J. Pharmacol.* **2014**, *171*, 636–645. [CrossRef]
19. Hengst, J.A.; Nduwumwami, A.J.; Raup-Konsavage, W.M.; Vrana, K.E.; Yun, J.K. Inhibition of Sphingosine Kinase Activity Enhances Immunogenic Cell Surface Exposure of Calreticulin Induced by the Synthetic Cannabinoid 5-epi-CP-55,940. *Cannabis Cannabinoid Res.* **2021**, *7*, 637–647. [CrossRef]
20. Legare, C.A.; Raup-Konsavage, W.M.; Vrana, K.E. Therapeutic Potential of Cannabis, Cannabidiol, and Cannabinoid-Based Pharmaceuticals. *Pharmacology* **2022**, *107*, 131–149. [CrossRef]
21. Gaoni, Y.; Mechoulam, R. Isolation, Structure, and Partial Synthesis of an Active Constituent of Hashish. *J. Am. Chem. Soc.* **1964**, *86*, 1646–1647. [CrossRef]
22. Citti, C.; Linciano, P.; Russo, F.; Luongo, L.; Iannotta, M.; Maione, S.; Laganà, A.; Capriotti, A.L.; Forni, F.; Vandelli, M.A.; et al. A novel phytocannabinoid isolated from *Cannabis sativa* L. with an in vivo cannabimimetic activity higher than Δ9-tetrahydrocannabinol: Δ9-Tetrahydrocannabiphorol. *Sci. Rep.* **2019**, *9*, 20335. [CrossRef]
23. Linciano, P.; Citti, C.; Russo, F.; Tolomeo, F.; Laganà, A.; Capriotti, A.L.; Luongo, L.; Iannotta, M.; Belardo, C.; Maione, S.; et al. Identification of a new cannabidiol n-hexyl homolog in a medicinal cannabis variety with an antinociceptive activity in mice: Cannabidihexol. *Sci. Rep.* **2020**, *10*, 22019. [CrossRef]
24. Linciano, P.; Citti, C.; Luongo, L.; Belardo, C.; Maione, S.; Vandelli, M.A.; Forni, F.; Gigli, G.; Laganà, A.; Montone, C.M.; et al. Isolation of a High-Affinity Cannabinoid for the Human CB1 Receptor from a Medicinal *Cannabis sativa* Variety: Δ9-Tetrahydrocannabutol, the Butyl Homologue of Δ9-Tetrahydrocannabinol. *J. Nat. Prod.* **2020**, *83*, 88–98. [CrossRef]

25. Nachnani, R.; Raup-Konsavage, W.M.; Vrana, K.E. The Pharmacological Case for Cannabigerol. *J. Pharmacol. Exp. Ther.* **2021**, *376*, 204–212. [CrossRef]
26. Nomura, S.; Endo-Umeda, K.; Aoyama, A.; Makishima, M.; Hashimoto, Y.; Ishikawa, M. Styrylphenylphthalimides as Novel Transrepression-Selective Liver X Receptor (LXR) Modulators. *ACS Med. Chem. Lett.* **2015**, *6*, 902–907. [CrossRef]
27. Kavarana, M.; Peet, R. Bioenzymatic Synthesis of THCV, CBV, and CBN and Their Use as Therapeutic Agents. Patent US-2017283837-A1, 4 April 2016.
28. Filer, C. Cannabinoid Derivatives. 2021.
29. Chiurchiù, E.; Sampaolesi, S.; Allegrini, P.; Ciceri, D.; Ballini, R.; Palmieri, A. A Novel and Practical Continuous Flow Chemical Synthesis of Cannabidiol (CBD) and its CBDV and CBDB Analogues. *Eur. J. Org. Chem.* **2021**, *2021*, 1286–1289. [CrossRef]
30. Papahatjis, D.P.; Nahmias, V.R.; Nikas, S.P.; Andreou, T.; Alapafuja, S.O.; Tsotinis, A.; Guo, J.; Fan, P.; Makriyannis, A. C1′-cycloalkyl side chain pharmacophore in tetrahydrocannabinols. *J. Med. Chem.* **2007**, *50*, 4048–4060. [CrossRef]
31. Zhu, Y.; Soroka, D.N.; Sang, S. Synthesis and inhibitory activities against colon cancer cell growth and proteasome of alkylresorcinols. *J. Agric. Food Chem.* **2012**, *60*, 8624–8631. [CrossRef]
32. Bloemendal, V.R.L.J.; Sondag, D.; Elferink, H.; Boltje, T.J.; van Hest, J.C.M.; Rutjes, F.P.J.T. A Revised Modular Approach to (−)-trans-Δ8-THC and Derivatives Through Late-Stage Suzuki–Miyaura Cross-Coupling Reactions. *Eur. J. Org. Chem.* **2019**, *2019*, 2289–2296. [CrossRef]
33. Abdur-Rashid, K.; Jia, W.; Abdur-rashid, K. Catalytic Cannabigerol Processes and Precursors. Patent WO2021195751A1, 31 March 2020.
34. Guindon, J.; Deng, L.; Fan, B.; Wager-Miller, J.; Hohmann, A.G. Optimization of a cisplatin model of chemotherapy-induced peripheral neuropathy in mice: Use of vitamin C and sodium bicarbonate pretreatments to reduce nephrotoxicity and improve animal health status. *Mol. Pain* **2014**, *10*, 56. [CrossRef]
35. Alonso, E.; Ramón, D.J.; Yus, M. Simple Synthesis of 5-Substituted Resorcinols: A Revisited Family of Interesting Bioactive Molecules. *J. Org. Chem.* **1997**, *62*, 417–421. [CrossRef] [PubMed]
36. Golliher, A.E.; Tenorio, A.J.; Dimauro, N.O.; Mairata, N.R.; Holguin, F.O.; Maio, W. Using (+)-carvone to access novel derivatives of (+)-ent-cannabidiol: The first asymmetric syntheses of (+)-ent-CBDP and (+)-ent-CBDV. *Tetrahedron Lett.* **2021**, *67*, 152891. [CrossRef] [PubMed]
37. Chemical, C. CBGV Cannabigerol. Available online: https://www.caymanchem.com/product/9002437/cannabigerovarin (accessed on 2 October 2022).
38. Available online: https://www.caymanchem.com/product/15293/cannabigerol (accessed on 2 October 2022).
39. Borrelli, F.; Pagano, E.; Romano, B.; Panzera, S.; Maiello, F.; Coppola, D.; De Petrocellis, L.; Buono, L.; Orlando, P.; Izzo, A.A. Colon carcinogenesis is inhibited by the TRPM8 antagonist cannabigerol, a Cannabis-derived non-psychotropic cannabinoid. *Carcinogenesis* **2014**, *35*, 2787–2797. [CrossRef]
40. De Petrocellis, L.; Ligresti, A.; Schiano Moriello, A.; Iappelli, M.; Verde, R.; Stott, C.G.; Cristino, L.; Orlando, P.; Di Marzo, V. Non-THC cannabinoids inhibit prostate carcinoma growth in vitro and in vivo: Pro-apoptotic effects and underlying mechanisms. *Br. J. Pharmacol.* **2013**, *168*, 79–102. [CrossRef] [PubMed]
41. Russo, C.; Lavorgna, M.; Nugnes, R.; Orlo, E.; Isidori, M. Comparative assessment of antimicrobial, antiradical and cytotoxic activities of cannabidiol and its propyl analogue cannabidivarin. *Sci. Rep.* **2021**, *11*, 22494. [CrossRef] [PubMed]
42. Salbini, M.; Quarta, A.; Russo, F.; Giudetti, A.M.; Citti, C.; Cannazza, G.; Gigli, G.; Vergara, D.; Gaballo, A. Oxidative Stress and Multi-Organel Damage Induced by Two Novel Phytocannabinoids, CBDB and CBDP, in Breast Cancer Cells. *Molecules* **2021**, *26*, 5576. [CrossRef] [PubMed]
43. Kennedy, M.F.; Tutton, P.J.; Barkla, D.H. Adrenergic factors regulating cell division in the colonic crypt epithelium during carcinogenesis and in colonic adenoma and adenocarcinoma. *Br. J. Cancer* **1985**, *52*, 383–390. [CrossRef]
44. Ban, J.O.; Kwak, D.H.; Oh, J.H.; Park, E.J.; Cho, M.C.; Song, H.S.; Song, M.J.; Han, S.B.; Moon, D.C.; Kang, K.W.; et al. Suppression of NF-kappaB and GSK-3beta is involved in colon cancer cell growth inhibition by the PPAR agonist troglitazone. *Chem. Biol. Interact.* **2010**, *188*, 75–85. [CrossRef]
45. Gupta, R.A.; Dubois, R.N. Controversy: PPARgamma as a target for treatment of colorectal cancer. *Am. J. Physiol. Gastrointest. Liver Physiol.* **2002**, *283*, G266–G269. [CrossRef]
46. Brockman, J.A.; Gupta, R.A.; Dubois, R.N. Activation of PPARgamma leads to inhibition of anchorage-independent growth of human colorectal cancer cells. *Gastroenterology* **1998**, *115*, 1049–1055. [CrossRef]
47. Thomas, A.; Stevenson, L.A.; Wease, K.N.; Price, M.R.; Baillie, G.; Ross, R.A.; Pertwee, R.G. Evidence that the plant cannabinoid Delta9-tetrahydrocannabivarin is a cannabinoid CB1 and CB2 receptor antagonist. *Br. J. Pharmacol.* **2005**, *146*, 917–926. [CrossRef] [PubMed]

molecules

MDPI

Article

Ent-Abietane Diterpenoids from *Euphorbia fischeriana* and Their Cytotoxic Activities

Qin-Feng Zhu †, Guo-Bo Xu †, Shang-Gao Liao * and Xue-Long Yan *

School of Pharmacy, Guizhou Medical University, Dongqing Road, Guiyang 550025, China
* Correspondence: lshangg@163.com (S.-G.L.); yanxlong54@163.com (X.-L.Y.)
† These authors contributed equally to this work.

Abstract: The roots of *Euphorbia fischeriana* have been used as a traditional Chinese medicine for the treatment of tuberculosis and ringworm. In the current study, diterpenoids from the ethyl acetate extract of the roots *E. fischeriana* and their cytotoxic effects against five cancer lines were investigated. Two new *ent*-abietane diterpenoids, euphonoids H and I (**1**–**2**), as well as their two analogues (**3**–**4**) were first isolated from this source. The structures of the two new compounds were elucidated on the basis of spectroscopic data and quantum chemical calculation. Their absolute configurations were assigned via ECD spectrum calculation. The isolated compounds were evaluated for their antiproliferative activities against five cancer cell lines. Compounds **1** and **2** exhibited significant inhibitory effects against human prostate cancers C4-2B and C4-2B/ENZR cell lines with IC_{50} values ranging from 4.16 ± 0.42 to 5.74 ± 0.45 μM.

Keywords: abietane-type; diterpenoid; *Euphorbia fischeriana*; antiproliferative activities

Citation: Zhu, Q.-F.; Xu, G.-B.; Liao, S.-G.; Yan, X.-L. *Ent*-Abietane Diterpenoids from *Euphorbia fischeriana* and Their Cytotoxic Activities. *Molecules* **2022**, *27*, 7258. https://doi.org/10.3390/molecules27217258

Academic Editors: Barbara De Filippis, Alessandra Ammazzalorso and Marialuigia Fantacuzzi

Received: 28 September 2022
Accepted: 21 October 2022
Published: 26 October 2022

1. Introduction

Natural products are promising sources for the discovery of novel agents/active templates for the development of effective agents against a variety of human diseases [1]. Due to their great structural diversity and wide range of bioactivities [2], diterpenoids have been a constant focus of drug discovery. Among the naturally occurring cyclic diterpenoids (e.g., abietane, labdane and clerodane diterpenoids), tricyclic abietane diterpenoids are of particular significance. These diterpenoids were reported to be present in species of Lamiaceae, Cupressaceae, Pinaceae and Euphorbiaceae as well as in several higher plants [3,4] and were shown to possess antitumor, antioxidant, antibacterial and anti-inflammatory effects [5]. Sugiol, an abietane diterpenoid previously isolated from *Metasequoia glyptostroboides* (Cupressaceae), has been developed as an advanced multimodal anti-inflammatory disease targeting tool [6]; Euphelionolides A, D, I and L, four *ent*-abietane diterpenoids isolated from *Euphorbia helioscopia* (Euphorbiaceae), were demonstrated to be effective free-radical scavengers acting via various reaction pathways [7]; 6-hydroxy-5,6-dehydrosugiol, a derivative of sugiol isolated from the stem bark of *Cryptomeria japonica*, was shown to be a potent androgen receptor antagonist in PCa cells [8].

The roots of *Euphorbia fischeriana* Steud have been used as a traditional Chinese medicine for the treatment of lymphoid tuberculosis and ringworm [9]. Previous phytochemical studies showed that polycyclic diterpenoids including *ent*-abietanes, *ent*-atisanes, *ent*-kauranes, *ent*-isopimaranes and *ent*-pimaranes possessing a common 6/6/6-tricyclic ring are the major constituents of *E. fischeriana* [10,11]. In our earlier study, a series of *ent*-abietane diterpenoids with significant cytotoxicity have been isolated from this plant [12]. As part of our continuing efforts toward novel antitumor diterpenoids, the chemical constituents of the roots of *E. fischeriana* were reinvestigated. As a result, two previously undescribed *ent*-abietanes and two known analogues were isolated from the roots of *E. fischeriana*. The new compounds showed significant cytotoxicity against human prostate cancer C4-2B and C4-2B/ENZR cell lines. Herein, the details of isolation, structure elucidation and cytotoxicity of these compounds are described.

2. Results and Discussion

The dry roots of *E. fischeriana* were repeatedly extracted with 95% EtOH at room temperature and the extract was successively partitioned with petroleum ether, ethyl acetate (EtOAc) and *n*-butanol. The EtOAc fraction was subjected repeatedly to column chromatography over silica gel, ODS gel, Sephadex LH-20 and semipreparative HPLC to yield two previously undescribed *ent*-abietane diterpenoids (**1–2**). In addition to the above new compounds, two known diterpenoids (Figure 1) were also obtained: raserranes A (**3**) and B (**4**). The structures of all compounds were well-characterized by NMR analysis and quantum chemical calculation.

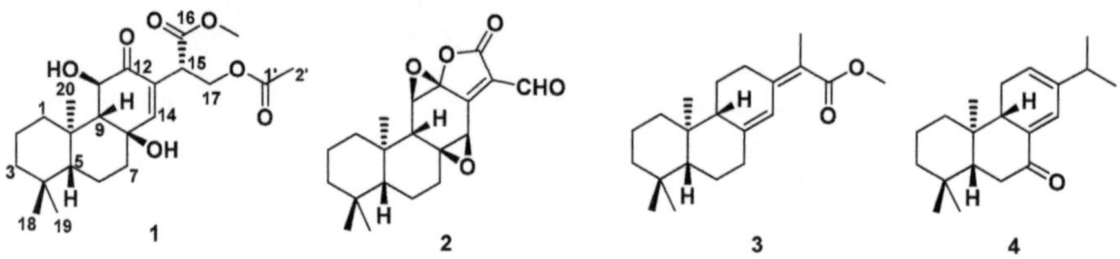

Figure 1. The structures of compounds **1–4**.

2.1. Structure Elucidation of Compounds 1 and 2

Euphonoid H (**1**) was obtained as a colorless oil and was shown to possess a molecular formula of $C_{23}H_{34}O_7$ based on its HRESIMS ion at 445.2213 $[M + Na]^+$ (calcd 445.2197). The ^1H spectrum (Supplementary Material) showed signals for an olefinic hydrogen (δ_H 6.71, H-14), one methoxyl (δ_H 3.68, 16-OCH_3) and four methyl groups (δ_H 2.02, 0.91, 0.79 and 0.69). The ^{13}C and HSQC NMR showed resonances assignable to one ketone (δ_C 196.0), two ester (δ_C 170.8 and 171.1), two olefinic carbons (δ_C 133.7 and 154.2), four methyl (δ_C 34.0, 22.1, 17.8 and 21.0), one methoxyl group (δ_C 34.0), three oxygenated carbons (δ_C 72.0, 69.5 and 62.5) and ten additional sp^3 carbons (δ_C between 18.5 and 60.4). Comprehensive analysis of the 1D and 2D-NMR data (Table 1) revealed that compound **1** possessed, except for an acetoxyl group and a methoxy group, an abietane diterpene skeleton similar to that of methyl-8β,11β-dihydroxy-12-oxo-ent-abietadi-13,15(17)-ene-16-oate previously isolated from this plant [13]. However, the ^{13}C NMR data for the $\Delta^{15(17)}$ (δ_C 137.3 for C-15 and 128.8 for C-17) of the latter were replaced by signals for a methine (δ_C 45.1, C-15) and an oxymethylene (δ_C 62.5, C-17). These observations implied that compound **1** was a hydrogenated derivative of the known compound.

Table 1. ^1H (400 MHz) and ^{13}C (100 MHz) NMR data for **1** and **2** in $CDCl_3$.

Position	1		2	
	δ_H (J in Hz)	δ_C, Type	δ_H (J in Hz)	Δ_c, Type
1	1.88 (1H, d, J = 13.0 Hz) 1.21–1.16 (1H, m)	39.7, CH_2	1.92 (1H, d, J = 12.5 Hz) 1.37–1.29 (1H, m)	39.2, CH_2
2	1.55 (1H, d, J = 13.5 Hz) 1.51–1.45 (1H, m)	18.5, CH_2	1.63–1.55 (1H, m) 1.56–1.51 (1H, m)	18.5, CH_2
3	1.43 (1H, d, J = 12.7 Hz) 1.26–1.19 (1H, m)	41.6, CH_2	1.47–1.43 (1H, m) 1.29–1.20 (1H, m)	41.4, CH_2
4		33.3, C		33.6, C
5	1.08 (1H, dd, J = 12.9, 2.6 Hz)	54.4, CH	1.12 (1H, dd, J = 12.3, 2.5 Hz)	53.6, CH

Table 1. *Cont.*

Position	1		2	
	δ_H (*J* in Hz)	δ_C, Type	δ_H (*J* in Hz)	Δ_c, Type
6	1.71–1.65 (1H, m) 1.16–1.12 (1H, m)	19.2, CH_2	1.88–1.80 (1H, m) 1.56–1.51 (1H, m), overlapped	20.9, CH_2
7	2.13–2.03(1H, m) 1.74–1.72 (1H, m)	41.4, CH_2	2.08–1.97 (1H, m) 1.51–1.48 (1H, m), overlapped	35.8, CH_2
8		69.5, C		71.7, C
9	2.13–2.03(1H, s)	60.4, CH	2.33 (1H, s)	48.1, CH
10		37.7, C		39.4, C
11	4.23 (1H, s)	72.0, CH	4.15 (1H, s)	64.8, CH
12		196.0, C		85.4, C
13		133.7, C		166.2, C
14	6.71 (1H, s)	154.2, CH	4.48 (1H, s)	55.3, CH
15	3.77 (1H, t, *J* = 7.2 Hz)	45.7, CH		127.5, C
16		170.8, C		165.8, C
17	4.41 (2H, d, *J* = 7.2 Hz)	62.5, CH_2	9.97 (1H, s)	185.0, CH
18	0.91 (3H, s)	34.0, CH_3	0.94 (3H, s)	33.6, CH_3
19	0.79 (3H, s)	22.1, CH_3	0.85 (3H, s)	22.0, CH_3
20	0.69 (3H, s)	17.8, CH_3	0.80 (3H, s)	15.6, CH_3
16-OCH_3	3.68 (3H, s)	52.4, CH_3		
1′		171.1, C		
2′	2.02 (3H, s)	21.0, CH_3		

Detailed 2D-NMR (^{1}H-^{1}H COSY, HSQC, HMBC and NOESY) data analysis further confirmed the above deduction and fulfilled the structural assignment. The ^{1}H-^{1}H COSY revealed four spin systems, CH_2-1/CH_2-2/CH_2-3, H-5/CH_2-6/CH_2-7, H-9/H-11 and H-15/CH_2-17 (Figure 2). HMBC correlations from H_3-20 (to C-1 and C-10), H_2-1 (to C-9), H_3-18 (to C-3, C-4 and C-5), H_2-6 (to C-4 and C-10), H-11 (to C-8 and C-13) and H-14 (to C-7, C-9 and C-12) to their corresponding carbons not only connected the former three fragments, but suggested that compound **2** shared the same ABC rings with methyl-8β,11β-dihydroxy-12-oxo-ent-abietadi-13,15(17)-ene-16-oate. In addition, HMBC correlations from H-15 to C-12, C-13 and C-14 and from H_2-17 to C-13 located the $\Delta^{15(17)}$ double bond at C-13. HMBC correlations from the methoxyl group to C-16 suggested the presence of a methoxyformyl group, while the HMBC correlation from H_2-17 to C-16 revealed its position at C-15. The acetoxyl group was connected to the abietane skeleton at C-17 by the key HMBC cross-peaks from H_2-17 and H_3-2′ to C-1′. Thus, the gross structure of **1** was established as depicted.

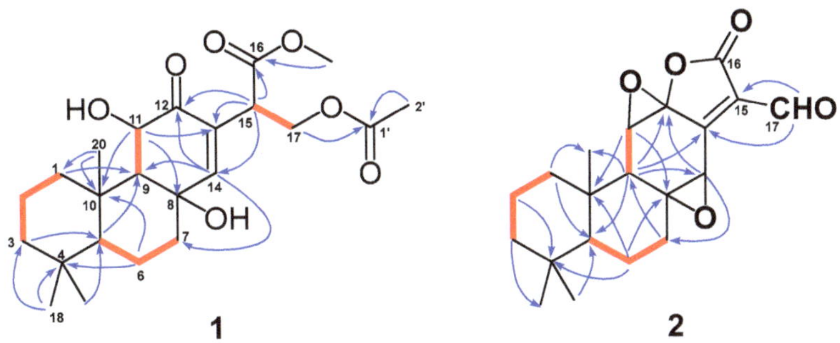

Figure 2. Key ^{1}H-^{1}H COSY (—) and HMBC (⌒) correlations of **1** and **2**.

The NOESY correlations (Figure 3) of H-5/H-9 indicated that these protons were cofacial and were arbitrarily assigned to be *β*-oriented, while the NOESY correlation of H_3-20/H-11 indicated that these protons were *α*-oriented. However, the NOESY spectrum did not give useful signals to determine the relative configuration of C-8 and C-15. To establish the relative configuration, the chemical shifts of four conformers were predicted at the B3LYP/6-311+G (d, p) level in chloroform (Figure 4). The results showed that the calculated chemical shifts of conformer **1b** was in the best agreement with the experimental values among those predicted for **1a, 1b, 1c** and **1d**. Further DP4+ analyses verified that conformer **1b** was assigned with a 99.99% probability among all the conformers (Figure 4). These results suggested that compound **1** had the structure of conformer **1b** with the relative stereochemistry of 5*R**, 8*R**, 9*R**, 10*R**, 11*R**, 15*S**.

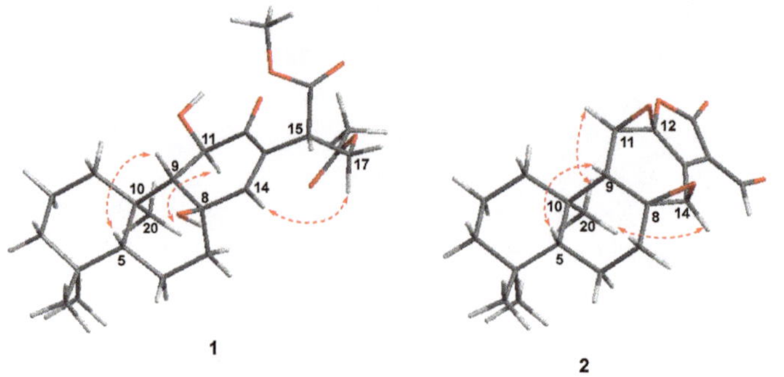

Figure 3. Key NOE correlations ( ) of compounds **1** and **2**.

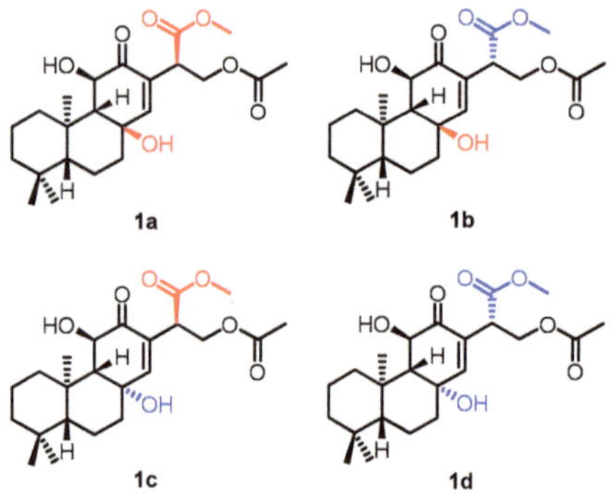

(**a**)

isomers	1a	1b	1c	1d
R^2	0.9986	0.9992	0.9986	0.9982
CLAD	6.63	3.38	5.33	4.96
CMAD	1.57	1.30	1.54	1.85
DP4+ (C data)	0.01%	99.99%	0.00%	0.00%

(**b**)

Figure 4. ^{13}C NMR calculation results of compound **1** at the mPW1PW91/6-311+G(d,p) level. (**a**) Structures of conformer **1a–1d**. (**b**) Key parameters of the calculated chemical shifts of conformers **1a–1d**.

The absolute configuration of **1** was established by comparing its experimental ECD spectrum with those calculated at the CAM-B3LYP/6-31+G(d) level in acetonitrile. As shown in Figure 5, the experimental ECD curve of **1** showed first negative and second positive Cotton effects around 250 and 213 nm, respectively, which matched well the calculated ECD spectrum of 5*R*, 8*R*, 9*R*, 10*R*, 11*R*, 15*S*-**1** (Figure 5a). Thus, compound **1**, as an *ent*-abietane diterpenoid, was established as depicted and named euphonoid H.

The molecular formula of **2** was determined to be $C_{20}H_{24}O_5$ by the HRESIMS ion peak at m/z 343.1550 ([M − H]$^-$, calcd 343.1551). The ^{1}H NMR data (Table 1) of **2** indicated the presence of three methyls [δ_H 0.98 (3H, Me-18), 0.85 (3H, Me-19), 0.80 (3H, Me-20)] and one aldehyde [δ_H 9.97 (s, H-17)]. The ^{13}C NMR (Table 1) and HSQC data of **2** revealed the presence of three methyls, five methylenes, five methines (including two oxygenated ones at δ_C 64.8 and 55.3 and seven quaternary carbons (including two olefinic ones at δ_C 166.2 and 127.5). The above NMR characteristic features of **2** resembled those of jolkinolide

B [14], the major differences being the replacement of the 17-CH_3 group in jolkinolide B by an aldehyde group (δ_C 185.0) in **2**. HMBC correlations from H-17 (δ_H 9.97, s) to C-13 (δ_C 166.2) and C-15 (δ_C 127.5) further confirmed the above deduction. The NOESY correlation H-5/H-9 suggested that H-5 and H-9 were β-oriented, whereas the NOESY correlations H_3-20/H-11 and H_3-20/H-14 indicated that H-11, H-14 and CH_3-20 were α-oriented. Subsequently, quantum chemical calculation of NMR chemical shifts was run on the proposed structure of **2**. As indicated by R^2 (^{13}C: 0.9979), CMAD (^{13}C: 1.88 ppm) and CLAD (^{13}C: 4.79 ppm) good consistency was observed between the theoretically predicted and experimental chemical shifts, which validated the proposed structure for **2** (Figure 6). Subsequently, ECD calculation (Figure 5b) of the two enantiomers of **2** enabled the establishment of the absolute configuration of **2** to be 5*S*, 8*S*, 9*R*, 10*R*, 11*R*, 12*R*, 14*R*. The structure of **2** was therefore established as depicted and named euphonoid I.

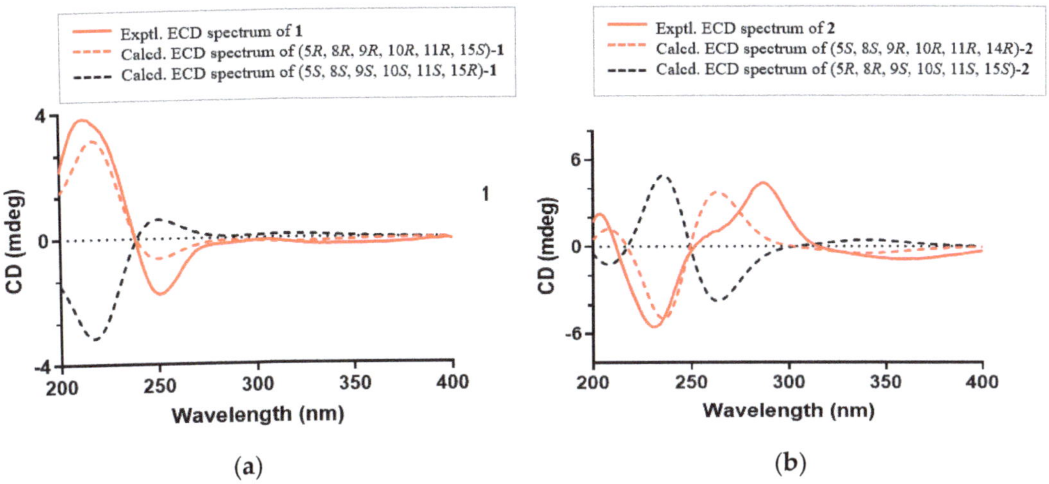

Figure 5. (**a**) Experimental and calculated ECD spectra of **1**; (**b**) Experimental and calculated ECD spectra of **2**.

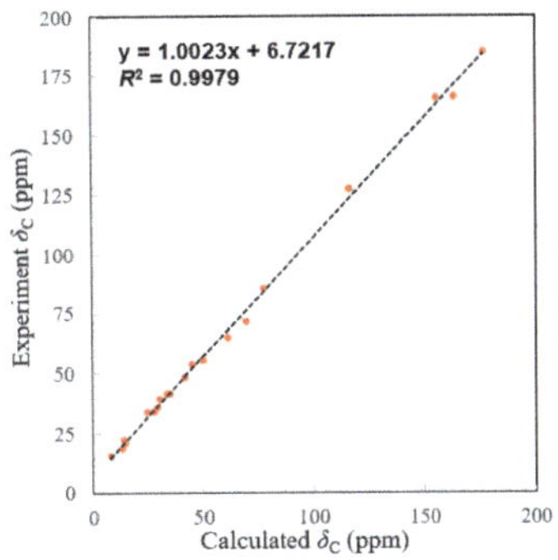

Figure 6. Linear correlation plots of predicted versus experimental ^{13}C NMR chemical shifts.

The other two known diterpenoids (**3–4**) were identified to be *ent*-abietane diterpenoids raserranes A (**3**) and B (**4**) by comparison of their NMR data with those reported in the literature, these four diterpenoids were discovered for the first time from this species [15].

2.2. *Biological Activity of Isolated Compounds*

The anticancer effects of the isolates **1–4** were evaluated against human breast cancer cells MDA-MB-231, human colon cancer cells HCT-15 and RKO and human prostate cancer cells C4-2B and C4-2B/ENZR (enzalutamide-resistant C4-2B cells). The IC_{50} values (Table 2) indicated that the two new compounds exhibited varying degrees of growth inhibition against the five cancer cell lines. Compound **1** showed significant inhibitory activities against C4-2B and C4-2B/ENZR cell lines with IC_{50} values of 5.52 ± 0.65 μM and 4.16 ± 0.42 μM, respectively. Compound **2** exhibited marked inhibitory activity towards the five human cancer cell lines (IC_{50} values ranging from 4.49 ± 0.78 to 12.45 ± 3.24 μM) and was particularly active against C4-2B and C4-2B/ENZR cell lines (IC_{50} values: 4.49 ± 0.78 and 5.74 ± 0.45, respectively).

Table 2. IC_{50} data of compounds **1–4** for the indicated cell lines.

Compound	IC_{50} [1] (μM)				
	MDA-MB-231	HCT-15	RKO	C4-2B	C4-2B/ENZR
1	21.80 ± 2.35	28.57 ± 1.16	20.46 ± 1.43	5.52 ± 0.65	4.16 ± 0.42
2	7.95 ± 0.82	12.45 ± 3.24	8.78 ± 2.45	4.49 ± 0.78	5.74 ± 0.45
3	>50	>50	>50	34.09 ± 7.78	>50
4	>50	>50	>50	23.34 ± 2.18	36.98 ± 6.18
DOX [2]	0.34 ± 0.16	0.72 ± 0.09	0.59 ± 0.29	0.11 ± 0.08	0.22 ± 0.18

[1] Each IC_{50} value was the mean ± standard deviation from three experiments; [2] Positive control: doxorubicin.

Macrocyclic and polycyclic diterpenes were usually encountered in the genus of *Euphorbia* and macrocyclic diterpenes were characteristic components of *Euphorbia* plants, while polycyclic diterpenes were nonspecific in this genus. Although polycyclic diterpenes were not the characteristic components of *Euphorbia* plants, some polycyclic diterpenes showed great potential in the development of anticancer drugs [16–18]. Jolkinolide B, a typical *ent*-abietane diterpene first isolated from *Euphorbia jolkini*, induced apoptosis and sensitized bladder cancer to mTOR inhibitors [19,20]; 17-hydroxy-jolkinolide B, a potent inhibitor of JAK/STAT3 signaling, is a promising anticancer drug candidate [21]. In this study, compounds **1–2** sharing the same abietane diterpene skeleton (6/6/6 carbon ring system) were shown to be promising anti-prostate cancer candidates. Among the four compounds isolated, compound **2** that possessed an α,β-unsaturated γ-lactone ring at C-12 and C-13, was very active against almost the test cancer cells. This observation was consistent with our previous discovery that such an α,β-unsaturated γ-lactone ring was beneficial for the anticancer activity of this type of diterpenoids [12]. Despite the fact that several antitumor abietane diterpenoids were reported in recent years, the pharmacophores and structure-activity relationship of abietane diterpenoids as anticancer agents were rarely investigated. Thus, synthesis of these diterpenoids and study of their structure–activity relationship and potential molecular mechanisms were of great significance for the design and development of anticancer agents.

3. Materials and Methods

3.1. *General Experimental Procedures*

Optical rotations were carried out on a Rudolph Autopol I automatic polarimeter (Rudolph Research Analytical, Hackettstown, NJ, USA). The UV spectra were measured at a Shimadzu UV-2450 spectrophotometer (Shimadzu Corporation, Kyoto, Japan). IR spectra were determined on a Bruker Tensor 37 infrared spectrophotometer (Bruker Optics, Ettlingen, Germany) with KBr disk. ECD spectra were measured on an Applied Photophysics Chirascan spectrometer (Applied Photophysics Ltd., England). NMR spectra were measured on Bruker AM-400 spectrometer with tetramethylsilane (TMS) as the internal standard. HR-ESIMS data were determined using a Waters Micromass Q-TOF spectrometer (Waters Corporation, Milford, MA, USA). The semi-preparative HPLC was performed on an Essentia LC-16 (Shimadzu, Suzhou, China). Column chromatography (CC) was used using silica gel (200–300 mesh, Qingdao Marine Chemical Factory, Qingdao, China).

3.2. Plant Material

The roots of *E. fischeriana* were collected in August 2015 from Tie ling city, Liaoning Province, P. R. China and identified by Prof. Qing-De Long (Guizhou Medical University). The specimens were deposited in School of Pharmaceutical Sciences, Guizhou Medical University (specimen no. 20150805).

3.3. Extraction and Isolation

The dried roots (10 kg) of *E. fischeriana* were crushed, extracted with 95% ethanol (50 L) at room temperature for three times (each for 24 h), the solvent was recovered under reduced pressure to obtain the crude extract. The crude extract was suspended in water (3 L) and then partitioned sequentially with petroleum ether, EtOAc and *n*-BuOH (saturated with water) and dried under reduced pressure to give their corresponding extracts (178.36, 220.82 and 205.43 g, respectively). The EtOAc fraction was subjected to CC (chromatographic column) on silica gel (1.3 kg, 100–200 mesh) using petroleum ether-CH_2Cl_2 (1:0 to 0:1) and CH_2Cl_2-MeOH (200:1 to 10:1) as eluents to give fractions 1–3 and 4–10, respectively. Fr. 5 (12.15 g) showed obvious brick-red spots in the TLC and was subjected to ODS CC eluted with MeOH-H_2O (40–100%) to obtain 6 fractions (Fr. 5A to Fr. 5F). Fr. 5C (2.42 g) was subsequently loaded on a Sephadex LH-20 column using CH_2Cl_2-MeOH (1:1) as eluent to obtain 3 fractions (Fr. 5C-a to Fr. 5C-c). Fr. 5C-a (0.69 g) was purified by semipreparative HPLC (ACN-H_2O, 87%, 3 mL/min) to obtain compound **3** (6.8 mg, t_R = 12.0 min). Compound **1** (4.3 mg, t_R = 18.5 min) was isolated from Fr. 5C-b (0.75 g) by preparative HPLC (ACN-H_2O, 85%, 3 mL/min). Fr. 5D (1.87 g) was firstly separated by silica gel CC (PE/EtOAc, 5:1) and then by semi-HPLC (ACN-H_2O, 90%, 3 mL/min) to afford **2** (3.5 mg, t_R = 13.2 min) and **4** (7.2 mg, t_R = 16.7 min), respectively.

Euphonoid H (**1**): colorless oil; $[\alpha]_D^{20}$ −43.2 (c 0.10, $CHCl_3$); UV (MeOH) λ_{max} (log ε) 230 (3.68) nm; IR (KBr) ν_{max} 3400, 2932, 1738, 1217, 1033 cm^{-1}; HRESIMS *m*/*z* 445.2213 (calcd. for $C_{23}H_{34}O_7Na^+$ $[M + Na]^+$, 445.2197); ^1H and ^{13}C NMR data see Table 1.

Euphonoid I (**2**): colorless oil; $[\alpha]_D^{20}$ + 2.8 (c 0.37, $CHCl_3$); UV (MeOH) λ_{max} (log ε) 266 (4.39) nm; IR (KBr) ν_{max} 2938, 1788, 1636, 1256, 968 cm^{-1}; HRESIMS *m*/*z* 343.1550 (calcd. for $C_{20}H_{23}O_5^-$ $[M - H]^-$, 343.1551); ^1H and ^{13}C NMR data see Table 1.

Raserrane A (**3**): colorless oil; $[\alpha]_D^{20}$ −42.8 (c 0.10, $CHCl_3$); HRESIMS *m*/*z* 339.2291 (calcd. for $C_{21}H_{32}O_2Na^+$ $[M + Na]^+$, 339.2295).

Raserrane B (**4**): colorless oil; $[\alpha]_D^{20}$ −133.4 (c 0.25, $CHCl_3$); HRESIMS *m*/*z* 287.2362 (calcd. for $C_{20}H_{31}O^+$ $[M + H]^+$, 287.2369).

3.4. Quantum Chemical NMR and ECD Calculations of Compound **1–2**

The random conformational searches were performed by SYBYL X 2.1.1 program using MMFF94s molecular force field. The obtained conformers were subsequently optimized by using Gaussion09 software at the B3LYP/6-31G(d) level in gas phase. The optimized stable conformers were selected for further NMR calculations at the mPW1PW91/6-311 + G(d,p) level in chloroform and ECD calculations at the CAM-B3LYP/6-31 + G(d) level in acetonitrile. The overall theoretical NMR data were analyzed by using linear regression and DP4+ probability. The overall ECD data were weighted by Boltzmann distribution and produced by SpecDis version 1.70.1 software (T. Bruhn; A. Schaumlöffel; Y. Hemberger; G. Pescitelli, Berlin, Germany).

3.5. Cell Culture

Five cancer cell lines, including human prostate cancer cells (C4-2B), enzalutamide-resistant C4-2B cells (C4-2B/ENZR), human breast cancer cells (MDA-MB-231) and human colon cancer cells (HCT-15 and RKO) used in this study were purchased from the Laboratory Animal Service Centre at Sun Yat-sen University (Guangzhou, China). Cell lines were cultured in Dulbecco's modified Eagle's medium (DMEM) with 10% fetal bovine serum (FBS) and antibiotics (100 units/mL penicillin and 100 g/mL streptomycin). These cells were incubated at 37 °C in an atmosphere of 5% CO_2.

3.6. Cytotoxicity Assay

The cells in logarithmic growth phase were seeded a in 96-well plates at a density of 5×10^3 cells/well for 24 h. Then, cells were treated with different concentrations of the compounds for an additional 48 h. Subsequently, 10 μL MTT (5 mg/mL) (Sigma, Saint Louis, MO, USA) were added to each well. After incubation in the incubator for 4 h, the suspension was discarded and the dark blue crystals were solubilized in dimethyl sulfoxide (DMSO). The absorbance of the solution was detected by a multifunction micro-plate reader (Molecular Devices, Flex Station 3, Molecular Devices, San Francisco, USA) at 450 nm. IC_{50} value was used to express the cytotoxic effect on the tested compounds.

4. Conclusions

In summary, two new highly oxygenated *ent*-abietane diterpenoids euphonoids H and I (**1–2**), together with two known analogues raserranes A (**3**) and B (**4**) were separated and identified from the EtOAc-soluble partition of the roots of *E. fischeriana*. Their structures were elucidated by comprehensive spectroscopic analysis, quantum chemical calculation and ECD calculations. All the compounds were isolated from *E. fischerian* for the first time. The two new compounds exhibited strong antiproliferative potency against the human prostate cancer cells C4-2B and C4-2B/ENZR, with IC_{50} values less than 10 μM. This study not only enriches the chemical diversity of *ent*-abietane diterpenoids in the *Euphorbia* species but also forms a basis for the discovery of bioactive natural products from Euphorbiaceae herbs.

The current results, together with others' previous discoveries, suggested that *ent*-abietane diterpenoids with certain structural motifs might possess very strong anticancer activity against prostate cancer cell lines and this type of diterpenoids provided a promising skeleton for the development of anti-cancer agents for the treatment of prostate cancers.

Supplementary Materials: The following supporting information can be downloaded online: https://www.mdpi.com/article/10.3390/molecules27217258/s1, Figures S1–S6: The 1D and 2D NMR (400 MHz) spectra of compound **1** in $CDCl_3$, Figure S7: The HRESIMS spectrum of compound **1**, Figure S8: The IR spectrum of compound **1**, Figures S9–S14: The 1D and 2D NMR (400 MHz) spectra of compound **2** in $CDCl_3$, Figure S15: The HRESIMS spectrum of compound **2**, Figure S16: The IR spectrum of compound **2**, Figures S17 and S18 and Tables S1–S9: NMR and ECD calculation method of compound **1**, Figures S19–S21 and Tables S10–S12: NMR and ECD calculation method of compound **2**, Figures S22–S25: ^{1}H NMR and HRESIMS spectra of compound **1–2**, Table S13: NMR Data for compounds **1–2** in $CDCl_3$.

Author Contributions: Original draft preparation, Q.-F.Z. and G.-B.X.; performing the experiments, Q.-F.Z. and X.-L.Y.; data analysis, G.-B.X.; review and editing, S.-G.L.; supervision, S.-G.L. and X.-L.Y. All authors have read and agreed to the published version of the manuscript.

Funding: This work was funded by the New-shoot Talents Project of Guizhou Medical University (19NSP077), the Scientific Research Foundation for Innovative Talent of Guizhou Province ([2020]6011), National Natural Science Foundation of China (22167009) and the Project of Science and Technology Department of Guizhou Province ([2020]5006, ZK [2021]554).

Institutional Review Board Statement: Not applicable.

Informed Consent Statement: Not applicable.

Data Availability Statement: The data are available in the Supporting Information of the article.

Conflicts of Interest: The authors declare no conflict of interest.

Sample Availability: Samples of the compounds are not available from the authors as the material has been used up for bioassays.

References

1. Newman, D.J.; Cragg, G.M. Natural products as sources of new drugs over the nearly four decades from 01/1981 to 09/2019. *J. Nat. Prod.* **2020**, *83*, 770–803. [CrossRef]
2. Hanson, J.R. Diterpenoids. *Nat. Prod. Rep.* **2009**, *26*, 1156–1171. [CrossRef] [PubMed]
3. Jian, B.; Zhang, H.; Liu, J. Structural diversity and biological activities of diterpenoids derived from *Euphorbia fischeriana* steud. *Molecules* **2018**, *23*, 935. [CrossRef] [PubMed]
4. Wu, Y.-B.; Ni, Z.-Y.; Shi, Q.-W.; Dong, M.; Kiyota, H.; Gu, Y.-C.; Cong, B. Constituents from *Salvia* species and their biological activities. *Chem. Rev.* **2012**, *112*, 5967–6026. [CrossRef] [PubMed]
5. Zhao, H.; Sun, L.; Kong, C.; Mei, W.; Dai, H.; Xu, F.; Huang, S. Phytochemical and pharmacological review of diterpenoids from the genus *Euphorbia* Linn (2012–2021). *J. Ethnopharmacol.* **2022**, *298*, 115574. [CrossRef] [PubMed]
6. Bajpai, V.K.; Sonwal, S.; Hwang, S.-K.; Shukla, S.; Khan, I.; Dey, D.K.; Chen, L.; Simal-Gandara, J.; Xiao, J.; Huh, Y.S.; et al. Sugiol, a diterpenoid: Therapeutic actions and molecular pathways involved. *Pharmacol. Res.* **2021**, *163*, 105313. [CrossRef] [PubMed]
7. Ngo, T.C.; Dao, D.Q.; Mai, T.V.T.; Nguyen, T.L.A.; Huynh, L.K. On the radical scavenging and DNA repairing activities by natural oxygenated diterpenoids: Theoretical insights. *J. Chem. Inf. Model.* **2022**, *62*, 2365–2377. [CrossRef] [PubMed]
8. Lin, F.-M.; Tsai, C.-H.; Yang, Y.-C.; Tu, W.-C.; Chen, L.-R.; Liang, Y.-S.; Wang, S.-Y.; Shyur, L.-F.; Chien, S.-C.; Cha, T.-L.; et al. A novel diterpene suppresses CWR22Rv1 tumor growth in vivo through antiproliferation and proapoptosis. *Cancer Res.* **2008**, *68*, 6634–6642. [CrossRef] [PubMed]
9. Chinese Pharmacopoeia Commission. *Pharmacopoeia of the People's Republic of China*; China Medical Science Press: Beijing, China, 2020; Volume 1, p. 298.
10. Shi, Q.-W.; Su, X.-H.; Kiyota, H. Chemical and pharmacological research of the plants in genus *Euphorbia*. *Chem. Rev.* **2008**, *108*, 4295–4327. [CrossRef] [PubMed]
11. Vasas, A.; Hohmann, J. Euphorbia diterpenes: Isolation, structure, biological activity, and synthesis (2008–2012). *Chem. Rev.* **2014**, *112*, 5967–6026. [CrossRef] [PubMed]
12. Yan, X.-L.; Zhang, J.-S.; Huang, J.-L.; Zhang, Y.; Chen, J.-Q.; Tang, G.-H.; Yin, S. Euphonoids A−G, cytotoxic diterpenoids from *Euphorbia fischeriana*. *Phytochemistry* **2019**, *166*, 112064. [CrossRef] [PubMed]
13. Morgenstern, T.; Bittner, M.; Silva, M.; Aqueveque, P.; Jakupovic, J. Diterpenes and phloracetophenones from *Euphorbia portulacoides*. *Phytochemistry* **1996**, *41*, 1149–1153. [CrossRef]
14. Uemura, D.; Hirata, Y. Two new diterpenoids, jolkinolides A and B, obtained from *Euphorbia jolkini* boiss. (Euphorbiaceae). *Tetrahedron Lett.* **1972**, *13*, 1387–1390. [CrossRef]
15. Liu, G.-L.; Xu, W.; Liu, X.-J.; Yan, X.-L.; Chen, J. Two new abietane diterpenoids from the leaves of *Rabdosia serra*. *J. Asian Nat. Prod. Res.* **2018**, *22*, 47–51. [CrossRef] [PubMed]
16. Jian, B.-Y.; Zhang, H.; Han, C.-C.; Liu, J.-C. Anti-cancer activities of diterpenoids derived from *Euphorbia fischeriana* Steud. *Molecules* **2018**, *23*, 387. [CrossRef] [PubMed]
17. Rosaria, A.; Giuseppe, A.M.; Monica, R.L.; Xiao, J.-B.; Simone, B.; Rosa, T. Advances on natural abietane, labdane and clerodane diterpenes as anti-cancer agents: Sources and mechanisms of action. *Molecules* **2022**, *27*, 4791.
18. Yan, X.-L.; Zou, M.-F.; Chen, B.-L.; Yuan, F.-Y.; Zhu, Q.-F.; Zhang, X.; Lin, Y.; Long, Q.-D.; Liu, W.-L.; Liao, S.-G. Euphorane C, an unusual C17-norabietane diterpenoid from *Euphorbia dracunculoides* induces cell cycle arrest and apoptosis in human leukemia K562 cells. *Arab. J. Chem.* **2022**, *15*, 104203. [CrossRef]
19. Sang, J.; Li, W.; Diao, H.-J.; Fan, R.-Z.; Huang, J.-L.; Gan, L.; Zou, M.-F.; Tang, G.-H.; Yin, S. Jolkinolide B targets thioredoxin and glutathione systems to induce ROS-mediated paraptosis and apoptosis in bladder cancer cells. *Cancer Lett.* **2021**, *509*, 13–25. [CrossRef] [PubMed]
20. Sang, J.; Gan, L.; Zou, M.-F.; Lin, Z.-J.; Fan, R.-Z.; Huang, J.-L.; Li, W.; Tang, G.-H.; Yin, S. Jolkinolide B sensitizes bladder cancer to mTOR inhibitors via dual inhibition of Akt signaling and autophagy. *Cancer Lett.* **2022**, *526*, 352–362. [CrossRef] [PubMed]
21. Wang, Y.; Ma, X.-Q.; Yan, S.-S.; Shen, S.-S.; Zhu, H.-L.; Gu, Y.; Wang, H.-B.; Qin, G.-W.; Yu, Q. 17-hydroxy-jolkinolide B inhibits signal transducers and activators of transcription 3 signaling by covalently cross-linking Janus kinases and induces apoptosis of human cancer cells. *Cancer Res.* **2009**, *69*, 7302–7310. [CrossRef] [PubMed]

molecules

MDPI

Article

Lactucin, a Bitter Sesquiterpene from *Cichorium intybus*, Inhibits Cancer Cell Proliferation by Downregulating the MAPK and Central Carbon Metabolism Pathway

Khandaker Md Sharif Uddin Imam [1], Yu Tian [2], Fengjiao Xin [1], Yingying Xie [1] and Boting Wen [1,*]

1 Laboratory of Biomanufacturing and Food Engineering, Institute of Food Science and Technology, Chinese Academy of Agricultural Sciences, Beijing 100193, China
2 Institute of Medicinal Plant Development, Chinese Academy of Medical Sciences & Peking Union Medical College, Beijing 100193, China
* Correspondence: wenboting@caas.cn; Tel.: +1-511-009-2600

Abstract: Lung cancer, especially adenocarcinoma, is the second most occurring and highest fatality-causing cancer worldwide. Many natural anticancer compounds, such as sesquiterpene lactones (SLs), show promising anticancer properties. Herein, we examined Lactucin, an SL from the plant *Cichorium intybus*, for its cytotoxicity, apoptotic-inducing, cell cycle inhibiting capacity, and associated protein expression. We also constructed a biotinylated Lactucin probe to isolate interacting proteins and identified them. We found that Lactucin stops the proliferation of A549 and H2347 lung adenocarcinoma cell lines while not affecting normal lung cell MRC5. It also significantly inhibits the cell cycle at G_0/G_1 stage and induces apoptosis. The western blot analysis shows that Lactucin downregulates the MAPK pathway, cyclin, and cyclin-dependent kinases, inhibiting DNA repair while upregulating p53, p21, Bax, PTEN, and downregulation of Bcl-2. An increased p53 in response to DNA damage upregulates p21, Bax, and PTEN. In an activity-based protein profiling (ABPP) analysis of A549 cell's protein lysate using a biotinylated Lactucin probe, we found that Lactucin binds PGM, PKM, and LDHA PDH, four critical enzymes in central carbon metabolism in cancer cells, limiting cancer cells in its growth; thus, Lactucin inhibits cancer cell proliferation by downregulating the MAPK and the Central Carbon Metabolism pathway.

Keywords: lung cancer; adenocarcinoma; NSCLC; apoptosis; cell cycle; ABPP

Citation: Imam, K.M.S.U.; Tian, Y.; Xin, F.; Xie, Y.; Wen, B. Lactucin, a Bitter Sesquiterpene from *Cichorium intybus*, Inhibits Cancer Cell Proliferation by Downregulating the MAPK and Central Carbon Metabolism Pathway. *Molecules* **2022**, 27, 7358. https://doi.org/10.3390/molecules27217358

Academic Editors: Barbara De Filippis, Alessandra Ammazzalorso and Marialuigia Fantacuzzi

Received: 27 September 2022
Accepted: 25 October 2022
Published: 29 October 2022

1. Introduction

Lung cancers are the second most occurring cancers and the primary cause of cancer-related death among both men and women worldwide [1]. In 2018, out of 9.6 million cancer-related deaths, 1.76 million were caused by lung cancers [2]. Non-Small Cell Lung Cancer (NSCLC) accounts for 85% of all lung cancers [3], and adenocarcinoma is the principal subtype makeup for 75–85% of lung cancer and related deaths [4].

Rapid metastasis of lung adenocarcinomata [5] are primarily responsible for their late diagnosis, significantly affecting patient survival [6]. Common causes of lung cancers include smoking, air pollution, occupational exposure, and genetics [6]. However, diet also plays a crucial chemoprophylactic role in lung cancers [7–9]. It is more evident from the increasing number of novel anticancer compounds discovered in common foods and drinks [10]. Besides rapid metastasis, the aggressive chemotherapeutic regimen often associated with late-stage lung cancer treatment also contributes to poor patient survival [11]. Natural products used as adjuvant therapy have promoted patient survival and quality of life [12,13]. These have created a demand for natural chemopreventive, chemoprotective, and adjuvant compounds in cancer treatment [3,12–14].

Natural products are an abundant source of novel therapeutics [14]. More than 67% of novel anticancer and antitumor drugs are natural compounds or their analog [14,15], and more than 200 compounds and derivatives are at different stages of drug development and trials [15]. Chicory (*Cichorium intybus* L.) is a widely distributed plant used as medicine, food, drink, and fodder [16]. It has been the subject of many pharmacological studies [16]. Recently, we reviewed the cytotoxic of Chicory [16], where 31 out of 87 *C. intybus* metabolites possess anticancer, antitumor, and related bioactivities. Lactucin is a phytometabolite from Chicory, phytochemically categorized as bitter Sesquiterpene Lactones (SLs). SLs have been a subject of interest in cancer research for decades, and many have reached clinical trials [15]. As indicated in Ghantous, Gali-Muhtasib, Vuorela, Saliba, and Darwiche [15] reviews, SLs bioactivity is strictly linked to three conserved structural features, e.g., (i) alkylating center reactivity, (ii) side chain and lipophilicity, and (iii) molecular geometry and electronic features. Since many of the structural features that lactucin shares with other SLs have shown antitumor bioactivity against NSCLC [15], Lactucin will likely possess these properties.

Some plants of the Asteraceae family commonly synthesize Lactucin. It is one of the ingredients of lactucarium, a milky white liquid secreted by several lettuce species, e.g., *Lactuca serriola, L. saligna, L. viminea, L. glareosa, L. sativa*, [17–19], etc. In 1970 Chicory root water extract was reported as a light-sensitive, highly potent antimalarial compound. Later Bischoff et al. [20] attributed it to Lactucin, making Chicory the most famous source of Lactucin. Besides antimalarial properties, Lactucin also exerts or potentially exerts anti-inflammatory [21], sedatives [17], anti-adipogenic [22], and anthelmintics [23] effects. Zhang et al. [24] reported Lactucin induces apoptosis and sub-G_1 cell cycle arrest in HL-60 (human leukemia cancer) cells. Ren et al. [25] reported similar effect on KB (human epidermoid carcinoma; IC_{50} = 75 μM), and Bel 7402 (human hepatocellular carcinoma; IC_{50} = 55 μM) cells. Apart from these reports, the anticancer effect of Lactucin, especially on lung cancer, remains largely unexplored. A structural activity study (SAR) by Ren, et al. [25] revealed the importance of an ester group (γ-butyrolactone) and one exocyclic methylene group for the antitumor activity of Lactucin-like Guanolides. Wang, et al. [22] reported that Lactucin inhibits adipogenesis by downregulating the JAK2/STAT3 signaling pathway and subsequent clonal expansion. However, the cellular target protein of Lactucin and the affected pathway in antitumor activity is still unknown. Herein, we evaluated the anticancer potency of Lactucin using A549 and H2347 lung adenocarcinoma cell lines in vitro to identify interacting proteins and underlying molecular mechanisms.

2. Results

2.1. Lactucin Inhibits Lung Adenocarcinoma Cells Proliferation

The effect of incrementing concentrations of Lactucin on normal lung cells and lung adenocarcinoma cells upon 24 h exposures was evaluated by 3-(4,5-dimethylthiazol-2-yl)-2,5-diphenyltetrazolium bromide (MTT) assay. Compared to respective control groups, higher Lactucin doses significantly inhibit A549 (IC_{50} = 79.87 μM) and H2347 (IC_{50} = 68.85 μM) lung adenocarcinoma cells' proliferation in a dose-dependent manner while not affecting MRC-5 cells' proliferation, Figure 1A. However, at different exposure periods (12, 24, and 28 h), Lactucin showed significant inhibitory activity on A549 cell proliferation at 24 h and 48 h exposures at higher doses only, Figure 1B. Given that Lactucin can significantly inhibit lung adenocarcinoma cell proliferation at 24 h, exposure at a higher amount without affecting normal lung cells, we used respective IC_{50} concentrations of Lactucin for treating A549 and H2347 cells in further cytological experiments. A549 and H2347 cells treated with incrementing doses of Lactucin for 24 h showed a significant dose-dependent increase in the expression of LC3-II (17 kDa) in H2347 cells; and LC3-I (19 kDa) in A549 and H2347 cells, Figure 1C,D.

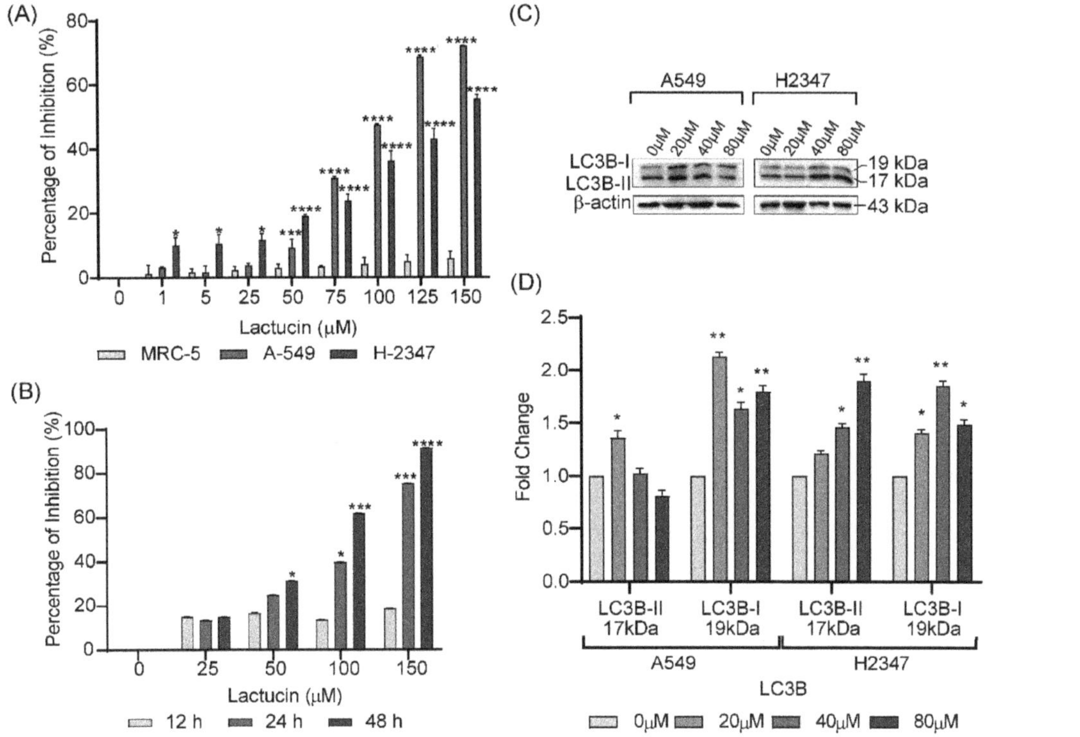

Figure 1. Lactucin significantly inhibits the proliferation of A549 and H2347 lung adenocarcinoma, while it doesn't inhibit MRC-5 normal lung cell growth in a dose (**A**) and time (**B**) dependent manner. Lactucin significantly induces dose-dependent expression of LC3-II in H2347 cells (**C**,**D**), detected by WB analysis. Here * $p < 0.05$, ** $p < 0.01$, *** $p < 0.001$, and **** $p < 0.0001$ indicate significantly different from control.

2.2. Effects of Lactucin on Cell Cycle Progression in Lung Adenocarcinoma Cells

Since Lactucin inhibited lung cancer cell proliferation, its cell cycle inhibitory property and related markers were analyzed. Cytometric analysis of DNA Content of 24 h lactucin treated (with respective IC_{50} concentrations) lung adenocarcinoma cells A549 and H2347 were performed. It revealed that Lactucin inhibits the cell cycle at the G_0/G_1 phase, Figure 2A. It was further supported by the western blot (WB) analysis of Lactucin-treated (24 h) adenocarcinoma (A549 and H2347) cell's protein, Figure 2B. Both cyclins (cyclin B1 and cyclin D1) and cyclin-dependent protein kinases (CDKs) (CDK2 and CDK4), which regulate the cell cycle through mutual interactions, were dose-dependently downregulated, Figure 2C,D. However, p21 and p53, the two CDKs inhibitors we tested, were dose-dependently upregulated. This result suggests Lactucin inhibits the cell cycle of lung adenocarcinoma cells at the G_0/G_1 phase by upregulating CDKs inhibitor p21 and p53, downregulating cyclins and CDKs expression.

2.3. Effects of Lactucin on Apoptosis in Lung Adenocarcinoma Cells

The apoptosis-inducing capacity of Lactucin was measured by flow cytometry analysis of treated A549 and H2347 cells. As shown in Figure 3A, after 24 h incubation with respective IC_{50} concentrations of Lactucin, A549 cell's apoptosis increased from 1.93% to 13.42%, and H2347 cell's apoptosis rose from 1.42% to 40.70%. We also observed significant induction of early apoptosis in A549 (from 3.86% to 18.35%) and H2347 (6.07% to 17.36%)

cells, Figure 3A. Apoptosis-related indicators such as Bax, Bcl-2 expression; and Caspase-3, and PARP activation, were also compared through WB, Figure 3B. We observed that Lactucin induced a dose-dependent increase in the concentration of both peptides of cleaved Caspase-3, Figure 3C, cleavage of PARP, expression of Bax, and inhibited the expression of Bcl-2, Figure 3D. The upregulation of Bax, downregulation of Bcl-2, and cleavage induction of Caspase-3 and PARP indicate that Lactucin has apoptosis-inducing properties.

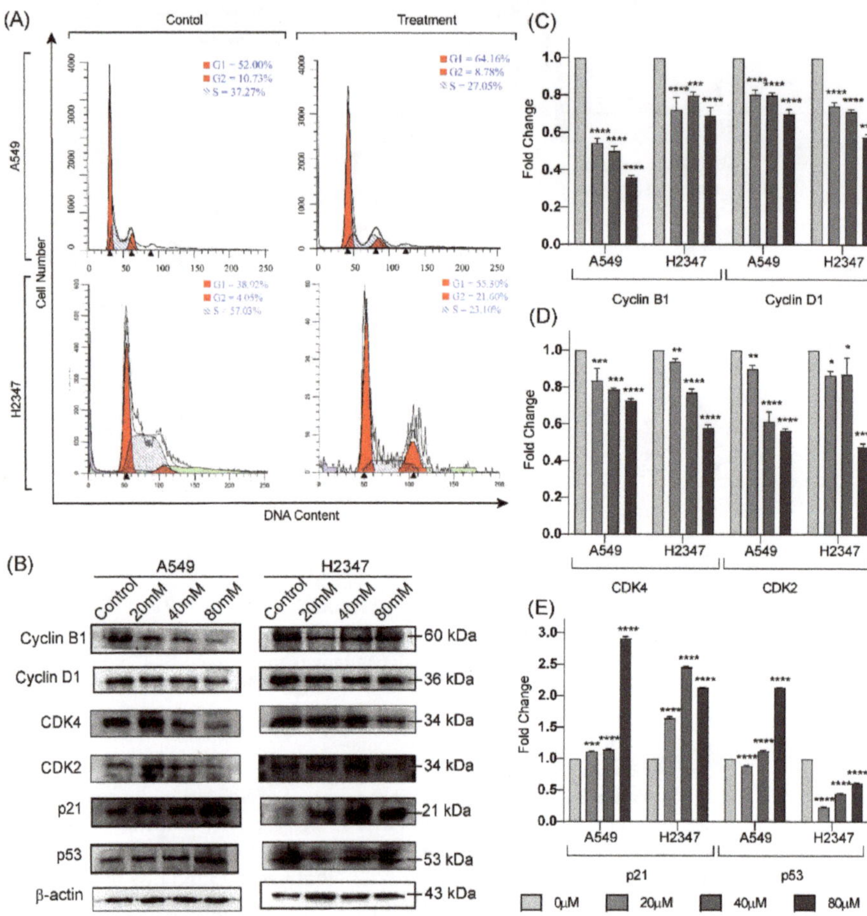

Figure 2. Lactucin and equivalent volume of vehicle (DMSO) exposure (24 h) induced cell cycle inhibition of lung adenocarcinoma A549 (80 μM), and H2347 (70 μM) cells (**A**) were measured by flow cytometry. WB analysis of cyclin B1, cyclin D1, CDK2, CDK4, p21, and p27 protein expression in A549 and H2347 cells after exposure to Lactucin at 0, 20, 40, and 80 μM for 24 h (**B**). Lactucin significantly downregulates Cyclin B1 and Cyclin D1 (**C**), CDK4, and CDK2 (**D**) and downregulates the p21 and p53 (**E**) expression in both A549 and H2347 cells in a dose-dependent manner. Data are expressed as the means ± standard deviation of triplicate experiments. * $p < 0.05$, ** $p < 0.01$, *** $p < 0.001$, and **** $p < 0.0001$ were considered significant.

2.4. Lactucin Affects the MAPK Signaling Pathway by Downregulating MEK, ERK Phosphorylation

Effects of Lactucin on metabolic markers of lung cancer cells were observed through WB, Figure 4A. Protein lysate from 24 h 80 μM Lactucin-treated A549 cells showed a different level of expression of metabolic markers, Figure 4B. Lactucin dose-dependently increased the expression of PTEN, a tumor suppressor protein that negatively regulates the activation of Akt to p-Akt, Figure 4 [26]. Dose-dependent MEK 1/2 and ERK activation inhibition indicate that Lactucin inhibits A549 cell proliferation by downregulating the MAPK/ERK pathway. We used a biotinylated Lactucin probe to confirm this and isolated Lactucin interaction proteins from A549 cells.

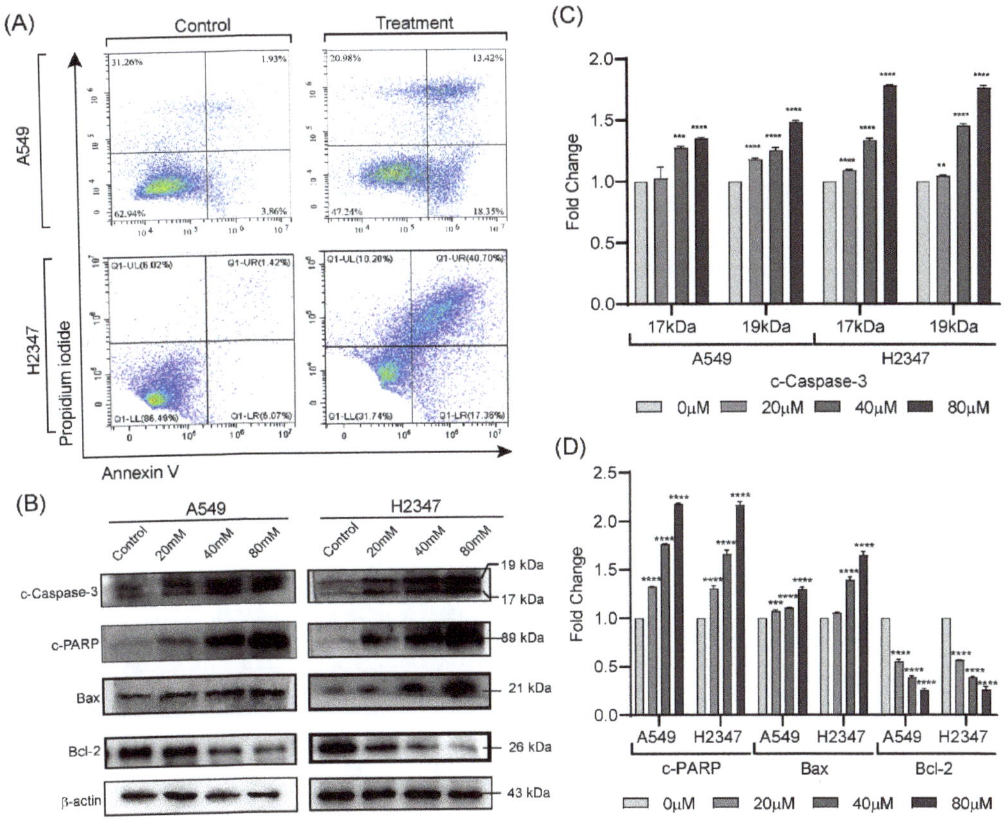

Figure 3. Effect of Lactucin on apoptosis induction of lung cancer cells. Lactucin and equivalent volume of the vehicle (DMSO) exposure (24 h) induced apoptosis of lung adenocarcinoma A549 (80 μM) and H2347 (70 μM) cells (**A**) were measured by flow cytometry. WB analysis of c-Caspase-3, c-PARP, Bax, and Bcl-2 protein expression was performed after A549 and H2347 cells were exposure to Lactucin at 0, 20, 40, and 80 μM for 24 h (**B–D**). Data are expressed as the means ± standard deviation of triplicate experiments. ** $p < 0.01$, *** $p < 0.001$, and **** $p < 0.0001$ indicate result's significant difference from the control.

2.5. Lactucin Inhibits A549 Cell Proliferation by Downregulating MAPK/ERK and Central Carbon Metabolism Pathways

Natural Lactucin was conjugated with Propargylamine through Michael's addition reaction. Structure of resulting Lactucin-Propargylamine conjugate [(3aR,4S,9aS,9bR)-4-hydroxy-9-(hydroxymethyl)-6-methyl-3-((prop-2-yn-1-ylamino)methyl)-3,3a,4,5,9a,9b-hexahydroazuleno[4,5-b]furan-2,7-dione] was confirmed using ^{1}H Nuclear Magnetic Resonance (NMR), Figure 5A. The yield of the probe was estimated at 50% using High Performance Liquid Chromatography (HPLC). Cytotoxicity of the Lactucin probe and Propargylamine showed that the Lactucin probe exerts similar antiproliferation activity on A549 cells as natural Lactucin does both, doses dependent (Figure 5B) and time-dependent (Figure 5C) manners. In contrast, Propargylamine does not exert any significant bioactivity.

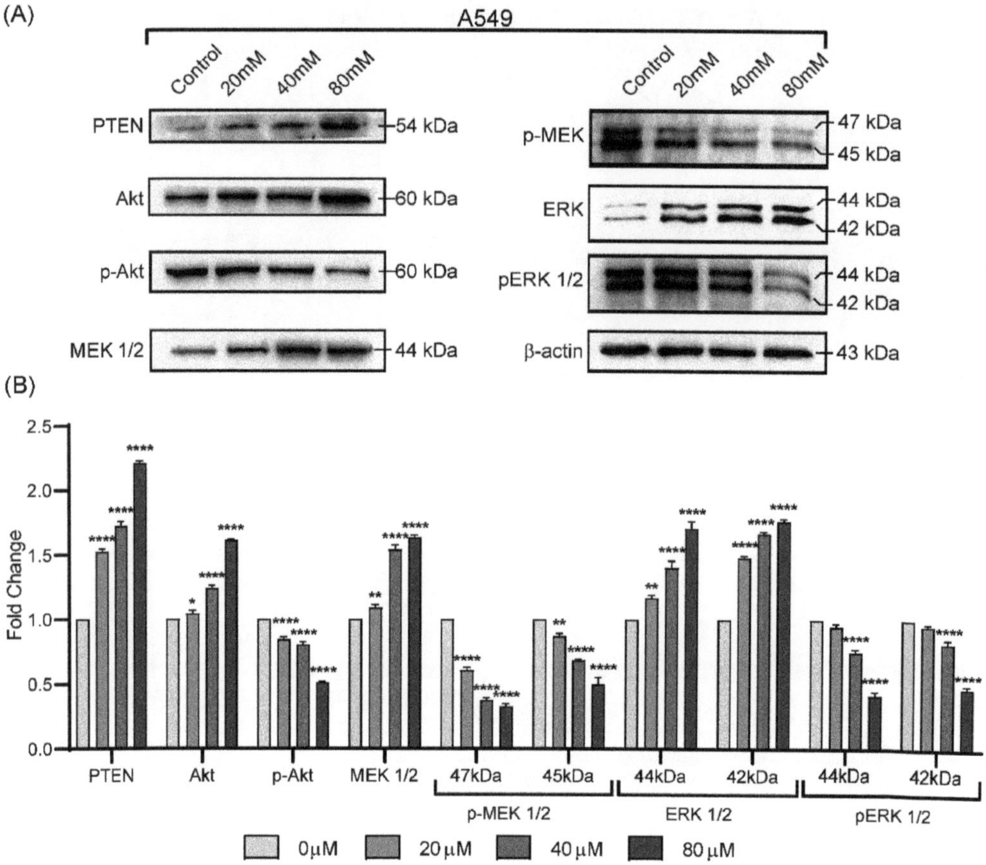

Figure 4. Lactucin inhibits A549 lung cancer cells by downregulating the MAPK/ERK pathway. (**A**) WB analysis of PTEN, Akt, p-Akt, MEK 1/2, p-MEK, ERK, and pERK 1/2 protein expression in A549 cell after exposure to Lactucin at 0, 20, 40, and 80 μM for 24 h. (**B**) Data are expressed as the means ± standard deviation of triplicate experiments. * $p < 0.05$, ** $p < 0.01$, and **** $p < 0.0001$ indicate result's significant difference from the control.

During the Activity-Based Protein Profiling (ABPP) assay, after Co-Immunoprecipitation (Co-IP), isolated protein lysate resolved on the Sodium Dodecyl Sulfate-Polyacrylamide Gel Electrophoresis (SDS-PAGE) showed five distinct bands in the treatment column after coomassie blue staining (Figure 6B). After testing these five bands using Liquid Chromatography with tandem Mass Spectrometry (LC-MS/MS) and analyzing them using MASCOT against 2019 human proteins. Many probable matches were found. Functional annotation clustering of LC-MS/MS results with the metabolic markers (upregulated and downregulated) data using DAVID Bioinformatics resources showed Lactucin interacts with several key enzymes of the "Central carbon metabolism in cancer" pathway (Kyoto Encyclopedia of Genes and Genomes, KEGG). These interacting proteins were identified as L01 = Phosphoglycerate mutase 1/2/4 (PGM, 70 kDa), L02 = Pyruvate kinase M1/2 (PKM, 58 kDa), L03 = Pyruvate dehydrogenase E1 subunit alpha 1/2 (PDH, 43 kDa), L04 = Lactate dehydrogenase A (LDHA, 37 kDa), but L05 was not identified. At the beginning of this manuscript, we defined cancer and tumor as proliferation disorders. However, they often show increased glucose and glutamine consumption, lactate secretion rate, glycolysis rate, and modified use of metabolic enzyme isoforms [27]. KEGG "Central carbon metabolism in cancer" pathway (Supplementary Material Figure S1 and Figure 6C) shows the difference in carbon metabolism between normal and malignant cells. Lactucin binding to PGM and PKM lower pyruvate synthesis, which binds to LDHA to lower Lactucin synthesis. Lactucin also binds to PDH, limiting the availability of Acetyl CoA entering the Tricarboxylic Acid (TCA) cycle and ultimately reducing lactate production, a hallmark of a metastasized tumor. Reducing PGM, PKM, and LDHA overexpression is attributed to the upregulation of p53 in response to DNA damage. From the KEGG pathway for NSCLC (Supplementary Material Figure S2 and Figure 6C), we see several oncogenes, such as p53, p21, and Bax, were upregulated; Cyclin D1, Akt, MEK, ERK, and CDK4 were downregulated.

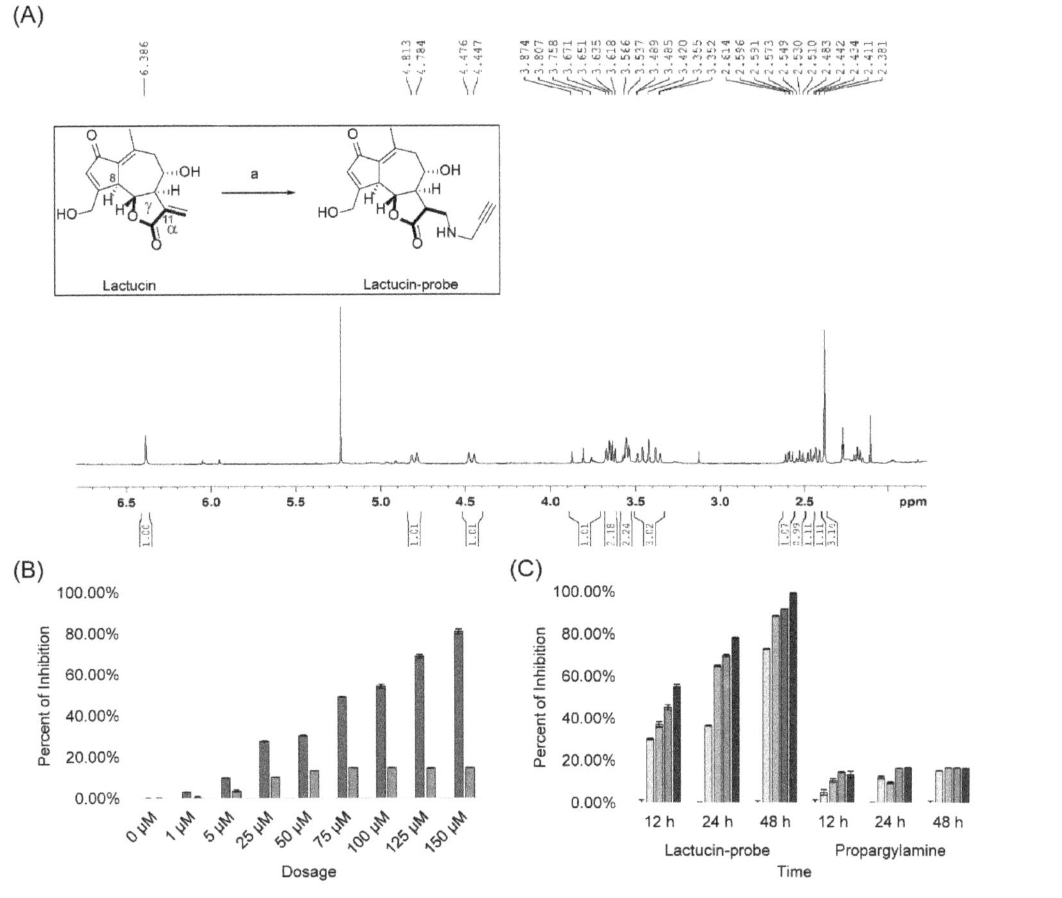

Figure 5. The structure of Lactucin-Propargylamine conjugate was confirmed using 1H NMR (**A**). Inset showing schematics of synthesis of Lactucin probe where reagents and conditions for synthesis were (a) propargylamine, pyridine, 0 °C, 36 h. Upon cytotoxicity evaluation on A549 cells, the Lactucin probe showed similar bioactivity as natural Lactucin compared to Propargylamine in incremental dose (**B**) and progressive dosing time (**C**) experiments.

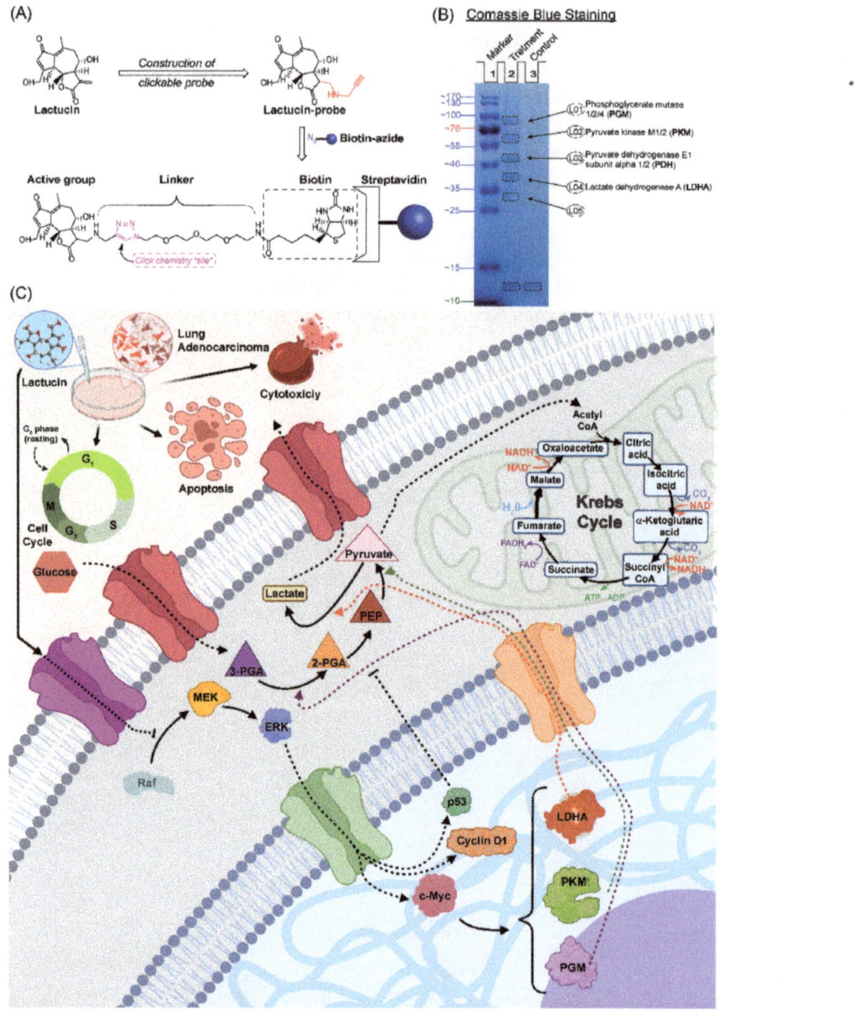

Figure 6. Lactucin downregulates Raf-MEK-ERK by inhibiting upstream trans-membrane peptides. Biotinylated Lactucin probes bound to targeted proteins are immobilized to streptavidin agarose through biotin, azide, and a linker molecule (**A**). Visualizing SDS resolved A549 protein lysate showed biotinylated Lactucin probe binds five peptides (**B**). Lactucin downregulates A549 lung adenocarcinoma cells Raf-MEK-ERK pathway and Central Carbon Metabolism in Cancer cells (**C**).

3. Discussion

In the present experiment, we observed that Lactucin has significant antiproliferative, G_0/G_1 cell cycle arrest, and apoptosis-inducing properties on A549 and H2347 lung adenocarcinoma, not on MRC-5 normal lung cells. Firstly, Lactucin-induced time and dose-dependent inhibition of A549 and H2347 cells were observed, and then their IC_{50} values were determined to be 79.87 μM and 68.85 μM, respectively. According to WHO [28], for L-6 (rat skeletal myoblast) cells, compounds with an IC_{50} above 90 μM are not cytotoxic, IC_{50} between 2–80 μM is moderately cytotoxic, and IC_{50} below 2 μM is cytotoxic. For natural compounds, Ren, et al. [25] described an IC_{50} below 100 μM to be cytotoxic and reported Lactucin inhibits KB and Bel 7402 cells with an IC_{50} value of 75 μM and 55 μM, respectively. Lima, et al. [29] considered IC_{50} of <40 μg/mL and <4 μg/mL for plant extract and pure compounds respectively to be cytotoxic. According to American National Cancer Institute (NCI), except for fibroblast, an IC_{50} of ≤30 μg/mL of plant extract is cytotoxic, but they did not specify pure natural compounds. IC_{50} values we observed in adenocarcinomas can thus be considered cytotoxic. The LC3-II and LC3-II/LC3-I ratio increase is a classic sign of autophagy [30]. However, this is not always the case due to the lower sensitivity of LC3-I than LC3-II in WB and the higher degradation rate of LC3-II in the presence of lysosomal protease inhibitor [30,31]. We observed a dose-dependent increase of LC3-II in H2347 and LC3-I in A549 and H2347 cells. It was probably due to the concomitant increase in LC3 production and LC3I to LC3II conversion, rapid degradation of LC3-II, or lower detection of LC3-I in WB. In conclusion, LC3 WB results didn't sufficiently indicate that Lactucin directly induces autophagy. LC3-I and LC3-II increase was probably due to autophagosome increase by some other means [30].

We found Lactucin induces G_0/G_1 cell cycle arrests from cell cycle analysis. Specific cell cycle-related proteins, such as cyclins and CDKs, positively upregulate the cell cycle, whereas CDKs inhibitors stop the Cyclins and CDKs unit assembly [32]. In this experiment, we observed the downregulation of Cyclin B1, Cyclin D1, CDK2, and CDK4, and the upregulation of p21 and p53. Downregulation of Cyclin D1 and upregulation of p53 were associated with G_0/G_1 cell cycle arrest and apoptosis [32], which coincides with our findings. Lactucin-induced inhibition of cell proliferation was also reported by Zhang, et al. [24] in human HL-60 leukemia cancer cells and by Wang, et al. [22] in mouse 3T3-L1 fibroblast cells. Though in 3T3-L1 G_0/G_1 cell cycle arrest was reported, [22] in HL-60 cells, Sub-G_1 cell cycle arrest was reported [24].

We also observed an increase in early and late apoptosis in A549 and H2347 cells induced by Lactucin. Lactucin induces apoptosis by upregulating the expression of mitochondrial apoptosis-related proteins, such as c-Caspase, c-PARP, and Bax, while downregulating the expression of Bcl-2. Zhang, et al. [24] reported Lactucin induces apoptosis in HL-60 cells by swelling up mitochondria and endoplasmic reticulum (ER) on the transition electron microscope (TEM). Jang, et al. [33] reported that Lactucin induces ROS-mediated apoptosis in human renal cancer cell Caki-1 by downregulating Bcl-2 expression and CFLARL stability where Bcl-2 downregulation was at a transcriptional level caused by inactivation of the NF-κB pathway. However, we observed concurrent upregulation of PTEN and downregulation of Akt, MEK, and ERK phosphorylation narrowed down the Lactucin-influenced NSCLC pathway to PI3K/Akt and MAPK/ERK. McCubrey, et al. [34] suggested that ERK can activate the NF-κB transcription factor (nuclear factor immunoglobulin κ chain enhancer-B cell) by phosphorylating and activating inhibitor κB kinase (IKK) through an indirect mechanism. We also performed an ABPP assay on A549 protein lysate using a Lactucin-Propargylamine probe. Structural activity relationship (SAR) studies by Ren, et al. [25] revealed that in SL, the position 8 ester group (γ-butyrolactone) and the methylene group at exocyclic position 11 (α), play a significant role in antitumor activities of Lactucin-like guaianolides (Figure 5A) [16]. α methylene γ lactone, the' enone' or unsaturated carbonyl system (O=C–C=CH_2) was also reported to increase the toxicity towards tumor cells [15]. While synthesizing the Lactucin-Propargylamine probe, we avoided the 8-ester group and 11 methylene group positions mentioned earlier. However, adding the alkynyl group to 11 (α), exocyclic methylene didn't hinder its cytotoxicity against A549 cells (Figure 5B,C). It also suggests that Lactucin may simultaneously exert its activity through different groups. Proteins isolated using this probe were analyzed in LC-MS/MS and combined with WB results for functional enrichment. In the DAVID functional enrichment of western blot and ABPP peptides, four were identified as key enzymes in central carbon metabolism in the cancer cell (Figure 6C). Overexpressed and modified central carbon metabolism enzymes are essential to support the exponential growth of the metastasized tumor. Regulating their expression will limit the available energy and thus control or seize tumor growth.

In anticancer therapy, oncogenes and tumor suppressors are two likely targets for inhibiting cancer cells [26]. From the KEGG pathway of NSCLEC by Kanehisa Laboratories, we know that in the case of NSCLC like A549 or H2347, we know the potential oncogene and tumor suppressors targets. DAVID enrichment results showed that in the NSCLC, Lactucin downregulates MEK-ERK pathway, resulting in the downregulation of CyclinD1, CDKs, and upregulation of the p53. p53, in turn, upregulates p21 and Bax. It doesn't show interaction with any of the upstream components of NSCLC. When DAVID enrichment for the KEGG pathway "Central Carbon Metabolism in Cancer" was plotted, it showed four Lactucin interacting enzymes besides the western blot findings. Downregulation of MAPK/ERK observed in Figure 6C also lowers the expression of c-Myc, a proto-oncogene involved in cell cycle progression, apoptosis, and cellular transformation. Low c-Myc inhibits uncontrolled DNA synthesis associated with cancer and thus lowers the expression of PGM, PKM, and LDHA, and eventually downregulates carbon consumption needed to sustain malignancy. Lactucin also binds to PDH, reducing its concentration, and decreasing Pyruvate to Acetyl CoA conversion, thus downregulating the TCA cycle and lactate production. Thus, Lactucin inhibits cell proliferation and simultaneously increases cell cycle arrest in lung adenocarcinoma by reducing the MAPK/ERK and lowering carbon metabolism-related enzyme availability.

4. Materials and Methods

Firstly, we tested the Lactucin for its cytotoxicity, cell cycle inhibiting, and apoptosis-inducing properties on lung adenocarcinoma cell lines. Then, its effect on cell cycle, apoptosis, and other related protein expression, was evaluated by WB analysis. Finally, we constructed a biotinylated Lactucin probe to extract Lactucin-interacting proteins, identified them using LC-MS/MS, and elucidated the molecular mechanisms.

4.1. Cell Materials

In the present study, we observed the effect of Lactucin (Shanghai Yuanye Biological Technology Co., Ltd., Shanghai, China) on two lung adenocarcinoma cell lines, namely, A549 (Cell Bank of Shanghai Institutes for Biological Sciences, Chinese Academy of Sciences, Shanghai, China), and H2347 (Chinese Academy of Medical Sciences and Peking Union Medical College, Beijing, China), as well as one normal lung cell line MRC-5 (National Infrastructure of Cell Line Resource, Beijing, China).

4.2. Cell Culture

Frozen (liquid-vapor) cell lines were cultured in complete growth media [A549 and H2347 cells in Roswell Park Memorial Institute 1640 (RPMI-1640) with 10% Fetal Bovine Serum (FBS) (Biological Industries, Kibbutz Beit Haemek, Israel) and 1% Penicillin/Streptomycin (Caisson Laboratories, Smithfield, VA, USA); MRC-5 in Minimum Essential Medium (MEM HyClone, Chicago, IL, USA), with 10% FBS, 1% Penicillin/Streptomycin, and 1% Nonessential Amino acids (10 mM 100×, Solarbio Biotechnology, Beijing, China) (EMEM)] [26]. For freezing A549, H2347, and MRC-5 cell line, 10% Dimethyl sulfoxide (DMSO, MP Biomedicals, Shanghai, China) in FBS, RPMI-1640, and MEM complete growth medium, respectively, was used. Adherent cells were detached using 1–3 mL of 0.25% Trypsin EDTA (Gibco, Thermo Fisher Scientific, Waltham, MA, USA) for 2–4 min at room temperature (RT).

4.3. Cell Viability Assay

Subconfluent cells (<90%) were aseptically trypsinized and diluted to 5×10^4 cell/mL using complete growth media RPMI-1640 (for A549 and H2347) or EMEM (for MRC-5). Cells were then seeded aseptically in 96 welled plates at 1×10^4 cells/well (200 μL/well) and incubated for 12 h at 37 °C in a 5% CO_2 incubator before dosing. After 12 h, we exposed the cells to different concentrations of Lactucin for 24 h. All Lactucin concentrations were prepared using complete growth media and contained equal vehicle volume DMSO

(v/v). Cell viability was determined using a MTT cell proliferation kit (M1020, Solarbio Biotechnology, Beijing, China) following the manufacturer's instructions. UV absorbance was scanned at 490 nm using a Spark microtitration plate reader (Tecan, Männedorf, Switzerland). Each experiment was repeated three times, the viability of the control group was set to 100%, and cell viability and IC_{50} values were calculated.

4.4. DNA Content/Cell Cycle Assay

Subconfluent A549 and H2347 cells (<90%) were cultured at 1×10^5 cell/mL concentration using complete growth media RPMI-1640 for 12 h at 37 °C in 5% CO_2. Cells were then treated with respective IC_{50} Lactucin solution or equivalent volume DMSO (v/v) solution and incubated for 24 h. After treatment, cells were trypsinized, washed, and fixed for 24 h. Fixed cells were washed and stained using a Propidium Iodide (PI) Flow Cytometry kit (Abcam, Cambridge, UK) following manufacturer instructions. The DNA contents were scanned using a flow cytometer (CytoFLEX, Beckman Coulter Inc., Miami, FL, USA).

4.5. Apoptosis Assay

Subconfluent A549 and H2347 cells (<90%) were cultured at 1×10^5 cell/mL concentration using complete growth media RPMI-1640 for 12 h at 37 °C in 5% CO_2. Cells were then treated with respective IC_{50} Lactucin solution or equivalent volume DMSO (v/v) solution and incubated for 24 h. After treatment, cells were trypsinized and washed. Following manufacturer instructions, cells were double-stained using the FITC Annexin V Apoptotic kit (BD Pharmingen, San Diego, CA, USA). Samples were filtered (70 μM Nylon cell strainer, Falcon, Corning, Durham, NC, USA) and scanned using a flow cytometer.

4.6. Protein Extraction

5×10^6 cell/mL untreated [A549 for Co-IP] and treated (Lactucin and DMSO in A549 and H2347 for WB) cells were washed (1× PBS chilled), scraped (cell scraper, Corning, Durham, NC, USA), collected in 1.5 mL centrifuge tubes, and then washed again twice (1× PBS chilled). Between each washing, cells were centrifuged at 600× g for 5 min at 4 °C. After the final centrifuge, 300–500 μL of chilled modified RIPA buffer (1% PMSF + 1% SDS in RIPA) was added to each tube, briefly vortexed and then homogenized using probe sonicator at 30% power of 3 × 5 s with a 10 s gap in between. Homogenized cells were then left to chill on ice for 1 h. After 1 h, cells were centrifuged at 14000× g at 4 °C for 10 min, and intact cells and nuclear materials were separated by pipetting the supernatant into new centrifuge tubes and stored at −20 °C. The protein concentrations were determined using the Bicinchoninic Acid (BCA) protein assay kit (Solarbio Biotechnology, Beijing, China) following manufacturer instructions. UV absorbance was scanned at 562 nm using a microtitration plate reader.

4.7. Western Blot Assay

Western blot was performed using the method adopted from Lu. et al. [26]. A549 and H2347 cells protein (10 μg/lane) along with a pre-stained page ruler (5 μg/lane) were resolved using 8, 10, and 12% SDS-PAGE, along with pre-stained protein ladder (#26617; Thermo Fisher Scientific, Carlsbad, CA, USA) and transferred to polyvinylidene fluoride (PVDF) transfer membrane (Immobilon®-P, Billerica, MA, USA) by wet transfer at 350 mA for 70–110 min (depending on targeted proteins molecular weight). PVDF membranes were washed thrice using Tris-buffered saline with 0.1% Tween® 20 Detergent (TBST) (10 min each) and blocked using 5% Bovine Serum Albumin (BSA) in TBST (10 mM Tris-HCl, 150 mM NaCl, 0.1% tween 20) at room temperature (RT) for 1 h. The PVDF was then washed thrice using TBST (10 min each), cut, and probed using primary antibodies at 4 °C overnight. The primary antibodies include anti-Akt (AA326), anti-Bax (AB026), anti-cleaved Caspase-3 (AC033), anti-CDK-4 (AC251-1), anti-Cyclin D1 (AC853-1), anti-p53 (AF0255), anti-ERK1/2 (AF1051), anti-MEK1/2 (AF1057), anti-cleaved-PARP-1 (AF1567), anti-mTOR (AF1648), anti-Ki67 (AF1738), anti-p-ERK (AF1891), anti-p-Akt1/2/3(Thr 308) (AF5734), anti-p21 (AP021-1), anti-PTEN (AP686) from Beyotime Biotechnology (Shanghai, China); anti-LC3B (NB100-2220) from Novus Biologicals (Littleton, CO, USA); anti-β-actin (SC47778), anti-Cdk-2 (SC6248), anti-Cyclin B1 (SC245), anti- p-MEK1/2 (SC81503), anti-Bcl-2 (SC7882) from Santa Cruz Biotechnology (Santa Cruz, CA, USA). Next, the PVDF was washed thrice using TBST (10 min each) and probed with appropriate goat anti-mouse (ab150113) or anti-rabbit (ab97051) secondary antibodies (Abcam, Cambridge, UK) for 1 h at RT. Finally, the PVDF was washed (thrice for 10 min each), exposed using luminol reagents (Millipore, Billerica, MA, USA), and photographed using the CLiNX Chemiluminescence imaging system (Shanghai, China).

4.8. Synthesis of Lactucin Probe

To synthesize the biotinylated Lactucin probe, Lactucin was conjugated with an alkynyl group through Michael's addition reaction, Figure 6A. To a solution of lactucin (5.0 mg, 0.018 mM) in dry pyridine (0.3 mL), Propargylamine (1.5 mg, 0.027 mM) (innochem, Beijing, China) was added and stirred at 0 °C for 36 h under N_2 air. The reaction was monitored by thin-layer chromatography (TLC). The solvent was concentrated and purified through column chromatography (Dichloromethane-CH_3OH, 15:1) and dried. For structural confirmation, the probe was analyzed using ^{1}H-NMR at 600 MHz (Oxford NMR AS600, Abingdon, UK) in deuterated DMSO (d-DMSO, Merck KGaA, Darmstadt, Germany), Figure 5A. The yield of the probe was estimated using HPLC.

4.9. Cytotoxicity Test and Protein Labelling by Lactucin Probe

Cytotoxicity of the Lactucin probe and Propargylamine was examined by incubating A549 cells with incriminating (0 to 150 μM) concentrations and incubation periods (12, 24, and 48 h) of each. The total A549 protein lysate was prepared using the method described in Section 4.6. The Lactucin binding proteins were labeled and pulled out using a biotinylated Lactucin probe following the ABPP method adopted from the method described by Speers and Cravatt [35]. Two 400 μL of protein lysate (2 mg/mL in PBS) were aliquoted into a 1.5mL microcentrifuge tube, and Lactucin-probe or Propargylamine was added (final concentration 100 μM). Both tubes were incubated at RT overnight in a shaker. It was followed by the addition of biotin-azide (Institute of Medicinal Plant Development, Beijing, China) (final concentration 100 μM), then Tris (2-carboxyethyl) phosphine (TCEP, T1656) (final concentration 1 mM), and Tris [(1-benzyl-1H-1,2,3-triazole-4-yl)methyl]-amine (TBTA, T2993) (final concentration 100 μM) (Tokyo Chemical Industry, Japan), and Copper sulfate pentahydrate ($CuSO_4 \cdot 5H_2O$) (final concentration 1 mM) (Merck KGaA, Darmstadt, Germany) to each tube with vortex after each addition. Both tubes were incubated at room temperature for 1 h with a vortex every 30 min. Then the tubes were centrifuged at 12,000× *g* for 10 min at 4 °C, and the supernatant was removed. Protein precipitate was dissolved by adding 750 μL of pre-cooled methanol and sonicating for 3–4 s at 4 °C using a probe sonicator (~30% power level). It was followed by methanol wash thrice with centrifugation (12,000× *g*, 4 °C for 10 min) in between.

4.10. Streptavidin Enrichment

Streptavidin enrichment was by method adopted from the method described by Speers and Cravatt [35]. Probed protein precipitates were dissolved in PBS using 600 μL of 0.2% SDS. Then 100 μL of streptavidin agarose resin (Pierce™ 20347, Thermo Fisher Scientific, Waltham, MA, USA) was added and mixed for 1 h in a shaker at RT. It is followed by washing with 1 mL of 1× PBS with centrifugation (for 1 min at 2500× *g*) in between and each time collection of supernatants. Finally, the streptavidin beads were eluted by adding 100 μL of 2× SDS-loading buffer, boiling in a water bath for 10 min. Cooling at 4 °C and centrifuging at 2500× *g* for 1 min. The supernatants were collected and stored at −20 °C until use.

4.11. SDS-PAGE and Staining

Protein samples collected from the previous step were resolved in 10% SDS-PAGE gel and visualized by boiling in 0.25% Coomassie Brilliant Blue (CBB) stain for 5 min [26]. The blue-stained gel was washed twice by boiling it with distilled water for 5–10 min. Protein bands from sample columns were cut and stored (at −20 °C) until the identification experiment.

4.12. LC-MS/MS Analysis

Resolved protein samples were analyzed using QTRAP® 6500 LC-MS/MS System (AB Sciex LLC, Framingham, MA, USA). Mass spectrometric data were searched against the NCBI database with a taxonomy restriction to 2019 human proteins (172,061 sequences; 53,783,369 residues, 27 July 2020) using MASCOT V2.0 (Matrix Sciences, London, UK).

4.13. Data Analysis

A bar diagram was plotted for the cytotoxicity test to visualize the "mean percent of inhibition ± standard error" of cell proliferation using Microsoft® Excel 2019 software. The significance of the lactucin doses was compared with control sample data and calculated by "one-way ANOVA" using "IBM® SPSS® Statistics 26". Significant difference at p 0.05, 0.01, 0.001, and 0.0001 was calculated and expressed with different Asterix "*" numbers on the chart or the data table legend. IC_{50} was calculated by plotting the Log10 dose on X-axis versus the Normalized response on the Y-axis in Graph Pad Prism 7. Cell cycle cytometry data were analyzed using ModFit LT™ (Version 5.0.9). Apoptosis compensation calculation and data analysis were done using CytExpert™ (Version 2.3.0.84). Protein concentrations were calculated in Microsoft® Excel 2019. WB bands were quantified using ImageJ® (Version 1.52a) and analyzed using Graph Pad Prism 7. NMR data was analyzed, the structure was predicted using MestReNova™, and the chemical structure was made using ChemDraw® Professional. LC-MS/MS results analyzed in MASCOT were combined with WB markers data, and functional enrichment was performed to predict the involved molecular pathway using DAVID Bioinformatics resources [36,37].

5. Conclusions

In developing anticancer therapy, discovering natural compounds and their mechanisms are the new frontier. They can concurrently affect multiple cell lines, and are helpful in attending to metastasized cancers, while still possessing molecular specificity towards different oncogenes and tumor suppressors. Herein, we reported cytotoxic, cell cycle inhibitory, and apoptosis-inducing properties of Lactucin in A549 and H2347 cells for the first time. We also narrowed down Lactucin's potential target in the A549 cell as MAPK/ERK pathway. Lactucin exerts its effect by lowering the carbon metabolism necessary for metastasized tumor development. To the best of our knowledge, this study was the first attempt at identifying Lactucin's anticancer mechanism in the lung cancer cell line.

Supplementary Materials: The following supporting information can be downloaded at: https://www.mdpi.com/article/10.3390/molecules27217358/s1, Figure S1: Functional enrichment of ABPP and WB peptides using DAVID Bioinformatics resources predicted Lactucin's interaction with several "Central carbon metabolism in cancer" pathways enzymes (the chart is from KEGG database); Figure S2: Downregulation of the MEK-ERK signaling pathway in NSCLC leads to upregulation of p53 and DNA repair, which downgrade increased carbon consumption-related enzymes (the chart is from KEGG database, red star $p < 0.05$).

Author Contributions: K.M.S.U.I. and Y.T. wrote the first draft and developed the figures and tables. F.X. contributed to the writing and argument development. Y.X. and B.W. jointly made critical revisions and approved the final version. All authors have read and agreed to the published version of the manuscript.

Funding: This work was supported by the Agricultural Science and Technology Innovation Program of Institute of Food Science and Technology, Chinese Academy of Agricultural Sciences (CAAS-ASTIP-G2022-IFST-07 fund; and the CAMS Innovation Fund for Medical Science (CIFMS), grant number 2021-1-I2M-028.

Institutional Review Board Statement: Not applicable.

Informed Consent Statement: Not applicable.

Data Availability Statement: The data presented in this study are available on request from the corresponding author.

Acknowledgments: We are incredibly grateful to Yu Tian for her help in constructing the Lactucin probe. We thank Boting Wen and Yulu Wang for the helpful discussion.

Conflicts of Interest: There are no conflict of interest to declare.

Sample Availability: Source of the compound Lactucin is described in the materials method section.

References

1. Cronin, K.A.; Lake, A.J.; Scott, S.; Sherman, R.L.; Noone, A.M.; Howlader, N.; Henley, S.J.; Anderson, R.N.; Firth, A.U.; Ma, J.; et al. Annual Report to the Nation on the Status of Cancer, part I: National cancer statistics. *Cancer* **2018**, *124*, 2785–2800. [CrossRef] [PubMed]
2. WHO Cancer—Fact Sheet. Available online: http://www.who.int/mediacentre/factsheets/fs297/en/ (accessed on 19 July 2020).
3. Zappa, C.; Mousa, S.A. Non-small cell lung cancer: Current treatment and future advances. *Transl. Lung Cancer Res.* **2016**, *5*, 288–300. [CrossRef] [PubMed]
4. Tsai, C.-M.; Sun, F.-M.; Chen, Y.-L.; Hsu, C.-L.; Yen, G.-C.; Weng, C.-J. Molecular mechanism depressing PMA-induced invasive behaviors in human lung adenocarcinoma cells by cis- and trans-cinnamic acid. *Eur. J. Pharm. Sci.* **2013**, *48*, 494–501. [CrossRef] [PubMed]
5. Walker, S. Updates in non-small cell lung cancer. *Clin. J. Oncol. Nurs.* **2008**, *12*, 587–596. [CrossRef] [PubMed]
6. Torre, L.A.; Siegel, R.L.; Jemal, A. Lung Cancer Statistics. In *Lung Cancer and Personalized Medicine*; Ahmad, A.G.S., Ed.; Springer: Cham, Switzerland, 2016; Volume 893, pp. 1–19. [CrossRef]
7. Malhotra, J.; Malvezzi, M.; Negri, E.; La Vecchia, C.; Boffetta, P. Risk factors for lung cancer worldwide. *Eur. Respir. J.* **2016**, *48*, 889–902. [CrossRef]
8. Donaldson, M.S. Nutrition and cancer: A review of the evidence for an anticancer diet. *Nutr. J.* **2004**, *3*, 19. [CrossRef]
9. Palmer, S. Diet, nutrition, and cancer. *Prog. Food Nutr. Sci.* **1985**, *9*, 283–341.
10. Lefranc, F.; Tabanca, N.; Kiss, R. Assessing the anticancer effects associated with food products and/or nutraceuticals using in vitro and in vivo preclinical development-related pharmacological tests. *Semin. Cancer Biol.* **2017**, *46*, 14–32. [CrossRef]
11. Harrington, S.E.; Smith, T.J. The role of chemotherapy at the end of life: "when is enough, enough?". *JAMA* **2008**, *299*, 2667–2678. [CrossRef]
12. Shah, S.K.; Walker, P.A.; Moore-Olufemi, S.D.; Sundaresan, A.; Kulkarni, A.D.; Andrassy, R.J. An evidence-based review of a *Lentinula edodes* mushroom extract as complementary therapy in the surgical oncology patient. *J. Parenter. Enter. Nutr.* **2011**, *35*, 449–458. [CrossRef]
13. Lin, S.-R.; Chang, C.-H.; Hsu, C.-F.; Tsai, M.-J.; Cheng, H.; Leong, M.K.; Sung, P.-J.; Chen, J.-C.; Weng, C.-F. Natural compounds as potential adjuvants to cancer therapy: Preclinical evidence. *Br. J. Pharm.* **2020**, *177*, 1409–1423. [CrossRef] [PubMed]
14. Prakash, O.; Kumar, A.; Kumar, P.; Ajeet, A. Anticancer Potential of Plants and Natural Products: A Review. *Am. J. Pharmacol. Sci.* **2013**, *1*, 104–115. [CrossRef]
15. Ghantous, A.; Gali-Muhtasib, H.; Vuorela, H.; Saliba, N.A.; Darwiche, N. What made sesquiterpene lactones reach cancer clinical trials? *Drug Discov. Today* **2010**, *15*, 668–678. [CrossRef] [PubMed]
16. Imam, K.M.S.U.; Xie, Y.; Liu, Y.; Wang, F.; Xin, F. Cytotoxicity of *Cichorium intybus* L. metabolites (Review). *Oncol. Rep.* **2019**, *42*, 2196–2212. [CrossRef] [PubMed]
17. Ilgün, S.; Küpeli Akkol, E.; Ilhan, M.; Çiçek Polat, D.; Baldemir Kılıç, A.; Coşkun, M.; Sobarzo-Sánchez, E. Sedative Effects of Latexes Obtained from Some *Lactuca* L. Species Growing in Turkey. *Molecules* **2020**, *25*, 1587. [CrossRef]
18. Assefa, A.D.; Choi, S.; Lee, J.E.; Sung, J.S.; Hur, O.S.; Ro, N.Y.; Lee, H.S.; Jang, S.W.; Rhee, J.H. Identification and quantification of selected metabolites in differently pigmented leaves of lettuce (*Lactuca sativa* L.) cultivars harvested at mature and bolting stages. *BMC Chem.* **2019**, *13*, 56. [CrossRef]
19. Abu-Reidah, I.M.; Contreras, M.M.; Arraez-Roman, D.; Segura-Carretero, A.; Fernandez-Gutierrez, A. Reversed-phase ultra-high-performance liquid chromatography coupled to electrospray ionization-quadrupole-time-of-flight mass spectrometry as a powerful tool for metabolic profiling of vegetables: Lactuca sativa as an example of its application. *J. Chromatogr. A* **2013**, *1313*, 212–227. [CrossRef]
20. Bischoff, T.A.; Kelley, C.J.; Karchesy, Y.; Laurantos, M.; Nguyen-Dinh, P.; Arefi, A.G. Antimalarial activity of Lactucin and Lactucopicrin: Sesquiterpene lactones isolated from *Cichorium intybus* L. *J. Ethnopharmacol.* **2004**, *95*, 455–457. [CrossRef]

21. Dang, T.; Zheng, G.; Zhang, Q.; Jin, P.; Zhang, H.; Su, L.; Qin, D.; Yao, G. Sesquiterpenoids with diverse carbon skeletons from the roots of *Cichorium glandulosum* and their anti-inflammatory activities. *Fitoterapia* **2019**, *136*, 104170. [CrossRef]
22. Wang, X.; Liu, M.; Cai, G.H.; Chen, Y.; Shi, X.C.; Zhang, C.C.; Xia, B.; Xie, B.C.; Liu, H.; Zhang, R.X.; et al. A Potential Nutraceutical Candidate Lactucin Inhibits Adipogenesis through Downregulation of JAK2/STAT3 Signaling Pathway-Mediated Mitotic Clonal Expansion. *Cells* **2020**, *9*, 331. [CrossRef]
23. Foster, J.G.; Cassida, K.A.; Turner, K.E. In vitro analysis of the anthelmintic activity of forage chicory (*Cichorium intybus* L.) sesquiterpene lactones against a predominantly *Haemonchus contortus* egg population. *Vet. Parasitol.* **2011**, *180*, 298–306. [CrossRef] [PubMed]
24. Zhang, F.-H.; Yan, Y.-L.; Wang, Y.; Liu, Z. Lactucin induces potent anticancer effects in HL-60 human leukemia cancer cells by inducing apoptosis and sub-G1 cell cycle arrest. *Bangladesh J. Pharmacol.* **2016**, *11*, 478. [CrossRef]
25. Ren, Y.; Zhou, Y.; Chen, X.; Ye, Y. Discovery, Structural Determination and Anticancer Activities of Lactucin like Guaianolides. *Lett. Drug Des. Discov.* **2005**, *2*, 444–450. [CrossRef]
26. Lu, X.-X.; Cao, L.-Y.; Chen, X.; Xiao, J.; Zou, Y.; Chen, Q. PTEN Inhibits Cell Proliferation, Promotes Cell Apoptosis, and Induces Cell Cycle Arrest via Downregulating the PI3K/AKT/hTERT Pathway in Lung Adenocarcinoma A549 Cells. *BioMed Res. Int.* **2016**, *2016*, 2476842. [CrossRef] [PubMed]
27. Coller, H. Is Cancer a Metabolic Disease? *Am. J. Pathol.* **2013**, *184*, 4–17. [CrossRef] [PubMed]
28. WHO. Cytotoxicity: In Vitro Determination. Available online: https://www.who.int/tdr/grants/workplans/en/cytotoxicity_invitro.pdf (accessed on 21 July 2020).
29. Lima, J.; Oliveira, R.; Silva, V.; Teixeira de Sousa, P., Jr.; Violante, I.; Macho, A.; Martins, D. Anti-inflammatory activity of 4′,6,7-trihydroxy-5-methoxyflavone from *Fridericia chica* (Bonpl.) L.G.Lohmann. *Nat. Prod. Res.* **2020**, *34*, 726–730. [CrossRef] [PubMed]
30. Giménez-Xavier, P.; Francisco, R.; Platini, F.; Pérez, R.; Ambrosio, S. LC3-I conversion to LC3-II does not necessarily result in complete autophagy. *Int. J. Mol. Med.* **2008**, *22*, 781–785. [PubMed]
31. Mizushima, N.; Yoshimori, T. How to Interpret LC3 Immunoblotting. *Autophagy* **2007**, *3*, 542–545. [CrossRef]
32. Xia, R.; Sheng, X.; Xu, X.; Yu, C.; Lu, H. Hesperidin induces apoptosis and G_0/G_1 arrest in human non-small cell lung cancer A549 cells. *Int. J. Mol. Med.* **2018**, *41*, 464–472. [CrossRef]
33. Jang, J.H.; Park, C.Y.; Sung, E.G.; Song, I.H.; Kim, J.Y.; Jung, C.; Sohn, H.Y.; Lee, T.J. Lactucin induces apoptosis through reactive oxygen species-mediated BCL-2 and CFLAR(L) downregulation in Caki-1 cells. *Genes Genom.* **2021**, *43*, 1199–1207. [CrossRef]
34. McCubrey, J.A.; Steelman, L.S.; Chappell, W.H.; Abrams, S.L.; Wong, E.W.T.; Chang, F.; Lehmann, B.; Terrian, D.M.; Milella, M.; Tafuri, A.; et al. Roles of the Raf/MEK/ERK pathway in cell growth, malignant transformation and drug resistance. *Biochim. Biophys. Acta* **2007**, *1773*, 1263–1284. [CrossRef] [PubMed]
35. Speers, A.E.; Cravatt, B.F. Activity-Based Protein Profiling (ABPP) and Click Chemistry (CC)-ABPP by MudPIT Mass Spectrometry. *Curr. Protoc. Chem. Biol.* **2009**, *1*, 29–41. [CrossRef] [PubMed]
36. Da Huang, W.; Sherman, B.T.; Lempicki, R.A. Bioinformatics enrichment tools: Paths toward the comprehensive functional analysis of large gene lists. *Nucleic Acids Res.* **2009**, *37*, 1–13. [CrossRef]
37. Da Huang, W.; Sherman, B.T.; Lempicki, R.A. Systematic and integrative analysis of large gene lists using DAVID bioinformatics resources. *Nat. Protoc.* **2009**, *4*, 44–57. [CrossRef] [PubMed]

marine drugs

Article

Anticancer Activity of Mannose-Specific Lectin, BPL2, from Marine Green Alga *Bryopsis plumosa*

Jei Ha Lee, Set Byul Lee, Heabin Kim, Jae Min Shin, Moongeun Yoon, Hye Suck An and Jong Won Han *

Department of Genetic Resources, National Marine Biodiversity Institute of Korea, Seocheon-gun 33662, Repulic of Korea
* Correspondence: jwhan@mabik.re.kr; Tel.: +82-419500913

Abstract: Lectin is a carbohydrate-binding protein that recognizes specific cells by binding to cell-surface polysaccharides. Tumor cells generally show various glycosylation patterns, making them distinguishable from non-cancerous cells. Consequently, lectin has been suggested as a good anticancer agent. Herein, the anticancer activity of *Bryopsis plumosa* lectins (BPL1, BPL2, and BPL3) was screened and tested against lung cancer cell lines (A549, H460, and H1299). BPL2 showed high anticancer activity compared to BPL1 and BPL3. Cell viability was dependent on BPL2 concentration and incubation time. The IC_{50} value for lung cancer cells was 50 μg/mL after 24 h of incubation in BPL2 containing medium; however, BPL2 (50 μg/mL) showed weak toxicity in non-cancerous cells (MRC5). BPL2 affected cancer cell growth while non-cancerous cells were less affected. Further, BPL2 (20 μg/mL) inhibited cancer cell invasion and migration (rates were <20%). BPL2 induced the downregulation of epithelial-to-mesenchymal transition-related genes (Zeb1, vimentin, and Twist). Co-treatment with BPL2 and gefitinib (10 μg/mL and 10 μM, respectively) showed a synergistic effect compared with monotherapy. BPL2 or gefitinib monotherapy resulted in approximately 90% and 70% cell viability, respectively, with concomitant treatment showing 40% cell viability. Overall, BPL2 can be considered a good candidate for development into an anticancer agent.

Keywords: mannose-binding lectin; BPL2; *Bryopsis plumosa*; anticancer; lung cancer

Citation: Lee, J.H.; Lee, S.B.; Kim, H.; Shin, J.M.; Yoon, M.; An, H.S.; Han, J.W. Anticancer Activity of Mannose-Specific Lectin, BPL2, from Marine Green Alga *Bryopsis plumosa*. *Mar. Drugs* **2022**, *20*, 776. https://doi.org/10.3390/md20120776

Academic Editors: Barbara De Filippis, Alessandra Ammazzalorso and Marialuigia Fantacuzzi

Received: 6 November 2022
Accepted: 7 December 2022
Published: 13 December 2022

1. Introduction

Lectin is a carbohydrate-binding protein that can agglutinate erythrocytes and cells by specifically binding to carbohydrate moieties on cells [1]. Owing to its carbohydrate-binding properties, it is often suggested for pharmacological applications such as antiviral, antimicrobial, and anticancer therapeutics [2–4].

Cancer has high death rates when compared to other human diseases, with over a million people globally newly diagnosed with the condition every year [5]. Although many researchers and countries have invested in anticancer agents, it remains an intractable disease.

Anticancer agents are most commonly developed from antibodies (based on the human immune system) [6], natural products (primarily secondary metabolites) [7], and proteins or peptides [8]. Chemotherapy is the most commonly used anti-cancer approach; however, it has some limitations, such as toxicity [9].

Tumor cells have shown various glycosylation patterns as a common feature, making them distinguishable from non-cancerous cells. Cellular glycosylation mechanisms are associated with physiological and pathological functions [10]. The alteration of glycans on the cancer cell surface affects the invasion and migration of cancer cells. Glycan is also involved in signal transduction, cell adhesion, and cell-substrate interactions [11]. Owing to this, biomarkers for diagnosis have been developed based on the glycosylation pattern of tumor cells [12].

Lectin can recognize tumor cells by binding to cell surface-altered carbohydrates [13]. Therefore, some lectins have been studied as diagnostic agents against tumor cells. Because lectins are also regulators of inflammation and the immune response toward tumor cells [10], they have been investigated as anticancer agents [14]. Lectin is a well-known protein that can inhibit tumor growth and induce cancer cell death. In the last several decades, several lectins with anticancer activities have been reported (e.g., ConA) [15]. Mistletoe (*Viscum album*) lectin is a well-known lectin that is effective against various neoplastic cells [16]. It induces apoptosis in colorectal cancer cells [17]. Moreover, RCA-I specifically binds to metastasis-associated cell surface glycans and inhibits cell invasion and migration [18].

Many marine algal lectins have been reported to be novel proteins. They are believed to have a unique feature compared with other lectins because marine algae have different carbohydrate complexes [19]. To date, various lectin or hemagglutination activities have been reported from the marine algal group [3,20], with various biomedical applications being proposed [21].

Bryopsis plumosa is a well-known coenocyte marine green alga containing abundant lectins involved in algal cell regeneration [22]. To date, *Bryopsis plumosa* lectins (BPLs), which specifically bind to different carbohydrates, have been reported. BPL1, 3, and 4 bind to GlcNAc and GalNAc, while BPL2 binds to D-mannose [22–25]. All *Bryopsis plumosa* lectins in literature were purified, and their amino acid sequences were determined. To date, the potential anticancer effect of *Bryopsis plumosa* lectin has been suggested [25]; however, few studies confirming this postulation have been reported.

In this study, the anticancer activity of BPLs (BPL1, 2, and 3) against lung cancer cell lines and their regulation of epithelial-to-mesenchymal transition (EMT) pathway-related genes were demonstrated.

2. Results

2.1. Preaparation of Bryopsis Plumosa Lectins

Bryopsis lectin was successfully isolated from the crude extract of Bryopsis plumosa. Combining GalNAc and D-Man affinity chromatography was performed to separate each lectin. Stepwise elution of lectins as different monosaccharides was effective in separating BPL1 and BPL3 (Figure 1). The flow-through fraction contained BPL2, which was successfully isolated using mannose affinity chromatography (Figure 1). The purity of each BPL was more than 95%. All the lectins showed similar hemagglutination activities, as previously reported [22–25].

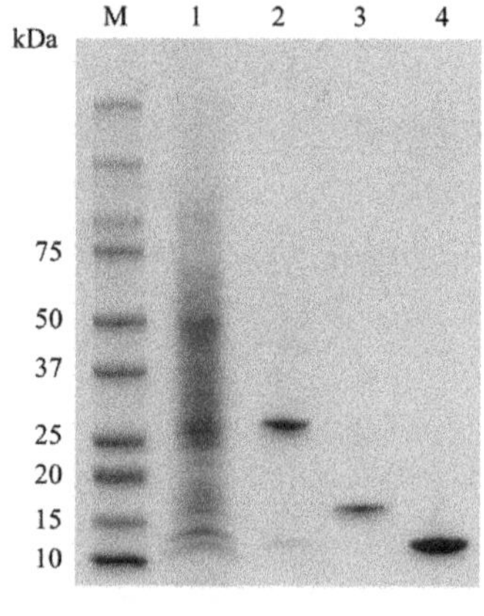

Figure 1. Purification of Bryopsis plumosa lectins (BPLs). M, Molecular weight marker; lane 1, crude extract; lane 2, BPL1; lane 3, BPL2; lane 4, BPL3.

2.2. Cell Viability of Lung Cancer Cells and Non-Cancerous Cells against BPLs

BPL2 inhibited the viability of lung cancer cell lines, whereas BPL1 and BPL3 did not show the inhibitory activity of the tested cell lines at any concentration (Supplementary

Figure S1). Cell viability was dependent on the BPL2 concentration and exposure time. BPL2 activity was most effective in the A549 and H1299 lung cancer cell lines, with cell viability being approximately 40% at 100 μg/mL of BPL2 after exposure for 24 h. However, weak toxicity towards non-cancerous cell lines (MRC5, HEK293T, and HaCaT) was observed at 100 μg/mL (~60–70% viability) (Figure 2A). The increase in the exposure time of BPL2 affected cell viability; cell viability was reduced to approximately 20% after 72 h of exposure (Figure 2B). Based on the cytotoxicity results in non-cancerous cell lines, subsequent experiments were performed at a BPL2 concentration of fewer than 25 μg/mL.

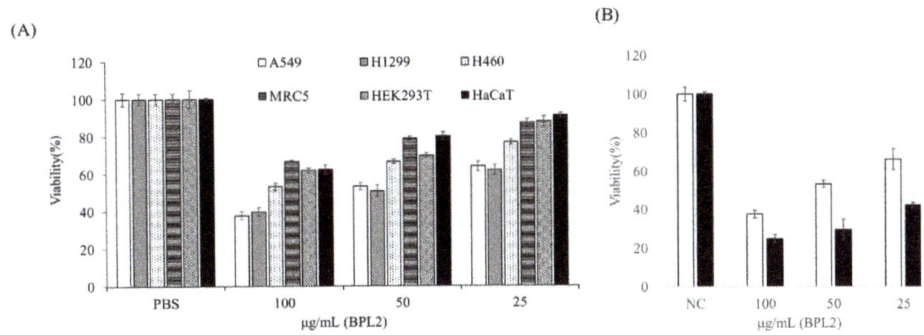

Figure 2. Effect of BPL2 on the viability of cell lines using MTT assays. (**A**) After 24 h of exposure to various cell lines, (**B**) After 24 (white bar) and 72 h (black bar) of exposure to the A549 cell line. Results are represented as the mean ± standard error.

According to the colony-forming assay, BPL2 was effective at low concentrations. All cancer cell lines disappeared after treatment with 20 μg/mL of BPL2. In addition, half of the colonies did not survive at 20 μg/mL BPL2 (Figure 3).

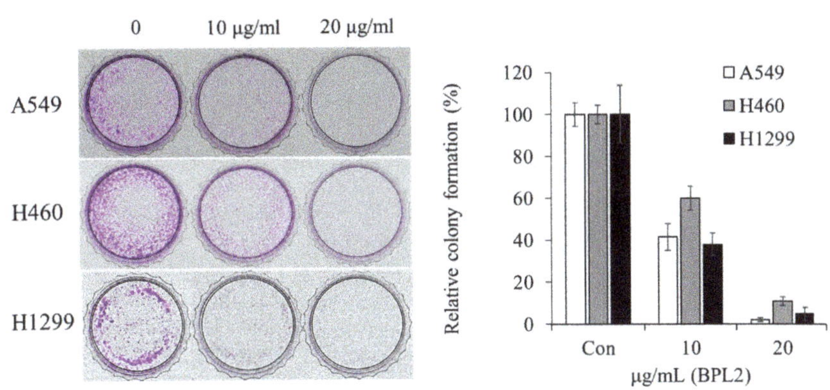

Figure 3. Colony-forming assay for the anticancer activity of BPL2. A549, H460, and H1299 cancer cell lines were used for these studies.

2.3. Determination of Migration and Invasion of Cancer Cells following BPL2 Treatment

BPL2 strongly inhibited the invasion and migration of lung cancer cells in the various cell lines (A549, H460, and H1299). A concentration-dependent effect was observed in both the cell migration and invasion assays. The migration of all cancer cell lines was reduced to less than 10% following treatment with 20 μg/mL of BPL2. The cell invasion rate of lung cancer cells also decreased to 20% at the same treatment conditions (Figure 4).

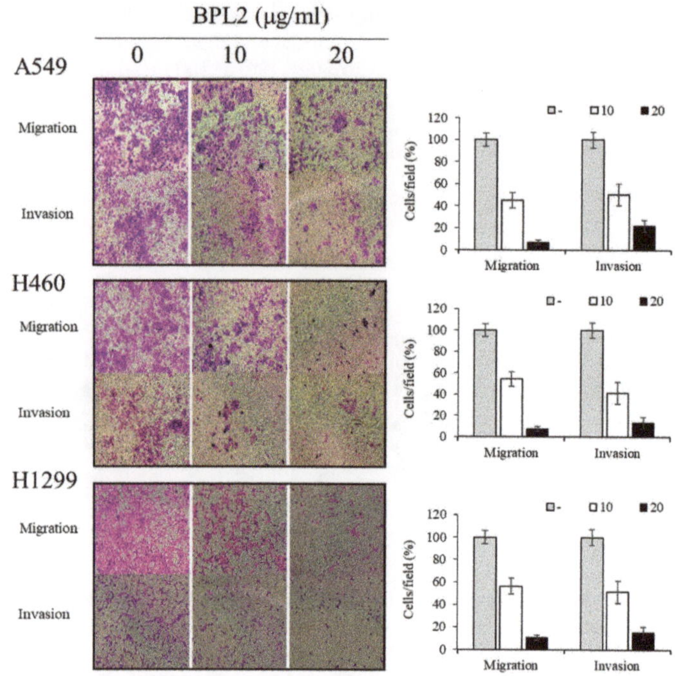

Figure 4. Effect of BPL2 on migration and invasion of cancer cells. Transwell migration (Upper images) and invasion assays (Bottom images) for A549, H460, and H1299 cell lines were performed using different concentrations of BPL2. Representative graphs are shown with the quantification of the randomly selected fields.

The expression levels of EMT-related genes (N-cadherin, E-cadherin, ZEB1, vimentin, and Twist) were investigated to understand the involvement of BPL2 in the EMT pathway. BPL2 induced the downregulation of ZEB1, Twist, vimentin, and N-cadherin and upregulated E-cadherin expression. Gene expression levels showed similar regulation in all tested cancer cell lines, viz. A549, H460, and H1299 (Figure 5A). The levels of EMT-related proteins (N-cadherin, ZEB1, vimentin, and snai1) showed the same trends as their corresponding gene expressions (Figure 5B).

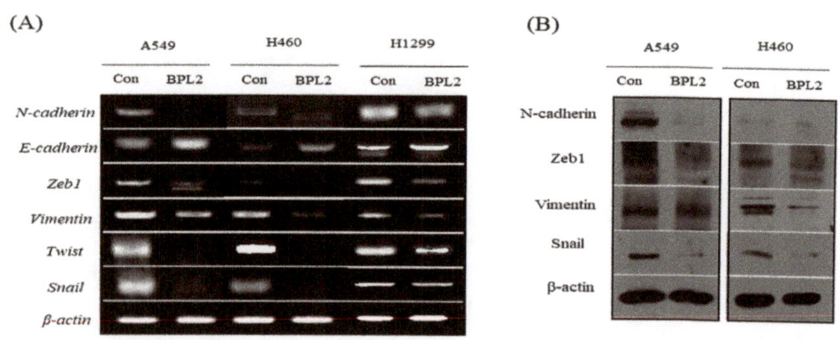

Figure 5. Levels of (**A**) EMT gene and (**B**) protein expression. (**A**) Gene expression in A549, H460, and H1299 cell lines following treatment with BPL2. (**B**) The protein expression in A549 cells following treatment with BPL2. β-actin was used as the control.

The levels of EGFR signaling-related protein expression were determined. EGFR in A549 and H460 cells decreased significantly upon BPL2 treatment. Activation of ERK and AKT, important downstream targets of the EGFR signaling pathway, reduced significantly (Figure 6).

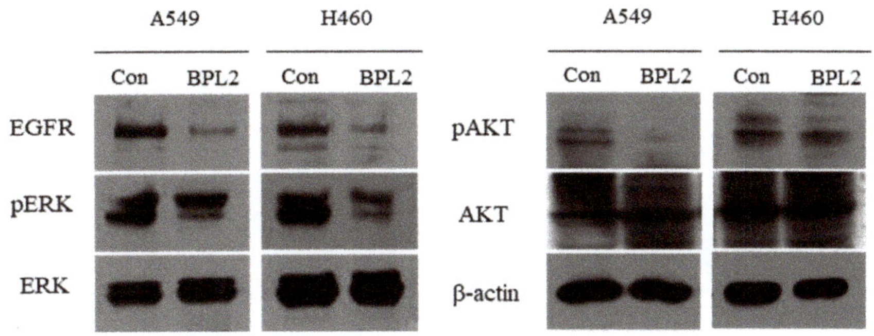

Figure 6. Levels of EGFR signaling-related protein expression. Level of proteins in A549 and H460 cell lines following treatment with BPL2 as determined by Western blot analysis. β-actin was used as the control.

2.4. *Analysis for Apoptosis in BPL2-Treated Lung Cancer Cell Lines*

To evaluate whether treatment with BPL2 induced apoptosis, an Annexin V/PI staining assay was performed. After treatment with BPL2 at 20 μg/mL for 48 h, significant apoptosis induction was observed. The apoptosis rate increased to 17.1% (early: 0.1%, late: 17.0%) in A549, 9.5% (early: 1.5%, late: 7.0%) in H460, and 18.8% (early: 9.7%, late: 9.1%) in H1299 cells after treatment with BPL2. Necrotic cell death was observed at 2.7% in A549 and 0.5% in H460 and H1299 cells (Figure 7).

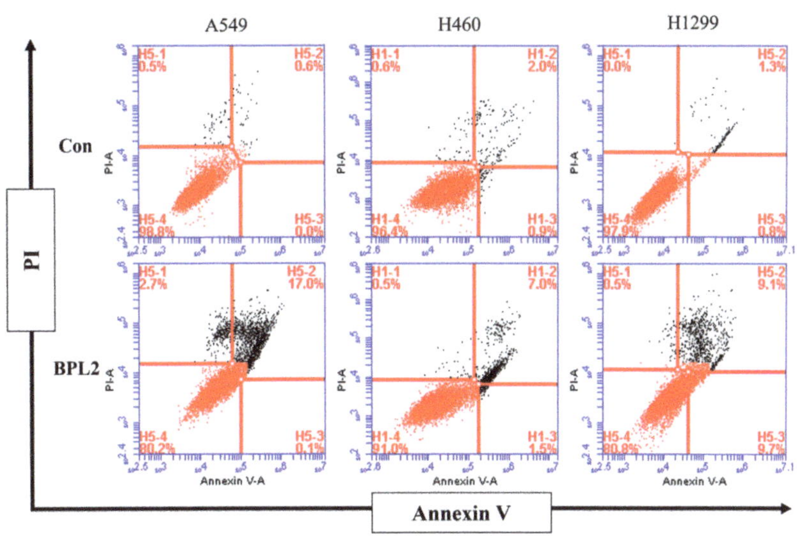

Figure 7. Analysis of apoptosis rates in BPL2-treated lung cancer cell lines. Lung cancer cells were incubated for 48 h with BPL2 and stained with Annexin V/PI for flow cytometric analysis. The upper left panel indicates necrotic cell death; the lower left panel indicates live cells; the upper right panel indicates late apoptosis, and the lower right panel indicates early apoptosis.

2.5. Effect of Concomitant Treatment with Gefitinib and BPL2 on Cell Viability

Concomitant treatment with gefitinib and BPL2 (10 μM and 10 μg/mL, respectively) showed a synergistic effect on the cancer cell lines compared with monotherapy. BPL2 or gefitinib monotherapy showed approximately 90% and 70% A549 cell viability, respectively, while concomitant therapy showed approximately 40% viability in the same cell line (Figure 8A). H460 cells treated with a combination of gefitinib-BPL2 did not show as much decrease in viability compared to A549 cells (Figure 8B). An increase in incubation time with the treatment agents led to a further 10% reduction in cell viability in both cell lines.

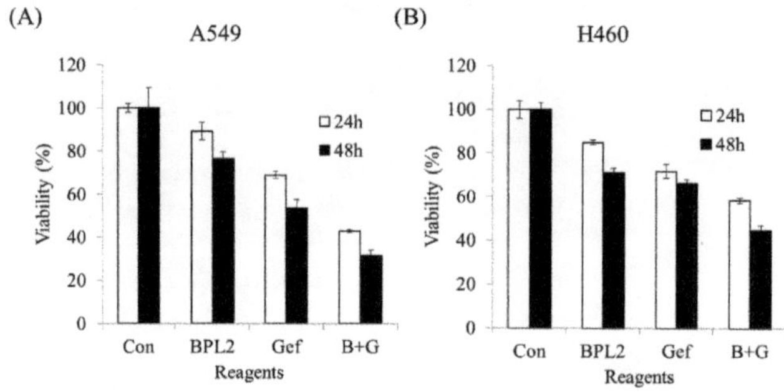

Figure 8. Concomitant treatment or monotherapy using gefitinib (10 μM) and BPL2 (10 μg/mL) on lung cancer cell lines. (**A**) A549, (**B**) H460. Con shows untreated cell lines. B+G shows cells treated with both agents.

3. Discussion

Similar to all other medicines, a lectin that is to be investigated for its therapeutic activity must be purified from its source [26]. Stepwise purification using two different affinity chromatographic techniques were successful in separating *Bryopsis plumosa* lectins. As previously reported [23,25], both GalNAc binding lectins (BPL1 and BPL3) were isolated by GalNAc affinity chromatography using a two-step elution method, and then the mannose-binding lectin (BPL2) was purified using D-mannose affinity chromatography [25]. The purity of the isolated lectins was sufficient to determine their effectiveness and mechanisms of action in cancer cell lines.

Several anticancer lectins from plants and animals have been reported in recent decades, such as galectin, C-type lectins, sialic acid binding, and Mistletoe lectin [14]. It is known that these lectins recognize carbohydrates on the cell surface and inhibit the survival of cancer cells by various mechanisms. A plant lectin has also been reported to affect apoptosis and autophagy by regulating a signal transduction pathway [14]. The specific binding of lectin to the cancer cell was well reported in targeting and imaging cancer cells. The alternation of cancer cell surface glycan was a well-known phenomenon and the carbohydrate recognition properties of lectin were often applied to cancer cell imaging [27]. Although the direct binding of BPL2 was not determined in this study, the binding of BPL2 on cancer cells could be assumed. The glycan binding specificity of BPL2 has been determined by hemagglutinating inhibition assay and it was specific to the α-methyl-D-mannose (Minimum inhibitory concentration, 3.9 mM), D-mannose (1.9 mM), L-fucose (7.8 mM), and D-glucose (125 mM) [25]. The abundance of high-mannose N-glycan or fucosylated on cancer cells has been reported [28,29]. Owing to the binding properties, lectins have been suggested as potential therapeutic agents that recognize the high-mannose N-glycans occurring at the membrane of various cancer cells [29]. Therefore, mannose-specific algal lectins such as Bryopsis lectin may have anti-cancer and anti-viral activity [29,30].

As expected, the D-mannose-specific lectin, BPL2, showed anticancer activity. However, GlcNAc- and GalNAc-binding lectins did not show any anticancer effects. It may be assumed that different lectins show specific cytotoxic effects against certain cancer cell lines and that the latter two lectins could have anticancer activity in other cancer cells (e.g., cutaneous cancer). The specificity of lectins for distinct cancer cells is a well-known phenomenon. Tian et al. reported the binding affinity and specificity of 27 different lectins in four distinct colorectal cancer cell lines. In addition to the different interactions of 27 lectins with colorectal cancer cell lines, the same lectin displayed differences in four distinct cell lines [31].

The viability of lung cancer cell lines was greatly decreased after exposure to BPL2. The IC_{50} value was approximately 50 μg/mL for A549 and H1299 cells. This is quite a low concentration compared with that of the red alga *Kappaphycus striatus* lectin, KSL, which was reported to have an IC_{50} value in the range of 0.80–1.94 μM (0.22–0.54 mg/mL) [32]. Owing to the cytotoxicity of BPL2 against non-cancerous cell lines, the minimum concentration of BPL2 (<20 μg/mL) for other experiments was determined based on the cell viability results that did not show cell toxicity.

Although the mechanisms underlying the anticancer activity of BPL2 were unclear, the molecule clearly showed effective inhibition of cell growth in a colony-forming assay at a low concentration (20 μg/mL). The reduction in cell growth may have been mediated by binding to the surface carbohydrates of cancer cells and inducing cytotoxicity. Mannose-binding plant lectin from *Remusatia vivipara* exhibits a strong glycan-mediated cytotoxic effect and inhibits the growth and motility of human breast cancer cells [33]. Cancer cells often exhibit alterations in the cell surface of polysaccharides that act as tumor-associated antigens. Lectin recognizes altered cell surface carbohydrates and inhibits cell growth through several mechanisms, such as the reactive oxygen species-dependent pathway [34] and an apoptosis-inducing mechanism [35]. Owing to this, BPL2 may have mechanisms that are similar to those of other plant lectins.

Inhibition of cancer invasion and migration is a priority in cancer therapy because most cancer deaths are caused by metastasis [36]. BPL2 clearly inhibited the invasion and movement of cancer cells in all the tested lung cancer cell lines. In general, cancer cell invasion and migration are affected by several mechanisms. For example, a lectin from *Bandeiraea simplicifolia* seeds (BS-I) inhibited cancer cells, hepatocellular carcinoma, invasion, and migration, mediated by inhibiting the activation of the AKT/GSK-3β/β-catenin pathway [37]. AKT/GSK3β/β-catenin signaling contributes to cell migration and the EMT pathway [38], which affects EMT gene expression patterns. EMT is a program of cells that are vital for embryonic development, wound healing, and the malignant progression of cancer [39]. Three of the EMT marker genes, viz. zinc-finger E-box binding protein 1 (ZEB1), vimentin, and Twist, among the reported genes (i.e., ZEB1, Snail, and Twist) for the EMT marker [40] were selected, and the gene expression patterns after or without exposure to BPL2 were determined. All the analyzed genes in the three tested lung cancer cell lines were downregulated following treatment with BPL2, which corresponds to cell migration and invasion experiments. The protein expression at the same conditions correlated significantly with the corresponding gene expression level, although, for vimentin, the trend was unclear. Therefore, the gene expression could be assumed to reflect the corresponding protein levels.

ZEB1 is a well-known transcription factor that is upregulated in various tumor cell lines and is related to the invasion and migration of cells in patients with lung cancer [41]. It is also a critical regulator of cell plasticity, DNA damage, cancer cell differentiation, and metastasis [42]. BPL2 suppresses ZEB1 gene regulation in lung cancer cell lines and induces cell death. Signal transduction and activation of ZEB1 in EMT plays an important role in embryonic development and malignant progression. It is also associated with resistance to cancer therapies [43]. Suppression of ZEB1 gene expression decreases cancer angiogenesis while eliciting continuous cancer vascular normalization [44]. BPL2 diminished ZEB1 expression, and it could be assumed that it inhibits cancer cell migration via the same mechanisms.

Twist and snail, key transcription factors, are involved in the EMT pathway and play an essential role in cell migration, invasion, and metastasis [45,46]. Although a slight difference was observed among the tested cancer cell lines, downregulation of the Twist and snail genes was clearly defined. Therefore, we assumed that the anticancer ability of BPL2 was related to the inhibition of the EMT pathway.

Vimentin expression is affected by the downregulation of ZEB1, in turn constraining tumor migration [47,48]. The regulation of Twist is also associated with the expression of membrane proteins (N-cadherin, fibronectin, and vimentin) involved in cell adhesion in cancer cells [49]. Because of the downregulation of transcription factors ZEB1 and Twist, a reduction in vimentin expression after treatment with BPL2 was expected. The expression of vimentin was reduced in the tested cell lines, although different expression levels were observed in each tested cell line. The membrane protein vimentin is widely distributed in the fibroblasts, white blood cells, and vascular endothelial cells. It supports cell membranes and organelles, and a lack of vimentin induces cell migration. BPL2 appears to affect the transcription factor of EMT, disturbs vimentin expression, and ultimately inhibits cancer cell growth, invasion, and migration. Therefore, BPL2 appears to be a candidate inhibitor of the EMT pathway. However, the mechanisms of BPL2 in cancer cell lines are still unclear, whether it is directly or indirectly related; therefore, further comprehensive studies are required to understand the inhibition mechanisms.

The regulation of N-cadherin and E-cadherin is switched during EMT signaling by a complex network of signaling pathways and transcription factors. Downregulation of E-cadherin is often observed in malignant epithelial cancers and is accepted as a tumor suppressor. In contrast to E-cadherin, N-cadherin is downregulated in tumor cells [50]. Similar to the regulation of N-cadherin and E-cadherin in the inhibition of tumor cell lines, treatment with BPL2 led to the upregulation of E-cadherin and downregulation of N-cadherin. The results of the EMT pathway involving marker gene regulation following treatment with BPL2 were well aligned with the suppression of the EMT pathway in tumor cell lines.

Cell surface glycan alteration during the EMT process has been observed in various cancer models. It has been reported that modification of the glycan on the cell surface plays a pivotal role in metastasis [51].

The mannan-binding lectin in the reduction of EMT has been reported to be related to the calcium entry machinery [52]. BPL2 does not require a divalent ion for its activity [25]; therefore, it could be assumed that BPL2 is not associated with calcium channels. There are few reports on the involvement of lectin in the EMT pathway. Although BPL2 has not been confirmed to directly contribute to the suppression of the EMT pathway, it could be assumed to inhibit the migration of cancer cells by recognizing the cell surface glycan alternations (high-mannose N-glycan) on cancer cells with metastatic ability.

Gefitinib, an epidermal growth factor receptor tyrosine kinase inhibitor (EGFR-TKI), is a well-known drug used for the treatment of non-small cell lung cancer [53]. Concurrent treatment with anticancer agents to attain therapeutic success is accepted as a common regimen. Simultaneous treatment with BPL2 and gefitinib resulted in synergistic effects. We confirmed that the level of total EGFR expression decreased following BPL2 treatment. BPL2 decreased the activation of ERK and AKT in A549 and H460 cells, followed by the downregulation of cellular EGFR levels. Similarly, a study reported decreased expression of EGFR by lectin protein from *Pseudomonas fluorescens* in gastric cancer cells [54,55]. Consistently, BPL2 significantly reduced the expression of EGFR along with the activation of ERK and AKT, downstream of the EGFR signaling pathway in lung cancer cells. Similarly, the synergistic effect of a combination treatment of gefitinib and docetaxel in EGFR-TKI-sensitive cells has been reported [56].

Polygonatum odoratum lectin elicits apoptosis and autophagy in cancer cells. Apoptosis is induced by the Akt-NF-κB pathway in lung cancer cells [57], and the EGFR-mediated Ras-Raf-MEK-ERK pathway in breast cancer cells [55]. Similar to *Polygonatum odoratum* lectin, BPL2 treatment resulted in differential expression of EGFR and EMT pathway-related proteins. Based on the results, it could be concluded that BPL2 could induce apoptosis by similar mechanisms.

The main role of gefitinib is to inhibit tyrosine kinase, involved in cellular proliferation [58] and promotes apoptosis [59]. Based on the results of the Annexin V/PI staining assay, BPL2 was found to induce apoptosis rather than necrosis in lung cancer cell lines. Like BPL2, induction of apoptosis by lectin has been reported, like mistletoe lectin [14,60], a lectin from *Dioclea lasiocarpa* [61], and lectin from *Sophora flavescens* [62]. The synergetic effect may have led to the induction of apoptosis. The combination of mistletoe lectin with other compounds showed a synergistic anti-cancer effect in breast cancer cells [63].

The anticancer activity of BPL2 was determined in this study, and it was related to the inhibition of the EMT pathway and induction of apoptosis. Furthermore, concurrent treatment with another anticancer agent, gefitinib, showed a synergistic effect in two lung cancer cell lines (A549 and H460). Therefore, the mannose-binding lectin, BPL2, could be a good candidate for drug development in anticancer therapeutics.

4. Materials and Methods

4.1. Preparation of Bryopsis plumosa Lectins (BPLs)

Bryopsis plumosa cultured in our laboratory was used to extract BPLs. BPLs were isolated following a previously reported method by Han et al. [23–25]. *Bryopsis plumosa* was harvested and washed with 1× Tris-buffered saline (TBS, pH 7.5) containing 1 mM $CaCl_2$ and 1 mM $MgCl_2$. The harvested samples were ground into a fine powder, after exposure to liquid nitrogen, using a mortar and pestle. Five volumes of ice-cold 1× TBS were added to the ground samples and incubated for 3 h at 4 °C. The incubated sample was centrifuged at 25,000× *g* for 30 min at 4 °C, and the cell debris was removed. The crude extract was loaded directly onto an affinity chromatography column. A Bio-Rad NGC FPLC system (Bio-Rad Laboratories, Hercules, CA, USA) was used for chromatographic analysis at a flow rate of 1 mL/min. First, GalNAc-agarose was used to purify BPL1, BPL3, and BPL4 using a stepwise elution method. The affinity column was washed with 10 volumes of 1× TBS. BPL3 and BPL4 were eluted using 0.2 M of GlcNAc in 1× TBS and then BPL1 was eluted using 50 mM GalNAc in 1× TBS. The flow-through from GalNAc-agarose, which contained mannose-binding lectin, was loaded onto the mannose-agarose. BPL2 was eluted with 0.5 M D-mannose dissolved in 1× TBS.

All lectins were confirmed using SDS-PAGE and UV spectrophotometry. The BPLs were dialyzed using 1× PBS and stored at −20 °C until use.

4.2. Cell Culture and Viability Assay (Determination of Viability of Tumo Cells)

Metastatic lung cancer cell lines (A549, H460, and H1299) were used to determine tumor cell viability. Non-cancerous and immortalized cells (MRC5, HEK293T, and HaCaT cells) were used as controls (Supplementary Table S1). All cells used for the cell viability test were cultured at 37 °C under atmospheric conditions of 5% CO_2 in fetal bovine serum (FBS) containing antibiotics (penicillin and streptomycin). The growth rate of the cells was determined by CCK-8 analysis. Aliquots of each cell line were added to 96-well plates to achieve a cell number of 5×10^3 cells per well and incubated in a 5% CO_2 atmosphere at 37 °C for 24 h. BPLs (BPL1, 2, and 3) at concentrations of 25, 50, and 100 μg/ml, respectively, were added to the cells and then incubated for 24–72 h. After incubation, the culture medium was removed and the cells were incubated in a fresh culture medium containing CCK-8 solution for 3 h. Cell viability was determined by measuring absorbance at 450 nm using a 96-well plate reader (Spectramax i3x; Molecular Devices, San Jose, CA, USA). Live cells were calculated as a percentage. All experiments were repeated at least three times.

4.3. Determination of Cell Growth Rate Based on BPL Treatments

The cell lines were cultured in the same manner as for the cell viability test. A colony-forming test was performed to compare the growth rate among cell lines treated with different concentrations of BPLs. Each cell line was divided into 1×10^3 cells per 30 mm dish and cultured at 37 °C in a CO_2 incubator for 24 h. The cell lines were treated with

BPLs at concentrations of 10 and 20 μg/mL. After being cultured for 7 days, the culture medium was discarded and stained with 0.5% crystal violet solution for 10 min. The stained cells were washed several times with 1× PBS and the growth rate was observed under a microscope.

4.4. Determination of Migration and Invasion of Cancer Cells

The migration and invasion assays were performed using a Transwell (Falcon, BD labware, Bedford, MA, USA) with a 0.8 μm pore size. The EMT protein marker was used to analyze the migration ability. The lung cancer cell lines were incubated at 37 °C for 48 h after inoculation into the migration well to obtain a density of 1×10^5 cells/well, which were stained using crystal violet solution.

4.5. Comparison of the Expression Level of Cell Migration and Invasion-Related Genes, and EGFR-Related Proteins

The expression levels of cancer cell-related genes (ZEB1, vimentin, and Twist) were analyzed using RT-PCR. Total RNA from each cell was isolated using the TRIzol RNA extraction solution. RNA quality was determined by gel electrophoresis using a UV-spectrophotometer. First-strand cDNA was synthesized using the Transcriptor First Strand cDNA Synthesis Kit (Roche Diagnostics, Penzberg, Germany). One microgram of total RNA was used for first-strand cDNA synthesis. Primer information for the RT-PCR is listed in Supplementary Table S2. Amplification was performed using an Applied Science PCR machine under the following conditions: pre-denaturation at 94 °C for 5 min, 30 cycles of denaturation at 94 °C for 5 min, annealing at 56 °C for 1 min, extension at 72 °C for 1.5 min; and final extension at 72 °C for 5 min. The relative expression levels of target genes were analyzed by gel electrophoresis.

For analysis of EMT-related protein levels, Western blot analysis was performed. Cells were lysed in a buffer with protease inhibitor cocktails (Sigma-Aldrich). Protein concentrations were determined by the Bradford assay (Bio-Rad, Hercules, CA, USA). Equal amounts of protein were separated on 10% sodium dodecyl sulfate-polyacrylamide gel (SDS-PAGE) and transferred onto NC membranes. Membranes were incubated with each antibody in a blocking solution overnight. After washing with Tris-buffered saline, membranes were incubated with mouse secondary antibody (Abcam, Cambridge, MA, USA) and visualized using a Supersignal west atto ultimate sensitivity substrate (Thermo Scientific, A38555). Antibodies specific for N-cadherin (59987), ZEB1 (515797), Vimentin (6260), Snail (271977), and β-actin (47778) were purchased from Santa Cruz Biotechnology.

The analysis of EGFR-related proteins was performed by the same procedure as for EMT-related proteins. The antibodies for EGFR (377547), pERK (7383), ERK (514302), AKT (5298), and pAKT (271966) were obtained from Santa Cruz Biotechnology.

4.6. The Effect of Concurrent Treatment (Gefitinib and BPL2) on Lung Cancer Cell Viability

Human cancer cell lines (A549 and H460) were used to determine the effect of concomitant drug administration. Cell lines were prepared following the method described above for cell viability. Concomitant gefitinib-BPL2 or BPL2 (10 μg/mL) and gefitinib (10 μM) monotherapy were used to treat the cell lines. The treated cancer cell lines were incubated for 24 or 48 h, and viability was measured using CCK-8 analysis kits.

4.7. Flow Cytometric Analysis for Apoptosis in BPL2-Treated Lung Cancer Cells

A549 and H1299 cell lines were treated with 20 μg/mL of BPL2 and incubated for 48 h in a CO_2 incubator. The cells were double stained using the AnnexinV/PI apoptosis detection kit (556547; BD Biosciences, San Jose, CA, UAS) following the manufacturer's instructions. Apoptosis was determined using a flow cytometer (Accuri C6 Plus; BD Biosciences.

5. Conclusions

The anticancer activity of algal lectins has been studied for several decades. Lectins from *Bryopsis plumosa* have been suggested as candidate antitumor agents. Herein, the anticancer activity of BPL2 was demonstrated in lung cancer cell lines, and the inhibition of cell migration and invasion by BPL2 was presumed to be related to the EMT pathway. Concurrent treatment with BPL2 and gefitinib had a synergetic effect on investigated lung cancer cell lines. Therefore, BPL2 could be a good candidate anticancer agent for lung cancer therapy.

Supplementary Materials: The following are available online at https://www.mdpi.com/article/10.3390/md20120776/s1: Table S1: Cancer and non-cancerous cell lines used for the anticancer assay, Table S2: Primer sequences used for RT-PCR analyses. Figure S1: Effect of BPL on the viability of A549 and H460 cell lines using MTT assays.

Author Contributions: Conceptualization, J.W.H.; experimental design, J.W.H. and J.H.L.; experiments, J.W.H., J.H.L., S.B.L., H.K. and J.M.S.; data analysis, J.W.H. and J.H.L.; manuscript writing, J.W.H., M.Y., H.S.A. and J.H.L. All authors have read and agreed to the published version of the manuscript.

Funding: This work was supported by a grant from the Marine Biodiversity Institute of Korea (No. 2022M00400).

Conflicts of Interest: The authors declare no conflict of interest. The funders had no role in the study design; collection, analyses, or interpretation of data; writing of the manuscript; or decision to publish the results.

References

1. Sharon, N.; Lis, H. Lectins: Cell-agglutinating and sugar-specific proteins. *Science* **1972**, *177*, 949–959. [CrossRef] [PubMed]
2. Nabi-Afjadi, M.; Heydari, M.; Zalpoor, H.; Arman, I.; Sadoughi, A.; Sahami, P.; Aghazadeh, S. Lectins and lectibodies: Potential promising antiviral agents. *Cell. Mol. Biol. Lett.* **2022**, *27*, 37. [CrossRef] [PubMed]
3. Singh, R.S.; Walia, A.K. Lectins from red algae and their biomedical potential. *J. Appl. Phycol.* **2018**, *30*, 1833–1858. [CrossRef] [PubMed]
4. Han, J.; Jung, M.; Shim, E.; Shim, J.; Kim, Y.; Kim, G. Functional recombinants designed from a fetuin/asialofetuin-specific marine algal lectin, Rhodobindin. *Mar. Drugs* **2015**, *13*, 2183–2195. [CrossRef] [PubMed]
5. Sung, H.; Ferlay, J.; Siegel, R.L.; Laversanne, M.; Soerjomataram, I.; Jemal, A.; Bray, F. Global Cancer Statistics 2020: GLOBOCAN estimates of incidence and mortality worldwide for 36 cancers in 185 countries. *CA Cancer J. Clin.* **2021**, *71*, 209–249. [CrossRef]
6. Attarwala, H. Role of antibodies in cancer targeting. *J. Nat. Sci. Biol. Med.* **2010**, *1*, 53. [CrossRef]
7. Seca, A.; Pinto, D. Plant secondary metabolites as anticancer agents: Successes in clinical trials and therapeutic application. *Int. J. Mol. Sci.* **2018**, *19*, 263. [CrossRef]
8. Karpiński, T.; Adamczak, A. Anticancer activity of bacterial proteins and peptides. *Pharmaceutics* **2018**, *10*, 54. [CrossRef]
9. Gewirtz, D.A.; Bristol, M.L.; Yalowich, J.C. Toxicity issues in cancer drug development. *Curr. Opin. Investig. Drugs* **2010**, *11*, 612–614.
10. Pinho, S.S.; Reis, C.A. Glycosylation in cancer: Mechanisms and clinical implications. *Nat. Rev. Cancer* **2015**, *15*, 540–555. [CrossRef]
11. Rodrigues, J.G.; Balmaña, M.; Macedo, J.A.; Poças, J.; Fernandes, Â.; De-Freitas-Junior, J.C.M.; Pinho, S.S.; Gomes, J.; Magalhães, A.; Gomes, C.; et al. Glycosylation in cancer: Selected roles in tumour progression, immune modulation and metastasis. *Cell. Immunol.* **2018**, *333*, 46–57. [CrossRef] [PubMed]
12. Liu, S.; Yu, Y.; Wang, Y.; Zhu, B.; Han, B. COLGALT1 is a potential biomarker for predicting prognosis and immune responses for kidney renal clear cell carcinoma and its mechanisms of ceRNA networks. *Eur. J. Med. Res.* **2022**, *27*, 122. [CrossRef]
13. Rodrigues Mantuano, N.; Natoli, M.; Zippelius, A.; Läubli, H. Tumor-associated carbohydrates and immunomodulatory lectins as targets for cancer immunotherapy. *J. Immunother. Cancer* **2020**, *8*, e001222. [CrossRef] [PubMed]
14. Yau, T.; Dan, X.; Ng, C.; Ng, T. Lectins with Potential for Anti-Cancer Therapy. *Molecules* **2015**, *20*, 3791–3810. [CrossRef]
15. Shi, Z.; Chen, J.; Li, C.; An, N.; Wang, Z.; Yang, S.; Huang, K.; Bao, J. Antitumor effects of concanavalin A and Sophora flavescens lectin in vitro and in vivo. *Acta Pharmacol. Sin.* **2014**, *35*, 248–256. [CrossRef] [PubMed]
16. Saha, C.; Das, M.; Stephen-Victor, E.; Friboulet, A.; Bayry, J.; Kaveri, S. Differential effects of Viscum album preparations on the maturation and activation of human dendritic cells and CD4+ T cell responses. *Molecules* **2016**, *21*, 912. [CrossRef] [PubMed]
17. Twardziok, M.; Kleinsimon, S.; Rolff, J.; Jäger, S.; Eggert, A.; Seifert, G.; Delebinski, C.I. Multiple active compounds from Viscum album L. synergistically converge to promote apoptosis in Ewing sarcoma. *PLoS ONE* **2016**, *11*, e0159749. [CrossRef]

18. Zhou, S.-M.; Cheng, L.; Guo, S.-J.; Wang, Y.; Czajkowsky, D.M.; Gao, H.; Hu, X.-F.; Tao, S.-C. Lectin RCA-I specifically binds to metastasis-associated cell surface glycans in triple-negative breast cancer. *Breast Cancer Res.* **2015**, *17*, 36. [CrossRef]
19. Maliki, I.M.; Misson, M.; Teoh, P.L.; Rodrigues, K.F.; Yong, W.T.L. Production of lectins from marine algae: Current status, challenges, and opportunities for non-destructive extraction. *Mar. Drugs* **2022**, *20*, 102. [CrossRef]
20. Mu, J.; Hirayama, M.; Sato, Y.; Morimoto, K.; Hori, K. A novel high-mannose specific lectin from the green alga Halimeda renschii exhibits a potent anti-influenza virus activity through high-affinity binding to the viral hemagglutinin. *Mar. Drugs* **2017**, *15*, 255. [CrossRef]
21. Singh, R.S.; Thakur, S.R.; Bansal, P. Algal lectins as promising biomolecules for biomedical research. *Crit. Rev. Microbiol.* **2015**, *41*, 77–88. [CrossRef] [PubMed]
22. Kim, G.H.; Klochkova, T.A.; Yoon, K.-S.; Song, Y.-S.; Lee, K.P. Purification and characterization of a lectin, bryohealin, involved in the protoplast formation of a marine green alga *Bryopsis plumosa* (Chlorophyta) 1. *J. Phycol.* **2006**, *42*, 86–95. [CrossRef]
23. Han, J.W.; Yoon, K.S.; Klochkova, T.A.; Hwang, M.S.; Kim, G.H. Purification and characterization of a lectin, BPL-3, from the marine green alga Bryopsis plumosa. *J. Appl. Phycol.* **2011**, *23*, 745–753. [CrossRef]
24. Han, J.-W.; Yoon, K.-S.; Jung, M.-G.; Chah, K.-H.; Kim, G.-H. Molecular characterization of a lectin, BPL-4, from the marine green alga Bryopsis plumosa (Chlorophyta). *Algae* **2012**, *27*, 55–62. [CrossRef]
25. Han, J.W.; Jung, M.G.; Kim, M.J.; Yoon, K.S.; Lee, K.P.; Kim, G.H. Purification and characterization of a D-mannose specific lectin from the green marine alga, *Bryopsis plumosa. Phycol. Res.* **2010**, *58*, 143–150. [CrossRef]
26. Jiang, Q.-L.; Zhang, S.; Tian, M.; Zhang, S.-Y.; Xie, T.; Chen, D.-Y.; Chen, Y.-J.; He, J.; Liu, J.; Ouyang, L.; et al. Plant lectins, from ancient sugar-binding proteins to emerging anti-cancer drugs in apoptosis and autophagy. *Cell Prolif.* **2015**, *48*, 17–28. [CrossRef] [PubMed]
27. Wang, S.; Yin, D.; Wang, W.; Shen, X.; Zhu, J.-J.; Chen, H.-Y.; Zhen, L. Targeting and imaging of cancer cells via monosaccharide-imprinted fluorescent nanoparticles. *Sci. Rep.* **2016**, *6*, 22757. [CrossRef]
28. Shan, M.; Yang, D.; Dou, H.; Zhang, L. Fucosylation in cancer biology and its clinical applications. *Prog. Mol. Biol. Transl. Sci.* **2019**, *162*, 93–119.
29. Barre, A.; Simplicien, M.; Benoist, H.; Van Damme, E.J.; Rougé, P. Mannose-specific lectins from marine algae: Diverse structural scaffolds associated to common virucidal and anti-cancer properties. *Mar. Drugs* **2019**, *17*, 440. [CrossRef]
30. Hwang, H.-J.; Han, J.-W.; Kim, G.H.; Han, J.W. Functional expression and characterization of the recombinant N-acetyl-glucosamine/N-acetyl-galactosamine-specific marine algal lectin BPL3. *Mar. Drugs* **2018**, *16*, 13. [CrossRef]
31. Tian, R.; Zhang, H.; Chen, H.; Liu, G.; Wang, Z. Uncovering the binding specificities of lectins with cells for precision colorectal cancer diagnosis based on multimodal imaging. *Adv. Sci.* **2018**, *5*, 1800214. [CrossRef] [PubMed]
32. Hung, L.D.; Trinh, P.T.H. Structure and anticancer activity of a new lectin from the cultivated red alga, Kappaphycus striatus. *J. Nat. Med.* **2021**, *75*, 223–231. [CrossRef]
33. Sindhura, B.R.; Hegde, P.; Chachadi, V.B.; Inamdar, S.R.; Swamy, B.M. High mannose N-glycan binding lectin from Remusatia vivipara (RVL) limits cell growth, motility and invasiveness of human breast cancer cells. *Biomed. Pharmacother.* **2017**, *93*, 654–665. [CrossRef] [PubMed]
34. Panda, P.K.; Mukhopadhyay, S.; Behera, B.; Bhol, C.S.; Dey, S.; Das, D.N.; Sinha, N.; Bissoyi, A.; Pramanik, K.; Maiti, T.K.; et al. Antitumor effect of soybean lectin mediated through reactive oxygen species-dependent pathway. *Life Sci.* **2014**, *111*, 27–35. [CrossRef] [PubMed]
35. Liu, B.; Li, C.; Bian, H.; Min, M.; Chen, L.; Bao, J. Antiproliferative activity and apoptosis-inducing mechanism of Concanavalin A on human melanoma A375 cells. *Arch. Biochem. Biophys.* **2009**, *482*, 1–6. [CrossRef] [PubMed]
36. Yilmaz, M.; Christofori, G.; Lehembre, F. Distinct mechanisms of tumor invasion and metastasis. *Trends Mol. Med.* **2007**, *13*, 535–541. [CrossRef]
37. Jian, Q.; Yang, Z.; Shu, J.; Liu, X.; Zhang, J.; Li, Z. Lectin BS-I inhibits cell migration and invasion via AKT/GSK-3β/β-catenin pathway in hepatocellular carcinoma. *J. Cell. Mol. Med.* **2018**, *22*, 315–329. [CrossRef]
38. Song, N.; Zhong, J.; Hu, Q.; Gu, T.; Yang, B.; Zhang, J.; Yu, J.; Ma, X.; Chen, Q.; Qi, J.; et al. FGF18 enhances migration and the epithelial-mesenchymal transition in breast cancer by regulating Akt/GSK3β/B-catenin signaling. *Cell. Physiol. Biochem.* **2018**, *49*, 1060–1073. [CrossRef]
39. Huang, Z.; Zhang, Z.; Zhou, C.; Liu, L.; Huang, C. Epithelial–mesenchymal transition: The history, regulatory mechanism, and cancer therapeutic opportunities. *MedComm* **2022**, *3*, e144. [CrossRef]
40. Jung, A.R.; Jung, C.-H.; Noh, J.K.; Lee, Y.C.; Eun, Y.-G. Epithelial-mesenchymal transition gene signature is associated with prognosis and tumor microenvironment in head and neck squamous cell carcinoma. *Sci. Rep.* **2020**, *10*, 3652. [CrossRef]
41. Larsen, J.E.; Nathan, V.; Osborne, J.K.; Farrow, R.K.; Deb, D.; Sullivan, J.P.; Dospoy, P.D.; Augustyn, A.; Hight, S.K.; Sato, M.; et al. ZEB1 drives epithelial-to-mesenchymal transition in lung cancer. *J. Clin. Investig.* **2016**, *126*, 3219–3235. [CrossRef] [PubMed]
42. Drápela, S.; Bouchal, J.; Jolly, M.K.; Culig, Z.; Souček, K. ZEB1: A Critical Regulator of Cell Plasticity, DNA Damage Response, and Therapy Resistance. *Front. Mol. Biosci.* **2020**, *7*, 36. [CrossRef] [PubMed]
43. Zhang, P.; Sun, Y.; Ma, L. ZEB1: At the crossroads of epithelial-mesenchymal transition, metastasis and therapy resistance. *Cell Cycle* **2015**, *14*, 481–487. [CrossRef]

44. Fu, R.; Li, Y.; Jiang, N.; Ren, B.-X.; Zang, C.-Z.; Liu, L.-J.; Lv, W.-C.; Li, H.-M.; Weiss, S.; Li, Z.-Y.; et al. Inactivation of endothelial ZEB1 impedes tumor progression and sensitizes tumors to conventional therapies. *J. Clin. Investig.* **2020**, *130*, 1252–1270. [CrossRef] [PubMed]
45. Khan, M.A.; Chen, H.; Zhang, D.; Fu, J. Twist: A molecular target in cancer therapeutics. *Tumor Biol.* **2013**, *34*, 2497–2506. [CrossRef] [PubMed]
46. Zhuo, W.; Wang, Y.; Zhuo, X.; Zhang, Y.; Ao, X.; Chen, Z. Knockdown of Snail, a novel zinc finger transcription factor, via RNA interference increases A549 cell sensitivity to cisplatin via JNK/mitochondrial pathway. *Lung Cancer* **2008**, *62*, 8–14. [CrossRef] [PubMed]
47. Dou, J.; He, X.; Liu, Y.; Wang, Y.; Zhao, F.; Wang, X.; Chen, D.; Shi, F.; Wang, J. Effect of downregulation of ZEB1 on vimentin expression, tumour migration and tumourigenicity of melanoma B16F10 cells and CSCs. *Cell Biol. Int.* **2014**, *38*, 452–461. [CrossRef]
48. Caramel, J.; Ligier, M.; Puisieux, A. Pleiotropic roles for ZEB1 in cancer. *Cancer Res.* **2018**, *78*, 30–35. [CrossRef]
49. Inoue, K.; Fry, E.A. Novel Molecular Markers for Breast Cancer. *Biomark. Cancer* **2016**, *8*, BIC.S38394. [CrossRef]
50. Loh, C.-Y.; Chai, J.; Tang, T.; Wong, W.; Sethi, G.; Shanmugam, M.; Chong, P.; Looi, C. The E-cadherin and N-cadherin switch in epithelial-to-mesenchymal transition: Signaling, therapeutic implications, and challenges. *Cells* **2019**, *8*, 1118. [CrossRef]
51. Li, S.; Mo, C.; Peng, Q.; Kang, X.; Sun, C.; Jiang, K.; Huang, L.; Lu, Y.; Sui, J.; Qin, X.; et al. Cell surface glycan alterations in epithelial mesenchymal transition process of Huh7 hepatocellular carcinoma cell. *PLoS ONE* **2013**, *8*, e71273. [CrossRef]
52. Liu, Y.; Xie, X.; Wang, P.; Luo, J.; Chen, Y.; Xu, Q.; Zhou, J.; Lu, X.; Zhao, J.; Chen, Z.; et al. Mannan-binding lectin reduces epithelial-mesenchymal transition in pulmonary fibrosis via inactivating the store-operated calcium entry machinery. *J. Innate Immun.* **2022**, 1–13. [CrossRef]
53. Cho, S.; Yee, J.; Kim, J.Y.; Jeong Rhie, S.; Gwak, H.S. Effects of concomitant medication use on gefitinib-induced hepatotoxicity. *J. Clin. Pharmacol.* **2018**, *58*, 263–268. [CrossRef]
54. Sato, Y.; Kubo, T.; Morimoto, K.; Yanagihara, K.; Seyama, T. High mannose-binding *Pseudomonas fluorescens* lectin (PFL) downregulates cell surface integrin/EGFR and induces autophagy in gastric cancer cells. *BMC Cancer* **2016**, *16*, 63. [CrossRef]
55. Ouyang, L.; Chen, Y.; Wang, X.Y.; Lu, R.F.; Zhang, S.Y.; Tian, M.; Xie, T.; Liu, B.; He, G. *Polygonatum odoratum* lectin induces apoptosis and autophagy via targeting EGFR-mediated Ras-Raf-MEK-ERK pathway in human MCF-7 breast cancer cells. *Phytomedicine* **2014**, *21*, 1658–1665. [CrossRef]
56. Wu, M.; Yuan, Y.; Pan, Y.-Y.; Zhang, Y. Antitumor activity of combination treatment with gefitinib and docetaxel in EGFR-TKI-sensitive, primary resistant and acquired resistant human non-small cell lung cancer cells. *Mol. Med. Rep.* **2014**, *9*, 2417–2422. [CrossRef]
57. Li, C.; Chen, J.; Lu, B.; Shi, Z.; Wang, H.; Zhang, B.; Zhao, K.; Qi, W.; Bao, J.; Wang, Y. Molecular switch role of Akt in *Polygonatum odoratum* lectin-induced apoptosis and autophagy in human non-small cell lung cancer A549 cells. *PLoS ONE.* **2014**, *9*, e101526. [CrossRef]
58. Jotte, R.M.; Spigel, D.R. Advances in molecular-based personalized non-small-cell lung cancer therapy: Targeting epidermal growth factor receptor and mechanisms of resistance. *Cancer Med.* **2015**, *4*, 1621–1632. [CrossRef]
59. Zhao, Z.Q.; Yu, Z.Y.; Li, J.; Ouyang, X.N. Gefitinib induces lung cancer cell autophagy and apoptosis via blockade of the PI3K/AKT/mTOR pathway. *Oncol Lett.* **2016**, *12*, 63–68. [CrossRef]
60. Khil, L.Y.; Kim, W.; Lyu, S.; Park, W.B.; Yoon, J.W.; Jun, H.S. Mechanisms involved in Korean mistletoe lectin-induced apoptosis of cancer cells. *World J. Gastroenterol.* **2007**, *13*, 2811–2818. [CrossRef]
61. Gondim, A.C.S.; Romero-Canelón, I.; Sousa, E.H.S.; Blindauer, C.A.; Butler, J.S.; Romero, M.J.; Sanchez-Cano, C.; Sousa, B.L.; Chaves, R.P.; Nagano, C.S.; et al. The potent anti-cancer activity of *Dioclea lasiocarpa* lectin. *J. Inorg. Biochem.* **2017**, *175*, 179–189. [CrossRef] [PubMed]
62. Liu, Z.; Liu, B.; Zhang, Z.T.; Zhou, T.T.; Bian, H.J.; Min, M.W.; Liu, Y.H.; Chen, J.; Bao, J.K. A mannose-binding lectin from *Sophora flavescens* induces apoptosis in HeLa cells. *Phytomedicine* **2008**, *15*, 867–875. [CrossRef] [PubMed]
63. Hong, C.E.; Park, A.K.; Lyu, S.Y. Synergistic anticancer effects of lectin and doxorubicin in breast cancer cells. *Mol. Cell. Biochem.* **2014**, *394*, 225–235. [CrossRef] [PubMed]

Scientia Pharmaceutica

Article

Ethanolic Extract of *Ocimum sanctum* Linn. Inhibits Cell Migration of Human Lung Adenocarcinoma Cells (A549) by Downregulation of Integrin αvβ3, α5β1, and VEGF

Ulayatul Kustiati [1], Suleyman Ergün [2], Srikanth Karnati [2], Dwi Aris Agung Nugrahaningsih [3], Dwi Liliek Kusindarta [1] and Hevi Wihadmadyatami [1,*]

1 Department of Anatomy, Faculty of Anatomy of Veterinary Medicine, Universitas Gadjah Mada, Yogyakarta 55281, Indonesia
2 Institute of Anatomy and Cell Biology, Julius Maximillans University, 97070 Wuerzburg, Germany
3 Department of Pharmacology, Faculty of Medicine, Public Health, and Nursing, Universitas Gadjah Mada, Yogyakarta 55281, Indonesia
* Correspondence: heviwihadmadyatami@ugm.ac.id; Tel.: +62-82137067422

Abstract: Adenocarcinoma lung cancer is a type of non-small cell lung carcinoma (NSCLC), which accounts for 85% of lung cancer incidence globally. The therapies that are being applied, both conventional therapies and antibody-based treatments, are still found to have side effects. Several previous studies have demonstrated the ability of the ethanolic extract of *Ocimum sanctum* Linn. (EEOS) as an ethnomedicine with anti-tumor properties. The aim of this study was to determine the effect of *Ocimum sanctum* Linn. ethanolic extract in inhibiting the proliferation, angiogenesis, and migration of A549 cells (NSCLC). The adhesion as well as the migration assay was performed. Furthermore, enzyme-linked immunosorbent assay (ELISA) was used to measure the expression of αvβ3 integrins, α5β1 integrins, and VEGF. The cells were divided into the following treatment groups: control (non-treated/NT), positive control (AP3/inhibitor β3 80 μg/mL), cisplatin (9 μg/mL), and EEOS at concentrations of 50, 70, 100, and 200 μg/mL. The results showed that EEOS inhibits the adhesion ability and migration of A549 cells, with an optimal concentration of 200 μg/mL. ELISA testing showed that the group of A549 cells given EEOS 200 μg/mL presented a decrease in the optimal expression of integrin α5β1, integrin αvβ3, and VEGF.

Keywords: EEOS; A549 cell line; integrin α5β1; integrin αvβ3; VEGF

Citation: Kustiati, U.; Ergün, S.; Karnati, S.; Nugrahaningsih, D.A.A.; Kusindarta, D.L.; Wihadmadyatami, H. Ethanolic Extract of *Ocimum sanctum* Linn. Inhibits Cell Migration of Human Lung Adenocarcinoma Cells (A549) by Downregulation of Integrin αvβ3, α5β1, and VEGF. *Sci. Pharm.* **2022**, *90*, 69. https://doi.org/10.3390/scipharm90040069

Academic Editor: Barbara De Filippis

Received: 22 August 2022
Accepted: 10 October 2022
Published: 31 October 2022

1. Introduction

Lung cancer is one of the biggest causes of death around the world. The results of the International Agency for Research on Cancer Global Cancer Observatory related to Cancer Incidence and Mortality Worldwide in 2018 showed that 58.5% of the world's lung cancer cases occurred in Asia. More than 85% of all lung cancers are non-small cell lung carcinoma (NSCLC). Adenocarcinoma is one type of NSCLC and is the most common type of lung cancer, in all patients and among non-smokers, globally [1]. Surgery, radiotherapy, and chemotherapy are conventional therapies that are still applied to reduce or delay deaths from NSCLC [2]. In the last few decades, despite advances in antibody-based NSCLC treatment technology, applied in combination with conventional therapies, such as pembrolizumab, nivolumab, and ipilimumab, the administration of therapy has not been optimal [3,4].

The side effects of therapy have prompted scientists to find innovative sources of new anti-cancer compounds from natural sources, including traditional herbal plants [1,5]. Herbal plants can provide beneficial effects through natural bioactive compounds found in tumor cases, including helping to overcome side effects or intrinsic radioresistance, preventing metastases, and improving quality of life and patient survival rates [6]. Holy basil (*Ocimum sanctum* Linn.) is a native Indonesian plant that is often found in the yards of houses, and it is widely consumed by the community as a complement to cuisine. Previous research on the ethanolic extract of *Ocimum sanctum* Linn. showed its ability to induce in vitro apoptosis in A-549 cells (human lung adenocarcinoma) [7,8] and inhibit angiogenesis [9]. In vivo, the ethanolic extract of *Ocimum sanctum* Linn. was shown to induce apoptosis [7] and inhibit metastasis [10] in Lewis lung carcinoma (LLC) cells.

2. Materials and Methods

2.1. Preparation of Ocimum sanctum Linn. Ethanolic Extract (EEOS)

The leaves of *Ocimum sanctum* Linn. simplisia were obtained from CV. Merapi Herbal, Yogyakarta, Indonesia, and the species was identified at the Department of Biology, Gadjah Mada University (Yogyakarta, Indonesia). The ethanolic extract was obtained by a maceration technique. A total of 4000 mL of 96% ethanol (Merck, Darmstadt, Germany) was added to 300 g simplicia *Ocimum sanctum* Linn. The filtration results were concentrated using a vacuum rotary evaporator (Heidolph, Schwabach, Germany), and 8.82% *w/w* of *Ocimum sanctum* Linn. ethanol extract was obtained in the form of a paste.

2.2. Cell Maintenance

A-549 cells were grown in DMEM high-glucose medium (Gibco, Oslo, Norway) with 10% FBS (Gibco, Oslo, Norway) supplementation, penicillin–streptomycin 2% (Gibco, Oslo, Norway), and amphotericin B 0.5% (Gibco, Oslo, Norway) in T25/T75 flasks (Greiner, Frickenhausen, Germany) and then stored in an incubator (Sanyo, Tokyo, Japan) at 37 °C, with 5% CO_2. The medium was changed every three days and subcultured when in confluent conditions. Cells were harvested by accutase cell detachment (0.5 mM EDTA.4Na) (Gibco, Oslo, Norway) and grown in new flasks. Confluent cells that were not used for the experiment were stored frozen with a composition of 10% DMSO (Santa Cruz Biotechnology, Dallas, TX, USA) and 90% medium in a 1 mL cryo-vial, and then stored in a −80 °C freezer or cryotank.

2.3. Adhesion Assay Using Cell Counting Kit-8 Assay

The CCK test was carried out according to the manual of the CCK-8 Kit (Abbkine, Hubei, China). A quantity of 1.5 × 104 A-549 cells/100 mL was grown on a culture test 96-well plate (Greiner, Frickenhausen, Germany). Cells were incubated for 24 h, then divided into five groups, including the non-treated group (NT); AP3 80 µg/mL; ethanol extract of *Ocimum sanctum* Linn. (EEOS) at 50, 70, 100, or 200 g/mL; and cisplatin 9 g/mL. Each treatment was replicated three times. The treatments were incubated for 24 h, then 100 mL of water-soluble tetrazolium (WST-8) reagent was added to each sample and incubated for 4 h (in the dark). Then, the reaction was stopped by adding 100 mL/well of DMSO (Santa Cruz Biotechnology, Dallas, TX, USA). The results were read using an ELISA Reader (BioRad, Hercules, CA, USA) at a wavelength (λ) of 460 nm. The absorbance results obtained were then calculated using the following formula to obtain the percentage of viability.

$$\text{cell viability}(\%) = \frac{\text{treatment absorbsion} - \text{media absorbsion}}{\text{absorbsion cell control} - \text{media absorbsion}} \times 100\%$$

The final data were analyzed via one-way ANOVA using GraphPad Prism 7 software (La Jolla, CA, USA).

2.4. A549 Cell Lysate Preparation

A-549 cell lysate preparation was carried out according to the kit manual (Biomol, Hamburg, Germany). A total of 5 × 10^5 A-549 cells/mL were grown in each well on a tissue culture test 6-well plate and then incubated for 1 hour. The treatments in each well consisted of non-treatment (NT); AP3 80 µg/mL; ethanol extract of *Ocimum sanctum* Linn. (EEOS) at 50, 70, 100, or 200 g/mL; or cisplatin 9 g/mL, all followed by incubation for

24 h. The medium was aspirated and the plate was washed using Dulbecco's PBS (Gibco, Oslo, Norway), then 900 L of RIPA lysis buffer was added (Santa Cruz Biotechnology, Dallas, TX, USA), and the plate was shaken for 15 min. A cell scraper was used to remove the cells from the bottom of the plate. The lysate was transferred to 1.5 mL microtubes (Eppendorf, Hamburg, Germany). The lysate was centrifuged at 10,000× *g* for 10 min at 4 °C. The supernatant was transferred to 1.5 mL microtubes.

2.5. *Enzyme-Linked Immunosorbent Assay (ELISA)*

2.5.1. Integrin Human ITG αvβ3 dan VEGF

This test was carried out using sandwich ELISA for both human integrin αvβ3 and VEGF (Fine Test, Wuhan, China). The procedure was performed according to the manual in the kit (Fine Test, Wuhan, China). The plate was washed twice before adding the sample in the form of lysate, along with the negative control, to a 96-well plate. A total of 100 mL of sample and standard was added to each well and incubated for 90 min at 37 °C. The plate then washed for 2 times. A volume of 100 uL of biotin-labeled antibody was added to each well and incubated for 60 min at 37 °C. The plate then washed 3 times. Working solution of 100 mL HRP–streptavidin conjugate (SABC) was added to each well and incubated for 30 min at 37 °C, and the plate was then washed for 5 times. TMB substrate (90 mL) was added and incubated for 15–30 min at 37 °C. A 50 mL stop solution was added, and the well plates were immediately read at a wavelength of 450 nm (BioRad, Hercules, CA, USA).

2.5.2. Integrin Human ITG α5β1

The test was performed using competitive ELISA human integrin α5β1 (MyBiosource, San Diego, CA, USA). The procedure was carried out according to the manual in the kit (MyBiosource, San Diego, CA, USA). A total of 100 mL of standard and lysate sample was added to each, then 10 mL of balanced solution was added and homogenized; no bubbles were formed. A total of 50 mL of the conjugate was added in the well, then homogenized, and incubated at 37 °C for 60 min. After 60 min, we drained the liquid on the plate and washed it with wash buffer 5 times, for 1 minute each time. Volumes of 50 mL of substrates A and B were added to the wells. The plates were then closed tightly and incubated at 37 °C for 15 min. Stop solution (50 mL) was added, and the well plate was immediately read at a wavelength of 450 nm (BioRad, Hercules, CA, USA).

2.5.3. Enzyme-Linked Immunosorbent Assay (ELISA) Data Analysis

ELISA data analysis of human ITG αvβ3, human ITG α5β1, and vascular endothelial growth factor (VEGF) was carried out quantitatively using an ELISA reader to determine the optical density value of each test, then the concentration values were calculated based on the standard value. Data were analyzed via one-way ANOVA using the GraphPad Prism 7 software (La Jolla, CA, USA).

2.6. *Scratch Wound Healing Assay*

The scratch wound healing assay procedure was carried out based on [11]. A-549 cells at 2.5 × 104 cells/500 mL were grown on a culture test 12-well plate (Greiner, Frickenhausen, Germany). Cells were incubated for 24 h. Cells were rinsed with DMEM high-glucose three times. A sterile 200 mL pipette tip (Vertex, Boston, MA, USA) was used to make a scratch on the cell surface, then they were treated in groups, namely non-treated (NT); AP3 80 µg/mL; ethanol extract of *Ocimum sanctum* Linn. (EEOS) at graded concentrations of 50, 70, 100, and 200 g/mL; and cisplatin 9 g/mL. The treatments were incubated for 24 h in a CO_2 incubator at 37 °C, then observed after 24 h via inverted microscopy. Data analysis of the scratch wound healing assay to determine cell migration was carried out by measuring the surface area of the treated cells. Areas were calculated using the free software ImageJ (https://imagej.nih.gov/ij/, accessed on 4 April 2022) (National institute of Health-NIH,

Bethesda, MD, USA). We then calculated the percentage of the area covered according to the following formula:

$$\text{closing area} = \frac{(\text{area of 0th hour} - \text{24th hour area})}{\text{area of 0th hour}} \times 100\%$$

The final data were analyzed via one-way ANOVA using GraphPad Prism 7 software (La Jolla, CA, USA).

3. Results

3.1. *EEOS Inhibited the Adhesion of A549 (Non-Small Cell Lung Carcinoma)*

To analyze the ability of EEOS to inhibit cell attachment, A459 cells were cultured on a well plate and treated for 24 h with different concentrations of EEOS (50, 70, 100, and 200 µg/mL). Cisplatin was used as a positive control and to provide a comparison with commercial drugs. Our results show that EEOS inhibited the cell attachment of A549 cells in a dose-dependent manner. EEOS showed significant inhibition at the optimum concentration of 200 µg/mL, but the inhibition was not significant with 50 µg/mL of EEOS (Figure 1).

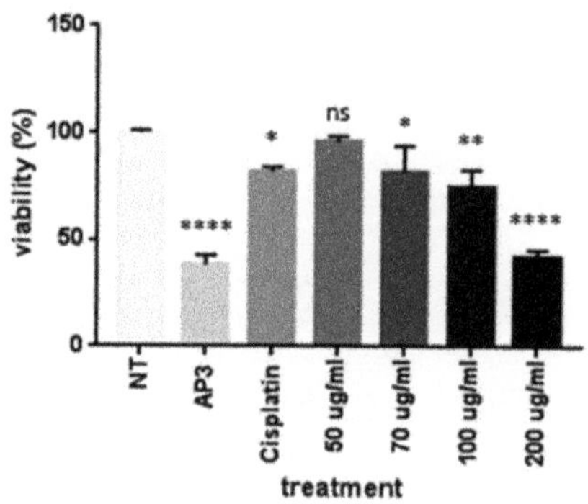

Figure 1. The ethanolic extract of *Ocimum sanctum* Linn. (EEOS) inhibited the adhesion of A549 cells (non-small cell lung carcinoma). The cells were cultivated in the presence of an inhibitor (AP3) as the positive control, cisplatin as the commercial drug comparison, and EEOS at concentrations of 50, 70, 100, and 200 µg/mL. After 24 h, EEOS's inhibitory effect was visualized using MTT reagent at a wavelength of 450 nm (NT: non-treated; * significant $p = 0.0332$; ** significant $p = 0.026$; **** significant $p < 0.0001$; ns = not significant).

3.2. *EEOS Inhibited the Cell Migration of A549 (Non-Small Cell Lung Carcinoma) after 24 h of Treatment*

The scratch wound healing assay is one of the most commonly used assays for assessing therapeutic impacts on cell migration. In this study, we found that EEOS significantly suppressed the cell migration of NSCLC (A549 cell line). We examined cell migration in response to the mechanical scratch wound. The cells were cultured in a well plate, and after confluence, the cells were treated with EEOS. After 24 h, the cell culture was observed under inverted microscopy. Images of scratch areas after 24 h (Figure 2) indicate that the untreated wounds were half closed within 24 h. To quantify the effects of putative migration inhibitors, the percentage of the open wound area after 24 h was determined (Figure 2). Our data clearly show that treatment with EEOS caused a significant inhibition of cell migration in a concentration-dependent manner.

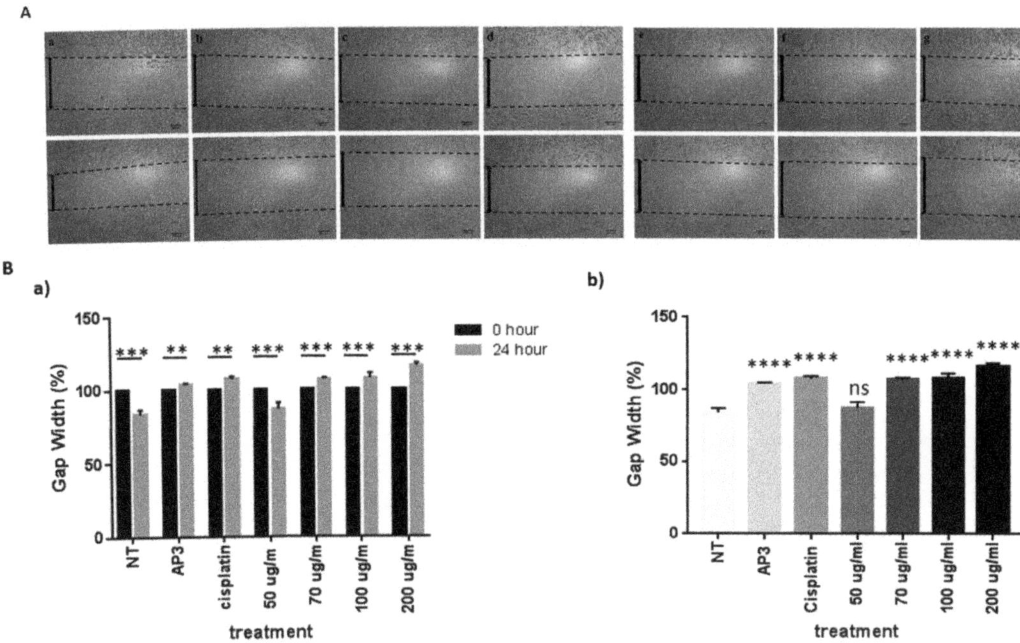

Figure 2. (**A**) Photomicroscopic images of A549 cells during the scratch wound healing assay. The cells were cultivated under normal conditions as non-treated cells (**a**), in the presence of an inhibitor (AP3) as the positive control (**b**), with cisplatin as the commercial drug comparison (**c**), and with EEOS at concentrations of 50 (**d**), 70 (**e**), 100 (**f**), and 200 g/mL (**e**). The wound healing was observed at the 0th hour and after 24 h. (**B**) Ethanolic extract of *Ocimum sanctum* Linn. reduced the migration ability of non-small cell lung carcinoma (A549), as shown by the scratch wound assay. The cells were cultivated in the presence of an inhibitor (AP3) as the positive control, cisplatin as the commercial drug comparison, and EEOS at concentrations of 50, 70, 100, and 200 g/mL. (**a**). The wound healing was observed at 0 h and after 24 h. (**b**). The wound healing after 24 h. Statistical analysis was performed via one-way ANOVA, followed by post hoc Tukey test (NT: non-treated; ** significant $p < 0.0060$; *** significant $p < 0.0009$; **** significant $p < 0.0001$; ns = not significant).

3.3. EEOS Inhibited Cell Migration of the A549 Cell Line (Non-Small Cell Line Carcinoma) by Suppressing the Concentrations of Integrin αvβ3, Integrin α5β1, and Vascular Endothelial Growth Factor (VEGF)

To strengthen the evidence regarding the effect of EEOS on cell migration, we performed ELISA on A549 cell lysates. The representative parameters observed were integrin αvβ3, integrin α5β1, and VEGF. The untreated A549 cells produced the highest concentration of integrin αvβ3, integrin α5β1, and VEGF. Additional treatment of A549 with EEOS diminished the integrin αvβ3, integrin α5β1, and VEGF concentrations in a dose-dependent manner. The integrin αvβ3 (Figure 3A), integrin α5β1 (Figure 3B), and VEGF (Figure 3C) concentrations were significantly suppressed under the optimum concentration of EEOS (200 μg/mL) and under cisplatin.

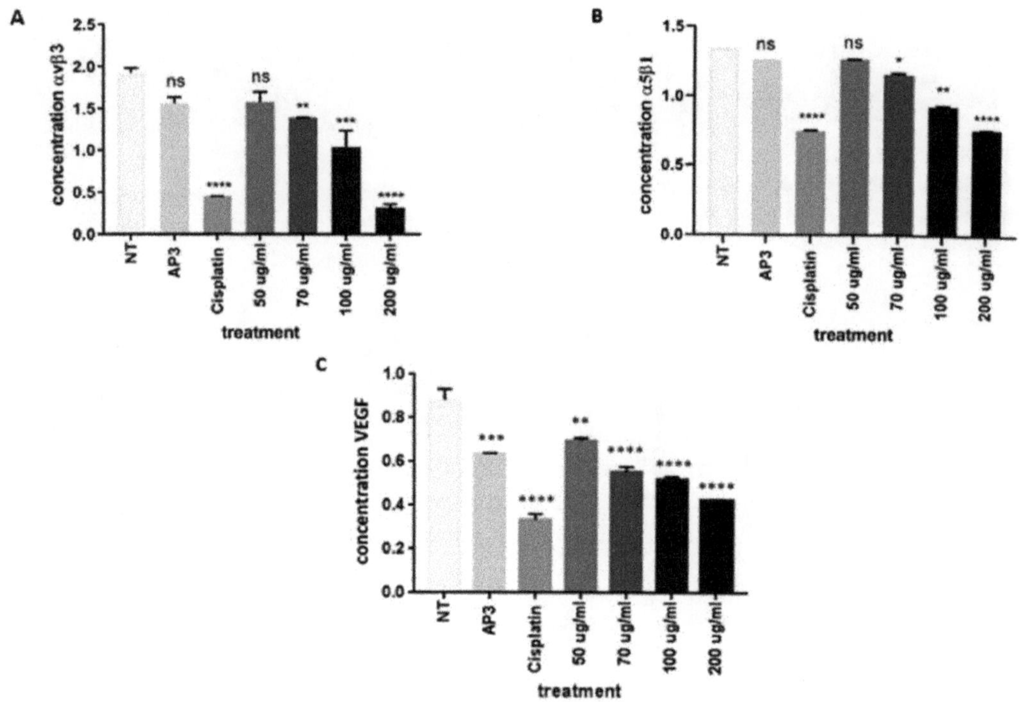

Figure 3. (**A**) The ethanolic extract of *Ocimum sanctum* Linn. decreased expression of non-small cell lung cancer (A549) integrin αvβ3, as shown by sandwich ELISA. The cells were cultivated in the presence of an inhibitor (AP3) as the positive control, cisplatin as the commercial drug comparison, and EEOS at concentrations of 50, 70, 100, and 200 g/mL for 24 h. A549 cells were then lysed and analyzed via ELISA for the concentration of αvβ3 integrin (ug/mL). Statistical analysis was performed via one-way ANOVA, followed by post hoc Tukey test (NT: non-treated; **, ***, and **** indicate statistically significant values for the non-treated group as a negative control compared with treatment, with *p*-values of 0.0085, 0.0004, and <0.0001, respectively; ns = not significant). (**B**) Ethanolic extract of *Ocimum sanctum* Linn. decreased expression of integrin α5β1 in non-small cell lung cancer (A549), as shown by competitive ELISA. The cells were cultivated in the presence of an inhibitor (AP3) as the positive control, cisplatin as the commercial drug comparison, and EEOS at concentrations of 50, 70, 100, and 200 g/mL for 24 h. A549 cells were then lysed and analyzed via ELISA for the concentration of α5β1 integrin (ug/mL). Statistical analysis was performed via one-way ANOVA, followed by post hoc Tukey test (NT: non-treated; *, **, and **** indicate statistically significant values for the non-treated group as a negative control compared with treatment, with *p*-values of 0.0348, 0.0027, and <0.0001, respectively; ns = not significant). (**C**) Ethanolic extract of *Ocimum sanctum* Linn. decreased expression of the non-small cell lung cancer (A549) integrin VEGF, as shown by sandwich ELISA. The cells were cultivated in the presence of an inhibitor (AP3) as the positive control, cisplatin as the commercial drug comparison, and EEOS at concentrations of 50, 70, 100, and 200 g/mL for 24 h. A549 cells were then lysed and analyzed via ELISA for the concentration of VEGF ((ug/mL). Statistical analysis was performed via one-way ANOVA, followed by post hoc Tukey test (NT: non-treated; **, *** and **** indicate statistical significance of the non-treated group as a negative control compared with treatment, with *p*-values of 0.0012, 0.0002, and <0.0001, respectively; ns = not significant).

4. Discussion

Cancer has properties such as evading cell death, sustaining proliferation, inducing vasculature, and activating invasion and metastasis [12]. In the process of malignancy, tumor cells will migrate to other organs through blood vessels and lymph vessels and grow in the appropriate organs; this process is called metastasis. Cell–cell and cell–extracellular matrix (ECM) adhesions play a fundamental role in governing the structural integrity of healthy tissue and in regulating cellular morphology, migration, proliferation, survival, and differentiation events [13]. In the classic view of malignant transformation in the epithelium, cells lose their dependence on integrin-mediated interactions with the extracellular matrix and the resulting signaling [14]. In the process of metastasis, tumor cells will migrate to find the best place to maintain their function. Cell migration, invasion, and adhesion are pivotal steps in this process [15,16].

In this study, we observed the ability of EEOS to prevent the adhesion of the A549 cell line. The CCK-8 test chart showed a decrease in the adhesion ability of A549 cells treated with EEOS (Figure 1). The results of this study add to the information from previous studies that EEOS can reduce the adhesion ability of A549 cells, as shown via adhesion assay [8]. We also performed scratch wound healing assay to investigate the migration ability of the A549 cell line. Our data show that EEOS also has the ability to inhibit A549 cell migration (Figure 2A,B). The ability of tumor cells to adhere and migrate is closely related to the process of tumor progression and metastasis, which is responsible for 90% of cancer-related deaths [17]. The phytochemical compounds in EEOS were previously dialyzed using thin-layer chromatography (TLS) and UV–vis spectrophotometry. The results of the analysis showed that EEOS contains several active compounds, such as flavonoids, phenols, saponins, alkaloids, tannins, terpenoids, and steroids [18]. Flavonoids and phenols have important roles as anti-cancer and cytotoxic agents, inducing apoptosis in cancer cells [19]. In silico molecular docking was also performed to predict the chemical binding between active compounds and protein. In silico molecular docking analysis of the flavonoid compounds (quercetin) and flavonoids (eugenol) showed that these active compounds can bind to the active site of integrins and VEGF, thereby inhibiting the activity of integrins and VEGF for adhesion, cell spread, and blood vessel formation [20]. The inhibition of active compounds with integrin complexes will have an impact on the inhibition of the extracellular matrix (ECM) adhesion process and result in a decrease in tumor cell invasion. In vitro results on the cell line A549 also showed consistent results that the content of active compounds in EEOS can reduce the viability of the A549 cell line.

To elucidate this mechanism, we also examined the expression of integrin $\alpha v\beta 3$, integrin $\alpha 5\beta 1$, and VEGF as biochemical cues for blood vessel formation, adhesion, and migration of cancer cells. We found that EEOS reduced the concentrations of integrin $\alpha v\beta 3$, integrin $\alpha 5\beta 1$, and VEGF in the A549 cell line (Figure 3A–C). Integrins are transmembrane adhesion receptors for the extracellular matrix (ECM) and have essential roles, including sensing and adhering to the extracellular environment to maintain global tissue architecture and multicellularity [21]. Integrins are the major class of receptors in adhesive events, acting by bi-directionally (inside-out and outside-in) transducing biochemical signals and mechanical force across the plasma membrane [22]. Integrins play a key role in single-cell migration and act via conformational changes in the extracellular matrix (outside-in) or intracellular protein that are triggered by altering the affinity of integrins (inside-out). These changes recruit cytoskeletal linker proteins to remodel nascent or focal adhesions and generate tension; these adherent structures generate forces of cellular movement. There are several pathways by which integrin can mediate cell spreading and migration and one of them involves focal adhesion kinase and the capacity of tyrosine-protein kinase Src to up-regulate integrin expression [23].

The integrins αvβ3 and α5β1 have roles as adhesion molecules in cell-to-cell interactions and motility-supporting roles that promote cell migration during nervous system development, and they also promote metastatic spread [24]. Integrin αvβ3 is mostly expressed on angiogenic endothelial cells in remodeling and pathological tissues. Expression of the αvβ3 integrin by endothelial cells promotes cell adhesion to the ECM, cell migration, and angiogenesis, along with angiogenic growth factors, including VEGF/VEGFR [25]. The α5β1 integrin is also overexpressed in, and closely related with, metastatic events. In normal endothelial cells, α5β1 will be expressed at very low levels, but this expression will be significantly increased in endothelial cells during cancer cell angiogenesis [26]. Integrin expression and activation directly influence human malignancies. Due to their broad impact in malignant transformations, they are considered potential targets for cancer therapy [27]. Integrins are considered as pharmacological targets for drugs by inhibiting several key processes in cancer development, such as cell proliferation, survival, and migration. Targeting integrins to enhance the delivery of anti-tumor agents or to delineate cancerous lesions is a new and promising approach. Integrin-inhibiting anticancer drugs have been conceived for their ability to impair ligand binding [28].

In addition to integrin expression, VEGF expression has been confirmed to be a critical pathological factor in the occurrence of NSCLC by increasing vascular permeability and increasing angiogenesis [29]. This study confirmed that EEOS has the ability to inhibit A549 cell angiogenesis by inhibiting tube formation, as shown through the angiogenesis assay [9] and reducing VEGF concentrations. During angiogenesis, VEGF has an associated mechanism with integrins, as integrins are overexpressed on the endothelial cell surface to facilitate the growth and survival of new vessels [25]. The supply of oxygen and nutrients to cells through blood vessels is the most important aspect in the survival of cells, including cancer cells. Vascular endothelial growth factor (VEGF) is a homodimeric glycoprotein from the endothelial growth factor family and is an important factor in the formation and regulation of angiogenesis processes [30]; in addition, VEGF has biological roles in the regulation of vascular permeability, metabolism, immune system, inflammation, and neurological function [31]. Tumors can generate their own vascular system. VEGF acts as an angiogenic factor by promoting their proliferation, migration, adhesion, and survival. VEGF may, thus, play a role in vascular invasion [32]. Furthermore, VEGF also play role in targeting other cells in the tumor microenvironment, as well as initiating the function of growth factors and integrin, mainly svb3 and a5b1 [33–35]. In recent years, the inhibition expression of VEGF has been utilized in tumor-targeted therapy [34].

Taken together, our findings underline the ability of the ethanolic extract of *Ocimum sanctum* Linn. to prevent the migration and metastasis of human lung adenocarcinoma cells (A549); however, more research and discussion are required, since our research was limited only to the role of integrin αvβ3, integrin α5β1, and VEGF. Moreover, the data derived from the in vitro analysis demonstrate the direct impact on the cells (Figure 4). Furthermore, in vivo experiments are needed as basic data to complete the preclinical phase of this analysis.

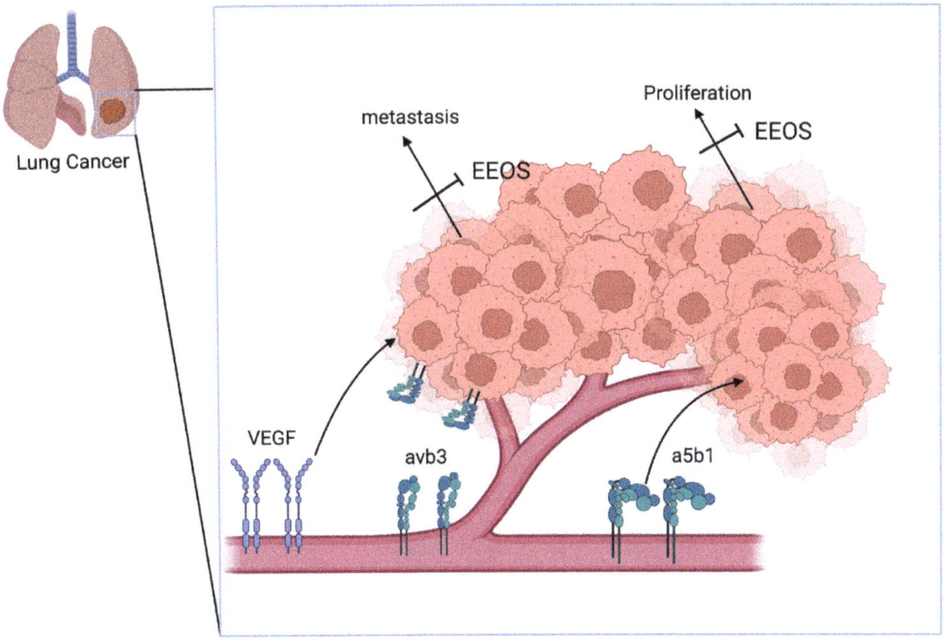

Figure 4. Schematic overview of the mechanism of *Ocimum sanctum* Linn. ethanolic extract, inhibiting the adhesion, proliferation, and migration of A549 human lung adenocarcinoma, mediated by the downregulation of $\alpha v\beta 3$, $\alpha 5\beta 1$, and VEGF. Overall, inhibition by EEOS will mitigate angiogenesis and metastasis of human lung adenocarcinoma cells.

5. Conclusions

Our findings demonstrate that EEOS disturbed the proliferation, angiogenesis, and migration of A549 cells, which may result from the disruption of cell adhesion and migration, as shown by the CCK-8 assay and scratch wound healing assay, as a consequence of the downregulation of $\alpha v\beta 3$ integrins, $\alpha 5\beta 1$ integrins, and VEGF. As a result, EEOS may represent a good therapeutic candidate for the treatment of lung adenocarcinoma. Further studies using in vivo methods are required to fully validate our findings in human lung adenocarcinoma growth.

Author Contributions: Conceptualization, H.W. and D.L.K.; Methodology, H.W. and D.L.K.; Software, U.K.; Validation, H.W. and U.K.; formal analysis, U.K., H.W. and S.K.; Investigation, U.K., H.W. and D.A.A.N.; Resources, H.W., D.L.K. and D.A.A.N.; Data Curation, U.K., D.L.K. and H.W.; Writing—Original Draft Preparation, H.W. and U.K.; Writing—Review and Editing, H.W., S.E., S.K., D.A.A.N. and D.L.K.; Visualization, H.W.; Supervision, H.W. and D.L.K. Project Administration, H.W. and D.L.K.; Funding Acquisition, H.W. All authors have read and agreed to the published version of the manuscript.

Funding: The research was funded by the Ministry of Education, Culture, Research and Technology for the PDUPT Grant Universitas Gadjah Mada, with the grant number 1703/UN1/DITLIT/DITLIT/PT.01.02/2022.

Institutional Review Board Statement: The experimental procedures were approved by the Ethical Committee of the Faculty of Veterinary Medicine, Universitas Gadjah Mada, Yogyakarta, Indonesia (approval number 00057/EC-FKH/Int./2021).

Informed Consent Statement: Not applicable.

Data Availability Statement: Not applicable.

Acknowledgments: The authors would like to thank the Ministry of Education, Culture, Research and Technology for the research funding (Basic Research) with the grant number 1703/UN1/DITLIT/DITLIT/PT.01.02/2022. The authors also thank the Pharmacology Laboratory, Faculty of Medicine, Public Health and Nursing, Universitas Gadjah Mada, and Mosa Rini Nurul H. for their excellent technical assistance.

Conflicts of Interest: The authors declare no conflict of interest.

References

1. Wulandari, L.; Febriani, A.; Fatmawati, F.; Soegiarto, G. Evaluation of Patients with Lung Cancer Treated with Epidermal Growth Factor Receptor–Tyrosine Kinase Inhibitor. *Asian J. Oncol.* **2018**, *4*, 48–53. [CrossRef]
2. Saba, N.; Khuri, F. The Role of Bisphosphonates in the Management of Advanced Cancer with a Focus on Non-Small-Cell Lung Cancer—Part I: Mechanisms of Action, Role of Biomarkers and Preclinical Applications. *Oncology* **2005**, *68*, 10–17. [CrossRef] [PubMed]
3. Hellmann, M.D.; Paz-Ares, L.; Bernabe Caro, R.; Zurawski, B.; Kim, S.-W.; Carcereny Costa, E.; Park, K.; Alexandru, A.; Lupinacci, L.; de la Mora Jimenez, E.; et al. Nivolumab plus Ipilimumab in Advanced Non–Small-Cell Lung Cancer. *N. Engl. J. Med.* **2019**, *381*, 2020–2031. [CrossRef]
4. Park, J.; Jeong, D.; Song, M.; Kim, B. Antioxidants Recent Advances in Anti-Metastatic Approaches of Herbal Medicines in 5 Major Cancers: From Traditional Medicine to Modern Drug Discovery. *Antioxidants* **2021**, *10*, 527. [CrossRef] [PubMed]
5. Garcia-Oliveira, P.; Fraga-Corral, M.; Pereira, A.G.; Lourenço-Lopes, C.; Jimenez-Lopez, C.; Prieto, M.A.; Simal-Gandara, J. Scientific Basis for the Industrialization of Traditionally Used Plants of the Rosaceae Family. *Food Chem.* **2020**, *330*, 127197. [CrossRef]
6. Redondo-Blanco, S.; Fernández, J.; Gutiérrez-del-Río, I.; Villar, C.J.; Lombó, F. New Insights toward Colorectal Cancer Chemotherapy Using Natural Bioactive Compounds. *Front. Pharmacol.* **2017**, *8*, 109. [CrossRef]
7. Magesh, V.; Lee, J.-C.; Ahn, K.S.; Lee, H.-J.; Lee, H.-J.; Lee, E.-O.; Jung, H.J.; Kim, J.S.; Kim, D.K.; Choi, S.-H.; et al. *Ocimum sanctum* Induces Apoptosis in A549 Lung Cancer Cells and Suppresses the In Vivo Growth of Lewis Lung Carcinoma Cells. *Phytother. Res.* **2009**, *23*, 1385–1391. [CrossRef]
8. Wihadmadyatami, H.; Karnati, S.; Hening, P.; Tjahjono, Y.; Rizal; Maharjanti, F.; Kusindarta, D.L.; Triyono, T.; Supriatno. Ethanolic Extract *Ocimum sanctum* Linn. Induces an Apoptosis in Human Lung Adenocarcinoma (A549) Cells. *Heliyon* **2019**, *5*, e02772. [CrossRef]
9. Wihadmadyatami, H.; Hening, P.; Kustiati, U.; Kusindarta, D.L.; Triyono, T.; Supriatno, S. *Ocimum sanctum* Linn. Ethanolic Extract Inhibits Angiogenesis in Human Lung Adenocarcinoma (A549) Cells. *Vet. World* **2020**, *13*, 2028–2032. [CrossRef]
10. Kim, S.C.; Magesh, V.; Jeong, S.J.; Lee, H.J.; Ahn, K.S.; Lee, H.J.; Lee, E.O.; Kim, S.H.; Lee, M.H.; Kim, J.H.; et al. Ethanol Extract of *Ocimum sanctum* Exerts Anti-Metastatic Activity through Inactivation of Matrix Metalloproteinase-9 and Enhancement of Anti-Oxidant Enzymes. *Food Chem. Toxicol.* **2010**, *48*, 1478–1482. [CrossRef]
11. Martinotti, S.; Ranzato, E. Scratch Wound Healing Assay. In *Methods in Molecular Biology*; Humana Press: Totowa, NJ, USA, 2020; Volume 2109, pp. 225–229.
12. Hanahan, D. Hallmarks of Cancer: New Dimensions. *Cancer Discov.* **2022**, *12*, 31–46. [CrossRef] [PubMed]
13. Abduljauwad, S.N.; Ahmed, H.u.R. Enhancing Cancer Cell Adhesion with Clay Nanoparticles for Countering Metastasis. *Sci. Rep.* **2019**, *9*, 5935. [CrossRef] [PubMed]
14. Janiszewska, M.; Primi, M.C.; Izard, T. Cell Adhesion in Cancer: Beyond the Migration of Single Cells. *J. Biol. Chem.* **2020**, *295*, 2495–2505. [CrossRef] [PubMed]
15. Pijuan, J.; Barceló, C.; Moreno, D.F.; Maiques, O.; Sisó, P.; Marti, R.M.; Macià, A.; Panosa, A. In Vitro Cell Migration, Invasion, and Adhesion Assays: From Cell Imaging to Data Analysis. *Front. Cell Dev. Biol.* **2019**, *7*, 107. [CrossRef]
16. Xu, L.; Gordon, R.; Farmer, R.; Pattanayak, A.; Binkowski, A.; Huang, X.; Avram, M.; Krishna, S.; Voll, E.; Pavese, J.; et al. Precision Therapeutic Targeting of Human Cancer Cell Motility. *Nat. Commun.* **2018**, *9*, 2454. [CrossRef]
17. Campbell, K.; Rossi, F.; Adams, J.; Pitsidianaki, I.; Barriga, F.M.; Garcia-Gerique, L.; Batlle, E.; Casanova, J.; Casali, A. Collective Cell Migration and Metastases Induced by an Epithelial-to-Mesenchymal Transition in Drosophila Intestinal Tumors. *Nat. Commun.* **2019**, *10*, 2311. [CrossRef]
18. Kustiati, U.; Wihadmadyatami, H.; Kusindarta, D.L. Dataset of Phytochemical and Secondary Metabolite Profiling of Holy Basil Leaf (*Ocimum sanctum* Linn) Ethanolic Extract Using Spectrophotometry, Thin Layer Chromatography, Fourier Transform Infrared Spectroscopy, and Nuclear Magnetic Resonance. *Data Brief* **2022**, *40*, 107774. [CrossRef]
19. Abotaleb, M.; Samuel, S.M.; Varghese, E.; Varghese, S.; Kubatka, P.; Liskova, A.; Büsselberg, D. Flavonoids in Cancer and Apoptosis. *Cancers* **2019**, *11*, 28. [CrossRef]
20. Kustiati, U.; Dewi Ratih, T.S.; Dwi Aris Agung, N.; Kusindarta, D.L.; Wihadmadyatami, H. In Silico Molecular Docking and in Vitro Analysis of Ethanolic Extract *Ocimum sanctum* Linn.: Inhibitory and Apoptotic Effects against Non-Small Cell Lung Cancer. *Vet. World* **2021**, *14*, 3175–3187. [CrossRef]
21. Kadry, Y.A.; Calderwood, D.A. Chapter 22: Structural and Signaling Functions of Integrins. *Biochim. Biophys. Acta Biomembr.* **2020**, *1862*, 183206. [CrossRef]

22. Bachmann, M.; Kukkurainen, S.; Hytönen, V.P.; Wehrle-Haller, B. Cell adhesion by integrins. *Physiol. Rev.* **2019**, *99*, 1655–1699. [CrossRef] [PubMed]
23. de Pascalis, C.; Etienne-Manneville, S. Single and Collective Cell Migration: The Mechanics of Adhesions. *Mol. Biol. Cell* **2017**, *28*, 1833–1846. [CrossRef] [PubMed]
24. Sökeland, G.; Schumacher, U. The Functional Role of Integrins during Intra- and Extravasation within the Metastatic Cascade. *Mol. Cancer* **2019**, *18*, 12. [CrossRef]
25. Weis, S.M.; Cheresh, D.A. Av Integrins in Angiogenesis and Cancer. *Cold Spring Harb. Perspect. Med.* **2011**, *1*, a006478. [CrossRef]
26. Zhu, H.; Chen, A.; Li, S.; Tao, X.; Sheng, B.; Chetry, M.; Zhu, X. Predictive Role of Galectin-1 and Integrin A5β1 in Cisplatin-Based Neoadjuvant Chemotherapy of Bulky Squamous Cervical Cancer. *Biosci. Rep.* **2017**, *37*, BSR20170958. [CrossRef] [PubMed]
27. Harjunpää, H.; Asens, M.L.; Guenther, C.; Fagerholm, S.C. Cell Adhesion Molecules and Their Roles and Regulation in the Immune and Tumor Microenvironment. *Front. Immunol.* **2019**, *10*, 1078. [CrossRef]
28. Valdembri, D.; Serini, G. The Roles of Integrins in Cancer. *Fac. Rev.* **2021**, *10*, 45. [CrossRef]
29. Zhang, J.; Liu, J.; Zhu, C.; He, J.; Chen, J.; Liang, Y.; Yang, F.; Wu, X.; Ma, X. Prognostic Role of Vascular Endothelial Growth Factor in Cervical Cancer: A Meta-Analysis. *Oncotarget* **2017**, *8*, 24797–24803. [CrossRef]
30. Chen, Y.; Mathy, N.W.; Lu, H. The Role of VEGF in the Diagnosis and Treatment of Malignant Pleural Effusion in Patients with Non-Small Cell Lung Cancer (Review). *Mol. Med. Rep.* **2018**, *17*, 8019–8030. [CrossRef]
31. Yang, Y.; Cao, Y. The Impact of VEGF on Cancer Metastasis and Systemic Disease. *Semin. Cancer Biol.* **2022**, *86*, 251–261. [CrossRef]
32. Zhang, L.; Wang, J.N.; Tang, J.M.; Kong, X.; Yang, J.Y.; Zheng, F.; Guo, L.Y.; Huang, Y.Z.; Zhang, L.; Tian, L.; et al. VEGF Is Essential for the Growth and Migration of Human Hepatocellular Carcinoma Cells. *Mol. Biol. Rep.* **2012**, *39*, 5085–5093. [CrossRef] [PubMed]
33. Lino, R.; Dos Santos, L.B.; Pisani, P.K.; Altei, G.F.D.; Cominetti, W.F.; Selistre-de-Araújo, H.S. Alphavbeta3 integrin blocking inhibits apoptosis and induces autophagy in murine breast tumor cells. Biochimica et Biophysica Acta (BBA)—Molecular Cell Research. *Biochim. Biophys. Acta Mol. Cell Res.* **2019**, *12*, 118536. [CrossRef] [PubMed]
34. Goel, H.L.; Mercurio, A.M. VEGF targets the tumour cell. *Nat. Rev. Cancer* **2013**, *12*, 871–882. [CrossRef] [PubMed]
35. Hou, J.; Yan, D.; Liu, Y.; Huang, P.; Cui, H. The Roles of Integrin α5β1 in Human Cancer. *Onco Targets Ther.* **2020**, *13*, 13329–13344. [CrossRef] [PubMed]

cancers

MDPI

Article

Libertellenone T, a Novel Compound Isolated from Endolichenic Fungus, Induces G2/M Phase Arrest, Apoptosis, and Autophagy by Activating the ROS/JNK Pathway in Colorectal Cancer Cells

Chathurika D. B. Gamage [1], Jeong-Hyeon Kim [2], Yi Yang [1], İsa Taş [1], So-Yeon Park [1], Rui Zhou [1], Sultan Pulat [1], Mücahit Varlı [1], Jae-Seoun Hur [3], Sang-Jip Nam [2,*] and Hangun Kim [1,*]

[1] College of Pharmacy and Research Institute of Life and Pharmaceutical Sciences, Sunchon National University, 255 Jungang-ro, Sunchon, Jeonnam 57922, Republic of Korea
[2] Department of Chemistry and Nanoscience, Ewha Womans University, Seoul 03760, Republic of Korea
[3] Korean Lichen Research Institute, Sunchon National University, 255 Jungang-ro, Sunchon, Jeonnam 57922, Republic of Korea
* Correspondence: sjnam@ewha.ac.kr (S.-J.N.); hangunkim@sunchon.ac.kr (H.K.)

Simple Summary: Libertellenone T (**B**) is a natural product derived from the secondary metabolites of the endolichenic fungus, *Pseudoplectania* sp. In this study, we investigated the underlying molecular mechanisms that induce the apoptotic cell death of the colorectal cancer cell line, Caco2, in response to **B**. Our findings demonstrate that **B** induces Caco2 cell apoptosis via G2/M phase arrest and activation of ROS/JNK signaling. Moreover, **B** exhibited excellent synergistic effects when combined with the known and novel anticancer agents 5-FU and compound D, respectively. In light of this investigation, we propose that **B** is a promising potential chemotherapeutic agent against colorectal cancer.

Abstract: Colorectal cancer (CRC) is the third most deadly type of cancer in the world and continuous investigations are required to discover novel therapeutics for CRC. Induction of apoptosis is one of the promising strategies to inhibit cancers. Here, we have identified a novel compound, Libertellenone T (**B**), isolated from crude extracts of the endolichenic fungus from *Pseudoplectania* sp. (EL000327) and investigated the mechanism of action. CRC cells treated by **B** were subjected to apoptosis detection assays, immunofluorescence imaging, and molecular analyses such as immunoblotting and QRT-PCR. Our findings revealed that **B** induced CRC cell death via multiple mechanisms including G2/M phase arrest caused by microtubule stabilization and caspase-dependent apoptosis. Further studies revealed that **B** induced the generation of reactive oxygen species (ROS) attributed to activating the JNK signaling pathway by which apoptosis and autophagy was induced in Caco2 cells. Moreover, **B** exhibited good synergistic effects when combined with the well-known anticancer drug, 5-FU, and another cytotoxic novel compound D, which was isolated from the same crude extract of EL000327. Overall, Libertellenone T induces G2/M phase arrest, apoptosis, and autophagy via activating the ROS/JNK pathway in CRC. Thus, **B** may be a potential anticancer therapeutic against CRC that is suitable for clinical applications.

Keywords: CRC; Libertellenone T; G2/M phase arrest; apoptosis; autophagy; ROS/JNK signaling

Citation: Gamage, C.D.B.; Kim, J.-H.; Yang, Y.; Taş, İ.; Park, S.-Y.; Zhou, R.; Pulat, S.; Varlı, M.; Hur, J.-S.; Nam, S.-J.; et al. Libertellenone T, a Novel Compound Isolated from Endolichenic Fungus, Induces G2/M Phase Arrest, Apoptosis, and Autophagy by Activating the ROS/JNK Pathway in Colorectal Cancer Cells. *Cancers* **2023**, *15*, 489. https://doi.org/10.3390/cancers15020489

Academic Editors: Barbara De Filippis, Alessandra Ammazzalorso and Marialuigia Fantacuzzi

Received: 28 November 2022
Revised: 10 January 2023
Accepted: 11 January 2023
Published: 12 January 2023

1. Introduction

An abnormal cell growth that occurs in the colon or rectum is simply recognized as colorectal cancer (CRC). A noncancerous cell growth, known as a polyp, can develop in the mucosal layer of the colon or rectum, and may develop into CRC. Less than 10% of polyps have a high potential to progress into invasive cancer over 10–20 years. CRC occurs predominantly in adults aged 50 and older [1]. In 2020, CRC was recognized as the third most common cancer type worldwide and the second most common cause of cancer death. Geographically, the occurrence of CRC is highest in Asian regions. The International Agency for Research on Cancer (IARC) estimated that the global burden of CRC will increase by 56%, and CRC related mortality will increase by 69% between 2020 and 2040 [2]. Therefore, a strong research focus on the discovery of novel anticancer therapeutics is urgently required.

Many scientists have focused their attention on the development of innovative drugs derived from natural sources such as plants, lichens, and micro-organisms over a few decades. A lichen is a symbiotic living form associated with a fungus (mycobiont) and a cyanobacterium or green alga (the photobiont), or both [2]. Some endolichenic fungi (ELF) reside inside the lichen thalli and produce bioactive secondary metabolites with medicinal and economic potential. These secondary metabolites show cytotoxic, antioxidant, antifungal, and antibacterial bioactivities, which are crucial in drug development in the pharmaceutical industry [3,4]. Therefore, the ability of ELF to produce unique secondary metabolites with anti-cancer properties provides a novel opportunity to identify effective cancer therapeutics [5–7]. Libertellenone T (**B**) is a novel cytotoxic compound isolated from secondary metabolites extracted from the endolichenic fungus, EL000327, from *Pseudoplectania* sp. found in the lichen *Graphis*, collected from Hallasan in Jeju Island, South Korea in 2009.

Many chemotherapeutics exert cytotoxicity and trigger cancer cell death via inducing apoptosis in cells. Apoptosis, or programmed cell death, is a cell suicide process that activates when their continuous survival is blocked [8]. Morphological and biochemical changes such as chromatin condensation, nuclear fragmentation, cell shrinkage, membrane blebbing, DNA, protein breakdown, and caspase activation can be observed in apoptotic cells. Cancer cells evade natural cell death as a result of genetic mutations acquired during transformation from normal cells to malignant cells. Disruption of the balance between pro-apoptotic and anti-apoptotic proteins, reduction in caspase function, and impairment of death receptor signaling all cause apoptosis resistance in cancer cells [9]. Therefore, restoration of these functions by therapeutics can successfully prevent cancer progression. Furthermore, alterations that occur in cell cycle regulators at check points cause abnormal cell proliferation in cancers [10]. Thus, the induction of G2/M phase arrest is another target of many anti-cancer agents. Controlling cell progression through the cell cycle by regulating related proteins or disrupting tubulin organization eventually leads cells to G2/M phase arrest and subsequent cell death [11,12].

Autophagy (macroautophagy) mainly involves the formation of an autophagosome by engulfing damaged organelles, fusion with lysosome, and degradation of cellular debris by lysosomal hydrolase [13,14]. Autophagy plays a paradoxical role in cancer progression. In the early stage of many cancers, autophagy acts as a tumor suppressor by protecting cell homeostasis. Conversely, autophagy promotes tumor growth in more advanced stages of cancer by increasing stress tolerance [15]. Many anticancer therapeutics are known to activate autophagy concurrently with apoptosis. This activation of autophagy can either promote or suppress cancer cell survival. Therefore, the role of autophagy is crucial in anticancer drug development [16]. Furthermore, the relationship between autophagy and apoptosis is unclear and yet to be investigated.

Reactive oxygen species (ROS) are highly reactive and short-lived small molecules in the form of free radicals [17]. ROS support many physiological functions in cells under optimum conditions. However, the over production of ROS can have a deleterious effect on cells and trigger oxidative stress. The generation of ROS can be triggered by both endogenous and exogenous sources such as mitochondrial transport chain leakage, high metabolic rate, environmental pollutants, radiation, and drugs [18]. ROS are responsible for activating many cellular signaling pathways that lead to cell survival or cell death including autophagy, apoptosis, and necrosis. c-Jun N-terminal kinase (JNK) signaling is activated in response to ER stress or activation of the mitochondrial pathway of apoptosis by ROS [19].

In this study, we investigated the possible mechanisms underlying the impact of **B** on CRC cells. We selected four CRC cell lines, HCT116, DLD1, HT29, and Caco2, harboring different genetic mutations and status of microsatellite instability, to evaluate the effect of **B** on them. HCT116 is a microsatellite instable (MSI) cell line with KRAS and PIK3CA mutations. DLD1 is the MSI cell line, harboring KRAS, PIK3CA, and TP53 mutations. HT29 is microsatellite stable (MSS), and BRAF and PIK3CA are muted cell lines, while Caco2 is MSS and the wild type of KRAS PIK3CA, TP53 [20]. Furthermore, we demonstrated that **B** induced mitotic arrest, apoptosis, and autophagy via activating the ROS/JNK signaling pathway. In addition, we found that **B**-induced autophagy promotes cell survival. Furthermore, **B** exhibited synergy not only with the known anticancer drug *5-Fluorouracil* (5-FU), but also with a novel compound D. Collectively, our data suggest that **B** is a potential candidate as an anticancer therapeutic with clinical application.

2. Materials and Methods

2.1. Fungal Strain

Lichen specimens of *Graphis* were collected from Hallasan in Jeju Island, South Korea in 2009. Voucher specimen was deposited in the Korean Lichen Research Institute, Sunchon National University, Korea. The endolichenic fungus EL000327 was isolated with the surface sterilization method [21].

2.2. ITS Sequencing

EL000327 was cultured for 2–3 weeks on potato dextrose agar (PDA) medium at 25 °C. The total DNA was extracted following the manufacturer's instructions from EL000327 using the DNeasy Plant Mini Kit (Qiagen, Hilden, Germany). Universal primers ITS1F (5'-CTTGGTCATTTAGAGGAAGTAA-3') [22] and LR5 (5'-ATCCTGAGGGAAACTTC-3') [23] were amplified with the internal transcribed spacer (ITS) region of the rDNA gene of EL000327 and ITS sequencing was performed as described [5] (Table S1).

2.3. Preparation of Secondary Metabolite Extract of EL000327

EL000327 was cultured on potato dextrose agar (PDA) medium at 25 °C for approximately 2–3 weeks until visible colonies were evident. ELF mycelia grown on agar were cut and inoculated into 200 mL potato dextrose broth (PDB) in 500 mL Erlenmeyer flasks (3 L) and incubated at 25 °C in a shaking incubator at 150 rpm for approximately 3–4 weeks. Then, 200 mL ethyl acetate (EA) was added to each flask, and the flask was shaken for approximately 2 h. Each culture was then filtered to separate the filtrate and mycelia. The filtrate was separated into water- and EA-soluble layers by allowing the filtrate to stand in a separating funnel. A total of 5.8 g of crude extracts of EL000327 was obtained by evaporating EA to dryness under a vacuum using a rotary evaporator. The crude extract was dissolved in 100% DMSO for use in experiments.

2.4. Isolation, Purification, and Identification of Chemical Structure of Compound B

The crude extract (5.8 g) was subjected to open column chromatography purification on a RP C18 flash column by the step gradient elution of methanol/H_2O from 20% to 100% of methanol, subsequently, to afford eight fractions (labeled 327-F1 ~ 327-F8). Fraction 327-F2 (360 mg) (H_2O:MeOH = 60:40) was purified by reversed-phase HPLC (Phenomenex Luna C-18 (2), 250 × 100 mm, 2.0 mL/min, 5 μm, 100 Å, UV = 254 nm) (Figure S8) using an isocratic solvent system with 47% acetonitrile in water to yield 7β-9α-dihydroxy-1,8(14),15-pimaratrien-3,11-dione (B, 95 mg, purity: 96.7%) as pink oil. ^{1}H NMR (400 MHz, CD_3OD) δ: 7.25 (d, J = 10.4 Hz, 1H), 6.02 (d, J = 2.2 Hz, 1H), 5.93 (d, J = 10.4 Hz, 1H), 5.74 (dd, J = 17.2, 10.4 Hz, 1H), 4.99 (dd, J = 17.3, 0.9 Hz, 1H), 4.95 (dd, J = 10.4, 0.9 Hz, 1H), 4.40 (m, 1H), 1.29 (s, 3H), 1.20 (s, 3H), 1.18 (s, 3H); ^{13}C NMR (100 MHz, CD_3OD) δ: 212.1, 206.3, 159.5, 145.4, 141.5, 130.9, 128.8, 69.6, 54.0, 45.7, 45.3, 43.2, 42.9, 33.2, 28.5, 28.1, 22.8, 20.8. HR-FAB-MS m/z $[M+H]^+$ 331.1904 (calcd. for $C_{20}H_{27}O_4$, 331.1909) (Figures S6 and S7).

2.5. Cell Culture

Human CRC cell lines HT29, HCT116, DLD1, Caco2, colon stemness cancer cell line; CSC221, human gastric cancer cell lines; AGS, TMK1, human prostate cancer cell line; RV1, human lung cancer cell line; A549, mouse colon cancer cell line; CT26 and canine kidney epithelial cell line; and MDCK were purchased from the Korean Cell Line Bank (Seoul, Korea). Cells were cultured in DMEM or RPMI culture medium (GenDEPOT, Katy, TX, USA) supplemented with 10% fetal bovine serum (FBS) (GenDEPOT, Katy, TX, USA) and 1% penicillin–streptomycin solution, and incubated in a humidified atmosphere at 37 °C in 5% CO_2.

2.6. Cell Viability Assay

The viability of the cells was determined using the 3-(4,5-dimethylthiazol-2-yl)-2,5-diphenyltetrazolium bromide (MTT) colorimetric assay (Sigma-Aldrich, St. Louis, MO, USA). The 2×10^4–4×10^4 cells/mL were seeded in 96-well plates. After the attachment, cells were treated with different concentrations of **B**, EL000327, D, and 5-FU for 48 h in the presence or absence of various inhibitors (Z-VAD-FMK (10 μM) (R&D System, Inc, McKinley Place N.E, MN, USA), 3-MA (1mM), CQ (10 μM), NAC (5 mM) (Sigma-Aldrich, St. Louis, MO, USA), and SP600125 (10 μM) (Cell Signaling Technology, MA, USA). Cells treated with 0.01% of DMSO were used as the control. Next, 15 μL of the MTT reagent was added to each well and incubated for 4 h at 37 °C. The medium was aspirated completely and 150 μL of DMSO (Sigma-Aldrich, St. Louis, MO, USA) was added to the cells before the absorbance was measured at 540 nm by a microplate reader (Bio Tek Instruments, Winooskim, VT, USA) using Gen 5 (2.03.1) software. SPSS statistical software 23 was used for the IC_{50} calculation. Synergic effects of **B** with D or 5-FU were assessed by compuSyn software.

2.7. Cell Cycle Analysis by Flow Cytometry

Caco2, HCT116, DLD1, and HT29 cells were seeded in 6-well plates at the density of 1.5–2×10^5 cells/well, incubated overnight, and treated with 0.01% of DMSO, various concentrations of **B**, and 60 μg/mL of EL000327 for 24 h, 48 h, or 72 h. Cells were harvested and washed with FACS washing buffer, incubated with trypsin solution, followed by RNase A for 10 min at room temperature. Cells were centrifuged and pellets were collected and stained with 100 mL of 4 mg/mL PI (Sigma-Aldrich, St. Louis, MO, USA) for 2 h in the dark at 4 °C. Cell cycle analysis was performed on a CytoFLEX instrument (Beckman Coulter Life Sciences, Indianapolis, IN, USA).

2.8. Western Blotting

Caco2 cells were cultured in 6-well plates at the density of 2×10^5 cells/well overnight and treated with 0.01% of DMSO, different concentrations of **B**, and 60 μg/mL of EL000327 for 24 h or 48 h in the presence or absence of various inhibitors (Z-VAD-FMK (10 μM), 3-MA (1 mM), CQ (10 μM), NAC (5 mM), and SP600125 (10 μM). Cells were harvested and lysed, and the protein concentrations were determined by the BCA protein assay following the manufacturer's instructions. Then, 25 or 50 μg of the total extract was separated by SDS-PAGE (12%) and transferred to a blotting membrane at 1.2 A for 6 h. Membranes were blocked with 5% of skim milk for 1 h followed by incubation with various primary antibodies (Cyclin B1, D1, p-Cdc2, BAX, Bcl-XL, PARP, caspase-3, Beclin 1, P-62, LC3B I/II, p-JNK, JNK, p-Akt, Akt, NF-κB, Actin purchased from Cell Signaling Technology, MA, USA) for 2 h at room temperature (RT). Blots were washed and incubated with horseradish peroxidase-conjugated secondary antibodies (Thermo Fisher Scientific, Waltham, MA, USA) for 30 to 60 min at RT. Specific antibody binding was detected under chemiluminescence imaging (iBright FL1000 Imaging System, Thermo Fisher Sciences, biomolecular imager, Amersham ImageQuantTM 800 Western Blot Imaging System) and measured by Multi Gauge 3.0. software. Relative density was calculated against the density of the actin bands.

2.9. Tubulin Polymerization Assay

The effect of **B** on tubulin organization was detected using the Tubulin Polymerization Assay Kit (Cytoskeleton, Inc., Denver, CO, USA) according to the manufacturer's instructions. In brief, tubulin proteins (>99% pure) were suspended at a final concentration of 3.0 mg/mL in ice-cold TP, and the tubulin solution was incubated at 37 °C with a general tubulin buffer with or without **B** (3.3, 20, 60 μg/mL). Paclitaxel and vinblastine (10 μM) were used as positive controls for the stabilization or destabilization of the microtubules, respectively. Tubulin polymerization was measured by continuously monitoring the change in turbidity at 340 nm by a microplate reader using Gen 5 (2.03.1) software.

2.10. Quantitative Real-Time PCR

Total RNA of 0.01% of DMSO, **B** (20, 60 μg/mL), and EL000327 (60 μg/mL) treated Caco2 cells were extracted using RNAiso Plus (TaKaRa, Kusatsu, Shiga, Japan) according to the manufacturer's instructions. cDNA was reverse transcribed from 3 μg of total RNA of each treated group using the M-MLV Reverse Transcriptase Kit (Invitrogen, Carlsbad, CA, USA). mRNA levels of stathmin and MAP4 was measured using stathmin (forward) 5-GGTGGCGGCAGGACTTTCCTTATCCCAGTTGATT-3 and (reverse) 5-TTCTCGTGCTCTCGTTTCTCAGCCAGCTGCTTC-3; MAP4 (forward) 5-CCCTTTCTGAG GTAGCGTGCCTTGTGGAGGT -3 and (reverse) 5-CTGGCTCCCTCATGTTCTTGGCACAG CAGA-3 primers and SYBR green (Enzynomics). qRT-PCR reaction and analysis were performed using CFX (Bio-Rad, Hercules, CA, USA).

2.11. Immunofluorescence (IF) Imaging

Caco2 cells were cultured on cover slips at the density of 1×10^5 in a 12-well plate. After the adherence, cells were treated with 0.01% of DMSO, different concentrations of **B**, paclitaxel (100 nM), vinblastine (50 nM), and deoxyphodophyllotoxin (DPT) (25 nM) for 24 h. Cells were washed with phosphate-buffered saline (PBS) three times, followed by fixation with 4% paraformaldehyde in PBS for 10 min, permeabilization with 0.1% Triton™ X-100 for 10 min at RT, and blocking with 1% BSA in PBS for 1 h at RT. The cells were labeled with alpha tubulin (B-5-1-2) Alexa Fluor 488 Mouse Monoclonal Antibody, at 2 μg/mL in 0.1% BSA, and incubated for 3 h at RT. Cells were washed three times with PBS for 5 min after every step. Then, the cells were blocked again with blocking solution containing 1% BSA for 30–45 min at RT. Cells were stained again with fluorescent phalloidin staining solution and incubated for 30–60 min at RT. After washing with PBS, cover slips were mounted on glass slides with prolong gold with DAPI and left overnight at RT. Images were taken using a K1-Fluo Confocal Laser Scanning Microscope (Nanoscope Systems, Daejeon, Republic of Korea).

2.12. Hoechst Staining

Caco2, HCT116, DLD1, and HT29 cells were seeded in a 12-well plate containing cover slips at a density of 1×10^5 cells/well. After overnight incubation, cells were treated with 0.01% of DMSO, **B** (20, 60 μg/mL), and EL000327 (60 μg/mL) for 12 or 24 h. Cells were washed with PBS, followed by fixation with 4% paraformaldehyde for 15 min. After washing again with PBS, cells were permeabilized in 0.1% Triton X-100 (Sigma-Aldrich) for 30 min, and stained with Hoechst 33258 (Sigma-Aldrich) for 1 h in the dark at room temperature. Cells were assessed by Nikon Eclipse 400 fluorescence microscope (Nikon Instech Co. Ltd., Kawasaki, Japan) to identify the morphological changers in the nuclei.

2.13. IncuCyte™ Caspase-3/7 and Annexin v Apoptosis Assay

Caco2 cells were seeded in a 96-well plate at a density of 2.5×10^3 cells/well. Cells were grown overnight to 25–30% confluence at the start of the assay. Media were supplemented with 5 μM of Caspase-3/7 (green) reagent (4440, Essen Bioscience, Morgan Rd, Ann Arbor, MI, USA) or Annexin V (red) reagent (4641, Essen Bioscience, Morgan Rd, Ann Arbor, MI, USA) diluted to 1:200 and added to the cells treated with 0.01% of

DMSO, different concentrations of **B**, and EL000327 for 48 h in the presence or absence of Z-VAD-FMK (10 μM). The apoptosis of cells was determined by fluorescence scanning performed every 2 h for 48 h by the IncuCyte Zoom® instrument with a 10× objective and analyzed with the Standard Scan Type.

2.14. *Apoptosis Analysis by Flow Cytometry*

Caco2, HCT116, DLD1, and HT29 cells were cultured in a 6-well plate at the density of 2×10^5 cells/well until adherence. Cells were treated with 0.01% of DMSO, different concentrations of **B**, and EL000327 for 48 h in the presence or absence of Z-VAD-FMK (10 μM). Cells were harvested and washed with PBS, resuspended in 100 μL of 1x binding buffer followed by staining with 5 μL of 50 μg/mL propidium iodide (PI; BD Biosciences, San Jose, CA, USA) and 3 μL of Annexin V–FITC (BD, Biosciences, San Jose, CA, USA), for 30 min in the dark. Death cells were detected by flow cytometry on a CytoFLEX instrument (Beckman Coulter Life Sciences, Indianapolis, IN, USA).

2.15. *Measurement of ROS Generation*

Caco2 cells were seeded in a 6-well plate at the density of 2×10^5 cells/well overnight and treated with 0.01% of DMSO, different concentrations of **B**, and EL000327 for 12 h in the presence or absence of NAC (5 mM). Cells were incubated with DCFH-DA (10 μM) in DMEM medium without FBS for 30 min at 37 °C and washed three times with DMEM. ROS generation was determined by fluorescence microscopy (K1-Fluo Confocal Laser Scanning Microscope, Nanoscope Systems, Daejeon, Republic of Korea) and flow cytometry (CytoFLEX; Beckman Coulter Life Sciences, Indianapolis, IN, USA) using peroxide-sensitive fluorescence probe DCFH-DA.

2.16. *Statistical Analysis*

All experiments were performed at least three times. Data are expressed as means ± standard deviation (SD). All statistical analyses were performed using Sigma Plot version 12.5. The Student's *t*-test was used to compare the statistical significance between two groups. Unless indicated otherwise, a p-value < 0.05 was considered significant.

3. Results

3.1. *The Novel Compound,* **B***, Isolated from Crude Extract, EL000327, Exerts Cytotoxicity on the CRC Cells*

The endolichenic fungus EL000327 (Figure 1a) was isolated from lichen specimen Graphis, collected from Hallasan in Jeju Island, South Korea in 2009 using the surface sterilization method. EL000327 was identified as a *Pseudoplectania* sp. according to a BLAST search of the GeneBank Database (Table S1). The cytotoxicity of the crude extract of EL000327 was tested against several human cancer cell lines: HT29, HCT116, Caco2, DLD1, CSC221, AGS, TMK1, RV1, A549, a mouse colon cancer cell line CT26, and non-cancerous cell lines HaCaT and MDCK. Among the cancer cell lines, EL000327 showed the highest cytotoxicity toward the human CRC cell line, Caco2 (IC_{50} = 52.2 μg/mL) and the mouse colon cancer cell line, CT26 (IC_{50} = 33.12 μg/mL). Cytotoxicity on the spontaneously transformed human keratinocyte cell (HaCaT) was similar to that of the Caco2 cells (IC_{50} = 48.7 μg/mL) (Figure 1b). The extract of EL000327 was subjected to a purification process to isolate and identify active compounds from the crude extract. First, the extract of EL000327 was separated into seven fractions, and Fr.2 (IC_{50} = 24.35 μg/mL) was identified as the fraction with the strongest cytotoxicity against Caco2 cells. In a further purification of Fr.2, six purified compounds (A′, A, **B**, B′, C, D) were isolated, as indicated in Figure 1c.

Compound **B** was isolated as a pink oil, and its molecular formula was deduced as $C_{20}H_{26}O_4$, based on the HR-FAB-MS data. The chemical structure of **B** was determined to be a novel compound 7β-9α-dihydroxy-1,8(14),15-pimaratrien-3,11-dione (Libertellenone T), based on intensive interpretation of MS, UV, and NMR spectroscopic data (Figure 1d).

Furthermore, the stereo-configurations of compound **B** were determined by comparing the NMR spectroscopic data and the values of optical rotation with the literature [24].

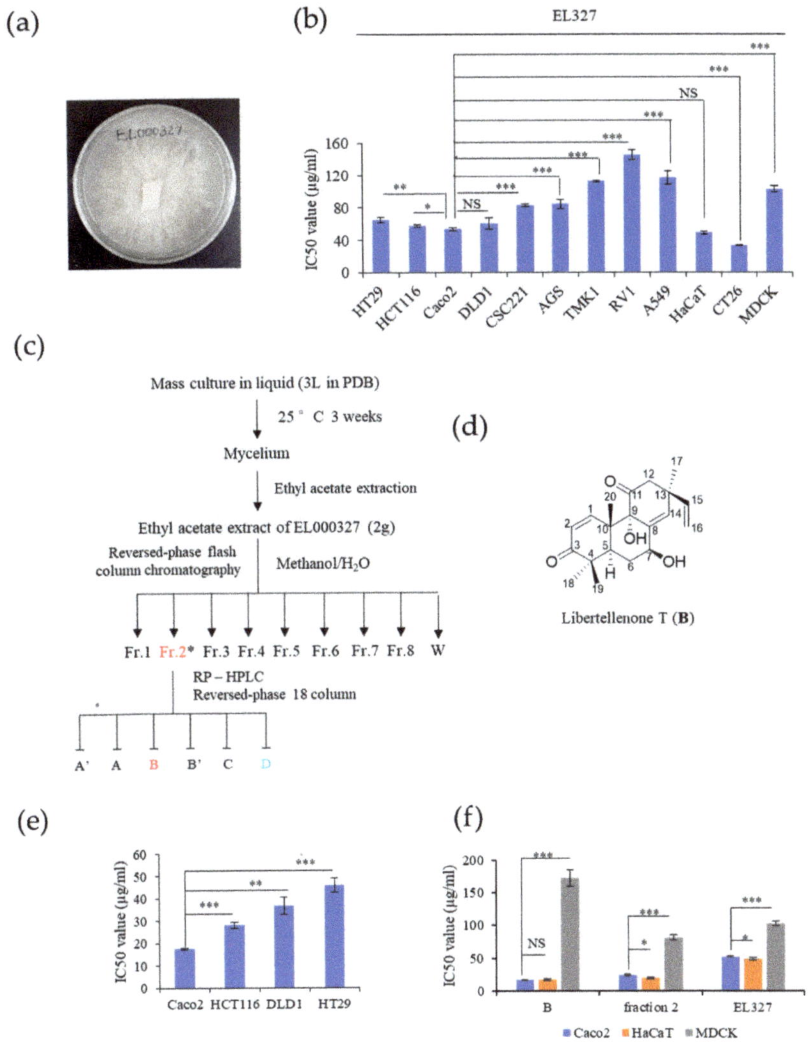

Figure 1. Compound **B** isolated from the crude extract of EL000327 exhibited cytotoxicity toward the human CRC cell line, Caco2. (**a**) Image of the endolichenic fungus, EL000327, belonging to *Pseudoplectania* sp. isolated from the lichen Graphis. (**b**) IC_{50} values of EL000327 in HT29, HCT116, Caco2, DLD1, CSC221, TMK1, RV1, A549, HaCaT, CT26, and MDCK cells. (**c**) Schematic representation of the process for the purification of compound **B** from the crude extract, EL000327. (**d**) Chemical structure of the novel compound, **B**. (**e**) IC_{50} values of human CRC cells Caco2, HCT116, DLD1, and HT29 after treatment with **B** for 48 h. (**f**) Comparison of IC_{50} values of the CRC cells Caco2 and non-cancer cell lines HaCaT and MDCK treated with single compound **B**, fraction 2, or crude extract, EL000327 for 48 h. Results are representative of three independent experiments. Data represent the mean ± S.D. * $p < 0.05$, ** $p < 0.01$, *** $p < 0.001$, NS: no significant difference ($p > 0.05$) compared with the Caco2 cells.

The cytotoxicity of purified compound **B** on Caco2, HCT116, DLD1, HT29, HaCaT, and MDCK cell lines was evaluated. **B** was toxic to the Caco2 (IC_{50} = 17.5 μg/mL) cell line at much lower doses than the HCT116 (IC_{50} = 28 μg/mL), DLD1 (IC_{50} = 36.6 μg/mL), and HT29 (IC_{50} = 28 μg/mL) cell lines and the non-cancer cell lines, HaCaT (IC_{50} = 17.6 μg/mL) and MDCK (IC_{50} = 171.8 μg/mL) (Figure 1e). Furthermore, for MDCK cells, the IC_{50} of **B** was significantly higher than those of Fr.2 (IC_{50} = 81.35 μg/mL) or the crude extract EL000327 (IC_{50} = 102.5 μg/mL) (Figure 1f). Thus, **B** was identified as a novel chemical compound, which exerted the highest cytotoxicity toward Caco2 among the tested human CRC cell lines, and was suitable for further investigation of its mechanism of action.

3.2. *B Induces G2/M Phase Arrest in CRC Cells as a Result of Microtubule Stabilization*

To determine whether **B** inhibits CRC cell growth by regulating the cell cycle, the cell cycle distribution of Caco2, HCT116, DLD1, and HT29 cells was analyzed by flow cytometry after treatment with **B**. Caco2 cells were treated with cytotoxic concentrations of **B** (20, 60 μg/mL) or EL000327 (60 μg/mL) for 24 h, 48 h, and 72 h. **B** markedly increased the proportion of cells at the G2/M phase in a dose-dependent manner after 24 h of treatment. At 48 h and 72 h after treatment, the proportion of cells at the G2/M phase decreased in a time-dependent manner, accompanied by an increase in the sub G1 population, indicating cell death after G2/M phase arrest. Treatment with EL000327 caused some accumulation of cells in the G2/M phase, but to a lesser extent than the treatment with **B** (Figures 2a and S1a). Analysis of the expression of known cell cycle regulatory proteins by Western blotting demonstrated that the expression of Cyclin B1, Cyclin D1, and p-Cdc2 was upregulated after treatment with **B** or EL000327 for 48 h (Figures 2b and S5a). To compare the effect of **B** on cell cycles of other CRC cell lines, the HCT116, DLD1, and HT29 cells were treated with 20 μg/mL of **B** for 24 h and the distribution of the cell cycle was analyzed. Cells accumulated in the G2/M phase was increased in all cell lines compared to the control (Figure S1b,c).

The dynamics of microtubules play a vital role in the progression of the cell cycle through the G2/M phase because microtubules form mitotic spindles, which provide structural support for chromosome segregation during mitosis. Therefore, tubulin polymerization assays were performed to evaluate the effect of **B** on tubulin polymerization in vitro. Treatment with the well-known microtubule stabilizer paclitaxel (10 μM) enhanced tubulin polymerization, whereas the microtubule destabilizer, vinblastine (10 μM) impaired tubulin polymerization. In untreated conditions, microtubules self-assembled to form tubulin polymers in a time dependent manner. Treatment with **B** (3.3, 20, 60 μg/mL) had a similar effect to paclitaxel and enhanced tubulin polymerization in a dose- and time-dependent manner (Figure 2c). qRT-PCR analysis demonstrated that the tubulin destabilizing gene *Satathmin* was significantly downregulated upon treatment with **B** or EL000327 (Figure 2d). The changes in mitotic spindle organization in Caco2 cells seen after treatment with **B** were visualized by immunofluorescence staining to confirm the results described above. Immunofluorescence microscopy demonstrated that **B** had a similar effect on the microtubules to paclitaxel (100 nM) by inducing multipolar mitotic spindles as a result of enhanced tubulin polymerization. Treatment with high concentrations of **B** (20, 60, 100 μg/mL) increased the bundling and stabilization of microtubules in Caco2 cells in a dose dependent manner. In contrast, the known microtubule destabilizers, vinblastine (50 nM) and DPT (25 nM), resulted in disrupted microtubule organization (Figure 2e). These data suggest that **B** induced G2/M phase arrest by regulating the cell cycle related protein and by stabilizing the microtubules. Furthermore, **B** was identified as a microtubule stabilizing agent, which has a functional effect that is similar to that of paclitaxel.

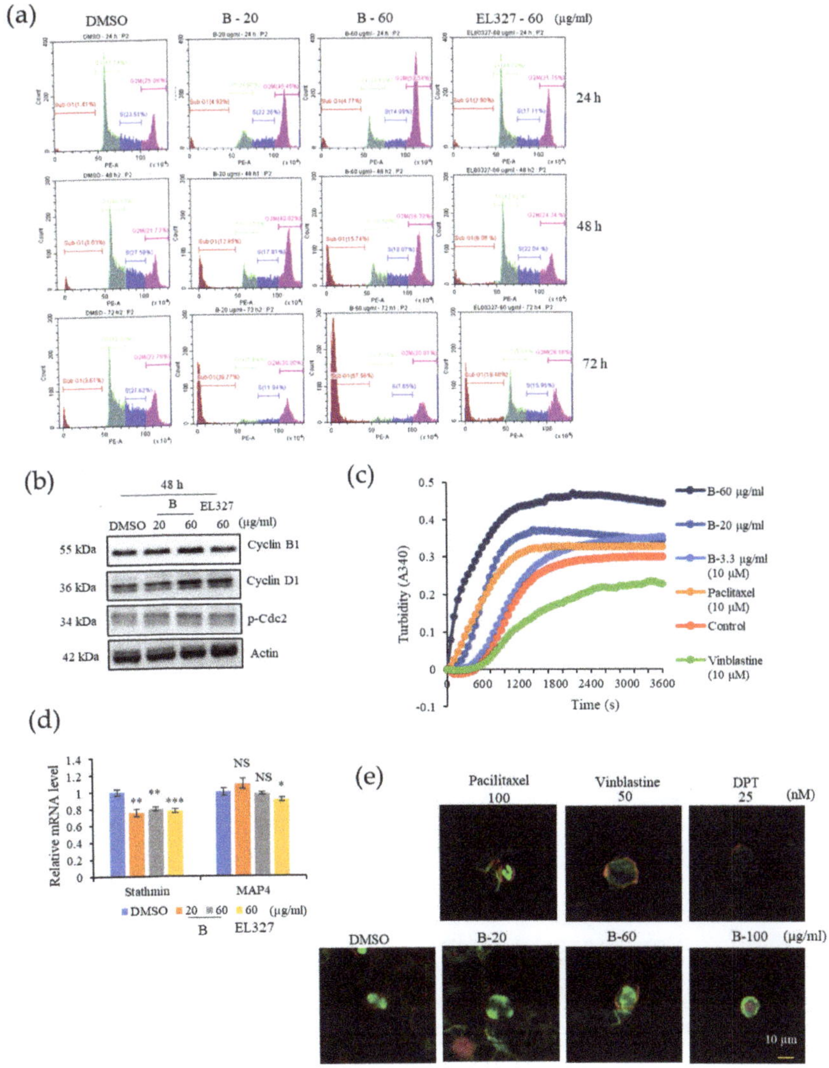

Figure 2. **B** induces G2/M phase arrest in Caco2 cells by inducing tubulin polymerization. (**a**) The cell-cycle distribution of Caco2 cells treated with **B** (20, 60 μg/mL) or EL000327 (60 μg/mL) for 24 h, 48 h, and 72 h as assessed by flow cytometry. (**b**) Western blot analysis of cell cycle regulating proteins, Cyclin B1, D1, and p-Cdc2 after treatment with **B** (20, 60 μg/mL) or EL000327 (60 μg/mL) for 24 h, 48 h, and 72 h. (**c**) Effect of **B** on tubulin polymerization in vitro, at concentrations of 20, 60, and 3.3 μg/mL. DMSO, paclitaxel, microtubule stabilizer (10 μM), and vinblastine microtubule destabilizer (10 μM) were used as the controls. (**d**) Relative mRNA levels of stathmin and MAP4, which are associated with microtubule destabilization and stabilization, respectively, after treatment with **B** (20, 60 μg/mL) or EL000327 (60 μg/mL) for 48 h. (**e**) Immunofluorescence microscopy of the microtubule organization in the Caco2 cells after treatment with **B** (20, 60, 100 μg/mL), paclitaxel (100 nM), vinblastine (50 nM) or DPT microtubule destabilizer (25 nM) for 24 h. Actin was stained with Alexa Fluor 568 phalloidin (red), microtubules were stained with α-tubulin antibodies (green), and DNA was stained with DAPI (blue). Results are representative of three independent experiments. Data represent the mean ± S.D. * $p < 0.05$, ** $p < 0.01$, *** $p < 0.001$, NS: no significant difference ($p > 0.05$) compared with the DMSO-treated control group.

3.3. B Induces Apoptotic Cell Death in CRC Cells

We next wished to determine whether the cytotoxicity exerted by **B** on CRC cells was due to the induction of apoptosis. Thus, Caco2, HCT116, DLD1, and HT29 cells were stained with Hoechst 33258 after treatment with cytotoxic concentrations of **B** or EL000327 for 12 h or 24 h to examine the morphological changes in the nuclei of cells. Cells treated with both **B** and EL000327 exhibited condensed chromatin, indicative of the initiation of apoptosis (Figures 3a and S2a,b). The number of condensed nuclei significantly increased in all CRC cell lines (Figures 3b and S2c). Furthermore, cell death induced by treatment with **B** was analyzed using the IncuCyte^{TM} apoptosis assay, which employs Caspase 3/7 (green) and Annexin V (red) dyes, in the presence or absence of the caspase inhibitor, Z-VAD-FMK. The level of Caspase-3/7 fluorescent green signal in Caco2 cells was markedly increased upon treatment with **B** or EL000327 for 48 h (Figure 3c,d). In this assay, the Annexin V dye emits a red fluorescent signal upon binding to the exposed phosphatidylserines (PS) of apoptotic cells. The number of red-labeled apoptotic cells increased after exposure to **B** in a dose-dependent manner. However, the suppression of caspases by Z-VAD-FMK significantly decreased the number of apoptotic cells detected by Annexin V staining (Figure 3e,f). To confirm the induction of caspase dependent apoptosis by **B** in Caco2 cells, flow cytometric analysis of apoptosis was also carried out. Cells were double stained with PI and Annexin V following treatment with **B** or EL000327 in the presence or absence of Z-VAD-FMK. Dose-dependently increasing numbers of apoptotic cells were observed after 48 h of treatment. Moreover, the inhibition of caspase significantly decreased apoptosis in the Caco2 cells (Figures 3g,h and S3a). In addition, the flow cytometric analysis revealed that **B** significantly induced the apoptosis of other CRC cell lines HCT116, DLD1, and HT29 as well as at the concentration of 20 µg/mL (Figure S3b,c). Taken together, both **B** and EL000327 induced apoptotic cell death in CRC cells.

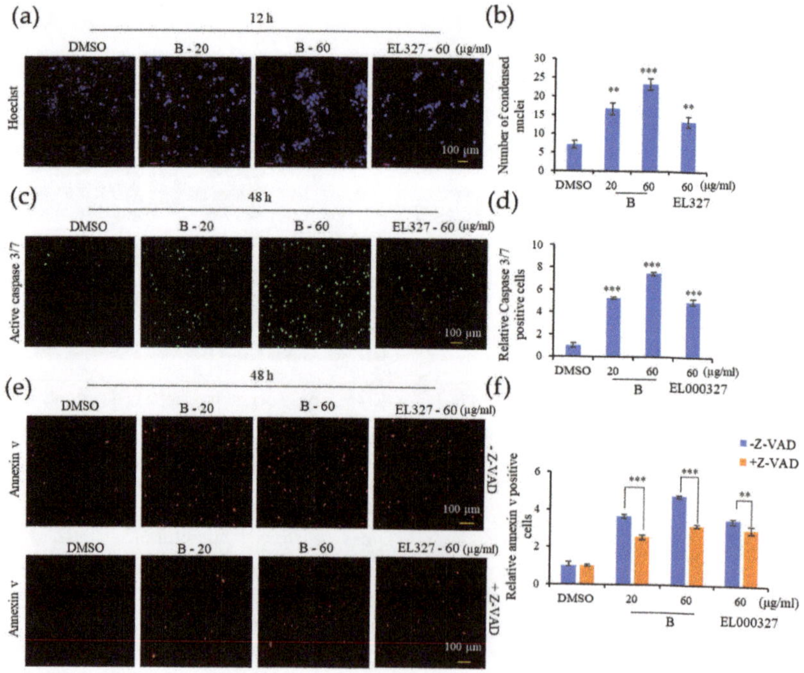

Figure 3. *Cont.*

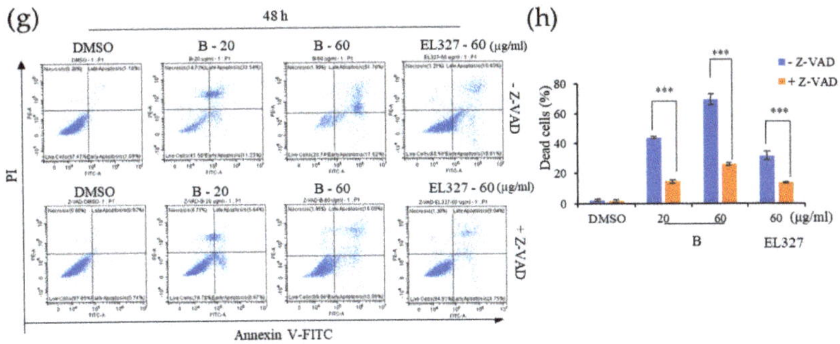

Figure 3. B induces caspase dependent apoptosis in Caco2 cells. (**a**) Nuclei condensation of Caco2 cells upon treatment with **B** (20, 60 μg/mL) or EL000327 (60 μg/mL) for 12 h, as determined by Hoechst staining. Arrowheads indicate nuclear condensation in cells. (**b**) Quantification of condensed nuclei in Caco2 cells treated with indicated concentrations of **B** or EL000327. (**c**) Caspase 3/7 (green) staining of Caco2 cells treated with **B** (20, 60 μg/mL) or EL000327 (60 μg/mL) for 48 h. (**d**) Quantification of apoptotic cells stained with Caspase 3/7 after treatment with the indicated concentrations of **B** or EL000327. (**e**) Annexin V staining of Caco2 cells treated with **B** (20, 60 μg/mL) or EL000327 (60 μg/mL) for 48 h in the presence or absence of the caspase inhibitor Z-VAD-FMK (10 μM). (**f**) Quantification of apoptotic cells stained with Annexin V after treatment with the indicated concentrations of **B** or EL000327 in the presence or absence of Z-VAD-FMK (10 μM). (**g**) Flow cytometric analysis of dead cells stained by Annexin v-FITC (apoptotic cells) and PI (necrotic cells) upon the treatment of **B** (20, 60 μg/mL) or EL000327 (60 μg/mL) for 48 h in the presence or absence of Z-VAD-FMK (10 μM). (**h**) Quantification of the percentage of apoptotic cells treated with indicated concentrations of **B** and EL000327 and analyzed by flow cytometry in the presence or absence of Z-VAD-FMK (10 μM). Results are representative of three independent experiments. Data represent the mean ± S.D. ** $p < 0.01$, *** $p < 0.001$; compared with the DMSO-treated control or Z-VAD-FMK treated group.

3.4. *B Induces Caspase-Dependent Apoptosis and Autophagy in Caco2 Cells*

Activation of the caspase dependent apoptosis by **B** in Caco2 cells was further confirmed by Western blot analysis in the presence or absence of Z-VAD-FMK. The level of the pro apoptotic protein BAX was significantly increased upon treatment with **B** or EL000327 at cytotoxic concentrations for 12 h. However, a significant change in the levels of BAX were not observed in cells that had been pretreated with Z-VAD-FMK. In contrast, the expression level of the anti-apoptotic protein Bcl-xL was decreased in the Caco2 cells after treatment with **B** or EL000327 for 24 h, but no change in the presence of Z-VAD-FMK (Figure 4a,b). Clear cleavage of the main apoptotic markers PARP and caspase-3 was detected after treatment with **B** (20, 60 μg/mL) or EL000327 (60 μg/mL) for 48 h in the absence of Z-VAD-FMK (Figure 4c). The effect of **B** and EL000327 on the activation of the JNK/c-jun and Akt signaling pathways was assessed, as these pathways eventually lead to the induction of apoptosis as well as autophagy in cells. Phosphorylation of JNK and c-jun was markedly induced upon treatment with **B** at IC_{50} concentrations for 48 h and decreased the phosphorylation of Akt. However, no significant changes in protein levels were detected in cells treated with EL000327 (Figure 4d). Regulation of the autophagy related proteins Beclin 1, p62, and LC3BI/II was also examined in the presence or absence of Z-VAD-FMK. Upregulation of Beclin 1 and LC3BI/II and downregulation of the p62 protein levels were observed in Caco2 cells upon treatment with cytotoxic concentrations of **B** or EL000327, indicating the inhibition of autophagosome degradation in these cells. However, consistent regulation patterns were not observed for these autophagy markers in the presence of Z-VAD-FMK (Figure 4e,f).

In order to confirm the major cell death pathway induced by **B** and crude extract EL000327, cell viability was assessed after pretreatment with apoptotic and autophagic inhibitors. Treatment with Z-VAD-FMK significantly increased the cell viability in Caco2 cells in response to treatment with **B** or EL000327. In contrast, the application of 3MA (3-methylladenine), a blocker of autophagosome formation, and CQ (chloroquine), an inhibitor of lysosomal acidification and autophagosome degradation, resulted in a dose dependent decrease in cell viability, indicating that the inhibition of autophagy enhanced the cytotoxicity of **B** toward Caco2 cells (Figure 4g). Of the autophagy blockers, CQ had a more potent effect on the induction of cell death than 3MA. Application of CQ markedly increased the levels of cleaved PARP and caspase-3 and decreased the level of Bcl-xL in the cells treated with **B** for 48 h (Figures 4h and S5b). These data suggest that **B** induced caspase dependent apoptosis mainly via the activation of the JNK/c-jun pathway in Caco2 cells. Furthermore, the observed induction of autophagy by **B** may activate the protective mechanism in cells.

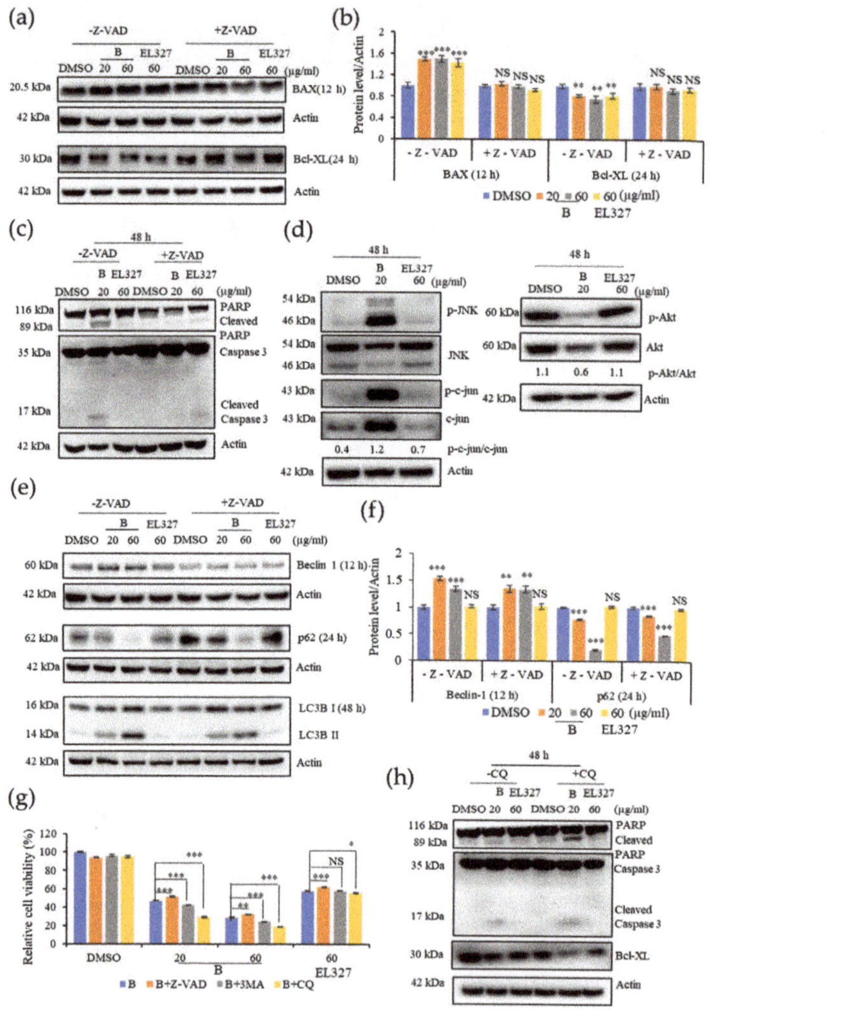

Figure 4. Inhibition of **B** induced autophagy increases apoptosis in Caco2 cells. (**a**) Western blot analysis of the pro-apoptotic protein BAX and the anti-apoptotic protein Bcl-xL treated by **B** (20 or 60 μg/mL) or EL000327 (60 μg/mL) for 12 or 24 h in the presence or absence of Z-VAD-FMK (10 μM).

(**b**) Quantification of BAX and Bcl-XL protein expressions. (**c**) Western blot of apoptotic proteins; PARP, Caspase-3treated by **B** (20 or 60 μg/mL) or EL000327 (60 μg/mL) for 48 h in the presence or absence of Z-VAD-FMK. (**d**) Expressions of the apoptotic signaling pathway related proteins p-JNK, JNK, p-c-jun, c-jun, p-AKT, and AKT in Caco2 cells treated with **B** (20 μg/mL) or EL000327 (60 μg/mL) for 48 h, as analyzed by Western blotting. (**e**) Western blot of autophagy related proteins; Beclin 1 (12 h), p62 (24 h), and LC3BI/II (48 h) in Caco2 cells pre-incubated with or without Z-VAD-FMK, and treated with **B** (20, 60 μg/mL) or EL000327 (60 μg/mL). (**f**) Quantification of Beclin 1 and p62 protein expressions. (**g**) The relative percentage cell viability of Caco2 cells treated with **B** (20, 60 μg/mL) or EL000327 (60 μg/mL) for 48 h, with or without Z-VAD-FMK (10 μM) and autophagy inhibitors 3 MA (1 mM) and CQ (10 μM). (**h**) Expression levels of PARP, caspase-3, and Bcl-xL determined by Western blot analysis after treatment with **B** (20, μg/mL) or EL000327 (60 μg/mL) for 48 h in the presence or absence of CQ (10 μM). Data represent the mean ± S.D. * $p < 0.05$, ** $p < 0.01$, *** $p < 0.001$; NS: no significant difference ($p > 0.05$), compared with the Z-VAD-FMK, 3MA, and CQ treated groups or the DMSO-treated control.

*3.5. **B** Activates JNK/c-Jun Signaling Pathway via Triggering ROS Generation*

Intracellular ROS play a vital role in activating cellular apoptotic and autophagic functions. To assess the effect of **B** on ROS generation, cells were treated with **B** or EL000327 at toxic concentrations for 12 h in the presence or absence of the antioxidant N-acetyl cysteine (NAC), and ROS were detected by staining cells with DCFH-DA, followed by fluorescence microscopy or flow cytometry. While exposure of Caco2 cells to **B** dramatically increased the green fluorescent signals indicative of ROS generation, pretreatment with NAC significantly reduced the fluorescent signals, suggesting a block in ROS generation (Figure 5a). The number of fluorescently labeled cells decreased upon treatment with NAC, as detected by flow cytometry. No significant change in fluorescence emission was detected in the EL000327 treated cells after 12 h compared to the control cells (Figure 5b,c). Thus, pretreatment with NAC decreased the expression of apoptotic and autophagy markers and rescued cells from **B**-induced apoptosis and autophagy. Furthermore, NAC reversed the phosphorylation of JNK and c-jun in cells treated with IC_{50} concentrations of **B** (Figure 5d,e). Collectively, these results indicate that **B** activates the ROS/JNK signaling pathway in Caco2 cells.

(a)

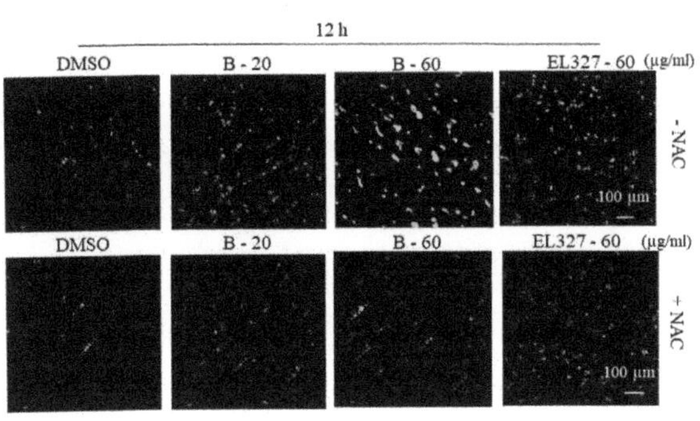

Figure 5. *Cont.*

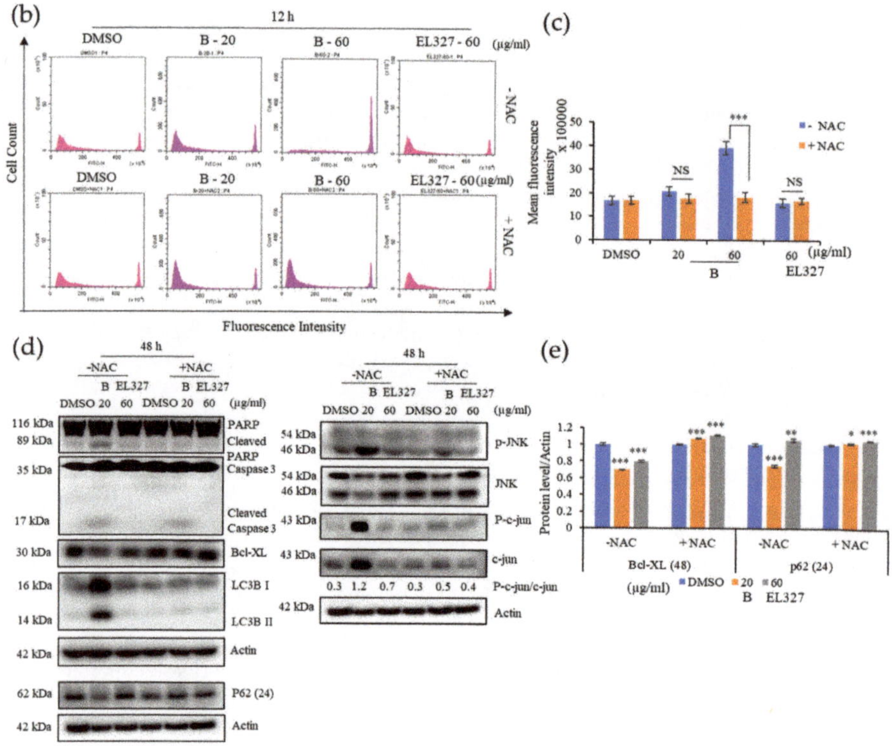

Figure 5. B induces ROS generation and activates JNK signaling in Caco2 cells. (**a**) Intracellular ROS generation was detected by fluorescence microscopy using DCFH-DA (10 µM) in Caco2 cells treated with **B** (20, 60 µg/mL) or EL000327 (60 µg/mL) for 12 h with or without the ROS inhibitor NAC (5 mM). (**b**) Flow cytometric analysis of the fluorescence intensity of Caco2 cells preincubated with DCFH-DA (10 µM) and treated with **B** (20, 60 µg/mL) or EL000327 (60 µg/mL) for 12 h with or without NAC (5 mM). (**c**) Quantification of the mean fluorescence intensity of Caco2 cells preincubated with DCFH-DA (10 µM) and treated with the indicated concentrations of **B** for 12 h in the presence or absence of NAC. (**d**) Western blot analysis of PARP, caspase-3, Bcl-xL, p62, LC3BI/II, p-JNK, JNK, p-c-jun, and c-jun protein expression after treatment with **B** (20, µg/mL) or EL000327 (60 µg/mL) for 24 or 48 h, with or without NAC (5 mM). (**e**) Quantification of Bcl-XL and p62 protein expressions in the presence or absence of NAC. Data represent the mean ± S.D. * $p < 0.05$, ** $p < 0.01$, *** $p < 0.001$; NS: no significant difference ($p > 0.05$) compared with the NAC-treated group or the DMSO-treated control.

3.6. *B Induces Apoptosis and Autophagy in Caco2 Cells by Activating ROS/JNK Signaling Pathways*

The involvement of ROS and JNK activation for the induction of apoptosis and autophagy by **B** and EL000327 was further investigated. Pretreatment of Caco2 with NAC or the JNK inhibitor SP600125 significantly reduced the sensitivity to **B** and EL000327 compared to the cells treated with **B** or EL000327 in the absence of inhibitors (Figure 6a). Flow cytometric analysis detected very low numbers of apoptotic cells in the presence of NAC or SP600125, confirming that ROS and JNK inhibitors rescued **B**-induced cell death in the Caco2 cells (Figures 6b,c and S4a). Moreover, the application of SP600125 significantly decreased the expression of apoptotic and autophagy markers as well as JNK pathway related proteins, as analyzed by Western blotting after treatment with **B** for 24 or 48 h (Figure 6d,e). Taken together, these results reveal that triggering the generation of ROS by

B activates JNK/c-jun signaling and leads to the induction of apoptosis and autophagy in Caco2 cells.

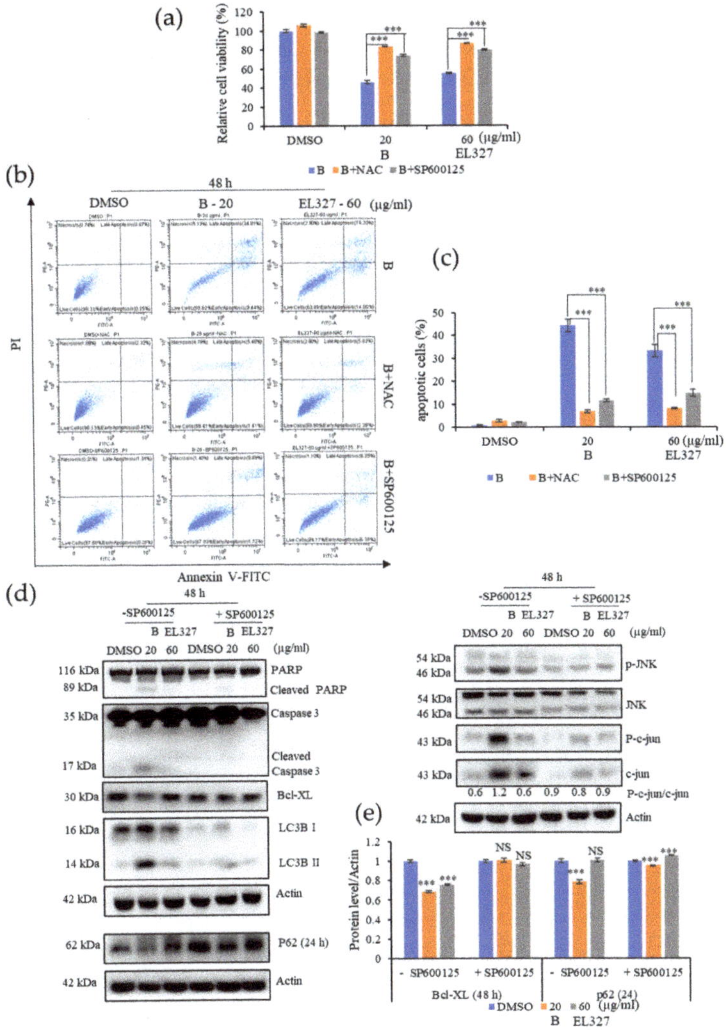

Figure 6. B activates ROS/JNK mediated apoptosis and autophagy in Caco2 cells. (**a**) The relative percentage cell viability of Caco2 cells detected after treatment with **B** (20 μg/mL) or EL000327 (60 μg/mL) for 48 h, with or without NAC (5 mM) or the JNK inhibitor SP600125 (10 μM). (**b**) Flow cytometric analysis of dead cells stained by Annexin V-FITC and PI after treatment with **B** (20 μg/mL) or EL000327 (60 μg/mL) for 48 h, with or without NAC (5 mM) or SP600125 (10 μM). (**c**) Quantification of the percentage of apoptotic cells after treatment with the indicated concentrations of **B** or EL000327 for 48 h with or without NAC and SP600125 and analyzed by flow cytometry. (**d**) Western blot analysis of apoptosis, autophagy, and the JNK signaling pathway related protein expression in Caco2 cells treated with **B** (20 μg/mL) or EL000327 (60 μg/mL) for 24 or 48 h, with or without SP600125 (10 μM). (**e**) Quantification of Bcl-XL and p62 protein expressions in the presence or absence of SP600125. Data represent the mean ± S.D. *** $p < 0.001$ compared with the NAC- and SP600125-treated groups or the DMSO-treated control. NS: no significant difference.

3.7. *B Exhibits Synergy with 5-FU and Compound D on CRC Cells*

To investigate the potential of **B** as an anticancer therapeutic drug in the clinic, we analyzed its effect when used in combination with 5-FU, a well-known chemotherapeutic that is used to treat several types of cancers including colorectal cancers, and D (IC_{50} = 10 μg/mL), another cytotoxic compound isolated from EL000327 (Figure 1c). The chemical structure of D is yet to be determined. Caco2 were treated with **B**, 5-FU, and D singly or 5-FU combined with **B** or D, and the HCT116 cells were treated with **B**, and 5-FU singly or 5-FU combined with **B** at various concentrations for 48 h; cell survival was analyzed using a MTT assay, The Chou–Talalay method was used to calculate the combination index (CI) of synergy using compuSyn software. Anti-cancer agents with synergism have a CI value of <1, and those with the smallest CI value are considered to be more suitable for cancer therapy. The combination of 2 μg/mL of **B** with 4 μg/mL (**1**; CI = 0.4) or 6 μg/mL of 5-FU (**2**; CI = 0.6), the combination of 4 μg/mL of **B** with 4 μg/mL of 5-FU (**3**; CI = 0.41), and the combination of 6 μg/mL of **B** with 2 μg/mL of 5-FU (**3**; CI = 0.23) all produced CI values of less than 1 on Caco2 cells. Furthermore, **B** exhibited good synergism with 5FU on HCT116 cells as well as when combined with 2 μg/mL of **B** with 4 μg/mL of 5-FU (**1**; CI = 0.96), 4 μg/mL of **B** with 2 μg/mL (**2**; CI = 0.52), or 4 μg/mL of 5-FU (**3**; CI = 0.54) and 6 μg/mL of **B** with 2 μg/mL of 5-FU (**4**; CI = 0.45) (Figure 7a). Western blot analysis demonstrated that the combination of **B** and 5-FU at the concentrations that provided a CI value of <1 considerably increased the cleaved PARP and Caspase-3expressions and decreased the level of anti-apoptotic protein Bcl-XL compared to treatment with **B** and 5-FU individually. Decreased level of p62 was observed after the combination treatments (Figure 7b,c). Furthermore, 2 μg/mL of **B** combined with 5 μg/mL (**1**; CI = 0.27), 5 μg/mL of **B** with 5 μg/mL of D (**2**; CI = 0.47), and 10 μg/mL of **B** with 1 μg/mL of D (**3**; CI = 0.19) (Figure 7d). Expression of cleaved PARP, caspase-3, and LC3BI/II was elevated when the cells were subjected to combined **B** and D treatments, as demonstrated by Western blotting. Furthermore, the levels of anti-apoptotic protein Bcl-XL and autophagy related protein p62 were downregulated by the combination treatment with **B** and D (Figure 7e,f). These results suggest that **B** acts synergistically with both 5-FU and compound D to significantly increase its cytotoxic effects on CRC cells at low concentrations. Therefore, **B** shows a high potential to act synergistically with other anticancer therapeutics to enhance their effect by increasing the cytotoxicity.

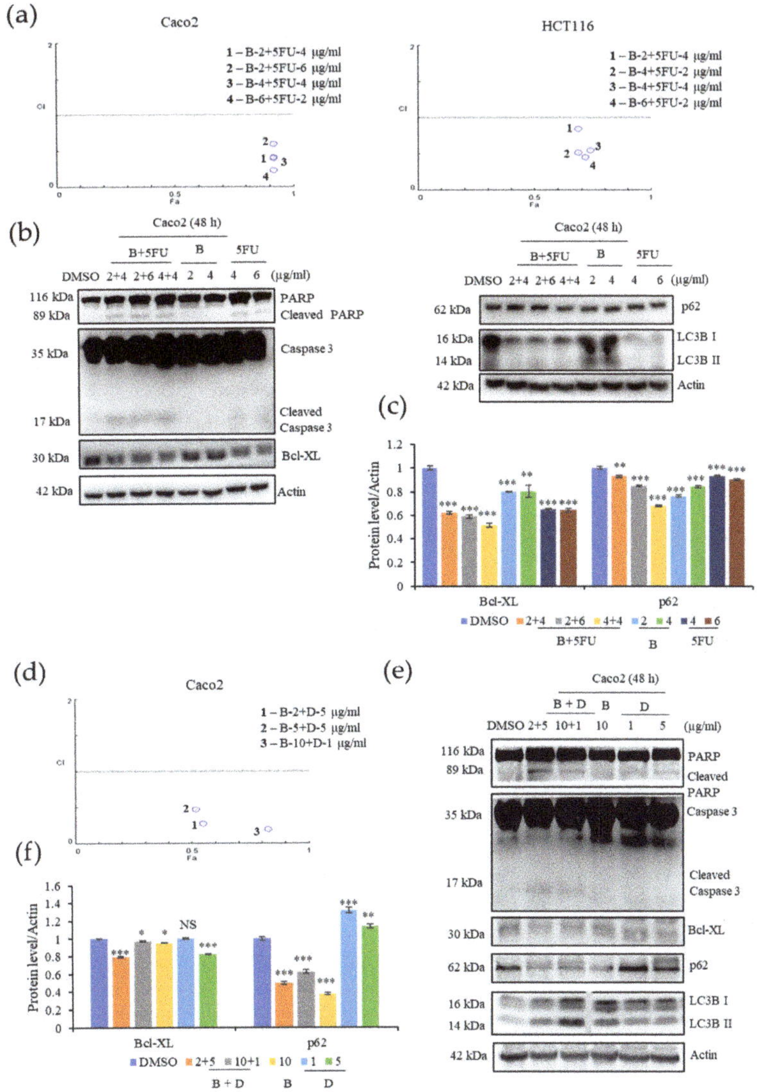

Figure 7. **B** shows synergy with 5-FU and with D, a compound isolated from the crude extract of EL000327 on the CRC cells. (**a**) Fa-CI plot of combination treatment with 5-FU (2, 4 or 6 μg/mL) and **B** (2, 4 or 6 μg/mL) on the Caco2 cells and the Fa-CI plot of combination treatment with 5-FU (2 or 4 μg/mL) and **B** (2, 4 or 6 μg/mL) on the HCT116 cells. (**b**) Expression of apoptosis and autophagy related protein in Caco2 cells after combination treatment with 5-FU (4 or 6 μg/mL) and **B** (2 or 4 μg/mL) or **B** (2 or 4 μg/mL) or 5FU (4 or 6 μg/mL) individually for 48 h, as detected by Western blotting. (**c**) Quantification of Bcl-XL and p62 protein expression after the treatment with **B**+5FU or **B** or 5FU at the indicated concentrations. (**d**) Fa-CI plot of combination treatment with D (5 or 1 μg/mL) and **B** (2, 5 or 10 μg/mL) on the Caco2 cells. (**e**) Western blot analysis of apoptosis and autophagy related protein expression in the Caco2 cells after combination treatment with D (5 or 1 μg/mL) and **B** (2 or10 μg/mL) or **B** (10 μg/mL) or D (1 or 5 μg/mL) individually for 48 h. (**e**) Quantification of Bcl-XL and p62 protein expression after the treatment with **B** + D or **B** or D at the indicated concentrations. Data represent the mean ± S.D. * $p < 0.05$, ** $p < 0.01$, *** $p < 0.001$; NS: no significant difference ($p > 0.05$) compared with the NAC-treated group or the DMSO-treated control.

4. Discussion

Natural products have been highly recognized as rich reservoirs of bioactive compounds with the potential to lead to the discovery of novel anticancer therapeutics. As a result of the tremendous efforts by scientists, many naturally derived anticancer agents have been discovered and successfully developed into drugs within the last 30 years. Such compounds account for approximately 25% of newly approved anticancer drugs [25]. Lichen substances and the secondary metabolites of endolichenic fungi have also been proven to have a wide range of anticancer activities against various types of cancers [5,26–31]. Therefore, it is essential to carry out a thorough investigation of bioactive compounds derived from the rich bioresources of lichens. Libertellenone T **(B)** is a novel cytotoxic compound, isolated as a pink oil from a secondary metabolite extract of the endolichenic fungi EL000327. Its molecular formula was determined to be $C_{20}H_{26}O_4$, based on HR-FAB-MS, coupled with the analysis of the NMR data. As the crude extract of EL000327 exerted comparatively high cytotoxicity on CRC, which is considered to be the second most lethal cancer type in the world [32], the cytotoxicity of **B** on CRC was assessed. Interestingly, the effect of **B** on the CRC cells was much stronger than EL000327 and the Caco2 cells were highly sensitive to the treatment of **B** compared to the HCT116, DLD1, and HT29 cells. Furthermore, the effect of **B** on the non-cancerous cell line Madin–Darby canine kidney epithelial cells (MDCK) was very low and the human non-cancerous cell line HaCaT was similar to the Caco2 cells. In the current study, the mechanisms underlying **B**-induced cell death were comprehensively investigated. We found that **B** induced mitotic arrest in CRC cells by stabilizing microtubules and preventing their depolymerization. Moreover, **B** activated apoptosis and autophagy via the ROS/JNK signaling pathway. **B**-induced autophagy had a protective effect on Caco2 cells. Most importantly, **B** showed synergy with the well-known chemotherapeutic 5-FU and another novel compound D isolated from the same crude extract of EL000327. Here, we mainly used Caco2 cells to study the mechanism of action of **B**, but our results revealed that **B** has an effect on other CRC cells such as HCT116, DLD1, and HT29. The induction of apoptosis in these cells upon the treatment of **B** was confirmed by the results of Hoechst staining and flow cytometry.

Check points prevent cells with damaged DNA from entering the next phase of the cell cycle. This phenomenon is highly regulated by a series of proteins, and the G2/M transition is mainly regulated by the Cyclin B/Cdc2 (Cdk1) complex. Phosphorylation of Cdc2 negatively regulates cell cycle progression from the G2 phase to M phase [11]. Furthermore, the Cyclin B/Cdk1 complex is highly activated in the metaphase as it supports the assembly of the mitotic apparatus and chromosome alignment. Once chromosomes are properly attached to spindles, the APC/C is activated and promotes progression to anaphase.

Degradation of cyclin B by the activation of the APC/C complex leads to Cdk1 inactivation [33]. Flow cytometric analysis of cell cycle progression in our study indicated a clear accumulation of Caco2 cells in the G2/M phase than other CRC cell lines HCT116, DLD1, and HT29 after treatment with **B** for 24 h. However, increasing G2/M cell populations compared to the control indicated that HCT116, DLD1, and HT29 cells require longer treatment to induce G2/M phase arrest. Furthermore, treatment with **B** resulted in the upregulation of Cyclin B1 and p-Cdc-2 expression. Therefore, we continued our studies to investigate whether **B** affected the microtubule dynamics in cells. According to the results of our in vitro tubulin polymerization assay, **B** stabilized microtubules in a manner similar to the clinically approved microtubule stabilizer, paclitaxel. These results were further confirmed by the immunofluorescence staining of cells treated with **B** and paclitaxel. Microtubule targeting agents in anticancer therapy can be classified into two groups based on their mode of action. Microtubule destabilizers prevent microtubule formation by inhibiting tubulin dimerization. In contrast, microtubule stabilizers promote tubulin dimerization and stabilize microtubules [34]. Both the stabilization and destabilization of microtubules lead to mitotic catastrophe followed by cell death due to failure to form the spindle required for chromosome segregation in the M phase of the cell cycle. Similarly, our compound, **B**, induced cell death after prolonged mitotic arrest, as shown by the appearance of a sub G1 population in cell cycle analysis.

Apoptosis is the process of programmed cell death and the most popular target of many anticancer therapies. Dysregulation of apoptosis signals in cancers promotes abnormal cell growth and tumorigenesis [9]. Restoring the lost apoptotic function in cancer cells is the main objective of much of the research into cancer treatments. The initiation of apoptosis in cells can be identified by morphological changes such as nuclear fragmentation, chromatin condensation, cell shrinkage, and membrane blebbing [35,36]. Hoechst, Caspase 3/7, and Annexin V staining demonstrated the initiation of apoptosis in CRC cells upon treatment with **B**. Apoptosis can be classed as either caspase-dependent or caspase-independent. Many anticancer agents mainly activate the caspase-dependent mitochondrial pathway. In addition, the death receptor mediated, and endoplasmic reticulum pathways also activate caspases at the final phase of apoptosis. Disruption of the mitochondrial membrane potential followed by translocation of AIF and endonuclease G to the nucleus induces caspase-independent apoptosis [37]. Data from the IncuCyte apoptosis assay and flow cytometric analysis of apoptosis demonstrated that treatment with the caspase inhibitor Z-VAD-FMK significantly reduced the extent to which **B** induced apoptosis in cells, indicating that apoptosis induced by **B** is caspase-dependent. Furthermore, Western blot analysis showed the activation of the proapoptotic protein BAX, the anti-apoptotic protein Bcl-xL, and eventually, Caspase-3and PARP cleavage in response to **B** treatment. Caspase-3 is the executioner caspase in all caspase dependent apoptosis pathways. Caspase-3 can be cleaved and activated by the upstream caspase, caspase-8, in the extrinsic pathway as well as by caspase-9, an initiating caspase, in the intrinsic pathway [38]. Cleavage of PARP by caspases is considered as a hallmark of apoptosis and an indicator that caspase dependent apoptosis has been accomplished [39]. Here, as predicted, Z-VAD-FMK treatment significantly impaired the expression of apoptotic markers in cells treated with **B**. Interestingly, the expression of the autophagic proteins Beclin 1 and LC3BI/II slightly decreased while p62 expression slightly increased upon treatment with **B** in the presence of Z-VAD-FMK. However, this result is not sufficient to assess the action of **B** toward autophagy in the presence of Z-VAD-FMK.

Autophagy plays a dual role in cancer treatment by either supporting or preventing cancer cell survival. In the current study, **B** induced autophagy in the Caco2 cells. Moreover, treatment with the autophagy inhibitors 3MA and CQ significantly increased **B**-induced cell death, suggesting that the activation of autophagy promotes CRC cell survival. Western blot analysis further confirmed that the inhibition of autophagy enhanced the activation of apoptosis, as demonstrated by elevated cleaved caspase-3 and PARP levels in the presence of CQ. Beclin 1, P62, and LC3BI/II are key regulators of the autophagic process. Beclin 1 regulates autophagosome formation at the beginning of autophagy. During autophagosome formation, cytosolic LC3B-I is converted to the membrane-bound LC3B-II form. Binding of LC3B to the adapter protein p62/SQSTM1 facilitates autophagic degradation [40]. In the present study, we observed increased the expressions of Beclin 1 and, LC3B-II and decreased p62 upon treatment with **B**. While elevated expression of Beclin 1 and, LC3B is indicative of the activation of autophagy in CRC cells, generally, activation of autophagy results in reduced expression of p62. However, under some circumstances, p62 expression can be elevated by upregulation of p62 transcription during starvation of cells, regardless of the effect of autophagy. Under prolonged starvation, p62 expression is restored to basal levels by transcriptional regulation, even, when its expression has been decreased by autophagic activities at earlier time points [41,42]. Furthermore, p62 transcription is modulated by oxidative stress (Nrf2), the Ras/MAPK pathway, and the JNK/c-Jun pathway as well as some chemicals, including autophagy inducers [43]. Following treatment with **B**, cell viability was lower in the presence of CQ than 3MA. Furthermore, the level of LC3B-II was significantly increased upon treatment with CQ in western blot analysis. CQ inhibits autophagy by inhibiting fusion of the autophagosome and lysosome, and by degradation of the autophagolysosome [44]. These results suggest that **B** may induce autophagy by promoting late phase autophagy, fusion, and degradation. Moreover, the expression of autophagy related proteins was decreased when apoptosis was suppressed by Z-VAD-FMK. In contrast, expression of apoptotic markers was increased when autophagy was blocked by CQ. This leads to the hypothesis that **B** predominantly induces apoptosis in CRC cells, and that autophagy is activated as a counter mechanism to protect the cells from apoptosis. However, this potential interconnection between activation of apoptosis and autophagy by **B** needs further, detailed investigation.

Our study revealed that ROS generation is highly induced upon the treatment with **B**. Excess levels of ROS can be deleterious to cells due to the induction of oxidative stress within cells. Blocking ROS generation using the antioxidant NAC decreased expression of both apoptotic and autophagy markers in response to treatment with **B**, as demonstrated by western blot analysis. Furthermore, NAC significantly decreased the phosphorylation of JNK and expression of c-JUN. Given that ROS generation began after 12 h of treatment with **B**, while apoptotic markers were detected after 48 h, it seems likely that **B** induced apoptosis is initiated by ROS. ROS activate many signaling pathways (PI3K/Akt, MAPK, Nrf2) and transcription factors (NF-κB, p53) that eventually induce apoptosis, autophagy, or necrosis. Oxidants like $OH^{\bullet}$, $ONOO^{-}$, and H_2O induce apoptosis and/or necrosis, while $O_2^{\bullet-}$ and H_2O_2 induce autophagy and mostly trigger cell survival.

Cell viability upon treatment with **B** was markedly increased in the presence of the NAC and JNK inhibitor, SP600125, while apoptosis was significantly decreased, according to flow cytometric and western blot analysis. Furthermore, levels of LC3B were also reduced in the presence of SP600125, indicating that autophagy was inhibited. Taken together, this suggests that JNK plays a significant role in the apoptosis and autophagy activated by treatment with **B**. Induction of c-jun/JNK signaling by ROS blocks the antiapoptotic protein, Bcl-2, and activates the proapoptotic proteins in the Bcl-2 family, which are critical for the release of cytochrome c to the cytosol. Activation of caspase-9 and the effector caspase-3 by cytochrome c eventually leads to cell death via the mitochondrial apoptotic pathway. ROS can also activate the extrinsic apoptotic pathway by directly causing damage to DNA [45]. Taken together, the above results suggest that **B** induces apoptosis and autophagy in CRC via activation of ROS/JNK signaling (Figure 8).

EL000327 is the crude extract from which **B** was isolated. This crude extract contained six compounds, including **B** and another highly cytotoxic compound, D. In our study, we compared the effect of our isolated compound on CRC cells with that of the crude extract, EL000327. Initiation of apoptosis upon treatment with EL000327 was detected by Hoechst staining, the incucyte apoptosis assay, and flow cytometric analysis of apoptosis. However, apoptotic markers were not clearly detected by western blot analysis at the same time points as **B**. Induction of cell cycle arrest, activation of autophagy, or the ROS/JNK pathway related proteins in Caco2 cells were also not observed upon treatment with EL000327. These results suggest that interactions between different compounds in the crude extract may alter the activity of EL000327. Alternatively, the effects of EL000327 and **B** may have been detected at different time points because EL000327 was either faster or slower to act than **B**.

5-Fluorouracil (*5-FU*) is a first-line treatment for many cancers, including CRC. 5-FU leads cells to death by preventing DNA replication and RNA synthesis through inhibition of cellular thymidylate synthase (TS) [46,47]. Combination treatments in which 5-FU is combined with different anticancer agents, enhance the anticancer effect and response rate of these treatments. Similarly, combination of **B** with 5-FU enhanced the cytotoxicity of **B** toward Caco2 and HCT116 cells at significantly lower treatment concentrations [48,49]. Combination of **B** and 5-FU induced apoptosis in Caco2 cells by enhancing the expression of cleaved caspase-3and PARP. Further investigations are required to understand the mechanism by which cytotoxicity is increased in the synergy between **B** and 5-FU. Furthermore, **B** exhibited excellent synergic effects with compound D. A combination of **B** and D induced apoptosis and autophagy in the Caco2 cells at comparatively low concentrations. These results provide evidence that **B** may act synergistically with a range of different anticancer agents to enhance their cytotoxic effect.

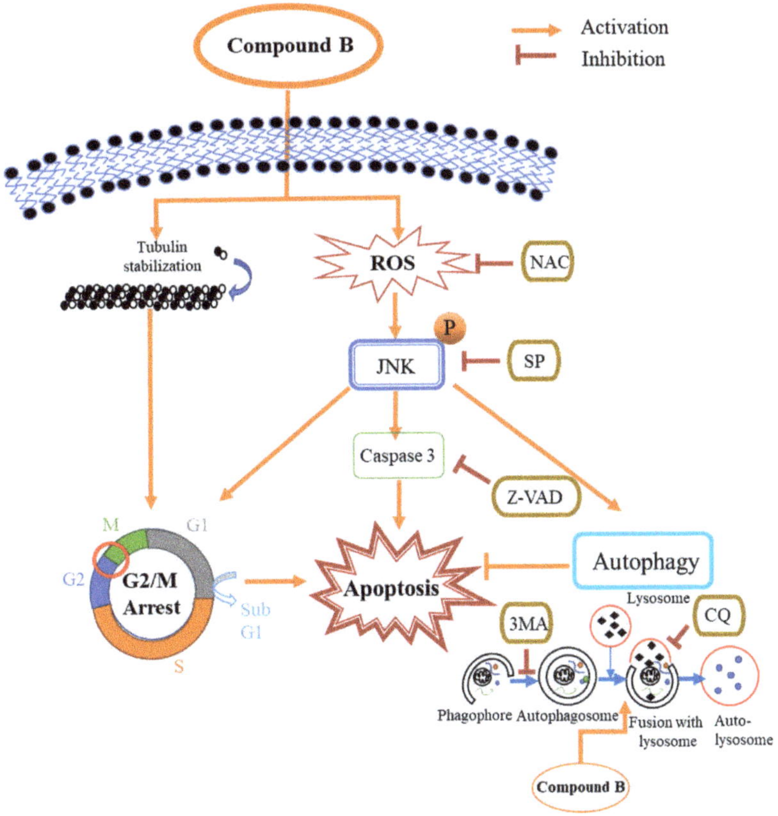

Figure 8. Schematic representation of the proposed mechanism for **B**-induced apoptosis and autophagy in the Caco2 cells. **B** induces apoptosis in Caco2 cells through the induction of G2/M phase arrest caused by tubulin stabilization. Simultaneously, **B** induces apoptosis and autophagy in Caco2 cells via the ROS/JNK signaling pathway. Inhibition of ROS, JNK, and caspases by NAC, SP600125, and Z-VAD-FMK, respectively, decreases **B** induced caspase-dependent apoptosis in Caco2 cells. 3MA and CQ inhibit autophagy in the Caco2 cells. The inhibition of autophagy by preventing the fusion of lysosomes with autophagosomes by CQ significantly increases the induction of caspase-dependent apoptosis by **B** in the Caco2 cells.

B is a novel naturally-derived compound, and this is the first study of the activity of **B** on CRC cells. We thoroughly investigated the mechanisms by which **B** induces apoptotic cell death and have laid the groundwork for a detailed analysis of the clinical usefulness of **B**. Moreover, we have demonstrated that the combination of **B** with known and novel anticancer agents may provide effective new treatment options for patients with CRC, which warrants further investigation.

5. Conclusions

The results of this study demonstrate that **B** induced caspase dependent apoptosis and autophagy in Caco2 cells via activating the ROS/JNK signaling pathway in vitro. In addition, **B** stabilized the microtubule dynamics and disrupted cell cycle progression by inducing G2/M phase arrest. Moreover, **B** exhibited synergism with known chemotherapeutic 5FU and novel compound D on the CRC cells. Together, **B** shows great potential as a novel drug candidate that can be used for further research to develop into an anticancer therapeutic against CRC.

Supplementary Materials: The following supporting information can be downloaded at: https://www.mdpi.com/article/10.3390/cancers15020489/s1, Table S1: Nucleotide sequence of EL000327. Figure S1: B induces G2/M phase arrest in the CRC cells; Figure S2: **B** induces nuclei condensation in the CRC cells; Figure S3: **B** induces apoptosis in CRC cells; Figure S4: **B** decreased apoptosis in the Caco2 cells in the presence of ROS and JNK inhibitors; Figure S5: **B** modulated cell cycle related protein expressions and anti-apoptotic protein Bcl-XL; Figure S6: ^{1}H NMR spectrum of Libertellenone T (**B**) in MeOD; Figure S7: ^{13}C NMR spectrum of Libertellenone T (**B**) in MeOD; Figure S8: Percentage purity of Libertellenone T (**B**); Figure S9: The raw data of Western blotting.

Author Contributions: H.K. and C.D.B.G. conceived and designed the experiments. C.D.B.G., S.-Y.P., M.V., R.Z., S.P., Y.Y. and İ.T. performed the experiments. J.-S.H. contributed the materials. J.-H.K. and S.-J.N. isolated the single compounds. C.D.B.G. and H.K. analyzed the data and wrote the manuscript. All authors have read and agreed to the published version of the manuscript.

Funding: This work was supported by the National Research Foundation of Korea grant (NRF-2020R1C1C1007832) funded by the Korean government (MSIP).

Institutional Review Board Statement: Not applicable.

Informed Consent Statement: Not applicable.

Data Availability Statement: All of the data generated or analyzed during this study are included in the published article and its Supplementary files.

Conflicts of Interest: The authors declare no conflict of interest.

References

1. ACS. Colorectal Cancer Facts and Figures 2020–2022. *Am. Cancer Soc.* **2020**, *66*, 48.
2. Honegger, R.; Axe, L.; Edwards, D. Bacterial epibionts and endolichenic actinobacteria and fungi in the Lower Devonian lichen Chlorolichenomycites salopensis. *Fungal Biol.* **2013**, *117*, 512–518. [CrossRef] [PubMed]
3. Kellogg, J.J.; Raja, H.A. Endolichenic fungi: A new source of rich bioactive secondary metabolites on the horizon. *Phytochem. Rev.* **2017**, *16*, 271–293. [CrossRef]
4. Suryanarayanan, T.S.; Thirunavukkarasu, N. Endolichenic fungi: The lesser known fungal associates of lichens. *Mycology* **2017**, *8*, 189–196. [CrossRef] [PubMed]
5. Yang, Y.; Bae, W.K.; Nam, S.J.; Jeong, M.H.; Zhou, R.; Park, S.Y.; Taş, İ.; Hwang, Y.H.; Park, M.S.; Chung, I.J.; et al. Acetonic extracts of the endolichenic fungus EL002332 isolated from Endocarpon pusillum exhibits anticancer activity in human gastric cancer cells. *Phytomedicine* **2018**, *40*, 106–115. [CrossRef]
6. Solárová, Z.; Liskova, A.; Samec, M.; Kubatka, P.; Büsselberg, D.; Solár, P. Anticancer Potential of Lichens' Secondary Metabolites. *Biomolecules* **2020**, *10*, 87. [CrossRef]
7. Majchrzak-Celińska, A.; Kleszcz, R.; Studzińska-Sroka, E.; Łukaszyk, A.; Szoszkiewicz, A.; Stelcer, E.; Jopek, K.; Rucinski, M.; Cielecka-Piontek, J.; Krajka-Kuźniak, V. Lichen Secondary Metabolites Inhibit the Wnt/β-Catenin Pathway in Glioblastoma Cells and Improve the Anticancer Effects of Temozolomide. *Cells* **2022**, *11*, 84. [CrossRef]
8. Gerl, R.; Vaux, D.L. Apoptosis in the development and treatment of cancer. *Carcinogenesis* **2005**, *26*, 263–270. [CrossRef]
9. Wong, R.S.Y. Apoptosis in cancer: From pathogenesis to treatment. *J. Exp. Clin. Cancer Res.* **2011**, *30*, 87. [CrossRef]
10. Kasibhatla, S.; Tseng, B. Why target apoptosis in cancer treatment? *Mol. Cancer Ther.* **2003**, *2*, 573–580.
11. Choi, Y.H.; Yoo, Y.H. Taxol-induced growth arrest and apoptosis is associated with the upregulation of the Cdk inhibitor, p21WAF1/CIP1, in human breast cancer cells. *Oncol. Rep.* **2012**, *28*, 2163–2169. [CrossRef]
12. Arora, S.; Wang, X.I.; Keenan, S.M.; Andaya, C.; Zhang, Q.; Peng, Y.; Welsh, W.J. Novel microtubule polymerization inhibitor with potent antiproliferative and antitumor activity. *Cancer Res.* **2009**, *69*, 1910–1915. [CrossRef]
13. Yang, Z.J.; Chee, C.E.; Huang, S.; Sinicrope, F.A. The role of autophagy in cancer: Therapeutic implications. *Mol. Cancer Ther.* **2011**, *10*, 1533–1541. [CrossRef]
14. Sun, K.; Deng, W.; Zhang, S.; Cai, N.; Jiao, S.; Song, J.; Wei, L. Paradoxical roles of autophagy in different stages of tumorigenesis: Protector for normal or cancer cells. *Cell Biosci.* **2013**, *3*, 35. [CrossRef]
15. Grácio, D.; Magro, F.; Lima, R.T.; Máximo, V. An overview on the role of autophagy in cancer therapy. *Hematol. Med. Oncol.* **2017**, *2*, 1–4. [CrossRef]
16. Sui, X.; Chen, R.; Wang, Z.; Huang, Z.; Kong, N.; Zhang, M.; Han, W.; Lou, F.; Yang, J.; Zhang, Q.; et al. Autophagy and chemotherapy resistance: A promising therapeutic target for cancer treatment. *Cell Death Dis.* **2013**, *4*, e838. [CrossRef]
17. Sies, H.; Jones, D.P. Reactive oxygen species (ROS) as pleiotropic physiological signalling agents. *Nat. Rev. Mol. Cell Biol.* **2020**, *21*, 363–383. [CrossRef]
18. Cosentino, G.; Plantamura, I.; Cataldo, A.; Iorio, M.V. MicroRNA and Oxidative Stress Interplay in the Context of Breast Cancer Pathogenesis. *Int. J. Mol. Sci.* **2019**, *20*, 5143. [CrossRef]

19. Redza-Dutordoir, M.; Averill-Bates, D.A. Activation of apoptosis signalling pathways by reactive oxygen species. *Biochim. Biophys. Acta-Mol. Cell Res.* **2016**, *1863*, 2977–2992. [CrossRef]
20. Ahmed, D.; Eide, P.W.; Eilertsen, I.A.; Danielsen, S.A.; Eknæs, M.; Hektoen, M.; Lind, G.E.; Lothe, R.A. Epigenetic and genetic features of 24 colon cancer cell lines. *Oncogenesis* **2013**, *2*, e71. [CrossRef]
21. Guo, L.D.; Huang, G.R.; Wang, Y.; He, W.H.; Zheng, W.H.; Hyde, K.D. Molecular identification of white morphotype strains of endophytic fungi from Pinus tabulaeformis. *Mycol. Res.* **2003**, *107*, 680–688. [CrossRef] [PubMed]
22. Gardes, M.; Bruns, T.D. ITS primers with enhanced specificity for basidiomycetes-application to the identification of mycorrhizae and rusts. *Mol. Ecol.* **1993**, *2*, 113–118. [CrossRef] [PubMed]
23. Vilgalys, R.; Hester, M. Rapid genetic identification and mapping of enzymatically amplified ribosomal DNA from several Cryptococcus species. *J. Bacteriol.* **1990**, *172*, 4238–4246. [CrossRef] [PubMed]
24. Seca, A.M.L.; Pinto, D.C.G.A.; Silva, A.M.S. Structural Elucidation of Pimarane and Isopimarane Diterpenoids: The 13C NMR Contribution. *Nat. Prod. Commun.* **2008**, *3*, 1934578X0800300317. [CrossRef]
25. Huang, M.; Lu, J.J.; Ding, J. Natural Products in Cancer Therapy: Past, Present and Future. *Nat. Products Bioprospect.* **2021**, *11*, 5–13. [CrossRef] [PubMed]
26. Nguyen, T.T.; Yoon, S.; Yang, Y.; Lee, H.B.; Oh, S.; Jeong, M.H.; Kim, J.J.; Yee, S.T.; Crişan, F.; Moon, C.; et al. Lichen secondary metabolites in Flavocetraria cucullata Exhibit anti-cancer effects on human cancer cells through the induction of apoptosis and suppression of tumorigenic potentials. *PLoS ONE* **2014**, *9*, e111575. [CrossRef]
27. Yang, Y.; Park, S.Y.; Nguyen, T.T.; Yu, Y.H.; Van Nguyen, T.; Sun, E.G.; Udeni, J.; Jeong, M.H.; Pereira, I.; Moon, C.; et al. Lichen secondary metabolite, physciosporin, inhibits lung cancer cell motility. *PLoS ONE* **2015**, *10*, e0137889. [CrossRef]
28. Taş, İ.; Han, J.; Park, S.Y.; Yang, Y.; Zhou, R.; Gamage, C.D.B.; Van Nguyen, T.; Lee, J.Y.; Choi, Y.J.; Yu, Y.H.; et al. Physciosporin suppresses the proliferation, motility and tumourigenesis of colorectal cancer cells. *Phytomedicine* **2019**, *56*, 10–20. [CrossRef]
29. Taş, İ.; Varlı, M.; Son, Y.; Han, J.; Kwak, D.; Yang, Y.; Zhou, R.; Gamage, C.D.B.; Pulat, S.; Park, S.Y.; et al. Physciosporin suppresses mitochondrial respiration, aerobic glycolysis, and tumorigenesis in breast cancer. *Phytomedicine* **2021**, *91*, 153674. [CrossRef]
30. Yang, Y.; Bhosle, S.R.; Yu, Y.H.; Park, S.-Y.; Zhou, R.; Taş, I.; Gamage, C.D.B.; Kim, K.K.; Pereira, I.; Hur, J.-S.; et al. Tumidulin, a lichen secondary metabolite, decreases the stemness potential of colorectal cancer cells. *Molecules* **2018**, *23*, 2968. [CrossRef]
31. Zhou, R.; Yang, Y.; Park, S.-Y.; Nguyen, T.T.; Seo, Y.-W.; Lee, K.H.; Lee, J.H.; Kim, K.K.; Hur, J.-S.; Kim, H. The lichen secondary metabolite atranorin suppresses lung cancer cell motility and tumorigenesis. *Sci. Rep.* **2017**, *7*, 8136. [CrossRef]
32. Xie, Y.H.; Chen, Y.X.; Fang, J.Y. Comprehensive review of targeted therapy for colorectal cancer. *Signal Transduct. Target. Ther.* **2020**, *5*, 22. [CrossRef]
33. Zachos, G. Regulating Cytokinesis. In *Encyclopedia of Cell Biology*; Bradshaw, R.A., Stahl, P.D., Eds.; Academic Press: Waltham, MA, USA, 2016; pp. 494–503. ISBN 978-0-12-394796-3.
34. Rohrer Bley, C.; Furmanova, P.; Orlowski, K.; Grosse, N.; Broggini-Tenzer, A.; McSheehy, P.M.J.; Pruschy, M. Microtubule stabilising agents and ionising radiation: Multiple exploitable mechanisms for combined treatment. *Eur. J. Cancer* **2013**, *49*, 245–253. [CrossRef]
35. Elmore, S. Apoptosis: A review of programmed cell death. *Toxicol. Pathol.* **2007**, *35*, 495–516. [CrossRef]
36. Hassan, M.; Watari, H.; AbuAlmaaty, A.; Ohba, Y.; Sakuragi, N. Apoptosis and Molecular Targeting Therapy in Cancer. *Biomed. Res. Int.* **2014**, *2014*, 150845. [CrossRef]
37. Lee, T.J.; Kim, E.J.; Kim, S.; Jung, E.M.; Park, J.W.; Jeong, S.H.; Park, S.E.; Yoo, Y.H.; Kwon, T.K. Caspase-dependent and caspase-independent apoptosis induced by evodiamine in human leukemic U937 cells. *Mol. Cancer Ther.* **2006**, *5*, 2398–2407. [CrossRef]
38. Liu, P.-F.; Hu, Y.-C.; Kang, B.-H.; Tseng, Y.-K.; Wu, P.-C.; Liang, C.-C.; Hou, Y.-Y.; Fu, T.-Y.; Liou, H.-H.; Hsieh, I.-C.; et al. Expression levels of cleaved caspase-3 and caspase-3 in tumorigenesis and prognosis of oral tongue squamous cell carcinoma. *PLoS ONE* **2017**, *12*, e0180620. [CrossRef]
39. Chaitanya, G.V.; Alexander, J.S.; Babu, P.P. PARP-1 cleavage fragments: Signatures of cell-death proteases in neurodegeneration. *Cell Commun. Signal.* **2010**, *8*, 31. [CrossRef]
40. Park, J.M.; Huang, S.; Wu, T.T.; Foster, N.R.; Sinicrope, F.A. Prognostic impact of Beclin 1, p62/sequestosome 1 and LC3 protein expression in colon carcinomas from patients receiving 5-fluorouracil as adjuvant chemotherapy. *Cancer Biol. Ther.* **2013**, *14*, 100. [CrossRef]
41. Sahani, M.H.; Itakura, E.; Mizushima, N. Expression of the autophagy substrate SQSTM1/p62 is restored during prolonged starvation depending on transcriptional upregulation and autophagy-derived amino acids. *Autophagy* **2014**, *10*, 431–441. [CrossRef]
42. Duran, A.; Amanchy, R.; Linares, J.F.; Joshi, J.; Abu-Baker, S.; Porollo, A.; Hansen, M.; Moscat, J.; Diaz-Meco, M.T. p62 is a key regulator of nutrient sensing in the mTORC1 pathway. *Mol. Cell* **2011**, *44*, 134–146. [CrossRef] [PubMed]
43. Liu, W.J.; Ye, L.; Huang, W.F.; Guo, L.J.; Xu, Z.G.; Wu, H.L.; Yang, C.; Liu, H.F. p62 links the autophagy pathway and the ubiqutin–proteasome system upon ubiquitinated protein degradation. *Cell. Mol. Biol. Lett.* **2016**, *21*, 29. [CrossRef] [PubMed]
44. Mulcahy Levy, J.M.; Thorburn, A. Autophagy in cancer: Moving from understanding mechanism to improving therapy responses in patients. *Cell Death Differ.* **2020**, *27*, 843–857. [CrossRef] [PubMed]
45. Zhou, Y.Y.; Li, Y.; Jiang, W.Q.; Zhou, L.F. MAPK/JNK signalling: A potential autophagy regulation pathway. *Biosci. Rep.* **2015**, *35*, e00199. [CrossRef]

46. Longley, D.B.; Harkin, D.P.; Johnston, P.G. 5-Fluorouracil: Mechanisms of action and clinical strategies. *Nat. Rev. Cancer* **2003**, *3*, 330–338. [CrossRef]
47. Ghafouri-Fard, S.; Abak, A.; Tondro Anamag, F.; Shoorei, H.; Fattahi, F.; Javadinia, S.A.; Basiri, A.; Taheri, M. 5-Fluorouracil: A Narrative Review on the Role of Regulatory Mechanisms in Driving Resistance to This Chemotherapeutic Agent. *Front. Oncol.* **2021**, *11*, 1210. [CrossRef]
48. Sethy, C.; Kundu, C.N. 5-Fluorouracil (5-FU) resistance and the new strategy to enhance the sensitivity against cancer: Implication of DNA repair inhibition. *Biomed. Pharmacother.* **2021**, *137*, 111285. [CrossRef]
49. Țigu, A.B.; Toma, V.-A.; Moț, A.C.; Jurj, A.; Moldovan, C.S.; Fischer-Fodor, E.; Berindan-Neagoe, I.; Pârvu, M. The Synergistic Antitumor Effect of 5-Fluorouracil Combined with Allicin against Lung and Colorectal Carcinoma Cells. *Molecules* **2020**, *25*, 1947. [CrossRef]

International Journal of *Molecular Sciences*

MDPI

Article

New Affordable Methods for Large-Scale Isolation of Major Olive Secoiridoids and Systematic Comparative Study of Their Antiproliferative/Cytotoxic Effect on Multiple Cancer Cell Lines of Different Cancer Origins

Aikaterini Papakonstantinou [1,2], Petrina Koumarianou [1,3,†], Aimilia Rigakou [2,†], Panagiotis Diamantakos [2], Efseveia Frakolaki [4,‡], Niki Vassilaki [4], Evangelia Chavdoula [5], Eleni Melliou [2,6], Prokopios Magiatis [2,*] and Haralabia Boleti [1,3,*]

1 Intracellular Parasitism Laboratory, Microbiology Department, Hellenic Pasteur Institute, 11521 Athens, Greece
2 Laboratory of Pharmacognosy and Natural Products Chemistry, Department of Pharmacy, National and Kapodistrian University of Athens, Panepistimiopolis Zografou, 15771 Athens, Greece
3 Light Microscopy Unit, Hellenic Pasteur Institute, 11521 Athens, Greece
4 Molecular Virology Laboratory, Microbiology Department, Hellenic Pasteur Institute, 11521 Athens, Greece
5 Biomedical Research Division, Institute of Molecular Biology and Biotechnology, Foundation for Research and Technology, 45110 Ioannina, Greece
6 World Olive Center for Health, Imittou 76, 11634 Athens, Greece
* Correspondence: magiatis@pharm.uoa.gr (P.M.); hboleti@pasteur.gr (H.B.); Tel.: +30-210-7274052 (P.M.); +30-210-6478879 (H.B.)
† These authors contributed equally to this work.
‡ Deceased.

Citation: Papakonstantinou, A.; Koumarianou, P.; Rigakou, A.; Diamantakos, P.; Frakolaki, E.; Vassilaki, N.; Chavdoula, E.; Melliou, E.; Magiatis, P.; Boleti, H. New Affordable Methods for Large-Scale Isolation of Major Olive Secoiridoids and Systematic Comparative Study of Their Antiproliferative/Cytotoxic Effect on Multiple Cancer Cell Lines of Different Cancer Origins. *Int. J. Mol. Sci.* **2023**, *24*, 3. https://doi.org/10.3390/ijms24010003

Academic Editors: Barbara De Filippis, Marialuigia Fantacuzzi and Alessandra Ammazzalorso

Received: 25 October 2022
Revised: 12 December 2022
Accepted: 14 December 2022
Published: 20 December 2022

Abstract: Olive oil phenols (OOPs) are associated with the prevention of many human cancers. Some of these have been shown to inhibit cell proliferation and induce apoptosis. However, no systematic comparative study exists for all the investigated compounds under the same conditions, due to difficulties in their isolation or synthesis. Herein are presented innovative methods for large-scale selective extraction of six major secoiridoids from olive oil or leaves enabling their detailed investigation. The cytotoxic/antiproliferative bioactivity of these six compounds was evaluated on sixteen human cancer cell lines originating from eight different tissues. Cell viability with half-maximal effective concentrations (EC_{50}) was evaluated after 72 h treatments. Antiproliferative and pro-apoptotic effects were also assessed for the most bioactive compounds ($EC_{50} \leq 50$ μM). Oleocanthal (**1**) showed the strongest antiproliferative/cytotoxic activity in most cancer cell lines (EC_{50}: 9–20 μM). The relative effectiveness of the six OOPs was: oleocanthal (**1**) > oleuropein aglycone (**3a,b**) > ligstroside aglycone (**4a,b**) > oleacein (**2**) > oleomissional (**6a,b,c**) > oleocanthalic acid (**7**). This is the first detailed study comparing the bioactivity of six OOPs in such a wide array of cancer cell lines, providing a reference for their relative antiproliferative/cytotoxic effect in the investigated cancers.

Keywords: olive oil phenols; olive secoiridoids; oleocanthal; oleacein; antiproliferative bioactivity; cytotoxic bioactivity; pro-apoptotic effect; human cancer cells; health protection

1. Introduction

Epidemiological data support the hypothesis that the Mediterranean diet (MD) may have an important role in preventing several types of cancer [1–4]. Furthermore, a clinical trial in which the diet was modified toward an improved adherence to MD showed a reduced total mortality and cancer risk after a 4-year follow-up [2]. A particular characteristic of the MD is that olive oil is the primary source of dietary lipids. The importance of olive oil in cancer prevention began to be highlighted by several epidemiological studies initiated in the mid-nineties which showed a decreased risk of cancer in different sites associated with the uptake of olive oil [5]. Although these results have to be confirmed by extensive clinical trials, a recent pilot clinical trial with patients suffering from chronic lymphocytic leukemia demonstrated, for the first time, the anti-cancer therapeutic properties of olive oil containing high amounts of the polyphenols oleocanthal (**1**) and oleacein (**2**) [6]. Although the term polyphenols is not chemically accurate when used for olive oil phenols, it is widely used in the formal legislation regarding the health claims of olive oil in the EU and for this reason it is also used herein.

The cancer-preventive capacity of olive oil could be mediated at least in part by the presence of minor components which include more than 230 chemical compounds present in a small amount (about 2% of oil weight). Among these components, of particular interest are the different classes of phenolic compounds represented by phenolic acids, phenolic alcohols, flavonoids, secoiridoids and lignans. In particular, the phenolic alcohols hydroxytyrosol and tyrosol are abundantly present in olives, olive leaves and olive oil as both free compounds and linked to either elenolic acid (EA) or its dialdehydic form (EDA) giving rise to the secoiridoid derivatives oleuropein aglycone (3,4, DHPEA-EA) (**3a,b**), ligstroside aglycone (*p*-HPEA-EA) (**4a,b**), oleocanthal (*p*-HPEA-EDA) (**1**) and oleacein (3,4, DHPEA-EDA) (**2**) [7]. These compounds are not generally present in other types of oil and in other foods of vegetable origin. Their concentration in olive oil varies and depends upon several factors such as the variety of the olive tree, the agronomic conditions during cultivation and the maturity of the fruit during harvesting as well as the technological aspects of olive oil production, especially the time and temperature of malaxation [8]. Moreover, although compounds (**1–4**) are also found in other plants, olive oil is the only edible source providing them. The polyphenols found in olive oil have well-established beneficial effects on human health and metabolism [9–12].

A cancer chemo-preventive activity of olive oil has been attributed to hydroxytyrosol and tyrosol and their secoiridoid derivatives oleocanthal (**1**), oleacein (**2**), oleuropein aglycone (**3a,b**) and ligstroside aglycone (**4a,b**) [7,9,13–19]. Several studies have demonstrated that certain of these compounds can inhibit proliferation and induce apoptosis in different tumor cell lines and most animal studies have confirmed the ability of certain olive oil polyphenols (OOPs) to inhibit carcinogenesis both in the initiation and in the promotion/progression phases [19–33]. However, further investigations are necessary to clarify the real chemo-preventive potential of OOPs in humans, such as performing intervention studies on populations at high cancer risk [7]. This shows the urgency of performing in-depth investigations on the mechanism(s) of action of OOPs, in cell- and animal-based cancer models. Additionally, it is important to investigate the safety/toxicity issues of all the main phenolic ingredients of olive oil.

Recent advances in the development of a simple and rapid methodology for the direct identification and concentration measurement of each phenol in olive oil using quantitative ^{1}H-nuclear magnetic resonance spectroscopy (qNMR) have offered a new perspective on the quality control of the health-protecting properties of olive oil [34,35]. During the last few years, several chromatographic techniques have been established for the isolation of each OOP, enlarging the spectrum of these natural products identified in olive oil [30,34–41]. In addition, several methods for their chemical synthesis have been published [42,43]. However, at present, there are no available methods based on selective extraction that could override the need for chromatographic purification. All existing methods are quite complicated or expensive for large-scale application, thus limiting the availability of OOPs as material for research or commercial purposes. In the present work, a variety of new methods for OOPs' isolation are presented which are easily applicable on a large scale, permitting the compounds' acquisition at appropriate amounts for further investigation of their bioactivities or for the production of commercial products.

Most studies concerning the cytotoxic or antitumor properties of OOPs have been performed so far with olive oil extracts, [16,25,44] hydroxytyrosol and tyrosol [13,45,46] and their secoiridoid derivatives oleocanthal (**1**) [20,24,29,31,47–49], oleacein (**2**) [19,26,50], oleuropein aglycone (**3a,b**) [17,27,51] and ligstroside aglycone (**4a,b**) [23,52,53]. No studies have been performed with the other polyphenols available today in pure form (i.e., oleokoronal (**5a,b,c**), oleomissional (**6a,b,c**) and oleocanthalic acid (**7**) [34,40]). Moreover, all these studies have been conducted with only one or a maximum of two compounds on one or up to very few cancer cell lines from one or a maximum of two cancer types by the same research team. Interestingly, all studies on the bioactivity of OOPs on cancer cell lines have been performed under the atmospheric O_2 tension (20% (v/v)) used in cell culture and traditionally applied in drug screening. The O_2 tensions, which in the body tissues and tumors are <5% (v/v) (tissue normoxia and hypoxia), have important effects in the bioenergetic metabolism of the cells affecting the sensitivity/response of tumors to anti-cancer agents [54–63].

The present study contributes to the current knowledge and fills gaps in the understanding of the potential antiproliferative/cytotoxic properties of OOPs by studying six different representatives of these phenols. These in turn are produced in the same laboratory specializing in the isolation and characterization of OOPs from olive oil or olive leaves coming from Greek varieties of olive trees, ensuring thereby the reproducibility of results for each tested compound [34,40,64,65]. Moreover, herein are presented results from the analysis of the antiproliferative/cytotoxic effects of six OOPs on a large number of cancer cell lines from eight different tissue origins and at conditions resembling the tumor microenvironment (i.e., hypoxia and serum starvation). This allows a systematic and reliable comparative analysis of their bioactivity on different tumors since the same methodology was applied and the OOPs were isolated by the same laboratory following standardized protocols. Finally, the test results of the antiproliferative/cytotoxic OOPs' action on non-tumorigenic cell lines are presented, contributing thereby to the search for the most effective ones with the fewest side effects on non-cancer cells.

2. Results and Discussion

2.1. Large-Scale Isolation of OOPs

The property of secoiridoid phenolic aldehydes such as oleocanthal (**1**) that allows them to react with water and generate water-soluble hydrates such as oleocanthadiol (**8**) [66] was used to develop methods of selective extraction without the application of a final chromatographic purification. The avoidance of chromatography is a very important advantage in comparison with the known methods of isolation [30,34–41], permitting the easy and cost-effective scale-up of the isolation procedure.

2.2. Isolation of Oleocanthal (1)

Oleocanthal (**1**) can be easily extracted from olive oil using water [30,67]. Oleocanthadiol (**8**), the product of oleocanthal's (**1**) reaction with water, is a water-soluble compound while the rest of the olive oil's lipophilic ingredients remain in the oil-containing phase. Evaporation of the aqueous phase as a next step in the procedure provided pure oleocanthal (**1**). It is important to note that successful application of this method requires that the starting material of olive oil does not contain secoiridoid phenolic aldehydes other than oleocanthal (**1**). Screening of thousands of olive oil samples using qNMR [35] led to the identification of an olive fruit variety (i.e., the Kalamon variety), which under appropriate milling conditions gives olive oil containing only oleocanthal (**1**) as secoiridoid phenolic aldehyde [8,68]. Starting with this type of olive oil, the described method provides pure oleocanthal (**1**) in one extraction step. When the starting material is an olive oil containing additional secoiridoid phenolic aldehydes, the water extraction step leads to a mixture of oleocanthal (**1**), oleacein (**2**), oleuropein aglycone (**3a,b**) and ligstroside aglycone (**4a,b**) that can be further purified using classic chromatographic methods, as previously reported [35].

2.3. Isolation of Oleacein (2)

The above-described property of the secoiridoid phenolic aldehydes of reacting reversibly with water led us to investigate the possibility of extracting secoiridoid phenolic aldehydes from olive leaves using cold water at temperatures ranging between 15 and 25

°C. In contrast to the common extraction using hot water at boiling temperature that leads to extracts with oleuropein (**9**) as the main phenolic ingredient [69,70], the cold-water extraction led to pure oleacein (**2**). In fact, when the intact leaves are shredded in the presence of cold water, the enzymes of oleuropein glucosidase [71] and demethylase [72] come into contact with their substrate oleuropein (**9**) and transform it to oleacein (**2**). When hot water is used, the enzymes are deactivated and oleuropein (**9**) remains intact. The cold-water extract contains oleaceinediol (**10**) together with several other hydrophilic ingredients such as sugars (i.e., mannitol, glucose, etc.). However, among them, only oleaceinediol (**10**) can be reversibly transformed back to the dialdehyde form of oleacein (**2**) when it comes in contact with solvents such as ethyl acetate (EtOAc) or dichloromethane (CH_2Cl_2). A simple re-extraction step of the cold-water extract led directly to pure oleacein (**2**) (purity > 95%).

2.4. *Isolation of Oleomissional (**6a,b,c**)*

Surprisingly, when intact olive leaves or olive fruits came in contact with organic solvents such as CH_2Cl_2, the obtained extract contained only oleomissional (**6a,b,c**) together with lipophilic triterpenoids. Oleomissional (**6a,b,c**) is the enolic form of the open-ring type of oleuropein aglycone (**6a**), which is in equilibrium with two isomeric oleuropeindials (**6b,c**) and is the first product arising from the action of oleuropein glucosidase on oleuropein. Solvents such as CH_2Cl_2 disrupt the cell membranes permitting the partial activity of glucosidase, which is a very resistant enzymatic system, but do not permit the action of the demethylase. The obtained oleomissional (**6a,b,c**) can be easily separated from the rest of the lipophilic compounds based on its ability to react with water and be reversibly transformed into a hydrophilic diol (oleomissionadiol). Re-extraction of the water solution using EtOAc or CH_2Cl_2 led to pure oleomissional (**6a,b,c**).

2.5. *Conversion of Oleomissional (**6a,b,c**) to Closed-Type Oleuropein Aglycone (**3a,b**)*

Oleomissionadiol (**11a,b**) in aqueous solutions is stable only when the pH is slightly acidic. When the pH becomes slightly alkaline then the molecule rearranges from the open form to the closed-ring form of the oleuropein aglycone (**3a,b**). This molecule exists as a mixture of two isomers (R, S) which can be easily obtained by a simple extraction of the alkaline aqueous solution using organic solvents.

2.6. *Effect of Six OOPs on the Proliferation/Viability of Cancer Cells*

The potential anticancer properties of OOPs have been extensively investigated during the last two decades, mainly for tyrosol, hydroxytyrosol and less often with oleocanthal (**1**) or other OOPs. The establishment of the aforementioned new methods for OOPs' isolation has enabled further studies on the biological properties of each one of them on a wide array of cancer cell models. The present study investigated the antiproliferative and/or cytotoxic effect of oleocanthal (**1**), oleacein (**2**), oleuropein aglycone (**3a,b**), ligstroside aglycone (**4a,b**) and the newly identified major phenolic ingredients oleomissional (**6a,b,c**) and oleocanthalic acid (**7**) [34,40] (Figure 1). The six compounds analyzed in this study were isolated as described in the Experimental Section. Their bioactivity was evaluated on sixteen human tumor-derived cell lines, sensitive or resistant to certain chemotherapy agents, from eight different tissue origins. Moreover, the bioactivity of the six OOPs was tested on five non-tumorigenic cell lines (Table S1).

The antiproliferative/cytotoxic effects of the selected OOPs on each cell line were assessed by measuring the cellular ATP levels after 72 h treatments using an ATP-based luminescence assay [73]. This assay, initially developed as a tumor chemosensitivity assay, has shown considerable promise as a general in vitro toxicity assay due to its high sensitivity that allows the detection of a small number of cells. Consequently, it can be applied to both cancer cell lines and primary tissue cells. To evaluate the dose–response effect of each OOP, concentrations of 1–100 μM were used and the bioactivity strength of the six OOPs was compared on the basis of their effective concentration (EC_{50s}; i.e., concentrations that inhibited the proliferation of the cell population by 50% as compared to control cells treated just with the solvent (i.e., DMSO)). The EC_{50} values were calculated by nonlinear regression (curve fit) using a sigmoidal dose–response equation (Figures 2A and S2).

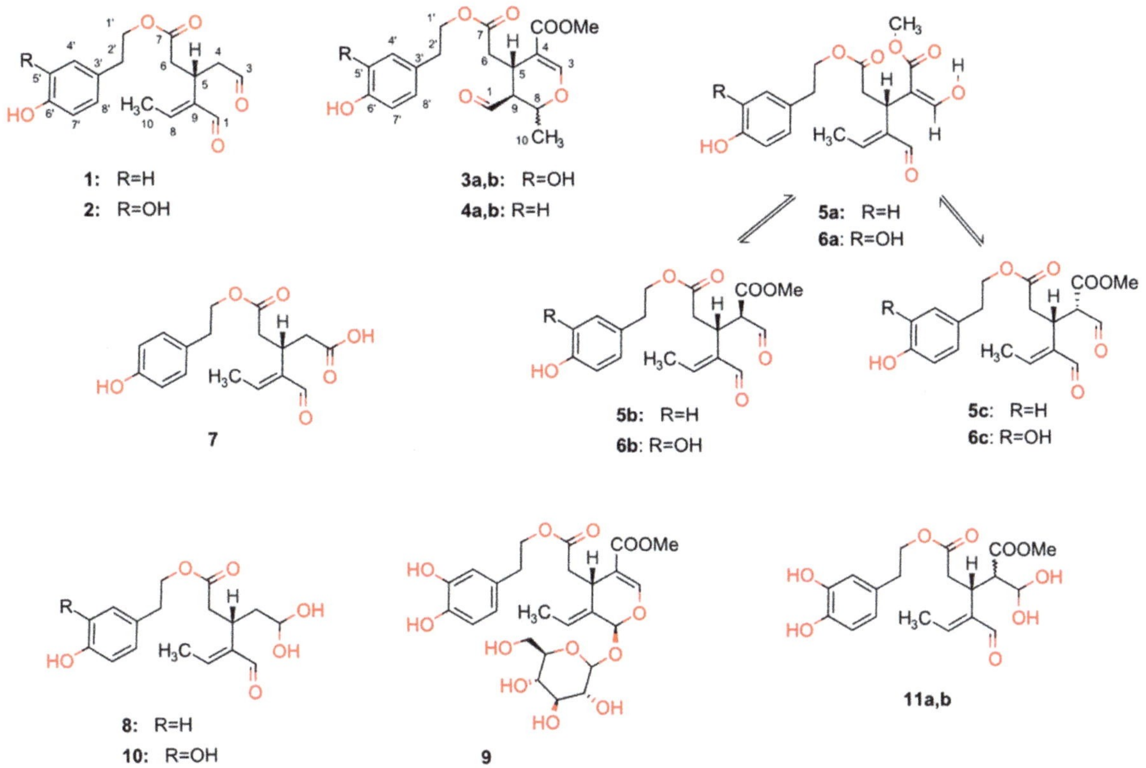

Figure 1. Structures of the studied OOPs and related compounds: oleocanthal (**1**), oleacein (**2**), oleuropein aglycone (**3a,b**), ligstroside aglycone (**4a,b**), oleomissional (**6a,b,c**), oleokoronal (**7a,b,c**), oleocanthalic acid (**7**), oleocanthadiol (**8**), oleuropein (**9**), oleaceinediol (**10**) and oleomissionadiol (**11a,b**).

The relative antiproliferative/cytotoxic activity of OOPs on cancer cells after 72 h treatment was: oleocanthal (**1**) > oleuropein aglycone (**3a,b**) > ligstroside aglycone (**4a,b**) > oleacein (**2**) > oleomissional (**6a,b,c**) > oleocanthalic acid (**7**) (Figure 2B and Table 1). The calculated EC_{50} values ranged between 9.1–100 μM (Table 1). The bioactivity of the oleocanthalic acid (**7**), studied here for the first time for its antiproliferative/cytotoxic activity, was initially evaluated systematically in the three breast cancer cell lines using a concentration range of 10–100 μM. In all cases, the viability measured was ≥80%, predicting EC_{50} values > 100 μM. Since this study was focused on OOPs with EC_{50} values < 100 μM, which would be promising for future use in cancer prevention or cancer treatment, the range of concentrations tested for all six compounds analyzed was below 100 μM. For this reason, oleocanthalic acid (**7**) was excluded from the rest of this study.

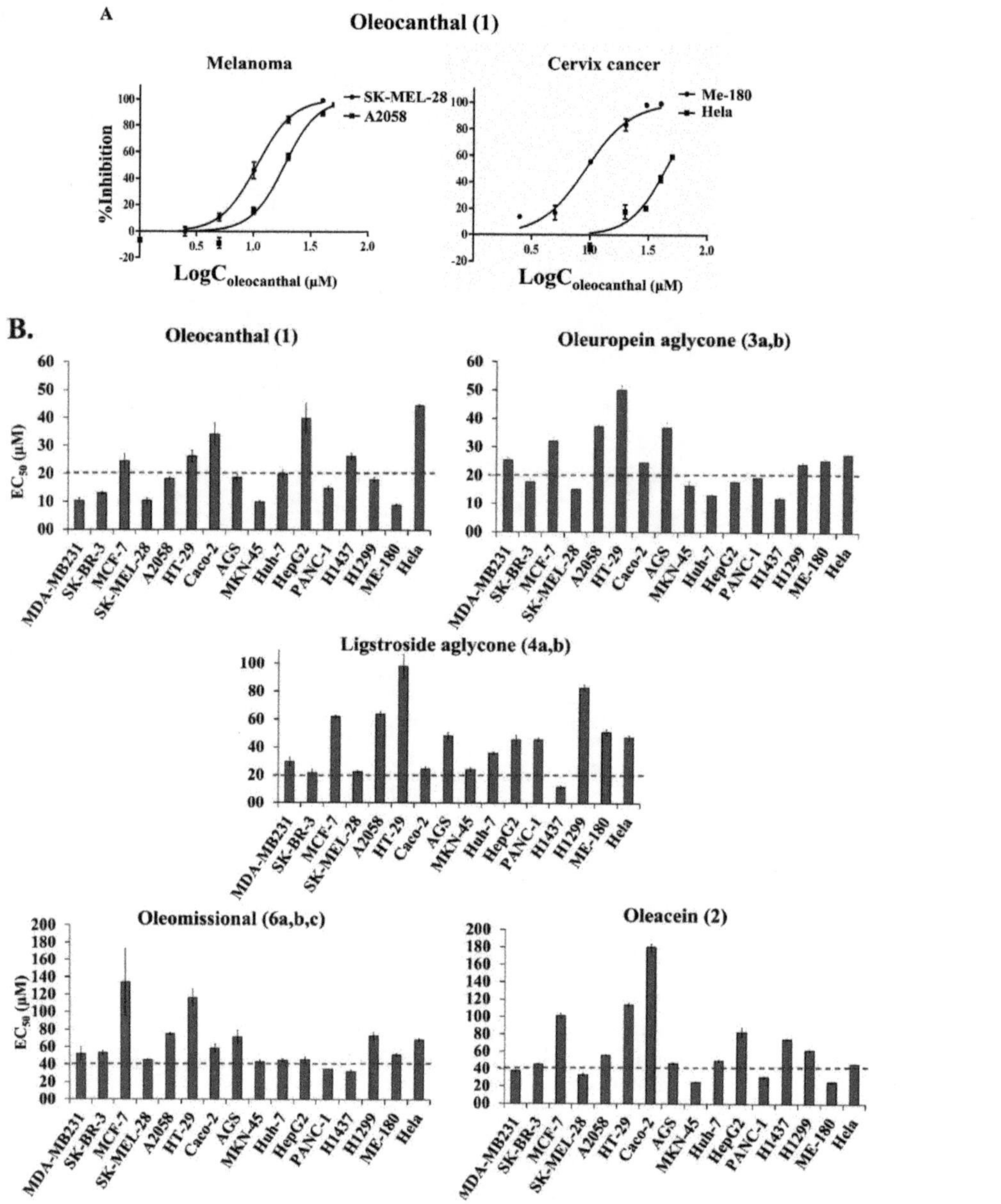

Figure 2. OOPs reduce cell numbers/viability of several cancer cell lines. (**A**) The effect of different concentrations of oleocanthal on four cancer cell lines is shown as sigmoidal dose–response curves in two representative panels. Cell numbers/viability was measured using the ATP-based luminescence assay after 72 h treatment. The results shown are from two or three independent experiments performed in triplicates. Data are represented as mean cell count ± SE in each treatment group normalized to the control group (i.e., cells treated only with 0.2% (*v*/*v*) DMSO). (**B**) Effects of different concentrations of oleocanthal (**1**), oleacein (**2**), oleuropein aglycone (**3a,b**), ligstroside aglycone (**4a,b**) and oleomissional (**6a,b,c**) on cell numbers/viability. Bar graphs representing the mean EC_{50} values for the studied compounds on the cell numbers/viability of a panel of sixteen cancer cell lines from

eight different tissue origins. Mean EC_{50} values ± SE are from two or three independent experiments performed in triplicate. The EC_{50} values were calculated using the GraphPad Prism software.

Table 1. EC_{50} values of OOPs (i.e., oleocanthal (**1**), oleacein (**2**), oleuropein aglycone (**3a,b**), ligstroside aglycone (**4a,b**), oleomissional (**6a,b,c**) and oleocanthalic acid (**7**)). Their effect on the proliferation or the viability of cancer and non-tumorigenic transformed cell lines or normal cell lines was determined by the ATP assay. EC_{50} values were calculated after 72 h treatments for each experiment using GraphPad Prism software and were then used to calculate the average and the SE values. The results presented are from two or three independent experiments performed in triplicate.

		EC_{50} Values of Olive Oil Polyphenols					
Cell Origin	**Cell Line**	**1**	**2**	**3a,b**	**4a,b**	**6a,b,c**	**7**
Human Breast cancer cell lines	MDA-MB 231	10.4 ± 0.8	37.7 ± 2.2	25.4 ± 0.8	31.6 ± 2.7	52.0 ± 7.6	>100
	SK-BR-3	13.0 ± 0.6	45.6 ± 2.2	17.7 ± 1.4	21.5 ± 2.5	53.4 ± 2.0	>100
	MCF-7	24.6 ± 2.6	>100	32.2 ± 1.1	61.8 ± 1.2	>100	>100
Skin melanoma cell lines	SK-MEL-28	10.4 ± 1.1	33.4 ± 2.4	15.1 ± 0.9	22.2 ± 1.2	45.1 ± 0.5	–
	A2058	18.4 ± 0.4	55.7 ± 3.4	37.2 ± 0.8	63.6 ± 1.6	74.9 ± 1.4	–
Colon and gastric cancer cell lines	HT-29	26.3 ± 2.0	>100	50.1 ± 1.5	98.2 ± 8.4	>100	–
	Caco-2	34.3 ± 4.1	>100	24.5 ± 0.9	24.4 ± 1.6	58.9 ± 4.6	–
	AGS	18.3 ± 1.0	46.2 ± 2.3	35.9 ± 1.4	48.5 ± 2.5	75.2 ± 5.2	–
	MKN-45	10.2 ± 0.4	25.0 ± 2.1	16.4 ± 1.6	24.0 ± 1.2	43.7 ± 1.5	–
Liver cancer cell lines	Huh-7	20.2 ± 1.5	49.6 ± 0.5	13.0 ± 0.1	36.0 ± 0.9	44.9 ± 1.6	–
	HepG-2	40.0 ± 5.3	82.8 ± 0.7	17.7 ± 0.5	45.8 ± 3.4	45.5 ± 3.5	–
Pancreatic cancer cell line	PANC-1	14.9 ± 0.9	30.9 ± 0.2	19.1 ± 0.6	45.7 ± 1.4	34.8 ± 0.1	–
Lung Cancer cell lines	H1437	26.5 ± 1.1	74.6 ± 2.1	11.9 ± 0.6	11.6 ± 1.1	32.1 ± 1.1	–
	H1299	18.2 ± 0.9	61.7 ± 1.3	24.1 ± 0.9	83.3 ± 1.9	73.4 ± 4.5	–
Cervical Cancer cell lines	ME-180	9.1 ± 0.3	25.2 ± 0.2	25.5 ± 0.5	51.1 ± 2.2	51.9 ± 1.5	–
	Hela	44.6 ± 0.4	46.3 ± 4.9	27.6 ± 0.3	47.6 ± 1.8	69.0 ± 1.6	–
Non cancer cell line derived from lung	MRC-5	2.0 ± 0.1	7.0 ± 0.9	8.6 ± 0.4	13.2 ± 0.9	24.2 ± 1.2	–
Spontaneously transformed aneuploidy immortal keratinocytes	HaCaT	19.3 ± 0.3	51.8 ± 4.2	36.6 ± 0.0	55.6 ± 1.0	63.7 ± 4.6	–
Human non-tumorigenic epithelial cell	MCF 10A	7.0 ± 0.3	24.7 ± 2.7	9.5 ± 0.4	55.8 ± 2.7	35.4 ± 1.9	–
Mesenchymal Cells	WJ-MSC	19.1 ± 5.6	28.2 ± 11.1	28.7 ± 0.3	39.3 ± 3.8	92.7 ± 38.5	–
Normal Human Dermal Fibroblasts	NHDF	24.7 ± 0.4	49.0 ± 1.2	42.7 ± 0.5	46.5 ± 5.0	64.2 ± 1.9	–

Oleomissional (**6a,b,c**), which was also studied here for the first time, presented EC_{50s} > 50 μM for the cell lines from breast cancer (i.e., MDA-MB 231, MCF-7 and SK-BR-3), skin melanoma (i.e., A2058), colon and gastric epithelium cancer (i.e., HT-29, Caco-2, AGS) and cervical cancer (i.e., ME-180, Hela). However, for the MKN-45 gastric cancer, SK-MEL-28 melanoma, liver and pancreas cancer cell lines (i.e., Huh-7, HepG-2 and PANC-1) and the H1437 lung cancer cell line, the EC_{50} values exhibited by oleomissional (**6a,b,c**), were <50 μM (Table 1). Significant variation was observed in the OOPs' EC_{50} values for cancer cell lines with different tissue tumor origin but also amongst cell lines of the same tissue origin but with different genetic identities (Figure 3, Table 1).

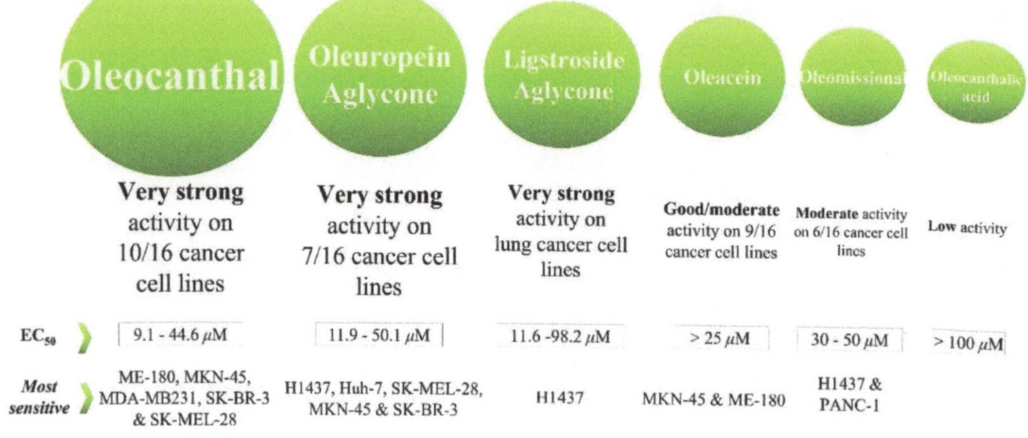

Figure 3. Bioactivity range of OOPs on several cancer cell lines from eight different tissue origins.

With respect to breast cancer, the MDA-MB-231, SK-BR-3 and MCF-7 cell lines were selected as representative for this study. The highly metastatic, triple-negative MDA-MB-231 cells lack the expression of estrogen receptor (ERα)—the target for hormonal therapy—and overexpress c-Met—a breast cancer molecular target of oleocanthal (**1**). The SK-BR-3 cell line overexpresses human epidermal growth factor receptor 2 (HER2) while the MCF-7 cells express ERα and c-Met [28,47,74]. Oleocanthal (**1**) was the most effective OOP on all three breast cancer cell lines (EC_{50} = 10.5–24.6 μM) and oleuropein aglycone (**3a,b**) followed in potency (EC_{50} = 17.7–32.2 μM). The MCF-7 cancer cells proved to be the most resistant to oleocanthal (**1**) of all three cell lines, with EC_{50s} > 25 μM.

The cytotoxic effect of oleocanthal (**1**) on breast cancer cells and its potential mechanism of action have been investigated under different conditions in several studies, mostly on MDA-MB 231 and MCF-7 cells. Until now, the reported EC_{50} values for oleocanthal (**1**) in the three breast cancer cell lines used in this study have varied between 10–18.5 μM for MDA-MB 231 and 18–40 μM for MCF-7 estimated after 48 or 72 h treatment with the OOP in different culture conditions (i.e., serum-free, FBS 0.5% (*v*/*v*), HGF-supplemented media and EGF-supplemented media) [28,47,74,75]. The corresponding EC_{50} values calculated in this study were close to the lowest values of these ranges. Siddique et al. (2019) determined the EC_{50} value of oleocanthal (**1**) on SK-BR-3 cells to be 27.3 μM (after 48 h treatment in HGF- and EGF-supplemented media), while in this study, the EC_{50} value was calculated to be 13 μM [76].

Similar studies on the oleuropein aglycone (**3a,b**) bioactivity are still limited. Menendez et al. (2007) reported that the concentration of oleuropein aglycone (**3a,b**) reducing cell viability by 50% after five days of treatment was 47 μM for the SK-BR-3 cells and >100 μM for the MCF-7 cells [17]. A very recent study by Mazzei et al. (2020) showed that the calculated EC_{50} values for MCF-7/TR (tamoxifen-resistant) and MDA-MB 231 cells were 70 μM and 53 μM, respectively [27]. These EC_{50} values are twice to three times higher than the values calculated in the present study (i.e., for MDA-MB 231, EC_{50} = 24.5 μM; for SK-BR-3, EC_{50} = 17.7 μM; for MCF-7, EC_{50} = 32.2 μM). The differences in these results may be due to variations in the experimental conditions or differences in the purity of the compound used.

As for ligstroside aglycone (**4a,b**), Busnena et al. (2013) reported an EC_{50} value for MDA-MB 231 of approximately 80 μM after 48 h treatment, while in the present study ligstroside aglycone (**4a,b**) was found to be much more effective (EC_{50} = 31.6 μM) [23]. Moreover, similar to the results presented herein, previous studies have shown that SK-BR-3 cells were sensitive to ligstroside aglycone (**4a,b**) (EC_{50} = 26 ± 6 μM after 5 day treatment) [53].

With respect to skin cancer, A2058 and SK-MEL-28 melanoma-derived cell lines were included in the present study. The calculated EC_{50} values for oleocanthal (**1**) were 10.4 μM and 18.4 μM in the SK-MEL-28 and A2058 cells, respectively. These EC_{50} values are similar to those observed for the breast cancer cell lines. The EC_{50} values for oleuropein aglycone (**3a,b**) were 15.1 μM and 37.2 μM, respectively, for the two cell lines. Interestingly, SK-MEL-28 cells were more sensitive to all OOPs than the A2058. To our knowledge, no data have been reported until now for the antiproliferative/cytotoxic effect of these two OOPs (**1** and **3a,b**) on the aforementioned cancer cell lines. However, oleocanthal (**1**) has been shown to inhibit cell viability in several human melanoma cell lines, including the A375, 501Mel and G361 cells at low concentrations [21,22]. Moreover, for oleocanthal (**1**) and oleacein (**2**), much higher EC_{50} values were reported recently on A375 cells (i.e., 67.5 ± 1.9 and 112.9 ± 4.9 μM, respectively) after 72 h treatment [50].

In the hepatic cancer cell lines, oleuropein aglycone (**3a,b**) was almost twice as effective than oleocanthal (**1**), with the Huh-7 being more sensitive to all OOPs than the HepG-2 cells. It is noteworthy that in two previous reports on the antiproliferative/cytotoxic activity of oleocanthal (**1**) against hepatocellular carcinoma [29,48], the calculated EC_{50} values were similar to those presented in this study; however, in one study, the Huh-7 cells were found to be more resistant than HepG-2 to treatment with oleocanthal (**1**) while in another they responded similarly [29]. Moreover, the pancreatic cancer cell line PANC-1 was almost equally sensitive to oleocanthal (**1**) and oleuropein aglycone (**3a,b**) but more sensitive to the rest of OOPs than the hepatic cancer cell lines.

The Caco-2 colon cancer cells were more sensitive to oleuropein (**3a,b**) and ligstroside (**4a,b**) aglycones than to oleocanthal (**1**) while for the HT-29 colon cancer cells the opposite was observed. It is worth noting that while in this study oleocanthal (**1**) was found to have moderate activity (EC_{50} = 33.4 μM, after 72 h treatment), others have reported that it had no cytotoxic effect on Caco-2 cells (EC_{50} > 150 μM) [75]. For the stomach cancer cell lines oleocanthal (**1**) was the most effective OOP, with oleuropein aglycone (**3a,b**) being the second most effective in both cell lines. Moreover, MKN-45 stomach cancer cells were more sensitive to all OOPs than the AGS cells.

The two lung cancer cell lines showed different sensitivities to oleocanthal (**1**) and the two aglycones (**3a,b** and **4a,b**). While oleocanthal (**1**) and oleuropein aglycone (**3a,b**) were the most effective OOPs on H1299 cells, the H1437 cells were more sensitive to the two aglycones (**3a,b** and **4a,b**) with oleocanthal (**1**) following in effectiveness. Moreover, they were more sensitive to the rest of the OOPs than the H1299 cells. Until now, only oleocanthal (**1**) has been shown in one report to inhibit the cell viability of several human lung cancer cell lines, including A549 and NCI-H322M cells [31].

Finally, the ME-180 cervical cancer cells were more sensitive than the Hela to all OOPs with oleocanthal (**1**) the most effective and oleuropein aglycone (**3a,b**) the second. Once more, the EC_{50} value reported in the present study for the activity of oleocanthal (**1**) on Hela cells was 44.6 μM, while in another study, an EC_{50} value >150 μM was calculated for oleocanthal [75].

To summarize, for most cancer cell lines tested herein, oleocanthal (**1**) was the most effective OOP in its antiproliferative/cytotoxic effect while oleuropein aglycone (**3a,b**) ranked second. The only exceptions where oleuropein or ligstroside aglycones (**3a,b** and **4a,b**) were more effective than oleocanthal (**1**) were on (a) the two hepatic cell lines, Huh-7 and HepG-2 ((**3a,b**) > (**1**)), and (b) on the H1437 lung cells (both aglycones (**3a,b** and **4a,b**) > (**1**))—results that merit further investigation. A detailed analysis of the bioactivity of the six OOPs highlighted their differential activity on cells of different cancer origin but also on cell lines of the same tissue origin but with different genetic backgrounds. With respect to the EC_{50} values of the OOPs studied until now, the majority of the EC_{50} values calculated in this study were either considerably lower or similar to the values already reported.

2.7. *Effect of Six OOPs on the Viability of Non-Tumorigenic Human Cells Lines; Selectivity of OOPs' Bioactivity*

The OOPs analyzed above, except oleocanthalic acid (**7**), were also tested for their antiproliferative/cytotoxic effect on non-cancer immortalized or normal human cell lines of different tissue origins. Human mesenchymal stem cells derived from umbilical cord

(Wharton's jelly stem cells (WJSCs)) were also used as an alternative cell model [77–79]. Two out of the five cell types (i.e., MRC-5 derived from lung and MCF-10A non-tumorigenic breast epithelial cells) were more sensitive than the cancer cell lines of similar tissue origin in all OOPs tested (Table 1). However, the skin-derived cells (i.e., HaCaT spontaneously transformed immortal keratinocytes and the NHDF Normal Human Dermal Fibroblasts) were either as sensitive as the A2058 melanoma cells (i.e., the HaCaT cells) or more resistant to oleocanthal (**1**) treatment than both the A2058 and SK-MEL-28 melanoma cell lines tested (i.e., the NHDF cells). The WJSCs were found to be as sensitive as NHDF to oleocanthal treatment, but more sensitive to oleacein (**2**) and the two aglycones (**3a,b** and **4a,b**).

To evaluate the anti-cancer potential of a compound, its cytotoxicity against non-tumorigenic cell lines must be determined in order to calculate the selectivity index value (SI). Comparison of the OOPs' selectivity indexes for the cell lines (cancer and non-tumorigenic transformed cells) of the same tissue origin (i.e., the ratio of EC_{50} for non-tumorigenic cells/EC_{50} for cancer cells) summarized in Table S3 indicated that the SIs ranged between 0.1–2.8 [80]. Oleocanthal (**1**) and the two aglycones (**3a,b** and **4a,b**) displayed SI > 2 for the melanoma cell line SK-MEL-28 (2.4, 2.8 and 2.1, respectively) while ligstroside aglycone (**4a,b**) showed moderately good selectivity for some breast cancer cell lines, as well (Table S3). According to Weerapreeyakul et al. (2012), a SI value $\geq$3 is required for classifying a compound as prospectively anti-cancer [81], but others consider SI values >2 as a positive indication for further investigation of a compound's anti-cancer potential [82,83]. The results presented in this study concerning the sensitivity of MCF-10A and HaCaT cells to treatment with OOPs do not correlate with previously reported studies in which the MCF-10A cells were found resistant to treatment with oleocanthal (**1**), ligstroside aglycone (**4a,b**) and oleuropein aglycone (**3a,b**) at concentrations of 40 μM, 50 μM and 150 μM, respectively [23,27,28,30]. Moreover, other studies have demonstrated that the HaCaT cells were resistant to treatment with oleocanthal (**1**) and oleacein (**2**), while EGF-stimulated HaCaT cells were found to be more sensitive to these OOPs [22,50]. Since we obtained the MCF-10A cells directly from the ATCC cell bank and evaluated their sensitivity to OOPs in parallel with the respective cancer cell lines using the same methodology and the same compounds, the results reported herein bear validity. The HaCaT cells were found as sensitive to A2058 melanoma cells. More specifically, they were more sensitive to oleocanthal (**1**) and oleuropein aglycone (**3a,b**) treatment, but the EC_{50} values of oleacein (**2**), ligstroside aglycone (**4a,b**) and oleomissional (**6a,b,c**) were higher than 50 μM.

Therefore, the above results, although encouraging with respect to the selectivity indexes estimated for oleocanthal (**1**) and the two aglycones (**3a,b** and **4a,b**) for some cancer types, raise questions concerning the validity of using transformed/immortalized cell lines to evaluate the potential use of OOPs or other natural products for anticancer treatments. They may not be representative cell models of normal tissues. Two-dimensional or 3D cell culture systems utilizing human primary cells from different tissues may provide more physiologically relevant information and more predictive data in in vitro assays testing the selectivity of OOPs' anti-cancer effect [84,85].

2.8. Kinetics of Antiproliferative/Cytotoxic Effect of OOPs

To examine the time dependence of the OOPs' effect on cancer cell lines, treatments were performed for different time lengths and the reductions in cell numbers were compared. The MDA-MB 231 and SK-MEL-28 breast cancer and melanoma cell models, respectively, were treated for 24, 48 and 72 h with OOP concentrations lower, higher or close to the EC_{50} values of the most active compounds (i.e., oleocanthal (**1**), oleacein (**2**), oleuropein aglycone (**3a,b**) and ligstroside aglycone (**4a,b**)). Cell numbers were assayed using the ATP assay.

As expected, the highest cell numbers in the treated cultures (i.e., the weakest effect of OOPs) were observed at 24 h, while the lowest (i.e., the strongest effect of OOPs) at 72 h treatments. Interestingly, treatments with some OOPs (i.e., ligstroside aglycone (**4a,b**) and oleacein (**2**)) had a similar effect to that observed at 24 h independently of the OOPs concentration used. By contrast, others ((i.e., oleocanthal (**1**) and oleuropein aglycone (**3a,b**)) acted earlier than 48 h, but reached the highest levels of effect at 72 h, when the used concentrations in the treatments were close to or higher than their EC_{50} values. Apparently, some OOPs exert their antiproliferative/cytotoxic effect earlier than 48 h while others act slower (Figure 4). On the basis of these results, it was decided to determine the EC_{50} values for all of OOPs tested in all the cell lines at 72 h of treatment.

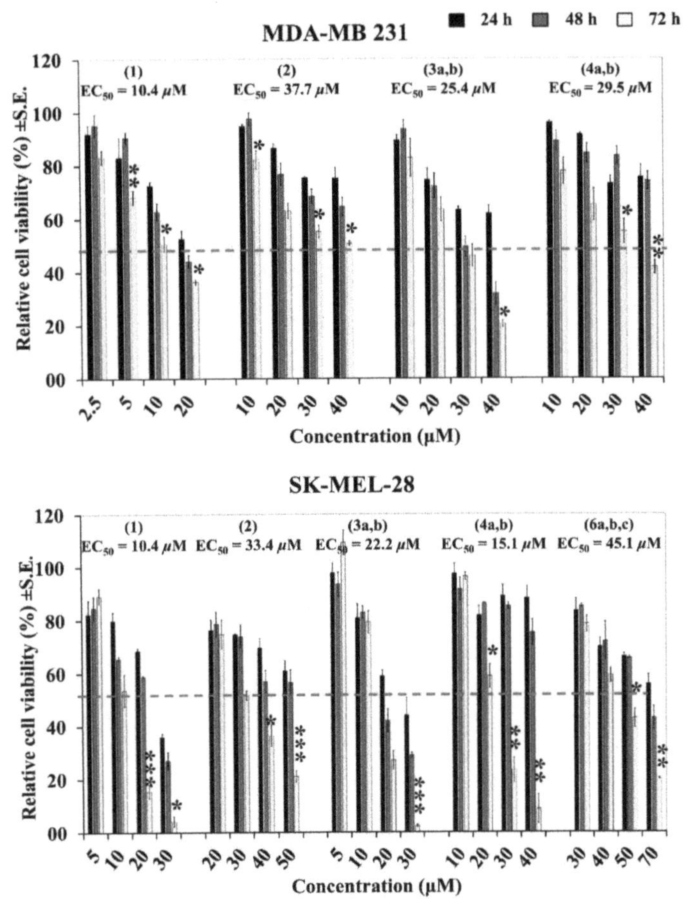

Figure 4. Time- and dose-dependent effect of OOPs on MDA-MB231 and SK-MEL 28 cell lines. Cells were treated with different concentrations (2.5–70 μM) of oleocanthal (**1**), oleacein (**2**), oleuropein aglycone (**3a,b**), ligstroside aglycone (**4a,b**) and oleomissional (**6a,b,c**). Cell viability was measured using the ATP-based luminescence assay at the end of 24, 48 and 72 h treatment. Results from two independent experiments performed in triplicate. Bar graphs represent the mean cell count ± SE in each treatment group normalized to the control group (i.e., cells treated only with 0.2% (*v*/*v*) DMSO). * $p < 0.05$; ** $p \leq 0.01$; *** $p \leq 0.001$ (*t*-test) comparing viability in the treatments for 48 h and 72 h.

2.9. Effect of the OOPs' Stability in the Calculation of EC_{50} Values

A very important observation made in this study pertains to the instability of oleocanthal (**1**) in the cell culture medium. Representative results from the treatment of SK-BR-3 cells for 48 h with two different concentrations of oleocanthal (**1**) added to the cells directly or after a 15 min pre-incubation in a culture medium are shown in Figure 5. Oleocanthal (**1**) was partially deactivated when its addition was delayed by the 15 min pre-incubation step and this was time- and dose-dependent (Figure S3A). The other OOPs tested were not affected similarly (Figure S3B). The low stability of oleocanthal (**1**) in the culture medium resulted in a strong local antiproliferative/cytotoxic effect (i.e., in the vicinity of the positions where it was added) while cells located in the tissue culture wells distant from the site of oleocanthal (**1**) addition were less affected. These results raised questions about the chemical form of the active oleocanthal (**1**) and the ways of handling it in our assays. It was therefore decided for all the experiments presented in this manuscript and the assays performed to calculate the EC_{50} values to add all the OOPs tested directly to the culture medium. A recent study showed that oleocanthal (**1**) spontaneously reacts with amino acids, with high preferential reactivity to glycine, which is found in abundance in culture media. A glycine derivative with a tetrahydropyridinium skeleton was identified as the product of this reaction and was called oleoglycine [66]. This type of reaction with amino acids or generally peptides and proteins may be one of the reasons for the variations observed in the EC_{50} values reported for oleocanthal (**1**) by different laboratories for the same cancer cell lines.

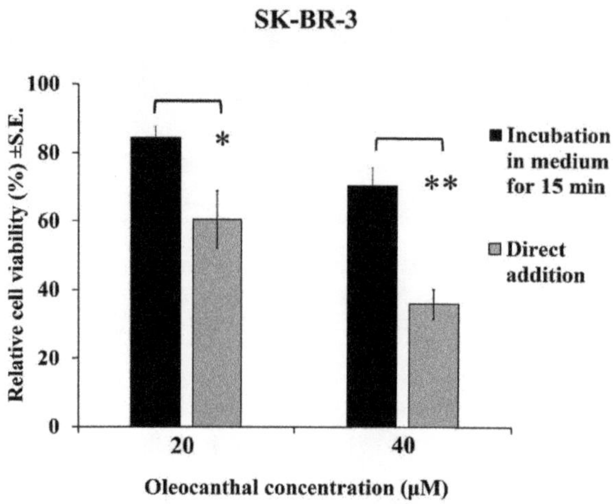

Figure 5. Partial deactivation of oleocanthal (**1**) in culture medium. SK-BR-3 cells were treated with two different concentrations of oleocanthal (**1**) at two different concentrations (20 and 40 μM) for 48 h. Viable cell numbers were determined using the ATP-based luminescence assay after 48 h of treatment. The compound was added to the cells either directly or after incubation with the culture medium for 15 min. The results presented are from four independent experiments performed in triplicate. Bar graphs represent the mean cell count ± SE in each treatment group normalized to the control group (i.e., cells treated only with 0.2% (v/v) DMSO). * $p < 0.05$; ** $p \leq 0.01$ (t-test) comparing the two different treatment methods.

2.10. Correlation of EC_{50} Values with the Doubling Times of the Cell Lines

Examination of the EC_{50} values for each OOP showed significant variations in the analyzed cancer cell lines of different tissue origin but also amongst cell lines of the same tissue origin but with different genetic characteristics (Table 1) To examine if the speed of proliferation of each cell line correlated to these results, the doubling time of each cell line was calculated (Table S2A) using the MTT assay (Experimental Section) which gave similar results to those obtained with the ATP assay (Figure S4). Overall, no clear correlation was detected between the EC_{50} values for each OOP and the doubling time of the cell lines.

In more detail, for the breast cell lines presented as representative examples (Table S2B), the slower-growing cell line SK-BR-3 was more sensitive to treatment with all OOPs as compared to the MCF-7 cell line with approximately the same doubling time. However, when compared with the faster-growing MDA-MB 231 cell line, the SK-BR-3 cells seemed to be more resistant to oleocanthal (**1**) and oleacein (**2**) treatment and more sensitive to treatment with the aglycones (i.e., (**3a,b**), (**4a,b**)). As for the skin cell lines, although they had comparable doubling times, the SK-MEL-28 was the most sensitive. It is worth mentioning that for the stomach cancer cell lines studied (i.e., the AGS and MKN-45 cells), the slower-growing cell line (i.e., AGS) seemed to be more resistant to treatment with all OOPs (higher EC_{50} values) as compared to the MKN-45 cells. The same trend was followed in the results for the colon cancer cell lines, but only for the treatment with the two aglycones ((**3a,b**) and (**4a,b**)) and oleomissional (**6a,b,c**) while for oleocanthal (**1**) and oleacein (**2**) the opposite trend was observed (Table 1 and Table S2). Moreover, the exact opposite trend was observed with regard to the lung cancer cell lines. Specifically, the H1437 cells growing faster than the H1299 cells seemed to be more resistant to treatment with oleocanthal (**1**) or oleacein (**2**) than the H1299 cell line. On the other hand, the H1437 cells were more sensitive to treatment with the other three OOPs (i.e., ligstroside aglycone (**4a,b**), oleuropein aglycone (**3a,b**) and oleomissional (**6a,b,c**)) in comparison to the other cell line of the same tissue origin. Finally, concerning the cervical cancer cell lines, it seemed that Hela, a highly proliferative cell line, is more resistant to OOPs treatment as compared to the ME-180 cancer cervical cells.

In summary, the above-commented results indicated that the EC_{50} values calculated in this study for each OOP tested (Table 1 and Figure 3) were cell type-specific and did not correlate with the doubling time of the cell lines (Table S2B).

2.11. *Effect of O_2 Concentration on the OOPs' Antiproliferative/Cytotoxic Activity*

The effects of drugs on cancer cell lines are usually tested under atmospheric conditions (20% (v/v) O_2). However, the O_2 content in tissues (normoxia) and solid tumors (hypoxia) is $\leq$ 5% (v/v). In some tumors (i.e., pancreatic tumors) the % O_2 is even $\leq$ 1% (v/v) [54,86,87]. This affects cell metabolism and signaling pathways which depend on the hypoxia-induced Factor 1A (HIF1A) and it could affect the activity of certain drugs [59,63,88–90]. To examine if low O_2 levels modify the activity of OOPs, oleocanthal (**1**), oleuropein aglycone (**3a,b**) and ligstroside aglycone (**4a,b**) were tested under low O_2 concentration (i.e., 1% (v/v) (hypoxia)) in comparison to 20% (v/v) (atmospheric O_2 levels in tissue culture) at three different concentrations close to the EC_{50} value for each OOP for the cell lines analyzed (Figure 6). The effects of these three OOPs were tested on the MDA-MB 231, SK-BR-3 and MCF-7 breast cancer and on the AGS stomach cancer cell lines.

O_2 concentration did not affect in the same way the antiproliferative/cytotoxic bioactivity of the three OOPs on all four cancer cell lines tested (Figure 6). Treatment with oleuropein or ligstroside aglycones (**3a,b** and **4a,b**) at low oxygen O_2 tension (i.e., 1% (v/v) (hypoxia)) rendered some cell lines more resistant. Ligstroside aglycone (**4a,b**) appeared to be less effective under hypoxic conditions on the AGS stomach cancer cells, while the bioactivity of oleocanthal (**1**) and oleuropein aglycone (**3a,b**) in the same cells was similar. Similarly to AGS cells, the MDA-MB 231 cells in hypoxia were more resistant to treatment with both aglycones ((**3a,b**), (**4a,b**)). Finally, the MCF-7 cells and SK-BR-3 breast cancer cells appeared to respond similarly to treatment with the three OOPs under hypoxic and atmospheric O_2 conditions. These results indicated once more the variability observed in the bioactivity of each OOP in each cell line, as described in the previous paragraphs. Overall, oleocanthal (**1**), oleuropein aglycone and ligstroside aglycone (**3a,b** and **4a,b**) were equally or less effective at low oxygen O_2 tension (i.e., 1% (v/v) (hypoxia)) as compared to atmospheric O_2 levels. This is an important piece of information for the design of future in vivo experiments aiming at the evaluation of the OOPs' anti-tumor properties.

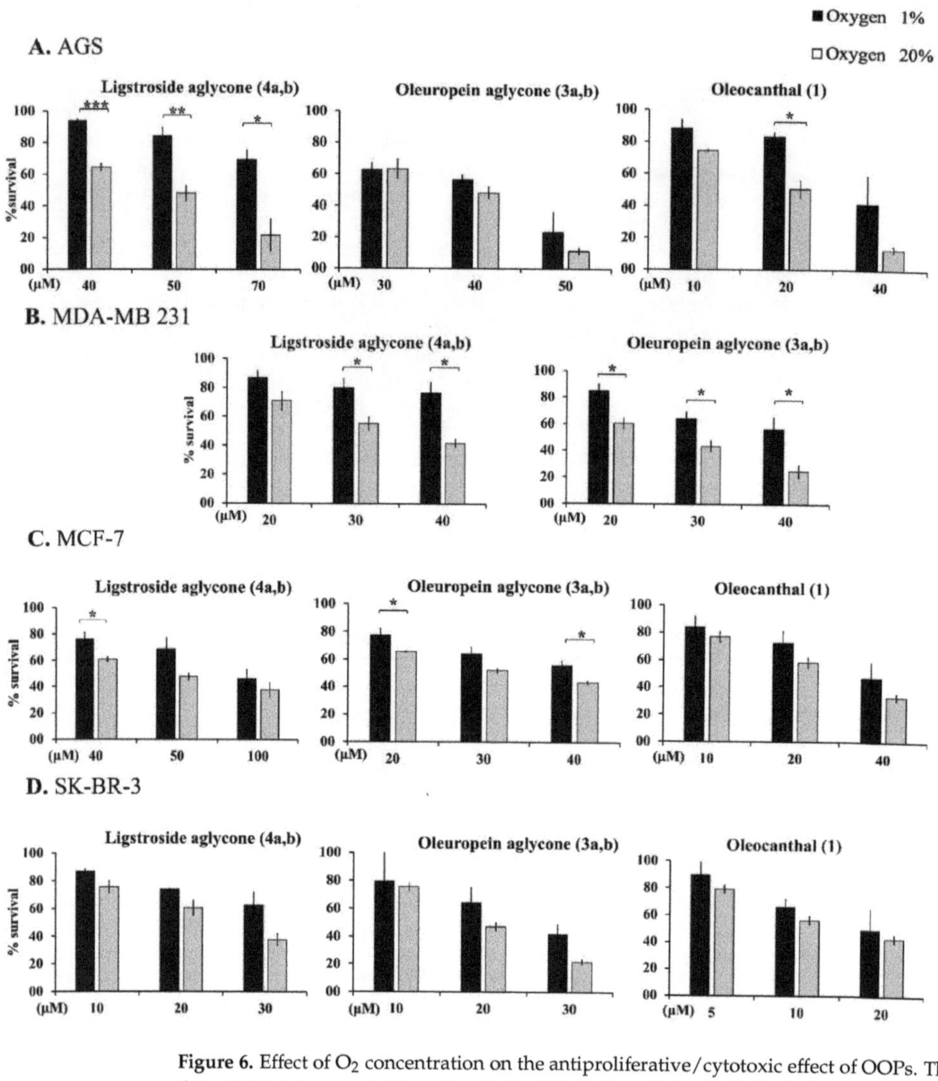

Figure 6. Effect of O_2 concentration on the antiproliferative/cytotoxic effect of OOPs. The effect of three different concentrations close to the EC_{50} value of oleocanthal (**1**), oleuropein aglycone (**3a,b**) and ligstroside aglycone (**4a,b**) was evaluated after 72 h treatment under either 1% (v/v) O_2 or 20% (v/v) O_2. Cell viability was determined on (**A**) AGS, (**B**) MDA-MB 231, (**C**) MCF-7 and (**D**) SK-BR-3 cell lines using ATP-based luminescence assay. The results presented are from two independent experiments performed in triplicate. Bar graphs represent the mean cell count ± SE in each treatment group normalized to the control group (i.e., cells treated only with 0.2% (v/v) DMSO). * $p < 0.05$; ** $p \leq 0.01$; *** $p \leq 0.001$ (t-test) comparing the two different conditions.

2.12. *Anti-Proliferative Effect of OOPs on Different Cancer Cell Lines*

The ATP and MTT assays utilized to assess cell viability in the experiments described above do not provide information about the OOPs' mechanism(s) of action. To distinguish if the observed reduction in cell numbers upon treatment with OOPs was due to a proliferation arrest or to a cytotoxic effect, the levels of DNA replication arrest were evaluated after treatment with each of the five OOPs (i.e., oleocanthal (**1**), oleacein (**2**), oleuropein aglycone

(**3a,b**), ligstroside aglycone (**4a,b**) and oleomissional (**6a,b,c**)). DNA replication, as a key determinant of chromosome segregation and stability in eukaryotes, is directly related to cell proliferation [91].

For this purpose, ten cancer cell lines (i.e., MDA-MB 231, SK-BR-3, MCF-7, A2058, SK-MEL-28, AGS, HepG-2, PANC-1, H1299 and Hela) originating from breast, melanoma, stomach, hepatic, pancreatic, lung and cervical tumors were analyzed in parallel with control samples (i.e., the same cells treated only with 0.2% (v/v) DMSO). They were treated for 24 h with OOPs having EC_{50} values $\leq$ 50 μM at concentrations equal to the EC_{50} of each one. Subsequently, the treated cells were allowed to incorporate 5-ethynyl-2′-deoxyuridine (EdU) into replicating DNA according to the protocol described in detail in the Experimental Section. EdU, a thymidine analog, can be incorporated into DNA in vivo and detected later by using copper-catalyzed azide–alkyne cycloaddition (click reaction) without prior DNA denaturation [91]. The pool of cells in the S phase can be then easily detected by fluorescence (FL) microscopy or by flow cytometry by analyzing the incorporation of EdU in replicating DNA of single cells [92]. In this study, after EdU incorporation, the nuclei of the entire cell population were stained with Hoechst and imaged by confocal microscopy (Experimental Section). EdU-positive nuclei, marked by green FL, as well as the total number of nuclei, marked by blue FL, were enumerated by applying the Icy image analysis algorithm on the digital images acquired by confocal microscopy. Treatment of the cell lines analyzed for 24 h with OOPs as single compounds (i.e., oleocanthal (**1**), oleacein (**2**), oleuropein aglycone (**3a,b**), ligstroside aglycone (**4a,b**) or oleomissional (**6a,b,c**)) resulted in inhibition of proliferation ranging from 4.7–47.8% (Figure 7 and Figure S5, Tables 2 and 3). Oleacein (**2**), oleuropein aglycone (**3a,b**) and oleomissional (**6a,b,c**) appeared as the most effective OOPs in the SK-MEL-28 melanoma cells (20.3–27.6% inhibition of proliferation), with (**3a,b**) and (**6a,b,c**) demonstrating very significant (p < 0.0001) inhibition of cell proliferation (Tables 2 and 3). Oleocanthal (**1**), oleacein (**2**) and the two aglycones (**3a,b** and **4a,b**) were the strongest proliferation inhibitors in the AGS stomach cancer cells (28.9–31.6% inhibition of proliferation), giving statistically significant results (p < 0.01) as compared to control samples (Tables 2 and 3). The strongest antiproliferative effect (47.0–47.8% inhibition) was observed in the treatment of H1299 lung cancer cells with oleocanthal (**1**) and oleacein (**2**), while in the PANC-1 pancreatic cancer cells, oleacein (**2**), oleuropein aglycone (**3a,b**), ligstroside aglycone (**4a,b**) and oleomissional (**6a,b,c**) had a similar effect (21.9–23.7% inhibition of DNA replication) (Tables 2 and 3).

Table 2. OOPs' antiproliferative effect. S-phase cells (i.e., % EdU +ve) are presented for each OOP treatment in each cell line. The effect of the most effective OOPs ($EC_{50} \leq 50$ μM) on cell proliferation was evaluated on all the breast cancer (i.e., MDA-MB 231, SK-BR-3 and MCF-7) and skin melanoma (SK-MEL-28, A2058) cell lines. Moreover, the antiproliferative effect of OOPs was tested on the most resistant cell line of the other tissue origins (i.e., AGS, HepG-2, PANC-1, H1299 and Hela cells). For this, the Cell proliferation kit III (EdU-488; FM) was used after 24 h treatments with the OOPs. The doubling times for each cell line are presented as well. The results are means ± SE from two (or three) independent experiments (total no. of cells ≥ 300). * p < 0.05, ** $p \leq 0.01$, *** $p \leq 0.001$, **** $p \leq 0.0001$ (t-test) compared to the corresponding control samples (i.e., cells treated with 0.2% (v/v) DMSO).

Compounds		DMSO	1		2		4a,b		3a,b		6a,b,c	
Cell Line	Doubling Time (Hours ± SE)	% EdU +ve ± SE	% EdU +ve ± SE	Significance	% EdU +ve ± SE	Significance	% EdU +ve ± SE	Significance	% EdU +ve ± SE	Significance	% EdU +ve ± SE	Significance
MDA-MB 231 [a]	26.2 ± 3.7	41.2 ± 1.8	29.1 ± 2.3	*	25.5 ± 4.1	*	33.0 ± 2.8	ns	19.7 ± 3.1	**	-	-
SK-BR-3	40.0 ± 4.2	23.5 ± 1.8	9.5 ± 3.9	ns	7.4 ± 0.7	*	18.8 ± 1.3	ns	6.6 ± 3.5	*	8.3 ± 0.9	*
MCF-7	34.5 ± 2.8	40.4 ± 1.6	21.6 ± 4.0	*	-	-	-	-	21.1 ± 2.0	*	-	-
A2058	28.6 ± 2.8	38.8 ± 4.5	25.5 ± 5.3	ns	-	-	-	-	23.7 ± 5.8	ns	-	-

Table 2. *Cont.*

Compounds		DMSO	1		2		4a,b		3a,b		6a,b,c	
Cell Line	Doubling Time (Hours ± SE)	% EdU +ve ± SE	% EdU +ve ± SE	Significance	% EdU +ve ± SE	Significance	% EdU +ve ± SE	Significance	% EdU +ve ± SE	Significance	% EdU +ve ± SE	Significance
SK-MEL-28	27.9 ± 0.7	25.4 ± 1.0 [a]	15.0 ± 4.8 [a]	ns	1.8 ± 0.4	**	20.8 ± 5.1 [a]	ns	0.7 ± 0.3 [a]	****	2.8 ± 1.0 [a]	****
AGS	33.7 ± 0.4	47.3 ± 2.5 [a]	16.2 ± 4.4 [a]	**	14.7 ± 0.4	**	14.0 ± 0.5	**	18.4 ± 1.5 [a]	***	-	-
HepG-2	37.2 ± 2.0	39.0 ± 3.2	26.4 ± 1.5	ns	-	-	12.0 ± 2.0	*	10.6 ± 3.1	*	31.7 ± 4.9	ns
PANC-1	16.4 ± 0.7	45.5 ± 4.5	23.6 ± 5.8	ns	37.6 ± 7.1	ns	22.1 ± 7.2	ns	21.9 ± 5.3	ns	21.7 ± 2.2	*
H1299	20.2 ± 6.4	61.0 ± 0.7	14.0 ± 1.9	**	13.2 ± 3.5	**	-	-	31.9 ± 5.9	*	-	-
Hela	15.5 ± 2.4	45.3 ± 1.4	-	-	21.7 ± 6.5	ns	31.2 ± 4.9	ns	20.9 ± 3.5	*	-	-

[a] Results from three independent experiments. The rest of values are from two independent experiments.

A

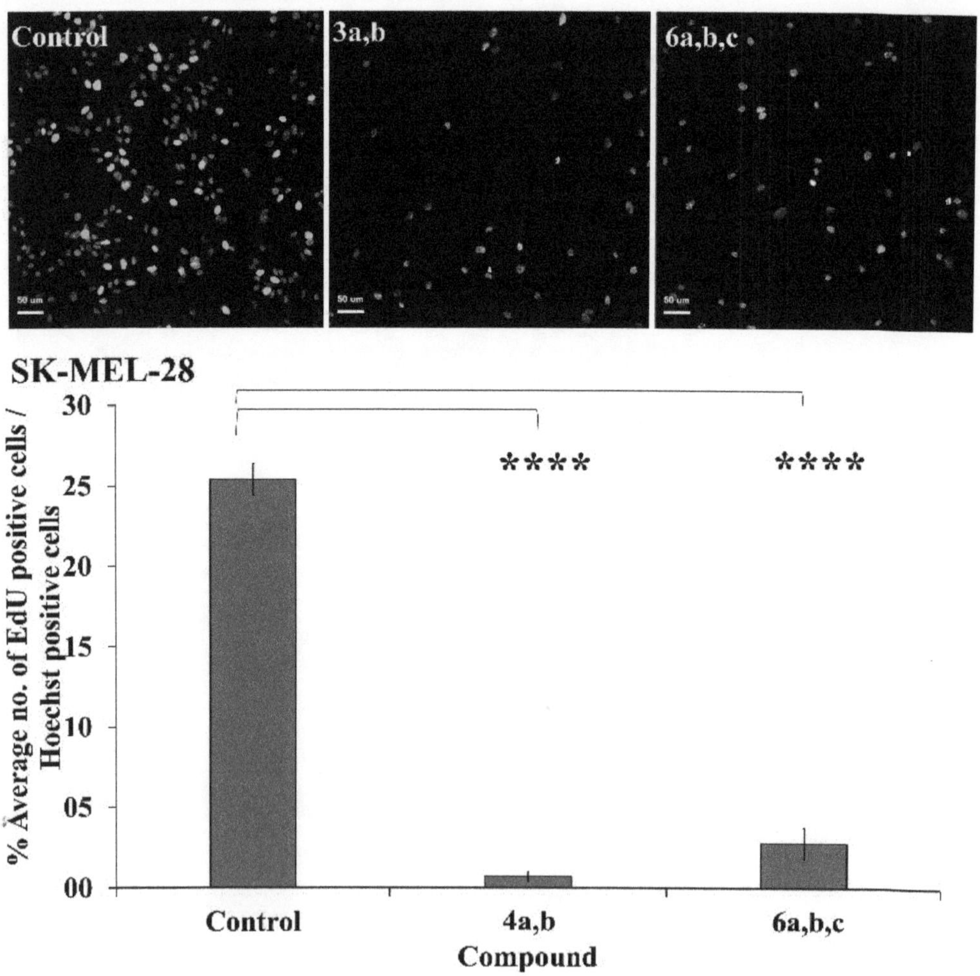

Figure 7. *Cont.*

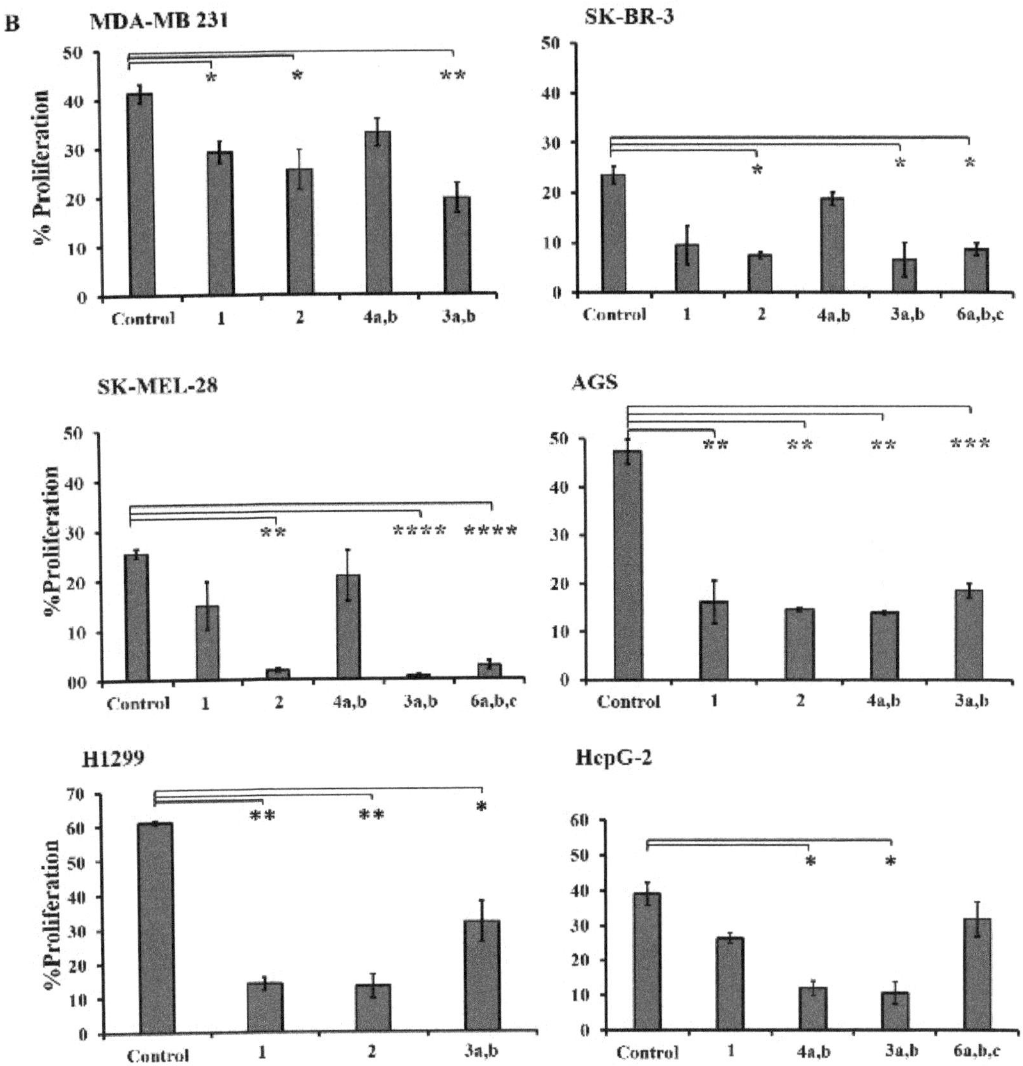

Figure 7. OOPs' effect on cell proliferation. (**A**) Confocal microscopy images of SK-MEL-28 cells evaluated for proliferation 24 h after treatment with oleuropein aglycone (**3a,b**) and oleomissional (**6a,b,c**) using concentrations equal to EC_{50} values (μM) for each cell line. S-phase cell nuclei were stained with EdU (green fluorescence) and all nuclei with Hoechst (Blue fluorescence, grey pseudo-color). Bar graphs represent the % of cells in S Phase (proliferating) calculated by the quantification of the EdU-positive cells divided by the number of Hoechst-positive cells. (**B**) Cell proliferation was determined after 24 h treatment with the EC_{50} values (μM) of oleocanthal (**1**), oleacein (**2**), oleuropein aglycone (**3a,b**), ligstroside aglycone (**4a,b**) and/or oleomissional (**6a,b,c**) on MDA-MB 231, SK-BR-3, SK-MEL-28, AGS, H1299 and HepG-2. Graphs represent the quantification of EdU incorporation by counting the number of EdU +ve cells/Hoechst +ve cells. The results are means ± SE from two or three independent experiments (total no. of cells ≥ 300). * $p < 0.05$; ** $p \leq 0.01$; *** $p \leq 0.001$; **** $p \leq 0.0001$ (t-test) compared to the corresponding control samples (i.e., cells treated with 0.2% v/v DMSO).

Table 3. OOPs' antiproliferative effect. The data from Table 2 expressed as levels of % inhibition of cell proliferation after normalization with the control. The doubling times for each cell line are presented as well. The results are means ± SE from two (or three) independent experiments (total no. of cells ≥ 300).

		% Inhibition ± SE				
Cell Line	**Doubling Time (Hours ± SE)**	**1**	**2**	**4a,b**	**3a,b**	**6a,b,c**
MDA-MB 231 [a]	26.2 ± 3.7	12.1 ± 1.0	15.7 ± 2.4	8.2 ± 1.8	21.5 ± 2.1	-
SK-BR-3	40.0 ± 4.2	14.1 ± 2.1	16.2 ± 2.4	4.8 ± 3.1	16.9 ± 1.7	14.8 ± 0.5
MCF-7	34.5 ± 2.8	19.1 ± 2.1	-	-	19.3 ± 0.5	-
A2058	28.6 ± 2.8	13.3 ± 0.8	-	-	15.0 ± 10.3	-
SK-MEL-28	27.9 ± 0.7	10.4 ± 5.7 [a]	20.3 ± 4.0	4.7 ± 4.6 [a]	24.7 ± 0.7 [a]	22.6 ± 1.3 [a]
AGS	33.7 ± 0.4	31.2 ± 4.5 [a]	31.0 ± 3.5	31.6 ± 2.6	28.9 ± 1.5 [a]	-
HepG-2	37.2 ± 2.0	12.7 ± 1.7	-	27.0 ± 1.1	28.4 ± 0.1	7.3 ± 1.7
PANC-1	16.4 ± 0.7	21.9 ± 1.3	7.9 ± 2.6	23.4 ± 2.7	23.6 ± 0.8	23.7 ± 6.7
H1299	19.4 ± 5.4	47.0 ± 2.5	47.8 ± 4.1	-	29.1 ± 6.5	-
Hela	15.5 ± 2.4	-	23.6 ± 7.9	14.1 ± 6.3	24.3 ± 2.1	-

[a] Results from three independent experiments. The rest of values are from two independent experiments.

In summary, all OOPs analyzed in this study with $EC_{50} \leq 50$ μM exert antiproliferative effect already detectable at 24 h treatment in all cell lines tested. Interestingly, each OOP caused different levels of cessation in DNA replication in each cell line.

Antiproliferative effect in vitro has mainly been reported for oleocanthal (**1**) and less for oleacein (**2**) and oleuropein aglycone (**3a,b**). Oleocanthal (**1**) was shown to suppress breast cancer cell proliferation detected by G0/G1 cell cycle arrest via inhibition of HGF-induced phosphorylation of c-Met and by modulating Ca^{2+} entry through TRPC6 [20,28]. Moreover, oleocanthal (**1**) was described to act as a dual inhibitor of c-MET and COX-2 on lung cancer cells [31]. As for melanoma and hepatocellular carcinoma cells it has been reported that oleocanthal (**1**) suppressed cell growth by inhibiting the phosphorylation of STAT3 (signal transducer and activator of transcription 3) [22,29]. On the other hand, oleacein (**2**) treatment induced G1/S phase arrest and downregulated the expression of pro-proliferative proteins (i.e., c-KIT, K-RAS, PIK3R3, mTOR) [26]. Moreover, oleacein (**2**) was found to suppress the proliferation of neuroblastoma cells by blocking the cell cycle in the S phase [19]. With respect to breast cancer cell lines, oleuropein aglycone (**3a,b**) induced cell cycle arrest in the G0/G1 phase and reduction of cells in the S phase as well as a significant down-regulation of cyclin D1 and cyclin E expression [27]. No reports were retrieved on the mechanisms by which ligstroside aglycone (**4a,b**) or oleomissional (**6a,b,c**) exert antiproliferative action.

2.13. Pro-Apoptotic Activity of OOPs on Different Cancer Cell Lines

Oleocanthal (**1**) has been shown to cause apoptosis in several cancer cell lines [21,28,29,38,48,93]. Moreover, a few studies have also reported the pro-apoptotic effect of oleacein (**2**), ligstroside aglycone (**4a,b**) and oleuropein aglycone (**3a,b**) [19,27,53].

To discern whether cell death triggered by OOPs treatment occurred via apoptosis or necrosis under the experimental conditions applied in this study, live cells treated with OOPs were stained simultaneously with FITC-conjugated annexin V and propidium iodide (PI). Annexin V binds to phosphatidylserine (PS) translocating from the inner to the outer leaflet of the plasma membrane in apoptotic cells. Therefore, annexin V-FITC binding to PS labels live apoptotic cells with green FL. PI stains DNA only in late apoptotic or necrotic cells since it does not permeate the intact membrane of live cells [94]. PS exposure to the extracellular space and cell membrane permeability were analyzed by flow cytometry as described in detail in the Experimental Section. Single OOPs with $EC_{50s} \leq 50$ μM were used to treat cells from nine cancer cell lines for 48 h (i.e., SK-BR-3, MDA-MB 231, MCF-7, SK-MEL-28, A2058, AGS, HT-29, PANC-1 and H1299) originating from breast, melanoma, stomach, pancreatic and lung tumors. OOP concentrations used were equal to the EC_{50} values for each cell line (Table 1). annexin V and PI staining discriminated between early- (i.e., annexin V +ve and PI −ve) and late-apoptotic cells (i.e., annexin V +ve and PI +ve), as well as between necrotic (i.e., annexin V −ve and PI +ve) and live (i.e., annexin V −ve and PI −ve) cells (Table 4) [95].

Table 4. OOPs' apoptotic effect on a panel of cancer cell lines. Flow cytometry analysis of apoptotic cells after 24 and 48 h treatment with specific OOPs (EC_{50} values). Live cells were labelled with annexin V-FITC and PI as described in the Experimental Section. Control samples (i.e., treated only with 0.2% (*v*/*v*) DMSO) were analyzed in parallel. The percentage cell population of annexin V +ve cells (early apoptotic) and that of both annexin V and PI +ve cells (late apoptotic) over the whole cell population were determined using the FlowJo software. The results are the means% ± SE from two or three independent experiments. L.A. = late apoptotic.

Cell Lines	OOP	Treatment Duration (h)	Early Apoptotic (% ± S.D.)	Late Apoptotic (% ± S.D.)	Total Apoptotic (%)	% Cell Viability
Breast cancer cells						
SK-BR-3	**1**	48	7.45 ± 4.4	1.26 ± 0.7	8.71 ± 5.1	59
	2		5.78 ± 0.9	No L.A.	5.78 ± 0.9	60
	3a,b		7.63 ± 1.9	No L.A.	7.63 ± 1.9	59
	4a,b		1.30 ± 0.3	No L.A.	1.30 ± 0.3	87
	6a,b,c		3.13 ± 0.7	No L.A.	3.13 ± 0.7	68
MDA-MB 231	**1**	48	1.19 ± 0.01	1.38 ± 0.1	2.56 ± 0.1	85
	2	48	1.89 ± 0.03	1.49 ± 0.3	3.38 ± 0.2	73
		72	3.65 ± 0.5	1.64 ± 0.5	5.29 ± 1.0	70
	3a,b	48	4.17± 0.4	3.87 ± 3.7	8.04 ± 4.1	69
MCF-7	**1**	48	6.30 ± 2.3	3.77 ± 0.8	10.07 ± 3.1	65
	3a,b		7.03 ± 0.3	1.29 ± 0.8	8.31 ± 1.2	69
Melanoma cells						
SK-MEL-28	**1**	48	4.10 ± 0.2	2.47 ± 0.7	6.57 ± 0.5	68
	2	48	5.87 ± 1.1	No L.A.	5.87 ± 1.1	76
		72	6.70 ± 1.0	1.34 ± 0.3	8.04 ± 0.7	72
	3a,b	48	8.33 ± 1.9	4.91 ± 1.7	13.24 ± 3.7	68
	4a,b		1.86 ± 0.8	No L.A.	1.86 ± 0.8	82
	6a,b,c	48	10.06 ± 0.7	1.31 ± 0.9	11.37 ± 0.3	76
		72	12.72 ± 0.6	2.23 ± 1.1	14.95 ± 0.4	63
A2058	**1**	48	5.05 ± 2.7	2.35 ± 1.7	7.40 ± 4.4	36
	3a,b		11.88 ± 2.3	7.26 ± 1.6	19.14 ± 0.7	24
Gastrointestinal cancer cells						
AGS	**1**	48	18.42 ± 4.4	4.94 ± 3.1	23.36 ± 1.4	33
	2		10.00 ± 1.3	4.55 ± 1.8	14.55 ± 3.1	41
	3a,b		19.40 ± 0.6	8.08 ± 2.0	27.48 ± 1.4	31
	4a,b		16.03 ± 0.8	7.77 ± 1.8	23.79 ± 2.6	36

Table 4. *Cont.*

Cell Lines	OOP	Treatment Duration (h)	Early Apoptotic (% ± S.D.)	Late Apoptotic (% ± S.D.)	Total Apoptotic (%)	% Cell Viability
HT-29	**1**	48	5.53 ± 1.1	6.10 ± 4.3	11.63 ± 5.4	66
	3a,b		6.95 ± 1.5	1.55 ± 1.5	8.50 ± 1.8 [a]	41 [a]
Pancreatic cancer cells						
PANC-1	**1**	48	4.47 ± 0.8	No L.A.	4.47 ± 0.8	60
	2		4.39 ± 1.8	No L.A.	4.39 ± 1.8	58
	3a,b		8.52 ± 2.3	3.01 ± 2.0	11.52 ± 4.3	40
	4a,b		12.37 ± 2.7	4.42 ± 0.4	16.78 ± 3.1	34
	6a,b,c		3.38 ± 1.3	No L.A.	3.38 ± 1.3	49
Lung cancer cells						
H1299	**1**	48	4.77 ± 0.9	7.27 ± 0.2	12.04 ± 1.1	57
	2		5.96 ± 1.6	3.07 ± 1.8	9.03 ± 0.2	40
	3a,b		9.14 ± 3.1	5.44 ± 2.2	14.58 ± 5.3	40

[a] Results from one experiment.

As shown in Figure 8A for the breast cancer cell lines, the apoptotic events increased as a result of treatment with OOPs, a result reflected in the decrease in live cell numbers (Table 4). In more detail, treatment of the breast cancer cell lines SK-BR-3, MDA-MB-231 and MCF-7 with oleuropein aglycone (**3a,b**) for 48 h resulted in similar levels of apoptotic events in all three cell lines (Table 4). Oleocanthal (**1**) was most effective in the SK-BR-3 and MCF-7 cells and triggered a similar percentage of apoptotic cells as oleuropein aglycone, while oleacein (**2**) had a low pro-apoptotic effect on SK-BR-3 and MDA-MB 231 cells (Table 4). In the melanoma cells, oleuropein aglycone (**3a,b**) was highlighted to induce higher levels of apoptosis than oleocanthal (**1**) at 48 h treatments. Most interestingly, oleomissional (**6a,b,c**) exerted a significant pro-apoptotic effect only in the SK-MEL-28 cells ($p < 0.01$, Table 4).

Among all the cancer cell lines studied, the highest amount of apoptotic cells was observed in the stomach cancer AGS, with the strongest pro-apoptotic effect (34.2% ± 2.7 cells of the total population) induced by oleocanthal (**1**) treatment (Figure 8A,B). The two aglycones (i.e., (**3a,b**) and (**4a,b**)) also caused the highest numbers of apoptotic events in AGS as compared to the other cell lines tested (Table 4, Figure 8A). Moreover, both aglycones had the most prominent pro-apoptotic action in the PANC-1 pancreatic cancer cells compared to the rest of the OOPs (Table 4). Observing the effect of oleocanthal (**1**) in the colon-originated HT-29 and the lung H1299 cancer cells (Table 4), it appeared that around 12% of the total cell population were apoptotic in both, including similar levels of early and late apoptotic events. Comparing the action of oleuropein aglycone (**3a,b**) between the two lines, a stronger apoptotic effect was observed in the H1299 cells than the effect of oleocanthal (**1**) and oleacein (**2**) (Table 4).

In summary, treatment with all five OOPs induced apoptotic events in all the cancer cells analyzed after 48 h treatment at concentrations equal to the EC_{50} of each compound for each cell line. Only the cases where OOPs had $EC_{50s} \leq 50$ μM were selected for this analysis. Not all OOPs were analyzed in each cell line and not all OOPs caused similar levels of apoptosis in the same cell line within the time window of analysis. The results presented in Table 4 confirmed the data already reported for the pro-apoptotic activity of oleocanthal (**1**), oleacein (**2**) and oleuropein aglycone (**3a,b**) but they additionally highlighted for the first time the significant pro-apoptotic activity of oleomissional (**6a,b,c**) in the SK-MEL-28 melanoma cells. Moreover, oleuropein aglycone (**3a,b**) appeared to have the strongest pro-apoptotic effect in all cell lines tested in the time window within which the apoptotic events were analyzed. The pro-apoptotic effect was more pronounced in the AGS cells, and it was also confirmed by morphological alterations characteristic of apoptotic cells observed by BF brightfield microscopy (Figure S6). Cell changes at early apoptosis include membrane blebbing, cell shrinkage and pyknosis while necrotic cells appear as round or oval masses with nuclear fragmentation and chromatin condensation [94].

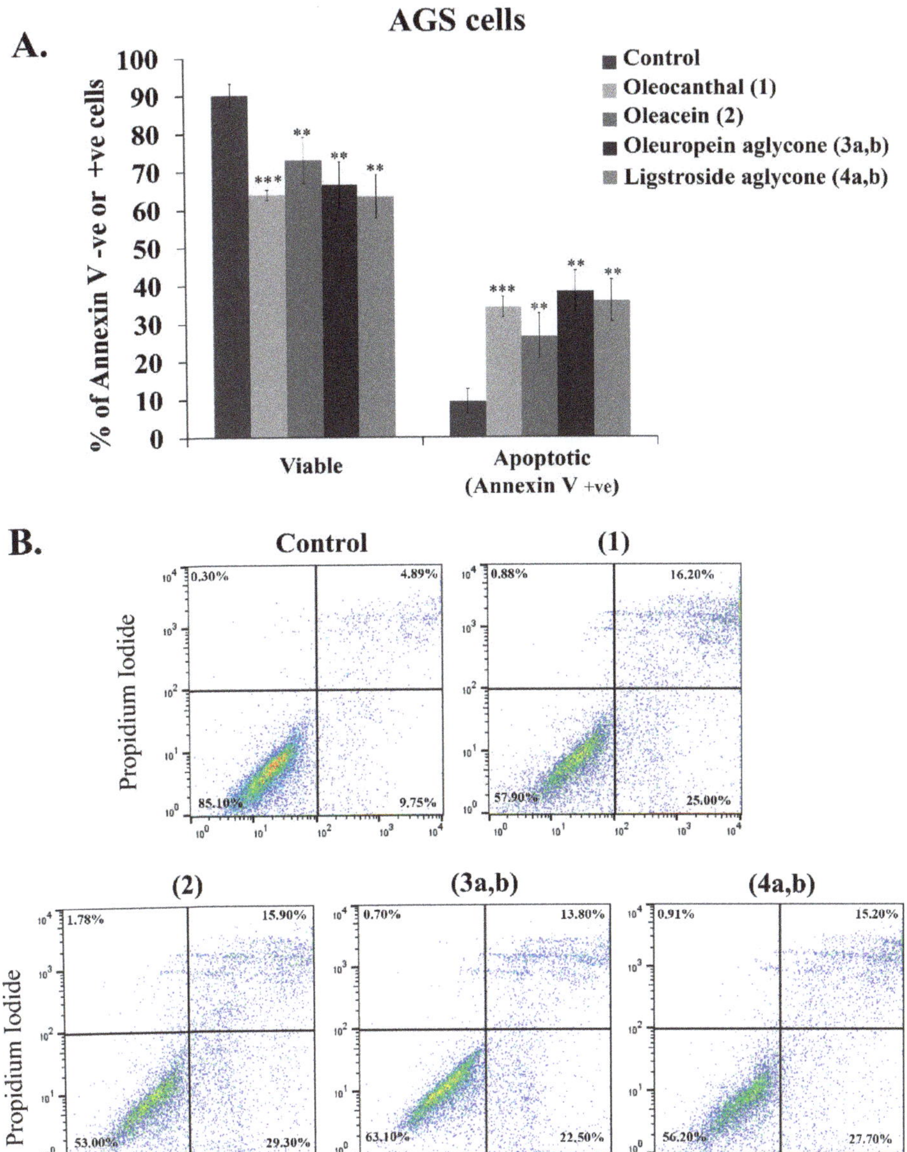

Figure 8. Treatment with OOPs generate apoptotic events in AGS stomach cancer cells. AGS cells were either left untreated (control) or treated with oleocanthal (**1**), oleuropein aglycone (**3a,b**), oleacein

(**2**) and ligstroside aglycone (**4a,b**) at concentrations of EC_{50} values for 48 h. At the end of the treatments, cells were stained with annexin V-FITC and propidium iodide (*Experimental Section*) and were analyzed by FACS. (**A**) The results are presented in bar diagrams as mean values of % annexin V-negative (−ve) for the viable cells and positive (+ve) for the apoptotic cells ± SE The results are from two or three independent experiments performed in duplicate. Differences compared to untreated cells were considered significant at $p < 0.01$ (**) and $p < 0.001$ (***). (**B**) Representative flow cytometry dot plots demonstrating the % of necrotic (upper left), late apoptotic (upper right), early apoptotic (lower right) or viable (lower left) cell populations in the respective quadrants.

It is worth noting that the scope of this study was to systematically investigate if the treatment of the cancer cell lines with the five OOPs under the experimental conditions used in this study could result in detectable apoptotic events. The mechanisms by which the different OOPs analyzed herein cause apoptosis were not the focus of this work.

Most reports on the pro-apoptotic effect of OOPs have mainly focused on oleocanthal (**1**) and breast cancer cell lines and less on cancer cell lines originating from other tissues. Several mechanisms have been proposed as the cause of apoptosis in the studied cell lines which in some cases coincide but in others differ [21,22,28,38,48,75]. Interestingly, in two reports by Legendre et al. and Goren et al., oleocanthal (**1**) induced lysosomal membrane permeabilization (LMP), thus compromising lysosomal integrity in a variety of cancer cells lines [96,97]. These results suggested that the apoptotic and necrotic events detected in oleocanthal-treated (**1**) cells are downstream of the observed LMP and depend on the corresponding degree of LMP [97]. The pro-apoptotic effects of oleacein (**2**) and oleuropein aglycone (**3a,b**) have been much less studied. Both OOPs were reported to trigger apoptosis by altering signaling events exerted by members of the BCL-2 protein family due to the up-regulation of pro-apoptotic factors (i.e., BAX protein) and down-regulation of anti-apoptotic ones (i.e., BCL2 and MCL1) [19,26,27].

3. Materials and Methods

3.1. Chemicals and Culture Media

The Dulbecco's modified Eagle's medium (DMEM) (LM-D1109), fetal bovine serum (FBS) (FB-1001), trypsin-EDTA 0.05% (*w*/*v*) in PBS without (*w*/*o*) calcium and magnesium with phenol red (LM-T1705), Dulbecco's phosphate-buffered saline (PBS) *w*/*o* calcium and magnesium (LM-S2041), HEPES buffer (LM-S2030/100) and penicillin/streptomycin (P/S) (LM-A4118) were purchased from Biosera (Nuaillé, France). RPMI 1640 GlutaMAX (LMR 1640/500), DMEM GlutaMAX™ (21885025), DMEM/F12 with GlutaMAX™ supplement (31331028), MEM Alpha Media (22561-021) and Horse Serum (HS) heat-inactivated New Zealand origin (26050088) were obtained from Gibco/Thermo Fisher Scientific (Waltham, MA, USA). The Mammary Epithelial Cell Growth Medium BulletKit was from Promega (C21110, Madison, WI, USA). Sodium pyruvate solution 100 mM (SH30239.01), L-Glutamine 200 mM (SH30034.01) and non-essential amino acids (SH30238.01) were purchased from Hyclone (Logan, UT, USA). Thiazolyl blue tetrazolium bromide (MTT, M5655) and dimethyl sulfoxide for cell culture (DMSO, D2650) were from Sigma-Aldrich (Darmstadt, Germany). The Vialight Plus Assay Kit used for the determination of cell viability was purchased from Lonza (Basel, Switzerland). The Cell Proliferation Kit III (EdU-488; FM) was from Promocell (PK-CA724-488FM, Heidelberg, Germany). Annexin V-FITC (#640945) and propidium iodide (PI) (#421301) were from Biolegend (San Diego, CA, USA). Hoechst was from Thermofisher (H3570, Waltham, MA, USA). Bovine Pituitary Extract (BPE), epidermal growth factor (EGF), insulin and hydrocortisone were purchased from Promega (C21110, Madison, WI, USA).

3.2. Isolation and Characterization of OOPs

The OOPs used in this study were purified by the methodology described in the sections below. The identity and purity of all the isolated compounds were confirmed using NMR spectroscopy with a Bruker Avance DRX 400 MHz. The ^{1}H NMR spectra of the isolated OOPs are presented in Figure S1 and the NMR data in Table S4. The ^{1}H NMR spectra were processed using either the MNova 6.0.2 (Mestrelab Research) or the TOPSPIN 4.1.4 software (Bruker, Billerica, MA, USA). The MS spectra and the optical rotation values are presented in Figure S7 and Table S5 respectively. The purified compounds were dissolved in DMSO and stored at −20 °C until use.

3.3. Isolation of Oleomissional (**6a,b,c**) from Unripe Intact Olive Fruits

Oleomissional (**6a,b,c**) was isolated from unripe (green) intact olive fruits collected in September–October. More specifically, 15 Kg of intact olive fruits (Lianolia Corfu variety) were immersed into 15 L of CH_2Cl_2 for thirty minutes and then the liquid phase (15 L) was collected and evaporated to dryness under vacuum in a rotary evaporator affording 80 g of a mixture which comprised mainly oleomissional (**6a,b,c**) and triterpenes. After that, 2.8 L of distilled water (pH = 6) was added, and the mixture was agitated for one hour. The mixture was heterogeneous and comprised the aqueous liquid phase and the solid terpenes, mainly oleanolic and maslinic acid, which could not be dissolved in water. The mixture was filtered, and the liquid aqueous phase (2.8 L) was collected and further extracted with 5.6 L of EtOAc. The organic phase was collected and evaporated to dryness under vacuum. The residue consisted of oleomissional (**6a,b,c**) (15 g) with >95% purity as measured by ^{1}H-NMR in $CDCl_3$ and NMR data in accordance with those previously described [34].

3.4. Conversion of Oleomissional (**6a,b,c**) to Closed-Type Oleuropein Aglycone (**3a,b**)

Oleomissional (**6a,b,c**) (3.5 g) isolated using the procedure described above was added to 2.5 L of water which contained $NaHCO_3$ for the adjustment of pH to 7.8. After 24 h stirring at room temperature, the mixture became a homogenous solution that was further subjected to extraction by EtOAc (5 L). The organic phase was collected, washed with distilled water and evaporated to dryness under vacuum. The residue consisted of pure closed-type oleuropein aglycone (mixture of two isomers (**3a** and **3b**) as revealed by ^{1}H-NMR in $CDCl_3$ and NMR data in accordance with those previously described [35].

3.5. Isolation of Oleacein (**2**) from Olive Tree Leaves

Freshly dried olive tree leaves (1 Kg of Kalamon variety) with moisture content <10% (*v*/*v*) were mixed with water (10 L) at 25 °C and cut into small pieces in the presence of water using a blender. The mixture was allowed to stand for 30 min. Then, it was filtered, and the aqueous phase was collected and extracted with EtOAc (8 L). The organic phase was collected and evaporated using a rotary evaporator under reduced pressure affording a viscous liquid (10 g) containing oleacein (**2**) (purity 95% (*w*/*w*)) with NMR data in accordance with those previously described [98].

3.6. Isolation of Oleocanthal (**1**) from Olive Oil

Olive oil (10 kg) produced from olives of Kalamon variety, specifically selected to contain only oleocanthal (**1**) (1 g/kg) without other phenols, was mixed with distilled and deionized water (10 L) and stirred mechanically for 24 h. Subsequently, the mixture was left to stand for 24 h and the two layers were separated by gravity. The heavier aqueous layer was collected, filtered to remove insoluble substances, and re-extracted with EtOAc (1 L). The organic layer was collected and evaporated, affording oleocanthal (**1**) 7.5 g (purity > 95%) with NMR data in accordance with those previously described [98].

3.7. Isolation of Ligstroside Aglycone (**4a,b**) and Oleocanthalic Acid (**7**)

Both compounds were isolated from olive oil extracts as previously described by Karkoula et al. [35] and Tsolakou et al. [40].

3.8. Cell Lines, Cell Culture Conditions and Treatment Protocols with OOPs

The human breast cancer cell line MDA-MB-231 was kindly donated by Dr. P. Lymberi (Hellenic Institute Pasteur, Athens, Greece) and the MCF-7 cell line by Dr. Kletsas (Institute of Biosciences and Applications, NCSR Democritus, Athens, Greece). The lung cancer cell lines H1437 and H1299 were kindly provided by Prof. E. Kolettas (University of Ioannina Medical School & IMBB, Ioannina, Greece). The human gastric cancer cell lines MKN-45 and AGS as well as the human colon cancer cell lines HT-29 and Caco-2 were donated by Dr. D. Sgouras (Hellenic Institute Pasteur, Athens, Greece). The Huh-7 cells (Registry No. JCRB0403) were kindly provided by Prof. R. Bartenschlager (Heidelberg University, Germany) [99]. The HepG-2 hepatocarcinoma cells were a gift from Professor George Notas (University of Crete School of Medicine and University Hospital of Heraklion Emergency Department) and the PANC-1 human pancreatic epithelioid carcinoma cells from Dr. Ioannis Papasotiriou (Research Genetic Cancer Centre, RGCC SA, Florina, Greece). The non-tumorigenic epithelial cell line MCF 10A, and the human skin melanoma cell lines SK-MEL-28 and A2058 were purchased from ATCC (Manassas, VA,USA), while the human immortalized keratinocytes HaCaT were from CLS (Eppelheim, Germany) (https://www.clsgmbh.de/p800_HaCaT.html, accessed on 6 August 2019). The NHDF human dermal fibroblasts isolated from human adult skin were obtained from Dr. Sophia Letsiou (APIVITA R&D department, Athens, Greece), the human mesenchymal stem cells derived from umbilical cord (Wharton's jelly stem cells (WJSCs)) were provided by Dr. Zoumpourlis (Institute of Chemical Biology, National Hellenic Research Foundation (NHRF), Athens, Greece) and the MRC-5 human fetal lung fibroblasts from Dr. Vassilis Aidinis (Institute of Immunology, Biomedical Sciences Research Center Alexander Fleming, Athens, Greece).

All cell lines were incubated at 37 °C and 5% (*v*/*v*) CO_2 and supplemented with 1% (*w*/*v*) antibiotic (final concentrations 100 U/mL penicillin and 100 μg/mL streptomycin). MDA-MB 231, MCF-7, SK-BR-3, A2058, NHDF, Huh-7 and AGS were cultured in high glucose (4500 mg/L) DMEM supplemented with 10% (*v*/*v*) FBS, 1 mM sodium pyruvate and non-essential amino acids, according to the manufacturer's recommendations (Dilution 1:100)—henceforth called "DMEM complete medium". The HaCaT cells were cultured in the same above-mentioned medium without the addition of sodium pyruvate and non-essential amino acids. Caco-2 cells were maintained in DMEM high glucose with 20% (*v*/*v*) FBS supplemented with 1 mM sodium pyruvate. PANC-1 cells were cultured in DMEM high glucose with 10% (*v*/*v*) FBS and 2 mM glutamine. SK-MEL-28, ME-180, H1437 and H1299 cells were cultured in RPMI GlutaMAX with 10% (*v*/*v*) FBS and 1 mM sodium pyruvate, while MKN-45 and HT-29 were maintained in RPMI GlutaMAX just with 10% (*v*/*v*) FBS. DMEM GlutaMAX with 10% (*v*/*v*) FBS plus 1 mM sodium pyruvate was used for the Hela and HepG-2 cell lines. MCF 10A was cultured in Mammary Epithelial Cell Growth Medium supplemented with 5% (*v*/*v*) HS, 0.004 mL/mL BPE, 10 ng/mL EGF, 5 μg/μL insulin and 500 ng/mL hydrocortisone. WJSCs were cultured in DMEM/F12 GlutaMAX™ supplemented with 10% (*v*/*v*) FBS, non-essential amino acids (Dilution 1:100) and HEPES buffer at a final concentration of 15 mM. Finally, the MRC-5 cell line was cultured with MEM Alpha Medium with 10% FBS.

The OOPs tested in this study were first dissolved in an appropriate DMSO volume such as to prepare a final stock solution of 50 mM, which was further used to prepare various compound concentrations in DMSO-based solutions. The final DMSO concentration in the cell culture was maintained constant in all treated groups of any given experiment and never exceeded the value of 0.2% (*v*/*v*). For the treatment experiments, cells were plated in 96-well culture plates, in 100 μL of complete medium at a seeding density of 5000–10,000 cells/well—depending on cells' size and doubling time—and were allowed to adhere overnight (~16 h). The next day, 150 μL of complete medium was added to each well and the cells were treated with various concentrations of OOPs. Each concentration was tested in triplicate and was repeated 2–3 times. To prepare the final concentration solutions, 0.5 μL of a 500× stock of each tested compound in DMSO was added directly into each well in a final volume of 250 μL culture medium and was gently mixed by pipetting. Control wells were prepared under the same experimental conditions by adding only DMSO at a final concentration of 0.2% (v/v). Compounds were not renewed during the entire period of cell exposure. All cells were cultured at 37 °C in a 5% (v/v) CO_2 for 24, 48 or 72 h.

3.9. Cell Viability Assays and Determination of the OOPs' EC_{50} Values

For the determination of the EC_{50} values, cell viability was assayed after 72 h treatment using the ViaLight^{TM} Cell Proliferation and Cytotoxicity BioAssay Kit according to the supplier's protocol with slight modifications. Briefly, after the treatment with OOPs, the adapted medium was removed from the dish wells and the cells were washed twice with medium without FBS. Then, the C-lysis (LT27-076) was diluted in PBS (1:2) and a volume of 50 μL was added to each well. Cells were incubated with C-lysis for at least 10 min. Finally, an equal volume of lysed cells from each well and ATP monitoring reagent (AMR; LT27-212) was transferred to the wells of a white-walled illuminometer plate (Greiner bio-one; 655074). Cell viability was quantified by measuring luminescence using a multi-mode microplate reader Safire^2 Tecan (software Magellan V6.00 STD.2PC WIN.20000/XP). EC_{50} values were calculated after 72 h treatment using the GraphPad Prism 6 software.

For the assessment of cell viability after treatment with OOPs the 3-(4, 5-dimethylthiazol-2yl)-2,5-diphenyl tetrazolium bromide (MTT) colorimetric assay was also used. MTT solution was added in cells at a final concentration of 0.5 mg/mL and the cells were incubated for 3 h. The MTT solution was subsequently discarded, and a 100 μL volume of DMSO was added into each well to dissolve the generated formazan crystals. Each sample's optical density was measured at 570 nm on a microplate reader (Dynatech Laboratories MRX Microplate Reader, Chantilly, VA, USA). Results from two or three independent experiments performed in triplicate were presented either in tables or in bar graphs as mean cell count ± SE for each treatment group normalized to the control group (cells treated with 0.2% (v/v) DMSO).

3.10. Cell Proliferation Assay—Cell Preparation and Staining

Human cancer cells were plated onto sterile glass coverslips (10-mm diameter, 5161063, ThermoFisher Scientific, Waltham, MA, USA) in 24-well tissue culture plates, at a density 5 times the density of cells seeded in 96-well plate and at a final medium volume of 500 μL. In order to obtain homogeneous plating, 250 μL of the medium was added directly to the wells already containing coverslips. Using a tip perpendicularly, coverslips were pressed in order to ensure their attachment to the bottom of the well. The cells were then seeded by adding 250 μL of single-cell suspension drop by drop following a cross path. Immediately after seeding, the plate was shaken back and forth at least ten times to achieve homogeneous plating. The cells were allowed to adhere overnight (~16 h) at 37 °C and 5% (v/v) CO_2. The next day, a volume of 500 μL fresh medium was added to each well and the treatment with OOPs was initiated by adding directly to the wells 2 μL of OOPs from the 500× stock in DMSO and immediately mixed afterward by pipetting. The concentration of each OOP used was its EC_{50} value and the treatment lasted 24 h. Control cells were prepared under the same experimental conditions using DMSO instead of the OOPs' solutions in DMSO at the same final concentration (0.2% (v/v) DMSO). Only the compounds with $EC_{50} \leq 50$ μM were tested for antiproliferative effect. Each condition was performed in duplicate. After treatment with the OOPs, live proliferating mammalian cells were labeled with 5-ethynyl-2′-deoxyuridine (EdU), a nucleoside analog of thymidine, using the Cell proliferation kit III (EdU-FM, PK-CA724-488FM, Promokine, Heidelberg, Germany). More specifically, a 20 μM EdU solution from a 10 mM stock in DMSO was prepared in a fresh culture medium. Culture supernatant was removed from treated cells to leave only 250 μL. An equal volume of 20 μM EdU solution was added and mixed with the medium to obtain a 10 μM EdU final concentration. The treated cells were incubated for the desired time of pulse length (2–4 h) under conditions optimal for each cell type depending on each cell line's doubling time. Following incubation, cells were washed twice with PBS, then fixed with 4% (*w*/*v*) paraformaldehyde in PBS for 15 min at room temperature (RT), and subsequently washed twice with 3% (*w*/*v*) BSA for 5 min each time. Cells were permeabilized by incubation (20 min, RT, in the dark) with 0.5% (*v*/*v*) Triton-X 100 in PBS. Following permeabilization the cells were washed twice with 3% (*w*/*v*) BSA in PBS and incubated for 30 min with the reaction cocktail, according to the instructions of the Cell proliferation kit III (EdU-488; FM). After staining for replicating DNA, the cells were washed three times with 3% (*w*/*v*) BSA in PBS, and were then incubated (10 min, at RT) with Hoechst 33342 in PBS (1:10.000) to visualize all the nuclei. The treated and stained cells on coverslips were washed twice with PBS, mounted on glass coverslips with Mowiol at RT and stored protected from light at 4 °C until analyzed by confocal microscopy imaging. Before imaging, glass slides with mounted coverslips were allowed to warm up at RT for proper emission of fluorophores. Additionally, the coverslips were carefully cleaned with 70% (*v*/*v*) EtOH in order to eliminate remaining mounting medium that could damage the objective lenses upon contact.

3.11. Image Acquisition by Confocal Microscopy and Digital Image Analysis

Cells were imaged with "sequential z scan" and "tile scan" modes of an SP8 confocal microscope using a 20× objective and a 512 × 512 pixel resolution format. The solid-state laser lines 405 and 488 nm were used in order to image the fluorescence of Hoechst and Alexa 488 emission signals respectively. Fluorescence signals for each fluorophore were collected separately. The same laser intensity and detector acquisition parameters of gain and offset were used in the OOP-treated and untreated samples. The Gain [V] was adjusted so that the brightest areas fall just below the limit for signal saturation. Each field size imaged consisted of 45 (9 × 5) tiles "stitched" with "seams smoothed" using the "Merge images" application after completion of the image acquisition. The z-stack was acquired 'Between Stacks' with a z-step size of 1 µm.

For further quantitative analysis of the digital images, a series of data from z-stacks were processed as follows: Eleven out of forty-five acquired series (25%) were analyzed using the open source image analysis software Icy Version 2.4.2.0 [100]. A Maximum Z Projection was applied to all of them and the HK-Means segmentation plugin [101] was used to extract objects corresponding to nuclei labeled with Hoechst (total cell population) and to proliferating cells' nuclei labeled with EdU488. Segmentation was performed simultaneously for both channels, or separately depending on the set-up for the channels. The number of Hoechst- and EdU-labelled nuclei was used to calculate the % of proliferating cells as the % of EdU positive/total number of nuclei labelled with Hoechst (% EdU +ve). At least 180 cells (181–2500) from two or three independent experiments were observed for each experimental group in most cases.

3.12. Annexin V/PI Staining and Analysis by Flow Cytometry

Apoptosis and necrosis were assessed by double staining with annexin V-FITC and propidium iodide (PI) and were analyzed using flow cytometry (FACS). Human cancer cells were plated in 96-well culture plates in 100 µL of complete medium and were allowed to adhere overnight (~16 h). The next day, 150 µL of fresh complete medium was added to each well and the cells were treated with OOPs at their EC_{50} concentration for 48 h (compounds with $EC_{50} \leq 50$ µM were tested). In detail, 0.5 µL of a 500× stock of each tested compound in DMSO was added directly into each well in a final volume of 250 µL culture medium and was gently mixed by pipetting. Control wells were prepared under the same experimental conditions by adding only DMSO at a final concentration of 0.2% (*v*/*v*). At the end of the treatment, the cells were detached by trypsinization, media with serum was added to deactivate trypsin, and the cells from three wells were pooled together by centrifugation (1000 rpm, 5 min, 24 °C), washed with cold PBS, centrifuged (1000 rpm, 5 min, 24 °C) and finally resuspended in cold 1× annexin V binding buffer (10 mM HEPES pH = 7.4, 150 mM NaCl, 2.5 mM $CaCl_2$) at a density of 10^4 cells/mL. Staining was performed by incubating with annexin V- FITC and propidium iodide (PI; BioLegend) for 15 min at room temperature in the dark, according to the manufacturer's instructions. Negative control samples consisted of cells treated only with 0.2% (*v*/*v*) DMSO for the same incubation time length (i.e., 48 h). Cells treated with Triton X-100 (0.25% (*v*/*v*)) for 5 min at 4 °C were used as controls for 100% permeabilization of the plasma membrane and maximum fluorescence staining with PI (positive control for cells in necrosis). The presence of live, apoptotic or necrotic cells was assessed with the FACS Calibur (Becton–Dickinson, San Jose, CA, USA). In total, 10,000 cells were analyzed per measurement and the acquired data were analyzed using the FlowJo V.10.0.8 software (Tree Star Inc., Ashland, OR, USA). Each condition was analyzed in duplicate, and the results presented are from 2 or 3 independent experiments.

3.13. Statistical Analysis

All data were derived from multiple experiments conducted at least in triplicate. Statistical analysis was performed using the GraphPad Prism v8 (GraphPad Software Inc., San Diego, CA, USA) and Office Excel 365 (Microsoft, Redmond, WA, USA). For the cell-viability assays, the data obtained from cells treated with OOPs were normalized to the average luminescence of the control group treated with the vehicle compound (i.e., DMSO), which was considered 100% viability, and the EC_{50s} were calculated using the GraphPad Prism algorithm.

Data showing OOPs' antiproliferative effect as the percentage of S-phase cells were derived from two or three independent experiments and were presented as mean values ± SE (Excel Formula applied for three experiments: SE = STDEV (A1, A2, A3)/SQRT(COUNT(A1, A2, A3)). Differences in proliferation levels between treated and untreated control cells were analyzed for significance using the unpaired two tailed Student's *t*-test, and *p* values were estimated using the GraphPad algorithm. Values were considered significant at a 0.05 level of confidence. The levels of antiproliferative effect shown as % inhibition of cell proliferation are presented as means ± SE after normalization, with the average proliferation levels of the control cells.

Data showing OOPs' apoptotic/necrotic effect were derived from two or three independent experiments and were presented as the means ± SE of the percentage (%) of both annexin V-positive cells (early apoptotic events) and % of annexin V/PI positive cells (late apoptotic events) over the whole cell population normalized to the corresponding events of the control cells, as determined using the FlowJo software.

4. Conclusions

The present work is the first systematic comparative ex vivo study evaluating the anti-cancer potential of extra virgin olive oil phenols. It was performed with secoiridoid phenols isolated in pure form (i.e., oleocanthal (**1**), oleacein (**2**), oleuropein aglycone (**3a,b**), ligstroside aglycone (**4a,b**), oleomissional (**6a,b,c**) and oleocanthalic acid (**7**)) using new methods for large-scale selective extraction from different olive plant parts. EC_{50} values of these OOPs' bioactivity on multiple cancer and non-cancer cell lines from different tissue origins were calculated. For this, the same experimental protocols were followed enabling thereby valid comparisons between the effects of all tested OOPs in either the same cell line or amongst different cell lines. The variability in the activity of the analyzed OOPs in different cell lines and different cancer types was clearly highlighted. The antiproliferative and pro-apoptotic bioactivity was confirmed for OOPs studied before, i.e., oleocanthal (**1**), [28–33] oleuropein aglycone (**3a,b**) [17,27,53], ligstroside aglycone (**4a,b**) [53] and oleacein (**2**) [19], and for the first time for oleomissional (**6a,b,c**). Important information was generated, encouraging further in vivo investigations of the OOPs presenting strong bioactivity in several cancer cell lines. Moreover, the important antiproliferative cytostatic effect of oleuropein and ligstroside aglycones ((**3a,b**) and (**4a,b**)) in the H1437 lung cancer and Caco-2 colon carcinoma cells, stronger than that of oleocanthal (**1**), which has been the most effective and well-studied OOP until now, highlights the selectivity in the action of the different OOPs on different cancer types.

To conclude, this study, besides the new methodologies for the isolation of olive oil secoiridoids, provides important information about the methodology of handling them for in vitro analysis of their bioactivity in cell culture models. The major messages from already performed studies converge to a conclusion that the analyzed secoiridoid phenols hold significant potential for further analysis in in vivo studies evaluating their anti-tumor properties [7]. However, a large variability exists in results already generated by others with respect to the EC_{50} values of each phenol as well as its activity in different cancer cell models. This is perhaps due to the fact that each compound was tested in one or very few cell lines, or in cell lines of only one cancer type. Moreover, the bioactivity of new phenols recently isolated (i.e., oleomissional (**6a,b,c**) and oleocanthalic acid (**7**)) had not been studied until now [34,40]. The present study aspires to fill gaps in knowledge such as the above-mentioned, and to become a reference report for the EC_{50} values of oleocanthal (**1**), oleacein (**2**), oleuropein aglycone (**3a,b**), ligstroside aglycone (**4a,b**), oleomissional (**6a,b,c**) and oleocanthalic acid (**7**) in the large array of cell lines analyzed herein, forming thereby a base for further in vivo studies in animal cancer models investigating their potential anti-tumoral effects.

Supplementary Materials: The following supporting information can be downloaded at: https://www.mdpi.com/article/10.3390/ijms24010003/s1. Refs [99,102] are cited in supplementary files.

Author Contributions: Conceived and designed the experiments: H.B., P.M., E.M., A.P., P.K. and N.V.; performed the experiments: A.P., P.K., A.R., P.D., E.F. and E.C.; analyzed the data: A.P., P.K., A.R., P.M. and H.B.; contributed reagents/materials/analysis tools: H.B., P.M. and E.M.; wrote the paper: A.P., P.K., P.M. and H.B.; edited the paper: E.C. and N.V. All authors have read and agreed to the published version of the manuscript.

Funding: This study was co-financed by Greece and the European Union (European Social Fund-ESF) through the Operational Program «Human Resources Development, Education and Lifelong Learning 2014-2020» in the context of the project "In vitro study of anticancer properties of olive oil polyphenols" (MIS 5048983).

Acknowledgments: The authors acknowledge the help of the World Olive Center for Health (https://worldolivecenter.com) and Leventis Foundation for the scholarship provided to A.P. and A.R. The authors also thank Evangelia Xingi at the Light Microscopy facility of the Hellenic Pasteur Institute for her assistance with the use of the SP8 confocal microscope, as well as all the scientists listed in the Experimental Section who donated cell lines used in this study, and Panagiotis Georgiadis at the National Research Foundation in Greece for the permission to use the multi-mode microplate reader Safire2/Tecan in his laboratory.

Conflicts of Interest: The authors P.M., E.M., A.R. and P.D. are inventors of the patents: "Method For Obtaining Oleocanthal Type Secoiridoids And For Producing Respective Pharmaceutical Preparations" WO/2020/165614 and "Method for obtaining of oleacein and oleomissional secoiridoids and method of producing pharmaceutical preparations thereof" WO/2020/165613. The remaining authors declare no conflicts of interest.

References

1. Morze, J.; Danielewicz, A.; Przybylowicz, K.; Zeng, H.; Hoffmann, G.; Schwingshackl, L. An updated systematic review and meta-analysis on adherence to mediterranean diet and risk of cancer. *Eur. J. Nutr.* **2021**, *60*, 1561–1586. [CrossRef]
2. Schwingshackl, L.; Schwedhelm, C.; Galbete, C.; Hoffmann, G. Adherence to Mediterranean Diet and Risk of Cancer: An Updated Systematic Review and Meta-Analysis. *Nutrients* **2017**, *9*, 1063. [CrossRef]
3. Mahamat-Saleh, Y.; Cervenka, I.; Al Rahmoun, M.; Savoye, I.; Mancini, F.R.; Trichopoulou, A.; Boutron-Ruault, M.C.; Kvaskoff, M. Mediterranean dietary pattern and skin cancer risk: A prospective cohort study in French women. *Am. J. Clin. Nutr.* **2019**, *110*, 993–1002. [CrossRef] [PubMed]
4. Couto, E.; Boffetta, P.; Lagiou, P.; Ferrari, P.; Buckland, G.; Overvad, K.; Dahm, C.C.; Tjonneland, A.; Olsen, A.; Clavel-Chapelon, F.; et al. Mediterranean dietary pattern and cancer risk in the EPIC cohort. *Br. J. Cancer* **2011**, *104*, 1493–1499. [CrossRef] [PubMed]
5. Psaltopoulou, T.; Kosti, R.I.; Haidopoulos, D.; Dimopoulos, M.; Panagiotakos, D.B. Olive oil intake is inversely related to cancer prevalence: A systematic review and a meta-analysis of 13,800 patients and 23,340 controls in 19 observational studies. *Lipids Health Dis.* **2011**, *10*, 127. [CrossRef]

6. Rojas Gil, A.P.; Kodonis, I.; Ioannidis, A.; Nomikos, T.; Dimopoulos, I.; Kosmidis, G.; Katsa, M.E.; Melliou, E.; Magiatis, P. The Effect of Dietary Intervention With High-Oleocanthal and Oleacein Olive Oil in Patients With Early-Stage Chronic Lymphocytic Leukemia: A Pilot Randomized Trial. *Front. Oncol.* **2021**, *11*, 810249. [CrossRef]
7. Fabiani, R. Anti-cancer properties of olive oil secoiridoid phenols: A systematic review of in vivo studies. *Food Funct.* **2016**, *7*, 4145–4159. [CrossRef]
8. Diamantakos, P.; Giannara, T.; Skarkou, M.; Melliou, E.; Magiatis, P. Influence of Harvest Time and Malaxation Conditions on the Concentration of Individual Phenols in Extra Virgin Olive Oil Related to Its Healthy Properties. *Molecules* **2020**, *25*, 2449. [CrossRef]
9. Han, X.Z.; Shen, T.; Lou, H.X. Dietary polyphenols and their biological significance. *Int. J. Mol. Sci.* **2007**, *8*, 950–988. [CrossRef]
10. Cicerale, S.; Conlan, X.A.; Sinclair, A.J.; Keast, R.S. Chemistry and health of olive oil phenolics. *Crit. Rev. Food Sci. Nutr.* **2009**, *49*, 218–236. [CrossRef]
11. Cicerale, S.; Lucas, L.; Keast, R. Biological activities of phenolic compounds present in virgin olive oil. *Int. J. Mol. Sci.* **2010**, *11*, 458–479. [CrossRef]
12. Boss, A.; Bishop, K.S.; Marlow, G.; Barnett, M.P.; Ferguson, L.R. Evidence to Support the Anti-Cancer Effect of Olive Leaf Extract and Future Directions. *Nutrients* **2016**, *8*, 513. [CrossRef]
13. Emma, M.R.; Augello, G.; Di Stefano, V.; Azzolina, A.; Giannitrapani, L.; Montalto, G.; Cervello, M.; Cusimano, A. Potential Uses of Olive Oil Secoiridoids for the Prevention and Treatment of Cancer: A Narrative Review of Preclinical Studies. *Int. J. Mol. Sci.* **2021**, *22*, 1234. [CrossRef]
14. Moral, R.; Escrich, E. Influence of Olive Oil and Its Components on Breast Cancer: Molecular Mechanisms. *Molecules* **2022**, *27*, 477. [CrossRef]
15. Casaburi, I.; Puoci, F.; Chimento, A.; Sirianni, R.; Ruggiero, C.; Avena, P.; Pezzi, V. Potential of olive oil phenols as chemopreventive and therapeutic agents against cancer: A review of in vitro studies. *Mol. Nutr. Food Res.* **2013**, *57*, 71–83. [CrossRef] [PubMed]
16. Corona, G.; Deiana, M.; Incani, A.; Vauzour, D.; Dessi, M.A.; Spencer, J.P. Inhibition of p38/CREB phosphorylation and COX-2 expression by olive oil polyphenols underlies their anti-proliferative effects. *Biochem. Biophys. Res. Commun.* **2007**, *362*, 606–611. [CrossRef]
17. Menendez, J.A.; Vazquez-Martin, A.; Colomer, R.; Brunet, J.; Carrasco-Pancorbo, A.; Garcia-Villalba, R.; Fernandez-Gutierrez, A.; Segura-Carretero, A. Olive oil's bitter principle reverses acquired autoresistance to trastuzumab (Herceptin) in HER2-overexpressing breast cancer cells. *BMC Cancer* **2007**, *7*, 80. [CrossRef]
18. El Haouari, M.; Quintero, J.E.; Rosado, J.A. Anticancer molecular mechanisms of oleocanthal. *Phytother. Res. PTR* **2020**, *34*, 2820–2834. [CrossRef]
19. Cirmi, S.; Celano, M.; Lombardo, G.E.; Maggisano, V.; Procopio, A.; Russo, D.; Navarra, M. Oleacein inhibits STAT3, activates the apoptotic machinery, and exerts anti-metastatic effects in the SH-SY5Y human neuroblastoma cells. *Food Funct.* **2020**, *11*, 3271–3279. [CrossRef]
20. Diez-Bello, R.; Jardin, I.; Lopez, J.J.; El Haouari, M.; Ortega-Vidal, J.; Altarejos, J.; Salido, G.M.; Salido, S.; Rosado, J.A. (-)-Oleocanthal inhibits proliferation and migration by modulating Ca(2+) entry through TRPC6 in breast cancer cells. *Biochim. Et Biophys. Acta. Mol. Cell Res.* **2019**, *1866*, 474–485. [CrossRef]
21. Fogli, S.; Arena, C.; Carpi, S.; Polini, B.; Bertini, S.; Digiacomo, M.; Gado, F.; Saba, A.; Saccomanni, G.; Breschi, M.C.; et al. Cytotoxic Activity of Oleocanthal Isolated from Virgin Olive Oil on Human Melanoma Cells. *Nutr. Cancer* **2016**, *68*, 873–877. [CrossRef] [PubMed]
22. Gu, Y.; Wang, J.; Peng, L. (-)-Oleocanthal exerts anti-melanoma activities and inhibits STAT3 signaling pathway. *Oncol. Rep.* **2017**, *37*, 483–491. [CrossRef] [PubMed]
23. Busnena, B.A.; Foudah, A.I.; Melancon, T.; El Sayed, K.A. Olive secoiridoids and semisynthetic bioisostere analogues for the control of metastatic breast cancer. *Bioorganic Med. Chem.* **2013**, *21*, 2117–2127. [CrossRef] [PubMed]
24. Unsal, U.U.; Mete, M.; Aydemir, I.; Duransoy, Y.K.; Umur, A.S.; Tuglu, M.I. Inhibiting effect of oleocanthal on neuroblastoma cancer cell proliferation in culture. *Biotech. Histochem. Off. Publ. Biol. Stain Comm.* **2020**, *95*, 233–241. [CrossRef]
25. Polini, B.; Digiacomo, M.; Carpi, S.; Bertini, S.; Gado, F.; Saccomanni, G.; Macchia, M.; Nieri, P.; Manera, C.; Fogli, S. Oleocanthal and oleacein contribute to the in vitro therapeutic potential of extra virgin oil-derived extracts in non-melanoma skin cancer. *Toxicol. Vitr. Int. J. Publ. Assoc. BIBRA* **2018**, *52*, 243–250. [CrossRef]
26. Carpi, S.; Polini, B.; Manera, C.; Digiacomo, M.; Salsano, J.E.; Macchia, M.; Scoditti, E.; Nieri, P. miRNA Modulation and Antitumor Activity by the Extra-Virgin Olive Oil Polyphenol Oleacein in Human Melanoma Cells. *Front. Pharmacol.* **2020**, *11*, 574317. [CrossRef]
27. Mazzei, R.; Piacentini, E.; Nardi, M.; Poerio, T.; Bazzarelli, F.; Procopio, A.; Di Gioia, M.L.; Rizza, P.; Ceraldi, R.; Morelli, C.; et al. Production of Plant-Derived Oleuropein Aglycone by a Combined Membrane Process and Evaluation of Its Breast Anticancer Properties. *Front. Bioeng. Biotechnol.* **2020**, *8*, 908. [CrossRef]
28. Akl, M.R.; Ayoub, N.M.; Mohyeldin, M.M.; Busnena, B.A.; Foudah, A.I.; Liu, Y.Y.; El Sayed, K.A. Olive Phenolics as c-Met Inhibitors: (-)-Oleocanthal Attenuates Cell Proliferation, Invasiveness, and Tumor Growth in Breast Cancer Models. *PLoS ONE* **2014**, *9*, e97622. [CrossRef]
29. Pei, T.; Meng, Q.; Han, J.; Sun, H.; Li, L.; Song, R.; Sun, B.; Pan, S.; Liang, D.; Liu, L. (-)-Oleocanthal inhibits growth and metastasis by blocking activation of STAT3 in human hepatocellular carcinoma. *Oncotarget* **2016**, *7*, 43475–43491. [CrossRef]

30. Siddique, A.B.; Ebrahim, H.; Mohyeldin, M.; Qusa, M.; Batarseh, Y.; Fayyad, A.; Tajmim, A.; Nazzal, S.; Kaddoumi, A.; El Sayed, K. Novel liquid-liquid extraction and self-emulsion methods for simplified isolation of extra-virgin olive oil phenolics with emphasis on (-)-oleocanthal and its oral anti-breast cancer activity. *PLoS ONE* **2019**, *14*, e0214798. [CrossRef]
31. Siddique, A.B.; Kilgore, P.C.S.R.; Tajmim, A.; Singh, S.S.; Meyer, S.A.; Jois, S.D.; Cvek, U.; Trutschl, M.; El Sayed, K.A. (-)-Oleocanthal as a Dual c-MET-COX2 Inhibitor for the Control of Lung Cancer. *Nutrients* **2020**, *12*, 1749. [CrossRef]
32. Siddique, A.B.; Ayoub, N.M.; Tajmim, A.; Meyer, S.A.; Hill, R.A.; El Sayed, K.A. (-)-Oleocanthal Prevents Breast Cancer Locoregional Recurrence After Primary Tumor Surgical Excision and Neoadjuvant Targeted Therapy in Orthotopic Nude Mouse Models. *Cancers* **2019**, *11*, 637. [CrossRef]
33. Qusa, M.H.; Abdelwahed, K.S.; Siddique, A.B.; El Sayed, K.A. Comparative Gene Signature of (-)-Oleocanthal Formulation Treatments in Heterogeneous Triple Negative Breast Tumor Models: Oncological Therapeutic Target Insights. *Nutrients* **2021**, *13*, 1706. [CrossRef]
34. Diamantakos, P.; Killday, K.; Gimisis, T.; Melliou, E.; Velkou, A.; Magiatis, P. Oleokoronal and oleomissional: New major phenolic ingredients of extra virgin olive oil. *Olivae* **2015**, *122*, 22–33.
35. Karkoula, E.; Skantzari, A.; Meliou, E.; Magiatis, P. Quantitative Measurement of Major Secoiridoid Derivatives in Olive Oil Using qNMR. Proof of the Artificial Formation of Aldehydic Oleuropein and Ligstroside Aglycon Isomers. *J. Agric. Food Chem.* **2014**, *62*, 600–607. [CrossRef] [PubMed]
36. Adhami, H.R.; Zehl, M.; Dangl, C.; Dorfmeister, D.; Stadler, M.; Urban, E.; Hewitson, P.; Ignatova, S.; Krenn, L. Preparative isolation of oleocanthal, tyrosol, and hydroxytyrosol from olive oil by HPCCC. *Food Chem.* **2015**, *170*, 154–159. [CrossRef]
37. Agalias, A.; Magiatis, P.; Skaltsounis, A.L.; Mikros, E.; Tsarbopoulos, A.; Gikas, E.; Spanos, I.; Manios, T. A new process for the management of olive oil mill waste water and recovery of natural antioxidants. *J. Agric. Food Chem.* **2007**, *55*, 2671–2676. [CrossRef]
38. Khanal, P.; Oh, W.K.; Yun, H.J.; Namgoong, G.M.; Ahn, S.G.; Kwon, S.M.; Choi, H.K.; Choi, H.S. p-HPEA-EDA, a phenolic compound of virgin olive oil, activates AMP-activated protein kinase to inhibit carcinogenesis. *Carcinogenesis* **2011**, *32*, 545–553. [CrossRef]
39. Paiva-Martins, F.; Gordon, M.H. Isolation and characterization of the antioxidant component 3,4-dihydroxyphenylethyl 4-formyl-3-formylmethyl-4-hexenoate from olive (Olea europaea) leaves. *J. Agric. Food Chem.* **2001**, *49*, 4214–4219. [CrossRef]
40. Tsolakou, A.; Diamantakos, I.P.; Kalaboki, I.; Mena-Bravo, A.; Priego-Capote, F.; Abdallah, I.M.; Kaddoumi, A.; Melliou, E.; Magiatis, P. Oleocanthalic Acid, a Chemical Marker of Olive Oil Aging and Exposure to a High Storage Temperature with Potential Neuroprotective Activity. *J. Agric. Food Chem.* **2018**, *66*, 7337–7346. [CrossRef]
41. Abuznait, A.H.; Qosa, H.; Busnena, B.A.; El Sayed, K.A.; Kaddoumi, A. Olive-oil-derived oleocanthal enhances beta-amyloid clearance as a potential neuroprotective mechanism against Alzheimer's disease: In vitro and in vivo studies. *ACS Chem. Neurosci.* **2013**, *4*, 973–982. [CrossRef] [PubMed]
42. Sarikaki, G.; Christoforidou, N.; Gaboriaud-Kolar, N.; Smith, A.B., 3rd; Kostakis, I.K.; Skaltsounis, A.L. Biomimetic Synthesis of Oleocanthal, Oleacein, and Their Analogues Starting from Oleuropein, A Major Compound of Olive Leaves. *J. Nat. Prod.* **2020**, *83*, 1735–1739. [CrossRef] [PubMed]
43. Guzmán, J.M.F.-B.; Castilla, I.M.; Benjumea., A.G. Use of Dmso for the Synthesis of Oleacein and Oleocanthal. WO2018162769, 9 March 2018.
44. Reboredo-Rodriguez, P.; Gonzalez-Barreiro, C.; Cancho-Grande, B.; Forbes-Hernandez, T.Y.; Gasparrini, M.; Afrin, S.; Cianciosi, D.; Carrasco-Pancorbo, A.; Simal-Gandara, J.; Giampieri, F.; et al. Characterization of phenolic extracts from Brava extra virgin olive oils and their cytotoxic effects on MCF-7 breast cancer cells. *Food Chem. Toxicol.* **2018**, *119*, 73–85. [CrossRef] [PubMed]
45. Imran, M.; Nadeem, M.; Gilani, S.A.; Khan, S.; Sajid, M.W.; Amir, R.M. Antitumor Perspectives of Oleuropein and Its Metabolite Hydroxytyrosol: Recent Updates. *J. Food Sci.* **2018**, *83*, 1781–1791. [CrossRef] [PubMed]
46. Lu, H.Y.; Zhu, J.S.; Zhang, Z.; Shen, W.J.; Jiang, S.; Long, Y.F.; Wu, B.; Ding, T.; Huan, F.; Wang, S.L. Hydroxytyrosol and Oleuropein Inhibit Migration and Invasion of MDA-MB-231 Triple-Negative Breast Cancer Cell via Induction of Autophagy. *Anti-Cancer Agent Me* **2019**, *19*, 1983–1990. [CrossRef] [PubMed]
47. Elnagar, A.Y.; Sylvester, P.W.; El Sayed, K.A. (-)-Oleocanthal as a c-Met inhibitor for the control of metastatic breast and prostate cancers. *Planta Med.* **2011**, *77*, 1013–1019. [CrossRef]
48. Cusimano, A.; Balasus, D.; Azzolina, A.; Augello, G.; Emma, M.R.; Di Sano, C.; Gramignoli, R.; Strom, S.C.; McCubrey, J.A.; Montalto, G.; et al. Oleocanthal exerts antitumor effects on human liver and colon cancer cells through ROS generation. *Int. J. Oncol.* **2017**, *51*, 533–544. [CrossRef]
49. Pang, K.L.; Chin, K.Y. The Biological Activities of Oleocanthal from a Molecular Perspective. *Nutrients* **2018**, *10*, 570. [CrossRef]
50. Kugic, A.; Dabelic, S.; Brala, C.J.; Dabelic, N.; Barbaric, M. Extra Virgin Olive Oil Secoiridoids Modulate the Metabolic Activity of Dacarbazine Pre-Treated and Treatment-Naive Melanoma Cells. *Molecules* **2022**, *27*, 3310. [CrossRef]
51. Menendez, J.A.; Joven, J.; Aragones, G.; Barrajon-Catalan, E.; Beltran-Debon, R.; Borras-Linares, I.; Camps, J.; Corominas-Faja, B.; Cufi, S.; Fernandez-Arroyo, S.; et al. Xenohormetic and anti-aging activity of secoiridoid polyphenols present in extra virgin olive oil: A new family of gerosuppressant agents. *Cell Cycle* **2013**, *12*, 555–578. [CrossRef]
52. Kikuchi, M.; Mano, N.; Uehara, Y.; Machida, K.; Kikuchi, M. Cytotoxic and EGFR tyrosine kinase inhibitory activities of aglycone derivatives obtained by enzymatic hydrolysis of oleoside-type secoiridoid glucosides, oleuropein and ligustroside. *J. Nat. Med.* **2011**, *65*, 237–240. [CrossRef] [PubMed]

53. Menendez, J.A.; Vazquez-Martin, A.; Garcia-Villalba, R.; Carrasco-Pancorbo, A.; Oliveras-Ferraros, C.; Fernandez-Gutierrez, A.; Segura-Carretero, A. tabAnti-HER2 (erbB-2) oncogene effects of phenolic compounds directly isolated from commercial Extra-Virgin Olive Oil (EVOO). *BMC Cancer* **2008**, *8*, 377. [CrossRef] [PubMed]
54. Knowles, H.J.; Harris, A.L. Hypoxia and oxidative stress in breast cancer. Hypoxia and tumourigenesis. *Breast Cancer Res. BCR* **2001**, *3*, 318–322. [CrossRef]
55. Jing, X.; Yang, F.; Shao, C.; Wei, K.; Xie, M.; Shen, H.; Shu, Y. Role of hypoxia in cancer therapy by regulating the tumor microenvironment. *Mol. Cancer* **2019**, *18*, 157. [CrossRef] [PubMed]
56. Byrne, M.B.; Leslie, M.T.; Gaskins, H.R.; Kenis, P.J.A. Methods to study the tumor microenvironment under controlled oxygen conditions. *Trends Biotechnol.* **2014**, *32*, 556–563. [CrossRef] [PubMed]
57. Yao, M.; Walker, G.; Gamcsik, M.P. A multiwell plate-based system for toxicity screening under multiple static or cycling oxygen environments. *Sci. Rep.* **2021**, *11*, 4020. [CrossRef]
58. Nam, H.; Funamoto, K.; Jeon, J.S. Cancer cell migration and cancer drug screening in oxygen tension gradient chip. *Biomicrofluidics* **2020**, *14*, 044107. [CrossRef]
59. Vassilaki, N.; Frakolaki, E. Virus-host interactions under hypoxia. *Microbes Infect* **2017**, *19*, 193–203. [CrossRef]
60. Wheaton, W.W.; Chandel, N.S. Hypoxia. 2. Hypoxia regulates cellular metabolism. *Am. J. Physiol. Cell Physiol.* **2011**, *300*, C385–C393. [CrossRef]
61. Solaini, G.; Baracca, A.; Lenaz, G.; Sgarbi, G. Hypoxia and mitochondrial oxidative metabolism. *Biochim. Et Biophys. Acta* **2010**, *1797*, 1171–1177. [CrossRef]
62. McKeown, S.R.; Cowen, R.L.; Williams, K.J. Bioreductive drugs: From concept to clinic. *Clin. Oncol.* **2007**, *19*, 427–442. [CrossRef] [PubMed]
63. Shannon, A.M.; Bouchier-Hayes, D.J.; Condron, C.M.; Toomey, D. Tumour hypoxia, chemotherapeutic resistance and hypoxia-related therapies. *Cancer Treat. Rev.* **2003**, *29*, 297–307. [CrossRef] [PubMed]
64. Karkoula, E.; Skantzari, A.; Melliou, E.; Magiatis, P. Direct Measurement of Oleocanthal and Oleacein Levels in Olive Oil by Quantitative H-1 NMR. Establishment of a New Index for the Characterization of Extra Virgin Olive Oils. *J. Agric. Food Chem.* **2012**, *60*, 11696–11703. [CrossRef] [PubMed]
65. Rigakou, A.; Diamantakos, P.; Melliou, E.; Magiatis, P. S-(E)-Elenolide: A new constituent of extra virgin olive oil. *J. Sci. Food Agric.* **2019**, *99*, 5319–5326. [CrossRef]
66. Darakjian, L.I.; Rigakou, A.; Brannen, A.; Qusa, M.H.; Tasiakou, N.; Diamantakos, P.; Reed, M.N.; Panizzi, P.; Boersma, M.D.; Melliou, E.; et al. Spontaneous In Vitro and In Vivo Interaction of (-)-Oleocanthal with Glycine in Biological Fluids: Novel Pharmacokinetic Markers. *ACS Pharmacol. Transl. Sci.* **2021**, *4*, 179–192. [CrossRef]
67. Magiatis, P.; Melliou, E.; Diamantakos, P.; Rigakou, A. Method for Obtaining Oleocanthal Type Secoiridoids and for Producing Respective Pharmaceutical Preparations. WO/2020/165614, 11 February 2020.
68. Diamantakos, P.; Ioannidis, K.; Papanikolaou, C.; Tsolakou, A.; Rigakou, A.; Melliou, E.; Magiatis, P. A New Definition of the Term "High-Phenolic Olive Oil" Based on Large Scale Statistical Data of Greek Olive Oils Analyzed by qNMR. *Molecules* **2021**, *26*, 1115. [CrossRef]
69. Agalias, A.; Melliou, E.; Magiatis, P.; Mitaku, S.; Gikas, E.; Tsarbopoulos, A. Quantitation of oleuropein and related metabolites in decoctions of Olea europaea leaves from ten Greek cultivated varieties by HPLC with diode array detection (HPLC-DAD). *J. Liq. Chromatogr. Relat. Technol.* **2005**, *28*, 1557–1571. [CrossRef]
70. EMA. *Assessment Report on Olea europaea L., Folium*; EMA: London, UK, 2017.
71. Koudounas, K.; Thomopoulou, M.; Rigakou, A.; Angeli, E.; Melliou, E.; Magiatis, P.; Hatzopoulos, P. Silencing of Oleuropein beta-Glucosidase Abolishes the Biosynthetic Capacity of Secoiridoids in Olives. *Front. Plant Sci.* **2021**, *12*, 671487. [CrossRef]
72. Volk, J.; Sarafeddinov, A.; Unver, T.; Marx, S.; Tretzel, J.; Zotzel, J.; Warzecha, H. Two novel methylesterases from Olea europaea contribute to the catabolism of oleoside-type secoiridoid esters. *Planta* **2019**, *250*, 2083–2097. [CrossRef]
73. Cree, I.A.; Andreotti, P.E. Measurement of cytotoxicity by ATP-based luminescence assay in primary cell cultures and cell lines. *Toxicol. Vitr.* **1997**, *11*, 553–556. [CrossRef]
74. Ayoub, N.M.; Siddique, A.B.; Ebrahim, H.Y.; Mohyeldin, M.M.; El Sayed, K.A. The olive oil phenolic (-)-oleocanthal modulates estrogen receptor expression in luminal breast cancer in vitro and in vivo and synergizes with tamoxifen treatment. *Eur. J. Pharmacol.* **2017**, *810*, 100–111. [CrossRef] [PubMed]
75. Khanfar, M.A.; Bardaweel, S.K.; Akl, M.R.; El Sayed, K.A. Olive Oil-derived Oleocanthal as Potent Inhibitor of Mammalian Target of Rapamycin: Biological Evaluation and Molecular Modeling Studies. *Phytother. Res. PTR* **2015**, *29*, 1776–1782. [CrossRef] [PubMed]
76. Siddique, A.B.; Ebrahim, H.Y.; Akl, M.R.; Ayoub, N.M.; Goda, A.A.; Mohyeldin, M.M.; Nagumalli, S.K.; Hananeh, W.M.; Liu, Y.Y.; Meyer, S.A.; et al. (-)-Oleocanthal Combined with Lapatinib Treatment Synergized against HER-2 Positive Breast Cancer In Vitro and In Vivo. *Nutrients* **2019**, *11*, 412. [CrossRef]
77. Christodoulou, I.; Goulielmaki, M.; Kritikos, A.; Zoumpourlis, P.; Koliakos, G.; Zoumpourlis, V. Suitability of Human Mesenchymal Stem Cells Derived from Fetal Umbilical Cord (Wharton's Jelly) as an Alternative In Vitro Model for Acute Drug Toxicity Screening. *Cells* **2022**, *11*, 1102. [CrossRef]
78. Christodoulou, I.; Goulielmaki, M.; Devetzi, M.; Panagiotidis, M.; Koliakos, G.; Zoumpourlis, V. Mesenchymal stem cells in preclinical cancer cytotherapy: A systematic review. *Stem Cell Res. Ther.* **2018**, *9*, 336. [CrossRef]

79. Christodoulou, I.; Kolisis, F.N.; Papaevangeliou, D.; Zoumpourlis, V. Comparative Evaluation of Human Mesenchymal Stem Cells of Fetal (Wharton's Jelly) and Adult (Adipose Tissue) Origin during Prolonged In Vitro Expansion: Considerations for Cytotherapy. *Stem Cells Int.* **2013**, *2013*, 246134. [CrossRef]
80. Indrayanto, G.; Putra, G.S.; Suhud, F. Validation of in-vitro bioassay methods: Application in herbal drug research. *Profiles Drug Subst. Excip. Relat. Methodol.* **2021**, *46*, 273–307.
81. Weerapreeyakul, N.; Nonpunya, A.; Barusrux, S.; Thitimetharoch, T.; Sripanidkulchai, B. Evaluation of the anticancer potential of six herbs against a hepatoma cell line. *Chin. Med.* **2012**, *7*, 15. [CrossRef]
82. Kaplanek, R.; Jakubek, M.; Rak, J.; Kejik, Z.; Havlik, M.; Dolensky, B.; Frydrych, I.; Hajduch, M.; Kolar, M.; Bogdanova, K.; et al. Caffeine-hydrazones as anticancer agents with pronounced selectivity toward T-lymphoblastic leukaemia cells. *Bioorganic Chem.* **2015**, *60*, 19–29. [CrossRef]
83. Artun, F.T.; Karagoz, A.; Ozcan, G.; Melikoglu, G.; Anil, S.; Kultur, S.; Sutlupinar, N. In vitro anticancer and cytotoxic activities of some plant extracts on HeLa and Vero cell lines. *J. Buon.* **2016**, *21*, 720–725.
84. Fang, Y.; Eglen, R.M. Three-Dimensional Cell Cultures in Drug Discovery and Development. *SLAS Discov.* **2017**, *22*, 456–472. [CrossRef] [PubMed]
85. Eglen, R.; Reisine, T. Primary cells and stem cells in drug discovery: Emerging tools for high-throughput screening. *Assay Drug Dev. Technol.* **2011**, *9*, 108–124. [CrossRef] [PubMed]
86. Yuen, A.; Diaz, B. The impact of hypoxia in pancreatic cancer invasion and metastasis. *Hypoxia* **2014**, *2*, 91–106. [PubMed]
87. McKeown, S.R. Defining normoxia, physoxia and hypoxia in tumours-implications for treatment response. *Br. J. Radiol.* **2014**, *87*, 20130676. [CrossRef]
88. Masson, N.; Ratcliffe, P.J. Hypoxia signaling pathways in cancer metabolism: The importance of co-selecting interconnected physiological pathways. *Cancer Metab.* **2014**, *2*, 3. [CrossRef]
89. Vassilaki, N.; Kalliampakou, K.I.; Kotta-Loizou, I.; Befani, C.; Liakos, P.; Simos, G.; Mentis, A.F.; Kalliaropoulos, A.; Doumba, P.P.; Smirlis, D.; et al. Low Oxygen Tension Enhances Hepatitis C Virus Replication. *J. Virol.* **2013**, *87*, 2935–2948. [CrossRef]
90. Frakolaki, E.G.E.; Feuillette-Cadenne, N.; Kaimou, P.; Niotis, G.; Bartenschlager, R.; Mavromara, P.; Zoidis, G.; Windisch, M.; Neuveut, C.; Vassilaki, N. The interplay between hepatotropic viruses and liver normoxia determines viral levels and response to therapeutics. In *From Basic Science to Biomarkers and Tools in Global Health*; Institut Pasteur: Paris, France, 2016.
91. Talarek, N.; Petit, J.; Gueydon, E.; Schwob, E. EdU Incorporation for FACS and Microscopy Analysis of DNA Replication in Budding Yeast. *Methods Mol. Biol.* **2015**, *1300*, 105–112.
92. Salic, A.; Mitchison, T.J. A chemical method for fast and sensitive detection of DNA synthesis in vivo. *Proc. Natl. Acad. Sci. USA* **2008**, *105*, 2415–2420. [CrossRef]
93. Scotece, M.; Gomez, R.; Conde, J.; Lopez, V.; Gomez-Reino, J.J.; Lago, F.; Smith, A.B., 3rd; Gualillo, O. Oleocanthal inhibits proliferation and MIP-1alpha expression in human multiple myeloma cells. *Curr. Med. Chem.* **2013**, *20*, 2467–2475. [CrossRef]
94. Elmore, S. Apoptosis: A review of programmed cell death. *Toxicol. Pathol.* **2007**, *35*, 495–516. [CrossRef]
95. Brauchle, E.; Thude, S.; Brucker, S.Y.; Schenke-Layland, K. Cell death stages in single apoptotic and necrotic cells monitored by Raman microspectroscopy. *Sci. Rep.* **2014**, *4*, 4698. [CrossRef] [PubMed]
96. LeGendre, O.; Breslin, P.A.; Foster, D.A. (-)-Oleocanthal rapidly and selectively induces cancer cell death via lysosomal membrane permeabilization. *Mol. Cell. Oncol.* **2015**, *2*, e1006077. [CrossRef] [PubMed]
97. Goren, L.; Zhang, G.; Kaushik, S.; Breslin, P.A.S.; Du, Y.N.; Foster, D.A. (-)-Oleocanthal and (-)-oleocanthal-rich olive oils induce lysosomal membrane permeabilization in cancer cells. *PLoS ONE* **2019**, *14*, e0216024. [CrossRef] [PubMed]
98. Montedoro, G.; Servilli, M.; Baldioli, M.; Selvaggini, R.; Miniati, E.; Macchioni, A. Simple and hydrolysable compounds in virgin olive oil. 3. Spectroscopic characterizations of the secoiridoid derivatives. *J. Agric. Food Chem.* **1993**, *41*, 2228–2234. [CrossRef]
99. Nakabayashi, H.; Taketa, K.; Miyano, K.; Yamane, T.; Sato, J. Growth of human hepatoma cells lines with differentiated functions in chemically defined medium. *Cancer Res.* **1982**, *42*, 3858–3863. [PubMed]
100. de Chaumont, F.; Dallongeville, S.; Chenouard, N.; Herve, N.; Pop, S.; Provoost, T.; Meas-Yedid, V.; Pankajakshan, P.; Lecomte, T.; Le Montagner, Y.; et al. Icy: An open bioimage informatics platform for extended reproducible research. *Nat. Methods* **2012**, *9*, 690–696. [CrossRef]
101. Dufour, A.; Meas-Yedid, V.; Grassart, A.; Olivo-Marin, J.C. Automated quantification of cell endocytosis using active contours and wavelets. In Proceedings of the 2008 19th International Conference on Pattern Recognition, Tampa, FL, USA, 8–11 December 2008.
102. Jang, J.W.; Song, Y.; Kim, K.M.; Kim, J.S.; Choi, E.K.; Kim, J.; Seo, H. Hepatocellular carcinoma-targeted drug discovery through image-based phenotypic screening in co-cultures of HCC cells with hepatocytes. *BMC Cancer* **2016**, *16*, 810. [CrossRef]

International Journal of
Molecular Sciences

MDPI

Article

Synthesis and Anti-Proliferative Evaluation of Arctigenin Analogues with C-9′ Derivatisation

Emily K. Paulin [1,2], Euphemia Leung [3,4], Lisa I. Pilkington [1] and David Barker [1,2,*]

1 School of Chemical Sciences, University of Auckland, Auckland 1010, New Zealand
2 The MacDiarmid Institute for Advanced Materials and Nanotechnology, Wellington 6012, New Zealand
3 Auckland Cancer Society Research Centre, University of Auckland, Auckland 1023, New Zealand
4 Department of Molecular Medicine and Pathology, University of Auckland, Auckland 1023, New Zealand
* Correspondence: d.barker@auckland.ac.nz; Tel.: +64-9-373-7599

Abstract: Dibenzylbutyrolactone lignans (DBLs) are a class of natural products with a wide variety of biological activities. Due to their potential for the development of human therapeutic agents, DBLs have been subjected to various SAR studies in order to optimise activity. Previous reports have mainly considered changes on the aromatic rings and at the benzylic carbons of the compounds, whilst the effects of substituents in the lactone, at the C-9′ position, have been relatively unexplored. This position has an unexploited potential for the development of novel dibenzyl butyrolactone derivatives, with previous preliminary findings revealing C-9′-hydroxymethyl analogues inducing programmed cell cycle death. Using the core structure of the bioactive natural product arctigenin, C-9′ derivatives were synthesised using various synthetic pathways and with prepared derivatives providing more potent anti-proliferative activity than the C-9′-hydroxymethyl lead compound.

Keywords: lignans; dibenzylbutyrolactone; arctigenin; prodrugs; anti-proliferative

Citation: Paulin, E.K.; Leung, E.; Pilkington, L.I.; Barker, D. Synthesis and Anti-Proliferative Evaluation of Arctigenin Analogues with C-9′ Derivatisation. *Int. J. Mol. Sci.* **2023**, *24*, 1167. https://doi.org/10.3390/ijms24021167

Academic Editors: Barbara De Filippis, Marialuigia Fantacuzzi and Alessandra Ammazzalorso

Received: 7 December 2022
Revised: 22 December 2022
Accepted: 4 January 2023
Published: 6 January 2023

1. Introduction

Lignans are a large natural product class of structurally and functionally diverse phenylpropanoids, isolated from over 70 known families of plants worldwide [1–4]. The lignan framework is derived from the oxidative dimerisation of two phenylpropane (C-6–C-3) moieties, which produces a linkage between each monomer's propyl side chains at the respective C-8 carbons [1,5].

Arctigenin is a natural product belonging to the dibenzylbutyrolactone subclass of lignans (Figure 1). These structures comprise a γ-lactone core, with dibenzyl substitution at the C-8 and C-8′ positions in an anti-relationship [6,7]. Arctigenin possesses a range of biological activities and consequently has been well-studied to determine structure-activity relationships of its derivatives [6–12]. Results from previous studies have confirmed the lignan's biological activities, with arctigenin analogues having cytotoxic, anti-tumour and hypoglycaemic activities, amongst others [10,12–14]. Many of these derivatives have explored modifications of the aromatic rings, and to a slightly lesser extent the benzylic positions, [9,11,13,15,16], but there is a large underrepresentation of lactone ring modifications.

To date, only one synthetic derivative of arctigenin with C-9′ modification has been reported—a compound containing a methylenehydroxy group at C-5 in the lactone ring (C-9′ according to lignan nomenclature, Figure 1 right) [17,18]. This compound showed the induction of apoptosis in Jurkat T cells with only 2% necrosis. This derivative was accessed using an acyl-Claisen rearrangement as the key step to establish the necessary *trans* relationship between C-8 and C-8′ groups. The prolific activities of arctigenin and lack of SAR information at the C-9′ position inspired this work to synthesise additional C-9′ analogues. Herein, we report the synthesis of 15 arctigenin derivatives with different C-9′ substitution, and their anti-proliferative activities.

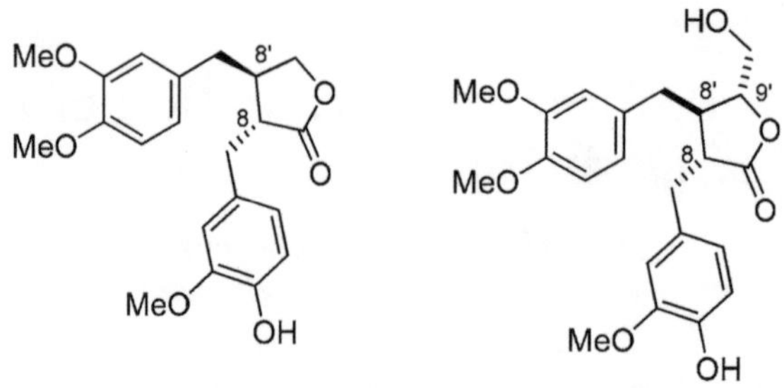

Figure 1. Arctigenin (**left**) and racemic C-9′ methylenehydroxy analogue (**right**).

2. Results and Discussion

2.1. Retrosynthetic Analysis of C-9′ Arctigenin Analogues

The proposed pathway to access the targeted arctigenin analogues also exploited an acyl-Claisen rearrangement [17] to introduce the correct relative stereochemistry between benzyl groups in the morpholine pentenamide **1** and converged two parallel pathways (Scheme 1). Cyclisation of the rearrangement product was envisaged to establish the core DBL lactone framework and included the C-9′ substitution of a methylenehydroxy group, from which derivatisations could be prepared. The acyl-Claisen precursors, an acid chloride **2** and allylic morpholine **3**, could be prepared from vanillin **4** and 4-allyl-1,2-dimethoxybenzene **5**, respectively, through two separate routes.

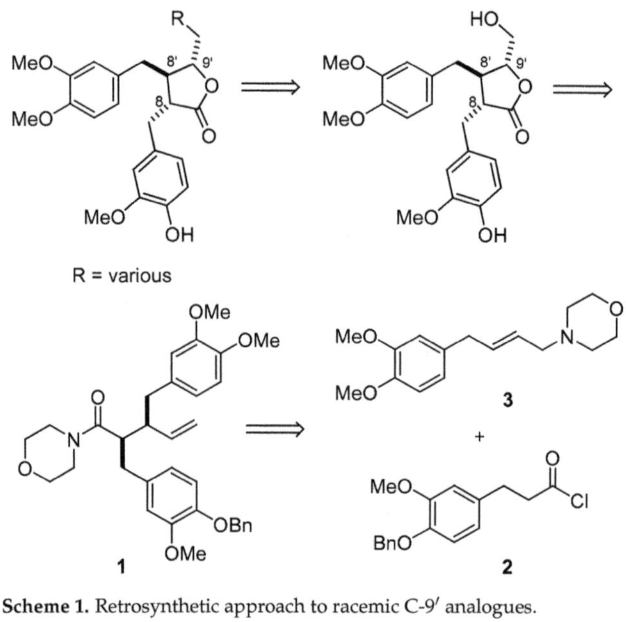

Scheme 1. Retrosynthetic approach to racemic C-9′ analogues.

2.2. Synthesis of Acid Chloride **2**

Acid chloride **2** was prepared when required from the more stable carboxylic acid **6**. Synthesis of **6** began from vanillin **4**, which was subjected to a Wittig olefination with (carbethoxymethylene)triphenylphosphorane, following literature methods [17] to give α,β-unsaturated ethyl ester **7** in 80% yield (*E*:*Z*, 92:8). The newly installed alkene was reduced by catalytic hydrogenation to give saturated ester **8** in quantitative yield (Scheme 2). With the saturated ester **8** in hand, the phenol substituent was protected as the benzyl ether to give **9** in 93% yield. Hydrolysis of the ester **9** gave carboxylic acid **6** in 92% yield and the resulting acid chloride was prepared in situ at the time of the successive step due to its instability.

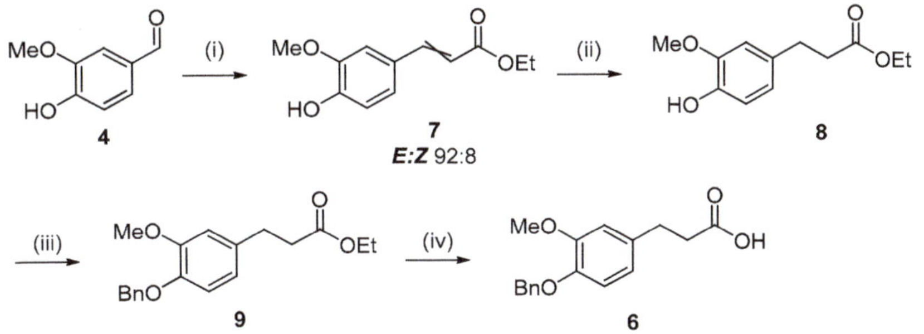

Scheme 2. Synthesis of acid **6**. Reagents and conditions: **(i)** Ph_3PCHCO_2Et (1.1 equiv.), CH_2Cl_2, rt, 21 h, **7** 80%; **(ii)** H_2, Pd/C (10% *w/w*), EtOAc, rt, 20 h, **8** quant.; **(iii)** BnBr (3 equiv.), K_2CO_3 (3 equiv.), MeCN, 80 °C, 46 h, **9** 93%; **(iv)** NaOH (4.5 equiv.), MeOH, rt, 2.5 h, **6** 92%.

2.3. *Synthesis of Allylic Morpholine* 3

To obtain allylic morpholine **3**, 4-allyl-1,2-dimethoxybenzene **5** was first dehydroxylated, under Upjohn conditions [19], to give diol **10** in 94% yield (Scheme 3). The newly formed diol moiety then underwent oxidative cleavage using $NaIO_4$ [17], to afford aldehyde **11** in 97% yield, which was used immediately, due to its tendency to degrade even stored at low temperatures. Thus, **11** underwent a Horner-Wadsworth-Emmons (HWE) reaction, forming the respective (*E*)-α,β-unsaturated ethyl ester **12** in 73% yield [20–22]. During repeated syntheses of α,β-unsaturated ester **12**, the *E*-selectivity of the Horner-Wadsworth-Emmons reaction was found to vary with the formation of both the *Z*-isomer and a third regioisomer, which was determined to be a β,γ-unsaturated ester **13** (Scheme 3). Separation of the desired *E*-isomer **12** on $AgNO_3$-treated silica was possible but poor, leading to diminished yields.

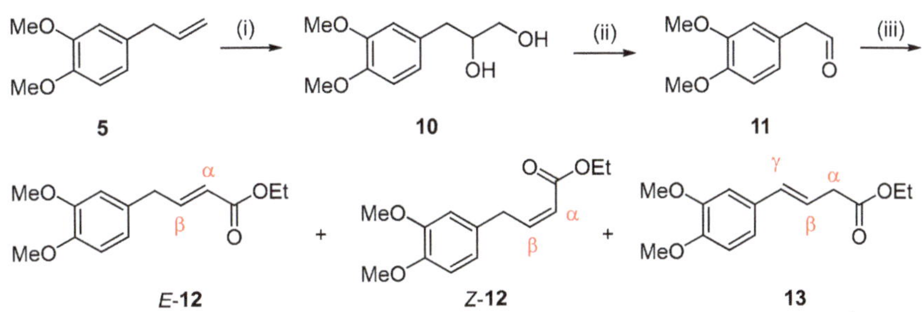

Scheme 3. Synthesis of allylic ester **12**. Reagents and conditions: **(i)** OsO_4 (2.5 mol-%), NMO (3 equiv.), *t*-BuOH/H_2O (1:1), rt, 4 days, **10** 94%; **(ii)** $NaIO_4$ (1.2 equiv.), MeOH/H_2O (3:1), rt, 3 days, **11** 97%; **(iii)** $(EtO)_2POCH_2CO_2Et$ (1.5 equiv.), NaH (2 equiv.), THF, 0 °C to rt, 18 h, *E*-**12**, 39%, *Z*-**12** 2%, **13** 7%.

2.4. *Prevention of Isomeric Esters*

Only *E*-isomer *E*-**12** was required for further steps, therefore, in order to prevent double bond migration to form **13**, different conditions were trialled for the formation of allylic ester **12**. While the mechanism of rearrangement was not confirmed, it was proposed to be base-mediated, through abstraction of the γ-proton after formation of the initial α,β-unsaturated product (Scheme 3), with the resulting β,γ-unsaturated product **13** stabilised by increased conjugation. As a result, different bases were screened. The migrated isomer was observed to a lesser extent under kinetic control or with the use of hindered bases, such as DBU under Masamune-Roush conditions [23], but unfortunately, these reactions still had poor *E*/*Z* stereocontrol. After reports of MeMgBr use to suppress isomerisation in $PhCH_2CHO$ aldehydes, this was applied as a base in the HWE reaction between triethylphosphonoacetate and aldehyde **11** [24]. As a result, neither the migrated species **13** nor *Z*-isomer *Z*-**12** were observed. On a larger scale, good selectivity was maintained (9:1 *E*:*Z*), but unfortunately, the yield was poor (10%), so the exploration of other methods was resumed.

2.5. Grubbs Cross Metathesis Pathway; Revised Route to 3

An alternative route which did not involve a HWE reaction was then developed by implementing a cross metathesis [25] approach between 4-allyl-1,2-dimethoxybenzene **5** and ethyl acrylate. Using Grubb's second-generation catalyst at a loading of 5 mol-% and three equivalents of ethyl acrylate, full conversion to the *E* product *E*-**12** took place in 91% yield. No migrated product **13** was observed, allowing large scale synthesis of ester *E*-**12**.

Ester *E*-**12** was then fully reduced to primary allylic alcohol **14** using DIBAL-H (Scheme 4). The final step towards allylic morpholine **3** involved substitution of the hydroxyl group in **14** for a morpholine moiety. The reaction was attempted using various strategies, including via mesylation, tosylation and bromination with all giving the desired product **3**, but in poor yields.

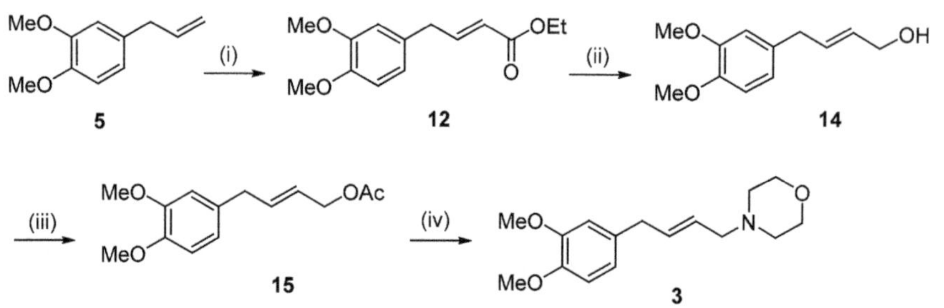

Scheme 4. Synthetic pathway to allylic morpholine **3** using cross metathesis approach. Reagents and conditions: (**i**) Ethyl acrylate (3 equiv.), Grubbs II (1.9 mol-%), CH_2Cl_2, rt, 24 h, **12** 91%; (**ii**) DIBAL-H (2.9 equiv.), PhMe, −10 °C to rt, 20 h, **14** quant.; (**iii**) Ac_2O (2.2 equiv.), Et_3N (3 equiv.), DMAP (10 mol-%), CH_2Cl_2, 0 °C to rt, 25 h, **15**; (**iv**) morpholine (1.9 equiv.), $Pd(PPh_3)_4$ (5 mol-%), THF, reflux, 5 days, **3** 83% (two steps).

In an alternate approach, acetate **15** was then synthesised from alcohol **14**, then subjected to Tsuji-Trost allylation conditions, using palladium tetrakis $Pd(PPh_3)_4$ and morpholine. With the possibility of two regioisomers of the allylic amine product, thermodynamic control was implemented to ensure the desired linear isomer was obtained over the possible kinetic branched product [26]. Over two steps from the allylic alcohol **14**, the desired allylic morpholine **3** was achieved in 83% yield as solely the *E*-isomer, linear product (Scheme 4).

2.6. Synthesis of 9′-CH2OH Lactones

With **3** and **6** prepared, acid **6** was then converted to acid chloride **2** in situ using oxalyl chloride, before undergoing a $TiCl_4$.2THF induced acyl-Claisen rearrangement [17,27] with (*E*)-allylic morpholine **3**. One equivalent of $TiCl_4$.2THF was required, as we have previously shown acyl-Claisen rearrangements with aromatic substituents require stochiometric amounts of Lewis acid to occur [27]. The rearrangement successfully took place to give racemic morpholine amide **1** in 85% yield as a single *syn*-diastereomer. Dihydroxylation, again under Upjohn conditions, cyclised amide **1** in situ to γ-lactone **16** in 88% yield (Scheme 5). The cyclisation proceeds through a diol intermediate, from which anti-**17** spontaneously formed lactone **16**. *Syn*-diol **17** was also formed in 12% yield and did not undergo cyclisation. This allowed *syn*-**17** to be isolated and treated with 2 M HCl to give the epimeric lactone **18** with a *trans,cis* relationship between the C-8, C-8′ and C-9′ stereocentres. Under both sets of conditions, the respective diastereomer (**16** or **18**) was afforded as the sole product. The benzyl ether in each diastereomer was deprotected to their respective phenol, in 56% yield as *trans,cis* isomer **19** and *trans,trans* isomer **20** in quantitative yields (Scheme 5).

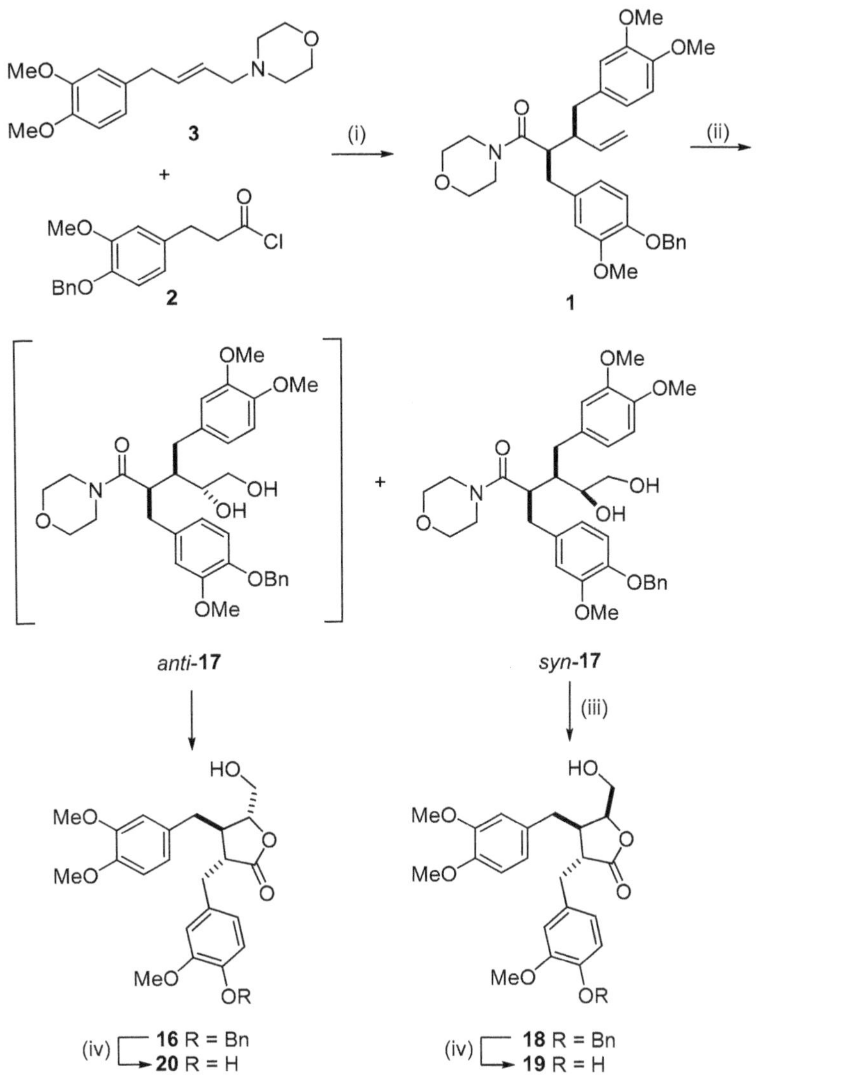

Scheme 5. Acyl-Claisen rearrangement and cyclisation. Reagents and conditions: **(i)** $TiCl_4$.2THF (1 equiv.), *i*-Pr_2NEt (1.5 equiv.), CH_2Cl_2, rt, 24 h, **1** 85%; **(ii)** OsO_4 (2.5 mol-%), NMO (3 equiv.), *t*-BuOH/H_2O (1:1), rt, 4 days, *syn*-**17** 12%, **16** 88%; **(iii)** 2M HCl, MeOH, reflux, 4 h, **18** 94%; **(iv)** Pd/C (10% *w*/*w*), H_2, EtOAc, rt, 19 h, **19** 56%. **20** quant.

2.7. Synthesis of Lactone Derivatives

With lactone **16** successfully synthesised, a range of C-9′ functionalised derivatives were targeted to explore the effects of modifications at this position on the anti-proliferative activity.

2.7.1. Ester Derivatives

A series of ester derivatives was completed to add prodrug-like groups, capable of being cleaved by cellular esterases [28]. Differing ester groups were installed using the addition of acid chlorides to lactone **16** with Et_3N and catalytic DMAP. Differing chain lengths and aromaticity were accessed with the synthesis of acetate **21**, propionate **22**, and benzoate **23** esters (Scheme 6). An additional benzoate ester **24** was synthesised from isomer **19**, in 48% yield, to provide an example of the epimeric *trans,cis* form. Following derivatisation of the 9′-CH_2OH functionality, the benzylic ether at C-4 was removed via catalytic hydrogenation to give the free phenol, a directly comparable analogue of arctigenin. The synthesis of **21–24** was achieved in yields ranging from 72–88%. Deprotection of the benzyl ether in all the ester analogues gave C-4 phenols **25–27**, in yields of 64% to quantitative (Scheme 6).

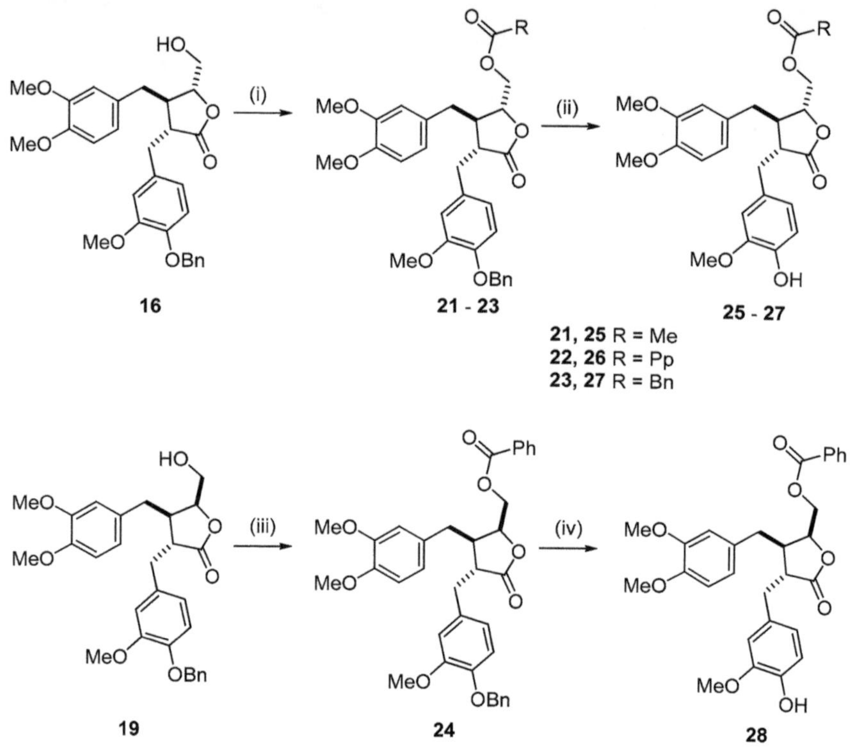

Scheme 6. Synthesis of esters. Reagents and conditions: **(i)** Et_3N (2 equiv.), DMAP (5 mol-%), RCOCl (1.2 equiv.), CH_2Cl_2, 0 °C to rt, 4–23 h, **21–23** 72–88%; **(ii)** Pd/C (10% *w*/*w*), H_2, EtOAc, rt, 22–24 h, **25–27** (64%–quant.); **(iii)** Et_3N (2 equiv.), DMAP (5 mol-%), BzCl (1.2 equiv.), CH_2Cl_2, 0 °C–rt, 21 h, **24** 48%; **(iv)** Pd/C (10% *w*/*w*), H_2, EtOAc, rt, 19 h, **28** quant.

2.7.2. Azido Derivatives

In addition to the obtained ester derivatives, it was decided to install a triazole scaffold due to its presence in clinically used drugs, with a range of pharmacological activities and ability to enhance solubility [29–31]. As a preliminary example of triazole derivatised arctigenin, the simple 4-phenyl-1*H*-1,2,3-triazole moiety was accessed through a copper-catalysed azide-alkyne 1,3-dipolar cycloaddition (CuAAC) click reaction between azide-containing arctigenin analogue **29** and phenylacetylene.

Azide **29** was afforded through a two-step approach of mesylation and subsequent displacement using sodium azide, affording azide **29** in 78% yield over two steps (Scheme 7).

This process also saw formation of a minor alkyl chloride side product **30** through halide displacement.

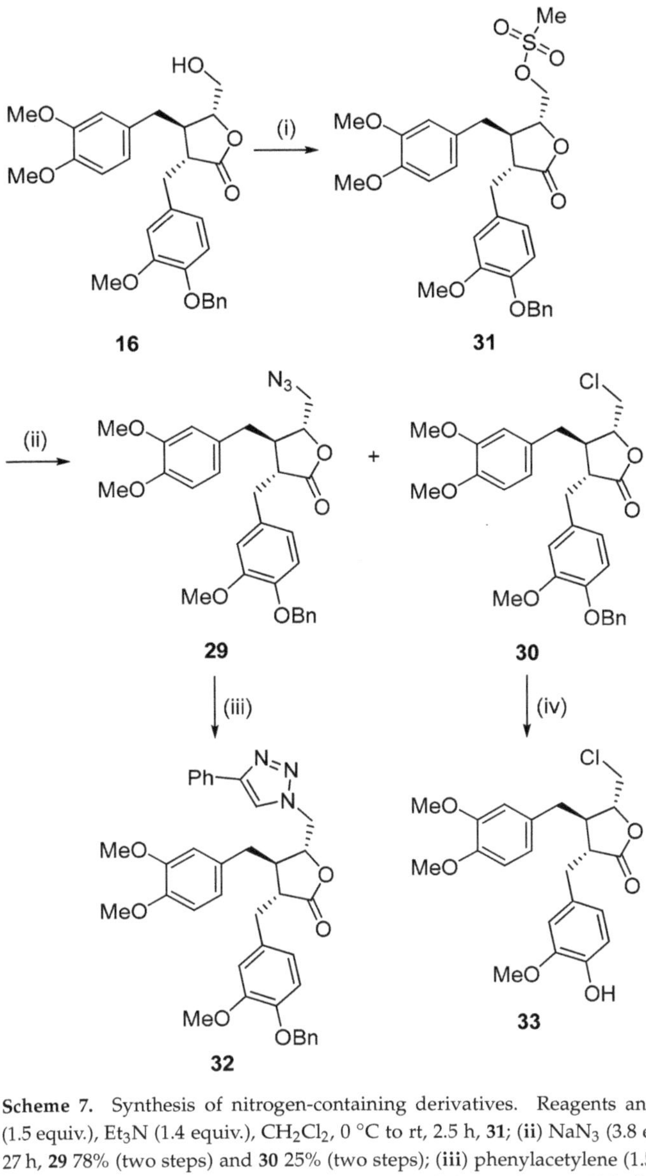

Scheme 7. Synthesis of nitrogen-containing derivatives. Reagents and conditions: **(i)** MsCl (1.5 equiv.), Et_3N (1.4 equiv.), CH_2Cl_2, 0 °C to rt, 2.5 h, **31**; **(ii)** NaN_3 (3.8 equiv.), DMF, 85–100 °C, 27 h, **29** 78% (two steps) and **30** 25% (two steps); **(iii)** phenylacetylene (1.5 equiv.), $Cu_2SO_4.5H_2O$ (0.16 equiv.), sodium L-ascorbate (0.2 equiv.), MeCN, rt, 4 days, **32** 74%; **(iv)** Pd/C (10% *w*/*w*), H_2, EtOAc, rt, 5 days, **33** 29%.

The reaction of azide **29** and phenylacetylene was achieved using sodium ascorbate and copper sulfate pentahydrate in acetonitrile and after four days obtained the 1,4-disubstituted triazole **32** in 74% yield (Scheme 7).

Chloride **30** was stable to catalytic hydrogenation conditions and the benzyl ether removed cleanly through hydrogenolysis to give **33** in 29% yield. However, hydrogenation of triazole **32** was found to be surprisingly difficult and the desired phenol could not be obtained even after using a variety of conditions.

2.8. Anti-Proliferative Activity

Following the synthesis of the arctigenin derivatives, their anti-proliferative activities were evaluated against colorectal cancer HCT-116 and triple negative breast cancer MDA-MB-231 cell lines (Table 1). Arctigenin has previously been shown to affect the growth of MDA-MB-231 [32] whilst the HCT-116 has been used for the anti-proliferative assessment of polyphenolic natural products [33,34]. All of the compounds showed improved activity in the HCT-116 cell line over MDA-MB-231 cells. Five of the fifteen compounds had better activity than the previously prepared hydroxylmethylene derivative **16** in the MDA-MB-231 cell line, and 10 out of the 15 compounds had better activity than that reported for arctigenin itself [32]. It was found that compounds with aromatic benzylic ethers tended to outperform their phenol counterparts, and *trans,trans* stereochemistry between C-8, C-8′ and C-9′ was favourable over a *trans,cis* relationship. The most potent four compounds, based upon their ability to inhibit cell growth at 10 μM, were the same across both cell lines; **24, 29, 32,** and **33**, and their IC_{50} values were determined. All of the tested compounds, **24, 29, 32** and **33** produced similar inhibition–with mean IC_{50} values ranging between 5.79–7.45 μM (MDA-MB-231) and 3.27–6.10 μM (HCT-116) (Table 2).

Table 1. Anti-proliferative activities when cells treated with compound (10 μM). Values are given as the average ± standard error of three experimental replicates. Most active compounds, selected for IC_{50} determination, in highlighted rows.

Compound	Relative Thymidine Uptake at 10 μM (%)	
	HCT-116	MDA-MB-231
16	42.70 ± 1.47	54.48 ± 2.17
18	67.44 ± 8.16	86.62 ±3.64
19	90.01 ± 0.97	100.40 ± 2.66
20	87.83 ± 1.20	92.22 ± 2.66
21	48.92 ± 1.48	60.60 ± 1.68
22	44.64 ± 1.08	50.69 ± 2.37
23	42.31 ± 0.93	60.45 ± 0.47
24	34.80 ± 0.15	44.15 ± 1.78
25	86.01 ± 0.65	104.00 ± 3.48
26	90.38 ± 2.00	105.19 ± 5.09
27	55.86 ± 0.86	75.04 ± 3.06
29	23.72 ± 1.54	36.53 ± 1.32
30	76.48 ± 3.97	96.57 ± 2.88
32	28.02 ± 2.17	44.80 ± 0.37
33	16.48 ± 0.29	34.09 ± 1.58
Arctigenin *	-	84.81 ± 5.96 [32]

* = determined using MTT assay, after 24 h [32].

Table 2. IC_{50} values. Values are given as the average ± standard error of three experimental replicates. Most active compounds in highlighted rows.

Compound	Mean IC_{50} ± Standard Error (μM)	
	HCT-116	MDA-MB-231
24	6.10 ± 1.53	6.90 ± 0.10
29	5.17 ± 1.13	6.23 ± 0.63
32	3.27 ± 1.13	6.89 ± 0.20
33	5.29 ± 1.17	7.45 ± 0.70

3. Materials and Methods

3.1. Synthesis

General experimental details: All reactions were carried out under an inert atmosphere using distilled anhydrous solvents unless otherwise specified. Triethylamine and diisopropylethylamine were each distilled and stored over activated 4 Å Molecular Sieves. All NMR spectra were recorded on a Bruker Avance DRX 400 MHZ spectrometer at ambient temperature. Chemical shifts are reported relative to the solvent peak of $CDCl_3$ (δ 7.26 for ^{1}H and δ 77.16 for ^{13}C) or DMSO (δ 2.50 for ^{1}H and δ 39.52 for ^{13}C). ^{1}H NMR data are reported as position (δ), relative integral, multiplicity (s, singlet; d, doublet; dd, doublet of doublets; ddd, doublet of doublet of doublets; dt, doublet of triplets; dq, doublet of quartets; t, triplet; td, triplet of doublets; q, quartet; m, multiplet), coupling constant (*J*, Hz), and the assignment of the atom. Proton-decoupled ^{13}C NMR data are reported as position (δ) and assignment of the atom. NMR assignments were performed using HMBC, COSY and HSQC, experiments. ^{1}H and ^{13}C NMR spectra for all precursor and final compounds (Figures S1–S45) are found in the supplementary material. The numbering of arctigenin analogues was done according to lignan nomenclature, with the two C-6-C-3 units numbered 1–9 and 1′–9′ [18]. All melting points for solid compounds are given in degrees Celsius (°C), were measured using a Reicher-Kofler block, and are uncorrected. A Perkin-Elmer Spectrum 1000 series Fourier Transform Infrared ATR spectrometer was used to record infrared spectra. Absorption maxima are expressed in wavenumbers (cm^{-1}). High-resolution mass spectroscopy (HRMS) was carried out by electrospray ionisation (ESI^+) on a MicroTOF-Q II mass spectrometer. Fétizon's reagent was prepared following a literature procedure [35]. Unless noted, chemical reagents were used as purchased. General procedures, synthetic experimental methods, and full characterisation data (including copies of NMR spectra for all synthesised final compounds) can be found in the Supplementary Materials.

3.2. Cell Proliferation Assays

The synthesised arctigenin derivatives were measured for anti-proliferative activity against colorectal cancer HCT-116 and triple negative breast cancer MDA-MB-231 cell lines using ^{3}H-thymidine incorporation assays. Cell lines were purchased from the American Type Culture Collection (ATCC). The anti-proliferative assays were conducted according to our previously reported methods. [36–38]. In short, cells were seeded in 96 well plates with 3000 cells per well and incubated with 10 μM of arctigenin-derived compounds for three days. An amount of 0.04 μCi of ^{3}H-thymidine was added per well and incubated for 5 h before cells were harvested and counted. All experiments were performed in duplicate wells on separate plates with three repeats. The percentage of cells which showed incorporation of ^{3}H-thymidine into the DNA relative to the control samples directly measured the cell proliferation. Two known previously active compounds were used as positive controls [39], alongside a negative control, with no compounded added.

4. Conclusions

In this study, fifteen novel C-9′ derivatives of arctigenin with C-9′ substitution were successfully synthesised, and analysed for their anti-proliferative activities, for the first time. This study demonstrated the use of acyl-Claisen rearrangement as an effective method to access a dibenzylbutyrolactone framework as a single *trans* diastereomer between C-8 and C-8′ and to provide C-9′ analogues with a *trans,trans* C-8, C-8′, C-9′ configuration. The benefits of this divergent strategy are evident through the preparation of these derivatives. Anti-proliferative testing of the synthesised compounds showed IC_{50} values as low as 3.27 μM in HCT-116 (compound **32**) and 5.79 μM (compound **29**) in MDA-MB-231 cancer cell lines, which were improved over the natural product, arcitgenin, itself. These results highlight that C-9′ substitution of dibenzylbutyrolactone lignans can improve the biological activity compared to the unsubstituted natural products. Furthermore, as the C-9′ is rarely substituted in other lignan natural products, this work suggests the potential that other classes of lignans could be similarly modified to increase their biological activity.

Supplementary Materials: The following supporting information can be downloaded at: https://www.mdpi.com/article/10.3390/ijms24021167/s1. Synthetic procedures for all novel compounds, ^{1}H and ^{13}C NMR spectra for all precursor and final compounds (Figures S1–S45). References [17,40–49] are cited in supplementary materials.

Author Contributions: Conceptualization, D.B.; methodology, E.K.P., E.L., L.I.P. and D.B.; validation, E.K.P. and E.L.; investigation, E.K.P. and E.L.; resources, E.L., L.I.P. and D.B.; writing—original draft preparation, E.K.P.; writing—review and editing, E.K.P., L.I.P. and D.B.; supervision, D.B. and L.I.P.; project administration, L.I.P. and D.B.; funding acquisition, D.B. All authors have read and agreed to the published version of the manuscript.

Funding: This research received no external funding.

Data Availability Statement: Data are contained within the article.

Acknowledgments: The authors would like to acknowledge financial support for this work from the University of Auckland (doctoral scholarship for E.K.P.).

Conflicts of Interest: The authors declare no conflict of interest.

Sample Availability: Samples of the compounds are available from the authors.

References

1. Tsopmo, A.; Awah, F.M.; Kuete, V. 12—Lignans and stilbenes from african medicinal plants. In *Medicinal Plant Research in Africa*; Kuete, V., Ed.; Elsevier: Oxford, UK, 2013; pp. 435–478. [CrossRef]
2. Barker, D. Lignans. *Molecules* **2019**, *24*, 1424. [CrossRef]
3. Gordaliza, M.; Castro, M.A.; del Corral, J.M.; Feliciano, A.S. Antitumor Properties of Podophyllotoxin and Related Compounds. *Curr. Pharm. Des.* **2000**, *6*, 1811–1839. [CrossRef] [PubMed]
4. Pan, J.-Y.; Chen, S.-L.; Yang, M.-H.; Wu, J.; Sinkkonen, J.; Zou, K. An Update on Lignans: Natural Products and Synthesis. *Nat. Prod. Rep.* **2009**, *26*, 1251–1292. [CrossRef] [PubMed]
5. Haworth, R.D. The Chemistry of the Lignan Group of Natural Products. *J. Chem. Soc.* **1942**, 448–456. [CrossRef]
6. Solyomváry, A.; Boldizsar, I.; Beni, S. Dibenzylbutyrolactone Lignans—A Review of Their Structural Diversity, Biosynthesis, Occurrence, Identification and Importance. *Mini-Rev. Med. Chem.* **2017**, *17*, 1053–1074. [CrossRef] [PubMed]
7. Srivastava, D. Arctigenin, a Plant Lignan with Tremendous Potential: A Review. *Int. J. Curr. Res.* **2017**, *9*, 6.
8. Kamlage, S.; Sefkow, M.; Pool-Zobel, B.L.; Peter, M.G. A Short Synthesis of Biologically Active Lignan Analogues. *Chem. Commun.* **2001**, 331–332. [CrossRef]
9. Duan, S.; Huang, S.; Gong, J.; Shen, Y.; Zeng, L.; Feng, Y.; Ren, W.; Leng, Y.; Hu, Y. Design and Synthesis of Novel Arctigenin Analogues for the Amelioration of Metabolic Disorders. *ACS Med. Chem. Lett.* **2015**, *6*, 386–391. [CrossRef]
10. Shen, S.; Zhuang, J.; Chen, Y.; Lei, M.; Chen, J.; Shen, X.; Hu, L. Synthesis and Biological Evaluation of Arctigenin Ester and Ether Derivatives as Activators of AMPK. *Bioorg. Med. Chem.* **2013**, *21*, 3882–3893. [CrossRef]
11. Eich, E.; Pertz, H.; Kaloga, M.; Schulz, J.; Fesen, M.R.; Mazumder, A.; Pommier, Y. (−)-Arctigenin as a Lead Structure for Inhibitors of Human Immunodeficiency Virus Type-1 Integrase. *J. Med. Chem.* **1996**, *39*, 86–95. [CrossRef]
12. Awale, S.; Kato, M.; Dibwe, D.F.; Li, F.; Miyoshi, C.; Esumi, H.; Kadota, S.; Tezuka, Y. Antiausterity Activity of Arctigenin Enantiomers: Importance of (2R,3R)-Absolute Configuration. *Nat. Prod. Commun.* **2014**, *9*, 79–82. [CrossRef]
13. Kudou, N.; Taniguchi, A.; Sugimoto, K.; Matsuya, Y.; Kawasaki, M.; Toyooka, N.; Miyoshi, C.; Awale, S.; Dibwe, D.F.; Esumi, H.; et al. Synthesis and Antitumor Evaluation of Arctigenin Derivatives Based on Antiausterity Strategy. *Eur. J. Med. Chem.* **2013**, *60*, 76–88. [CrossRef] [PubMed]
14. Wang, L.; Zhao, F.; Liu, K. [Induction of apoptosis of the human leukemia cells by arctigenin and its mechanism of action]. *Yao Xue Xue Bao* **2008**, *43*, 542–547. [PubMed]
15. Alizadeh, B.H.; Foroumadi, A.; Kobarfard, F.; Saeedi, M.; Shafiee, A. Synthesis of Novel Dibenzylbutyrolactones as Dimethylmatairesinol Analogues. *J. Heterocycl. Chem.* **2014**, *52*, 1693–1698. [CrossRef]
16. Želazková, J. Total synthesis of arctigenin derivatives as potential anticancer agents. In Proceedings of the 15th International Electronic Conference on Synthetic Organic Chemistry (ECSOC-15), Online, 1–30 November 2011; p. 9. [CrossRef]
17. Davidson, S.J.; Pilkington, L.I.; Dempsey-Hibbert, N.C.; El-Mohtadi, M.; Tang, S.; Wainwright, T.; Whitehead, K.A.; Barker, D. Modular Synthesis and Biological Investigation of 5-Hydroxymethyl Dibenzyl Butyrolactones and Related Lignans. *Molecules* **2018**, *23*, 3057. [CrossRef]
18. Moss, G.P. Nomenclature of Lignans and Neolignans (IUPAC Recommendations 2000). *Pure Appl. Chem.* **2000**, *72*, 1493–1523. [CrossRef]
19. VanRheenen, V.; Kelly, R.C.; Cha, D.Y. An Improved Catalytic OsO4 Oxidation of Olefins to Cis-1,2-Glycols Using Tertiary Amine Oxides as the Oxidant. *Tetrahedron Lett.* **1976**, *17*, 1973–1976. [CrossRef]

20. Molnár, K.; Takács, L.; Kádár, M.; Faigl, F.; Kardos, Z. Z- and E-Selective Horner–Wadsworth–Emmons Reactions. *Synth. Commun.* **2017**, *47*, 1214–1224. [CrossRef]
21. Carruthers, J.E.; Carruthers, W.; Coldham, I. *Modern Methods of Organic Synthesis*; Cambridge University Press: Cambridge, UK, 2004.
22. Wadsworth, W.S.; Emmons, W.D. The Utility of Phosphonate Carbanions in Olefin Synthesis. *J. Am. Chem. Soc.* **1961**, *83*, 1733–1738. [CrossRef]
23. Blanchette, M.A.; Choy, W.; Davis, J.T.; Essenfeld, A.P.; Masamune, S.; Roush, W.R.; Sakai, T. Horner-Wadsworth-Emmons Reaction: Use of Lithium Chloride and an Amine for Base-Sensitive Compounds. *Tetrahedron Lett.* **1984**, *25*, 2183–2186. [CrossRef]
24. Claridge, T.D.W.; Davies, S.G.; Lee, J.A.; Nicholson, R.L.; Roberts, P.M.; Russell, A.J.; Smith, A.D.; Toms, S.M. Highly (*E*)-Selective Wadsworth−Emmons Reactions Promoted by Methylmagnesium Bromide. *Org. Lett.* **2008**, *10*, 5437–5440. [CrossRef]
25. Ogba, O.M.; Warner, N.C.; O'Leary, D.J.; Grubbs, R.H. Recent Advances in Ruthenium-Based Olefin Metathesis. *Chem. Soc. Rev.* **2018**, *47*, 4510–4544. [CrossRef] [PubMed]
26. Dubovyk, I.; Watson, I.D.G.; Yudin, A.K. Achieving Control over the Branched/Linear Selectivity in Palladium-Catalyzed Allylic Amination. *J. Org. Chem.* **2013**, *78*, 1559–1575. [CrossRef]
27. Barker, D.; Dickson, B.; Dittrich, N.; Rye, C.E. An Acyl-Claisen Approach to the Synthesis of Lignans and Substituted Pyrroles. *Pure Appl. Chem.* **2012**, *84*, 1557–1565. [CrossRef]
28. Yang, Y.; Aloysius, H.; Inoyama, D.; Chen, Y.; Hu, L. Enzyme-Mediated Hydrolytic Activation of Prodrugs. *Acta Pharm. Sin. B* **2011**, *1*, 143–159. [CrossRef]
29. Kharb, R.; Sharma, P.C.; Yar, M.S. Pharmacological Significance of Triazole Scaffold. *J. Enzyme Inhib. Med. Chem.* **2011**, *26*, 1–21. [CrossRef] [PubMed]
30. Hein, J.E.; Fokin, V.V. Copper-Catalyzed Azide–Alkyne Cycloaddition (CuAAC) and beyond: New Reactivity of Copper(I) Acetylides. *Chem. Soc. Rev.* **2010**, *39*, 1302–1315. [CrossRef] [PubMed]
31. Liang, L.; Astruc, D. The Copper(I)-Catalyzed Alkyne-Azide Cycloaddition (CuAAC) "Click" Reaction and Its Applications. An Overview. *Coord. Chem. Rev.* **2011**, *255*, 2933–2945. [CrossRef]
32. Lou, C.; Zhu, Z.; Zhao, Y.; Zhu, R.; Zhao, H. Arctigenin, a Lignan from Arctium Lappa L., Inhibits Metastasis of Human Breast Cancer Cells through the Downregulation of MMP-2/-9 and Heparanase in MDA-MB-231 Cells. *Oncol. Rep.* **2017**, *37*, 179–184. [CrossRef]
33. Paulin, E.K.; Leung, E.; Pilkington, L.I.; Barker, D. The enantioselective total syntheses of (+)-7-oxohinokinin, (+)-7-oxoarcitin, (+)-conicaol B and (−)-isopolygamain. *Org. Biomol. Chem.* **2022**, *20*, 4324–4330. [CrossRef]
34. Lo, S.; Leung, E.; Fedrizzi, B.; Barker, D. Syntheses of mono-acylated luteolin derivatives, evaluation of their antiproliferative and radical scavenging activities and implications on their oral bioavailability. *Sci. Rep.* **2021**, *11*, 12595. [CrossRef]
35. Kakis, F.J.; Fetizon, M.; Douchkine, N.; Golfier, M.; Mourgues, P.; Prange, T. Mechanistic Studies Regarding the Oxidation of Alcohols by Silver Carbonate on Celite. *J. Org. Chem.* **1974**, *39*, 523–533. [CrossRef]
36. Leung, E.; Kim, J.E.; Rewcastle, G.W.; Finlay, G.J.; Baguley, B.C. Comparison of the Effects of the PI3K/MTOR Inhibitors NVP-BEZ235 and GSK2126458 on Tamoxifen-Resistant Breast Cancer Cells. *Cancer Biol. Ther.* **2011**, *11*, 938–946. [CrossRef]
37. Hung, J.M.; Arabshahi, H.J.; Leung, E.; Reynisson, R.; Barker, D. Synthesis and cytotoxicity of thieno[2,3-b]pyridine and furo[2,3-b]pyridine derivatives. *Eur. J. Med. Chem.* **2014**, *86*, 420–437. [CrossRef]
38. Haverkate, N.A.; Leung, E.; Pilkington, L.I.; Barker, D. Tethered Aryl Groups Increase the Activity of Anti-Proliferative Thieno[2,3-*b*]Pyridines by Targeting a Lipophilic Region in the Active Site of PI-PLC. *Pharmaceutics* **2021**, *13*, 2020. [CrossRef] [PubMed]
39. Rees, S.W.P.; Barker, D.; Pilkington, L.I.; Leung, E.; Reynisson, J. Development of 2-Morpholino-N-Hydroxybenzamides as Anti-Proliferative PC-PLC Inhibitors. *Bioorg. Chem.* **2021**, *114*, 105152. [CrossRef] [PubMed]
40. Xia, Y.; Mo, Z.; Sun, L.; Zou, L.; Zhang, W.; Zhang, J.; Wang, L. First Total Synthesis of Quiquesetinerviusin A. *J. Chem. Res.* **2017**, *41*, 296–300. [CrossRef]
41. Hattori, H.; Mitsunaga, T.; Clive, D.L.J. Synthesis of Phenolic Components of Grains of Paradise. *Tetrahedron Lett.* **2019**, *60*, 1989–1991. [CrossRef]
42. Purushotham Reddy, S.; Chinnababu, B.; Venkateswarlu, Y. First Stereoselective and Concise Synthesis of Rhoiptelol C. *Helv. Chim. Acta* **2014**, *97*, 999–1003. [CrossRef]
43. Mane, B.B.; Kumbhar, D.D.; Waghmode, S.B. Enantioselective Total Synthesis of Ligraminol D and Ligraminol E. *Synlett* **2019**, *30*, 2285–2289. [CrossRef]
44. Kikuzaki, H.; Hara, S.; Kawai, Y.; Nakatani, N. Antioxidative Phenylpropanoids from Berries of Pimenta Dioica. *Phytochemistry* **1999**, *52*, 1307–1312. [CrossRef]
45. Davies, S.G.; Goddard, E.C.; Roberts, P.M.; Russell, A.J.; Smith, A.D.; Thomson, J.E.; Withey, J.M. Strategies for the Construction of Morphinan Alkaloid AB-Rings: Regioselective Friedel-Crafts-Type Cyclisations of γ-Aryl-β-Benzoylamido Acids with Asymmetrically Substituted γ-Aryl Rings. *Tetrahedron Asymmetry* **2016**, *27*, 274–284. [CrossRef]
46. Sun, R.; Song, W.; Ma, C.; Zhang, H.; Yu, X. Titanium(IV) Chloride-Mediated Stereoselective α-Alkylidenation to Efficiently Assemble Multisubstituted 1,3-Dienes. *Adv. Synth. Catal.* **2016**, *358*, 3977–3982. [CrossRef]
47. Hryniewicka, A.; Misztalewska, I.; Czajkowska-Szczykowska, D.; Urbańczyk-Lipkowska, Z.; Morzycki, J.W.; Witkowski, S. New Olefin Metathesis Catalysts Bearing Polyether Clamp in N-Heterocyclic Carbenes Ligands. *Tetrahedron* **2014**, *70*, 6810–6816. [CrossRef]

48. Parpal, F.; Pandolfi, E.; Heguaburu, V. (π-Allyl)Palladium Coupling of 2-(Tributylstannyl)cyclopent-2-enone for the Synthesis of Jasmonoid Analogs. *Tetrahedron Lett.* **2017**, *58*, 1965–1968. [CrossRef]
49. Dittrich, N.; Pilkington, L.I.; Leung, E.; Barker, D. Synthesis of N-Benzyl-des-D-ring Lamellarin K via an Acyl-Claisen/Paal-Knorr Approach. *Tetrahedron* **2017**, *73*, 1881–1894. [CrossRef]

International Journal of
Molecular Sciences

MDPI

Article

Trichosanthin Promotes Anti-Tumor Immunity through Mediating Chemokines and Granzyme B Secretion in Hepatocellular Carcinoma

Kaifang Wang [1,2,†], Xiaona Wang [3,†], Minghuan Zhang [3], Zhenguang Ying [1], Zeyao Zhu [4], Kin Yip Tam [5], Chunman Li [6], Guowei Zhou [3], Feng Gao [1], Meiqi Zeng [1], Stephen Cho Wing Sze [2], Xia Wang [3,*] and Ou Sha [1,*]

1 School of Dentistry, Shenzhen University Medical School, Shenzhen 518000, China; wangkaifang@hkbu.edu.hk (K.W.); yzgop@hotmail.com (Z.Y.); gaofeng@szu.edu.cn (F.G.); mqzeng@szu.edu.cn (M.Z.)
2 Department of Biology, Faculty of Science, Hong Kong Baptist University, Hongkong 999077, China; scwsze@hkbu.edu.hk
3 Department of Anatomy and Histology, School of Basic Medical Sciences, Shenzhen University Medical School, Shenzhen 518000, China; 2060243056@email.szu.edu.cn (X.W.); 2060243027@szu.edu.cn (M.Z.); zhougw@szu.edu.cn (G.Z.)
4 Department of Biology, School of Life Sciences, Southern University of Science and Technology, Shenzhen 518000, China; zhuzy@sustech.edu.cn
5 Faculty of Health Sciences, University of Macau, Macau, China; kintam@um.edu.mo
6 Guangdong Provincial Key Laboratory of Infectious Diseases and Molecular Immunopathology, Shantou University Medical College, Shantou 515000, China; cmli@stu.edu.cn
* Correspondence: xia.wang@szu.edu.cn (X.W.); shaou@szu.edu.cn (O.S.)
† These authors contributed equally to this work.

Abstract: Trichosanthin (TCS) is a type I ribosome-inactivating protein extracted from the tuberous root of the plant *Trichosanthes*. TCS shows promising potential in clinical drug abortion, anti-tumor and immunological regulation. However, the molecular mechanisms of its anti-tumor and immune regulation properties are still not well discovered. In the present study, we investigated the anti-tumor activity of TCS in hepatocellular carcinoma (HCC), both in vitro and in vivo. Both HCC cell lines and xenograft tumor tissues showed considerable growth inhibition after they were treated with TCS. TCS provoked caspase-mediated apoptosis in HCC cells and xenograft tumor tissues. The recruitment of $CD8^+$ T cells to HCC tissues and the expression of chemokines, CCL2 and CCL22, were promoted upon TCS treatment. In addition, TCS induced an upregulation of Granzyme B (GrzB), TNF-α and IFN-γ in HCC tissues, which are the major cytotoxic mediators produced by T cells. Furthermore, TCS also resulted in an increase of mannose-6-phosphate receptor (M6PR), the major receptor of GrzB, in HCC tissues. In summary, these results suggest that TCS perhaps increases T-cell immunity via promoting the secretion of chemokines and accelerating the entry of GrzB to HCC cells, which highlights the potential role of TCS in anti-tumor immunotherapy.

Keywords: Trichosanthin (TCS); hepatocellular carcinoma (HCC); T cell; chemokine; Granzyme B (GrzB); apoptosis

Citation: Wang, K.; Wang, X.; Zhang, M.; Ying, Z.; Zhu, Z.; Tam, K.Y.; Li, C.; Zhou, G.; Gao, F.; Zeng, M.; et al. Trichosanthin Promotes Anti-Tumor Immunity through Mediating Chemokines and Granzyme B Secretion in Hepatocellular Carcinoma. *Int. J. Mol. Sci.* **2023**, *24*, 1416. https://doi.org/10.3390/ijms24021416

Academic Editors: Barbara De Filippis, Marialuigia Fantacuzzi and Alessandra Ammazzalorso

Received: 30 November 2022
Revised: 4 January 2023
Accepted: 10 January 2023
Published: 11 January 2023

1. Introduction

Hepatocellular carcinoma (HCC) is the second most common cause of cancer mortality worldwide [1]. Since HCC is highly aggressive and metastatic, only about 10% of patients have limited options, such as surgical resection, liver transplantation and local ablation [2]. HCC is also one of the most common chemotherapy-resistant tumors. The continuous administration of conventional chemotherapeutic agents and antitumor immune agents causes side effects, such as tumor resistance and poor prognosis. Therefore, it is imperative to explore new drugs or therapeutic strategies targeting HCC [3]. Researchers have identified numerous plant-derived extracts with potent antitumor properties, and representative ones include paclitaxel [4], curcumin [5], millipedium [6], Trichosanthin [7], etc.

Trichosanthin (TCS), a single-chain ribosome-inactivating protein extracted from the tuberous root of the traditional Chinese herb *Trichosanthes*, exhibits prospective application in clinical drug abortion, anti-virus, anti-tumor and immune regulation [8]. Numerous studies have shown that TCS could directly inhibit the proliferation and apoptosis of cancer cells by regulating the expression of Bcl-2 [9], inducing S-phase cell cycle arrest in cancer cells [10], inhibiting tumor dysplasia-related signaling pathways [11], increasing the expression or activation of caspase family proteins [12–14], etc. In physiological conditions, TCS could regulate the immune status of the body by regulating the $CD4^+/CD8^+$ T-cell ratio and producing related immune cytokines in peripheral blood [15]. Studies have shown that TCS could enhance the sensitivity of tumors to chemotherapeutic drug treatment [13,16]. Recombinant TCS has shown potent anti-tumor effects [17–19]. It is crucial to investigate the anti-tumor mechanisms and potential applications of TCS.

Granzyme B (GrzB) is an extremely high anti-tumor bioactive protein produced mainly by $CD8^+$ T cells and NK cells [20]. Numerous studies have shown that GrzB can rapidly activate caspase 3-related signaling pathways in target cells [21], which in turn promote cancer cell apoptosis or inflammatory death [22]. Our previous works on immunodeficient nude mice found that the combination of TCS and GrzB had a positive effect in inhibiting HCC, and TCS enhanced the translocation of GrzB from mannose-6-phosphate receptors (M6PR) to HCC cells [23]. However, whether TCS could inhibit HCC by regulating anti-tumor immunity has not been examined yet. In this study, we used TCS to treat HCC cells and a xenograpft tumor model to investigate the mechanism of TCS regulating the recruitment of T cells in the host immune response against HCC.

2. Results

2.1. TCS Reduces the Viability of HCC Cells in Culture

To test if TCS was able to inhibit HCC cell growth in culture, TCS (concentration ranged from 1.5625 to 400 μg/mL) was administered to the H22 HCC cell line for 24, 48 and 72 h. TCS inhibited H22 cell viability in a dose-dependent manner (Figure 1A). The IC50 of HCC cells treated with TCS for 48 h and 72 h was approximately 25 μg/mL (Figure 1A). Then, we treated HCC cells with 25 μg/mL TCS and assayed cell viability at multiple time points, and we observed a significant decrease of cell viability after 36 h (Figure 1B). The Calcein-AM/PI assay also showed a significant and time-dependent increase of dead HCC cells after TCS treatment (Figure 1C). PARP, a nucleus polymerase that appears to be involved in DNA repair and that is a common apoptosis marker cleaved by Caspase-3 [24], was also induced by TCS in a dose-dependent manner (Figure 1F). To further confirm TCS might impair cell viability, the apoptosis inhibitor Z-VAD-FMK was applied to treat HCC cells for 48 h, combined with TCS at multiple concentrations. Z-VAD-FMK significantly inhibited the cell death and PARP cleavage induced by TCS (Figure 1E,F). This suggested that TCS triggered HCC cell death mainly by promoting caspase activities.

2.2. TCS Promoted HCC Cell Death via Apoptosis

Apoptosis and autophagy are common modes of tumor cell death [25,26]. It has been reported that TCS can promote the death of Oral squamous cell carcinoma SCC25 by inducing cell apoptosis [9]. In order to better understand the mechanisms of TCS-induced cell death, HCC cells were treated with 25 μg/mL TCS, total protein was extracted and the expression levels of apoptosis- and autophagy-related proteins were detected by Western blot. Apoptosis usually involves the activation of a series of caspase enzymes. The upstream caspase of the intrinsic pathway is caspase 9, while the exogenous pathway is caspase 8; after that, internal and external pathways converge to caspase 3 [27]. Western blot analysis showed that Caspase 9, Caspase 8 and Caspase 3 were all decreased in HCC cells after 72 h of TCS treatment (Figure 2A). Instead, the level of Cleaved-caspase 9, Cleaved-caspase 8 and Cleaved-caspase 3 were all elevated after 48 h of TCS treatment (Figure 2A).

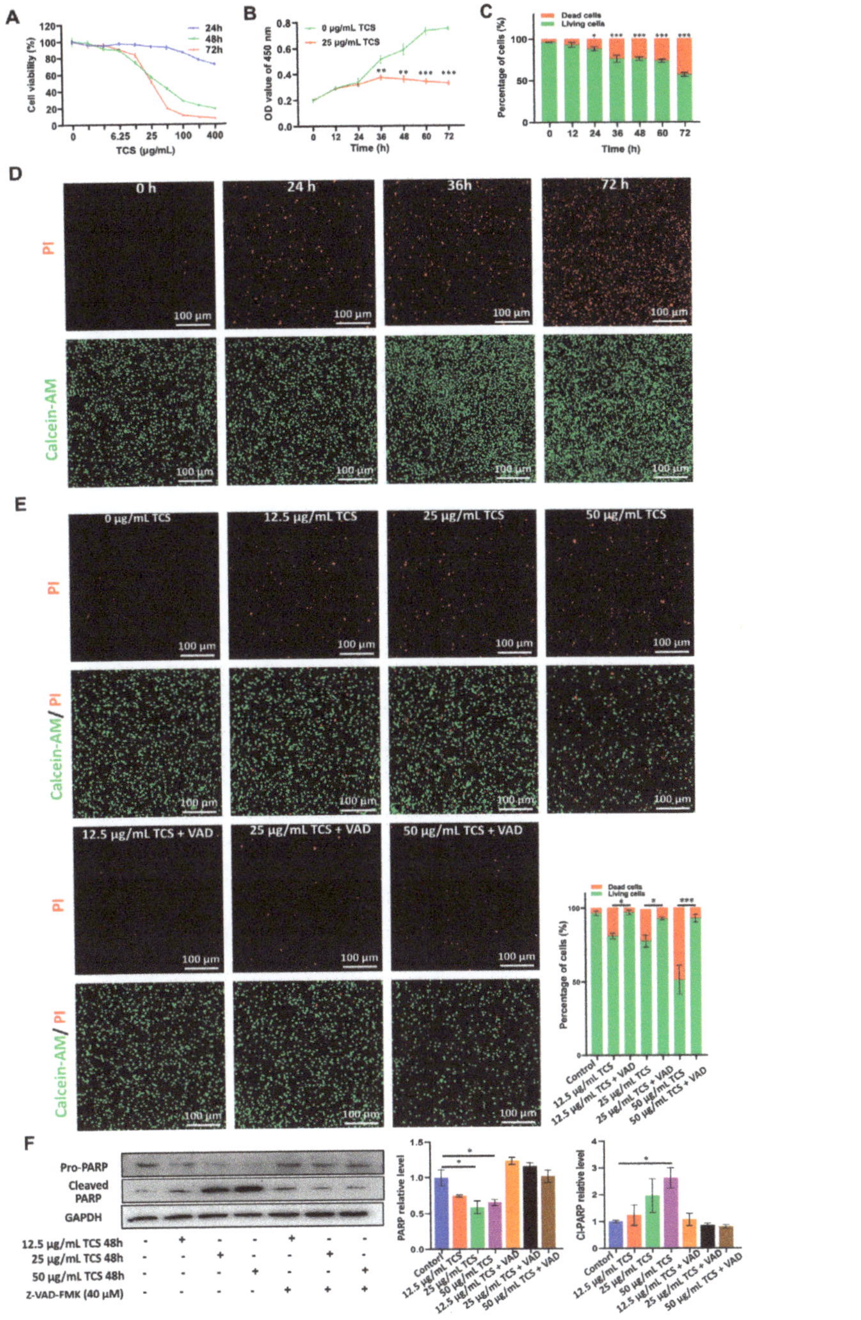

Figure 1. Effects of TCS on the cell viability and death of HCC cells. (**A**) H22 HCC cells were treated with different doses of TCS for 24 h, 48 h and 72 h. CCK-8 assay with absorbance at 450 nm was used

to evaluate the cell viability; (**B**) IC50 dose of TCS (25 μg/mL) was used to treat H22 HCC cells for 12 h, 24 h, 36 h, 48 h, 60 h and 72 h. CCK-8 assay with absorbance at 450 nm was used to evaluate the cell viability; (**C**) 25 ug/mL TCS treated HCC cell lines at different times with the ratio of dead cells to live cells; (**D**) IC50 dose of TCS (25 μg/mL) was used to treat H22 HCC cells for 0 h, 24 h, 36 h and 72 h. The Calcein-AM/PI method was used to detect dead or alive cells, with green as live cells and red as dead cells. Bar = 100 μm; (**E**) H22 HCC cells were treated with different doses (0, 12.5, 25 and 50 μg/mL) of TCS. Meanwhile, 40 μM caspase inhibitor (Z-VAD-FMK) was used in combination. Calcein-AM/PI assay was used to detect dead or alive cells; green is live cells, red is dead cells. Bar = 100 μm; (**F**) Western blot assay for PARP and Cleaved-PARP protein expression after 48 h of TCS and Z-VAD-FMK coadministration. *, $p < 0.05$; **, $p < 0.01$; ***, $p < 0.001$.

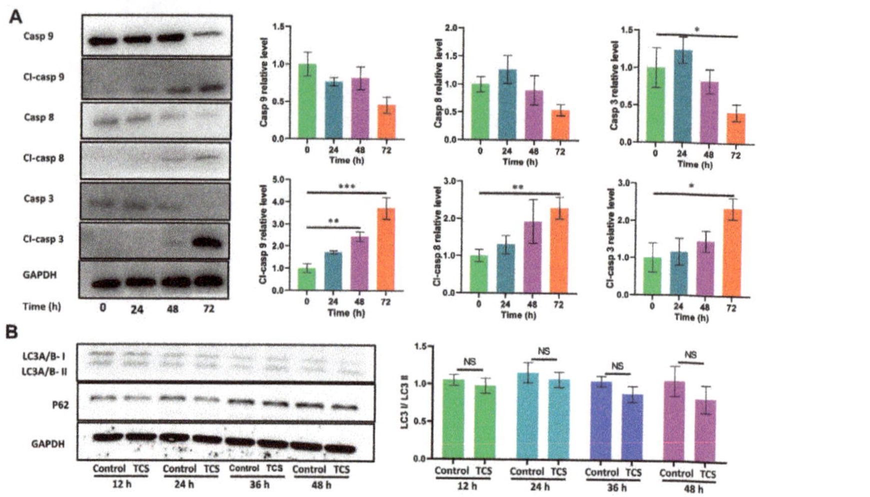

Figure 2. Effects of TCS on apoptosis and autophagy of HCC cells. (**A**) H22 HCC cells were treated with 25 μg/mL TCS for 24 h, 48 h and 72 h. Western blot assayed the levels of key apoptosis proteins Caspase 9, Cleaved-caspase 9, Caspase 8, Cleaved-caspase 8, Caspase 3 and Cleaved-caspase 3; (**B**) H22 HCC cells were treated with 25 μg/mL TCS for 12 h, 24 h, 36 h and 48 h. Western blot assayed the levels of key autophagy proteins P62 and LC3A/B. NS means no significant difference, *, $p < 0.05$; **, $p < 0.01$; ***, $p < 0.001$.

Studies have also shown that TCS can inhibit the growth of gastric cancer cell MKN-45 by inducing autophagy [28]. In the process of autophagosome formation, LC3I is lipidized to form LC3II; therefore, LC3I/LC3-II is considered a marker of autophagosome. In addition, the autophagic receptor p62 is also commonly used as an autophagic marker [29]. However, our results show that the level of the autophagy markers P62 and LC3I/LC3II were not significantly different between the control and TCS-treated groups (Figure 2B). This indicated that TCS did not induce significant autophagy in HCC cells. Therefore, TCS induced HCC cell death, mainly via apoptosis.

2.3. TCS Inhibits HCC Tumor Growth In Vivo

To investigate the therapeutic effect of TCS on HCC in vivo, an H22 HCC xenograpft model was established subcutaneously in BALB/c mice, which were treated with TCS at Day 5, 7, 9, 11, 13, 15 and 17 (Figure 3A). TCS treatment significantly inhibited the growth of HCC tumors in mice in a dose-dependent manner (Figure 3B). The application of TCS at the highest concentration of 2 μg/g achieved a tumor volume inhibition rate of about 52.91% (Figure 3C) and a tumor mass inhibition rate of about 55.01% (Figure 3D,E). Although the mice treated with TCS exhibited a decreasing trend in body weight, there was no significant difference compared to the control group. These results suggested that TCS could inhibit HCC cell growth in vivo.

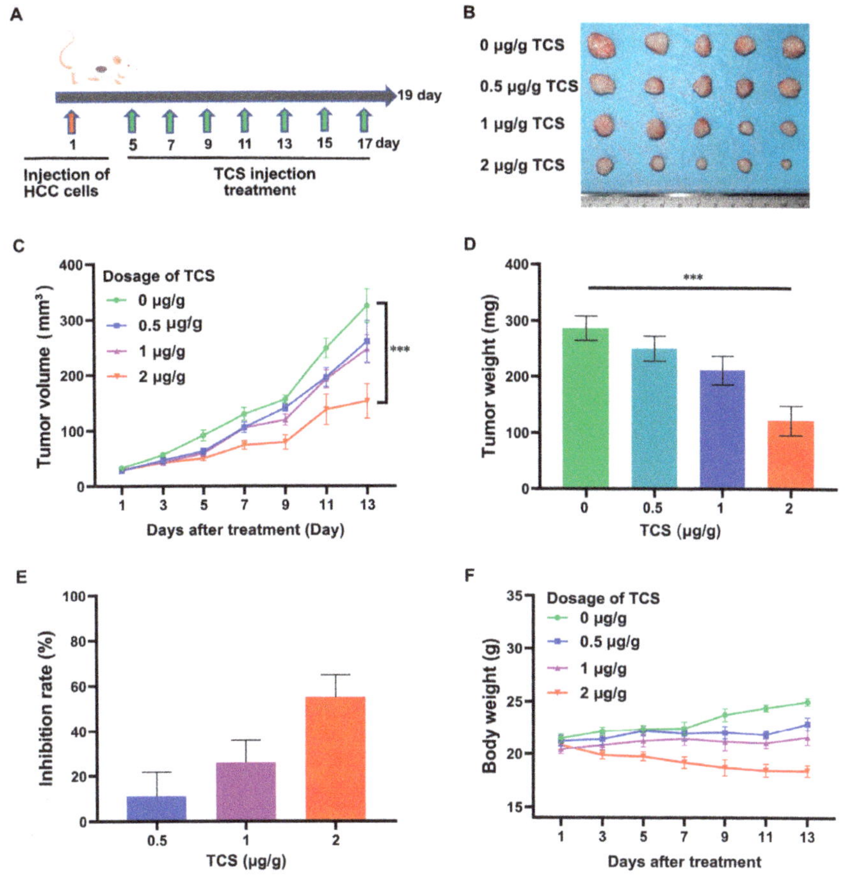

Figure 3. Effects of TCS on apoptosis and autophagy of HCC cells. (**A**) Timeline schedule of mice injected with HCC cells and treated with TCS; (**B**) On day 19, mice were euthanized and tumor tissues were obtained as shown in the figure; (**C–E**) Quantitation of data showed the volume of tumors, weight and the inhibition rate of TCS on the weight of tumor tissue; (**F**) Quantitation of data showed the weight changes in mice treated with varying doses of TCS. ***, $p < 0.001$.

Next, we assayed Ki67, a tumor proliferation marker [30], by immunohistochemical fluorescence. The number of Ki67-positive cells decreased in the TCS-treated group in a dose-dependent manner (Figure 4A). TCS significantly promoted the activation of Caspase 9, Caspase 8 and Caspase 3 in tumor tissues. The levels of Cleaved-caspase 9, Cleaved-caspase 8 and Cleaved-caspase 3 were significantly increased (Figure 4B). Therefore, TCS could inhibit the progression of HCC malignancy in mice, mainly through activation of the caspase pathway.

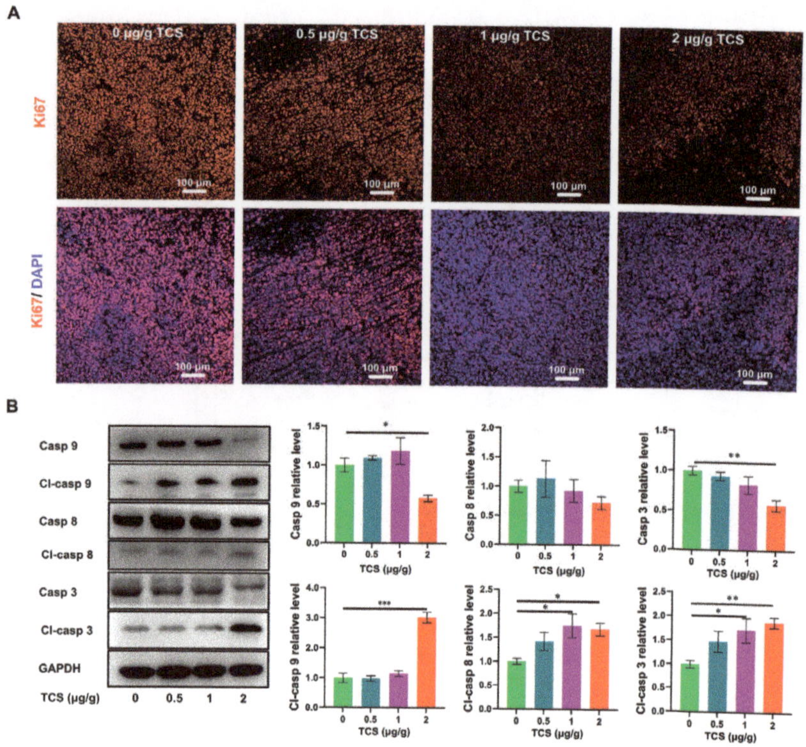

Figure 4. Effects of TCS on proliferation and apoptosis of HCC in vivo. (**A**) Immunofluorescence method detected nuclear proliferation factor Ki67 (Ki67: red, DAPI: blue). Bar = 100 μm; (**B**) Western blot method detected the protein levels of Caspase 9, Cleaved-caspase 9, Caspase 8, Cleaved-caspase 8, Caspase 3 and Cleaved-caspase 3 in HCC tissues. *, $p < 0.05$; **, $p < 0.01$; ***, $p < 0.001$.

2.4. TCS Promotes Infiltration of CD8+ T Cells into HCC

TCS promoted $CD8^+$ T-cell infiltration in cancer tissues [15]. Therefore, we investigated the level of the infiltration of $CD8^+$ T cells in mouse HCC xenograft tissues. The number of $CD8^+$ T cells in HCC tumor tissues increased with the doses of TCS (Figure 5A). Interestingly, enrichment of $CD8^+$ T cells could be seen at the edge of tumor tissues (Figure 5B).

Chemokines are signaling molecules necessary for normal T-cell transport and function [31], and the interleukin family plays an important role in immune regulation and inflammatory responses [32]. In addition, the increased secretion of TNF-α and IFN-γ contributes to the antitumor interaction with T cells [33]. Therefore, mRNA expressions of chemokines CCL2, CCL17 and CCL22, as well as IL-6, IL-18, TNF-α and IFN-γ, in tumor tissues and H22 cells were detected by RT-qPCR. The results of RT-qPCR showed that the expression levels of CCL2, CCL22, TNF-α and IFN-γ in tumor tissues were significantly increased after TCS treatment. Additionally, CCL2, CCL17, CCL22 and TNF-α were also increased in H22 cells after TCS treatment (Figure S1). Furthermore, according to the results of RT-qPCR, four cytokines with significant differences, CCL2, CCL22, TNF-α and IFN-γ, were detected for protein levels by ELISA. The results of tumor tissue samples showed that the protein levels of chemokines CCL2 and CCL22, as well as TNF-α and IFN-γ, were significantly increased upon TCS treatment (Figure 5C). Serum levels of CCL22, TNF-α and IFN-γ were elevated after TCS treatment, although only IFN-γ statistically significantly increased (Figure 5D). In addition, the expression levels of chemokines CCL2 and CCL22 in HCC cell culture fluid were also significantly increased upon TCS treatment (Figure 5E).

These results suggested that TCS could enrich $CD8^{+}$ T cells to tumor tissues and promote the expression of chemokines in HCC cells, which would enhance the anti-tumor immune response of the organism.

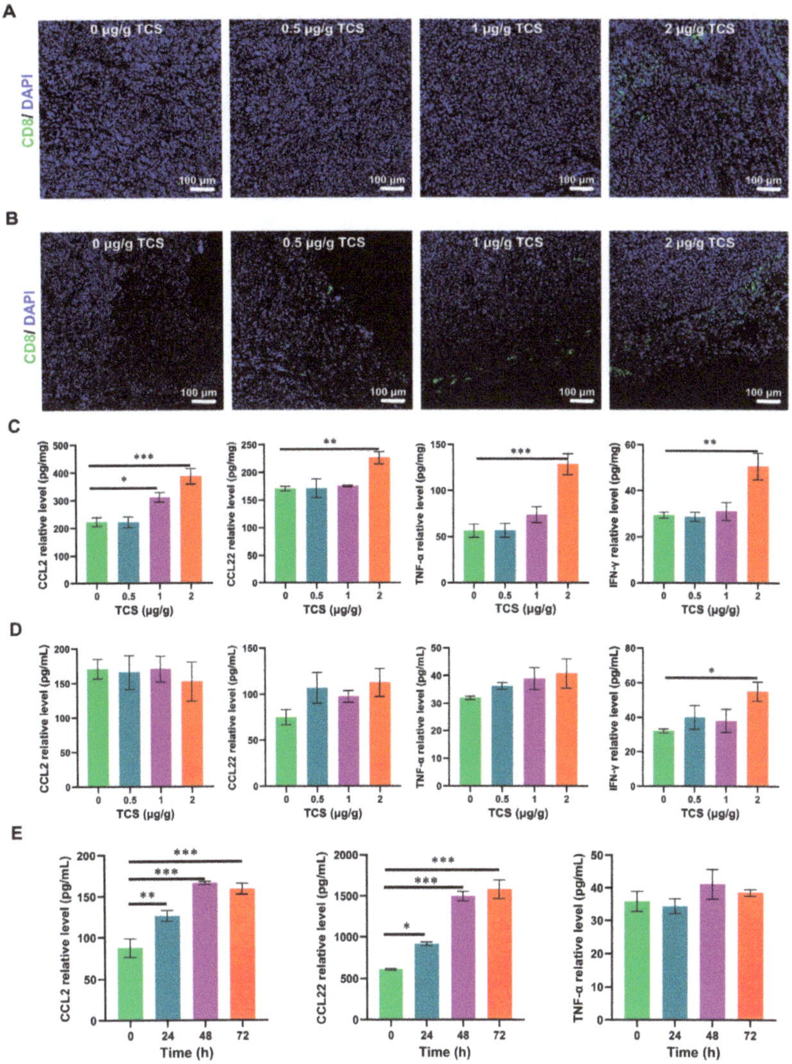

Figure 5. Effects of TCS on chemotactic enrichment. (**A**) Immunofluorescence method detected CD8-positive cells in the center of HCC tissues. Bar = 100 μm; (**B**) Immunofluorescence method detected CD8-positive cells at the edge of HCC tissues. Bar = 100 μm; (**C**) ELISA method detected the protein levels of CCL2, CCL22, TNF-α and IFN-γ in HCC tissues treated with different doses of TCS (0, 0.5, 1 and 2 μg/g); (**D**) ELISA method detected the protein levels of CCL2, CCL22, TNF-α and IFN-γ of mouse serum; (**E**) ELISA method detected the protein levels of CCL2, CCL22 and TNF-α in H22 HCC cells treated with 25 μg/g TCS after 24 h, 48 h and 72 h, GAPDH as the internal reference gene. *, $p < 0.05$; **, $p < 0.01$; ***, $p < 0.001$.

2.5. TCS Enhances the Expression of Granzyme B and M6PR

GrzB, a serine proteinase released by cytotoxic T cells and NK cells, mediates cell apoptosis in target cells [34,35]. Since TCS could recruit $CD8^{+}$ T cells to xenograft tumor tissues, we next examined whether the expression and transportation of GrzB were affected by TCS. As expected, GrzB was elevated in HCC tissues in TCS-treated mice in a dose-dependent manner (Figure 6A–C). The proportion of $TUNEL^{+}/GrzB^{+}$ cells in tumor tissues significantly increased as TCS dosages were raised (Figure 7A–C). We also confirmed that the alterations in the number of $TUNEL^{+}$ and $TUNEL^{+}/GrzB^{+}$ cells were positively correlated with TCS dosages (Figure 7B,C). Our previous studies showed the translocation of GrzB from mannose-6-phosphate receptors (M6PR) to HCC cells was enhanced by TCS [23]. Therefore, we next examined the level of M6PR, both in cell lines and xenograft tumor tissues. We showed that TCS promoted the expression level of M6PR in tumor tissues and HCC cells (Figure 8C,D). As TCS dosages were augmented, the proportion of $TUNEL^{+}/M6PR^{+}$ cells in tumor tissues also significantly increased (Figure 8A,B). The number of M6PR and TUNEL double-positive cells showed a positive correlation with the TCS dose (Figure 8A,B). These data indicated that TCS could inhibit HCC growth by inducing the upregulation of GrzB and promote HCC cell apoptosis in vivo by encouraging M6PR to deliver GrzB into HCC cells.

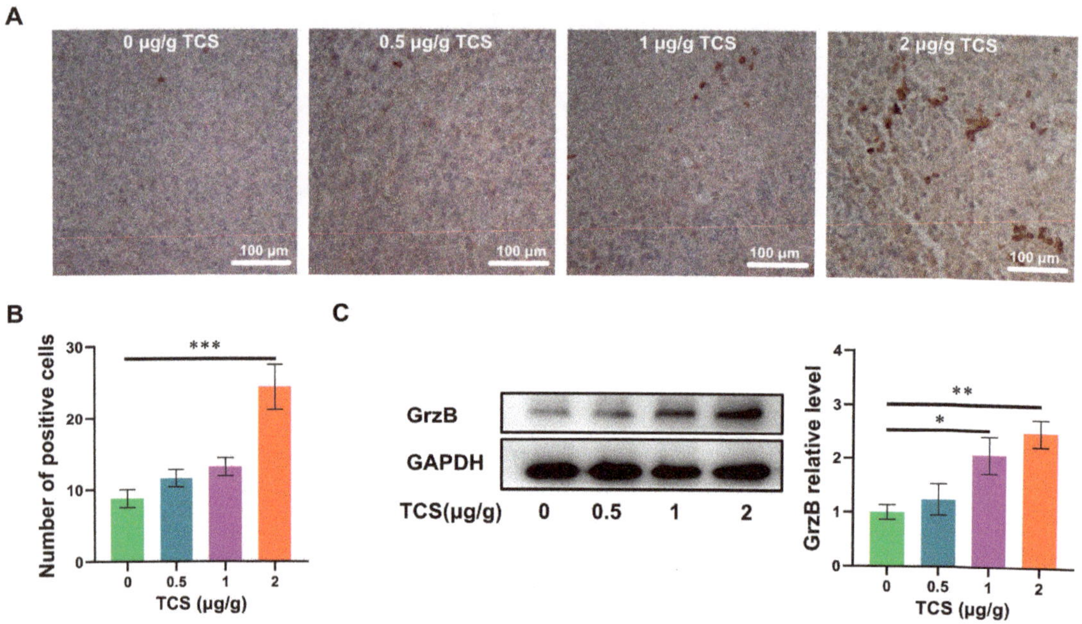

Figure 6. Effects of TCS on GrzB expression in vivo. (**A**,**B**) Immunochemical method detected GrzB in hepatocellular carcinoma tissues. Bar = 100 μm; (**C**) Western blot method detected the level of GrzB in HCC tissues treated with different doses of TCS. *, $p < 0.05$; **, $p < 0.01$; ***, $p < 0.001$.

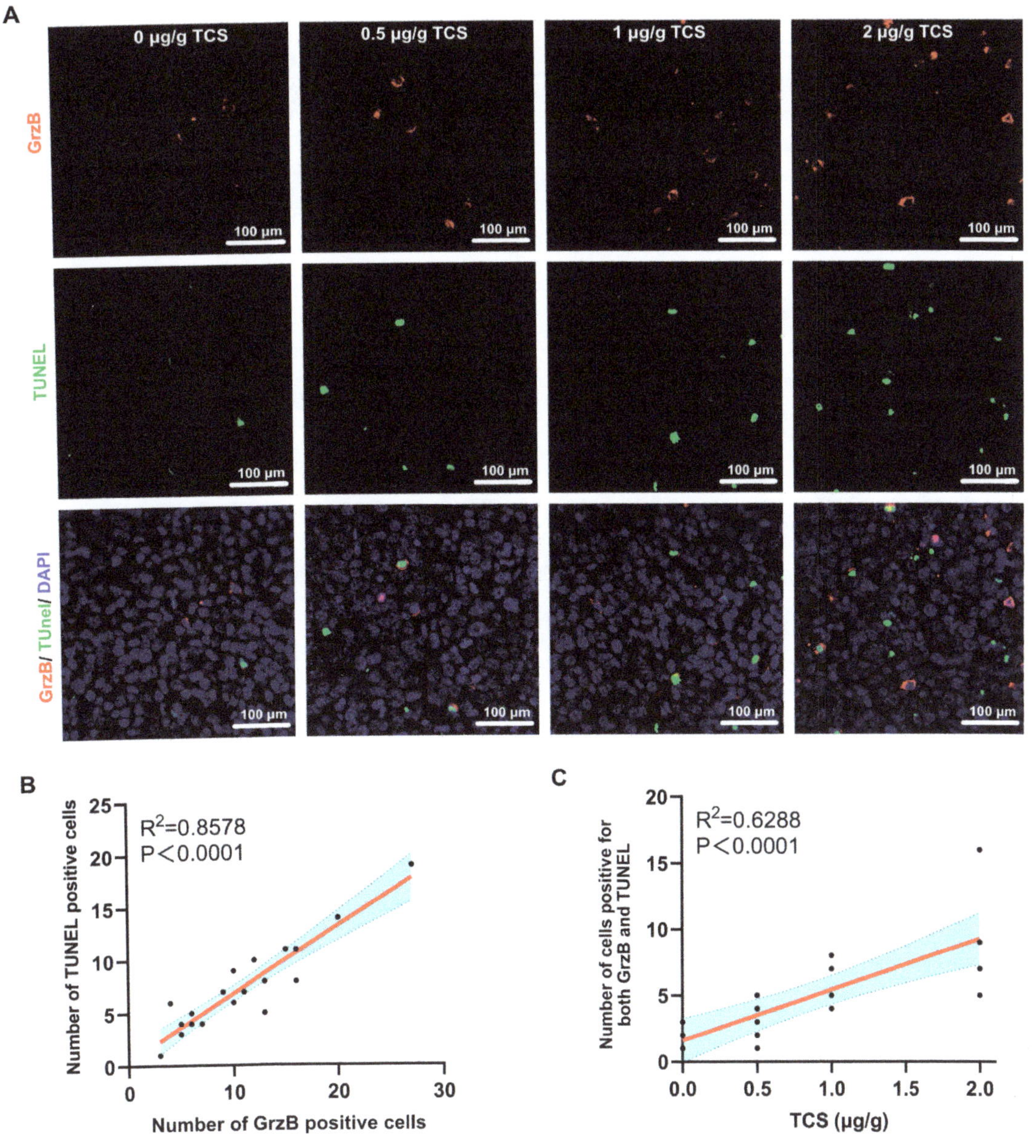

Figure 7. TCS promotes GrzB-induced apoptosis in hepatocellular carcinoma. (**A**) Immunochemical method detected TUNEL and GrzB in HCC tissues after TCS treatment. Bar = 100 μm; (**B**) Correlation analysis of GrzB positivity with the number of positive signals for TUNEL; and (**C**) Correlation analysis of the number of simultaneous positive signals for GrzB and TUNEL with the dose of TCS.

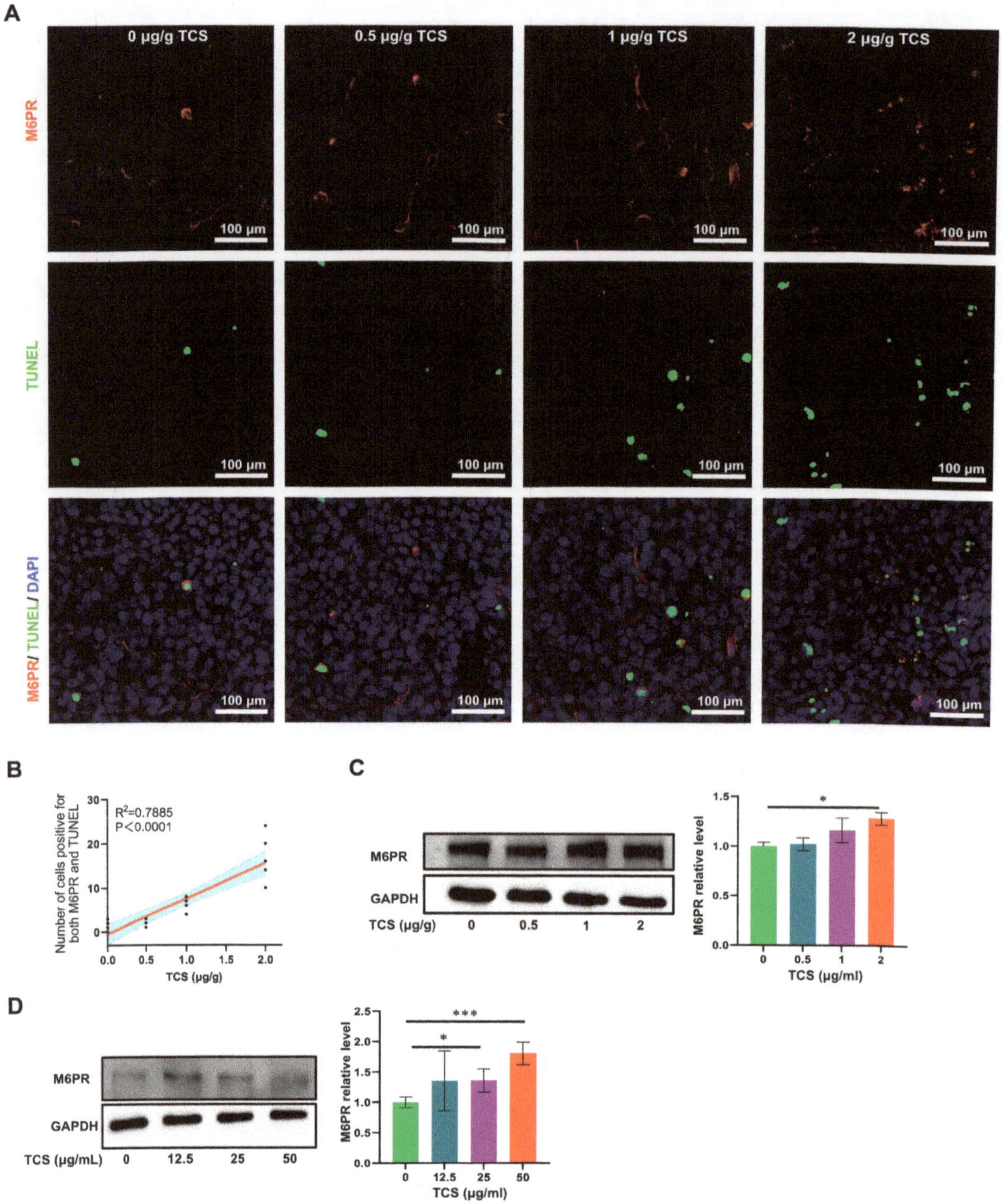

Figure 8. TCS promotes M6PR expression in vivo and in vitro. (**A**) Immunochemical method detected GrzB and M6PR in HCC tissues upon TCS treatment. Bar = 100 μm; (**B**) Correlation analysis of the number of simultaneous positive signals of GrzB and M6PR with the dose of TCS; (**C**) Western blot method detected the levels of M6PR in HCC tissues treated with different doses of TCS (0, 0.5, 1 and 2 μg/g); (**D**) Western blot method detected the levels of M6PR in H22 HCC cells treated with different doses of TCS (0, 12.5, 25 and 50 μg/mL). *, $p < 0.05$; ***, $p < 0.001$.

3. Discussion

TCS is the major active ingredient of *Trichosanthes Kirilowii* [36]. Previous studies reported TCS alone showed an excellent inhibitory effect on cancer cell proliferation in vitro [9,23,37]. However, TCS alone had not significantly inhibited tumor growth in immunodeficient nude mice in vivo [23]. In the present study, we constructed tumor models in BALB/c mice with a functional immune system. We found that TCS not only activated caspase family proteins in tumor tissues, but also promoted T-cell immunity. Chemotactic enrichment of T cells in HCC tissues and elevated levels of GrzB were observed in vivo. This suggests that TCS has considerable promise as an immunotherapy tool and may increase the effectiveness of anti-tumor treatments.

TCS induced cell cycle block, autophagic death and caspase-mediated apoptosis in cancer cells [28,38]. Proper levels of autophagy remove damaged organelles from cells and contribute to the maintenance of normal cell survival, while inducing excessive autophagy causes cell death [39,40]. TCS induced ROS production in gastric cancer cells, which in turn promoted the autophagic death of gastric cancer cells [28]. However, in the present study, TCS barely promoted the autophagic death of HCC cells. Recently, Hu et al. detected by proteomics that TCS inhibited nuclear proliferation factors in human choriocarcinoma cell lines, mainly inducing caspase-mediated apoptosis in cancer cells [41]. Caspase 8 is a key protease in apoptosis caused by exogenous factors [42]. Caspase 9 is an endogenous apoptosis-related protease activated by damage to organelles, such as endoplasmic reticulum or mitochondria [43]. Both cleaved-caspase 8 and cleaved-caspase 9 activate caspase 3 to form cleaved-caspase 3, which in turn degrades the DNA repair-associated protein PARP and induces apoptosis in cancer cells [44,45]. The results of our study showed that apoptosis inhibitor (Z-VAD-FMK) was able to inhibit TCS-induced HCC cell death, and caspase proteins were significantly activated. Thus, TCS mainly activated caspase-mediated endogenous and exogenous apoptotic pathways to inhibit HCC cells.

TCS can regulate the immune functions of macrophages [46], DC cells [47] and T cells [48]. However, variable effects of TCS on the regulation of immune cell function have been observed in different diseases, such as physiological conditions [48], inflammation [46], HIV infection [49] and cancer [15]. Enhancement of the antitumor response of T cells would be one of the effective ways to inhibit HCC [50]. T cells can induce cancer cell death through both receptor and non-receptor mediated pathways [51]. TCS could enhance the immune effect of T cells against lung cancer through the receptor pathway by enhancing the expression of class I, restricted, T cell-associated molecules in $CD8^+$ T cells [15]. A recent study showed that tonics containing the Chinese herb *Trichosanthes* significantly elevated the serum levels of cytokines, such as IFN-γ, IL-6 and TNF-α, which would be beneficial in enhancing the immune effect of the lymphocyte system [52]. Numerous immune subpopulations, including T cells, natural killer (NK) cells and B cells, can produce IFN-γ in the tumor microenvironment [53]. $CD8^+$ cytotoxic T lymphocytes (CTL) are known to be the main producers of IFN-γ and one of the indicators of activation of the T-cell antitumor function [54]. Studies have shown that IFN-γ could induce apoptosis or scorch death of cancer cells through IFN-γ receptors on the surface of cancer cells [55,56]. TNF-α plays different roles in the pre-cancerous and cancer microenvironments. Despite a sustained inflammatory response possibly being detrimental to suppressing precancerous lesions, increased TNF-α in a tumor microenvironment could effectively activate TNFR1 to trigger cancer cell suppression [57,58]. Tumor-infiltrating lymphocytes are an important prognostic factor for cancer progression and a key player in cancer immunotherapy. CCL2, CCL17 and CCL22 are cytokines with a role in T-cell recruitment [59,60]. Despite the role of CCL2 in recruiting both cytotoxic T cells (CTL) and monocytes to tumor sites [61,62], studies have shown that enhancement of the CCL2/CCR2 axis [63] or inhibition of CCL2 nitration [64] in antitumor therapy significantly promotes T-cell infiltration and exerts antitumor effects. Binding of CCL22 with CCR4 enhances T-cell dendritic cell binding and increases CTL activation [65], while enhancing tumor cell responses to IFN-γ [66]. GrzB, the cytokine secreted by $CD8^+$ T cells, has the greatest killing effect on cancer cells by directly or indirectly activating caspases to inhibit cancer cell proliferation and induce apoptosis [67]. GrzB could be transported by M6PR into cancer cells [68]. Previous studies by our group demonstrated that the combination of TCS and GrzB in the treatment of nude mice implanted with HCC significantly inhibited the growth of HCC, and TCS promoted the transport of GrzB by M6PR into HCC cells [23]. In the present study, we examined the anti-tumor mechanisms of TCS by facilitating the xenograft tumor model within BALB/c mice with a functional immune system. We observed that $CD8^+$ T cells were recruited into the HCC tissues in the TCS-treated group in a dose-dependent manner. The expression level of chemokines was elevated in HCC tissues, a favorable condition for T cells to kill HCC cells through the receptor or cytokine pathway. Additionally, TCS directly elevated GrzB levels in tumor tissues, which were significantly and positively correlated with apoptotic cancer cells. This implies that TCS can enhance T-cell anti-tumor immunity against HCC by encouraging T-cell enrichment, elevating the expression of chemokines in tumor cells and promoting their production of GrzB. These results provide supporting information for the study of TCS to enhance anti-tumor immunity.

4. Materials and Methods

Recombinant TCS protein extraction and purification: The recombinant TCS plasmid was constructed by Tsingke Biotechnology Co., Ltd. (Guangzhou, China). The rTCS sequence was inserted between the EcoRI site and the XhoI site of pet-28a+. *E.coli* BL21 (DE3) was used to induce the expression of recombinant TCS protein (when OD600 = 0.60, add a final concentration of 2 mM IPTG). Centrifuge the prokaryotic expression induced bacterial solution at 4 °C, 12,000 rpm, 2 min; discard the supernatant; then, add the lysis buffer (50 mM NaH2PO4, 300 mM NaCl, 10 mM imidazole, pH 8.0); blow repeatedly; and perform ultrasonic lysis on ice (power: 30%, ultrasound: 5 s, stop: 10 s, total working time: 30 min); and then collect the supernatant at 4 °C, 12,000 rpm, 30 min. After the supernatant containing the target protein is filtered and sterilized, it is purified by the protein purifier (GE, AKTA purifier, Boston, MA, USA). The obtained recombinant TCS protein was freeze-dried and stored at −30 °C.

Cell culture: Mouse HCC cell line (H22) (Procell, CL-0341) was cultured in Roswell Park Memorial Institute 1640 (RPMI-1640) medium containing 10% fetal bovine serum, 100 U/mL of penicillin and 100 μg/mL of streptomycin. HCC cells were cultured in a 5% CO_2 incubator at a constant temperature of 37 °C.

HCC cell viability assay: H22 cells were inoculated in 96-well plates at a density of 5×10^3, with 100 μL cell culture solution per well. For a concentration-dependent assay, TCS (0, 1.5625, 3.125, 6.25, 12.5, 25, 50, 100, 200 and 400 μg/mL) was added to the treatment for 24 h, 48 h and 72 h. For a time-dependent assay, TCS (0, 25 μg/mL) was added to the treatment for 0 h, 12 h, 24 h, 36 h, 48 h, 60 h and 72 h. Cell viability was then determined by the method of CCK-8. Briefly, at the end of the intervention, 10 μL of CCK-8 solution was added to each well of the 96-well plate and mixed, and the reaction plates were incubated at 37 °C for 1–3 h. The absorbance of each well solution was measured, using the microplate reader (BioTek, Epoch, Winooski, VT, USA) at 450 nm wavelength detection light.

Calcein-AM/PI staining: Unspecific esterases present in living cells can metabolize Calcein-AM and emit green fluorescence. Propidium iodide (PI) will label the nuclei of dead cells. H22 cells were inoculated in 6-well plates at a concentration of 1×10^5/mL culture medium per well. Cells were treated with different doses of TCS, then Calcein-AM and PI were added and incubated for 5 min, and fluorescent pictures were collected under a confocal microscope. Cell death index calculation: percentage of dead cells = number of dead cells/total number of cells.

Antibodies: The antibody information in this study is shown in Table S1.

Reagents: Z-VAD-FMK (Beyotime, Nanjing, China, cat# C1202), Calcein-AM (MCE, Monmouth Junction, NJ, USA, cat# HY-D0041), PI (MCE, Monmouth Junction, NJ, USA, cat# HY-D0815), DAPI (Solarbio, Beijing, China, cat# D8200) DeadEnd™ Fluorometric TUNEL System (Beyotime, Nanjing, China, cat# C1088). IHC Reagent Kit (Solarbio, Beijing,

China, cat# SP0021), Total Mrna Extraction Kit (Promega, Madison, WI, USA, cat# LS1040), Hifair III 1st Strand cDNA Synthesis SuperMix for qPCR (gDNA digester plus) (Yeasen, Shanghai, China, cat# 11141ES60), GoldenstarTM RT6 cDNA Synthesis Kit (TSINGKE, Xi'an, China, cat# TSG302M), ELISA MAX™ Standard Set Mouse MCP-1 (BioLegend, San Diego, CA, USA, cat# 432701), ELISA MAX™Deluxe Set Mouse IFNγ (BioLegend, San Diego, CA, USA, cat# 430804), Mouse TNF-α ELISA kit (Jianglaibio, Shanghai, China, cat# JL10484), Mouse MDC/CCL22 ELISA kit (Jianglaibio, Shanghai, China, cat# JL11125), etc.

Apoptosis inhibition test assay: Z-VAD-FMK is a pan-caspase inhibitor that prevents the cleavage degradation of DNA repair enzyme PARP by Caspase family proteins [69]. H22 cells were inoculated in 6-well plates at a concentration of 1×10^5/mL culture medium per well. Z-VAD-FMK was intervened according to the following protocol: control (no TCS), TCS (12.5 μg/mL), TCS (25 μg/mL), TCS (50 μg/mL), TCS (12.5 μg/mL) + Z-VAD-FMK (40 μM), TCS (25 μg/mL) + Z-VAD-FMK (40 μM), TCS (50 μg/mL) + Z-VAD-FMK (40 μM) for 48 h of continuous intervention, and cells were analyzed by Calcein-AM/PI staining and immune-blotting for PARP-related proteins.

Xenograft tumor model: The procedure of the animal experiments performed in the study fulfilled the requirements of the ethical review committee. Male BALB/c mice (5-week-old, 20 ± 2 g, Guangdong Medical Laboratory Animal Center, Guangzhou) were housed in an SPF-grade environment with a 12 h light/dark cycle and maintained on free diets. Mice were injected subcutaneously with 5×10^5 H22 HCC cells in the right axilla. Beginning on the fifth day after implantation, mice with H22 HCC were randomly divided into four groups of five mice each and treated according to the following treatment protocols: phosphate-buffered saline (PBS) control group, 0.5 μg/g (TCS weight/mouse body weight) TCS group, 1 μg/g body weight TCS group, 2 μg/g body weight TCS group. Body weight TCS group. Control group was injected with 100 μL of PBS, and drug treatment was injected on the 4, 6, 8, 10, 12, 14 and 16 days after implantation of HCC cells. Tumor volume and body weight were measured, and tumor size was estimated according to the following formula: tumor volume = 0.5 × maximum diameter × shortest diameter × shortest diameter.

Immunohistochemistry (IHC) assay: Immunohistochemical staining of mouse tumor tissues was performed using the IHC kit and GrzB polyclonal antibody. Tumor tissues embedded in paraffin blocks were cut into 5 μm thick sections. The paraffin sections were dewaxed and hydrated, following 3% hydrogen peroxide treatment and antigen repair boiling in sodium citrate solution for 10 min. After incubation with normal goat serum at room temperature for 20 min, the tissue sections were incubated with anti-GrzB antibody (1:500) overnight at 4 °C. Then, samples were incubated with biotinylated goat anti-rabbit serum immunoglobulin G (IgG) antibody (1:100) for 30 min at 37 °C. After thorough washing, streptavidin-POD working solution was added and incubated for 30 min at 37 °C. Sections were counter-stained with hematoxylin. Morphological images were collected using an Olympus microscope. For immunofluorescence assay, tissue sections were incubated with antibodies against Ki67 (1:500), M6PR (1:500), GrzB (1:500) and CD8 (1:500) overnight at 4 °C. Samples were then incubated with appropriate FITC, Alexa Fluor 555 or Horseradish Peroxidase-conjugated secondary antibodies for 3 h. Nuclei were stained with DAPI or hematoxylin, followed by observation and image capture under a confocal microscope.

TUNEL apoptosis assay: Tumor tissues were examined using the Beyotime one-step TUNEL apoptosis assay kit. After dewaxing and hydration of the tumor tissues, the TUNEL staining procedure was performed, according to the manufacturer's instructions. The nuclei were stained with DAPI.

Western blot assay: Protein extraction and Western blot assay were performed, as described in the previous report [23]. The following antibodies were used for detection: anti-Caspase 3 (1:1000), anti-Caspase 8 (1:1000), anti-Caspase 9 (1:1000), anti-Cleaved-caspase 3 (1:1000), anti-Cleaved-caspase 8 (1:1000), anti-Cleaved-caspase 9 (1:1000), anti-GrzB (1:1000), anti-M6PR (1:1000), anti-LC3B (1:1000), anti-P62 (1:1000), anti-GAPDH

(1:5000). They were incubated overnight at 4 °C and then incubated with horseradish peroxidase (HRP)-conjugated counterpart secondary antibody (1:5000) at room temperature. Chemiluminescence was performed using ECL Ultra HRP substrate and photographed under the SAGECREATION ChemiMini™ Imaging System.

Quantitative real-time PCR: Total RNA from HCC cells and tumor tissues was extracted using the Total RNA Extraction Kit. Using the GoldenstarTM RT6 cDNA Synthesis Kit, mRNA was reversed into cDNA by reverse transcription procedure. Quantitative PCR amplification was performed using the Hifair III 1st Strand cDNA Synthesis Super Mix for qPCR in Quantstudio™ 7 Flex Real-Time PCR System (ABI). The expression of target genes was normalized against GAPDH using the $2^{-\Delta\Delta Ct}$ assay. Primer oligos were synthesized by TSINGKE Biological Co., Ltd. (Beijing, China) and are listed in Table S2.

Enzyme linked immunosorbent assay (ELISA): Cell culture supernatants, mouse serum and tumor tissues were collected. Then, the levels of TNF-α, IFN-γ, CCL22 and CCL2 were assessed using ELISA kits, according to the manufacturer's instructions. Absorbance was measured using a microplate reader (BioTek Instruments, Inc., Winooski, VT, USA).

Statistical analysis: Statistical analyses were performed using SPSS 26.0 software (SPSS Inc., Chicago, IL, USA). The error bars in the graphical data represent means ± Standard Error of Mean (SEM). Three or more comparisons were compared using one-way ANOVA, followed by the least significant difference (LSD) test. Unpaired two-tailed Student's t-test was used to compare two sets of data. A value of $p < 0.05$ was considered a statistically significant difference between the data groups. *, $p < 0.05$; **, $p < 0.01$; ***, $p < 0.001$.

5. Conclusions

In conclusion, the results of this study demonstrated that TCS inhibited HCC cells by activating caspase, recruiting CD8$^+$ T cells, enhancing the expression of chemokines and up-regulating M6PR genes to transport GrzB (Figure 9). This also indicates that TCS is a natural drug with great potential to enhance anti-tumor immunity, which is valuable for further in-depth pharmacological studies.

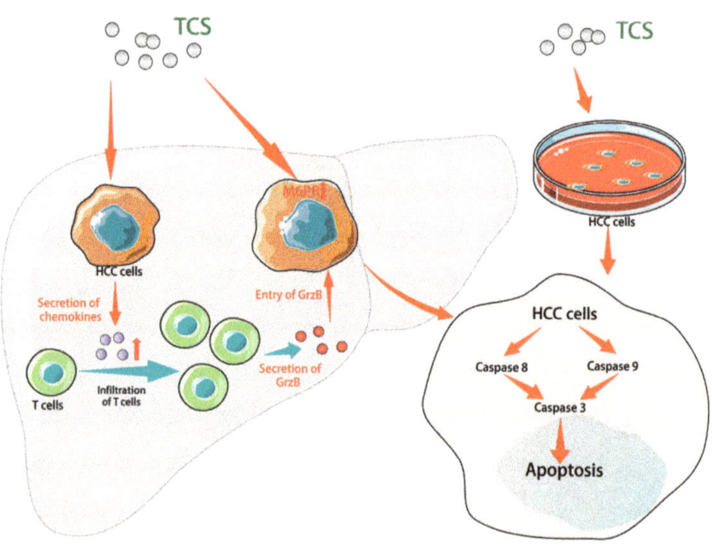

Figure 9. Diagram showing the molecular mechanism of TCS on anti-tumor activity. TCS stimulated the expression of chemokines CCL2, CCL17 and CCL22, which may encourage the enrichment of CD8$^+$ T cells within HCC tissue. GrzB secreted by the T cells were transported into the HCC cells by cellular M6PR and facilitated cell apoptosis. TCS-induced caspases mediated apoptosis both in vivo and in vitro.

Supplementary Materials: The following supporting information can be downloaded at: https://www.mdpi.com/article/10.3390/ijms24021416/s1.

Author Contributions: O.S., K.W. and C.L. designed this study. K.W., X.W. (Xiaona Wang), M.Z. (Minghuan Zhang), Z.Y. and Z.Z. performed the experiments and statistical analysis. K.W. and X.W. (Xiaona Wang) prepared figures and wrote the manuscript. K.Y.T., G.Z., F.G., M.Z. (Meiqi Zeng) and S.C.W.S. participated in the discussion and provided suggestions. X.W. (Xia Wang) and O.S. reviewed and edited the manuscript. All authors have read and agreed to the published version of the manuscript.

Funding: This study was financially supported by the National Natural Science Foundation of China (81773939) and the Technology Foundation of Shenzhen City (JCYJ20210324094005015).

Institutional Review Board Statement: The animal study protocol was approved by the Animal Ethical and Welfare Committee of SZU (AEWXC-202200024 and 20220104).

Informed Consent Statement: Not applicable.

Data Availability Statement: Not applicable.

Conflicts of Interest: The authors declare no conflict of interest.

References

1. Sung, H.; Ferlay, J.; Siegel, R.L.; Laversanne, M.; Soerjomataram, I.; Jemal, A.; Bray, F. Global Cancer Statistics 2020: GLOBOCAN Estimates of Incidence and Mortality Worldwide for 36 Cancers in 185 Countries. *CA Cancer J. Clin.* **2021**, *71*, 209–249. [CrossRef] [PubMed]
2. Maki, H.; Hasegawa, K. Advances in the surgical treatment of liver cancer. *Biosci. Trends* **2022**, *16*, 178–188. [CrossRef]
3. Anwanwan, D.; Singh, S.K.; Singh, S.; Saikam, V.; Singh, R. Challenges in liver cancer and possible treatment approaches. *Biochim. et Biophys. Acta (BBA)-Rev. Cancer* **2020**, *1873*, 188314. [CrossRef]
4. Zhu, L.; Chen, L. Progress in research on paclitaxel and tumor immunotherapy. *Cell. Mol. Biol. Lett.* **2019**, *24*, 40. [CrossRef] [PubMed]
5. Weng, W.; Goel, A. Curcumin and colorectal cancer: An update and current perspective on this natural medicine. *Semin. Cancer Biol.* **2022**, *80*, 73–86. [CrossRef]
6. Shen, L.-W.; Jiang, X.-X.; Li, Z.-Q.; Li, J.; Wang, M.; Jia, G.-F.; Ding, X.; Lei, L.; Gong, Q.-H.; Gao, N. Cepharanthine sensitizes human triple negative breast cancer cells to chemotherapeutic agent epirubicin via inducing cofilin oxidation-mediated mitochondrial fission and apoptosis. *Acta Pharmacol. Sin.* **2022**, *43*, 177–193. [CrossRef]
7. Zhu, C.; Zhang, C.; Cui, X.; Wu, J.; Cui, Z.; Shen, X. Trichosanthin inhibits cervical cancer by regulating oxidative stress-induced apoptosis. *Bioengineered* **2021**, *12*, 2779–2790. [CrossRef]
8. Lu, J.-Q.; Wong, K.-B.; Shaw, P.-C. A Sixty-Year Research and Development of Trichosanthin, a Ribosome-Inactivating Protein. *Toxins* **2022**, *14*, 178. [CrossRef] [PubMed]
9. Zhu, Z.; Ying, Z.; Zeng, M.; Zhang, Q.; Liao, G.; Liang, Y.; Li, C.; Zhang, C.; Wang, X.; Jiang, W.; et al. Trichosanthin cooperates with Granzyme B to restrain tumor formation in tongue squamous cell carcinoma. *BMC Complement. Med. Ther.* **2021**, *21*, 88. [CrossRef]
10. Zhang, D.; Chen, B.; Zhou, J.; Zhou, L.; Li, Q.; Liu, F.; Chou, K.-Y.; Tao, L.; Lü, L.-M. Low concentrations of trichosanthin induce apoptosis and cell cycle arrest via c-Jun N-terminal protein kinase/mitogen-activated protein kinase activation. *Mol. Med. Rep.* **2015**, *11*, 349–356. [CrossRef]
11. Chen, Y.; Han, L.; Bai, L.; Tang, H.; Zheng, A. Trichosanthin inhibits the proliferation of cervical cancer cells and downregulates STAT-5/C-myc signaling pathway. *Pathol.-Res. Pract.* **2019**, *215*, 632–638. [CrossRef]
12. Li, M.; Li, X.; Li, J.-C. Possible Mechanisms of Trichosanthin-Induced Apoptosis of Tumor Cells. *Anat. Rec.* **2010**, *293*, 986–992. [CrossRef]
13. You, C.; Sun, Y.; Zhang, S.; Tang, G.; Zhang, N.; Li, C.; Tian, X.; Ma, S.; Luo, Y.; Sun, W.; et al. Trichosanthin enhances sensitivity of non-small cell lung cancer (NSCLC) TRAIL-resistance cells. *Int. J. Biol. Sci.* **2018**, *14*, 217–227. [CrossRef]
14. Tan, Y.; Xiang, J.; Huang, Z.; Wang, L.; Huang, Y. Trichosanthin inhibits cell growth and metastasis by promoting pyroptosis in non-small cell lung cancer. *J. Thorac. Dis.* **2022**, *14*, 1193–1202. [CrossRef]
15. Cai, Y.; Xiong, S.; Zheng, Y.; Luo, F.; Jiang, P.; Chu, Y. Trichosanthin enhances anti-tumor immune response in a murine Lewis lung cancer model by boosting the interaction between TSLC1 and CRTAM. *Cell. Mol. Immunol.* **2011**, *8*, 359–367. [CrossRef] [PubMed]
16. Zhang, K.; Xu, J.; Huang, X.; Wu, L.; Wen, C.; Hu, Y.; Su, Y.; Chen, Y.; Zhang, Z. Trichosanthin down-regulated p210Bcr-Abl and enhanced imatinib-induced growth arrest in chronic myelogenous leukemia cell line K562. *Cancer Chemother. Pharmacol.* **2007**, *60*, 581–587. [CrossRef]
17. Wu, A.; Chen, Y.; Wang, H.; Chang, Y.; Zhang, M.; Zhao, P.; Tang, Y.; Xu, Q.; Zhu, Z.; Cao, Y.; et al. Genetically-engineered "all-in-one" vaccine platform for cancer immunotherapy. *Acta Pharm. Sin. B* **2021**, *11*, 3622–3635. [CrossRef] [PubMed]

18. Chang, Y.; Yao, S.; Chen, Y.; Huang, J.; Wu, A.; Zhang, M.; Xu, F.; Li, F.; Huang, Y. Genetically-engineered protein prodrug-like nanoconjugates for tumor-targeting biomimetic delivery *via* a SHEATH strategy. *Nanoscale* **2019**, *11*, 611–621. [CrossRef] [PubMed]
19. Chen, Y.; Zhang, M.; Jin, H.; Tang, Y.; Wu, A.; Xu, Q.; Huang, Y. Prodrug-Like, PEGylated Protein Toxin Trichosanthin for Reversal of Chemoresistance. *Mol. Pharm.* **2017**, *14*, 1429–1438. [CrossRef] [PubMed]
20. Hiroyasu, S.; Zeglinski, M.R.; Zhao, H.; Pawluk, M.A.; Turner, C.T.; Kasprick, A.; Tateishi, C.; Nishie, W.; Burleigh, A.; Lennox, P.A.; et al. Granzyme B inhibition reduces disease severity in autoimmune blistering diseases. *Nat. Commun.* **2021**, *12*, 302. [CrossRef]
21. Liu, Y.; Fang, Y.; Chen, X.; Wang, Z.; Liang, X.; Zhang, T.; Liu, M.; Zhou, N.; Lv, J.; Tang, K.; et al. Gasdermin E–mediated target cell pyroptosis by CAR T cells triggers cytokine release syndrome. *Sci. Immunol.* **2020**, *5*, eaax7969. [CrossRef]
22. Arias, M.; Martínez-Lostao, L.; Santiago, L.; Ferrandez, A.; Granville, D.J.; Pardo, J. The Untold Story of Granzymes in Oncoimmunology: Novel Opportunities with Old Acquaintances. *Trends Cancer* **2017**, *3*, 407–422. [CrossRef] [PubMed]
23. Li, C.; Zeng, M.; Chi, H.; Shen, J.; Ng, T.-B.; Jin, G.; Lu, D.; Fan, X.; Xiong, B.; Xiao, Z.; et al. Trichosanthin increases Granzyme B penetration into tumor cells by upregulation of CI-MPR on the cell surface. *Oncotarget* **2017**, *8*, 26460–26470. [CrossRef] [PubMed]
24. Galia, A.; Calogero, A.; Condorelli, R.A.; Fraggetta, F.; La Corte, A.; Ridolfo, F.; Bosco, P.; Castiglione, R.; Salemi, M. PARP-1 protein expression in glioblastoma multiforme. *Eur. J. Histochem.* **2012**, *56*, 9. [CrossRef] [PubMed]
25. Su, Z.; Yang, Z.; Xu, Y.; Chen, Y.; Yu, Q. Apoptosis, autophagy, necroptosis, and cancer metastasis. *Mol. Cancer* **2015**, *14*, 48. [CrossRef]
26. Russo, M.; Russo, G.L. Autophagy inducers in cancer. *Biochem. Pharmacol.* **2018**, *153*, 51–61. [CrossRef]
27. Wong, R.S.Y. Apoptosis in cancer: From pathogenesis to treatment. *J. Exp. Clin. Cancer Res.* **2011**, *30*, 87. [CrossRef] [PubMed]
28. Wei, B.; Huang, Q.; Huang, S.; Mai, W.; Zhong, X. Trichosanthin-induced autophagy in gastric cancer cell MKN-45 is dependent on reactive oxygen species (ROS) and NF-κB/p53 pathway. *J. Pharmacol. Sci.* **2016**, *131*, 77–83. [CrossRef]
29. Sirohi, K.; Swarup, G. Defects in autophagy caused by glaucoma-associated mutations in optineurin. *Exp. Eye Res.* **2016**, *144*, 54–63. [CrossRef]
30. Kałuza, J.; Adamek, D.; Pyrich, M. Ki-67 as a marker of proliferation activity in tumor progression of recurrent gliomas of supratentorial localization. Immunocytochemical quantitative studies. *Pol. J. Pathol* **1997**, *48*, 31–36.
31. Strazza, M.; Mor, A. Consider the Chemokines: A Review of the Interplay Between Chemokines and T Cell Subset Function. *Discov. Med.* **2017**, *24*, 31–39. [PubMed]
32. Opal, S.M.; DePalo, V.A. Anti-Inflammatory Cytokines. *Chest* **2000**, *117*, 1162–1172. [CrossRef] [PubMed]
33. Sucker, A.; Zhao, F.; Pieper, N.; Heeke, C.; Maltaner, R.; Stadtler, N.; Real, B.; Bielefeld, N.; Howe, S.; Weide, B.; et al. Acquired IFNγ resistance impairs anti-tumor immunity and gives rise to T-cell-resistant melanoma lesions. *Nat. Commun.* **2017**, *8*, 15440. [CrossRef]
34. Turner, C.T.; Hiroyasu, S.; Granville, D.J. Granzyme B as a therapeutic target for wound healing. *Expert Opin. Ther. Targets* **2019**, *23*, 745–754. [CrossRef] [PubMed]
35. Krepela, E. Granzyme B-induced apoptosis in cancer cells and its regulation (Review). *Int. J. Oncol.* **2010**, *37*, 1361–1378. [CrossRef]
36. Mondal, A. A novel extraction of trichosanthin from *Trichosanthes kirilowii* roots using three-phase partitioning and its in vitro anticancer activity. *Pharm. Biol.* **2014**, *52*, 677–680. [CrossRef]
37. Zhu, Y.; Sun, Y.; Cai, Y.; Sha, O.; Jiang, W. Trichosanthin reduces the viability of SU-DHL-2 cells via the activation of the extrinsic and intrinsic apoptotic pathways. *Mol. Med. Rep.* **2016**, *13*, 403–411. [CrossRef]
38. Wang, P.; Huang, S.; Wang, F.; Ren, Y.; Hehir, M.; Wang, X.; Cai, J. Cyclic AMP-Response Element Regulated Cell Cycle Arrests in Cancer Cells. *PLoS ONE* **2013**, *8*, e65661. [CrossRef]
39. Li, X.; He, S.; Ma, B. Autophagy and autophagy-related proteins in cancer. *Mol. Cancer* **2020**, *19*, 12. [CrossRef]
40. Gao, W.; Wang, X.; Zhou, Y.; Wang, X.; Yu, Y. Autophagy, ferroptosis, pyroptosis, and necroptosis in tumor immunotherapy. *Signal Transduct. Target. Ther.* **2022**, *7*, 196. [CrossRef]
41. Asrorov, A.M.; Muhitdinov, B.; Tu, B.; Mirzaakhmedov, S.; Wang, H.; Huang, Y. Advances on Delivery of Cytotoxic Enzymes as Anticancer Agents. *Molecules* **2022**, *27*, 3836. [CrossRef]
42. Tummers, B.; Green, D.R. Caspase-8: Regulating life and death. *Immunol. Rev.* **2017**, *277*, 76–89. [CrossRef]
43. Avrutsky, M.I.; Troy, C.M. Caspase-9: A Multimodal Therapeutic Target With Diverse Cellular Expression in Human Disease. *Front. Pharmacol.* **2021**, *12*, 701301. [CrossRef] [PubMed]
44. Boulares, A.H.; Yakovlev, A.G.; Ivanova, V.; Stoica, B.A.; Wang, G.; Iyer, S.; Smulson, M. Role of poly(adp-ribose) polymerase (parp) cleavage in apoptosis. Caspase 3-resistant parp mutant increases rates of apoptosis in transfected cells. *J. Biol. Chem.* **1999**, *274*, 22932–22940. [CrossRef] [PubMed]
45. Creagh, E.; Conroy, H.; Martin, S.J. Caspase-activation pathways in apoptosis and immunity. *Immunol. Rev.* **2003**, *193*, 10–21. [CrossRef]
46. Jiandong, L.; Yang, Y.; Peng, J.; Xiang, M.; Wang, D.; Xiong, G.; Li, S. Trichosanthes kirilowii lectin ameliorates streptozocin-induced kidney injury via modulation of the balance between M1/M2 phenotype macrophage. *Biomed. Pharmacother.* **2019**, *109*, 93–102. [CrossRef]
47. Zhou, X.; Yang, N.; Lu, L.; Ding, Q.; Jiao, Z.; Zhou, Y.; Chou, K.-Y. Up-regulation of IL-10 expression in dendritic cells is involved in Trichosanthin-induced immunosuppression. *Immunol. Lett.* **2007**, *110*, 74–81. [CrossRef]
48. Zhao, S.; Wang, Y.; Wei, H. Trichosanthin induced Th2 polarization status. *Cell. Mol. Immunol.* **2006**, *3*, 297–301.

49. Zhao, J.; Ben, L.-H.; Wu, Y.-L.; Hu, W.; Ling, K.; Xin, S.-M.; Nie, H.-L.; Ma, L.; Pei, G. Anti-HIV Agent Trichosanthin Enhances the Capabilities of Chemokines to Stimulate Chemotaxis and G Protein Activation, and This Is Mediated through Interaction of Trichosanthin and Chemokine Receptors. *J. Exp. Med.* **1999**, *190*, 101–112. [CrossRef]
50. Sangro, B.; Chan, S.L.; Meyer, T.; Reig, M.; El-Khoueiry, A.; Galle, P.R. Diagnosis and management of toxicities of immune checkpoint inhibitors in hepatocellular carcinoma. *J. Hepatol.* **2020**, *72*, 320–341. [CrossRef] [PubMed]
51. Cao, X.; Cai, S.F.; Fehniger, T.A.; Song, J.; Collins, L.I.; Piwnica-Worms, D.R.; Ley, T.J. Granzyme B and Perforin Are Important for Regulatory T Cell-Mediated Suppression of Tumor Clearance. *Immunity* **2007**, *27*, 635–646. [CrossRef]
52. Han, N.-R.; Kim, K.-C.; Kim, J.-S.; Ko, S.-G.; Park, H.-J.; Moon, P.-D. The immune-enhancing effects of a mixture of Astragalus membranaceus (Fisch.) Bunge, Angelica gigas Nakai, and Trichosanthes Kirilowii (Maxim.) or its active constituent nodakenin. *J. Ethnopharmacol.* **2022**, *285*, 114893. [CrossRef] [PubMed]
53. Gocher, A.M.; Workman, C.J.; Vignali, D.A.A. Interferon-γ: Teammate or opponent in the tumour microenvironment? *Nat. Rev. Immunol.* **2022**, *22*, 158–172. [CrossRef] [PubMed]
54. Guan, X.; Polesso, F.; Wang, C.; Sehrawat, A.; Hawkins, R.M.; Murray, S.E.; Thomas, G.V.; Caruso, B.; Thompson, R.F.; Wood, M.A.; et al. Androgen receptor activity in T cells limits checkpoint blockade efficacy. *Nature* **2022**, *606*, 791–796. [CrossRef] [PubMed]
55. Gao, J.; Shi, L.Z.; Zhao, H.; Chen, J.; Xiong, L.; He, Q.; Chen, T.; Roszik, J.; Bernatchez, C.; Woodman, S.E.; et al. Loss of IFN-γ Pathway Genes in Tumor Cells as a Mechanism of Resistance to Anti-CTLA-4 Therapy. *Cell* **2016**, *167*, 397–404.e9. [CrossRef]
56. Angeli, J.P.F.; da Silva, T.N.X.; Schilling, B. CD8+ T cells PUF(A)ing the flames of cancer ferroptotic cell death. *Cancer Cell* **2022**, *40*, 346–348. [CrossRef]
57. Shen, J.; Xiao, Z.; Zhao, Q.; Li, M.; Wu, X.; Zhang, L.; Hu, W.; Cho, C.H. Anti-cancer therapy with TNFα and IFNγ: A comprehensive review. *Cell Prolif.* **2018**, *51*, e12441. [CrossRef]
58. Martínez-Reza, I.; Díaz, L.; García-Becerra, R. Preclinical and clinical aspects of TNF-α and its receptors TNFR1 and TNFR2 in breast cancer. *J. Biomed. Sci.* **2017**, *24*, 90. [CrossRef]
59. Henry, C.J.; Ornelles, D.A.; Mitchell, L.M.; Brzoza-Lewis, K.L.; Hiltbold, E.M. IL-12 Produced by Dendritic Cells Augments CD8+ T Cell Activation through the Production of the Chemokines CCL1 and CCL17. *J. Immunol.* **2008**, *181*, 8576–8584. [CrossRef]
60. Yamaguchi, H.; Hiroi, M.; Mori, K.; Ushio, R.; Matsumoto, A.; Yamamoto, N.; Shimada, J.; Ohmori, Y. Simultaneous Expression of Th1- and Treg-Associated Chemokine Genes and $CD4^+$, $CD8^+$, and $Foxp3^+$ Cells in the Premalignant Lesions of 4NQO-Induced Mouse Tongue Tumorigenesis. *Cancers* **2021**, *13*, 1835. [CrossRef]
61. Xu, M.; Wang, Y.; Xia, R.; Wei, Y.; Wei, X. Role of the CCL2-CCR2 signalling axis in cancer: Mechanisms and therapeutic targeting. *Cell Prolif.* **2021**, *54*, e13115. [CrossRef]
62. Lança, T.; Silva-Santos, B. Recruitment of γδ T lymphocytes to tumors. *Oncoimmunology* **2013**, *2*, e25461. [CrossRef]
63. Lança, T.; Costa, M.F.; Gonçalves-Sousa, N.; Rei, M.; Grosso, A.R.; Penido, C.; Silva-Santos, B. Protective Role of the Inflammatory CCR2/CCL2 Chemokine Pathway through Recruitment of Type 1 Cytotoxic γδ T Lymphocytes to Tumor Beds. *J. Immunol.* **2013**, *190*, 6673–6680. [CrossRef]
64. Molon, B.; Ugel, S.; Del Pozzo, F.; Soldani, C.; Zilio, S.; Avella, D.; De Palma, A.; Mauri, P.; Monegal, A.; Rescigno, M.; et al. Chemokine nitration prevents intratumoral infiltration of antigen-specific T cells. *J. Exp. Med.* **2011**, *208*, 1949–1962. [CrossRef]
65. Rapp, M.; Grassmann, S.; Chaloupka, M.; Layritz, P.; Kruger, S.; Ormanns, S.; Rataj, F.; Janssen, K.-P.; Endres, S.; Anz, D.; et al. C-C chemokine receptor type-4 transduction of T cells enhances interaction with dendritic cells, tumor infiltration and therapeutic efficacy of adoptive T cell transfer. *Oncoimmunology* **2016**, *5*, e1105428. [CrossRef]
66. Fialová, A.; Partlová, S.; Sojka, L.; Hromádková, H.; Brtnický, T.; Fučíková, J.; Kocián, P.; Rob, L.; Bartůňková, J.; Špíšek, R. Dynamics of T-cell infiltration during the course of ovarian cancer: The gradual shift from a Th17 effector cell response to a predominant infiltration by regulatory T-cells. *Int. J. Cancer* **2012**, *132*, 1070–1079. [CrossRef]
67. Afonina, I.S.; Cullen, S.P.; Martin, S.J. Cytotoxic and non-cytotoxic roles of the CTL/NK protease granzyme B. *Immunol. Rev.* **2010**, *235*, 105–116. [CrossRef] [PubMed]
68. Ahmed, K.A.; Xiang, J. mTORC1 regulates mannose-6-phosphate receptor transport and T-cell vulnerability to regulatory T cells by controlling kinesin KIF13A. *Cell Discov.* **2017**, *3*, 17011. [CrossRef] [PubMed]
69. Hirsch, T.; Marchetti, P.; Susin, S.A.; Dallaporta, B.; Zamzami, N.; Marzo, I.; Geuskens, M.; Kroemer, G. The apoptosis-necrosis paradox. Apoptogenic proteases activated after mitochondrial permeability transition determine the mode of cell death. *Oncogene* **1997**, *15*, 1573–1581. [CrossRef] [PubMed]

International Journal of *Molecular Sciences*

MDPI

Article

Camptothecin Effectively Regulates Germline Differentiation through Bam–Cyclin A Axis in *Drosophila melanogaster*

Jing Zhang [1,2], Shijie Zhang [1,2], Zhipeng Sun [1,2], Yu Cai [3,4], Guohua Zhong [1,2,*] and Xin Yi [1,2,*]

1 Key Laboratory of Crop Integrated Pest Management in South China, Ministry of Agriculture, South China Agricultural University, Guangzhou 510642, China
2 Key Laboratory of Natural Pesticide and Chemical Biology, Ministry of Education, South China Agricultural University, Guangzhou 510642, China
3 Temasek Life Sciences Laboratory, National University of Singapore, Singapore 119077, Singapore
4 Department of Biological Sciences, National University of Singapore, Singapore 119077, Singapore
* Correspondence: guohuazhong@scau.edu.cn (G.Z.); yixin2324@scau.edu.cn (X.Y.)

Abstract: Camptothecin (CPT), first isolated from Chinese tree *Camptotheca acuminate*, produces rapid and prolonged inhibition of DNA synthesis and induction of DNA damage by targeting topoisomerase I (top1), which is highly activated in cancer cells. CPT thus exhibits remarkable anticancer activities in various cancer types, and is a promising therapeutic agent for the treatment of cancers. However, it remains to be uncovered underlying its cytotoxicity toward germ cells. In this study we found that CPT, a cell cycle-specific anticancer agent, reduced fecundity and exhibited significant cytotoxicity toward GSCs and two-cell cysts. We showed that CPT induced GSC loss and retarded two-cell cysts differentiation in a niche- or apoptosis-independent manner. Instead, CPT induced ectopic expression of a differentiation factor, bag of marbles (Bam), and regulated the expression of cyclin A, which contributed to GSC loss. In addition, CPT compromised two-cell cysts differentiation by decreasing the expression of Bam and inducing cell arrest at G1/S phase via cyclin A, eventually resulting in two-cell accumulation. Collectively, this study demonstrates, for the first time in vivo, that the Bam–cyclin A axis is involved in CPT-mediated germline stem cell loss and two-cell cysts differentiation defects via inducing cell cycle arrest, which could provide information underlying toxicological effects of CPT in the productive system, and feature its potential to develop as a pharmacology-based germline stem cell regulation agent.

Keywords: camptothecin; germ cells; Bam; cell cycle

Citation: Zhang, J.; Zhang, S.; Sun, Z.; Cai, Y.; Zhong, G.; Yi, X. Camptothecin Effectively Regulates Germline Differentiation through Bam–Cyclin A Axis in *Drosophila melanogaster*. *Int. J. Mol. Sci.* **2023**, *24*, 1617. https://doi.org/10.3390/ijms24021617

Academic Editors: Barbara De Filippis, Alessandra Ammazzalorso and Marialuigia Fantacuzzi

Received: 30 November 2022
Revised: 9 January 2023
Accepted: 10 January 2023
Published: 13 January 2023

1. Introduction

Camptothecin (CPT) is a pentacyclic alkaloid that was first isolated from stem wood of *Camptotheca acuminate* [1]. The US National Cancer Institute screening program identified CPT as a promising therapeutic agent for the treatment of cancers because it specifically targets topoisomerase I (top1), which is highly activated in cancer cells [2]. CPT could prevent the re-ligation of the nicked DNA and dissociation of top1 from the DNA by binding to both of the top1 enzyme and the intact DNA strand through hydrogen bonding. During replication, this CPT-involved ternary complex could act as a roadblock for the replication fork to result in shear stress upon the intact DNA strand, and eventually leading to breakage, DNA damage, and cell death [3–5]. Previous pharmacological studies indicated that CPT could inhibit DNA and RNA (including ribosomal RNA) synthesis, induce DNA damage, and arrest cell cycle at both S and G2 phases [6–8]. To this end, CPT could induce G1/S phase arrest in oral squamous cancer cells, ovarian clear cell carcinoma, and was found to possess a wide spectrum of antitumor activities [9–11]. However, the severe side effects of CPT, such as nausea, vomiting, dermatitis, diarrhea, cystitis, leukopenia, precluded its initial clinical development as a chemotherapeutic drug [12]. Despite many pharmacokinetic studies, it remains to be unpredictable underlying its toxicity toward different systems.

Drosophila ovarian system has been considered as a fruitful in vivo system for studying cell biology and dissecting the cytotoxicity of CPT in productive system [13]. In females, the gametes are produced from a specialized tissue called germline stem cells (GSCs) [14]. As the source of gametes, the only cell type that can pass the genetic information to the next generation, GSCs play a fundamental role in maximizing the quantity of gametes that animals produce, while ensuring their highest quality [14]. The maintenance and differentiation of GSC is modulated by intrinsic and extrinsic signal pathways in the ovary to be instructive to specify cell fate [15]. As one of those identified intrinsic factors to be able to regulate GSCs [16–19], cell cycle control serves as a critical aspect in the decision between GSC maintenance and differentiation [20]. The new GSC daughter and the cystoblast (CB) remain connected throughout most of the cell cycle; consequently, changes to the cell cycle would be critical for promoting or hampering GSC differentiation [21]. For instance, loss of cyclin B (CycB), a late-G2 phase regulator to control the G2-M phase transition, could lead to GSC self-renewal and maintenance defects [20]. Additionally, following gamma irradiation, GSCs briefly pause the cell cycle and become 'quiescent', resulting in progeny loss [22,23]. Although a plethora of intrinsic factors have been identified for their roles in regulating stem cell fate via affecting the cell cycle [22,24], it remains largely unclear whether CPT, a cell cycle-specific anticancer agent, could affect GSC fate.

In this study, we unveiled the cytotoxicity of CPT in GSC loss and two-cell differentiation defects. Instead of niche and apoptosis, the differentiation factor, bag of marbles (Bam), directly received CPT signals to influence GSC numbers. In addition, CPT compromised germ cell differentiation by decreasing the expression of Bam and inducing cell arrest in G1/S phase via cyclin A (CycA), resulting in two-cell accumulation. Overall, this study demonstrates, for the first time in vivo, that the Bam–CycA axis is involved in CPT-mediated GSC loss and two-cell differentiation defects via inducing cell cycle arrest, and the results in this study highlight the toxicological role of CPT in germ cells and its potential to serve as a pharmacology-based GSC regulation agent.

2. Results

2.1. The Effects of CPT on Germ Cells

CPT showed strong cytotoxicity against a variety of tumor types in vitro and in vivo; we then sought to examine the mortality of flies following CPT treatment. We found that although CPT-treatment did not have noticeable impact on fly survival rate, the treated females produced significantly fewer eggs, compared to control-treated females (Figure 1a,b), suggesting that CPT may affect fly oogenesis. Indeed, while the ovariole of the control female contained 5–7 follicles, the CPT-treated female only possessed 1–2 follicles at the discontinued stage (Figure 1h). In addition, some phenotypes were also observed at the anterior tip of the ovariole—the germarial region in treated flies, which is the focus of this study. In the germarium, two to three GSCs (identified by pMad-positive cells) resided at the anterior tip, next to a cluster of cap cells [25], and contained an anteriorly-positioned spherical fusome (or spectrome) (Figure 1c), but CPT treatment led to a reduction in the number of GSCs (Figure 1d). The daughters of GSCs, namely cystoblasts (CBs), move posteriorly as they differentiate: each CB divides four times with incomplete cytokinesis to form an interconnected 16-cell cyst in which one of the cells adopts oocyte fate and the rest become supporting nurse cells [26]. We found that CPT also affected the early steps of the germ cell development process and blocked CB differentiation, resulting in accumulation of CB-like (Figure 1e,f) and two-cell (Figure 1g,h) in the germarium. Each cyst could be surrounded by a single layer of follicle cells to form egg chambers. However, CPT-treated flies possessed a significantly higher ratio of abnormal phenotypes of egg chamber (apparent failure of egg chamber budding leading to empty ovarioles) compared with control flies (Figure 1i,j). Those observations indicated that CPT treatment led to a GSC loss and also a delay in germ cell differentiation, consequently resulting in defects in egg production.

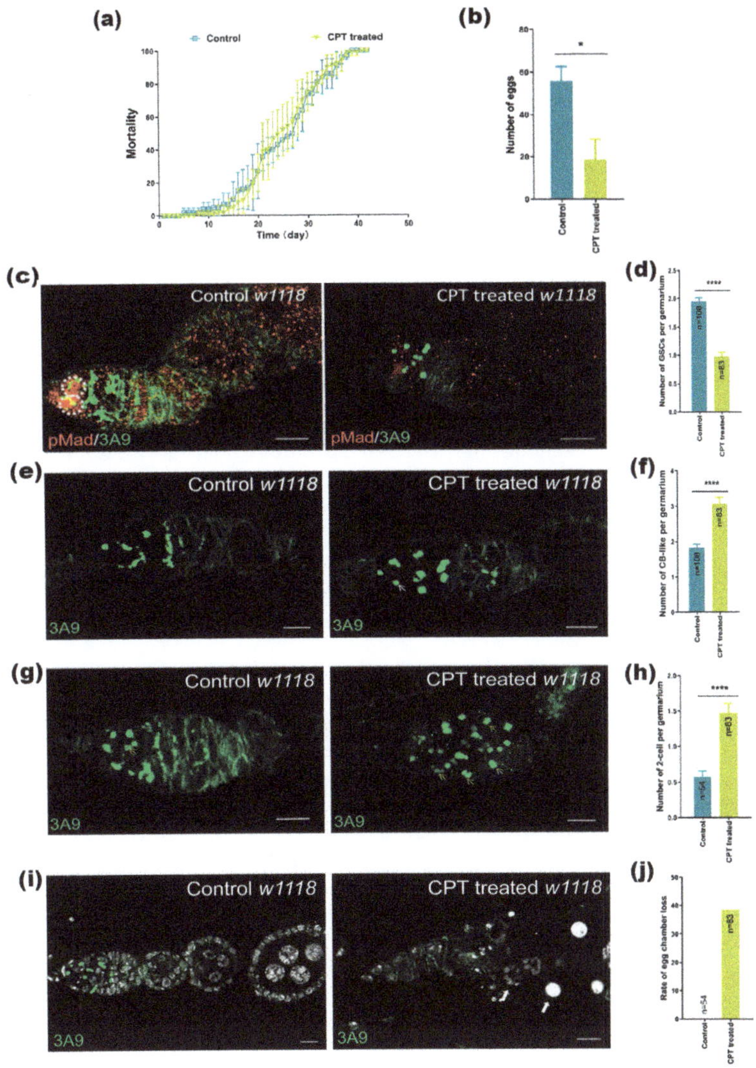

Figure 1. The effects of CPT on germ cells. (**a**) The mortality of flies after the flies were treated by CPT. (**b**) The number of eggs laid at the 9th d post CPT or DMSO solution treatment. (**c**) GSCs stained with anti-pMad and anti-3A9 antibodies in germarium at the 9th day post CPT or DMSO treatment. GSCs were indicated by white dashed circle. (**d**) Statistical data showing the GSC number from control and treated groups. (**e**) Germ cells stained with anti-3A9 antibody in germarium at the 9th day post CPT or DMSO treatment. CB-like cells were indicated by white arrow. (**f**) Statistical data showing the CB number from control and treated groups. (**g**) Representative DMSO- and CPT-treated images showing the effect of CPT on two-cell stained with anti-3A9. two-cell was indicated by yellow arrow. (**h**) Statistical data showing the two-cell number from control and treated groups. (**i**) Representative control and CPT-treated images showing CPT treatment blocked germ cell differentiation leading to accumulation of CB and two-cells and stained by Hoechst (white) and 3A9 (green). The white arrow indicated egg chamber loss. (**j**) The number of egg chambers showing abnormal phenotype, including apparent failure of egg chamber budding leading to empty egg chamber. Values are the means (±SEs) of replicates. Statistical comparisons were based on Students' s *t*-tests. The level of significance for the results was set at * $p < 0.05$, **** $p < 0.0001$. Scale bar, 10 μm.

2.2. CPT Treatment Fails to Cause Apoptosis and Influence Niche in Ovarian GSCs

In the *Drosophila* ovary, extrinsic signaling from niche and intrinsic translational machinery regulate the balance between GSC maintenance and differentiation of their daughters [27]. We investigated whether CPT-induced GSC loss was due to apoptosis by examining the expression of two cell death markers, including Terminal deoxynucleotidyl transferase-mediated dUTP Nick End Labeling (TUNEL) assays and cleaved Caspase-3 activities. We found no cleaved TUNEL signals and Caspase-3 activity detected in GSCs, CBs-like and two-cell, in both control and CPT treated ovaries (Figure 2a,b), indicating that the defects in GSC maintenance by CPT treatment are not a result of cell death. We next addressed whether the GSC loss is a consequence of premature differentiation. At the anterior tip of the ovary, terminal filament (TF) cells, cap cells (Cpc), and escort cells (ECs) could provide a physical location to house GSCs and form a GSC niche, which could send signals to GSCs, including Decapentaplegic (Dpp), Hedgehog (Hh), and Unpaired (Upd), to regulate their proliferation to maintain tissue homeostasis [28,29]. As the spatial organization of the GSC niche permits direct contacts between two or three CpCs and one GSC, which are anchored to the CpCs by adherent junctions, we then first examined whether the GSC loss induced by CPT attributed to the defects in Dpp expression by using *dpp-lacZ* in combination with anti-Engrailed (En) antibody to mark En and Dpp expression in Cpcs. We found that neither the protein accumulation of En nor the level of Dpp (Figure 2c) showed significant changes after CPT treatment. Since the expression of Dpp was unaffected, the number of Cpcs was measured by using anti-lacZ staining, and the results showed the number of Cpcs remained still after treatment (Figure 2e and Supplementary Figure S1), indicating CPT did not induce changes in Cpc number as well. We further confirmed the expression of *dpp* by in situ hybridization, which also showed no significant changes were observed at transcript level following CPT treatment (Figure 2d). In addition, armadillo (Arm) is concentrated at the interface between Cpcs and GSCs in the adult ovary, which supports a role of this adhesion system in anchoring GSCs to their niche [30,31]. Still, we found no changes in Arm expression level and pattern after CPT treatment (Figure 2f), suggesting CPT induced decline in the number of GSCs was independent of Arm. Together, these results suggest that CPT-induced GSC loss is likely not a result of defective niche activity. We then investigated how CPT-treatment affected CB and two-cell cyst differentiation. As EC-expressed Thickveins (Tkv) acts as a receptor sink to remove excess Cpc-expressed Dpp, thereby promoting GSC differentiation [32], we then examined Tkv expression by immunostaining with anti-Tkv to address whether the levels of Tkv in the germarium were affected by CPT and accounted for GSC loss. The results showed that similar fluorescence intensity and identical distribution patterns were observed in fly ovaries with or without CPT treatment, indicating CPT treatment could not trigger expression changes of Tkv at both protein and transcript level (Figure 2g). As EC cellular processes are also closely associated with differentiated germ cells, and the physical interactions between ECs and germ cells are essential for GSC differentiation [26], and Erk signaling has an important role in generating EC shapes and protrusive activity, we then examined the pErk activity in EC after exposure to CPT. The results showed that pErk was readily expressed in control EC, and CPT treatment did not induce significant changes in pErk expression. We noted that the expression of pErk increased in the early follicular cell, which unlikely contributed to GSC loss (Figure 2h). Moreover, we further investigated whether ECs could be influenced by CPT by using *pz1444* and anti-3A9 to identify ECs in the anterior region where GSCs are localized. For both control and CPT treated groups, we could observe positive signals for ECs in the region 1 or 2a (n = 83), while after CPT treatment, the localization of ECs expanded to the posterior regions (i.e., egg chamber) (Figure 2i). However, such abnormal phenotype of EC localization unlikely contributed to GSC loss. We thus excluded the roles of apoptosis and niche in CPT-induced GSC loss and differentiation defects.

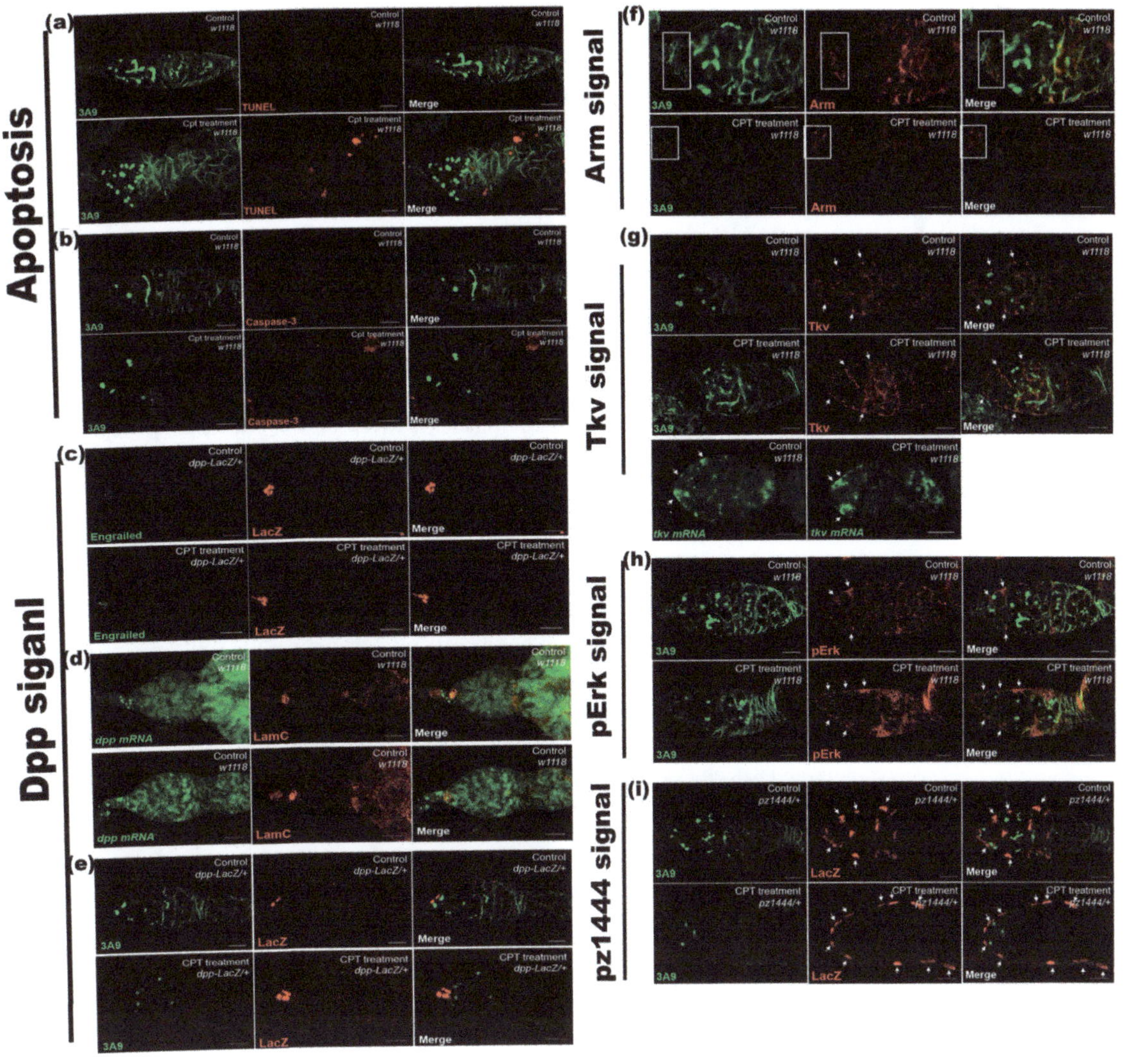

Figure 2. The roles of apoptosis and niche in CPT-induced GSCs loss. (**a**) Apoptotic signals from ovaries of control and CPT treated flies labeled with TUNEL (red) and stained with anti-3A9 (green). (**b**) Caspase-3 activity in CPT-treated and control germarium staining by Hoechst (white), Caspase-3 (red), and anti-3A9 (green). (**c**) Control and CPT-treated germaria with anti-En (green) and anti-LacZ (red) staining. (**d**) In situ hybridization examining *dpp* expression with anti-LamC (red) staining. (**e**) Control and CPT-treated germaria with anti-LacZ (red) and anti-3A9 (green) staining. (**f**) Arm immunoprecipitation with or without CPT exposure with Arm (red) and anti-3A9 (green) staining. Meanwhile, square flame indicated the expression of Arm. (**g**) Control and CPT-treated germaria with anti-Tkv (red) and anti-3A9 (green) staining, and in situ hybridization showing *tkv* mRNA expression in control and CPT-treated germaria. (**h**) Control and CPT-treated EC with anti-pErk (red) and anti-3A9 (green) staining. White arrow indicated the signal of pErk. (**i**) Control and CPT-treated EC with anti-LacZ (red) and anti-3A9 (green) staining. White dashed circle indicated ectopic location of ECs. Newly emerged flies (1 day post emergence) were treated with 100 mg/L CPT and control flies received equal amount of DMSO. The flies were dissected at the 9th day post treatment. Scale bar, 10 μm.

2.3. *Bam Signal Was Involved in CPT-Induced Toxicity in Germarium*

As Bam serves as a key factor to regulate GSC differentiation and germline cyst development, we then further examined whether Bam signaling was involved in CPT-induced GSC loss and two-cell accumulation. Germaria staining with Bam indicated that CPT treatment induced ectopic expression of Bam in GSCs, but suppressed the high expression of Bam in differentiation cells. In some germaria, the protein expression of Bam expanded to the posterior end of the tumorous germarium (Figure 3a). These results were further confirmed by staining with a Bam-GFP (GFP gene driven by the Bam promoter) reporter, which also showed ectopic GFP signals in GSCs but weaker fluorescence intensity in differentiating germ cells in CPT-treated germarium compared with control (Figure 3b,c). The transcriptional expression of *bam* was further confirmed by in situ hybridization. Consistent with changes in protein level, CPT induced ectopic *bam* expression in GSCs but decreased mRNA level of *bam* in differentiating germ cells (Figure 3d). To verify the role of Bam in CPT-induced two-cell accumulation, we checked the effects of Bam mutation on the phenotype of germaria with or without CPT treatment. Germarium bearing one copy of bam^{86} mutation contained a slight increase in the number of two-cell compared with wild type flies. Interestingly, CPT-treatment led to a drastic increase in CB and two-cell cyst in the germarium with copy bam^{86} mutation, leading to typical tumor-like germarium (Figure 4a). We thus recorded the number of two-cells, and found that CPT exposure in bam^{86} mutation germarium triggered an increase in the number of two-cells by 3.2-fold, compared with bam^{86} mutation germarium without CPT treatment (Figure 4b). We speculated that CPT could induce DNA damage and cell cycle arrest in two-cell phase by suppressing the expression of Bam to delay the differentiation of CB and two-cell cysts. To further determine whether increasing Bam expression could promote two-cell differentiation, we used the *hs-bam* transgene, in which Bam expression is under control of the heat-shock-inducible *hsp70* promoter to drive Bam expression in the ovaries, with or without CPT treatment. CPT-treated *hs-Bam* transgene germaria, without heat-shock, contained more two-cell cysts compared with DMSO-treated *hs-bam* transgene germaria without heat-shock (Figure 4c), indicating that the heat shock *bam* construct itself does not affect two-cell differentiation. Heat-shock-induced Bam expression with CPT treatment can sufficiently promote the differentiation of two-cell cysts into four-cell or eight-cell cysts, when compared with control flies of *hs-Bam* transgene germaria without heat shock (Figure 4d). These results demonstrated that CPT could influence the differentiation process by regulating Bam expression.

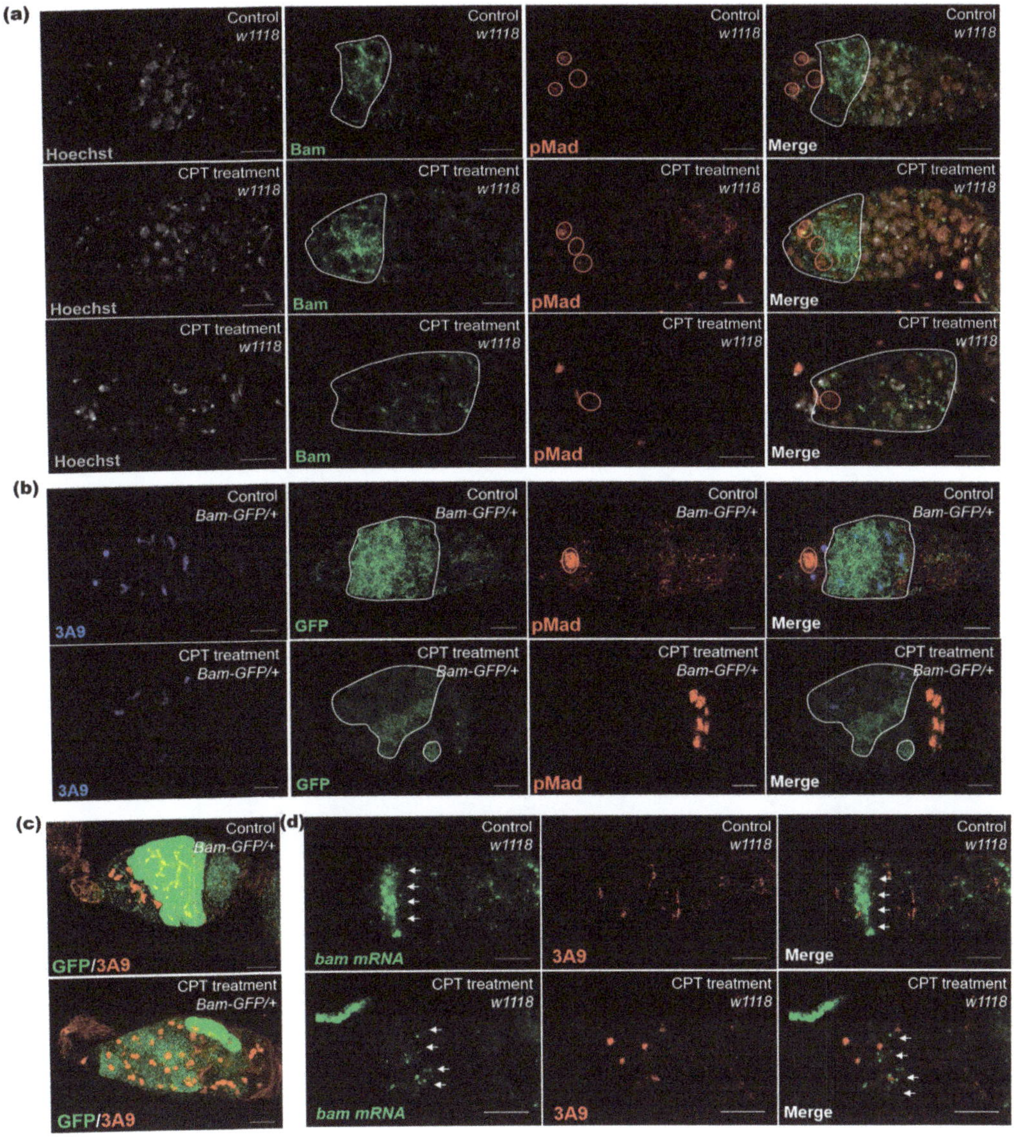

Figure 3. CPT could influence differentiation process by regulating Bam expression. (**a**) Control and CPT-treated germaria were labeled with Hoechst (white), anti-Bam (green) and anti-pMad (red) to examine Bam expression. White dashed circle indicated the location of Bam in control and CPT-treated germarium. (**b**) Germaria of female flies expressed GFP under the control of transcriptional of Bam stained with GFP (green), anti-3A9 (blue), and pMad (red). (**c**) Germaria of female flies expressed GFP under the control of transcriptional of Bam stained with GFP (green) and anti-3A9 (red). (**d**) In situ hybridization to examine *bam* expression at mRNA level with anti-3A9 (red) labeling with or without CPT treatment, white arrows indicated *bam mRNA* signal. Scale bar, 10 μm.

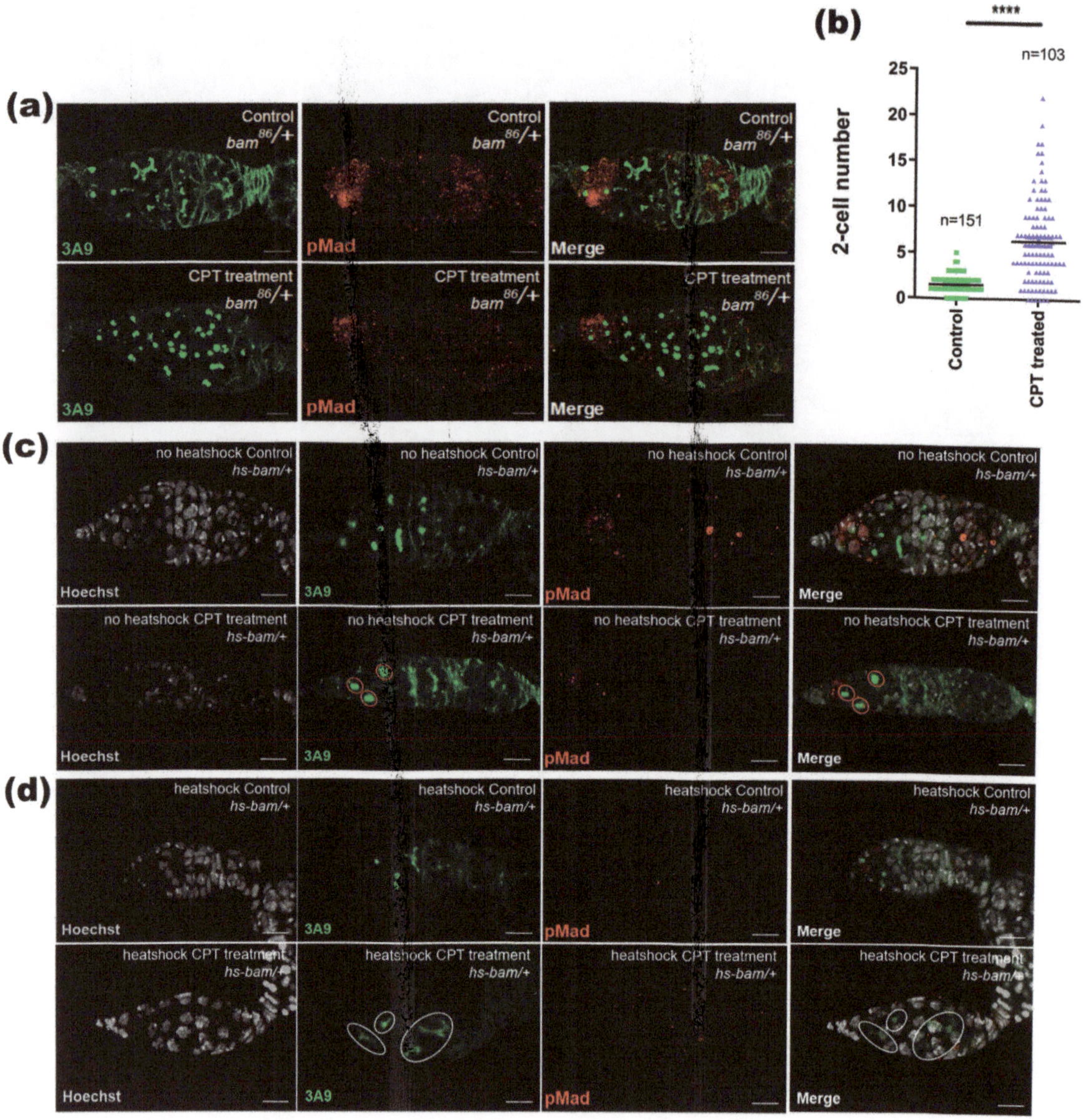

Figure 4. Bam can significantly rescue the two-cell accumulation caused by CPT. (**a**) *bam*^{86} with anti-pMad (red) and anti-3A9 (green) staining with or without CPT treatment. (**b**) Data summarized the number of two-cell cysts in (**a**), green indicated control, blue indicated CPT treatment. (**c**,**d**) Control and CPT-treated female flies with or without exposure to heat shock to drive *bam* expression and staining with anti-pMad (red) and anti-3A9 (green). Statistical comparisons were based on Students' s *t*-tests. The level of significance for the results was set at **** $p < 0.0001$. Scale bar, 10 μm.

2.4. The Role of Top1 in CPT-Induced Toxicology

To examine if top1 was also required for CPT-induced toxicology in GSCs, we used *nos-gal4*-driven RNAi expression to knock down *top1* gene expression specifically in germ cells. Our results showed that germline-specific *top1*^{RNAi} shrunk the germarium and led to rapid germ cell loss, and that CPT treatment could exacerbate such GSC loss phenotype, exhibiting similar but more severe abnormal germarium and triggering almost entire GSC and CB loss (Figure 5a,b). Control germaria maintained two or three GSCs and two CBs, and *top1*^{RNAi} germarium contained 1.4 GSCs and 1.5 CBs, respectively; however, *top1*^{RNAi} germarium with CPT treatment did not carry any GSCs or CBs (Figure 5c,d). The severity of GSC and CB loss phenotype in *top1*^{RNAi} germarium with CPT treatment suggested that top1 and CPT work in a linear pathway. Unexpectedly, germline-specific *top1* knockdown with CPT treatment also led to significant two-cell cyst loss compared with *top1*^{RNAi} germarium without CPT treatment (Figure 5e), which might be attributed to germ cell loss in some cases from *top1*^{RNAi} germarium with CPT treatment. We recounted the number of two-cell cysts by excluding the cases with complete germ cell loss, and found that *top1*^{RNAi} germarium with CPT treatment could lead to significant accumulation of two-cell, compared with *top1*^{RNAi} germarium without CPT treatment (Figure 5f). To further illuminate the relationship between top1 and the aforementioned differentiation factor, Bam, in CPT-induced GSC loss and two-cell accumulation, we examined Bam expression in *top1*^{RNAi} GSCs with or without CPT treatment. The results showed that CB and two-cell cysts expressed readily detectable levels of Bam; however, ectopic Bam expression occurred in a number of GSCs in *top1*^{RNAi} germarium without CPT treatment, or phenocopied CPT treatment. These data suggested that changes in top1 expression were sufficient to induce ectopic Bam expression in GSCs. CPT exposure in a *top1*^{RNAi} background also induced ectopic expression of Bam in GSCs (Figure 5g). These results indicated that top1 was involved in CPT-induced ectopic Bam expression, GSC loss, and two-cell accumulation. As DNA damage might be induced by CPT treatment via targeting top1, we examined p53 activity in early germ cells as its activity in *Drosophila* ovarian GSCs could be activated in response to DNA damage [33,34]. We could not find any obvious p53 signal in control of GSC, CB, and two-cell cysts, while CPT treatment could induce significant upregulation of p53 activities as evident by upregulated GFP signals in GSC, as well as in two-cells in CPT-treated germarium (Figure 5h). These data suggested that different degrees of DNA damage occurred in early germ cells in response to CPT treatment.

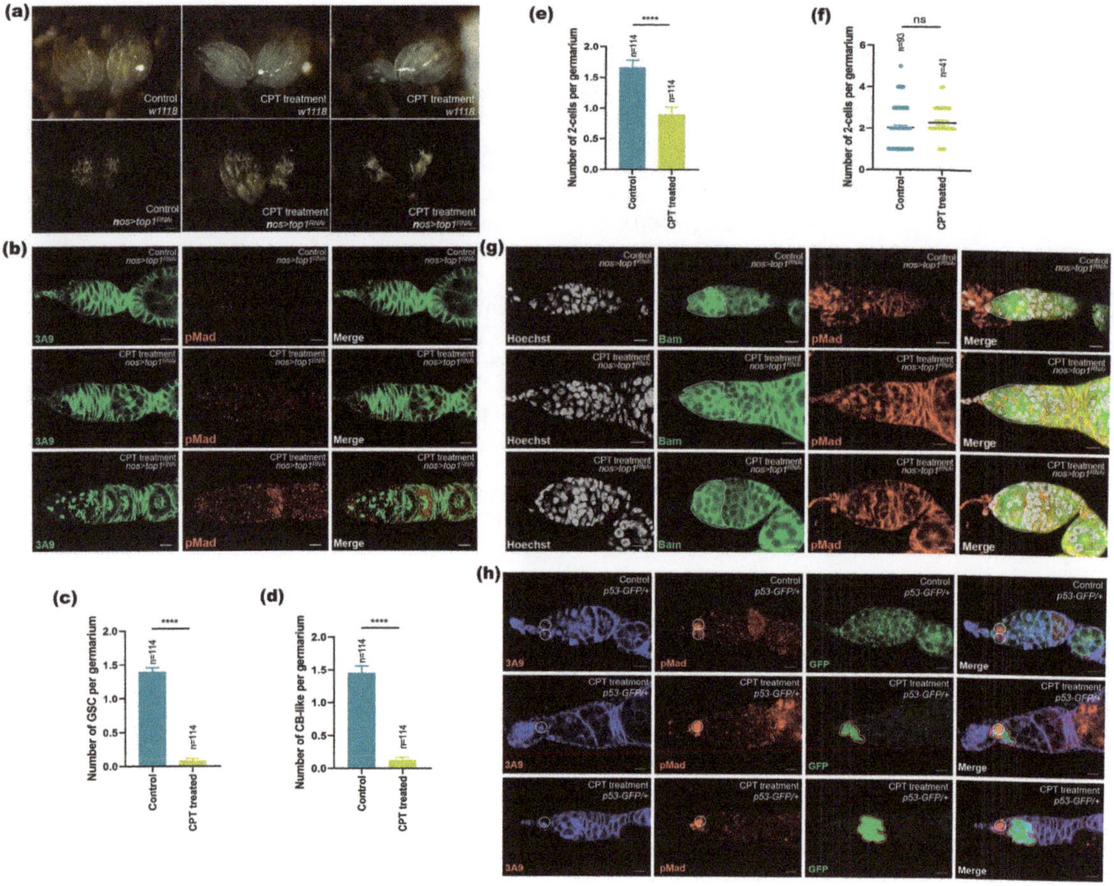

Figure 5. Top1 was involved in CPT-induced toxicity in germ cells. (**a**) Ovarian morphology from control and *top1*^{RNAi} germarium with or without CPT treatment. (**b**) Control and *top1*^{RNAi} germarium with or without CPT treatment and stained with anti-pMad (red) and anti-3A9 (green). (**c**) GSC quantification results are shown. (**d**) CB-like quantification results are shown. (**e**) Two-cell cysts quantification results are shown. (**f**) Two-cell cysts quantification results are shown by excluding the cases with germ cell loss. n is the number of the examined germaria; all the error bars represent SEMs; *p* values were calculated by comparing between *top1*^{RNAi} germarium with or without CPT treatment using Student's *t* test. Blue indicated control, yellow indicated CPT treatment in (**c**–**f**). (**g**) Bam expression pattern in *top1*^{RNAi} germarium with or without CPT treatment staining with anti-3A9 (red) and anti-Bam (green). (**h**) Germaria of female flies expressed GFP under the control of transcriptional of p53 stained with anti-3A9 (blue), anti-GFP (green), and anti-pMad (red). White dash circle indicated GFP signals. The level of significance for the results was set at **** $p < 0.0001$. Scale bar, 10 μm.

2.5. CPT Treatment Led to Cell Cycle Arrest

To monitor cell cycle progression of germ cells in the germarium, we used immunofluorescence combined FUCCI (fluorescent ubiquitylation cell cycle indicators) to identify cells in different phases of the cell cycle [35]. We then expressed *UASp-GFP-E2f1* (1–230) *UASp-mRFP1-cycB* (1–266) under control of *nos-gal4* to distinguish G1, S and G2 phases of interphase (Figure 6a). For CB in the control group, the fraction of proliferating G2/M and S cells accounted for 94.05% and 3.57% (n = 84), and after CPT treatment, the proportion of G2/M and S cells changed to 55.96% and 25.69%, respectively (n = 109) (Figure 6b). The same situation also occurred in two-cell, as the proportion of G2/M and S cells fluctuated from 87.95% and 10.84% (n = 83) to 48.26% and 28.36% (n = 201), respectively (Figure 6b). Additionally, the number of GSCs in phase G2/M transition accounted for 99.26% (n = 135) in the control group, and exhibited no significant change after exposure to CPT (the proportion of cells in phase G2/M was 90.48% in CPT treated group, n = 63) (Figure 6b). Consistent with a previous study, during cell division, high intensities of green and red fluorescence could be observed when nuclear envelope breakdown and degradation of the red probe (mRFP-NLS-CycB$_{1-166}$) occurred. Based on this fact, the intensity of the green signal (GFP-E2F1$_{1-230}$) would drop dramatically (as CRL4^{Cdt2} is activated at the G1-S transition) after a ~10 h steadily increase. After ~1 h gap period (without signal), the red fluorescence intensity would increase followed by reaccumulation of the green probe [35]. Our results showed that following CPT treatment, both the CycB and E2f1 signals were absent in 17.43% and 22.89% cells from CB-like and two-cell, significantly higher compared with control (2.38% and 1.20% from CB and two-cell in control group) (Figure 6b), which indicated that CPT treatment led to cells undergoing phase G1/S or S arrest, and such arrest might contribute to the previously observed increase in the number of two-cells after CPT treatment.

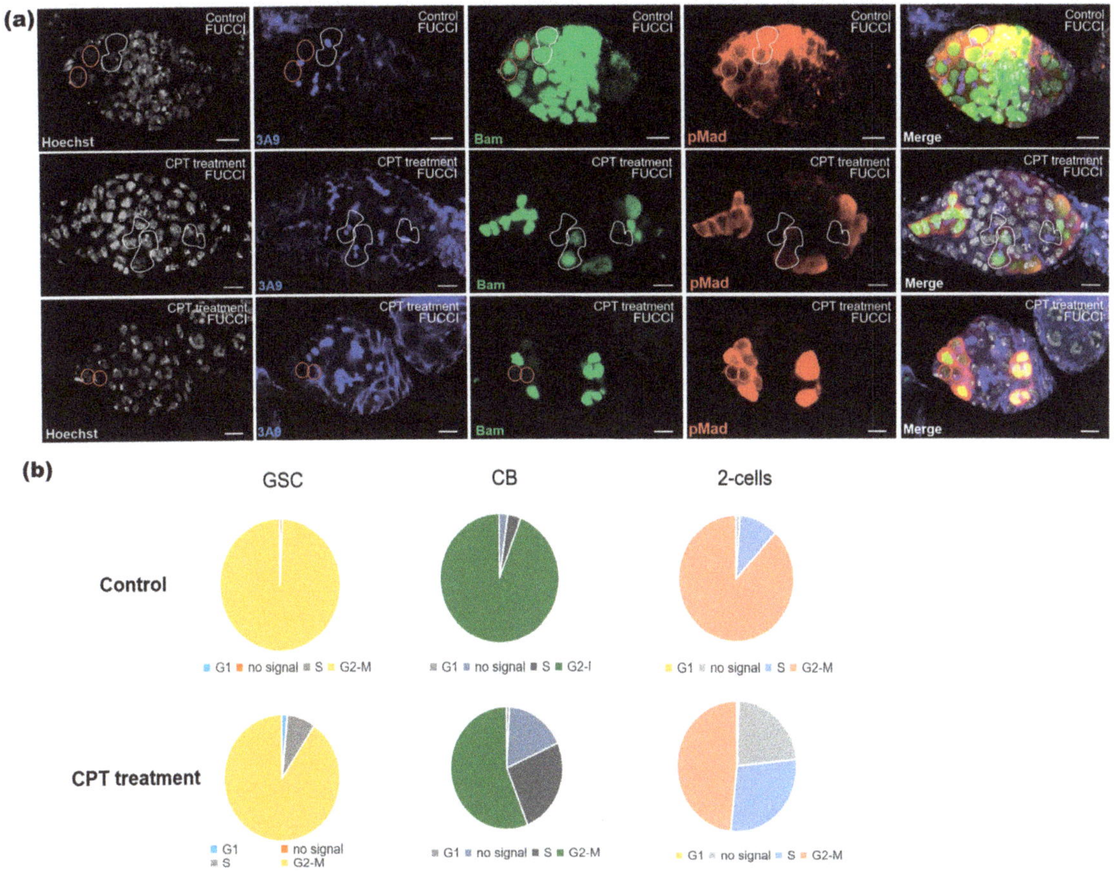

Figure 6. Cell cycle was determined by FUCCI system. (**a**) FUCCI were applied to identify cells in different phases of the cell cycle and stained with Hoechst (white), anti-3A9 (blue), anti-GFP (green), and anti-RFP (red). White dashed circle indicated two-cell without signals. (**b**) Quantification of cells in different phases of cell cycle.

2.6. *CycA Was Involved in CPT-Induced Differentiation Defects*

To illuminate the roles of cell-cycle regulators in CPT-induced differentiation defects, we examine the effects of CycA, cyclin B (CycB), and cyclin E (CycE) overexpression and RNAi on germ cells following CPT exposure. The results showed that overexpression of CycA with CPT exposure could enhance the toxicity of CPT exposure, exhibiting a higher rate of GSC loss and more two-cell accumulation (Figure 7a). These findings were consistent with a previous study, where ectopic expression of Bam in GSCs could be enhanced by co-expression of CycA [36]. However overexpression of *cycB* (Figure 7b) or *cycE* RNAi (Figure 7c) did not display expanded undifferentiated cell phenotypes. As one of the downstream targets of Bam in GSC [24], these results suggested that CycA expression might be involved in CPT-induced GSC loss and two-cell accumulation.

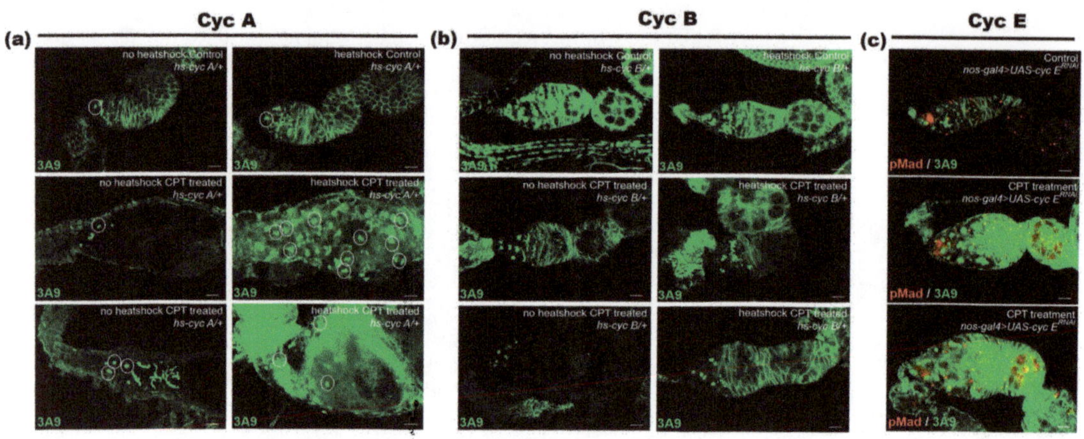

Figure 7. CycA was involved in CPT-induced GSC loss and two-cell accumulation. (**a**) Control and CPT-treated female flies with or without exposure to heat shock to drive *CycA* expression and staining with anti-3A9 (green). (**b**) Control and CPT-treated female flies with or without exposure to heat shock to drive *CycB* expression and staining with anti-3A9 (green). (**c**) Control and *CycE*^{RNAi} germarium and stained with anti-pMad (red) and anti-3A9 (green).

To further determine whether CycA is the direct cause of GSC loss and two-cell accumulation, we used *nos-gal4* to drive *CycA* gene overexpression specifically in germ cells. Immunostaining showed that *CycA* overexpression displayed a more severe phenotype of GSC loss in the germarium compared with CPT treatment (Figure 8a,e,f). However, *CycA* overexpression did not show a significant increase in the number of two-cell cysts (Figure 8b,e,f), which might be attributed to low efficiency of *nos-gal4*-driven overexpression in two-cell cysts and phenotype of germ cell loss induced by overexpression of *CycA*, overriding the two-cell accumulation phenotype. To confirm these observations, we used *nos-gal4* to drive down-regulation of the *CycA* gene specifically in germ cells. The genetic experiments revealed that the decreasing of *CycA* with CPT treatment can significantly restore GSC number, indicating that the down-regulation of *CycA* expression can rescue GSC loss phenotype caused by CPT treatment (Figure 8c,g,h). Moreover, the decline in the level of *CycA* can also abrogate two-cell accumulation induced by CPT (the number of two-cell cysts in the control group was 3.52, and the number in *CycA* RNAi germarium was 2.91) (Figure 8d,g,h). These results further confirmed that CycA participated in the CPT-induced GSC loss and two-cell accumulation.

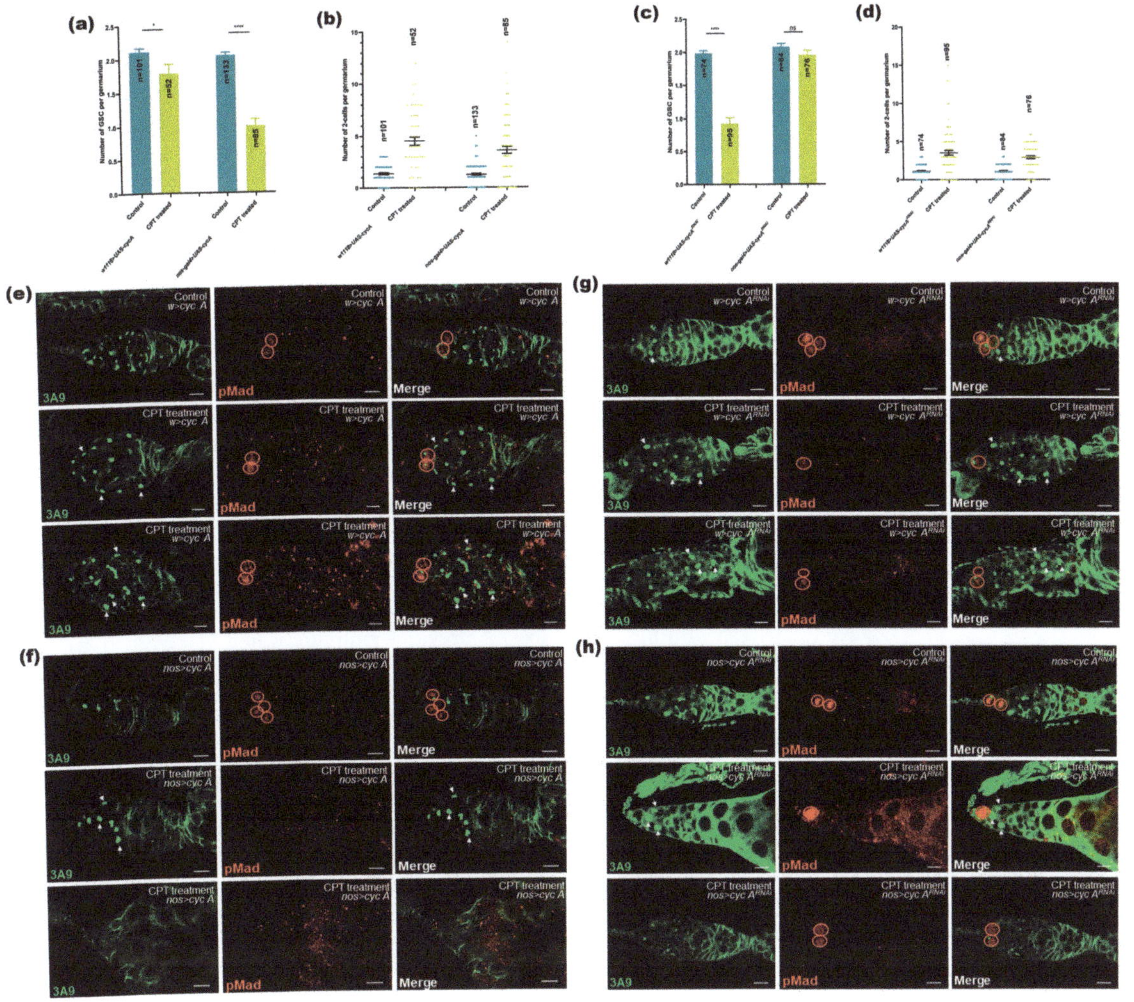

Figure 8. CycA is involved in GSC loss and two-cell accumulation induced by CPT treatment. (**a**) The GSC number of control and *CycA* overexpression germaria. (**b**) The number of two-cell cysts in control and *CycA* overexpression germaria. (**c**) The number of GSCs in control and $CycA^{RNAi}$ germaria. (**d**) The number of two-cell cysts in control and $CycA^{RNAi}$ germaria. (**e**,**f**) Control and *CycA* overexpression germaria with or without CPT treatment and stained with anti-pMad (red) and anti-3A9 (green). Blue indicated control, yellow indicated CPT treatment in (**c**–**f**). (**g**,**h**) Control and $CycA^{RNAi}$ germaria with or without CPT treatment and stained with anti-pMad (red) and anti-3A9 (green). Statistical comparisons were based on Students's *t*-tests. The level of significance for the results was set at * $p < 0.05$, **** $p < 0.0001$. Scale bar, 10 μm.

3. Discussion

It is well established that CPT-induced toxicity is dependent upon top1, which is capable of introducing a transient single-strand break in DNA, through which another strand can pass, thereby reducing DNA supercoiling [37,38]. Due to the specific function of top1, the single-strand cleavage/rejoining activity of top1 suggests that it may serve as a swivel for unwinding and rewinding of DNA helices associated with many critical cellular processes, including DNA replication, transcription, repair, and recombination induction of cell cycle arrest [39,40]. Therefore, CPT and CPT-derived chemicals were reported to cause severe toxicity in the hematopoietic system, lymphatic tissue, gastrointestinal tract, and reproductive organs, and have been developed for cancer therapy [41–43]. Our data demonstrated that CPT is deleterious to *D. melanogaster* germline development, and it leads to GSC loss and concomitantly blocks CB and two-cell cyst differentiation by ectopically inducing Bam expression and regulating CycA. Other than growing evidence on intrinsic factors-dependent mechanisms regulating the GSC lineage in *D. melanogaster* [44], we reported the toxicological effects of CPT on GSCs and two-cells for the first time, highlighting the potential of its pharmacophores to be developed in stem cell-based therapies.

It is well documented that top1 is the only cellular target of CPT [2]. Top1 activity is robust in malignant cells and correlates with disease progression in colorectal and ovarian cancers [45], making CPT a potent agent for anticancer chemotherapy. We found that the inhibition of the expression of *top1* led to a large number of germ cell loss without CPT treatment, and the phenotype is similar to that of CPT treatment. At the same time, $top1^{RNAi}$ flies with CPT treatment could exacerbate GSC loss and two-cell accumulation phenotypes induced by CPT treatment alone, exhibiting more severe abnormal germarium and triggering almost the entire GSC and CB loss. Therefore, we suggested CPT affected GSC maintenance and two-cell accumulation through inhibiting the expression of *top1*. Based on the current study, it is noteworthy that we found oral ingestion of CPT led to GSC loss in *D. melanogaster* probably via interfering with the cell cycle, which serves as a critical aspect in the decision between GSC maintenance and differentiation. Our results suggest that during germline differentiation, CPT-mediated changes in CycA expression have a role in reprogramming self-renewal, leading to precocious GSC differentiation, and eventually contributing to GSC loss. A previous study indicated that overexpression of a stable form of CycA led to severe *Drosophila* GSCs loss [46], and stabilized CycA could prevent exiting from the cell cycle and entering into G1 at an appropriate developmental stage [47]. Thus, CycA plays an important role in cell cycle in *Drosophila* GSCs, and we also found CycB overexpression has no detectable phenotype in GSCs. In addition, we found CycA regulated GSC differentiation in a Bam-dependent manner, which is evident by the results that ectopic expression of Bam in GSCs would increase the stability of CycA, and down-regulation of CycA antagonized the function of ectopic Bam in GSCs. These results suggested that changes in CycA level are sufficient to explain the loss of GSCs when expressing Bam ectopically. Consistent with the previous study, they found that ectopic expression of the stable form of CycA in germ cells caused GSC loss, which is similar to the phenotype resulting from ectopic expression of Bam in GSCs [36,48]. Ji et al. convincingly showed that ectopic expression of Bam in GSC could be enhanced by co-expression of CycA, and suppressed by CycA reduction [24]. Furthermore, they found CycA can be coimmunoprecipitated with Bam from S2 cells and ovarian extracts [24,46,49]. The relationship between Bam and CycA might be interpreted as the way that Bam functions as a ubiquitin-associated protein to deubiquitinate and stabilize CycA, thereby balancing GSC self-renewal [24]. The results in this study indicated that the Bam–CycA regulatory axis plays an important role in GSC differentiation and cell-cycle alterations in response to the cytotoxicity of CPT, but the detailed regulatory mechanism remains to be further elucidated.

In the female germline, Bam is a key intrinsic regulator of differentiation [50] because Bam RNA appeared shortly after the differentiation of a stem cell that produces new CBs [51]. In the absence of Bam activity, GSC daughters failed to differentiate, and ectopic expression of Bam in GSCs was sufficient to induce GSC loss and led to the accumulation of undifferentiated germ cell tumors [52,53]. In our study, CPT treatment also resulted in accumulation of two-cell cysts, and such differentiation defects were further enhanced by the heterozygous mutation of *bam*. By contrast, heat-shock-induced Bam expression can sufficiently promote the differentiation of two-cell cysts, while reducing CycA can rescue two-cell accumulation caused by CPT treatment, indicating the Bam–CycA axis might also contribute to the two-cell accumulation phenotype. Previous study revealed the *bam* gene was required for the differentiation of CBs from the stem cells, perhaps by altering the cell cycle and stabilizing differentiation factors, such as CycA [51]. Moreover, Bam-dependent deubiquitinase complex can disrupt GSC maintenance by targeting CycA, and DNA damage could disrupt Bam-dependent differentiation pathways and cause the accumulation of CB-like cells in a Lok-dependent manner [54]. Based on those facts, we hypothesized that CPT treatment could regulate the expression of Bam, and the alterations in Bam expression are sufficient to trigger the transcription program of the cysts following differentiation, leading to cell arrest at G1/S and two-cell accumulation probably via affecting CycA.

4. Materials and Methods

4.1. *Drosophila Stocks*

D. melanogaster was reared by standard *Drosophila* medium. All fly stocks were maintained at 25 °C and a related humidity of 60% with 1:1 (light:dark) photoperiod. For each treatment group, newly emerged adults (<24 h) were placed into a vial containing standard media and were applied 100 mg/L CPT for 9 days. DMSO treated flies were considered as the control. The genotypes of the mutant lines used in this study were: *w1118* (used as wild-type control), *dpp2.0-lacZ* [55], *Bam-GFP* [50], *pz1444*, *nos-gal4 vp16*, *hs-bam* (a gift from Yu Cai [Temasek Life Sciences Laboratory, National University of Singapore, Singapore), *uas-top1*^{RNAi} (Bloomington, BL#55314), *bam*^{86} (Bloomington, BL#5427), FUCCI (*UASp-GFP-E2F11–230*; *UASp-mRFP1-cycB1–266*, Bloomington, BL#55101), *hs-cycA* (Bloomington, BL#91660), *hs-cycB* (Bloomington, BL#91664), *UAS-cycE*^{RNAi} (Bloomington, BL#29314). All crosses were maintained at room temperature. For heat-shock stock, crosses were maintained at 25 °C. The flies were heat-shocked for 1 h at 37 °C following CPT treatment for 9 days, followed by 24 h recovery at room temperature. Additionally, the dissection and immunostaining were performed.

4.2. *Survival Analysis*

Twenty adult flies (male:female = 1:1, 24 h post emergence) were placed in vials with or without CPT and maintained at 25 °C. The number of flies was counted every day and the mortality was calculated after all the flies died.

4.3. *Fecundity Examination*

Twenty adult flies (male:female = 1:1, 24 h post emergence) were placed in vials with or without CPT and the number of eggs laid at the 9th d post treatment was collected and counted. The egg production was measured within 24 h and three independent trials were performed.

4.4. *Immunostaining*

After the ovaries of female flies were dissected in PBS, the tissues were fixed with 4% paraformaldehyde (PFA) for 20 min at room temperature, rinsed with PBT (0.1% Triton X-100 in PBS) three times for 10 min each, blocked in 5% NGS (Normal goat serum) for 1 h, and incubated with primary antibodies overnight. Then, the samples were washed three times with PBT for 10 min each. After incubation with secondary antibody for 3 h, the tissues were stained with Hoechst for 10 min, and washed again with PBT 3 times.

The primary antibodies used in this study were listed as follows: rabbit anti-pMad (1:800; Cell Signaling Technology, Danvers, MA, USA), rabbit anti-Caspase 3 (1:2000, Cell Signaling Technology, USA), rabbit anti-pErk (1:400; Cell Signaling Technology, USA) mouse anti-lacZ (1:10,000; abcam, Cambridge, UK), and rabbit anti-LacZ (1:10,000; abcam, UK). Other antibodies were purchased from Temasek Life Sciences Laboratory, including mouse anti-3A9, rabbit anti-α-Spectrin [56], mouse anti-Bam, chicken anti-GFP, rabbit anti-Tkv [32], guinea pig anti-Vasa, mouse anti-Arm, mouse anti-En, rat anti-Fluorescein (FITC), Cy3- and Cy5-goat against rabbit, mouse, chicken, rat and guinea pig secondary antibodies were purchased from Jackson Immuno Research Laboratories (West Grove, PA,

USA), Inc. The DNA dye used was Hoechst 33258 (1:5000; Cell Signaling Technology, USA). Samples were analyzed with an upright confocal microscopy.

For TUNEL (Roche, # 12156792910, Penzberg, Germany), the ovaries were dissected in PBS, and fixed in 4% PFA for 1 h. After washing three times with PBS for 10 min each, the tissues were incubated in Permeabilization solution for 2 min on ice. In total, 5 μL of enzyme solution was added to the 45 μL label solution to obtain 50 μL TUNEL reaction mixture, and this was shaken for 1 h at 37 °C, and then we continued with immunostaining procedures as mentioned previously.

4.5. In Situ Hybridization

For in situ hybridization, the probes were labeled by Roche DIG RNA labeling kit (Roche, #11175025910, Germany) following instructions of the manufacturer. Ovaries were dissected in PBS, and then fixed in 4% PFA overnight. After washing 3 times with PBT (PBS + 0.1% Tween 20), the tissues were again washed with methanol/PBT for 5 min and rinsed three times with PBT. After the samples were rinsed with 1:1 hybridization buffer/PBT for 5 min, 100% hybridization buffer for 5 min, and three times with PBT for 5 min each, respectively, the DIG-labeled RNA probes were pre-hybridized at 100 °C for 1 h prior to hybridization. For the hybridization, the tissues were incubated overnight with a probe at 60 °C. After hybridization, to wash off the unspecific binding, the tissues were rinsed with washing buffer four times for 30 min, and then washed with MABT buffer two times for 10 min. After blocking with 5% blocking solution, the tissues were incubated with anti-DIG-POD (1:200; Roche) in PBT (with 0.5% blocking solution) overnight. After washing with MABT for 1 h, we added 1 μL diluted fluo-dye (Roche) in amplification buffer into the tissue solution and kept it at room temperature for 1.5 h. Following the procedures of in situ hybridization, the immunostaining was carried out as previously mentioned [28]. Observations were carried out with an upright confocal microscopy.

4.6. Statistical Analysis

The data analyses were performed using SPSS software. The differences between two samples were analyzed by Student's *t*-test (* $p < 0.05$, ** $p < 0.01$, *** $p < 0.001$, **** $p < 0.0001$).

5. Conclusions

In this study, we unveiled the cytotoxicity of CPT in GSC loss and two-cell differentiation defects, which could provide information for its therapeutic application. CPT could induce ectopic expression of Bam in GSCs via top1, and such a phenotype could be enhanced by overexpression of CycA, which might contribute to the observed GSC loss. In addition, CPT can cause DNA damage in the early germline cell by regulating Bam expression at both transcript and protein level, thus leading to cell arrest at G1/S and two-cell accumulation. Collectively, the results in this study provided convincing results that CPT may have therapeutic potential as an anticancer agent in germ cells. Further study is needed to evaluate the safety of CPT in advanced models to confirm the mechanism in germline cells of other organisms.

Supplementary Materials: The following supporting information can be downloaded at: https://www.mdpi.com/article/10.3390/ijms24021617/s1.

Author Contributions: Conceptualization, J.Z. and Z.S.; methodology, J.Z., Z.S., S.Z. and Y.C.; validation, G.Z.; formal analysis, J.Z., G.Z. and X.Y.; investigation, J.Z., Z.S. and Y.C.; data curation, J.Z., Y.C. and X.Y.; writing—original draft, J.Z. and X.Y.; writing—review and editing, J.Z.; supervision, G.Z. All authors have read and agreed to the published version of the manuscript.

Funding: This research was funded by National natural science foundation of China (No. 31572335) and National natural science foundation of Guangdong Province (No. 2021A1515110795).

Institutional Review Board Statement: Not applicable.

Data Availability Statement: All data generated or analyzed during this study are included in this published article and its Supplementary Materials. Reagents used in this publication will be provided upon request.

Conflicts of Interest: The authors declare no conflict of interest.

Abbreviations

CPT, Camptothecin; GSC, germline stem cell; Bam, bag of marbles; CycA, cyclin A; top1, topoisomerase I; CB, cystoblast; TF, terminal filament; Cpc, cap cell; ECs, escort cells; Dpp, Decapentaplegic; Hh, Hedgehog; Upd, Unpaired; En, Engrailed; Arm, armadillo; CycB, cyclin B; CycE, cyclin E; PFA, paraformaldehyde; TUNEL, Terminal deoxynucleotidyl transferase-mediated dUTP Nick End Labeling.

References

1. Li, F.; Jiang, T.; Li, Q.; Ling, X. Camptothecin (CPT) and its derivatives are known to target topoisomerase I (Top1) as their mechanism of action: Did we miss something in CPT analogue molecular targets for treating human disease such as cancer? *Am. J. Cancer Res.* **2017**, *7*, 2350.
2. Morham, S.G.; Kluckman, K.D.; Voulomanos, N.; Smithies, O. Targeted disruption of the mouse topoisomerase I gene by camptothecin selection. *Mol. Cell. Biol.* **1996**, *16*, 6804–6809. [CrossRef]
3. Sloan, R.; Huang, S.N.; Pommier, Y.; Jinks-Robertson, S. Effects of camptothecin or TOP1 overexpression on genetic stability in Saccharomyces cerevisiae. *DNA Repair* **2017**, *59*, 69–75. [CrossRef] [PubMed]
4. Baker, N.M.; Rajan, R.; Mondragon, A. Structural studies of type I topoisomerases. *Nucleic Acids Res.* **2009**, *37*, 693–701. [CrossRef] [PubMed]
5. Ray Chaudhuri, A.; Hashimoto, Y.; Herrador, R.; Neelsen, K.J.; Fachinetti, D.; Bermejo, R.; Cocito, A.; Costanzo, V.; Lopes, M. Topoisomerase I poisoning results in PARP-mediated replication fork reversal. *Nat. Struct. Mol. Biol.* **2012**, *19*, 417–423. [CrossRef] [PubMed]
6. Jayasooriya, R.G.; Dilshara, M.G.; Molagoda, I.M.; Park, C.; Park, S.R.; Lee, S.; Choi, Y.H.; Kim, G.Y. Camptothecin induces G2/M phase arrest through the ATM-Chk2-Cdc25C axis as a result of autophagy-induced cytoprotection: Implications of reactive oxygen species. *Oncotarget* **2018**, *9*, 21744–21757. [CrossRef]
7. Pommier, Y. Repair of and checkpoint response to topoisomerase I-mediated DNA damage. *Mutat. Res. Fundam. Mol. Mech. Mutagen.* **2003**, *532*, 173–203. [CrossRef]
8. Goldwasser, F.; Shimizu, T.; Jackman, J.; Hoki, Y.; O'Connor, P.M.; Kohn, K.W.; Pommier, Y. Correlations between S and G2 arrest and the cytotoxicity of camptothecin in human colon carcinoma cells. *Cancer Res.* **1996**, *56*, 4430–4437.
9. Adachi, S.; Ogasawara, T.; Yamasaki, N.; Shibahara, H.; Kanazawa, R.; Tsuji, Y.; Takemura, T.; Koyama, K. A pilot study of CPT-11 and cisplatin for ovarian clear cell adenocarcinoma. *Jpn. J. Clin. Oncol.* **1999**, *29*, 434–437. [CrossRef]
10. Khaiwa, N.; Maarouf, N.R.; Darwish, M.H.; Alhamad, D.W.; Sebastian, A.; Hamad, M.; Omar, H.A.; Orive, G.; Al-Tel, T.H. Camptothecin's journey from discovery to WHO Essential Medicine: Fifty years of promise. *Eur. J. Med. Chem.* **2021**, *223*, 113639. [CrossRef]
11. Li, J.; Chen, W.; Zhang, P.; Li, N. Topoisomerase II trapping agent teniposide induces apoptosis and G2/M or S phase arrest of oral squamous cell carcinoma. *World J. Surg. Oncol.* **2006**, *4*, 41. [CrossRef]
12. Moertel, C.G.; Schutt, A.J.; Reitemeier, R.; Hahn, R. Phase Il Study of Camptothecin (NSC-100880) in the Treatment. *Cancer Chemother. Rep.* **1972**, *56*, 95–101. [PubMed]
13. Xia, L.; Jia, S.; Huang, S.; Wang, H.; Zhu, Y.; Mu, Y.; Kan, L.; Zheng, W.; Wu, D.; Li, X.; et al. The Fused/Smurf complex controls the fate of *Drosophila* germline stem cells by generating a gradient BMP response. *Cell* **2010**, *143*, 978–990. [CrossRef] [PubMed]
14. Nelson, J.O.; Chen, C.; Yamashita, Y.M. Germline stem cell homeostasis. *Curr. Top. Dev. Biol.* **2019**, *135*, 203–244.
15. Shen, R.; Weng, C.; Yu, J.; Xie, T. eIF4A controls germline stem cell self-renewal by directly inhibiting BAM function in the *Drosophila* ovary. *Proc. Natl. Acad. Sci. USA* **2009**, *106*, 11623–11628. [CrossRef]
16. Hsu, H.J.; Bahader, M.; Lai, C.M. Molecular control of the female germline stem cell niche size in *Drosophila*. *Cell. Mol. Life Sci.* **2019**, *76*, 4309–4317. [CrossRef] [PubMed]
17. Xi, R.; Doan, C.; Liu, D.; Xie, T. Pelota controls self-renewal of germline stem cells by repressing a Bam-independent differentiation pathway. *Development* **2005**, *132*, 5365–5374. [CrossRef]
18. Decotto, E.; Spradling, A.C. The *Drosophila* ovarian and testis stem cell niches: Similar somatic stem cells and signals. *Dev. Cell* **2005**, *9*, 501–510. [CrossRef] [PubMed]
19. Fu, Z.; Geng, C.; Wang, H.; Yang, Z.; Weng, C.; Li, H.; Deng, L.; Liu, L.; Liu, N.; Ni, J.; et al. Twin Promotes the Maintenance and Differentiation of Germline Stem Cell Lineage through Modulation of Multiple Pathways. *Cell Rep.* **2015**, *13*, 1366–1379. [CrossRef] [PubMed]

20. Wang, Z.; Lin, H. The division of *Drosophila* germline stem cells and their precursors requires a specific cyclin. *Curr. Biol.* **2005**, *15*, 328–333. [CrossRef]
21. Hsu, H.J.; Drummond-Barbosa, D. Insulin signals control the competence of the *Drosophila* female germline stem cell niche to respond to Notch ligands. *Dev. Biol.* **2011**, *350*, 290–300. [CrossRef]
22. Artoni, F.; Kreipke, R.E.; Palmeira, O.; Dixon, C.; Goldberg, Z.; Ruohola-Baker, H. Loss of foxo rescues stem cell aging in *Drosophila* germ line. *Elife* **2017**, *6*, e27842. [CrossRef]
23. Xing, Y.; Su, T.T.; Ruohola-Baker, H. Tie-mediated signal from apoptotic cells protects stem cells in *Drosophila melanogaster*. *Nat. Commun.* **2015**, *6*, 7058. [CrossRef] [PubMed]
24. Ji, S.; Li, C.; Hu, L.; Liu, K.; Mei, J.; Luo, Y.; Tao, Y.; Xia, Z.; Sun, Q.; Chen, D. Bam-dependent deubiquitinase complex can disrupt germ-line stem cell maintenance by targeting cyclin A. *Proc. Natl. Acad. Sci. USA* **2017**, *114*, 6316–6321. [CrossRef] [PubMed]
25. Shi, J.; Jin, Z.; Yu, Y.; Zhang, Y.; Yang, F.; Huang, H.; Cai, T.; Xi, R. A Progressive Somatic Cell Niche Regulates Germline Cyst Differentiation in the *Drosophila* Ovary. *Curr. Biol.* **2021**, *31*, 840–852. [CrossRef]
26. Kirilly, D.; Wang, S.; Xie, T. Self-maintained escort cells form a germline stem cell differentiation niche. *Development* **2011**, *138*, 5087–5097. [CrossRef] [PubMed]
27. Tastan, Ö.Y.; Maines, J.Z.; Li, Y.; Mckearin, D.M.; Buszczak, M. *Drosophila* Ataxin 2-binding protein 1 marks an intermediate step in the molecular differentiation of female germline cysts. *Development* **2010**, *137*, 3167–3176. [CrossRef]
28. Losick, V.P.; Morris, L.X.; Fox, D.T.; Spradling, A. *Drosophila* stem cell niches: A decade of discovery suggests a unified view of stem cell regulation. *Dev. Cell* **2011**, *21*, 159–171. [CrossRef]
29. Luo, L.; Siah, C.K.; Cai, Y. Engrailed acts with Nejire to control decapentaplegic expression in the *Drosophila* ovarian stem cell niche. *Development* **2017**, *144*, 3224–3231. [CrossRef]
30. Hamada-Kawaguchi, N.; Nore, B.F.; Kuwada, Y.; Smith, C.I.E.; Yamamoto, D. Btk29A Promotes Wnt4 Signaling in the Niche to Terminate Germ Cell Proliferation in *Drosophila*. *Science* **2014**, *343*, 294–297. [CrossRef]
31. Gonzalez-Reyes, A. Stem cells, niches and cadherins: A view from *Drosophila*. *J. Cell Sci.* **2003**, *116*, 949–954. [CrossRef]
32. Luo, L.; Wang, H.; Fan, C.; Liu, S.; Cai, Y. Wnt ligands regulate Tkv expression to constrain Dpp activity in the *Drosophila* ovarian stem cell niche. *J. Cell Biol.* **2015**, *209*, 595–608. [CrossRef] [PubMed]
33. Sperka, T.; Wang, J.; Rudolph, K.L. DNA damage checkpoints in stem cells, ageing and cancer. *Nat. Rev. Mol. Cell Biol.* **2012**, *13*, 579–590. [CrossRef] [PubMed]
34. Lord, C.J.; Ashworth, A. The DNA damage response and cancer therapy. *Nature* **2012**, *481*, 287–294. [CrossRef] [PubMed]
35. Zielke, N.; Korzelius, J.; van Straaten, M.; Bender, K.; Schuhknecht, G.F.; Dutta, D.; Xiang, J.; Edgar, B.A. Fly-FUCCI: A versatile tool for studying cell proliferation in complex tissues. *Cell Rep.* **2014**, *7*, 588–598. [CrossRef]
36. Mathieu, J.; Huynh, J. Bam and Otu can regulate stem cell fate by stabilizing cyclin A. *Proc. Natl. Acad. Sci. USA* **2017**, *114*, 6154–6156. [CrossRef]
37. Chen, G.; Wang, Z.W.; Wen, P.; Wei, W.; Chen, Y.; Ai, H.; Sun, W.B. Hydrocarbons mediate seed dispersal: A new mechanism of vespicochory. *New Phytol.* **2018**, *220*, 714–725. [CrossRef] [PubMed]
38. Pommier, Y. Topoisomerase I inhibitors: Camptothecins and beyond. *Nat. Rev. Cancer* **2006**, *6*, 789–802. [CrossRef]
39. Park, D.S.; Morris, E.J.; Greene, L.A.; Geller, H.M. G1/S cell cycle blockers and inhibitors of cyclin-dependent kinases suppress camptothecin-induced neuronal apoptosis. *J. Neurosci.* **1997**, *17*, 1256–1270. [CrossRef]
40. Walowsky, C.; Fitzhugh, D.J.; Castaño, I.B.; Ju, J.Y.; Levin, N.A.; Christman, M.F. The Topoisomerase-related Function Gene TRF4 Affects Cellular Sensitivity to the Antitumor Agent Camptothecin. *J. Biol. Chem.* **1999**, *274*, 7302–7308. [CrossRef]
41. Kroep, J.R.; Gelderblom, H. Diflomotecan, a promising homocamptothecin for cancer therapy. *Expert Opin. Investig. Drugs* **2009**, *18*, 69–75. [CrossRef] [PubMed]
42. Moukharskaya, J.; Verschraegen, C. Topoisomerase 1 Inhibitors and Cancer Therapy. *Hematol. Oncol. Clin. N. Am.* **2012**, *26*, 507–525. [CrossRef]
43. Bailly, C. Topoisomerase I poisons and suppressors as anticancer drugs. *Curr. Med. Chem.* **2000**, *7*, 39–58. [CrossRef] [PubMed]
44. Drummond-Barbosa, D. Local and Physiological Control of Germline Stem Cell Lineages in *Drosophila melanogaster*. *Genetics* **2019**, *213*, 9–26. [CrossRef]
45. Nishida, M.; Tsunoda, H.; Ichikawa, Y.; Yoshikawa, H. Complete response to irinotecan hydrochloride and nedaplatin in a patient with advanced ovarian clear cell carcinoma. *Int. J. Clin. Oncol.* **2004**, *9*, 403–405. [CrossRef] [PubMed]
46. Drummond-Barbosa, E.T.A.A. Cyclin E controls *Drosophila* female germline stem cell maintenance independently of its role in proliferation by modulating responsiveness to niche signals. *Development* **2013**, *140*, 530–540.
47. Novak, B.; Tyson, J.J.; Gyorffy, B.; Csikasz-Nagy, A. Irreversible cell-cycle transitions are due to systems-level feedback. *Nat. Cell Biol.* **2007**, *9*, 724–728. [CrossRef]
48. Lilly, M.A.; de Cuevas, M.; Spradling, A.C. Cyclin A associates with the fusome during germline cyst formation in the *Drosophila* ovary. *Dev. Biol.* **2000**, *218*, 53–63. [CrossRef]
49. Flora, P.; Schowalter, S.; Wong-Deyrup, S.; DeGennaro, M.; Nasrallah, M.A.; Rangan, P. Transient transcriptional silencing alters the cell cycle to promote germline stem cell differentiation in *Drosophila*. *Dev. Biol.* **2018**, *434*, 84–95. [CrossRef]
50. Chen, D.; McKearin, D.M. A discrete transcriptional silencer in the bam gene determines asymmetric division of the *Drosophila* germline stem cell. *Development* **2003**, *130*, 1159–1170. [CrossRef]

51. McKearin, D.M.; Spradling, A.C. bag-of-marbles: A *Drosophila* gene required to initiate both male and female gametogenesis. *Genes Dev.* **1990**, *4*, 2242–2251. [CrossRef] [PubMed]
52. Li, Y.; Minor, N.T.; Park, J.K.; McKearin, D.M.; Maines, J.Z. Bam and Bgcn antagonize Nanos-dependent germ-line stem cell maintenance. *Proc. Natl. Acad. Sci. USA* **2009**, *106*, 9304–9309. [CrossRef] [PubMed]
53. Ohlstein, B.; McKearin, D. Ectopic expression of the *Drosophila* Bam protein eliminates oogenic germline stem cells. *Development* **1997**, *124*, 3651–3662. [CrossRef] [PubMed]
54. Ma, X.; Han, Y.; Song, X.; Do, T.; Yang, Z.; Ni, J.; Xie, T. DNA damage-induced Lok/CHK2 activation compromises germline stem cell self-renewal and lineage differentiation. *Development* **2016**, *143*, 4312–4323. [PubMed]
55. Jiang, J.; Struhl, G. Protein kinase A and hedgehog signaling in *Drosophila* limb development. *Cell* **1995**, *80*, 563–572. [CrossRef]
56. Liu, Z.; Zhong, G.; Chai, P.C.; Luo, L.; Liu, S.; Yang, Y.; Baeg, G.H.; Cai, Y. Coordinated niche-associated signals promote germline homeostasis in the *Drosophila* ovary. *J. Cell Biol.* **2015**, *211*, 469–484. [CrossRef]

International Journal of
Molecular Sciences

MDPI

Article

JI017 Induces Cell Autophagy and Apoptosis via Elevated Levels of Reactive Oxygen Species in Human Lung Cancer Cells

Jin Mo Ku [1], Min Jeong Kim [2], Yu-Jeong Choi [2], Seo Yeon Lee [2], Ji-Yeong Im [3], Yong-Kyu Jo [4], Sanghoon Yoon [5], Ji-Hyun Kim [4], Jie Won Cha [5], Yong Cheol Shin [1] and Seong-Gyu Ko [1,*]

1 Department of Preventive Medicine, College of Korean Medicine, Kyung Hee University, 1 Hoegi, Seoul 130-701, Republic of Korea; saory_ykm@naver.com (J.M.K.); syc99@khu.ac.kr (Y.C.S.)
2 Department of Science in Korean Medicine, Graduate School, Kyung Hee University, Seoul 130-701, Republic of Korea; jung8328@hanmail.net (M.J.K.); ehowlqk11@naver.com (Y.-J.C.); dltjdus0225@naver.com (S.Y.L.)
3 Department of Clinical Korean Medicine, Graduate School, Kyung Hee University, Seoul 130-701, Republic of Korea; jyhani@naver.com
4 Department of Korean Medicine, Graduate School, Kyung Hee University, Seoul 130-701, Republic of Korea; ykcho0707@hanmail.net (Y.-K.J.); jhvoice@hanmail.net (J.-H.K.)
5 Department of Applied Korean Medicine, Graduate School, College of Korean Medicine, Kyung Hee University, Seoul 130-701, Republic of Korea; chin9yaaaa@gmail.com (S.Y.); goldfish310@hanmail.net (J.W.C.)
* Correspondence: epiko@khu.ac.kr; Tel.: +82-2-961-0329; Fax: +82-2-966-1165

Abstract: Lung cancer is one of the most common malignant tumors and a leading cause of cancer-related death in the worldwide. Various anticancer drugs, such as cisplatin and pemetrexed, have been developed for lung cancer treatment but due their drug resistance and side effects, novel treatments need to be developed. In this study, the efficacy of the natural drug JI017, which is known to have few side effects, was tested in lung cancer cells. JI017 inhibited A549, H460, and H1299 cell proliferation. JI017 induced apoptosis, regulated apoptotic molecules, and inhibited colony formation. Additionally, JI017 increased intracellular ROS generation. JI017 downregulated PI3K, AKT, and mTOR expression. JI017 increased the cytosolic accumulation of LC3. We found that JI017 promoted apoptosis through ROS-induced autophagy. Additionally, the xenograft tumor size was smaller in JI017-treated mice. We found that JI017 treatment increased MDA concentrations, decreased Ki-67 protein levels, and increased cleaved caspase-3 and LC3 levels in vivo. JI017 decreased cell proliferation and increased apoptosis by inducing autophagy signaling in H460 and H1299 lung cancer cells. Targeting JI017 and autophagy signaling could be useful in lung cancer treatment.

Keywords: autophagy; JI017; lung cancer; ROS

Citation: Ku, J.M.; Kim, M.J.; Choi, Y.-J.; Lee, S.Y.; Im, J.-Y.; Jo, Y.-K.; Yoon, S.; Kim, J.-H.; Cha, J.W.; Shin, Y.C.; et al. JI017 Induces Cell Autophagy and Apoptosis via Elevated Levels of Reactive Oxygen Species in Human Lung Cancer Cells. *Int. J. Mol. Sci.* **2023**, *24*, 7528. https://doi.org/10.3390/ijms24087528

Academic Editors: Barbara De Filippis, Marialuigia Fantacuzzi and Alessandra Ammazzalorso

Received: 5 April 2023
Revised: 15 April 2023
Accepted: 18 April 2023
Published: 19 April 2023

1. Introduction

Lung cancer is one of the most common malignant tumors and a leading cause of cancer-related death in the worldwide in both males and females, excluding sex-specific cancers [1]. Lung cancer is heterogenous in terms of pathological features: small-cell lung cancer (SCLC) accounts for ~14% of lung cancer patients and non-small cell lung cancer (NSCLC) accounts for ~82% of lung cancer patients [2,3]. The emergence of novel therapeutic methods has significantly improved the treatment of NSCLC, but the prognosis is still not good, and the overall 5-year survival rate of NSCLC patients is only 19.3% [4,5]. Various anticancer drugs, such as pemetrexed and cisplatin, have been used for the treatment of lung cancer, but these anticancer drugs cause acute kidney damage through nephrotoxicity and oxidative damage and cause side effects due to toxicity [6–9]. Therefore, the development of new therapeutic drugs with fewer side effects is necessary.

Autophagy is the process of removing damaged proteins and organelles within cells and recycling intracellular materials and energy, and this mechanism plays an important role in maintaining intracellular homeostasis [10–14]. Autophagy is activated in injury and disease in response to stresses such as nutrient deprivation, infection, and certain signaling pathways and contributes to cell survival [15,16]. Excessive autophagy is known to induce apoptosis [17]. For example, combined treatment with docetaxel and curcumin induces the apoptosis of malignant esophageal squamous cell carcinoma cells by increasing autophagy [18]. LC3 is a major participant in autophagy, and at initiation, the protein complex LC3-I is degraded to LC3-II, recruited into autophagosomes, and interacts with p62 [19]. Then, the formation of the lysosomal complex then leads to total proteolysis [20].

Reactive oxygen species (ROS) are highly reactive molecules formed from diatomic oxygen that are natural byproducts of normal oxygen metabolism, and they play an important role in homeostasis in the body [21]. Cellular stress caused by changes in the external environment dramatically increases intracellular ROS concentrations, which can cause severe damage to cellular structures, resulting in oxidative damage. Additionally, increased ROS levels are accompanied by apoptosis [22–24]. Therefore, ROS are an indicator of cellular stress and apoptosis [25,26]. Moreover, they are known to be important regulators of autophagy activation, and targeting increased autophagy and ROS production has been identified as a novel therapeutic approach for the treatment of several types of cancer [27,28].

Recently, studies on the anticancer effects of natural products have been conducted, and interest in natural product-derived medicines is increasing [29–32]. According to our previous report, *Angelica gigas* (*Ag*), *Zingiber officinale Roscoe* (*Zo*), and *Aconitum carmichaeli* (*Ac*) showed anticancer effects in the cell lines of several cancers, including brain, breast, prostate, colorectal, skin, and pancreatic cancer [33–38]. Furthermore, it is known that natural treatments for various inflammatory diseases and obesity have neuroprotective effects [39–41]. Decursin-inhibited tumor progression in head and neck squamous cell, as well as the active compound of *Ag*, induces apoptosis by inhibiting the PI3K–Akt axis in HeLa cells [42,43]. Among the active compounds of *Zo*, 6-gingerol suppresses tumor cell proliferation by blocking the nuclear translocation of HIF-1α in lung cancer [44].

Although the anticancer effects of JI017 are known, the efficacy of JI017 treatment for NSCLC has not yet been evaluated. In this study, we investigated whether JI017 exhibits NSCLC cell death and cell growth inhibitory effects. In addition, we analyzed the protein signaling pathway to elucidate the mechanism by which JI017 treats NSCLC.

2. Results

2.1. *JI017-Induced Apoptosis and Inhibited Proliferation in Lung Cancer Cells*

JI017 is known to be an effective anticancer drug for prostate, ovarian, and breast cancer [45–48]. Therefore, we investigated the effect of JI017 treatment on cell viability in several lung cancer cell lines. A549, H460, and H1299 cells were treated with different concentrations of JI017 for 24 h. Cell viability was then measured by MTS assay. We found that JI017 treatment significantly suppressed cell growth in a dose-dependent manner (Figure 1A). Additionally, JI017 treatment significantly reduced colony formation (Figure 1B). Moreover, cell migration was decreased in the JI017 treatment group compared to the control group (Figure 1C).

To investigate whether JI017 induces apoptosis, we performed an annexin V-FITC/PI assay in A549, H460, and H1299 cells. As expected, we found that the JI017 treatment group had an increased apoptosis rate in A549, H460, and H1299 cells, with apoptotic cell ratios of 9 to 56%, 10 to 88%, and 11 to 71%, respectively (Figure 1D). To confirm that caspase activation is induced by JI017 and is involved in apoptosis, we measured the expression of apoptotic molecules through Western blot analysis. We found that JI017 decreased the levels of Bcl-2 in A549, H460, and H1299 cells. Additionally, we found that JI017 increased the levels of Bax, cleaved caspase-3, cleaved caspase-8, cleaved caspase-9, and cleaved PARP in A549, H460, and H1299 cells (Figure 1E). These results confirmed that JI017 induced apoptosis through the apoptotic mechanisms of Bax, Bcl-2, caspase-3, caspase-8, and PARP in A549, H460, and H1299 cells.

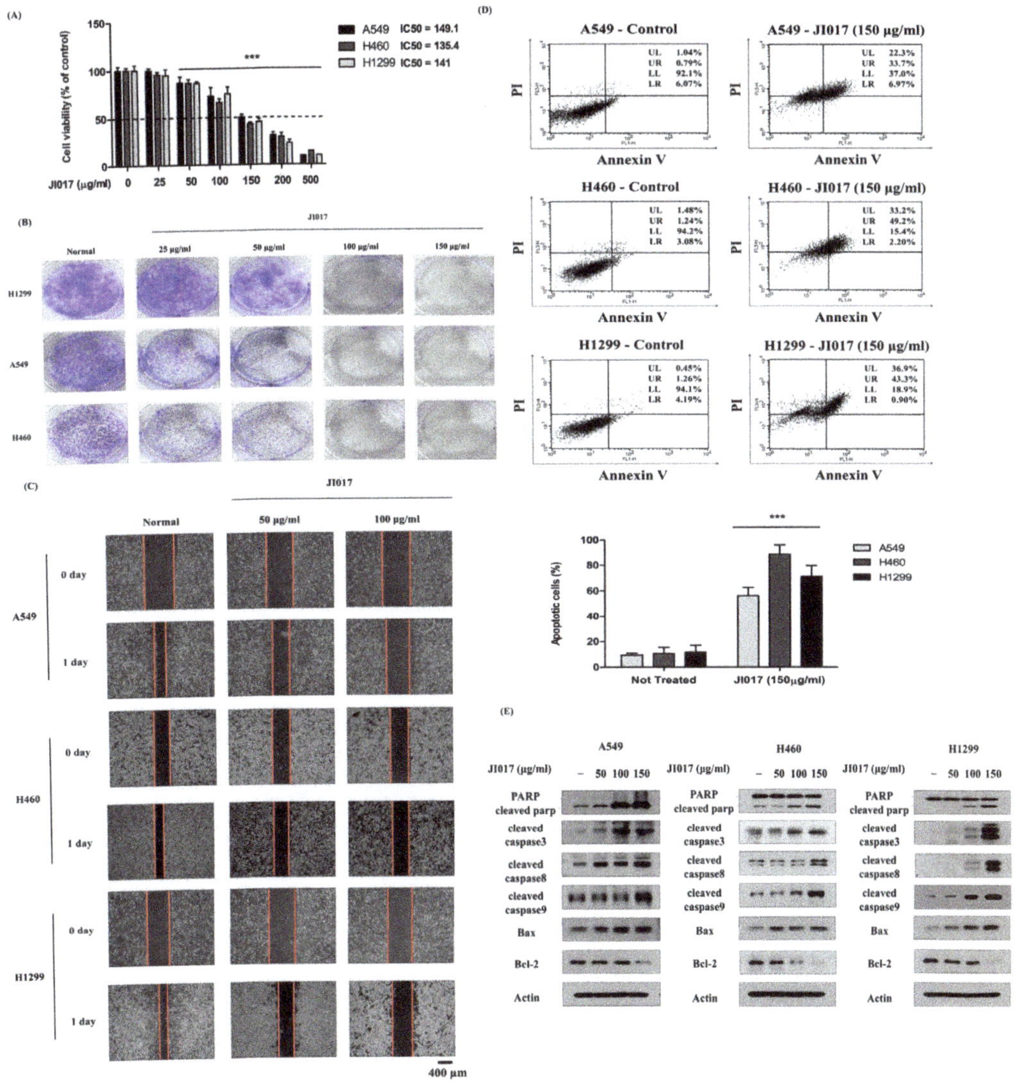

Figure 1. Effect of JI017 on A549, H460, and H1299 cell viability. (**A**) Cells were treated with different concentrations of JI017 for 24 h. (**B**) Cell viability was then measured using the MTS assay. H460, A549, and H1299 cells were treated with JI017 and exposed for 7 days, then the effect on cell growth was assessed using a colony formation assay. (**C**) The migration of JI017-treated cells was assessed using a wound-healing assay. Intervals between cells are marked with red lines. Scale bar = 400 μm. (**D**) H460 and H1299 cells were treated with JI017 for 24 h, stained with Annexin V/PI, and analyzed by flow cytometry. (**E**) Whole cell lysates were analyzed by Western blotting with anti-PARP; anti-cleaved caspase 3, -8, and -9; and anti-Bax, anti-Bcl-2, and anti-Actin antibodies. Data are presented as the mean ± SEM. *** $p < 0.001$ compared to untreated cells.

2.2. JI017 Increased the Generation of Intracellular ROS

ROS is a small molecule, and it is primarily involved in several signaling pathways, and excessive ROS accumulation can induce lipid, nucleic acid, protein, and DNA damage and affect cancer cells to promote apoptosis [23,24]. We used the fluorescent dye

2′,7′-dichlorofluorescein diacetate (DCFH-DA) to measure ROS levels in lung cancer cells. The cells were treated with JI017 (150 μg/mL) or pretreatment with the ROS inhibitor NAC and JI017 for 24 h and labeled with DCFH-DA. The analysis measured signal intensity using a flow cytometer. JI017 treatment increased the DCFH-DA signal intensity in lung cancer cells. JI017 treatment combined with NAC pretreatment decreased the signal intensity of DCFH-DA in H460 and H1299 cells (Figure 2A). As a result, we confirmed that JI017 induced intracellular ROS generation. Additionally, we investigated whether ROS generated by JI017 mediated apoptosis. We added JI017 (150 μg/mL) to H460 and H1299 cells pretreated with NAC and performed MTS. JI017 treatment combined with NAC pretreatment decreased cell death was compared with that of JI017 treatment alone in H460 and H1299 cells (Figure 2B). Moreover, the cells treated with both JI017 and NAC showed decreased levels of the apoptosis markers cleaved caspase3 and cleaved PARP compared with those in the cells treated with JI017 alone (Figure 2C). These results suggested that JI017 induced apoptosis by increasing ROS production in lung cancer cells.

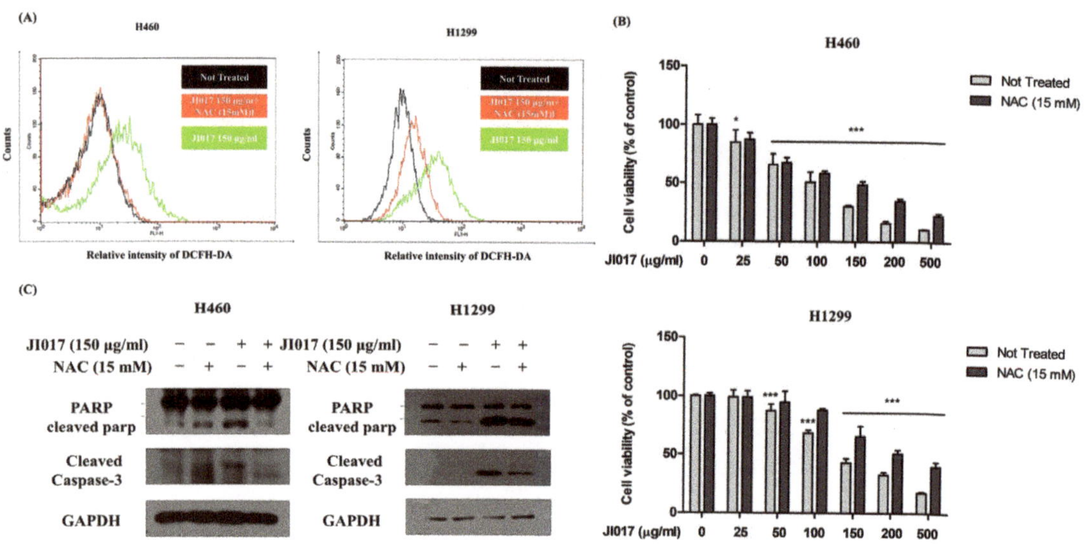

Figure 2. Effect of JI017 in A549, H460, and H1299 ROS accumulation. (**A**) Treatment with JI017 (150 μg/mL) in H460 and H1299 cells for 24 h; they were labeled with DCFH-DA (10 μM) for 30 min. Additionally, intracellular ROS levels were determined by flow cytometry. Pretreatment with NAC (15 mM) for 1 h was followed by treatment with various concentrations of JI017. (**B**) Cell viability was measured using the MTS assay. (**C**) Whole cell lysates were analyzed by Western blotting with anti-PARP, anti-cleaved caspase 3, and anti-GAPDH antibodies. Data are presented as the mean ± SEM. * $p < 0.05$ and *** $p < 0.001$ compared to untreated cells.

2.3. *JI017-Induced Autophagy by Increasing LC3 Levels in H460 and H1299 Cells*

We performed Western blot analysis to evaluate the expression of the PI3K-AKT-mTOR pathway and IF staining analysis to evaluate the expression of LC3. JI017 treatment decreased the levels of PI3K, AKT, and mTOR in H460 and H1299 cells (Figure 3A). The inhibition of mTOR is known to increase autophagy signaling [49]. To investigate whether JI017 induces autophagy, Western blot analysis was used, and it was confirmed in H460 and H1299 cells. The activation of the LC3 protein is a marker of autophagy, and we found that JI017 treatment increased the levels of LC3 A/B and p62 (Figure 3B). Additionally, the change in the LC3 level after JI017 treatment time was examined, and it was confirmed that both LC3 and cleaved PARP levels increased after 12 h of treatment with JI017 (Figure 3C). Additionally, the IF staining experiments showed that the cytoplasmic accumulation of

LC3 was increased through JI017 treatment (Figure 3D). The autophagy pathway plays an important role in cancer cell death, and these results suggest that JI017 induces autophagy in lung cancer cells.

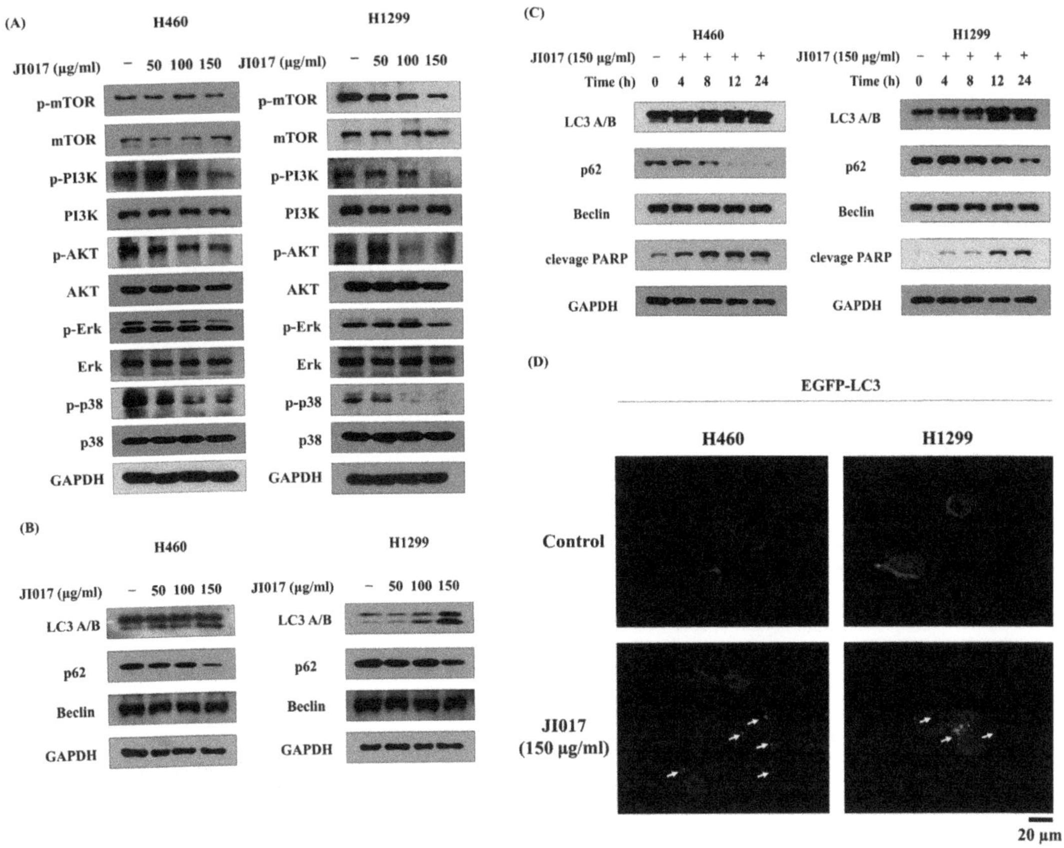

Figure 3. JI017 activated autophagy by suppressing the PI3K-AKT-mTOR pathway in H460 and H1299 cells. H460 and H1299 cells were treated with JI017 (50, 100, and 150 μg/mL) for 24 h. (**A**,**B**) Whole cell lysates were analyzed by Western blotting. (**C**) H460 and H1299 cells were treated with JI017 (150 ng/mL) for different times (4, 8, 12, and 24 h). (**D**) H460 and H1299 cells transfected with the pEGFP-LC3 vector were treated with JI017 (150 μg/mL) for 8 h. The Fluorescence microscopy analysis confirmed positive staining of LC3B puncta. LC3B puncta are indicated by white arrows. Scale bar = 20 μm.

2.4. *JI017 Induced Autophagy through Increased ROS Production in H460 and H1299 Cells*

3MA is known to inhibit the autophagy pathway in the early stage, and chloroquine and Bafilomycin in the late stage [50–52]. Therefore, we treated H460 and H1299 cells with 3MA (2 mM) or chloroquine (100 μM) in combination with JI017 (150 μg/mL) and performed Western blot analysis. We found that 3MA treatment reduced the elevated LC3 levels induced by JI017 administration. Moreover, cells treated with JI017 and 3MA or chloroquine exhibited reduced levels of caspase3 cleavage and PARP cleavage compared to cells treated with JI017 alone, confirming reduced apoptosis (Figure 4A). To investigate whether JI017-induced apoptosis is regulated by autophagy inhibition, we compared cell viability after treatment with 3MA, bafilomycin, and chloroquine. Compared with JI017 treatment alone, JI017 treatment combined with 3MA or Bafilomycin or chloroquine decreased cell death by approximately 20% in H460 and H1299 cells (Figure 4B). Moreover, cells treated with JI017 combined with NAC decreased the level of LC3 compared with the cells treated with JI017 alone (Figure 2C). These results suggested that JI017 promoted apoptosis through ROS-induced autophagy in H460 and H1299 cells.

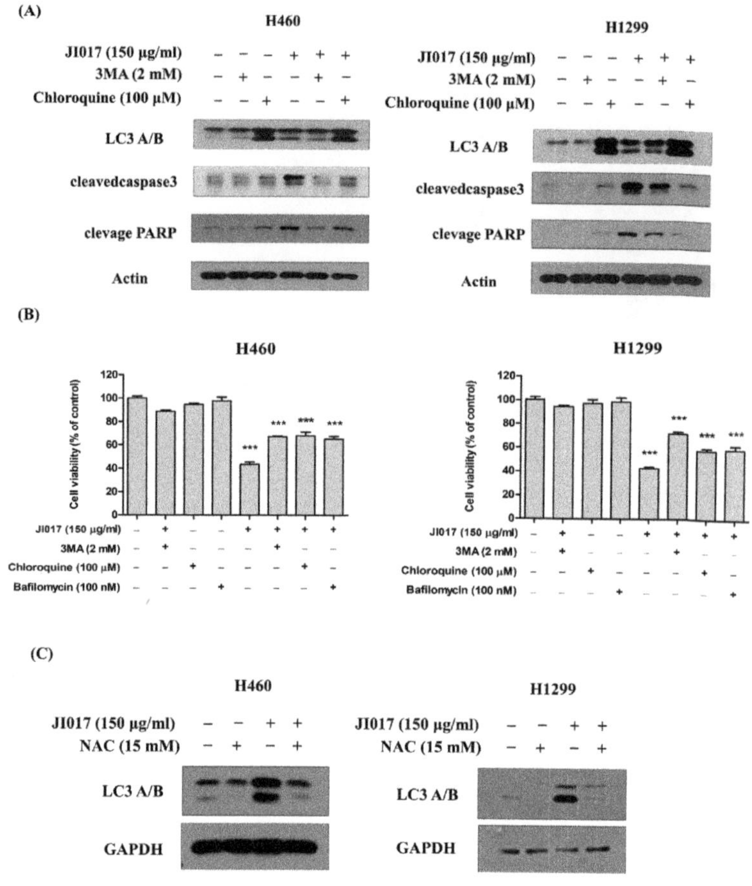

Figure 4. JI017 induced apoptosis through an autophagy pathway and ROS generation. (A) H460 and H1299 cells were treated with 3MA (2 mM) or chloroquine (100 μM) combined with JI017 (150 μg/mL). 3MA, chloroquine, or bafilomycin treatment was followed by treatment with JI017. (B) Cell viability was measured using MTS assay. (C) H460 and H1299 cells were treated with NAC (15 mM) and JI017 (150 μg/mL). Whole cell lysates were analyzed by Western blotting with anti-LC3 and anti-GAPDH antibodies. Data are presented as the mean ± SEM. *** $p < 0.001$ compared to untreated cells.

2.5. Effect of JI017 Suppressed Cell Growth In Vivo

To further confirm the efficacy of JI017 for inhibiting cell growth in animal experiments, H460 cells were subcutaneously injected into nude mice. We did not find any change in body weight in the control group and the JI017-treated group (Figure 5A). The sizes of xenograft tumors in the JI017-treated mice were smaller compared to the xenograft tumors in the control mice, and the tumor suppression rate was 79.2%. These results indicated JI107 treatment slowed the tumor growth rate (Figure 5B,C). Because ROS reacts easily with lipids, free radical formation can be confirmed through lipid peroxidation markers. The peroxidation of membrane lipids can alter physical properties, such as lipid interaction, ion gradient, membrane fluidity, and permeability [53]. We found that JI017 treatment increased MDA concentrations in vivo (Figure 5D). Moreover, the addition of JI017 increased the levels of LC3 and cleaved caspase3 (Figure 5E). These results showed that the protein levels of Ki-67 decreased and the protein levels of cleaved caspase-3 and LC3 increased in the JI017-treated group compared to the control group (Figure 5F). Overall, the above results show that JI017 induced ROS in vivo and inhibited lung cancer cell proliferation and tumor growth.

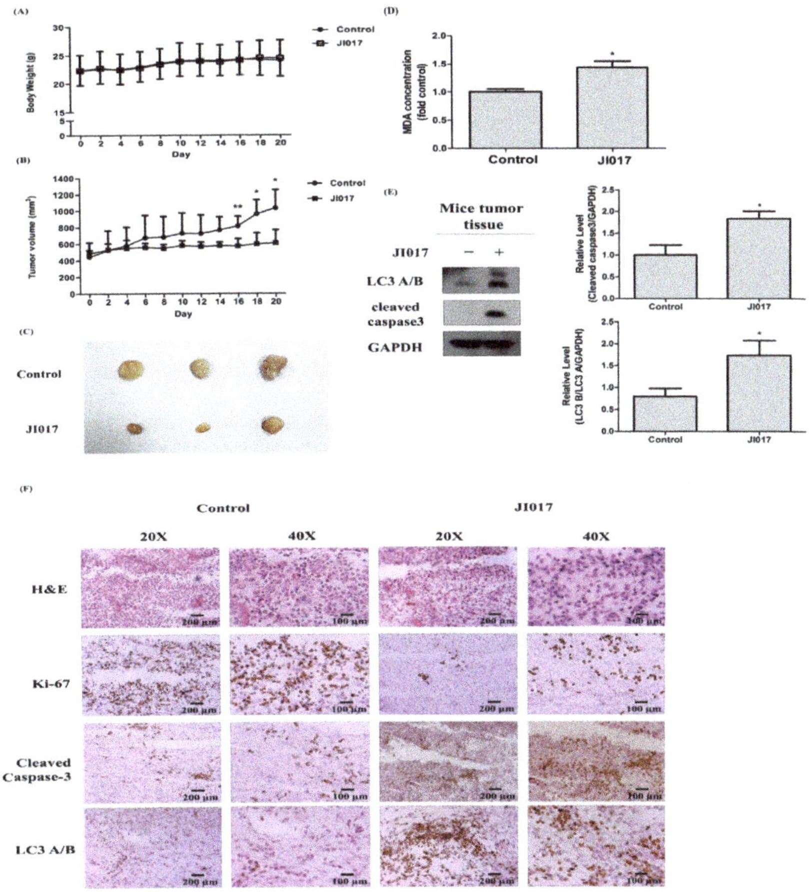

Figure 5. JI017 suppressed lung cancer cell growth in mice. BALB/c nude mice were subcutaneously injected with H460 cells. (**A**) The mouse body weight and (**B**) the tumor growth rate are shown. (**C**) Representative tumor images of the control group and the JI017-treated group. (**D**) The MDA concentration was assessed by a thiobarbituric reactive substance (TBARS) assay and normalized to the protein concentration. (**E**) Whole tissue lysates were analyzed by Western blotting with anti-LC3, anti-cleaved caspase 3, and anti-GAPDH antibodies. (**F**) The IHC staining of Ki-67 and cleaved caspase-3 and LC3 was carried out. Scale bar = 200 µm for 20× and Scale bar = 100 µm for 40×. The data are expressed as the mean ± SEM in all groups (n = 8–11). * $p < 0.05$ and ** $p < 0.01$ compared to the untreated group.

3. Discussion

In this study, we found that treatment with JI017 in H460 and H1299 cells induced apoptosis by increasing autophagy pathway signaling. Although various anticancer drugs have been developed to treat lung cancer, new therapies are needed due to their many side effects. Recently, many studies have investigated anticancer effects through autophagy activity [54,55].

Additionally, interest in natural product-derived drugs is increasing in the pharmaceutical industry because of their low side effects [29,30,32]. Thus, our drug is a good suitable candidate for the treatment of human lung cancer.

It was reported that JI017 exerts anticancer effects and, thus, has potential as a new drug that death of cancer cells and inhibits cancer cell growth [45,48]. JI017 is a combination of *Ag*, *Zo*, and *Ac*, and its anti-cancer treatment effects have been reported through various mechanisms. Unlike simply confirming the active compound of a natural product, in a new compound, as a natural product complex, various effects are shown, and as a result, the treatment mechanism is multi-faceted, so there are still many areas to be studied. Therefore, we investigated the effect of JI017 treatment on lung cancer cells. We investigated whether JI017 treatment affected cell viability in H460 and H1299 cells and found that JI017 treatment significantly inhibited cell growth. In addition, growth inhibition was accompanied by the inhibition of cell migration and colony formation. We confirmed cancer cell apoptosis using flow cytometry after staining with annexin V/PI and analyzed protein changes in the apoptosis mechanism through Western blotting experiments. We found that JI017 treatment decreased the levels of Bcl-2 in A549, H460, and H1299 cells. Additionally, we found that the JI017 treatment of A549, H460 and H1299 cells increased the levels of Bax, cleaved caspase-3, cleaved caspase-8, cleaved caspase-9, and cleaved PARP, known as the markers of apoptosis. These results suggested that JI017 induced apoptosis in lung cancer cells.

Excessive ROS accumulation is known to promote apoptosis [56]. We evaluated the level of ROS in lung cancer cells using the fluorescent dye 2′,7′-dichlorofluorescein diacetate (DCFH-DA). We confirmed that JI017 treatment increased intracellular ROS generation. In addition, pretreatment with NAC, a ROS inhibitor, and treatment with JI017 decreased the rate of apoptosis, and we confirmed that the levels of caspase 3 and cleaved PARP, which are markers of apoptosis, were reduced in H460 and H1299 cells. These results suggested that JI017 induced apoptosis by ROS production in lung cancers.

We investigated the pathway by which JI017 induced ROS accumulation and apoptosis in H460 and H1299 cells using Western blotting. The PI3K/Akt pathway is a representative regulator of growth, proliferation, the cell cycle, metastasis, apoptosis, and autophagy [57–59]. The inhibition of the PI3K/AKT/mTOR pathway can result in cell survival or death via autophagy or apoptosis, respectively [60–64]. JI017 decreased the levels of PI3K, AKT, and mTOR in H460 and H1299 cells. Therefore, we investigated whether JI017 induced autophagy using Western blot assay and IF staining analysis. We found that JI017 regulated LC3 A/B and p62 expression. The change in the LC3 level after JI017 treatment time was examined, and it was confirmed that the LC3 level and the cleavage of PARP increased after 12 h of treatment with JI017. Additionally, through IF staining results, it was confirmed that JI017 treatment increased the cytoplasmic accumulation of LC3 in cells. These results suggest that JI017 treatment induces autophagy and results in apoptosis in lung cancer. We treated JI017 with 3MA and chloroquine, which are autophagy inhibitors, to verify that JI017 induced apoptosis through the autophagy pathway. We found that 3MA reduced LC3 levels that increased with JI017 treatment. Moreover, cells treated with JI017 combined with 3MA or Bafilomycin or chloroquine showed decreased levels of apoptosis markers and cell death compared with those in cells treated with JI017 alone. In addition, cells treated with JI017 in combination with NAC exhibited reduced levels of LC3 compared to those in cells treated with JI017 alone, suggesting that JI017 promoted apoptosis through ROS-induced autophagy in H460 and H1299 cells (Figure 6). Moreover, we subcutaneously injected H460 cells into nude mice to confirm that JI017 has an inhibitory effect on lung cancer in vivo. Compared to control mice, the xenograft tumors in JI017-treated mice showed a lower growth rate and a TGI value of 79.2%. We found that JI017 treatment increased the MDA concentration in tumor tissues in vivo, and as a result, we determined that it induced ROS generation. Additionally, in the JI017 treatment group, the protein level of Ki-67 was decreased, and the protein levels of cleaved caspase-3 and LC3 were increased. Collectively, these findings suggested that JI017 inhibited lung cancer proliferation and tumor growth in vivo. JI017 clearly induced apoptosis in human lung cancer cells, making it a useful compound in the treatment of lung cancer. Additionally, targeting autophagy to treat lung cancer could be a useful therapeutic mechanism. Our study clearly demonstrates that the anticancer effect of JI017 in human lung cancer cells occurs through ROS-induced autophagy signaling. As a new natural compound anti-cancer treatment, we think that additional research on various mechanisms should be conducted.

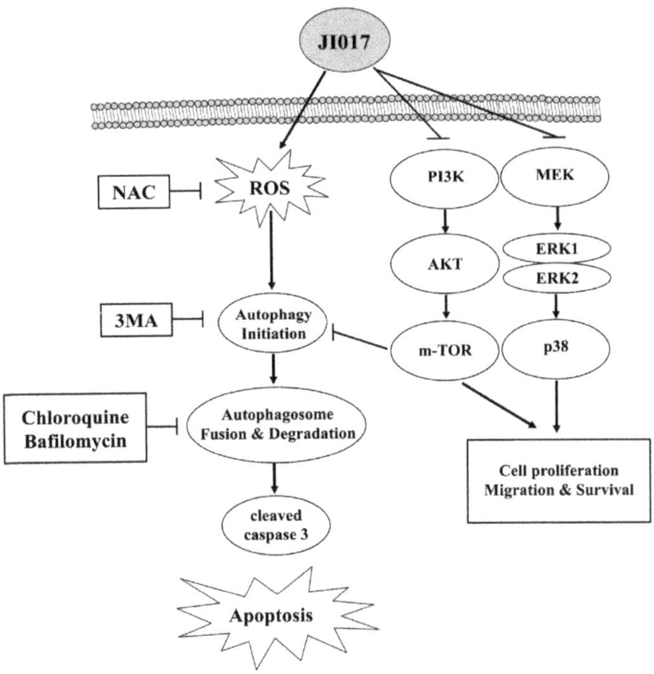

Figure 6. Mechanistic pathway diagram for the autophagy activation potency of JI017 through AKT, ERK inhibition, and ROS induction in lung cancer.

4. Materials and Methods

4.1. Reagents

JI017 consists of *Ag*, *Ac*, and *Zo* components that were supplied by the Jaseng Hospital of Korean Medicine (Seoul, Republic of Korea). The roots were boiled for 3 h in distilled 70% ethanol. The extract was filtrated twice through Whatman grade 2 qualitative filter paper (GE Healthcare Life Sciences, Marlborough, MA, USA) to remove any insoluble materials. The filtrated extract was lyophilized to a powder using a freeze dryer (IlShinBioBase, Dongducheonsi, Gyeonggi, Republic of Korea) and stored at 4 °C. The dried extract was then dissolved in dimethyl sulfoxide (DMSO).

4.2. Cell Culture

A549, H460, and H1299 human lung cancer cells obtained from the American Type Culture Collection (ATCC) were maintained in RPMI 1640 or F-12K medium supplemented with 10% heat-inactivated fetal bovine serum (Invitrogen, Carlsbad, CA, USA) and 100 U/mL antibiotics–antimycotics (Invitrogen). Cells were maintained at 37 °C in a humidified incubator with 5% CO_2.

4.3. Cell Viability Assay

An MTS assay was performed to determine cell viability. To accomplish this, cells (A549, H460, and H1299 cells) were seeded into a 96-well plate at a density of 3×10^3 cells per well and treated 24 h later with varying concentrations of JI017 (25–500 μg/mL) for an additional 24 h. Ten microliters of MTS solution was added to each well of the plate, which was incubated in the dark at 37 °C for another 1 h 30 min. Optical density was measured at 450 nm using an ELISA plate reader (Versa Max, Molecular Devices, San Jose, CA, USA).

4.4. Flow Cytometric Analysis

Flow cytometry was used to analyze cell cycle distribution. Cells were seeded in 60 mm dishes. After 24 h, cells were cultured for an additional 24 h in the absence (control) or presence of JI017 (50–150 μg/mL). Trypsinized cells were washed with PBS and fixed in 95% ethanol containing 0.5% Tween-20 overnight at −20 °C. After washing with PBS, the cells were then incubated with 1 U/mL RNase A and 10 μg/mL PI for 30 min at room temperature in the dark. The DNA content in each cell nucleus was determined by a FACSCalibur flow cytometer (Becton-Dickinson, San Jose, CA, USA), and the cell cycle was analyzed using ModFit LT V2.0 software.

4.5. Annexin V-FITC Apoptosis Assay

Flow cytometry was used to analyze cell apoptosis. Cells were cultured in 60 mm dishes. After 24 h, cells were cultured for an additional 24 h in the absence (control) or presence of JI017 (50–150 μg/mL). Annexin V-FITC/PI double staining Apoptosis Detection Kit was purchased from Invitrogen (Waltham, MA, USA), and apoptosis assay was performed using a flow cytometer according to the manufacturer's instructions.

4.6. Colony Formation Assay

The cells were plated into 6-well culture plates at a density of 1×10^3 cells/well. After 24 h, cells were cultured for an additional 10 d in the absence (control) or presence of JI017 (25, 50, 100, and 150 μg/mL) to allow colony formation. Colonies were stained with a 1% crystal violet solution (Amersco, Solon, OH, USA).

4.7. Western Blot Analysis

Cells were harvested, lysed with cell lysis buffer (50 mM Tris-Cl pH 7.4, 1% NP-40, 0.25% sodium deoxycholate, 0.1% SDS, 150 mM NaCl, 1 mM EDTA, and protease inhibitor) for 20 min and centrifuged at 13,000 rpm (4 °C) for 20 min. Twenty micrograms of protein were separated by SDS-polyacrylamide gel electrophoresis and transferred to a nitrocellulose membrane (Protran nitrocellulose membrane, Whatman, UK). The membrane was blocked with 5% nonfat milk, probed with specific primary antibodies, incubated with HRP-conjugated secondary IgG antibodies (Calbiochem, San Diego, CA, USA), and visualized using an enhanced chemiluminescence detection system (Amersham ECL kit, Amersham Pharmacia Biotech Inc., Piscataway, NJ, USA). Antibodies against cleaved caspase-8, -3, and -9; GAPDH; p38; phospho-Akt; phospho-mTOR; phospho-PI3K; and total Akt were obtained from Cell Signaling (Danvers, MA, USA). Antibodies against actin, Bax, Bcl-2, Beclin, PARP/p85, phospho-Erk, phospho-p38, total Erk, and total mTOR were obtained from Santa Cruz Biotechnology (Dallas, TX, USA). The anti-PI3K antibody was obtained from Merck Millipore (Burlington, MA, USA). The anti-LC3 antibody was obtained from Novus Biologicals (Centennial, CO, USA). The anti-p62 antibody was obtained from Abcam (Cambridge, UK).

4.8. Quantification of Autophagy

Autophagy was quantified by counting the percentage of cells showing the accumulation of GFP-LC3 in vacuoles. Cells presenting a mostly diffuse distribution of GFP-LC3 in the cytoplasm and nucleus were considered non-autophagic, whereas cells representing several intense punctate GFP-LC3 aggregates with no nuclear GFP-LC3 were classified as autophagic. Cells were fixed with paraformaldehyde (4% *w/v*) for GFP-LC3 and immunofluorescence assays. Images were acquired using confocal microscopy (Carl Zeiss, Oberkochen, Germany).

4.9. Lipid Peroxidation Measurement

Lipid peroxidation was measured using the Lipid Peroxidation (MDA) Assay Kit (Sigma-Aldrich, St. Louis, MO, USA) according to the manufacturer's instructions. Extensive oxidative species generation can lead to the formation of malondialdehyde (MDA) as a result of the peroxidation of polyunsaturated fatty acids (PUFAs), which contain at least three double bonds. MDA can react with thiobarbituric acid (TBA) to form a colorimetric, as well a fluorescent, product, which is a well-known biomarker of the peroxidation of polyunsaturated lipids [65]. The tissues were lysed on ice using MDA lysis buffer containing 3 μL of butylated hydroxytoluene (BHT), and the samples were centrifuged at 13,000× *g* for 10 min. Next, a TBA solution was added and incubated at 95 °C for 60 min. The samples were chilled to room temperature in an ice bath for 10 min and transferred to a black bottomed 96-well plate. Optical density was measured at 532 nm using an ELISA plate reader.

4.10. Animal Studies

All animal experiment procedures were approved by the Kyung Hee University Institutional Animal Care and Use Committee (KHSASP-20-250). Five-week-old male BALB/C nu/nu mice were obtained from Raonbio (Seoul, Republic of Korea). The mice were maintained for 1 week under controlled temperature (23 ± 3 °C) and humidity (55 ± 15%) in a 12 h light/12 h dark cycle before initiating the experiment. Then, H460 cells were harvested and injected subcutaneously (5.0×10^6 cells in 100 μL 1:1 PBS:Matrigel solution) into the right flank of the mice. When the xenografts reached a volume of 80–100 mm^3, the animals were randomized into 2 groups (n = 6): the control group (saline) and the JI017 treatment group (500 mg/kg). The animals in the JI017 treatment group were treated with JI017 by oral administration every 2 days. Tumor sizes were measured every 2 days for changes in tumor growth, and tumor volumes were calculated using a standard formula: 1/2 (length × $width^2$). Mice were sacrificed using carbon dioxide, followed by cervical dislocation, and the tumor tissue was isolated for further study, such as immunohistochemical (IHC) analyses.

4.11. IHC Analysis

To examine the protein expression of tumor-related genes in tumor tissue section samples, each serial frozen section was dried at RT for 20 min. After hydration, the samples were fixed with 4% paraformaldehyde and washed at 4 °C for 5 min. Then, the cells were blocked with bovine serum albumin (3% BSA) and probed with primary antibodies (1:100–1:400) overnight at 4 °C. Proteins were identified using anti-cleaved caspase3 and anti-LC3 and anti-Ki67 antibodies. The next day, the samples were washed and probed with secondary antibody for 30 min at RT. Then, the sections were incubated with Vectastain ABC reagent (Vector Laboratories, Inc., Burlingame, CA, USA, sk4100) for 30 min. Immune complexes were revealed via incubation with 3,3′-diaminobenzidine (DAB) at RT for 1 min based upon the targeted antigen. The sections were counterstained with hematoxylin and dehydrated on slides in 75%, 95%, and 100% ethanol for 1 min each, after which the sections were cleared in xylene for 5 min. Finally, the slides were mounted using mounting medium. Images were acquired using microscopy.

4.12. Statistical Analysis

All experimental data are expressed as the mean ± standard deviation (SD) or mean ± standard error of the mean (SEM) of at least three separate experiments. Statistical significance was determined using a one-way analysis of variance followed by the Tukey—Kramer multiple comparisons posttest to analyze differences between groups. A

p value < 0.05 was considered to indicate a statistically significant difference, and $p < 0.05$, $p < 0.01$, and $p < 0.001$ are assigned separate symbols in the figures. All experiments were performed at least three times. All statistical analyses were performed using PRISM 5 software (GraphPad Software Inc., La Jolla, CA, USA).

5. Conclusions

In this study, we analyzed the effect of JI017 on human lung cancer cells. JI017 treatment induced the activation of autophagy signaling by increasing the generation of intracellular ROS. As a result, JI017 treatment decreased cell viability and caused apoptotic cell death in lung cancer cells. These results support JI017 as a favorable candidate drug for the treatment of human lung cancer.

Author Contributions: J.M.K. carried out the experiments and drafted the manuscript. M.J.K., Y.-J.C. and S.Y.L. revised the research and manuscript and assisted in the research work. J.M.K., M.J.K., Y.-J.C., J.W.C. and S.Y.L. contributed to the design of this study and performed the data analysis. S.Y., J.-H.K., Y.-K.J., J.-Y.I. and J.W.C. assisted with the use of the software. Y.C.S. and S.-G.K. guided the research and revised and submitted the manuscript. S.-G.K. supervised the experiments and corrected the manuscript. All authors have read and agreed to the published version of the manuscript.

Funding: This work was supported by a National Research Foundation of Korea (NRF) grant funded by the Korean government (MSIT) (No. NRF-2020R1A5A2019413).

Institutional Review Board Statement: The animal study protocol was approved by the Kyung Hee University Institutional Animal Care and Use Committee (KHSASP-20-250).

Informed Consent Statement: Not applicable.

Data Availability Statement: All data and materials are contained and described within the manuscript.

Acknowledgments: We thank our colleagues from the Laboratory of Prevention Medicine for protocol assistance and useful discussions.

Conflicts of Interest: The authors declare no conflict of interest.

Abbreviations

Ac, *Aconitum carmichaeli*; *Ag*, *Angelica gigas*; BHT, butylated hydroxytoluene; DAB, 3,3′-Diaminobenzidine; DMSO, dimethyl sulfoxide; EDTA, ethylenediaminetetraacetic acid; FACS, fluorescence-activated cell sorter; FBS, fetal bovine serum; GAPDH, glyceraldehyde 3-phosphate dehydrogenase; IHC, immunohistochemistry; MDA, malondialdehyde; NSCLC, non-small-cell lung cancer; PARP, poly (ADP-ribose) polymerase; PBS, phosphate-buffered saline; PI, propidium iodide; PMSF, phenylmethylsulfonyl fluoride; PUFAs, polyunsaturated fatty acids; ROS, reactive oxygen species; SCLC, small-cell lung cancer; SD, standard deviation; SDS, sodium dodecyl sulphate, TBA, thiobarbituric acid; *Zo*, *Zingiber officinale Roscoe*.

References

1. Goodman, J.E.; Mayfield, D.B.; Becker, R.A.; Hartigan, S.B.; Erraguntla, N.K. Recommendations for further revisions to improve the International Agency for Research on Cancer (IARC) Monograph program. *Regul. Toxicol. Pharmacol.* **2020**, *113*, 104639. [CrossRef] [PubMed]
2. Griffin, R.; Ramirez, R.A. Molecular Targets in Non-Small Cell Lung Cancer. *Ochsner J.* **2017**, *17*, 388–392. [PubMed]
3. Miller, H.A.; van Berkel, V.H.; Frieboes, H.B. Lung cancer survival prediction and biomarker identification with an ensemble machine learning analysis of tumor core biopsy metabolomic data. *Metab. Off. J. Metab. Soc.* **2022**, *18*, 57. [CrossRef] [PubMed]
4. Iqbal, N.; Shukla, N.K.; Deo, S.V.; Agarwala, S.; Sharma, D.N.; Sharma, M.C.; Bakhshi, S. Prognostic factors affecting survival in metastatic soft tissue sarcoma: An analysis of 110 patients. *Clin. Transl. Oncol.* **2016**, *18*, 310–316. [CrossRef] [PubMed]
5. Jonna, S.; Subramaniam, D.S. Molecular diagnostics and targeted therapies in non-small cell lung cancer (NSCLC): An update. *Discov. Med.* **2019**, *27*, 167–170. [PubMed]
6. Farooqui, Z.; Shahid, F.; Khan, A.A.; Khan, F. Oral administration of Nigella sativa oil and thymoquinone attenuates long term cisplatin treatment induced toxicity and oxidative damage in rat kidney. *Biomed. Pharmacother.* **2017**, *96*, 912–923. [CrossRef]

7. Pierson-Marchandise, M.; Gras, V.; Moragny, J.; Micallef, J.; Gaboriau, L.; Picard, S.; Choukroun, G.; Masmoudi, K.; Liabeuf, S.; French National Network of Pharmacovigilance, C. The drugs that mostly frequently induce acute kidney injury: A case—Noncase study of a pharmacovigilance database. *Br. J. Clin. Pharmacol.* **2017**, *83*, 1341–1349. [CrossRef]
8. Rombola, G.; Vaira, F.; Trezzi, M.; Chiappini, N.; Falqui, V.; Londrino, F. Pemetrexed induced acute kidney injury in patients with non-small cell lung cancer: Reversible and chronic renal damage. *J. Nephrol.* **2015**, *28*, 187–191. [CrossRef]
9. Soni, S.; Basu, M.; Agrawal, P.; Kumar, N.; Bhatnagar, A.; Chhillar, N. Multiple parametric approaches to assess acute radiation lung injury of rats radiation lung injury of rats. *Ukr. Biochem. J.* **2016**, *88*, 22–30. [CrossRef]
10. Li, C.; Zhang, Y.; Liu, J.; Kang, R.; Klionsky, D.J.; Tang, D. Mitochondrial DNA stress triggers autophagy-dependent ferroptotic death. *Autophagy* **2021**, *17*, 948–960. [CrossRef]
11. Li, J.; Liu, J.; Xu, Y.; Wu, R.; Chen, X.; Song, X.; Zeh, H.; Kang, R.; Klionsky, D.J.; Wang, X.; et al. Tumor heterogeneity in autophagy-dependent ferroptosis. *Autophagy* **2021**, *17*, 3361–3374. [CrossRef] [PubMed]
12. Li, W.; He, P.; Huang, Y.; Li, Y.F.; Lu, J.; Li, M.; Kurihara, H.; Luo, Z.; Meng, T.; Onishi, M.; et al. Selective autophagy of intracellular organelles: Recent research advances. *Theranostics* **2021**, *11*, 222–256. [CrossRef] [PubMed]
13. Kuma, A.; Hatano, M.; Matsui, M.; Yamamoto, A.; Nakaya, H.; Yoshimori, T.; Ohsumi, Y.; Tokuhisa, T.; Mizushima, N. The role of autophagy during the early neonatal starvation period. *Nature* **2004**, *432*, 1032–1036. [CrossRef] [PubMed]
14. Kim, S.E.; Overholtzer, M. Autophagy proteins regulate cell engulfment mechanisms that participate in cancer. *Semin. Cancer Biol.* **2013**, *23*, 329–336. [CrossRef]
15. Chaudhary, K.; Shinde, R.; Liu, H.; Gnana-Prakasam, J.P.; Veeranan-Karmegam, R.; Huang, L.; Ravishankar, B.; Bradley, J.; Kvirkvelia, N.; McMenamin, M.; et al. Amino acid metabolism inhibits antibody-driven kidney injury by inducing autophagy. *J. Immunol.* **2015**, *194*, 5713–5724. [CrossRef]
16. Jiang, X.; Overholtzer, M.; Thompson, C.B. Autophagy in cellular metabolism and cancer. *J. Clin. Investig.* **2015**, *125*, 47–54. [CrossRef]
17. Chen, C.; Wang, D.; Yu, Y.; Zhao, T.; Min, N.; Wu, Y.; Kang, L.; Zhao, Y.; Du, L.; Zhang, M.; et al. Legumain promotes tubular ferroptosis by facilitating chaperone-mediated autophagy of GPX4 in AKI. *Cell Death Dis.* **2021**, *12*, 65. [CrossRef]
18. Deng, L.; Wu, X.; Zhu, X.; Yu, Z.; Liu, Z.; Wang, J.; Zheng, Y. Combination effect of curcumin with docetaxel on the PI3K/AKT/mTOR pathway to induce autophagy and apoptosis in esophageal squamous cell carcinoma. *Am. J. Transl. Res.* **2021**, *13*, 57–72.
19. Galluzzi, L.; Green, D.R. Autophagy-Independent Functions of the Autophagy Machinery. *Cell* **2019**, *177*, 1682–1699. [CrossRef]
20. Tanida, I.; Ueno, T.; Kominami, E. LC3 conjugation system in mammalian autophagy. *Int. J. Biochem. Cell Biol.* **2004**, *36*, 2503–2518. [CrossRef]
21. Whittington, K.; Harrison, S.C.; Williams, K.M.; Day, J.L.; McLaughlin, E.A.; Hull, M.G.; Ford, W.C. Reactive oxygen species (ROS) production and the outcome of diagnostic tests of sperm function. *Int. J. Androl.* **1999**, *22*, 236–242. [CrossRef] [PubMed]
22. Ullah, A.; Ullah, N.; Nawaz, T.; Aziz, T. Molecular Mechanisms of Sanguinarine in Cancer Prevention and Treatment. *Anti-Cancer Agents Med. Chem.* **2023**, *23*, 765–778. [CrossRef] [PubMed]
23. Joselin, A.P.; Hewitt, S.J.; Callaghan, S.M.; Kim, R.H.; Chung, Y.H.; Mak, T.W.; Shen, J.; Slack, R.S.; Park, D.S. ROS-dependent regulation of Parkin and DJ-1 localization during oxidative stress in neurons. *Hum. Mol. Genet.* **2012**, *21*, 4888–4903. [CrossRef] [PubMed]
24. Mehterov, N.; Balazadeh, S.; Hille, J.; Toneva, V.; Mueller-Roeber, B.; Gechev, T. Oxidative stress provokes distinct transcriptional responses in the stress-tolerant atr7 and stress-sensitive loh2 Arabidopsis thaliana mutants as revealed by multi-parallel quantitative real-time PCR analysis of ROS marker and antioxidant genes. *Plant Physiol. Biochem.* **2012**, *59*, 20–29. [CrossRef] [PubMed]
25. Shin, D.Y.; Kim, G.Y.; Li, W.; Choi, B.T.; Kim, N.D.; Kang, H.S.; Choi, Y.H. Implication of intracellular ROS formation, caspase-3 activation and Egr-1 induction in platycodon D-induced apoptosis of U937 human leukemia cells. *Biomed. Pharmacother.* **2009**, *63*, 86–94. [CrossRef] [PubMed]
26. Ullah, A.; Leong, S.W.; Wang, J.; Wu, Q.; Ghauri, M.A.; Sarwar, A.; Su, Q.; Zhang, Y. Cephalomannine inhibits hypoxia-induced cellular function via the suppression of APEX1/HIF-1alpha interaction in lung cancer. *Cell Death Dis.* **2021**, *12*, 490. [CrossRef] [PubMed]
27. Wang, L.; Fu, X.; Hyun, J.; Xu, J.; Gao, X.; Jeon, Y.J. In Vitro and In Vivo Protective Effects of Agaro-Oligosaccharides against Hydrogen Peroxide-Stimulated Oxidative Stress. *Polymers* **2023**, *15*, 1612. [CrossRef]
28. Yang, H.L.; Lin, Y.A.; Pandey, S.; Liao, J.W.; Way, T.D.; Yeh, Y.L.; Chen, S.J.; Hseu, Y.C. In vitro and in vivo anti-tumor activity of Antrodia salmonea against twist-overexpressing HNSCC cells: Induction of ROS-mediated autophagic and apoptotic cell death. *Food Chem. Toxicol.* **2022**, *172*, 113564. [CrossRef]
29. Hafeez, B.B.; Siddiqui, I.A.; Asim, M.; Malik, A.; Afaq, F.; Adhami, V.M.; Saleem, M.; Din, M.; Mukhtar, H. A dietary anthocyanidin delphinidin induces apoptosis of human prostate cancer PC3 cells in vitro and in vivo: Involvement of nuclear factor-kappaB signaling. *Cancer Res.* **2008**, *68*, 8564–8572. [CrossRef]
30. Hafeez, B.B.; Mustafa, A.; Fischer, J.W.; Singh, A.; Zhong, W.; Shekhani, M.O.; Meske, L.; Havighurst, T.; Kim, K.; Verma, A.K. alpha-Mangostin: A dietary antioxidant derived from the pericarp of *Garcinia mangostana* L. inhibits pancreatic tumor growth in xenograft mouse model. *Antioxid. Redox Signal.* **2014**, *21*, 682–699. [CrossRef]

31. Hafeez, B.B.; Fischer, J.W.; Singh, A.; Zhong, W.; Mustafa, A.; Meske, L.; Sheikhani, M.O.; Verma, A.K. Plumbagin Inhibits Prostate Carcinogenesis in Intact and Castrated PTEN Knockout Mice via Targeting PKCepsilon, Stat3, and Epithelial-to-Mesenchymal Transition Markers. *Cancer Prev. Res.* **2015**, *8*, 375–386. [CrossRef] [PubMed]
32. Lall, R.K.; Adhami, V.M.; Mukhtar, H. Dietary flavonoid fisetin for cancer prevention and treatment. *Mol. Nutr. Food Res.* **2016**, *60*, 1396–1405. [CrossRef] [PubMed]
33. Choi, H.S.; Cho, S.G.; Kim, M.K.; Kim, M.S.; Moon, S.H.; Kim, I.H.; Ko, S.G. Decursin in Angelica gigas Nakai (AGN) Enhances Doxorubicin Chemosensitivity in NCI/ADR-RES Ovarian Cancer Cells via Inhibition of P-glycoprotein Expression. *Phytother. Res.* **2016**, *30*, 2020–2026. [CrossRef] [PubMed]
34. Li, J.J.; Chen, W.L.; Wang, J.Y.; Hu, Q.W.; Sun, Z.P.; Zhang, S.; Liu, S.; Han, X.H. Wenshen Zhuanggu formula effectively suppresses breast cancer bone metastases in a mouse Xenograft model. *Acta Pharmacol. Sin.* **2017**, *38*, 1369–1380. [CrossRef] [PubMed]
35. Nedungadi, D.; Binoy, A.; Vinod, V.; Vanuopadath, M.; Nair, S.S.; Nair, B.G.; Mishra, N. Ginger extract activates caspase independent paraptosis in cancer cells via ER stress, mitochondrial dysfunction, AIF translocation and DNA damage. *Nutr. Cancer* **2021**, *73*, 147–159. [CrossRef]
36. Kweon, B.; Han, Y.H.; Kee, J.Y.; Mun, J.G.; Jeon, H.D.; Yoon, D.H.; Choi, B.M.; Hong, S.H. Effect of Angelica gigas Nakai Ethanol Extract and Decursin on Human Pancreatic Cancer Cells. *Molecules* **2020**, *25*, 2028. [CrossRef]
37. Hamza, A.A.; Heeba, G.H.; Hamza, S.; Abdalla, A.; Amin, A. Standardized extract of ginger ameliorates liver cancer by reducing proliferation and inducing apoptosis through inhibition oxidative stress/ inflammation pathway. *Biomed. Pharmacother.* **2021**, *134*, 111102. [CrossRef]
38. Nemoto, Y.; Satoh, K.; Toriizuka, K.; Hirai, Y.; Tobe, T.; Sakagami, H.; Nakashima, H.; Ida, Y. Cytotoxic and radical scavenging activity of blended herbal extracts. *In Vivo* **2002**, *16*, 327–332.
39. Semwal, R.B.; Semwal, D.K.; Combrinck, S.; Viljoen, A.M. Gingerols and shogaols: Important nutraceutical principles from ginger. *Phytochemistry* **2015**, *117*, 554–568. [CrossRef]
40. Zhou, G.; Tang, L.; Zhou, X.; Wang, T.; Kou, Z.; Wang, Z. A review on phytochemistry and pharmacological activities of the processed lateral root of Aconitum carmichaelii Debeaux. *J. Ethnopharmacol.* **2015**, *160*, 173–193. [CrossRef]
41. Sowndhararajan, K.; Kim, S. Neuroprotective and Cognitive Enhancement Potentials of Angelica gigas Nakai Root: A Review. *Sci. Pharm.* **2017**, *85*, 21. [CrossRef] [PubMed]
42. Zhu, M.L.; Li, J.C.; Wang, L.; Zhong, X.; Zhang, Y.W.; Tan, R.Z.; Wang, H.L.; Fan, J.M.; Wang, L. Decursin inhibits the growth of HeLa cervical cancer cells through PI3K/Akt signaling. *J. Asian Nat. Prod. Res.* **2021**, *23*, 584–595. [CrossRef] [PubMed]
43. Joo, M.; Heo, J.B.; Kim, S.; Kim, N.; Jeon, H.J.; An, Y.; Song, G.Y.; Kim, J.M.; Lee, H.J. Decursin inhibits tumor progression in head and neck squamous cell carcinoma by downregulating CXCR7 expression in vitro. *Oncol. Rep.* **2022**, *47*, 39. [CrossRef] [PubMed]
44. Kim, M.J.; Ku, J.M.; Choi, Y.J.; Lee, S.Y.; Hong, S.H.; Kim, H.I.; Shin, Y.C.; Ko, S.G. Reduced HIF-1alpha Stability Induced by 6-Gingerol Inhibits Lung Cancer Growth through the Induction of Cell Death. *Molecules* **2022**, *27*, 2106. [CrossRef]
45. Kim, T.W.; Ko, S.G. The Herbal Formula JI017 Induces ER Stress via Nox4 in Breast Cancer Cells. *Antioxidants* **2021**, *10*, 1881. [CrossRef] [PubMed]
46. Kim, T.; Ko, S.G. JI017, a Complex Herbal Medication, Induces Apoptosis via the Nox4-PERK-CHOP Axis in Ovarian Cancer Cells. *Int. J. Mol. Sci.* **2021**, *22*, 12264. [CrossRef]
47. Lee, J.H.; Ji, H.; Ko, S.G.; Kim, W. JI017 Attenuates Oxaliplatin-Induced Cold Allodynia via Spinal TRPV1 and Astrocytes Inhibition in Mice. *Int. J. Mol. Sci.* **2021**, *22*, 8811. [CrossRef]
48. Kim, M.J.; Ku, J.M.; Hong, S.H.; Kim, H.I.; Kwon, Y.Y.; Park, J.S.; Jung, D.H.; Shin, Y.C.; Ko, S.G. In vitro Anticancer Effects of JI017 on Two Prostate Cancer Cell Lines Involve Endoplasmic Reticulum Stress Mediated by Elevated Levels of Reactive Oxygen Species. *Front. Pharmacol.* **2021**, *12*, 683575. [CrossRef]
49. Wang, R.; Ha, K.Y.; Dhandapani, S.; Kim, Y.J. Biologically synthesized black ginger-selenium nanoparticle induces apoptosis and autophagy of AGS gastric cancer cells by suppressing the PI3K/Akt/mTOR signaling pathway. *J. Nanobiotechnol.* **2022**, *20*, 441. [CrossRef]
50. Vlahos, C.J.; Matter, W.F.; Hui, K.Y.; Brown, R.F. A specific inhibitor of phosphatidylinositol 3-kinase, 2-(4-morpholinyl)-8-phenyl-4H-1-benzopyran-4-one (LY294002). *J. Biol. Chem.* **1994**, *269*, 5241–5248. [CrossRef]
51. Powis, G.; Bonjouklian, R.; Berggren, M.M.; Gallegos, A.; Abraham, R.; Ashendel, C.; Zalkow, L.; Matter, W.F.; Dodge, J.; Grindey, G.; et al. Wortmannin, a potent and selective inhibitor of phosphatidylinositol-3-kinase. *Cancer Res.* **1994**, *54*, 2419–2423. [PubMed]
52. Blommaart, E.F.; Krause, U.; Schellens, J.P.; Vreeling-Sindelarova, H.; Meijer, A.J. The phosphatidylinositol 3-kinase inhibitors wortmannin and LY294002 inhibit autophagy in isolated rat hepatocytes. *Eur. J. Biochem.* **1997**, *243*, 240–246. [CrossRef] [PubMed]
53. Gaschler, M.M.; Stockwell, B.R. Lipid peroxidation in cell death. *Biochem. Biophys. Res. Commun.* **2017**, *482*, 419–425. [CrossRef] [PubMed]
54. Huang, J.; Ye, Y.; Xiao, Y.; Ren, Q.; Zhou, Q.; Zhong, M.; Jiao, L.; Wu, L. Geniposide ameliorates glucocorticoid-induced osteoblast apoptosis by activating autophagy. *Biomed. Pharmacother.* **2022**, *155*, 113829. [CrossRef] [PubMed]
55. Kong, W.; Zhu, H.; Zheng, S.; Yin, G.; Yu, P.; Shan, Y.; Liu, X.; Ying, R.; Zhu, H.; Ma, S. Larotrectinib induces autophagic cell death through AMPK/mTOR signalling in colon cancer. *J. Cell. Mol. Med.* **2022**, *26*, 5539–5550. [CrossRef]

56. She, Y.Y.; Lin, J.J.; Su, J.H.; Chang, T.S.; Wu, Y.J. 4-Carbomethoxyl-10-Epigyrosanoldie E Extracted from Cultured Soft Coral Sinularia sandensis Induced Apoptosis and Autophagy via ROS and Mitochondrial Dysfunction and ER Stress in Oral Cancer Cells. *Oxid. Med. Cell. Longev.* **2022**, *2022*, 3017807. [CrossRef]
57. Alzahrani, A.S. PI3K/Akt/mTOR inhibitors in cancer: At the bench and bedside. *Semin. Cancer Biol.* **2019**, *59*, 125–132. [CrossRef]
58. Pompura, S.L.; Dominguez-Villar, M. The PI3K/AKT signaling pathway in regulatory T-cell development, stability, and function. *J. Leukoc. Biol.* **2018**, *108*, 1065–1076. [CrossRef]
59. Li, H.; Prever, L.; Hirsch, E.; Gulluni, F. Targeting PI3K/AKT/mTOR Signaling Pathway in Breast Cancer. *Cancers* **2021**, *13*, 3517. [CrossRef]
60. Fang, S.; Wan, X.; Zou, X.; Sun, S.; Hao, X.; Liang, C.; Zhang, Z.; Zhang, F.; Sun, B.; Li, H.; et al. Arsenic trioxide induces macrophage autophagy and atheroprotection by regulating ROS-dependent TFEB nuclear translocation and AKT/mTOR pathway. *Cell Death Dis.* **2021**, *12*, 88. [CrossRef]
61. Han, X.; Zhong, Z.; Kou, J.; Zheng, Y.; Liu, Z.; Jiang, Y.; Zhang, Z.; Gao, Z.; Cong, L.; Tian, Y.; et al. ROS Generated by Upconversion Nanoparticle-Mediated Photodynamic Therapy Induces Autophagy Via PI3K/AKT/ mTOR Signaling Pathway in M1 Peritoneal Macrophage. *Cell. Physiol. Biochem.* **2018**, *48*, 1616–1627. [CrossRef] [PubMed]
62. Zhao, J.; Sun, Y.; Shi, P.; Dong, J.N.; Zuo, L.G.; Wang, H.G.; Gong, J.F.; Li, Y.; Gu, L.L.; Li, N.; et al. Celastrol ameliorates experimental colitis in IL-10 deficient mice via the up-regulation of autophagy. *Int. Immunopharmacol.* **2015**, *26*, 221–228. [CrossRef]
63. Lee, H.W.; Jang, K.S.; Choi, H.J.; Jo, A.; Cheong, J.H.; Chun, K.H. Celastrol inhibits gastric cancer growth by induction of apoptosis and autophagy. *BMB Rep.* **2014**, *47*, 697–702. [CrossRef] [PubMed]
64. Guertin, D.A.; Sabatini, D.M. Defining the role of mTOR in cancer. *Cancer Cell* **2007**, *12*, 9–22. [CrossRef] [PubMed]
65. Gueraud, F.; Atalay, M.; Bresgen, N.; Cipak, A.; Eckl, P.M.; Huc, L.; Jouanin, I.; Siems, W.; Uchida, K. Chemistry and biochemistry of lipid peroxidation products. *Free Radic. Res.* **2010**, *44*, 1098–1124. [CrossRef] [PubMed]

International Journal of
Molecular Sciences

MDPI

Article

α-Tocotrienol and Redox-Silent Analogs of Vitamin E Enhances Bortezomib Sensitivity in Solid Cancer Cells through Modulation of NFE2L1

Kyota Ishii [1], Mayuko Hido [2], Misaki Sakamura [2], Nantiga Virgona [3] and Tomohiro Yano [3,*]

1 Laboratory of Molecular Bromacology, Graduate School of Sports Health, Toyo University, Akabane City 115-8650, Japan; s4h202300016@toyo.jp
2 Department of Food and Nutritional Sciences, Faculty of Food and Nutritional Sciences, Toyo University, Itakura 374-0193, Japan; s1c112000217@toyo.jp (M.H.); s1c112000611@toyo.jp (M.S.)
3 Research Institute of Life Innovation, Toyo University, Akabane City 115-8650, Japan; nantigav@yahoo.com.au
* Correspondence: yano_t@toyo.jp; Tel.: +81-276-82-9143

Abstract: Proteasome inhibitors (PIs) have emerged as an attractive novel cancer therapy. However, most solid cancers are seemingly resistant to PIs. The activation of transcription factor Nuclear factor erythroid 2 related factor-1 (NFE2L1) has been characterized as a potential resistance response to protect and restore proteasome activity in cancer cells. In this study, we demonstrated that α-Tocotrienol (T3) and redox-silent analogs of vitamin E (TOS, T3E) enhanced the sensitivity of bortezomib (BTZ), a proteasome inhibitor, in solid cancers through modulation of NFE2L1. In BTZ treatment, all of T3, TOS, and T3E inhibited an increase in the protein levels of NFE2L1, the expression levels of proteasome-related proteins, as well as the recovery of proteasome activity. Moreover, the combination of one of T3, TOS, or T3E and BTZ induced a significant decrease in cell viability in solid cancer cell lines. These findings suggested that the inactivation of NFE2L1 by T3, TOS, and T3E is essential to potentiate the cytotoxic effect of the proteasome inhibitor, BTZ, in solid cancers.

Keywords: vitamin E; NFE2L1; proteasome inhibitor; bortezomib

Citation: Ishii, K.; Hido, M.; Sakamura, M.; Virgona, N.; Yano, T. α-Tocotrienol and Redox-Silent Analogs of Vitamin E Enhances Bortezomib Sensitivity in Solid Cancer Cells through Modulation of NFE2L1. *Int. J. Mol. Sci.* **2023**, *24*, 9382. https://doi.org/10.3390/ijms24119382

Academic Editors: Barbara De Filippis, Alessandra Ammazzalorso and Marialuigia Fantacuzzi

Received: 2 May 2023
Revised: 23 May 2023
Accepted: 24 May 2023
Published: 27 May 2023

1. Introduction

A proteasome is an enzyme complex that plays a role in degrading specific proteins and unnecessary proteins in the cells [1]. Since cancer cells have high expression of proteasome component proteins and higher proteasome activity than normal cells, proteasome may be important for cancer survival and proliferation [2–6]. In accordance with this, proteasome inhibitors (PIs) are known to induce effective cell death and anti-proliferation effect in some cancer cells, with some PIs in use as anticancer drugs for blood cancers like multiple myeloma [7]. Furthermore, PIs are also expected to have therapeutic effects against solid cancers, and the efficacy of PIs in several solid cancers has been investigated. However, some clinical studies have concluded that PIs are ineffectual in the treatment of solid cancers, and it is regarded that solid cancers have PI resistance [8–13].

Recently, Nuclear factor erythroid 2-related factor-1 (NFE2L1) has been identified as a protein involved in PI resistance in cancer cells [14–17]. NFE2L1 is initially present on the endoplasmic reticulum membrane (~120 kDa), and it is released from the endoplasmic reticulum to the cytoplasm by NGLY1, p97 and Hrd1 [18–20]. When proteasome activity is sufficient, cytoplasmic NFE2L1 is generally degraded by the proteasome. However, when the functions of proteasomes are impaired, cytoplasmic NFE2L1 is stabilized and processed into a mature form (~110 kDa) by DDI2 [15,16]. Mature NFE2L1 translocates to the nucleus and induces the expression of proteasome-related genes [21]. They then ultimately recover proteasome activity. Given these facts, the finding of inhibitors of NFE2L1 may lead to improved sensitivity to PI in solid tumors. However, the screening for inhibitors of NFE2L1 has not progressed well.

Vitamin E is a kind of phytochemical that has a long-term historical relationship to cancer. While vitamin E is well regarded as useful for cancer prevention due to its antioxidant effect, tocotrienols, a member of the vitamin E family, and redox-silent analogs of vitamin E such as α-tocopheryl succinate (TOS) and 6-O-Carboxypropyl-alpha-tocotrienol (T3E) are also known to exhibit anticancer effects via inhibition of specific cancer-related molecules such as HIF, Src, and STAT3 [22–27]. Furthermore, previous studies have reported that γ-tocotrienol and T3E modulate the expression levels of some proteasome-component proteins regulated by NFE2L1 [28,29]. Therefore, vitamin E and its redox-silent analogs may affect NFE2L1.

In this study, we demonstrate that α-tocotrienol (T3), TOS, and T3E enhance sensitivity to bortezomib, a proteasome inhibitor, in solid cancer cells through modulating protein levels of NFE2L1.

2. Results

2.1. T3, TOS, and T3E Suppressed the Increase in Protein Levels of NFE2L1 Induced by Bortezomib Treatment

NFE2L1 is known to stabilize and translocate from cytoplasm to nucleus under proteasome inhibition [30]. First, we confirmed the protein levels of NFE2L1 in the cytoplasm and nucleus by immunoblotting. For solid cancer, we used the malignant pleural mesothelioma, H2452, due to its reported resistance to bortezomib [13,31]. As shown in Figure 1a, two bands were identified in the cytoplasmic fraction under bortezomib treatment, and the lower band was clearly identified in the nuclear fraction. Therefore, we assumed that the upper band is unprocessed NFE2L1 without transcriptional activity and the lower band is processed NFE2L1 with transcriptional activity.

Next, we used an immunoblot to evaluate the effect of TP (α-tocopherol), T3, TOS, and T3E on the protein levels of NFE2L1 under bortezomib treatment. As shown in Figure 1b, bortezomib alone demonstrated a significant increase in protein levels of unprocessed and processed NFE2L1 compared to the control group, while the combination group with bortezomib and T3, TOS, and T3E did not show this increase. Also, TOS, and T3E alone groups showed a trend toward a decrease in NFE2L1 protein level. These results suggest that T3, TOS, and T3E modulate protein levels of NFE2L1 under proteasome inhibition.

2.2. T3, TOS, and T3E Suppressed the Increase in Expression Levels of Proteasome-Related Proteins Induced by Bortezomib Treatment

It is known that the expression levels of proteasome-related proteins are increased by NFE2L1 under proteasome inhibition [14,32]. We also speculated that T3, TOS, and T3E might also moderate expression levels of proteasome-related proteins under proteasome inhibition. Consequently, we next evaluated the effects of TP, T3, TOS, and T3E on the expression levels of the proteasome-component proteins, PSMA7, PSMB7, and PSMC4, as well as POMP, a proteasome maturing protein, under bortezomib treatment by RT-PCR assay. As demonstrated in Figure 2a, the bortezomib alone group showed a significant increase in the mRNA expression levels of each protein compared to the control group, while the combination groups of bortezomib with T3, TOS, and T3E did not show as significant an increase as that in the bortezomib alone group. These results suggest that T3, TOS, and T3E modulate the expression levels of proteasome-related proteins under proteasome inhibition.

All figure in this paper is my original.

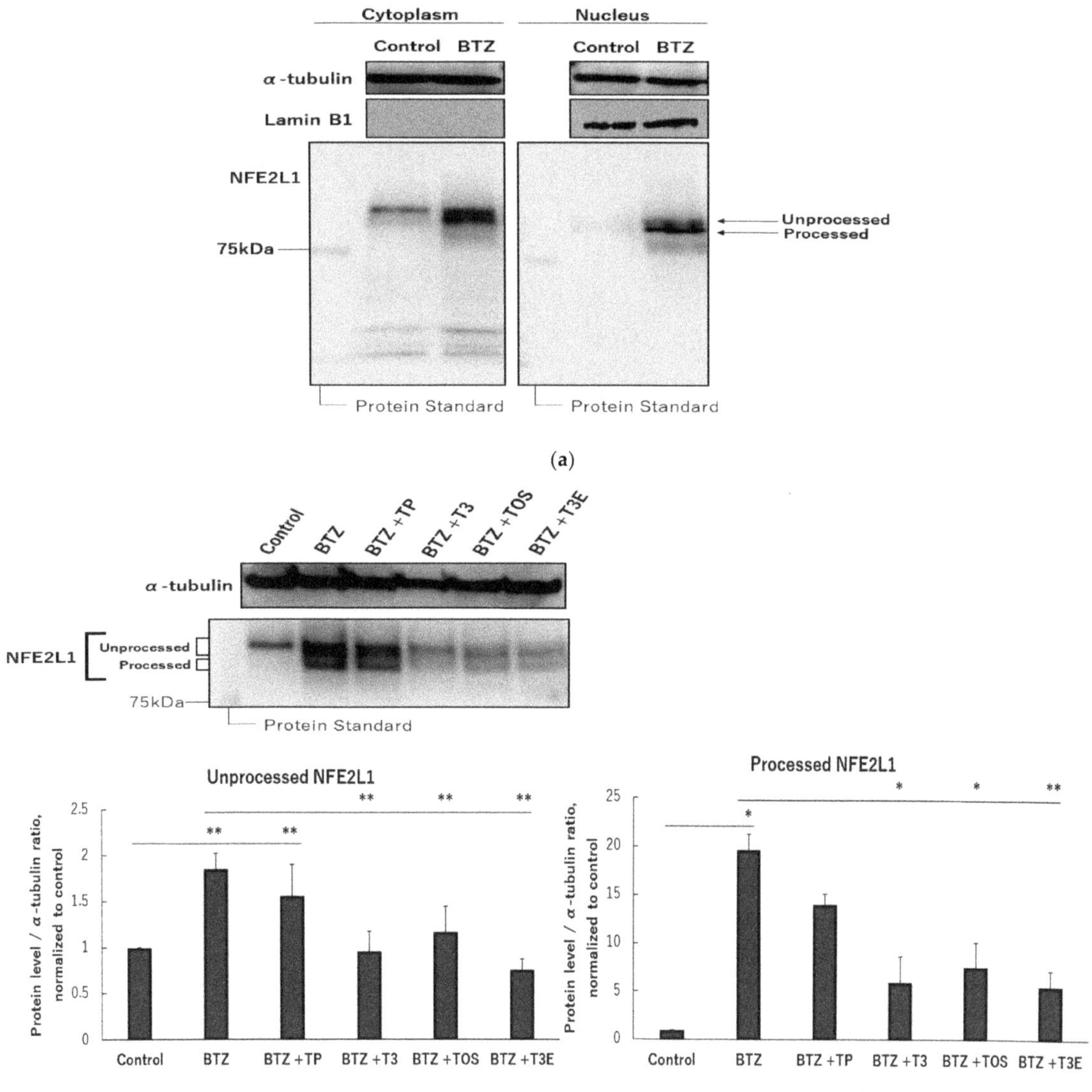

Figure 1. Effects of vitamin E on protein level of NFE2L1 in treatment of bortezomib. (**a**) H2452 cells were treated with bortezomib (50 nM) for 12 h and fractionated into cytoplasm and nucleus by NE-PER™ nuclear and cytoplasmic extract reagent kit. Protein levels in both fractions were assessed by immunoblotting. (**b**) H2452 cells were treated with bortezomib 50 nM or bortezomib 50 nM +TP 20 μM, T3 20 μM, TOS 20 μM, and T3E 20 μM for 12 h, and the protein levels were assessed of NFE2L1 by immunoblotting. α-Tubulin protein levels served as the loading control. A densitometric analysis was performed as described in the Materials and Methods section. Data are means ± SD, n = 3. * $p < 0.05$, ** $p < 0.01$ vs. as indicated. BTZ; bortezomib, TP; α-tocopherol, T3; α-tocotrienol, TOS; α-tocopheryl succinate, T3E; 6-O-Carboxypropyl-alpha-tocotrienol.

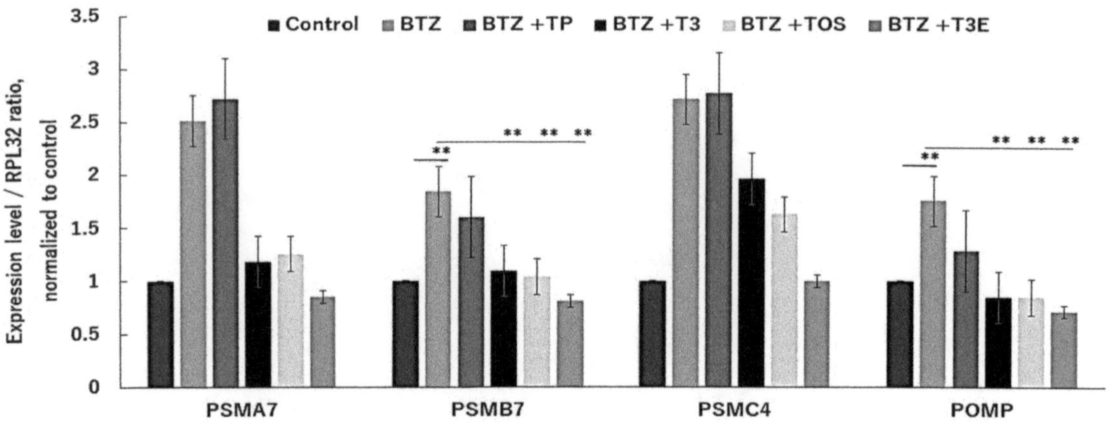

Figure 2. Effects of vitamin E on mRNA level of proteasome related proteins in the treatment of bortezomib. H2452 cells were treated with bortezomib 50 nM or bortezomib 50 nM +TP 20 μM, T3 20 μM, TOS 20 μM, T3E 20 μM for 12 h, and the mRNA levels of PSMA7, PSMB7, PSMC4, and POMP were assessed by real-time quantitative PCR as described in the Materials and Methods section. RPL32 mRNA levels served as the loading control. Data are means ± SD, n = 3. ** $p < 0.01$ vs. as indicated. BTZ; bortezomib, TP; α-tocopherol, T3; α-tocotrienol, TOS; α-tocopheryl succinate, T3E; 6-O-Carboxypropyl-alpha-tocotrienol.

2.3. T3, TOS, and T3E Suppressed the Recovery of Proteasome Activity under and after Bortezomib Treatment

Under or following proteasome inhibition, NFE2L1 is known to recover proteasome activity [14]. We hypothesized that T3, TOS, and T3E might inhibit the recovery of proteasome activity under or after proteasome inhibition. Subsequently, we next evaluated the effects of TP, T3, TOS, and T3E on the recovery of proteasomal chymotrypsin-like activity undergoing and following bortezomib treatment. Proteasome activity was significantly reduced in all treatment groups compared to the control group (Figure 3a). After removing bortezomib from each treatment group, proteasome activity recovered to approximately 60% in the bortezomib alone group, whereas it was less than 40% in the combination groups with bortezomib and T3, TOS, T3E (Figure 3b).

Since ubiquitinated proteins are well known to accumulate under proteasome inhibition, T3, TOS, and T3E may enhance the accumulation of ubiquitinated proteins induced by PIs via inhibition of the recovery in proteasome activity. For this reason, we next evaluated the effect of the combination of bortezomib with TP, T3, TOS, and T3E on the accumulation of ubiquitinated protein by an immunoblot. As seen in Figure 3c, the combination groups with bortezomib and T3, TOS, and T3E showed a more remarkable accumulation of ubiquitinated protein compared to the bortezomib alone group. These results suggest that T3, TOS, and T3E inhibit the recovery of proteasome activity under and after proteasome inhibition.

2.4. T3, TOS, and T3E Enhanced Sensitivity to Bortezomib in H2452

We next evaluated the effect of bortezomib in combination with TP, T3, TOS, and T3E on cell viability using a WST-8 assay. As shown in Figure 4, the combination groups with bortezomib and T3, TOS, and T3E showed a significant decrease in cell viability compared to the control group, bortezomib alone group, and respective alone groups, suggesting that T3, TOS, and T3E may enhance bortezomib sensitivity.

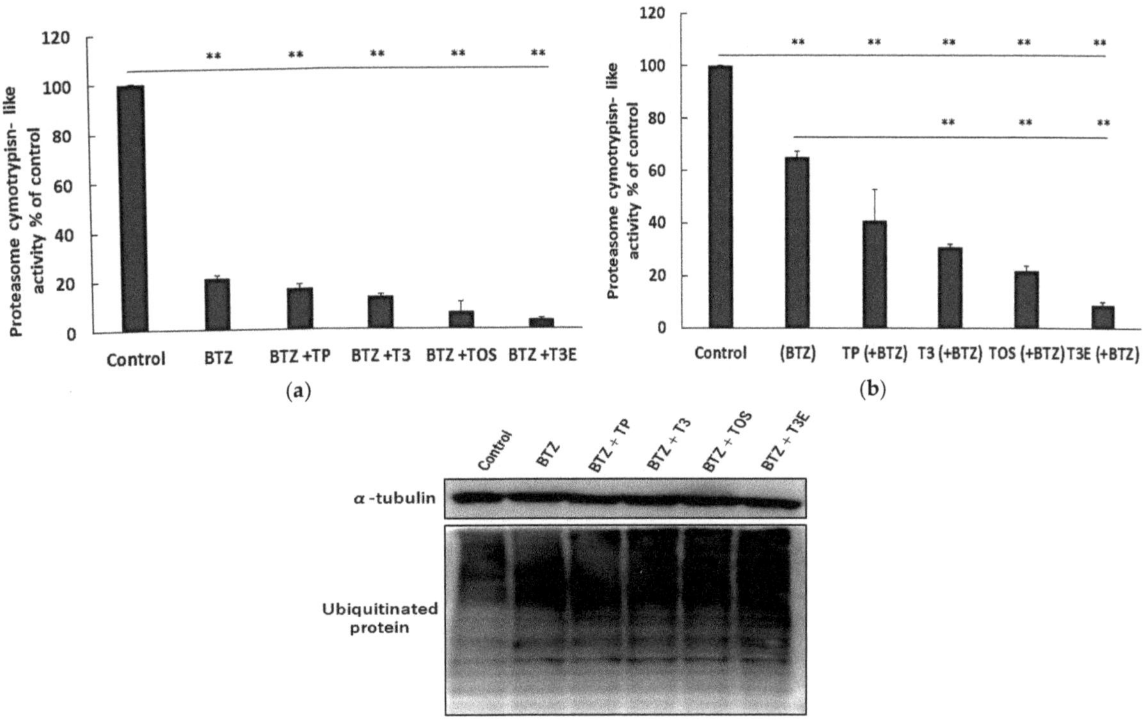

(c)

Figure 3. Effects of vitamin E on proteasome activities in the treatment of bortezomib. H2452 cells were treated with bortezomib 50 NM or bortezomib 50 nM +TP 20 μM, T3 20 μM, TOS 20 μM, T3E 20 μM for 6 h (**a**), and another 6 h except for bortezomib (**b**). After the treatment, chymotrypsin-like activity was assessed by a chemiluminescent method, as described in the Materials and Methods section. Data are means ± SD, n = 3. ** $p < 0.01$ vs. as indicated. (**c**) H2452 cells were treated with bortezomib 50 nM or bortezomib 50 nM + TP 20 μM, T3 20 μM, TOS 20 μM, and T3E 20 μM for 12 h. After the treatment, ubiquitinated protein levels in each sample were assessed by immunoblotting. α-Tubulin protein levels served as the loading control. Results are representative of three independent experiments. BTZ; bortezomib, TP; α-tocopherol, T3; α-tocotrienol, TOS; α-tocopheryl succinate, T3E; 6-O-Carboxypropyl-alpha-tocotrienol.

2.5. T3, TOS, and T3E Also Enhanced the Sensitivity to Bortezomib through Protein Levels of NFE2L1 and NRF3 in Other Solid Cancer Cell Lines

Based on our results, T3, TOS, and T3E may enhance the sensitivity to bortezomib in the H2452 cell line by modulating protein levels of NFE2L1. However, it is unclear whether the same effect can be achieved in other solid cancer cell lines. Therefore, we performed an evaluation of the effects of T3, TOS, and T3E on NFE2L1 and sensitivity to bortezomib in the lung adenocarcinoma cell line, A549, and the pancreatic cancer cell line, PANC1. As a result, the bortezomib alone group showed an increase in protein levels of unprocessed and processed NFE2L1 and mRNA expression levels of proteasome-related proteins compared to the control group, while the combination groups with bortezomib and T3, TOS, and T3E did not show a similar increasing tendency as bortezomib alone group in PANC1 and A549 (Figure 5a–d). In addition, the combination groups with bortezomib and T3, TOS, and T3E demonstrated a significant decrease in cell viability compared to the control group, bortezomib alone group, and the respective alone groups in PANC1 and A549 (Figure 5e,f).

These results suggest that T3, TOS, and T3E may enhance the sensitivity to bortezomib in different types of solid cancers by modulating protein levels of NFE2L1.

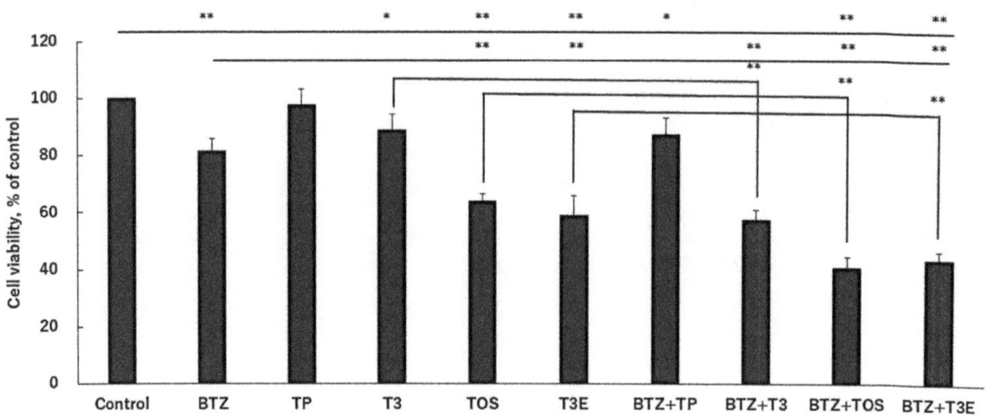

Figure 4. Effects of the combination of bortezomib and vitamin E on the viabilities. H2452 cells were treated with bortezomib 50 nM or bortezomib 50 nM +TP 20 μM, T3 20 μM, TOS 20 μM, T3E 20 μM for 24 h, and cell viability was evaluated by the WST-8 assay. Data are means ± SD, n = 5. * $p < 0.05$, ** $p < 0.01$ vs. as indicated. BTZ; bortezomib, TP; α-tocopherol, T3; α-tocotrienol, TOS; α-tocopheryl succinate, T3E; 6-O-Carboxypropyl-alpha-tocotrienol.

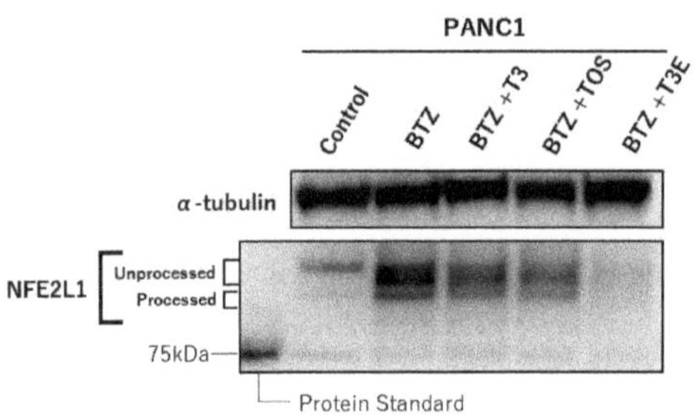

(a)

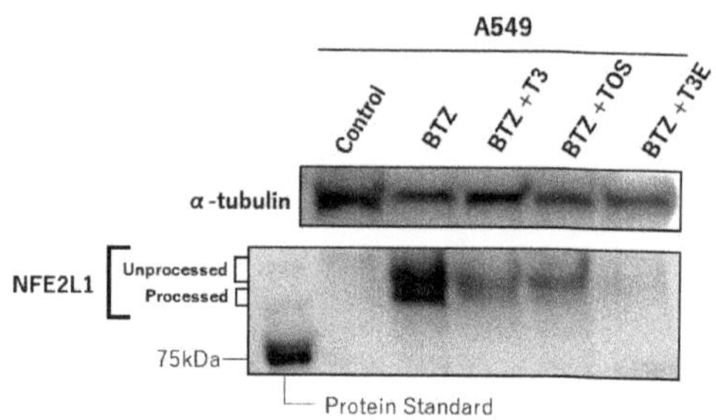

(b)

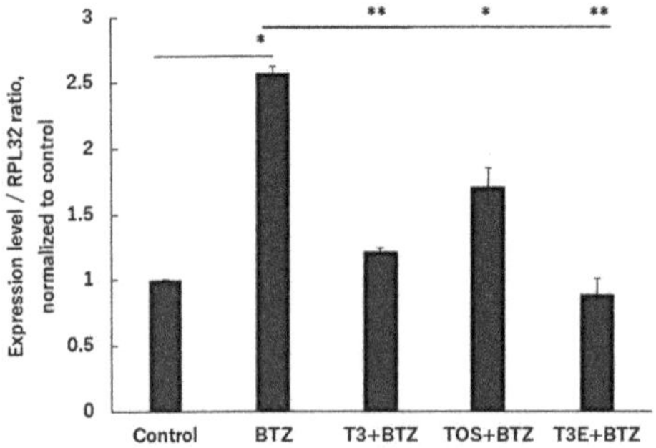

(c)

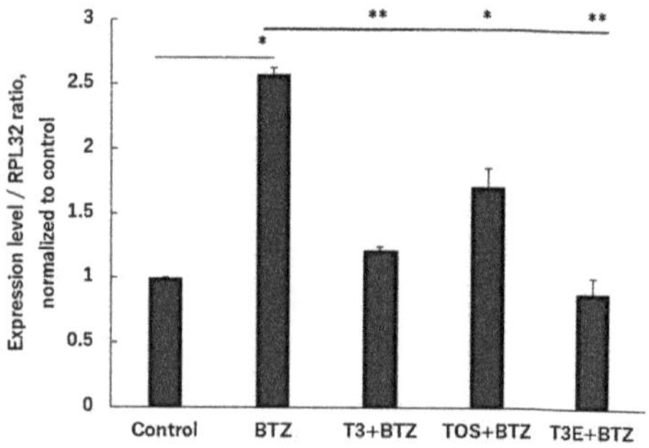

(d)

Figure 5. *Cont.*

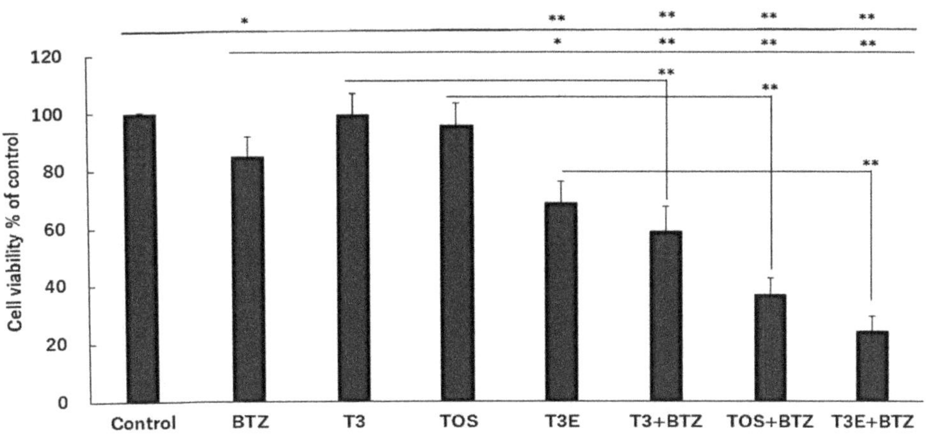

(e)

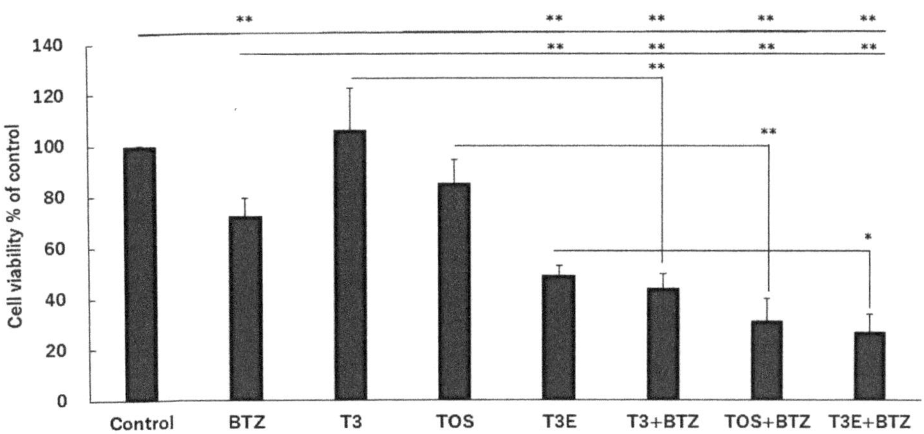

(f)

Figure 5. Effects of vitamin E on NFE2L1 in another solid cancer cells. PANC1 (**a**) and A549 (**b**) cells were treated with bortezomib 50 nM or bortezomib 50 nM +TP 20 μM, T3 20 μM, TOS 20 μM, T3E 20 μM for 12 h, and NFE2L1 protein levels were assessed by immunoblotting. Results are representative of three independent experiments. After PANC1 (**c**) and A549 cells (**d**) were treated with bortezomib 50 nM or bortezomib 50 nM +TP 20 μM, T3 20 μM, TOS 20 μM, T3E 20 μM for 12 h, and the mRNA levels of PSMB7 were assessed by real-time quantitative PCR as described in the Materials and Methods section. RPL32 mRNA levels served as the loading control. Data are means ± SD, n = 3. * p <0.05 ** $p < 0.01$ vs. the control. PANC1 (**e**) and A549 cells (**f**) were treated with bortezomib 50 nM or bortezomib 50 nM +TP 20 μM, T3 20 μM, TOS 20 μM, T3E 20 μM for 24 h. After the treatment, cell viability was evaluated by the WST-8 assy. Data are means ± SD, n = 5. * $p < 0.05$, ** $p < 0.01$ vs. as indicated. TP; α-tocopherol, T3; α-tocotrienol, TOS; α-tocopheryl succinate, T3E; 6-O-Carboxypropyl-alpha-tocotrienol.

2.6. *Atorvastatin Did Not Affect NFE2L1 and NRF3 under Bortezomib Treatment*

Vitamin E and its derivatives are well known to have a cholesterol-lowering effect. It also has been reported that NFE2L1 is involved in the regulation of cholesterol [33]. Based on these findings, we speculated that the cholesterol-lowering effect of T3, TOS, and T3E could moderate the protein levels of NFE2L1. Therefore, finally, we evaluated the effect of atorvastatin, a cholesterol-depleting agent, on NFE2L1 under bortezomib treatment. We observed no significant differences between the bortezomib alone group and the combination group with bortezomib and atorvastatin in protein levels of unprocessed and processed NFE2L1 (Figure 6a), mRNA expression levels of PSMB7 (Figure 6b) and the accumulation of ubiquitinated proteins (Figure 6c). These results suggest that the cholesterol-lowering effect does not affect NFE2L1 under proteasome inhibition.

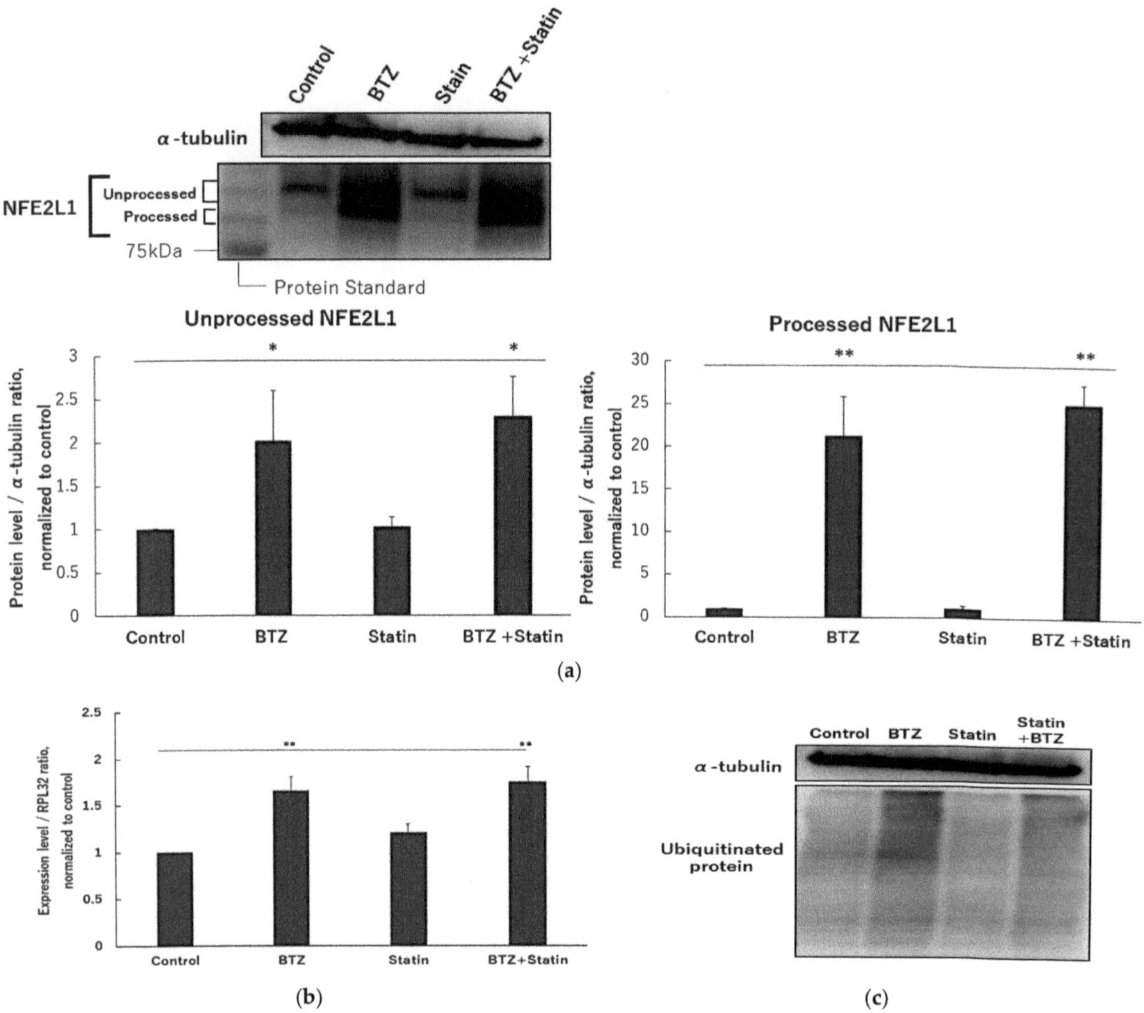

Figure 6. Effects of atorvastatin on NFE2L1 in treatment bortezomib. H2452 cells were treated with bortezomib 50 nM or bortezomib 50 nM +atorvastatin 10 μM for 24 h, and NFE2L1 (**a**) and ubiquitinated protein (**c**) levels were assessed by immunoblotting. α-Tubulin protein levels served as the loading control. A densitometric analysis was performed as described in the Materials and Methods section. (**b**) After H2452 cells were treated with bortezomib 50 nM or bortezomib 50 nM +atorvastatin 10 μM for 24 h, and the mRNA levels of PSMB7 were assessed by real-time quantitative PCR as described in the Materials and Methods section. RPL32 mRNA levels served as the loading control. Data are means ± SD, n = 3. * $p < 0.05$ ** $p < 0.01$ vs. the control. BTZ; bortezomib, statin; atorvastatin.

3. Discussion

In this study, we initially examined the effects of TP, T3, TOS, and T3E on NFE2L1 and proteasome homeostasis under bortezomib treatment. We observed that T3, TOS, and T3E (but not TP) suppressed the increase in protein levels of NFE2L1, as well as the expression levels of transcriptional target genes such as proteasome-component proteins (PSMA7, PSMB7, and PSMC4) and proteasome maturation proteins (POMP). Furthermore, it was observed that T3, TOS, and T3E inhibited the recovery of proteasome activity under and after bortezomib treatment and that the combination with bortezomib and T3, TOS, and T3E significantly reduced cell viability compared to them alone.

Under proteasome inhibition, NFE2L1 is known to synthesize new proteasomes by promoting the transcription of proteasome-related genes to maintain proteasome homeostasis. It has been reported that their inhibition prevented recovery of proteasome activity during proteasome inhibition and greatly enhanced the sensitivity to proteasome inhibitors in solid tumor cells such as breast cancer [14]. Since similar events to these reports were observed in the present study, T3, TOS, and T3E may also enhance sensitivity to bortezomib in solid cancer cells by targeting NFE2L1 under proteasome inhibition. This suggests that T3, TOS, and T3E may be candidate adjunctive agents for solid cancer treatment with bortezomib. On the other hand, NFE2L2 and NFE2L3, which is a transcription factor belonging to the leucine zipper family like NFE2L1, has also been reported to be involved in the recovery of proteasome activity under proteasome inhibition [5,14,34,35]. Since T3, TOS, and T3E strongly inhibited the recovery of proteasome activity, they may also affect NFE2L2 and NFE2L3. However, further studies are needed to clarify the effects of T3, TOS, and T3E on NFE2L2 and NFE2L3. We also observed the NFE2L1 inhibitory effects in T3, TOS, and T3E but not in TP. When comparing TP and T3, it is known that T3 is more readily taken up in cells than TP due to the presence of a double bond in the side chain [36,37]. Therefore, T3 may have a more immediate and full effect on NFE2L1 in comparison to TP. Additionally, TOS and T3E are derivatives that block the antioxidant group in vitamin E and are not consumed as antioxidants like TP and T3. Therefore, TOS and T3E may show stronger inhibitory effects on NFE2L1 than TP.

This study revealed that TOS and T3E, which are vitamin E derivatives with blocked antioxidant groups, also exerted inhibitory effects on NFE2L1, while atorvastatin, a cholesterol-lowering agent, did not exert inhibitory effects on NFE2L1. This suggests that T3, TOS, and T3E may exert inhibitory effects on NFE2L1 without implicating the antioxidant and cholesterol-lowering effects that have been identified in vitamin E. However, in this study, we did not confirm the effects of T3, TOS, and T3E on proteins such as NGLY, p97 and Hrd1, which are involved in the release of NFE2L1 from the endoplasmic reticulum into the cytoplasm, and additional investigations are needed to elucidate the mechanism of NFE2L1 inhibition by T3, TOS, and T3E.

DDI2 is a molecule which involve in the maturation of NFE2L1, and its inhibition suppress the function of NFE2L1 [15,16,38]. In the present study, we found that T3, TOS, and T3E suppressed the increase in protein levels of NFE2L1 under proteasome inhibition without affecting the protein level of DDI2 (Figure S1), suggesting that they are a new type of NFE2L1 inhibitor. Additionally, T3, TOS, and T3E may also affect molecules involved in NFE2L1 protein regulation, which suggests that T3, TOS, and T3E may be good tools for investigating NFE2L1 regulation.

4. Materials and Methods

4.1. Reagents

All cultures and chemicals were purchased from Nacalai Tesque (Kyoto, Japan) unless otherwise indicated. Fetal bovine serum (FBS) was purchased from Bio West (Nuaillé, France). Bortezomib (a protease inhibitor) was obtained from Wako Chemicals (Osaka, Japan). TP and TOS were purchased from Sigma Aldrich (St. Louis, MO, USA), and T3 was purchased from Tama Biochemicals (Tokyo, Japan). Antibodies for NFE2L1 (#8052), ubiquitin (#3936) and Lamin B1 (#13435) were purchased from Cell Signaling Technology

(Beverly, MA, USA). DDI2 antibody (sc-514004) is purchased from Santa Cruz Biotechnology (Dallas, TX, USA).

4.2. α-T3E Synthesis

α-T3E was synthesized from T3 according to a previously reported procedure [39]. The purity of α-T3E was confirmed by GC–MS, 1H NMR, 13C NMR, and IR. NMR and IR spectra were consistent with the structure of α-T3E. 1H NMR (CDCl3) spectrum: 1.27 (3H, s), 1.59 (9H, s), 1.67 (3H, s), 2.00 (3H, s), 2.09 (3H, s), 2.12 (3H, s), 1.70–2.15 (16H, m), 2.57 (2H, t, J = 7.8 Hz), 2.65 (2H, t, J = 6.5 Hz), 3.68 (2H, t, J = 7.7 Hz), 4.95–5.25 (3H, m), 8.5 (1H, broad). IR (KBr) spectrum: 3200–3400 cm^{-1} (carboxylic OH) and 1710 cm^{-1} (C6=O).

4.3. Cell Culture

H2452, PANC1, and A549 cells were purchased for ATCC (Manassas, VA, USA). PANC1 and A549 were routinely grown in RPMI1640 supplemented with 10% FBS, 50 IU/mL penicillin, and 50 μg/mL streptomycin, and H2452 cells were routinely grown in RPMI1640 supplemented with 10% FBS, 6.5 mg/mL glucose, 1 mM sodium pyruvate, 10 mM HEPES, 50 IU/mL penicillin, and 50 μg/mL streptomycin at 37 °C in a humidified atmosphere with 5% CO_2. Exponentially growing cells were used in experiments. Cells were plated on culture plates and cultured for 24 h to permit adherence. Cells were then cultured in RPMI1640 supplemented with 2% FBS for the indicated period, and each parameter was then examined.

4.4. Reagent Dissolution

TP, T3, TOS, and T3E were dissolved using ethanol. Bortezomib was dissolved with ethanol and sonication. Also, ethanol was added to the control group in each assay.

4.5. Cellular Fractionation

H2452 cells were cultured at a density of 1×10^6 cells in a 10 cm dish for 24 h and were then treated with each agent for 12 h. After the treatment, cells were collected and fractionated into cytoplasm and nucleus fractions using NE-PER™ nuclear and cytoplasmic extract reagent kit (Thermo Fisher Scientific, Waltham, MA, USA).

4.6. Cell Viability

The WST-8 assay was performed to evaluate the effects of each reagent on the viability of H2452, PANC1, and A549. Cells were seeded on a 96-well plate (5×10^3 cells/well), cultured for 24 h, and subsequently treated with each reagent for the indicated period as described in each figure legend. After each treatment, 10 μL of WST-8 solution was applied to each well containing 100 μL of the cell suspension and incubated at 37 °C for a further 30 min in 5% CO_2. Color development was monitored at 450 nm using a multi-well plate reader (SUNRISE Rainbow RC-R, Tecan Japan, Kanagawa, Japan).

4.7. Proteasome Activity

H2452 cells were seeded on a 96-well white plate (5×10^3 cells/100 μL/well), cultured for 24 h, and subsequently treated with bortezomib 50 nM or bortezomib 50 nM +TP 20 μM, T3 20 μM, TOS 20 μM, T3E 20 μM for 6 h, and another 6 h except for bortezomib. After the treatment, to assess chymotrypsin-like activity in cells, 50 μL of Proteasome-Glo™ Chymotrypsin-Like Cell-Based Assay Reagent (Promega Japan, Tokyo, Japan) was added to each well, and the plate was then incubated at room temperature for 20 min. The chymotrypsin-like activity was assessed based on estimated chemiluminescence intensity using a luminometer (Infinite M1000 PRO, TECAN Japan).

4.8. Isolation of mRNA and Real-Time Quantitative PCR

H2452, PANC1, and A549 cells were cultured at a density of 5×10^5 cells in a 60-mm dish for 24 h and were then treated with each agent for 12 to 24 h. After the treatment, cells were collected, and total RNA was isolated using the Tissue Total RNA Extraction Mini Kit (Favorgen Biotech Corp., Ping-Tung, Taiwan). Total RNA (300 ng for each sample) was used for cDNA synthesis with the ReverTra Ace qPCR RT Kit (Toyobo, Osaka, Japan). cDNA templates were analyzed by real-time PCR using Thermal Cycler Dice Real Time System Lite (TAKARA BIO INC., Shiga, Japan) and THUNDER-BIRD™ SYBR qPCR Mix (Toyobo, Osaka, Japan), with the following program: at 95°C for 10 s followed by 40 cycles at 95 °C for 15 s and at 60 °C for 1 min. Primer sets are shown in Table 1. Gene expression data were normalized to the expression of the reference gene ribosomal protein L32.

Table 1. List of PCR primers.

Gene Name	Primer	Sequence
60S ribosomal protein L32 (RPL32)	Forward	AACCCTGTTGTCAATGCCTC
	Reverse	CATCTCCTTCTCGGCATCA
Proteasome 20S Subunit Alpha 7 (PSMA7)	Forward	CTGTGCTTTGGATGACAACG
	Reverse	CGATGTAGCGGGTGATGTACT
Proteasome 20S Subunit Beta 4 (PSMB4)	Forward	TCAGTCCTCGGCGTTAAGTT
	Reverse	GCTTAGCACTGGCTGCTTCT
Proteasome 20S Subunit Beta 7 (PSMB7)	Forward	CGGCTGTGTCGGTGTATG
	Reverse	GCCAGTTTTCCGGACCTT
Proteasome 26S Subunit ATPase4 (PSMC4)	Forward	GGAAGACCATGTTGGCAAAG
	Reverse	AAGATGATGGCAGGTGCATT
Proteasome maturation protein (POMP)	Forward	AGGCAGTGCAGCAGGTTC
	Reverse	GGCTCTCCCATGACTTCG

4.9. Immunoblotting

H2452, PANC1, and A549 cells were cultured at a density of 5×10^5 cells in a 60-mm dish for 24 h and then treated with each agent for 12 to 24 h. After the treatment, cells were harvested and lysed in ice-cold Laemmli sample buffer (Bio-Rad, Berkeley, CA, USA) containing a protease inhibitor cocktail (Nakadai Tesque) and phosphatase inhibitor (Nacalai Tesque). Cells were incubated on ice for 20 min following centrifugation at 12,000 rpm at 4 °C for 10 min. Samples were electrophoresed through a 10% or 15% SDS–polyacrylamide gel and transferred to a polyvinylidene difluoride membrane using the iBlot 2 Dry Blotting System (Thermo Fisher Scientific, Waltham, MA, USA). Membranes were blocked with Blocking One P (Nacalai Tesque) for 1 h, incubated with primary antibodies for 1 h, and then incubated with the secondary antibody for 1 h. Detection was accomplished using Chemi-Lumi One Super (Nacalai Tesque) and C-DiGit (LI-COR, Lincoln, NE, USA). A densitometric analysis of each immune band was performed using Image Studio for C-DiGit (LI-COR). Molecular sizing was conducted using Protein Ladder One Plus, Triple-color for SDS-PAGE (Nacalai Tesque). Protein concentrations were assessed using the DC Protein Assay System (Bio-Rad).

4.10. Statistical Analysis

Differences among groups were analyzed by a one-way ANOVA followed by the Tukey test. All statistical analyses were performed using Ekuseru Toukei software ver 8.0 (Social Survey Research Information Co., Ltd., Tokyo, Japan). Differences with p-values of 0.05 or less were considered to be significant. All experiments were conducted with a minimum of three samples from three independent experiments, and data were expressed as means ± SD. The number of samples in each experiment is shown in the respective figure legends.

Supplementary Materials: The following supporting information can be downloaded at: https://www.mdpi.com/article/10.3390/ijms24119382/s1

Author Contributions: The contributions of individual authors to this manuscript are as follows: Conceptualization, T.Y.; performance of experiments, K.I., M.H. and M.S.; data analysis, K.I.; writing-draft, K.I., writing, K.I. and N.V.; supervision, T.Y. All authors have read and agreed to the published version of the manuscript.

Funding: Funding for this study was supported by the Inoue Enryou Memorial Foundation of Toyo University.

Institutional Review Board Statement: Not applicable.

Informed Consent Statement: Not applicable.

Data Availability Statement: All relevant data are within the manuscript.

Conflicts of Interest: The authors declare no conflict of interest.

References

1. Shen, M.; Schmitt, S.; Buac, N.; Dou, P. Targeting the ubiquitin-proteasome system for cancer therapy. *Expert Opin. Ther. Targets* **2013**, *17*, 1091–1108. [CrossRef]
2. Arlt, A.; Bauer, I.; Schafmayer, C.; Tepel, J.; Sebens, M.S.; Brosch, M.; Röder, C.; Kalthoff, H.; Hampe, J.; Moyer, M.P.; et al. Increased proteasome subunit protein expression and proteasome activity in colon cancer relate to an enhanced activation of nuclear factor E2-related factor 2 (NFE2L2). *Oncogene* **2009**, *28*, 3983–3996. [CrossRef]
3. Chen, L.; Madura, K. Increased proteasome activity, ubiquitin-conjugating enzymes, and eEF1A translation factor detected in breast cancer tissue. *Cancer Res.* **2005**, *65*, 5599–5606. [CrossRef]
4. Stoebner, P.-E.; Lavabre-Bertrand, T.; Henry, L.; Guiraud, I.; Carillo, S.; Dandurand, M.; Joujoux, J.-M.; Bureau, J.-P.; Meunier, L. High plasma proteasome levels are detected in patients with metastatic malignant melanoma. *Br. J. Dermatol.* **2005**, *152*, 948–953. [CrossRef] [PubMed]
5. Walter, R.F.H.; Sydow, S.R.; Berg, E.; Kollmeier, J.; Christoph, D.C.; Christoph, S.; Eberhardt, W.E.E.; Mairinger, T.; Wohlschlaeger, J.; Schmid, K.W.; et al. Bortezomib sensitivity is tissue dependent and high expression of the 20S proteasome precludes good response in malignant pleural mesothelioma. *Cancer Manag. Res.* **2019**, *11*, 8711–8720. [CrossRef]
6. Dutaud, D.; Aubry, L.; Henry, L.; Levieux, D.; Hendil, K.B.; Kuehn, L.; Bureau, J.P.; Ouali, A. Development and evaluation of a sandwich ELISA for quantification of the 20S proteasome in human plasma. *J. Immunol. Methods* **2002**, *260*, 183–193. [CrossRef]
7. Fricker, D.L. Proteasome Inhibitor Drugs. *Annu. Rev. Pharmacol. Toxicol.* **2020**, *60*, 457–476. [CrossRef]
8. Daniel, J.E. The ubiquitin-proteasome system: Opportunities for therapeutic intervention in solid tumors. *Endocr. Relat. Cancer* **2015**, *22*, T1.
9. Roeten, M.S.F.; Cloos, J.; Jansen, G. Positioning of proteasome inhibitors in therapy of solid malignancies. *Cancer Chemother. Pharmacol.* **2018**, *81*, 227–243. [CrossRef] [PubMed]
10. Hainsworth, J.D.; Meluch, A.A.; Spigel, D.R.; Barton, J.; Simons, L.; Meng, C.; Gould, B.; Greco, F.A. Weekly docetaxel and bortezomib as first-line treatment for patients with hormone-refractory prostate cancer: A Minnie Pearl Cancer Research Network phase II trial. *Clin. Genitourin. Cancer* **2007**, *5*, 278–283. [CrossRef] [PubMed]
11. Wang, H.; Cao, Q.; Dudek, A.Z. Phase II study of panobinostat and bortezomib in patients with pancreatic cancer progressing on gemcitabine-based therapy. *Anticancer. Res.* **2012**, *32*, 1027–1031. [PubMed]
12. Fanucchi, M.P.; Fossella, F.V.; Belt, R.; Natale, R.; Fidias, P.; Carbone, D.P.; Govindan, R.; Raez, L.E.; Robert, F.; Ribeiro, M.; et al. Randomized phase II study of bortezomib alone and bortezomib in combination with docetaxel in previously treated advanced non-small-cell lung cancer. *J. Clin. Oncol.* **2006**, *24*, 5025–5033. [CrossRef]
13. Fennell, D.A.; McDowell, C.; Busacca, S.; Webb, G.; Moulton, B.; Cakana, A.; O'Byrne, K.J.; Meerbeeck, J.V.; Donnellan, P.; McCaffrey, J.; et al. Phase II clinical trial of first or second-line treatment with bortezomib in patients with malignant pleural mesothelioma. *J. Thorac. Oncol.* **2012**, *7*, 1466–1470. [CrossRef] [PubMed]
14. Radhakrishnan, S.K.; Lee, C.S.; Young, P.; Beskow, A.; Chan, J.Y.; Deshaies, R.J. Transcription factor Nrf1 mediates the proteasome recovery pathway after proteasome inhibition in mammalian cells. *Mol. Cell* **2010**, *38*, 17–28. [CrossRef]
15. Op, M.; Ribeiro, S.T.; Chavarria, C.; Gassart, A.D.; Zaffalon, L.; Martinon, F. The aspartyl protease DDI2 drives adaptation to proteasome inhibition in multiple myeloma. *Cell Death Dis.* **2022**, *13*, 475. [CrossRef]
16. Chen, T.; Ho, M.; Briere, J.; Moscvin, M.; Czarnecki, P.G.; Anderson, K.C.; Blackwell, T.K.; Bianchi, G. Multiple myeloma cells depend on the DDI2/NRF1-mediated proteasome stress response for survival. *Blood Adv.* **2022**, *6*, 429–440. [CrossRef]
17. Sekine, H.; Okazaki, K.; Kato, K.; Alam, M.M.; Shima, H.; Katsuoka, F.; Tsujita, T.; Suzuki, N.; Kobayashi, A.; Igarashi, K.; et al. O-GlcNAcylation Signal Mediates Proteasome Inhibitor Resistance in Cancer Cells by Stabilizing NRF1. *Mol. Cell. Biol.* **2018**, *38*, e00252-18. [CrossRef]

18. Tomlin, F.M.; Gerling-Driessen, U.I.M.; Liu, Y.; Flynn, R.A.; Vangala, J.R.; Lentz, C.S.; Clauder-Muenster, S.; Jakob, P.; Mueller, W.F.; Ordoñez-Rueda, D.; et al. Inhibition of NGLY1 Inactivates the Transcription Factor Nrf1 and Potentiates Proteasome Inhibitor Cytotoxicity. *ACS Cent. Sci.* **2017**, *3*, 1143–1155. [CrossRef] [PubMed]
19. Steffen, J.; Seeger, M.; Koch, A.; Krüger, E. Proteasomal degradation is transcriptionally controlled by TCF11 via an ERAD-dependent feedback loop. *Mol. Cell* **2010**, *40*, 147–158. [CrossRef]
20. Radhakrishnan, S.K.; Besten, W.D.; Deshaies, R.J. p97-dependent retrotranslocation and proteolytic processing govern formation of active Nrf1 upon proteasome inhibition. *elife* **2014**, *3*, e01856. [CrossRef]
21. Koizumi, S.; Hamazaki, J.; Murata, S. Transcriptional regulation of the 26S proteasome by Nrf1. *Phys. Biol. Sci.* **2018**, *94*, 325–336. [CrossRef]
22. Abraham, A.; Kattoor, A.J.; Saldeen, T.; Mehta, J.L. Vitamin E and its anticancer effects. *Crit. Rev. Food Sci. Nutr.* **2019**, *59*, 2831–2838. [CrossRef]
23. Kaneko, S.; Sato, C.; Shiozawa, N.; Sato, A.; Sato, H.; Virgona, N.; Yano, T. Suppressive Effect of Delta-Tocotrienol on Hypoxia Adaptation of Prostate Cancer Stem-like Cells. *Anticancer. Res.* **2018**, *38*, 1391–1399.
24. Rajendran, P.; Li, F.; Manu, A.K.; Shanmugam, K.M.; Loo, Y.S.; Kumar, P.A.S. Gγ-Tocotrienol is a novel inhibitor of constitutive and inducible STAT3 signalling pathway in human hepatocellular carcinoma: Potential role as an antiproliferative, pro-apoptotic and chemosensitizing agent. *Br. J. Pharmacol.* **2011**, *163*, 283–298. [CrossRef]
25. Savitskaya, M.A.; Onischenko, G.E. α-Tocopheryl Succinate Affects Malignant Cell Viability, Proliferation, and Differentiation. *Biochemistry* **2016**, *81*, 806–818. [CrossRef] [PubMed]
26. Kashiwagi, K.; Virgona, N.; Harada, K.; Kido, W.; Yano, Y.; Ando, A.; Hagiwara, K.; Yano, T. A redox-silent analogue of tocotrienol acts as a potential cytotoxic agent against human mesothelioma cells. *Life Sci.* **2009**, *84*, 650–656. [CrossRef] [PubMed]
27. Shiozawa, N.; Sugahara, R.; Namiki, K.; Sato, C.; Ando, A.; Sato, A.; Virgona, N.; Yano, T. Inhibitory effect of a redox-silent analogue of tocotrienol on hypoxia adaptation in prostate cancer cells. *Anticancer. Drugs* **2017**, *28*, 289–297. [CrossRef]
28. Ramdas, P.; Radhakrishnan, A.K.; Sani, A.A.; Kumari, M.; Rao, J.S.; Rahman, P.S. Advancing the Role of Gamma-Tocotrienol as Proteasomes Inhibitor: A Quantitative Proteomic Analysis of MDA-MB-231 Human Breast Cancer Cells. *Biomolecules* **2019**, *10*, 19. [CrossRef]
29. Ishii, K.; Fusegi, M.; Mori, T.; Teshima, K.; Ninomiya, N.; Kohno, K.; Sato, A.; Ishida, T.; Miyakoshi, Y.; Yano, T. A Redox-Silent Analogue of Tocotrienol May Break the Homeostasis of Proteasomes in Human Malignant Mesothelioma Cells by Inhibiting STAT3 and NRF1. *Int. J. Mol. Sci.* **2022**, *23*, 2655. [CrossRef] [PubMed]
30. Nowak, K.; Taubert, R.M.; Haberecht, S.; Venz, S.; Krüger, E. Inhibition of calpain-1 stabilizes TCF11/Nrf1 but does not affect its activation in response to proteasome inhibition. *Biosci. Rep.* **2018**, *38*, BSR20180393. [CrossRef]
31. Arlt, A.; Sebens, S.; Krebs, S.; Geismann, C.; Grossmann, M.; Kruse, M.L.; Schreiber, S.; Schäfer, H. Inhibition of the NRF2 transcription factor by the alkaloid trigonelline renders pancreatic cancer cells more susceptible to apoptosis through decreased proteasomal gene expression and proteasome activity. *Oncogene* **2013**, *32*, 4825–4835. [CrossRef]
32. Waku, T.; Katayama, H.; Hiraoka, M.; Hatanaka, A.; Nakamura, N.; Tanaka, Y.; Tamura, N.; Watanabe, A.; Kobayashi, A. NFE2L1 and NFE2L3 Complementarily Maintain Basal Proteasome Activity in Cancer Cells through CPEB3-Mediated Translational Repression. *Mol. Cell Biol.* **2020**, *40*, e00010-20. [CrossRef]
33. Widenmaier, B.S.; Snyder, A.N.; Nguyen, B.T.; Arduini, A.; Lee, Y.G.; Arruda, P.A.; Saksi, J.; Bartelt, A.; Hotamisligil, S.G. NRF1 Is an ER Membrane Sensor that Is Central to Cholesterol Homeostasis. *Cell.* **2017**, *171*, 1094–1109. [CrossRef] [PubMed]
34. Chowdhury, A.M.; Katoh, H.; Hatanaka, A.; Iwanari, H.; Nakamura, N.; Hamakubo, T.; Natsume, T.; Waku, T.; Kobayashi, A. Multiple regulatory mechanisms of the biological function of NRF3 (NFE2L3) control cancer cell proliferation. *Sci. Rep.* **2017**, *7*, 12494. [CrossRef] [PubMed]
35. Waku, T.; Nakamura, N.; Koji, M.; Watanabe, H.; Katoh, H.; Tatsumi, C.; Tamura, N.; Hatanaka, A.; Hirose, S.; Katayama, H.; et al. NRF3-POMP-20S Proteasome Assembly Axis Promotes Cancer Development via Ubiquitin-Independent Proteolysis of p53 and Retinoblastoma Protein. *J. Mol. Cell Biol.* **2020**, *40*, e00597-19. [CrossRef] [PubMed]
36. Saito, Y.; Yoshida, Y.; Nishio, K.; Hayakawa, M.; Niki, E. Characterization of cellular uptake and distribution of vitamin E. *Ann. N. Y. Acad. Sci.* **2004**, *1031*, 368–375. [CrossRef]
37. Irías-mata, A.; Sus, N.; Flory, S.; Stock, D.; Woerner, D.; Podszun, M.; Frank, J. α-tocopherol transfer protein does not regulate the cellular uptake and intracellular distribution of α- and γ-tocopherols and -tocotrienols in cultured liver cells. *Redox Biol.* **2018**, *19*, 28–36. [CrossRef]
38. Fassmannová, D.; Sedlák, F.; Sedláček, J.; Špička, I.; Šašková, G.K. Nelfinavir Inhibits the TCF11/Nrf1-Mediated Proteasome Recovery Pathway in Multiple Myeloma. *Cancers* **2020**, *12*, 1065. [CrossRef]
39. Yano, Y.; Satoh, H.; Fukumoto, K.; Kumadaki, I.; Ichikawa, T.; Yamada, K.; Hagiwara, K.; Yano, T. Induction of cytotoxicity in human lung adenocarcinoma cells by 6-O-carboxypropyl-alpha-tocotrienol, a redox-silent derivative of alpha-tocotrienol. *Int. J. Cancer* **2005**, *115*, 839–846. [CrossRef]

International Journal of
Molecular Sciences

MDPI

Article

Modulation of the Endomembrane System by the Anticancer Natural Product Superstolide/ZJ-101

Phillip R. Sanchez [1,2], Sarah A. Head [2], Shan Qian [3], Haibo Qiu [3], Avishek Roy [3], Zhendong Jin [3], Wei Zheng [1,*] and Jun O. Liu [2,*]

[1] National Center for Advancing Translational Sciences (NCATS), National Institutes of Health, Rockville, MD 20892, USA; phillip.sanchez@nih.gov
[2] Department of Pharmacology & Molecular Sciences, Johns Hopkins School of Medicine, Baltimore, MD 21205, USA
[3] Department of Pharmaceutical Sciences and Experimental Therapeutics, College of Pharmacy, The University of Iowa, Iowa City, IA 52242, USA; zhendong-jin@uiowa.edu (Z.J.)
* Correspondence: wzheng@mail.nih.gov (W.Z.); joliu@jhu.edu (J.O.L.)

Abstract: Marine natural products represent a unique source for clinically relevant drugs due to their vast molecular and mechanistic diversity. ZJ-101 is a structurally simplified analog of the marine natural product superstolide A, isolated from the New Caledonian sea sponge *Neosiphonia Superstes*. The mechanistic activity of the superstolides has until recently remained a mystery. Here, we have identified potent antiproliferative and antiadhesive effects of ZJ-101 on cancer cell lines. Furthermore, through dose–response transcriptomics, we found unique dysregulation of the endomembrane system by ZJ-101 including a selective inhibition of O-glycosylation via lectin and glycomics analysis. We applied this mechanism to a triple-negative breast cancer spheroid model and identified a potential for the reversal of 3D-induced chemoresistance, suggesting a potential for ZJ-101 as a synergistic therapeutic agent.

Keywords: natural product; superstolide; glycomics; transcriptomics; phenotypic analysis; 3D spheroid

Citation: Sanchez, P.R.; Head, S.A.; Qian, S.; Qiu, H.; Roy, A.; Jin, Z.; Zheng, W.; Liu, J.O. Modulation of the Endomembrane System by the Anticancer Natural Product Superstolide/ZJ-101. *Int. J. Mol. Sci.* **2023**, *24*, 9575. https://doi.org/10.3390/ijms24119575

Academic Editors: Barbara De Filippis, Alessandra Ammazzalorso and Marialuigia Fantacuzzi

Received: 8 May 2023
Revised: 24 May 2023
Accepted: 29 May 2023
Published: 31 May 2023

1. Introduction

Neosiphonia Superstes is a species of marine sponge localized to the region of New Caledonia in the South Pacific [1]. Originally identified during the 1874 voyage of the HMS Challenger expedition, the sponge was resurrected in the early 1990s when D'auria et al. isolated novel macrolides they termed superstolides A and B, which were subsequently shown to display anticancer activity [2–4]. The unprecedented chemical structures of this group of marine natural products suggest they might have a unique cellular target(s) and a novel mechanism of action. However, the scarcity of natural products seriously hampered the biological investigation. In 2013, a truncated superstolide A was designed and synthesized (named ZJ-101) that maintains the potent anticancer activity of the original natural product, thereby solving the supply problem of superstolide A, albeit indirectly [5]. Subsequently, several analogs were produced with enhanced potency in the single-digit nanomolar range. However, the mechanism of action of ZJ-101 and other analogs has remained unknown.

Employing several phenotypic assays in cancer cell lines, we identified novel activities and phenotypes associated with ZJ-101 that have revealed a unique mechanism of action. Notably, an anti-adhesive effect was identified, which was approximately 30-fold more potent than the previously described anti-proliferative effect. Cell cycle and growth rate analysis revealed a strong cytostatic effect. Transcriptomic and lectin stain imaging analyses further converged on a dysregulation of glycosylation within the endomembrane system. Through this analysis, we identified a selectivity for dysregulation of *O*-linked glycosylation, which primarily occurs within the Golgi apparatus. The disruption of glycosylation by

ZJ-101 leads to pleiotropic effects on proliferation and adhesion, which synergize with etoposide in a 3D spheroid combination model. Taken together, these findings implicate a unique mechanism of action for the family of superstolides and other related analogs [3–6].

2. Results

2.1. *ZJ-101 Is Cytostatic*

The anti-adhesive effects of ZJ-101 (chemical structure shown in Figure 1A) were first observed using light microscopy. One micromole ZJ-101 overnight treatment of HEK293T cells causes a dramatic effect on morphology, with cells rounding and dislodging from the culture surface (Figure 1B). Although this effect is observed in every cell line tested at similar time points, HEK293T cells provide the clearest example of this morphological change due to their naturally spread appearance in 2D culture (Figure 1B). Treated MDA-MB-231 cells exhibiting the same morphological changes were harvested, and cell cycle analysis via propidium iodide staining was performed. No statistically meaningful differences between negative control and ZJ-101 treated cells were observed either at 24 or 48 h of sustained treatment; taxol, utilized as a positive control, caused a G2-phase arrest as expected (Figure 1C).

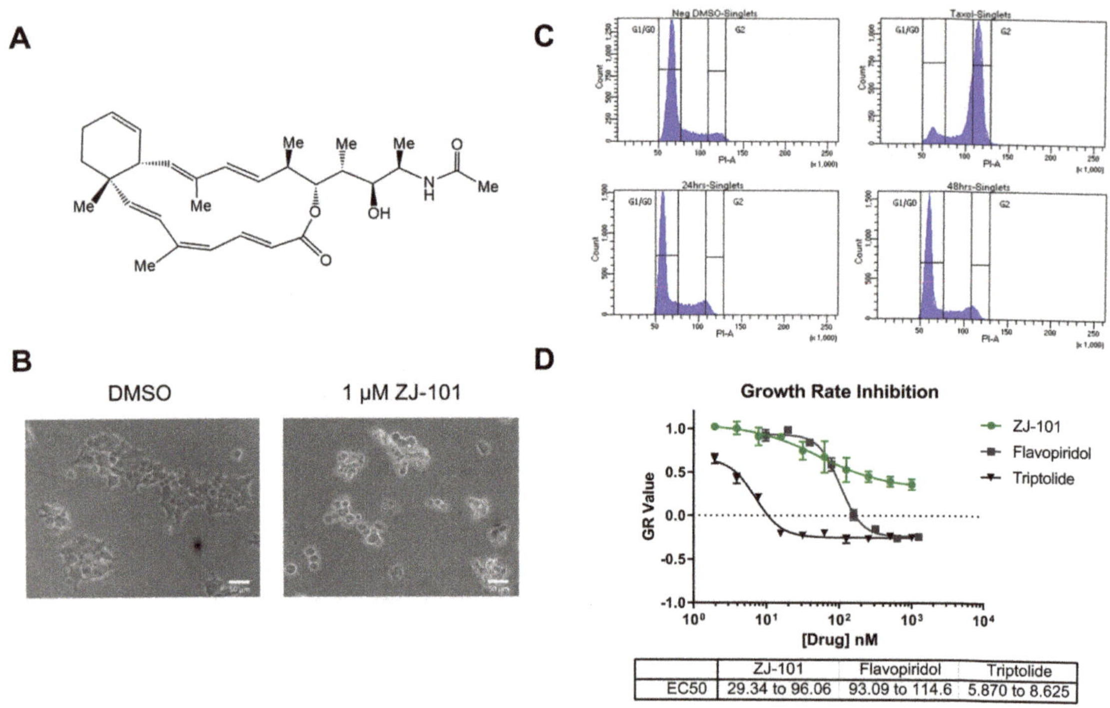

Figure 1. ZJ-101 is cytostatic and anti-adhesive. (**A**) Structure of ZJ-101. (**B**) Cell morphology after treatment with ZJ-101. (**C**) Cell cycle analysis via propidium iodide (PI) staining in MDA-MB-231 cells. Taxol utilized as a G2-phase block control. (**D**) Growth rate inhibition metrics assay (GR assay) determines that ZJ-101 is primarily cytostatic with an EC_{50} between 29 and 96 nM. when compared to known cytotoxic compounds.

To determine the extent to which ZJ-101 induced cell death, we used the growth rate normalized inhibition metrics assay (GR assay) [7]. The GR assay counts populations of live and dead cells using separate live-cell imaging dyes. We found that ZJ-101 acted in a purely cytostatic manner, consistent with a GR value greater than 0, with ZJ-101 achieving a GR of 0.5 at the highest dose after a 72 h treatment in MDA-MB-231 cells (Figure 1D). The EC_{50} of 29–96 nM as measured by the GR assay is nearly identical to that of traditional viability dyes such as resazurin (Figure S1A). Two known cytotoxic compounds, triptolide and flavopiridol, were utilized as controls and found to pass below the GR value of 0, indicating cytotoxicity. Additionally, the GR assay was used to evaluate the effect of ZJ-101 on isogenic p53 and p21 knockout HCT-116 cells (Figure S1B). $p53^{-/-}$ HCT-116 shared nearly identical GR and EC_{50} values for ZJ-101 with wild-type HCT-116. However, double knockout cells for p21 potentiated the anti-proliferative effect of ZJ-101, resulting in a lower GR value of 0.08 at the highest dose. Despite the observed enhanced suppression of cell growth, the EC_{50} for $p21^{-/-}$ cells is between 115 and 197 nM, compared to the WT values of 29–96 nM.

2.2. ZJ-101 Is a Potent Inhibitor of Cell–Cell Adhesion

To discern the effects of cell–surface vs. cell–cell adhesion, we performed a three-day 3D spheroid formation assay. We selected MDA-MB-231 cells for this assay due to their widely reported ability to form tight 3D spheroids in culture [8]. In this assay, cells are seeded at a density of 2×10^3 cells/well in 96-well ultra-low attachment (ULA) plates.

Cells will transition from monolayers at the bottom of each well into 3D spheroids over a period of 72 h, as noted in the negative control (Figure 2A). To measure the compactness of cells into spheroids, termed spheroidicity, we utilize the overall diameter of cellular distribution within the well. Concurrent treatment with ZJ-101 following cell seeding had a dose-dependent effect on spheroid formation at concentrations of up to 5 μM (Figure 2B). Measuring the overall diameter of the spheroid, relative to a negative control, we determined the EC_{50} for spheroid formation inhibition was between 0.69 and 1.16 nM (Figure 2B). We further assessed the ability of ZJ-101 to affect cell–cell contacts already established in 3D spheroids. Using pre-formed spheroids, grown for 72 h prior to drug addition, we observed an equally strong disruption of cell–cell adhesion. At concentrations above 20 nM, ZJ-101 was able to fully dissolve spheroids over 72 h, leaving individual cells to settle at the bottom of the well (Figure 2C). A rapid disassembly of spheroids can be seen even after the first 24 h of treatment (Figure 2C). Quantitation of spheroidicity at 72 h after addition results in an EC_{50} for spheroid disassembly between 2.37 and 12.05 nM. The discrepancy between approximate EC_{50}'s for spheroid formation versus disassembly is 4 nM. Both effects, however, remain an order of magnitude smaller than the cytostatic effect observed in the GR assay (Figure 1D).

2.3. Transcriptome Analysis Identifies a Dysregulation of the Endomembrane System

Transcriptome analysis has recently become a powerful method to discern drug mechanisms of action. We performed two sets of analyses with four logs of ZJ-101 dose (0.5, 5.0, 50.0, and 500 nM) each. This dose range provides the broadest context for the previously observed phenotypes. To identify differentially expressed genes before cellular morphology is typically affected by ZJ-101, we used a 6 h time point for 2D-cultured MDA-MB-231 cells. Additionally, we performed a 24 h time treatment in pre-formed 3D MDA-MB-231 spheroids to identify genes with altered expression following cell–cell adhesion loss. As previously observed in the spheroid disassembly assay (Figure 2C), this 24 h treatment results in moderate adhesion loss, which increases with dose. Both sets of transcriptome data shared dose-dependent effects on genes within the endomembrane system (GO:0012505), endoplasmic reticulum (GO:0005783), and cell adhesion (GO:0007155), as determined by GO term enrichment analysis via g:Profiler (Figure 3A,B) [9].

The most significantly upregulated genes shared between both sets of data were ATP6V0A1, GPRC5A, SLC3A2, EPHA2, and HSP90AA1 (Figure 3C,D) [10]. Notably,

ATP6V0A1, which encodes a V-type ATPase involved in endosome pH regulation, is significantly upregulated by ZJ-101 treatment. Cellular chaperones such as HSP90AA1 and various Hsp40 family members like DNAJB9 are likewise upregulated in both cellular contexts (Figure 3C,D). At 500 nM, the highest concentration assessed, an upregulation of heat-shock responsive genes was observed within the 6 h time point for the 2D cultured cells (Figure S3A). Unfolded protein response (UPR)-related target genes are simultaneously suppressed (Figure S3B).

Broadly, genes involved in cell adhesion and extracellular matrix organization are downregulated by ZJ-101 treatment (Figure 3C,D). These include the integrin ITGA5, integrin ligand ICAM1, Von Willibrand factor A (VWA1), and collagen type V alpha 1 (COL5A1). Genes involved in protein glycosylation found in the Golgi apparatus, such as B4GALT1 and GALNT1, were also suppressed (Figure 3C,D).

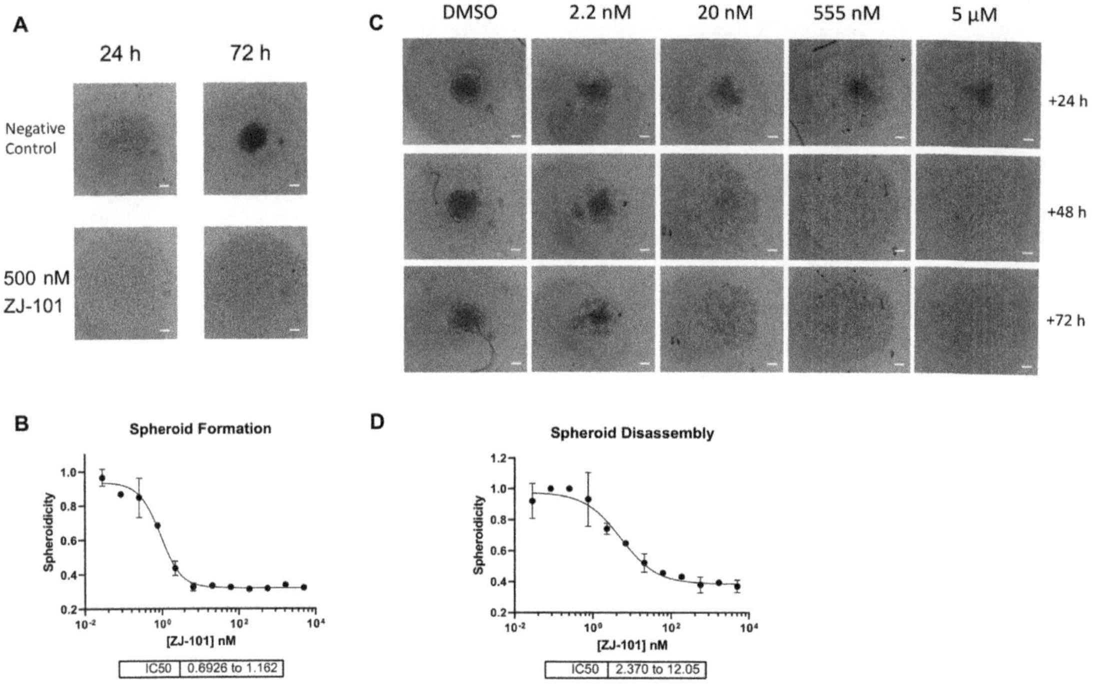

Figure 2. Three-dimensional cell adhesion is potently disrupted by ZJ-101. (**A**) MDA-MB-231 spheroid formation assay. Scale bar = 200 μm (**B**) Effect on spheroid formation is dose-dependent, with an IC_{50} of approximately 1 nM. (**C**) Representative images of pre-formed spheroids (72 h old), treated with ZJ-101 over the indicated times. (**D**) Effect on spheroid disassembly has an EC_{50} of approximately 5 nM.

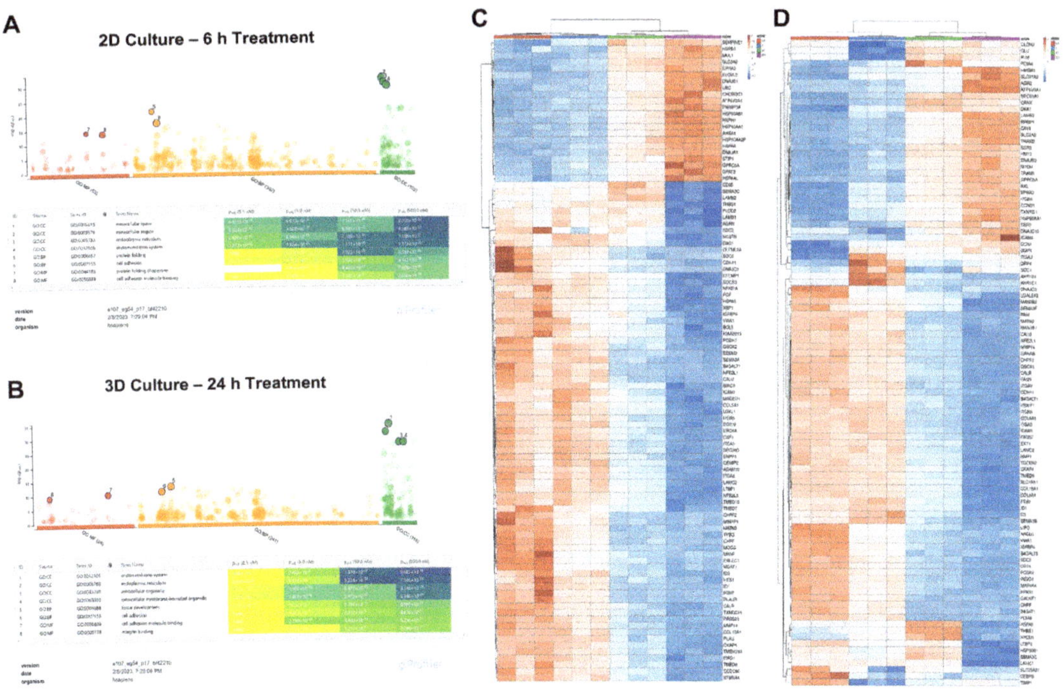

Figure 3. Endomembrane system genes differentially regulated independent of cellular context. (**A**) g:Profiler Gene Ontology (GO) term enrichment analysis after 6 h treatment of four ZJ-101 doses (0.5, 5.0, 50, 500 nM) in MDA-MB-231 cells cultured in 2D format ($n = 3$ biological replicates). The top significantly enriched GO terms from each category were selected and include the extracellular space, endoplasmic reticulum, and endomembrane system with increasing dose. Terms which do not reach significance at a particular dose are indicted by strikethrough (**B**) GO terms for 3D-cultured MDA-MB-231 cells ($n = 3$ biological replicates) treated with ZJ-101 for 24 h. (**C**) ClustVis heatmap for top differentially expressed genes after 6 h ZJ-101 dose–response in 2D-cultured MDA-MB-231 cells. (**D**) ClustVis heatmap for the 24 h ZJ-101 dose–response in 3D-cultured MDA-MB-231 cells.

2.4. Golgi Function Is Dysregulated by ZJ-101

Following transcriptome analysis, our focus narrowed to the endomembrane system, consisting of the ER, Golgi, and general secretory vesicles. We first performed immunostaining of the *cis*-Golgi marker GM130 in fixed HeLa cells to observe changes in Golgi morphology at short time points. In HeLa cells, GM130 assumes a compact perinuclear position, providing a simple marker for alterations in morphology. To minimize changes to overall cellular morphology from the cytotoxic positive control, Brefeldin A (BFA), a four-hour time point was chosen. As seen in Figure 4A, four hours of treatment with BFA drastically alters Golgi morphology by redistributing GM130 to the endoplasmic reticulum, while ZJ-101 at a dose of 1 µM does not (Figure S2A). Washout of BFA after pre-treatment with ZJ-101 also does not alter the ability of GM130 to recover its original morphology (Figure S2B). To interrogate Golgi function, we utilized the fluorescent conjugate of the lectin *Helix Pomatia* Agglutinin (HPA), which selectively binds O-GalNAc residues localized to the Golgi [11,12]. HPA lectin staining was dose-dependently suppressed by ZJ-101 following four hours of treatment in HeLa cells, with the EC_{50} for this effect being approximately 67 nM (Figure 4B). Other lectins, concanavalin A (ConA) and wheat germ agglutinin (WGA), which bind selectively to N-glycans, were unaffected by the treatment (Figure 4B).

Glycomics analysis was performed on both *N*- and *O*-glycans purified from cells treated with 500 nM ZJ-101 for 6 h. Generally, both *N*- and *O*-glycans decreased in relative abundance upon treatment with ZJ-101 (Figure 4C). Several high-molecular-weight *N*-glycans, containing complex polysialylated LacNAc chains, were increased (Table 1). Notable *O*-glycans that were increased include Core-2 *O*-glycans and Disalyl T-Antigen (Table 1).

Glycan incorporation was assessed using an image-based bioorthogonal click-chemistry assay. Azido-modified GlcNAc, GalNAc, and ManNAc, as well as alkynyl-modified Fucose, were added to the media during the 6 h treatment with increasing doses of ZJ-101. Significant decreases in GalNAz and fucose alkyne were observed at 500 nM treatment, with reductions of 12.8% and 25.5% for each, respectively (Figure 4D). No significant changes were observed for GlcNAz incorporation. ManNAz incorporation increased marginally by approximately 12% (Figure 4D).

Table 1. Upregulated glycans.

N-Linked Glycans			
Composition	**Proposed Structure**	**Observed *m/z***	**log2FC**
Hex:6 HexNAc:5 NeuAc:2	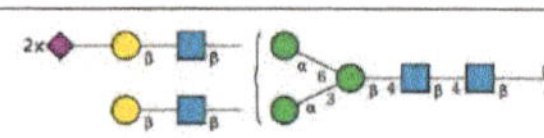	3241.6	0.579
Hex:7 HexNAc:6 Fuc:1	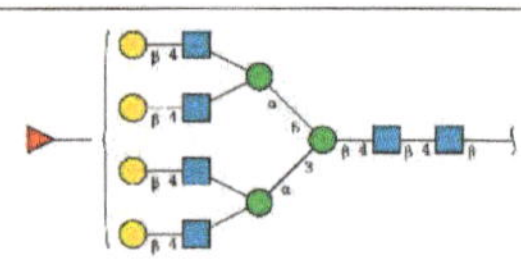	3142.6	0.341
Hex:6 HexNAc:5 Fuc:1 NeuAc:2	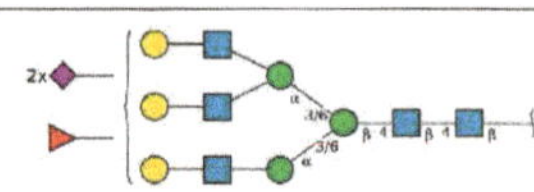	3415.7	0.249
Hex:6 HexNAc:5 NeuAc:3	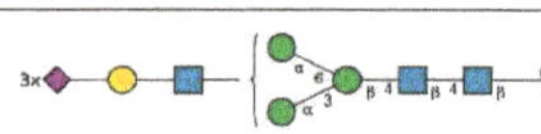	3602.8	0.241
Hex:6 HexNAc:5 Fuc:1 NeuAc:1	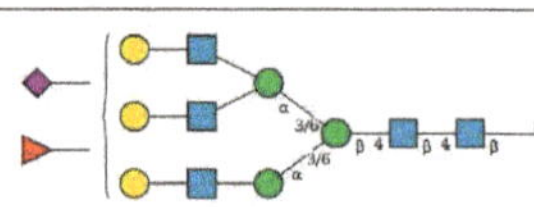	3054.5	0.183
***O*-Linked Glycans**			
Composition	**Proposed Structure**	**Observed *m/z***	**log2FC**
Hex:2 HexNAc:2 NeuAc:2	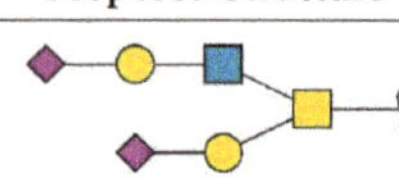	1705.9	0.883
Hex:2 HexNAc:3	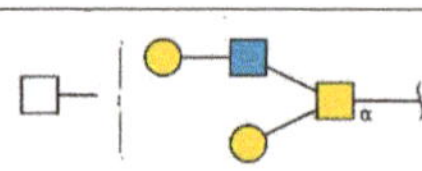	1228.6	0.338
Hex:1 HexNAc:1 NeuAc:2	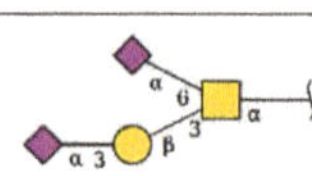	1256.6	0.229

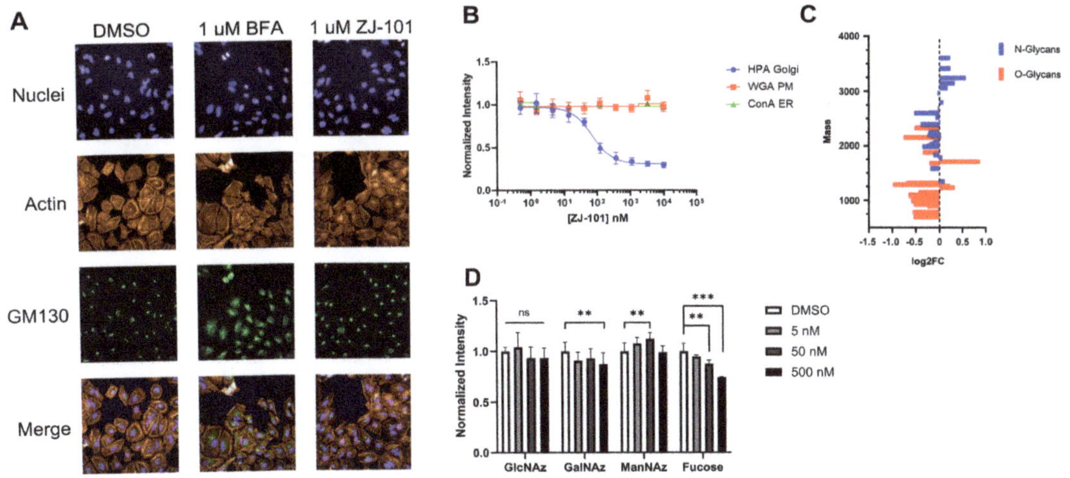

Figure 4. Golgi function is dysregulated by ZJ-101. (**A**) Golgi structure within HeLa cells, as visualized by GM130 immunofluorescence, is not altered by ZJ-101 treatment. Brefeldin A (BFA) has a dose-dependent effect on GM130 redistribution to the endoplasmic reticulum (ER) (n = 3). Scale bar: 20 µM. (**B**) Lectin staining imaging assay; helix pomatia agglutinin (HPA), wheat germ agglutinin (WGA), and concanavalin A (ConA). ZJ-101 selectively and dose-dependently decreases HPA staining intensity at 4 h of treatment. (n = 3). (**C**) Glycomics analysis sorted by mass for N- and O-glycans after 6 h treatment with 500 nM ZJ-101. Most N- and O-glycans are downregulated, notable high-molecular weight N-glycans and complex O-glycans are upregulated and noted in Table 1. (**D**) Glycan incorporation imaging assay performed using biorthogonal click chemistry of azide-modified glucosamine, galactosamine, mannosamine, and alkynyl-modified fucose. ZJ-101 treatment of 6 h results in significant decreases in alkynyl-Fuc and azido-GalNAc incorporation (n = 3). Data represent the mean ± SEM. n.s. = not significant, ** $p \leq 0.01$, *** $p \leq 0.001$.

2.5. ZJ-101 Modulates the Endolysosome

We found no disruption of Golgi structure by ZJ-101 treatment, as judged by GM130 staining (Figure 4A), and no dysregulation of endosome pH using lysotracker dye (Figure 5). We utilized multiple controls for the lysotracker assay to compare ZJ-101 with known modulators of the endomembrane system. Neither Kifunensine, an inhibitor of *N*-glycosylation, nor Brefeldin A, a disruptor of Golgi structure and function, decreased lysosome spot intensity relative to the negative control (Figure 5B) [13,14]. Bafilomycin A1, an inhibitor of V-ATPases found on endosomes, potently decreases lysotracker spot intensity, indicating increased endosome pH (Figure 5B) [15]. Although ZJ-101 does not affect lysosome staining intensity, the average lysosome puncta area is significantly (p = 0.02) decreased (Figure 5C) and is shared by brefeldin A and kifunensine treatments. Despite the decreased puncta size, the percentage of total area that lysosomes occupy in the cell was not changed by ZJ-101, indicating possible enhanced endolysosomal fission events (Figure 5D).

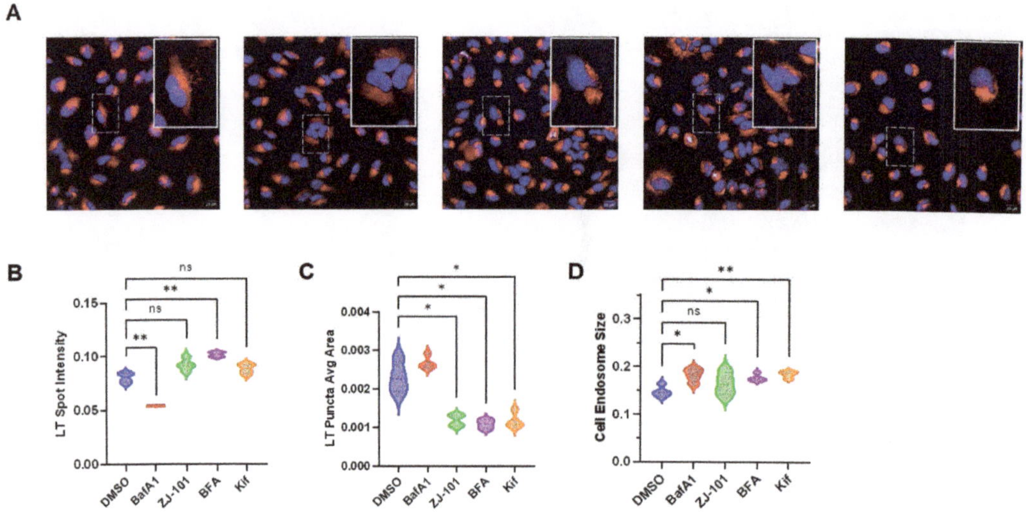

Figure 5. Endolysosomes are modulated by ZJ-101. (**A**) Representative images of lysotracker staining with LT dye in red, nuclei in blue. Cells were treated for 2 h with the following doses: 200 nM bafilomycin A1, 500 nM ZJ-101, 500 nM brefeldin A, 10 μM kifunensine. (**B**) LT spot intensity for each compound assessed. Bafilomycin A1 significantly decreases intensity relative to vehicle control. (**C**) LT puncta average size by area. Treatment with inhibitors of various endomembrane system components results in smaller than average LT puncta spot size, while cells treated with bafilomycin A1 do not have significantly changed LT puncta area relative to DMSO. (**D**) Total LT stained endolysosomal area within the cell. Small, but significant, increases in the total size of endolysosomal compartments are seen with brefeldin A, kifunensine, and bafilomycin A1. ZJ-101 treatment does not result in significant changes to overall endolysosomal area. n.s. = not significant, * $p < 0.05$, ** $p \leq 0.01$.

2.6. ZJ-101 Reverses Etoposide Resistance in 3D Spheroid Model

Resistance to common chemotherapeutics can arise from several factors, including cell–cell adhesion and cell–matrix interactions. To assess the potential for reversal of 3D-induced chemoresistance, we tested ZJ-101 in combination with etoposide in MDA-MB-231 spheroids. Using a modified spheroid disassembly assay incorporating the cellular dyes calcein AM, Hoechst 33342, and ethidium homodimer (EthD), we are able to evaluate the effect of ZJ-101 on cell adhesion and proliferation. Similar to the GR assay, EthD allows for the determination of cytotoxicity. Using an 8 × 8 matrix, 63 combinations of ZJ-101 and etoposide are assessed (Figure 6A). Etoposide was found to be synergistic with ZJ-101 for the induction of cell death, as stained by ethidium homodimer (Figure 6A,B). Synergy was assessed using the SynergyFinder web app (https://synergyfinder.fimm.fi/ (accessed on 19 November 2020)) which calculates a ZIP synergy score for 8 × 8 combination matrices [16]. Etoposide synergizes with ZJ-101 with an average δ-score for concentrations above 10 μM between 40 and 50, indicating 40–50% excess synergy with ZJ-101 over etoposide alone (Figure 6D).

A

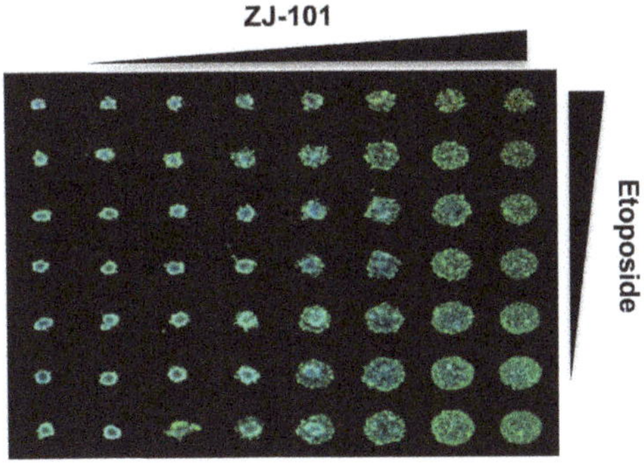

B

EthD Positive Counts

103	87	106	126	174	240	250	224
90	127	111	163	175	212	213	237
78	55	63	79	117	138	151	177
53	69	63	110	93	125	159	168
71	43	80	42	74	103	170	146
46	52	69	60	66	59	103	155
41	59	82	47	52	68	123	143

C

Spheroidicity

1.470588	1.25	1.136364	1	0.735294	0.5	0.462963	0.438596
1.136364	1	0.862069	0.625	0.471698	0.320513	0.301205	0.333333
1.086957	1.086957	1.041667	0.806452	0.543478	0.274725	0.252525	0.277778
1.25	1.136364	1	0.78125	0.543478	0.342466	0.245098	0.274725
1.086957	0.925926	0.925926	0.641026	0.357143	0.274725	0.215517	0.229358
1.136364	1	0.862069	0.657895	0.290698	0.213675	0.201613	0.211864
1	1.041667	0.543478	0.490196	0.280899	0.221239	0.192308	0.210084

D

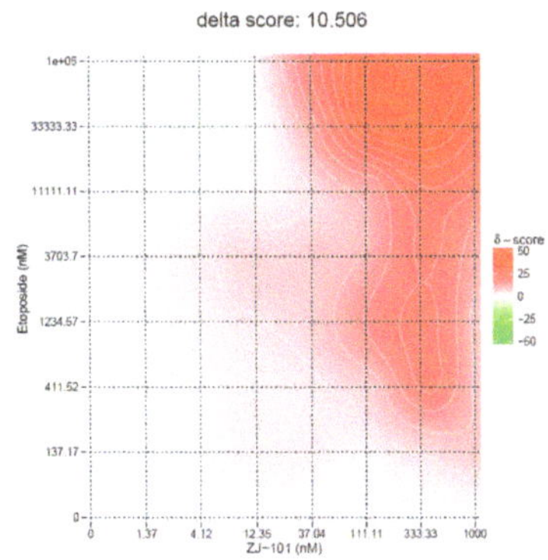

Figure 6. ZJ-101 reverses resistance to etoposide in combination with matrix spheroid assay. (**A**) Fluorescent live-cell images of MDA-MB-231 3D spheroid matrix of ZJ-101 and etoposide at 1:3 dilutions from their maximum concentrations of 1 µM and 100 µM respectively. (**B**) Ethidium homodimer (EthD) counts for each well shown. White–Red heatmap corresponds with increasing counts (**C**) Spheroidicity—the measurement of the diameter of each spheroid normalized to untreated wells. Lower spheroidicity indicates disruption of cell–cell adhesion caused by ZJ-101 treatment and is indicated by the White–Blue heatmap. (**D**) SynergyFinder graph of combinations of ZJ-101 and etoposide shows enhanced synergy above 10 µM etoposide. Green-Red heatmap of delta-scores indicate negative to positive regions of synergy respectively for all dose combination pairs.

3. Discussion

Our group has identified several key phenotypes that suggest a distinct mechanism of action for the compound ZJ-101 by acting through the endomembrane system. We first identified the clear ability of ZJ-101 to cause cell rounding and dislodging from a growth substrate within a few hours. Cellular adhesion occurs in primarily two modalities: cell–cell and cell–substrate adhesion. To determine if ZJ-101 had preferential activity for either of these, we assessed its activity in a 3D spheroid model. To our amazement, extremely low doses of ZJ-101 could halt the formation of spheroids. At approximately 1 nM of the compound, we observed a halt in the progression of standard spheroid formation in the triple-negative breast cancer cell line MDA-MB-231. The disparity in EC_{50s} for the antiproliferative effect previously established versus anti-adhesion in the spheroid model was approximately 30-fold. This unexpected enhancement in potency against the spheroid model challenged our previous assumptions about the molecule.

We utilized the growth rate normalized metric assay (GR assay) to minimize variation between experiments and dependence on cell growth rates. A major benefit of this assay is its ability to discern cytostatic versus cytotoxic effects by comparing cell viability to cellular proliferation. Since all cell types have their own intrinsic growth rate kinetics, we can accurately compare responses to drugs between cell types by normalizing them to this rate. Using this live/dead cell image-based assay, we were able to determine that the effect of ZJ-101 on cancer cells is entirely cytostatic. In GR metrics, cytotoxic compounds are identified by their ability to deplete cell populations below initial seeding densities, denoted by a GR value less than 0. At a GR value greater than 0 but less than 1, cellular proliferation is suppressed in a cytostatic manner. ZJ-101 suppresses cellular growth with a GR value of 0.5 at the highest concentration of 1 μM using the calcein-AM/ethidium homodimer dye staining assay. We obtained the same EC_{50} value (30–90 nM) for ZJ-101 using GR metrics as we previously determined using resazurin-based viability assays (Figure S1A). These results confirmed that one of ZJ-101′s primary novel phenotypes is cytostatic suppression of cellular proliferation.

Cytostasis is often a temporary cellular state induced by exogenous signals or chemicals that suppress cell division. Senescence, a physiological state of non-dividing cells that can be induced by oxidative stress or DNA damage, has all the hallmarks of cellular cytostasis. A key characteristic of senescence is a sharp increase in G1-phase cell populations. Because of the lack of change in any population (G1, S, or G2) during prolonged treatment with ZJ-101, cellular senescence could potentially be ruled out as a mechanism for the cytostatic activity. At time points of up to 48 h, MDA-MB-231 cells remained dislodged from their substrate under the sustained treatment of ZJ-101, further underscoring the distinct lack of any sub-G1 populations. Typically, cells will undergo apoptosis following sustained senescence or cell adhesion loss, a unique form of apoptosis termed anoikis [17]. To further explore senescence using GR metrics, we tested isogenic cell lines of HCT-116 containing knockouts of p21 and p53, key senescence potentiators [18]. We found no reversal of anti-proliferative activity under treatment with ZJ-101 in these knockout lines. Instead, p21 knockout potentiates the effect of ZJ-101′s suppression of cell proliferation. This result runs counter to an activation of senescence by ZJ-101, given that p21 expression is protective against cytostasis. Although the outcome of ZJ-101 treatment results in the halting of cellular proliferation, more work is required to determine the specific pathway(s) leading to this long-term cytostatic suppression.

To identify cellular pathways regulated by ZJ-101, transcriptome sequencing was undertaken across four doses in two contexts: before 2D adhesion loss at 6 h, and after adhesion loss at 24 h in 3D spheroids (Figure S4). Gene Ontology (GO) analysis identified increasing significance for the endoplasmic reticulum (GO:005783), cell adhesion (GO:007155), and the endomembrane system (GO:0012505) as the dose of ZJ-101 increases. Notably, endomembrane system genes represent the highest differentially expressed genes by significance between 2D and 3D culture formats. Genes related to the endoplasmic reticulum follow a paradoxical response to ZJ-101 treatment. Despite a general upregulation of heat-shock genes such as HSP90AA1, unfolded protein response (UPR) target genes were suppressed at 6 h. UPR-related genes remained suppressed at the 24 h time point as well, indicating a context-independent downregulation of ER-stress-responsive genes. Likewise, cell adhesion and extracellular matrix (ECM) genes were suppressed. Among these, several integrins, such as ITGA5, ITGAV, and ITGB5, were downregulated. These integrins are primarily responsible for cell–ECM adhesion and cannot solely explain the dual inhibition of cell–substrate and cell–cell adhesion caused by ZJ-101. Due to this unique transcriptional response, we reasoned that the stress caused by ZJ-101 may localize to a source within the wider endomembrane system, such as the Golgi and endosomes.

Genes involved in endosome homeostasis, such as ATP6V0A1, were significantly dysregulated by ZJ-101. V-type ATPases, such as ATP6V0A1, regulate endosome and vesicle pH. We compared ZJ-101 to the well-known inhibitor of V-type ATPases, Bafilomycin A1, through lysotracker staining, which fluoresces in the acidic compartments of endosomes and lysosomes. As observed in Figure 5B, bafilomycin A1 potently decreases lysotracker staining intensity relative to control, while ZJ-101 does not. Additionally, ZJ-101 treatment decreases endolysosome size in a similar manner to brefeldin A and kifunensine. Brefeldin A's unique mechanism of redistributing the Golgi membrane to the ER through uncompetitive inhibition of the Arf1 GDP exchange cycle poses the most curious parallel for ZJ-101′s potential mechanism of action [19]. Although ZJ-101 does not redistribute GM130 as BFA does, they both likely enhance endolysosomal fission events, leading to the decreased puncta size observed after treatment. It is possible that ZJ-101 inhibits a target in opposition to the BFA mechanism, preserving the Golgi structurally but resulting in similar outcomes. Kifunensine also affects endolysosomal size, though it acts through inhibition of the ER mannosidase I enzyme. By inhibiting N-glycan trimming in the ER, protein sorting through the ER-associated degradation (ERAD) pathway is increased, leading to a loss of successful traversal of cargo through the secretory pathway [20].

We initially identified a dysregulation of glycosylation localized to the Golgi apparatus through lectin staining assays. Lectin staining determined a selectivity for decreasing N-acetyl-galactosamine (GalNAc) residues, which are typically added to substrates by GalNAc transferases within the Golgi [21]. Despite no clear structural alteration to the Golgi itself, GalNAc accumulation was suppressed at short time points by ZJ-101. Glycomics analysis confirmed a general downregulation of *O*- and *N*-glycan-bearing proteins (Figure S5), with several exceptions. Poly-sialylated high-molecular-weight N-glycans, bearing N-acetyl-lactosamine (LacNAc), were upregulated to a relatively high degree. These glycans are produced by the enzyme βGALT4 in the *trans*-Golgi, which indicates this region remains active during ZJ-101 treatment [22]. This result is counter to that of the transcriptomic signature, where transcripts of B4GALT1 and other galactosyltransferases are found to be suppressed by ZJ-101. It is possible this downregulation is caused by a feedback loop from these LacNAc residues accumulating in the *trans*-Golgi. Additional poly-sialylated O-glycan residues, such as the sialyl-Tn antigen, known to be processed by ST6GalNAc, were also found to be upregulated (Table 1), indicating that sialyl-transferase activity in the Golgi also remained. Despite the global decrease in N-glycan abundance, lectin staining of both high-mannose and N-acetyl-glucosamine (GlcNAc) residues was unchanged by ZJ-101 treatment. This discrepancy may stem from the long half-lives of proteins bearing these residues, which may not yet have turned over. It's likely that new proteins exiting the Golgi, or held within the trans-Golgi network, bear the more complex LacNAc residues identified in the glycomics analysis. A similar accrual of poly-sialylated N-glycans in the trans-Golgi was recently observed by Kitano et al. following Rab11 knockdown, which may provide a possible explanation for ZJ-101′s effect [23]. Further inquiry is required to determine whether glycosyltransferase localization at the Golgi is affected by ZJ-101.

We performed a high-content 3D-spheroid drug combination synergy assay using a modified spheroid disassembly assay. Our objective was to identify whether the anti-adhesive effect of ZJ-101 could reverse a common mechanism of drug resistance mediated by tight cellular adhesion [24,25]. In a 2D context, etoposide treatment induces high BRCA1 expression in MDA-MB-231 cells, making them naturally resistant to etoposide's mechanism of action [26]. For MDA-MB-231 spheroids in particular, ECM interactions further limit drug accessibility, providing a key context to assess 3D-induced chemoresistance to topoisomerase II inhibitors [27]. Broad suppression of extracellular matrix and cell adhesion gene transcripts by ZJ-101 lends further support to a possible reversal of chemoresistance mediated by such factors. Our combination synergy assay utilizes the zero interaction potency (ZIP) synergy score, which evaluates individual drug combination pairs relative to their separate dose–response curves [28]. ZIP synergy normalizes drug response to assume a "zero interaction" or minimal shift in dose–response between combination pairs. Etoposide synergizes with ZJ-101 with an average δ score of 10.5 across all combination pairs, indicating positive synergy. δ-scores describe the excess percentage at which combination pairs are synergistic or antagonistic. For etoposide, the average δ-score for concentrations above 10 μM is between 40 and 50, indicating 40–50% excess synergy with ZJ-101 over etoposide alone.

In conclusion, we have identified several unique phenotypes produced by treatment with the marine natural product-derived compound, ZJ-101. We discovered a strongly cytostatic and antiadhesive phenotype at single-digit nanomolar concentrations, which is unique and unprecedented. Through transcriptomic analysis, we identified dysregulation of the endomembrane system, which was later confirmed by lectin staining and glycomics analysis. Our work has established a potential synergistic mechanism for the reversal of chemoresistance mediated by 3D cell adhesion. Other mechanisms of multidrug resistance mediated by endolysosomal trafficking provide a future direction for compounds such as ZJ-101, which dysregulate glycosylation [29]. Recent screens for regulators of cellular glycosylation have indicated potential use against SARS-CoV-2 viral entry, offering another potential path for further ZJ-101 investigation [30].

4. Materials and Methods

4.1. Cell Culture

Cells were cultured in DMEM media (Gibco Cat # 11885, Billings, MT, USA) supplemented with 10% fetal bovine serum and 1% penicillin/streptomycin.

4.2. Cell Cycle Analysis

Cell cycle analysis was performed using propidium iodide staining of fixed MDA-MB-231 cells treated with ZJ-101. Briefly, a 70% confluent 10 cm dish of MDA-MB-231 was collected via trypsinization and washed with 1× PBS. Pelleted cells were fixed by the dropwise addition of 2 mL of ice-cold 75% EtOH. Fixed cells were washed again with PBS and stained with 1 mg/mL propidium iodide solution prior to FACS analysis.

4.3. Growth-Rate Inhibition Metric Analysis

Control populations of MDA-MB-231 cells were prepared for growth rate normalization at seeding densities of 50, 200, 500, and 1000 cells per well in a 384-well flat bottom plate (Corning Inc., Corning, NY, USA). Following compound treatment, cells were stained with 1 μM Calcein AM (for live cells), 20 μg/mL Hoechst 33342 (for nucleus), and 1 μM ethidium homodimer (a cell membrane impermeable dye for dead cells) for 15 min at 37 °C prior to imaging. Imaging was performed using the 4× objective on the ImageXpress Micro (Molecular Devices, San Jose, CA, USA) with image-based focusing. Collected images were assessed using the live/dead program in MetaXpress (version 6.1), and data were organized and entered into grcalculator.org, where growth rate normalized inhibition calculations were performed for each compound tested.

4.4. 3D Spheroid Assays

Three-dimensional spheroid formation was assessed using Corning ultra-low attachment (ULA) plates. MDA-MB-231 cells were seeded in ULA plates at a density of 2×10^3 cells/well (96-well) or 5×10^2 cells/well (384-well) in DMEM media supplemented with 10% FBS and centrifuged for 5 min at 400× *g*. Cells were then left undisturbed in a 37 °C, 5% CO_2 incubator for 72 h to form spheroids. ZJ-101 was added at the indicated concentrations and incubated for a further 72 h. Pretreatment of ZJ-101 was also performed with basic light images taken every 24 h for up to 72 h. Spheroidicity was determined based on the overall diameter normalized to an untreated control using ImageJ (version 1.52r).

The 3D spheroid combination assay was performed as a spheroid disassembly assay requiring 72 h of pre-formed spheroids prior to a further 72 h of drug addition. ZJ-101 and etoposide were arranged with 1:3 dilutions in an 8 × 8 matrix format at the indicated concentrations. Fluorescent images were acquired after staining using the same protocol and instrumentation outlined in the GR assay. Laser-based focusing was utilized to obtain clear spheroid images from the bottom of each well. Ten z-stack images were taken and combined into a single maximum-intensity image. Images were processed with the live/dead program in MetaExpress.

4.5. Cell Staining and Imaging

Basic light microscopy was performed on HEK293T cells cultured in 6-well TC-treated plates (Greiner #657160, Kremsmünster, Austria) by capturing images through the 20X objective of a Zeiss Axiovert 25 (Carl Zeiss Microscopy, White Plains NY, USA) with a 12.2 megapixel camera. For MDA-MB-231 spheroid light microscopy, the same protocol was used with a 10X objective.

For all staining assays, HeLa cells were cultured on 96-well CellView TC-treated microplates (Greiner #655891, Kremsmünster, Austria). Cells were washed with cold PBS prior to fixation with 4% PFA for 10 min at RT. After fixation, cells were washed twice with PBS and permeabilized with 0.1% Triton-X for 10 min at RT. Cells were again washed twice with PBS and blocked with cell staining buffer for 30 min. Antibodies for GM130 (Cell Signaling #12480, Danvers, MA, USA) were added at 1:1000 in staining buffer for 1 h at RT. After three washes with PBS, secondary anti-rabbit AlexaFluor-488, or AlexaFluor-647 (ThermoFisher, Waltham, MA, USA) were added along with the indicated fluorescent lectin conjugates (HPA-647, WGA-488, and PNA-555 from ThermoFisher) at 1:1000 dilution for 1 h RT. Cells were again washed and stained with 1:10^4 Hoechst 33,342 for 3 min prior to imaging with an OperaPhenix (PerkinElmer, Waltham, MA, USA). Images were uploaded to the Columbus Analyzer (version 2.9.1.699) and processed for high-content analysis.

For the live cell lysotracker assay, HeLa cells were cultured as above during treatment with the specified compounds. Cells were loaded with DMEM media containing 100 nM Lysotracker Deep Red for 30 min at 37 °C. After lysotracker staining, media was exchanged for Live Cell Imaging Solution (Invitrogen #A14291DJ, Waltham, MA, USA) containing 1:10^4 Hoechst 33342 for nuclei staining. Images were uploaded to the Columbus Analyzer and processed for high-content analysis using default settings for spot detection and intensity calculation.

4.6. Transcriptome Analysis

MDA-MB-231 cells from 10 cm dishes were harvested through scraping (for 2D) or spheroids collected (for 3D) using a wide-gauge pipette and subjected to RNA extraction via the RNeasy mini kit using the manufacturer's instructions. Biological replicates of N = 3 were used for both sets of analyses, with N = 96 spheroids representing a single biological replicate for the 3D populations. RNA-sequencing was performed by Genewiz as paired-end 150 bp reads following poly-A selection to enrich mRNA transcripts. Paired-end FASTQ files were uploaded to Galaxy using the public server at usegalaxy.org (accessed on 7 April 2021) and aligned to hg38 using HISAT2. Transcripts were assembled and counted using htseq-count, and differential gene expression was evaluated with DESeq2 with default settings. Fold changes were assessed against the DMSO vehicle controls. Transcripts were annotated using the most current GENCODE release. Gene Ontology analysis was performed using g:Profiler at https://biit.cs.ut.ee/gprofiler/gost (accessed on 8 April 2021) by inputting the top 200 significant genes for each concentration of ZJ-101 and arranging them by descending order of significance [9]. Heatmaps and PCA plots were generated using ClustVis v1.0 at https://biit.cs.ut.ee/clustvis/ (accessed on 8 April 2021) [10].

The data discussed in this publication have been deposited in NCBI's Gene Expression Omnibus and are accessible through GEO accession number GSE231359 https://www.ncbi.nlm.nih.gov/geo/query/acc.cgi?acc=GSE231359 (accessed on 8 April 2021) [31].

4.7. Glycan Analysis

4.7.1. Glycan Incorporation Assay

Briefly, 50 µM azido-modified sugars (Invitrogen) tetraacetylated N-azidoacetylglucosamine (GlcNAz), tetraacetylated N-azidoacetylgalactosamine (GalNAz), tetraacetylated N-azidoacetyl-D-mannosamine (ManNAz), and 100 µM alkynyl-fucose (Invitrogen) were added to 96-well plates in combination with the indicated doses of ZJ-101. Cells were then washed, fixed, and permeabilized prior to the click reaction. Copper-catalyzed click reactions were performed using the Click-iT Cell Reaction Buffer Kit (Invitrogen C10269) per the manufacturer's instructions, containing 5 µM of either Fluor alkyne-647 (Invitrogen A10278) to label azido-incorporated sugars or Fluor Azide-488 to label incorporated alkynyl-fucose. Plates were washed five times before Hoechst counterstaining and imaging. Glycan incorporation was determined by the total intensity of each signal normalized to untreated control cells.

4.7.2. Glycome Profiling

Glycomics profiling was performed by Creative Proteomics. N-glycans were prepared from fresh cell pellets washed with PBS, resuspended in 1 mL of lysis buffer, and sonicated (5 pulses of 10 s). Samples were then dialyzed in 50 mM ammonium bicarbonate for 24 h at 4 °C, with the buffer changed three times. Following dialysis, the samples were lyophilized. To the lyophilized powder, 1 mL of 2 mg/mL DTT was added, and the solution was incubated at 50 °C for 2 h. Briefly, 1 mL of a 12 mg/mL IAA (iodoacetamide, Sigma, St. Louis, MO, USA) solution was then added and incubated at RT in the dark for 2 h. The DTT and IAA-treated proteins were then dialyzed against 50 mM ammonium bicarbonate (Sigma) for 24 h at 4 °C. Samples were next resuspended in 1 mL of 500 µg/mL TPCK-treated trypsin (Sigma) solution and incubated at 37 °C overnight. The trypsin reaction mixture was purified over C18 Sep-Pak columns (Waters, Milford, MA, USA) by 1-propanol elution. Fractions containing peptides were pooled and lyophilized. The lyophilized peptides were resuspended in 200 µL of 50 mM ammonium bicarbonate, to which 3 µL of PNGaseF (New England Biolabs, Ipswich, MA, USA) was added for a 4 h incubation at 37 °C. Following this initial incubation, another 5 µL of PNGaseF was added for overnight incubation at 37 °C. The enzymatic reaction was stopped by the addition of two drops of 5% acetic acid, and the released N-glycans were purified over C18 Sep-Pak columns. Flow-through and 5% acetic acid washing fractions containing the released N-glycans were pooled and lyophilized and were subject to permethylation. For O-glycan analysis, the PNGaseF-treated glycopeptides were eluted from the C18 column with 1-propanol. The lyophilized eluted peptides were subjected to *O*-glycan preparation.

O-glycan-containing powder was solubilized by 400 µL of a sodium borohydride (Sigma-Aldrich) solution in 0.1 M NaOH (55 mg NaBH4/1 mL 0.1 M NaOH) and incubated overnight at 45 °C. The reaction was stopped by adding drops of pure acetic acid until the fizzing stopped. The samples were passed through a Dowex 50W X8 resin (Sigma-Aldrich) column, and the pooled fractions were dried by lyophilization. The lyophilized samples were next resuspended in 1 mL of an acetic acid:methanol solution (1:9 *v*/*v*) and co-evaporated under nitrogen flow. This step was repeated 3 more times, and the dried samples were resuspended in 200 µL of 50% methanol prior to being loaded onto the C18 Sep-Pak column. Free *O*-glycans were collected in the flow-through and 5% acetic acid wash fractions. These fractions were pooled, lyophilized, and subjected to permethylation.

Permethylation was performed as follows. Seven pellets of NaOH in 3 mL of DMSO were ground with a mortar and pestle. One milliliter of this slurry solution was added to the dry sample in a glass tube with a screw cap. Five hundred microliters of iodomethane was then added to the slurry and shaken at RT for ~30 min. After the reaction reaches completion, noting the formation of white solids, the cap is released slowly to relieve the gas pressure that has built up. One milliliter of MilliQ water was added to stop the reaction, and the sample was vortexed until all solids were dissolved. To the sample, 1 mL of chloroform and an additional 3 mL of MilliQ water were added with continuous vortexing to mix both phases. The samples were then centrifuged briefly to separate the chloroform and the water phases (~5000 rpm, <20 s). The aqueous top layer was discarded, and washing was repeated twice with the addition of 3 mL of MilliQ water. The chloroform fraction was then dried with a SpeedVac (~20–30 min). A C18 Spe-Pak (200 mg) column was prepared with methanol, MiliQ water, acetonitrile, and MilliQ water. The dry sample was resuspended with 200 µL of 50% methanol and loaded onto the column. The column is then washed with 2 mL of 15% acetonitrile and eluted into a clean glass tube with 3 mL of 50% acetonitrile. Finally, the eluted fraction was subjected to MS analysis.

MS data were acquired on a Bruker UltraFlex II MALDI-TOF mass spectrometer instrument (Bruker Scientific LLC, Billerica, MA, USA). Reflective positive mode was used, and data were usually recorded between 500 *m*/*z* and 6000 *m*/*z* for *N*-linked glycans and between 500 *m*/*z* and 4000 *m*/*z* for *O*-glycans. For each MS N- and *O*-glycan profile, the aggregation of 20,000 laser shots or more was considered for data extraction. Mass signals with a signal/noise ratio of at least 2 were considered, and only MS signals matching an *N*- and *O*-glycan composition were considered for further analysis and annotation. Subsequent MS post-data acquisition analysis was made using mMass [32].

4.8. Statistical Analysis

Statistical tests were performed on GraphPad Prism version 9.5. The normalized data from $n = 3$ independent experiments were analyzed for significance using the Brown–Forsythe and Welch one-way ANOVA. Statistical significance is set for * $p < 0.05$, ** $p \leq 0.01$, *** $p \leq 0.001$.

Supplementary Materials: The following supporting information can be downloaded at: https://www.mdpi.com/article/10.3390/ijms24119575/s1.

Author Contributions: P.R.S. conceptualization, methodology, investigation, formal analysis, data curation, visualization, writing—original draft; S.A.H. supervision, methodology, writing—review and editing; S.Q. resources; H.Q. resources; A.R. resources; Z.J. resources; project administration, writing—review and editing; W.Z. conceptualization, supervision, project administration, funding acquisition, resources, writing—review and editing; J.O.L. conceptualization, supervision, project administration, funding acquisition, resources, writing—review and editing. All authors have read and agreed to the published version of the manuscript.

Funding: The work was supported by the intramural research program of the National Center for Advancing Translational Sciences (W.Z.). This work was also supported by a grant to Z.J. and J.O.L. from the National Institutes of Health (NIH Grant: 1R21CA204836-01). Work performed at JHMI was also supported by the FAMRI grant to J.O.L. P.R.S. received support from the National Institutes of Health (NIH Grant: 5T32GM008763) and the Postdoctoral Intramural Research Training Award (IRTA) of the NIH.

Data Availability Statement: Data are available upon request.

Conflicts of Interest: Zhendong Jin is the founder and a shareholder of InnoBioPharma, LLC, Piscataway, NJ, USA, which sponsored the project, "Development of novel anticancer agents based on natural products" at the University of Iowa. All other authors declare no conflict of interest.

References

1. Kelly, M. *The Marine Fauna of New Zealand: Porifera: Lithistid Demospongiae (Rock Sponges)*; NIWA: Auckland, New Zealand, 2007.
2. Sollas, W.J. Report on the Tetractinellida Collected by H.M.S. Challenger, During the Years 1873–1876. Report on the Scientific Results of the Voyage of H.M.S. Challenger during the Years 1873–1876. *Zoology* **1888**, *25*. [CrossRef]
3. D'Auria, M.V.; Debitus, C.; Paloma, L.G.; Minale, L.; Zampella, A. Superstolide A: A potent cytotoxic macrolide of a new type from the New Caledonian deep water marine sponge Neosiphonia superstes. *J. Am. Chem. Soc.* **1994**, *116*, 6658–6663.
4. D'Auria, M.V.; Paloma, L.G.; Minale, L.; Zampella, A.; Debitus, C. A novel cytotoxic macrolide, superstolide B, related to superstolide A, from the New Caledonian marine sponge Neosiphonia superstes. *J. Nat. Prod.* **1994**, *57*, 1595–1597. [CrossRef] [PubMed]
5. Chen, L.; Ahmed, K.B.R.; Huang, P.; Jin, Z. Design, synthesis, and biological evaluation of truncated superstolide A. *Angew. Chem. Int. Ed. Engl.* **2013**, *52*, 3446–3449. [CrossRef] [PubMed]
6. Maiga-Wandiam, B.; Corbu, A.; Massiot, G.; Sautel, F.; Yu, P.; Lin, B.W.-Y.; Houk, K.N.; Cossy, J. Intramolecular Diels-Alder Approaches to the Decalin Core of Verongidolide: The Origin of the exo-Selectivity, a DFT Analysis. *J. Org. Chem.* **2018**, *83*, 5975–5985. [CrossRef]
7. Hafner, M.; Niepel, M.; Chung, M.; Sorger, P.K. Growth rate inhibition metrics correct for confounders in measuring sensitivity to cancer drugs. *Nat. Methods* **2016**, *13*, 521–527. [CrossRef]
8. Benton, G.; DeGray, G.; Kleinman, H.K.; George, J.; Arnaoutova, I. In Vitro Microtumors Provide a Physiologically Predictive Tool for Breast Cancer Therapeutic Screening. *PLoS ONE* **2015**, *10*, e0123312.
9. Raudvere, U.; Kolberg, L.; Kuzmin, I.; Arak, T.; Adler, P.; Peterson, H.; Vilo, J. g:Profiler: A web server for functional enrichment analysis and conversions of gene lists (2019 update). *Nucleic Acids Res.* **2019**, *47*, W191–W198. [CrossRef]
10. Metsalu, T.; Vilo, J. ClustVis: A web tool for visualizing clustering of multivariate data using Principal Component Analysis and heatmap. *Nucleic Acids Res.* **2015**, *43*, W566–W570. [CrossRef]
11. Virtanen, I. Helix pomatia agglutinin binds specifically to the Golgi apparatus in cultured human fibroblasts and reveals two Golgi apparatus-specific glycoproteins. *Histochemistry* **1990**, *94*, 397–401. [CrossRef]
12. Sanchez, J.-F.; Lescar, J.; Chazalet, V.; Audfray, A.; Gagnon, J.; Alvarez, R.; Breton, C.; Imberty, A.; Mitchell, E.P. Biochemical and structural analysis of Helix pomatia agglutinin. A hexameric lectin with a novel fold. *J. Biol. Chem.* **2006**, *281*, 20171–20180. [CrossRef]

13. Lodge, E.K.; Bell, J.D.; Roloff, E.M.; Hamilton, K.E.; Louters, L.L.; Looyenga, B.D. Pharmacologic inhibition of N-linked glycan trimming with kifunensine disrupts GLUT1 trafficking and glucose uptake. *Biochimie* **2020**, *174*, 18–29.
14. Fujiwara, T.; Oda, K.; Yokota, S.; Takatsuki, A.; Ikehara, Y. Brefeldin A causes disassembly of the Golgi complex and accumulation of secretory proteins in the endoplasmic reticulum. *J. Biol. Chem.* **1988**, *263*, 18545–18552.
15. Bowman, E.J.; Siebers, A.; Altendorf, K. Bafilomycins: A class of inhibitors of membrane ATPases from microorganisms, animal cells, and plant cells. *Proc. Natl. Acad. Sci. USA* **1988**, *85*, 7972–7976.
16. Zheng, S.; Wang, W.; Aldahdooh, J.; Malyutina, A.; Shadbahr, T.; Tanoli, Z.; Pessia, A.; Tang, J. SynergyFinder Plus: Toward Better Interpretation and Annotation of Drug Combination Screening Datasets. *Genom. Proteom. Bioinform.* **2022**, *20*, 587–596. [CrossRef]
17. Paoli, P.; Giannoni, E.; Chiarugi, P. Anoikis molecular pathways and its role in cancer progression. *Biochim. Biophys. Acta* **2013**, *1833*, 3481–3498.
18. Waldman, T.; Kinzler, K.W.; Vogelstein, B. p21 is necessary for the p53-mediated G1 arrest in human cancer cells. *Cancer Res.* **1995**, *55*, 5187–5190.
19. Niu, T.K.; Pfeifer, A.C.; Lippincott-Schwartz, J.; Jackson, C.L. Dynamics of GBF1, a Brefeldin A-sensitive Arf1 exchange factor at the Golgi. *Mol. Biol. Cell* **2005**, *16*, 1213–1222.
20. Anelli, T.; Sitia, R. Protein quality control in the early secretory pathway. *EMBO J.* **2008**, *27*, 315–327. [CrossRef]
21. Wandall, H.H.; Nielsen, M.A.I.; King-Smith, S.; de Haan, N.; Bagdonaite, I. Global functions of O-glycosylation: Promises and challenges in O-glycobiology. *FEBS J.* **2021**, *288*, 7183–7212. [CrossRef]
22. Rabouille, C.; Hui, N.; Hunte, F.; Kieckbusch, R.; Berger, E.G.; Warren, G.; Nilsson, T. Mapping the distribution of Golgi enzymes involved in the construction of complex oligosaccharides. *J. Cell Sci.* **1995**, *108 Pt 4*, 1617–1627. [PubMed]
23. Kitano, M.; Kizuka, Y.; Sobajima, T.; Nakano, M.; Nakajima, K.; Misaki, R.; Itoyama, S.; Harada, Y.; Harada, A.; Myioshi, E.; et al. Rab11-mediated post-Golgi transport of the sialyltransferase ST3GAL4 suggests a new mechanism for regulating glycosylation. *J. Biol. Chem.* **2021**, *296*, 100354. [CrossRef] [PubMed]
24. Rebucci, M.; Michiels, C. Molecular aspects of cancer cell resistance to chemotherapy. *Biochem. Pharmacol.* **2013**, *85*, 1219–1226. [CrossRef] [PubMed]
25. Bukowski, K.; Kchiuk, M.; Kontek, R. Mechanisms of Multidrug Resistance in Cancer Chemotherapy. *Int. J. Mol. Sci.* **2020**, *21*, 3233. [CrossRef]
26. Zhang, X.; Hofmann, S.; Harbeck, N.; Jeschke, U.; Sixou, S. Impact of Etoposide on BRCA1 Expression in Various Breast Cancer Cell Lines. *Drugs R D* **2017**, *17*, 569–583. [CrossRef]
27. Lovitt, C.J.; Shelper, T.B.; Avery, V.M. Doxorubicin resistance in breast cancer cells is mediated by extracellular matrix proteins. *BMC Cancer* **2018**, *18*, 41.
28. Yadav, B.; Wennerberg, K.; Aittokallio, T.; Tang, J. Searching for Drug Synergy in Complex Dose-Response Landscapes Using an Interaction Potency Model. *Comput. Struct. Biotechnol. J.* **2015**, *13*, 504–513.
29. Hussein, N.A.; Malla, S.; Pasternak, M.A.; Terrero, D.; Brown, N.G.; Ashby, C.R., Jr.; Assaraf, Y.G.; Chen, Z.-S.; Tiwari, A.K. The role of endolysosomal trafficking in anticancer drug resistance. *Drug Resist. Updates* **2021**, *57*, 100769.
30. Sorensen, D.M.; Büll, C.; Madsen, T.D.; Lira-Navarette, E.; Clausen, T.M.; Clark, A.E.; Garretson, A.F.; Karlsson, R.; Pijnenborg, J.F.A.; Yin, X.; et al. Identification of global inhibitors of cellular glycosylation. *Nat. Commun.* **2023**, *14*, 948. [CrossRef]
31. Edgar, R.; Domrachev, M.; Lash, A.E. Gene Expression Omnibus: NCBI gene expression and hybridization array data repository. *Nucleic Acids Res.* **2002**, *30*, 207–210.
32. Strohalm, M.; Kavan, D.; Novák, P.; Volný, M.; Havlícek, V. mMass 3: A cross-platform software environment for precise analysis of mass spectrometric data. *Anal. Chem.* **2010**, *82*, 4648–4651. [CrossRef]

International Journal of
Molecular Sciences

MDPI

Article

Mitochondria-Targeting 1,5-Diazacyclooctane-Spacered Triterpene Rhodamine Conjugates Exhibit Cytotoxicity at Sub-Nanomolar Concentration against Breast Cancer Cells

Niels Heise [1], Selina Becker [1], Thomas Mueller [2], Matthias Bache [3], René Csuk [1,*] and Antje Güttler [3]

1 Organic Chemistry, Martin-Luther-University Halle-Wittenberg, Kurt-Mothes-Str. 2, 06120 Halle (Saale), Germany; niels.heise@chemie.uni-halle.de (N.H.); selinabecker11@googlemail.com (S.B.)
2 University Clinic for Internal Medicine IV, Hematology/Oncology, Martin-Luther-University Halle-Wittenberg, Ernst-Grube-Str. 40, 06120 Halle (Saale), Germany; thomas.mueller@medizin.uni-halle.de
3 Department of Radiotherapy, Martin-Luther-University Halle-Wittenberg, Ernst-Grube-Str. 40, 06120 Halle (Saale), Germany; matthias.bache@uk-halle.de (M.B.); antje.guettler@uk-halle.de (A.G.)
* Correspondence: rene.csuk@chemie.uni-halle.de; Tel.: +49-345-5525660

Abstract: 1,5-Diazacyclooctane was prepared by a simple synthetic sequence and coupled to pentacyclic triterpenoic acids oleanolic acid, ursolic acid, betulinic acid, platanic acid, and asiatic acid; these amides were activated with oxalyl chloride and reacted with rhodamine B or rhodamine 101 to yield conjugates. The conjugates were screened in SRB assays with various human breast cancer cell lines (MDA-MB-231, HS578T, MCF-7, and T47D) and found to exert cytotoxic activity even at a low concentration. Therefore, for an asiatic acid rhodamine 101 conjugate (28), an IC_{50} = 0.60 nM was determined and found to induce apoptosis in MDA-MB-231 and HS578T cells. Extra experiments showed the compound to act as a mitocan and to induce inhibition of proliferation or growth arrest in MDA-MB-231 cells at lower doses followed by an induction of apoptosis at higher doses. Furthermore, differential responses to proliferation inhibition and apoptosis induction may explain differential sensitivity of mammary cell lines to compound 28.

Keywords: asiatic acid; breast cancer; mitocans; rhodamine conjugates; triterpenoic acids

Citation: Heise, N.; Becker, S.; Mueller, T.; Bache, M.; Csuk, R.; Güttler, A. Mitochondria-Targeting 1,5-Diazacyclooctane-Spacered Triterpene Rhodamine Conjugates Exhibit Cytotoxicity at Sub-Nanomolar Concentration against Breast Cancer Cells. *Int. J. Mol. Sci.* **2023**, *24*, 10695. https://doi.org/10.3390/ijms241310695

Academic Editors: Barbara De Filippis, Alessandra Ammazzalorso and Marialuigia Fantacuzzi

Received: 4 June 2023
Revised: 20 June 2023
Accepted: 21 June 2023
Published: 27 June 2023

1. Introduction

Breast cancer is the most common type of tumor disease and, despite recent advances in cancer therapy, it remains the leading cause of tumor-related death in women [1–8]. While traditional treatments like surgery, chemotherapy, radiation, and hormone therapy are effective [9], they often cause severe side effects and may not be suitable for all patients. Therefore, there is a need to develop new and effective treatment options. One highly promising approach is the use of natural products derived compounds as anticancer agents, especially pentacyclic triterpenoids, which have emerged as a class of phytochemicals with potential anticancer activity. Several studies have demonstrated their ability to cause apoptosis, reduce clonogenic survival and migration, and enhance the radiosensitivity of human breast cancer cells [10–13]. These effects have been attributed to their ability to modulate various signaling pathways involved in cancer progression.

Pentacyclic triterpenoic acids linked with lipophilic cations, such as rhodamines [13–27], are known to act as mitocans even at low nanomolar concentrations by inhibiting their synthesis of ATP [21]. In this context, the mitochondrial targeting function of rhodamine seems particularly worth mentioning [28–30]. Therefore, the use of an amine spacer is crucial for enhancing their cytotoxicity, whereby secondary amines are favored over primary amines to prevent lactamization and maintain their cationic structures. Furthermore, incorporating a homopiperazinyl spacer leads to more cytotoxic compounds than those analogs with a piperazinyl spacer. Therefore, we have been interested in the use of a

1,5-diazacyclooctane spacer and its influence on the cytotoxicity of different pentacyclic triterpenoic acid conjugates of rhodamine B and rhodamine 101.

2. Results

Since the first preparation of octahydro-1,5-diazocine (**1**, 1,5-diazacyclooctane, a "bis-homo-piperazine", Scheme 1) in 1939 by W. L. C. Veer [31] several routes have been suggested to this compound, among them the ring cleavage reaction of 1,5-diaminobicyclo [3.3.0]octane, the condensation of propane-1,3-diamine with 1,3-dibromopropane, and the silica-supported intramolecular cyclization of propane-1,3-diamine at 350 °C [32–43].

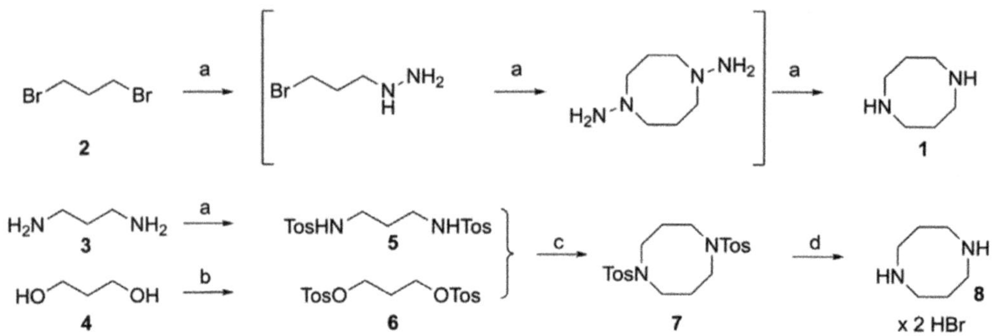

Scheme 1. Synthesis of octahydro-1,5-diazocine (**1**) and its dihydrobromide (**8**): Reactions and conditions: a: NH_2-NH_2, EtOH, reflux, 4 h; then HBr, benzaldehyde, 7.5%; b: TosCl, no solvent, 80 °C, 30 min, 83%; c: TosCl, pyridine, 0 °C, 30 min, 87%; d: NaOMe, MeOH, DMF, 80 °C, 12 h, 84%; then HBr (33% glacial AcOH), 80 °C, 3 h, 92%.

As an alternative, one could also imagine the reduction of the bis-lactam 1,5-diazocane-2,6-dione; the latter compound is accessible either via Staudinger ring closure reactions and Beckmann and Schmidt rearrangements, however, usually under very drastic conditions (e.g., fuming sulfuric acid) [44–48]. All these routes are not very suitable, since their mostly drastic conditions make the preparation of larger amounts on a laboratory scale quite difficult.

Special attention, therefore, is deserved for the only recently proposed [49] route starting from propane-1,3-diamine and propane-1,3-diol, two starting materials that are available in larger quantities and commercially cheap. In this process, both starting materials are first tosylated and then condensed by a double nucleophilic substitution. An alternative is the reaction of 1,3-dibromopropane (**2**) with hydrazine. This route would have the advantage of yielding the desired product in a one-pot procedure. However, it very quickly became apparent that many byproducts were formed in this reaction so that the maximum yield of pure **1** was 7.5% only. Working with larger quantities of hydrazine poses an additional risk.

However, the published synthesis using propane-1,3-diamine (**3**) and propane-1,3-diol (**4**) could not be reproduced in terms of the yields obtained either, so we decided to optimize this synthetic route on our own.

Thus, propane-1,3-diamine (**3**) was tosylated (Scheme 1) to yield **5** in an 83% yield, while the tosylation of propane-1,3-diol (**3**) gave 87% of the di-tosylate **6**. These two compounds were condensed in the presence of sodium methoxide (which proved to result in higher yields than using sodium ethoxide) to afford 84% of **7**. De-tosylation was performed with hydrobromic acid in the presence of thioanisole and the desired octahydro-1,5-diazocine was obtained as di-hydrobromide (**8**) in a 92% isolated yield.

The starting materials for the preparation of the spacered rhodamine conjugates were the triterpene carboxylic acids oleanolic acid (OA, Figure 1), ursolic acid (UA), and the lupanes betulinic acid (BA) and platanic acid (PA); in previous works, asiatic acid

(AA) had been shown to be particularly suitable with respect to cytotoxic activity and was, therefore, included in this study as a model featuring a tri-hydroxylated triterpene carboxylic acid [21].

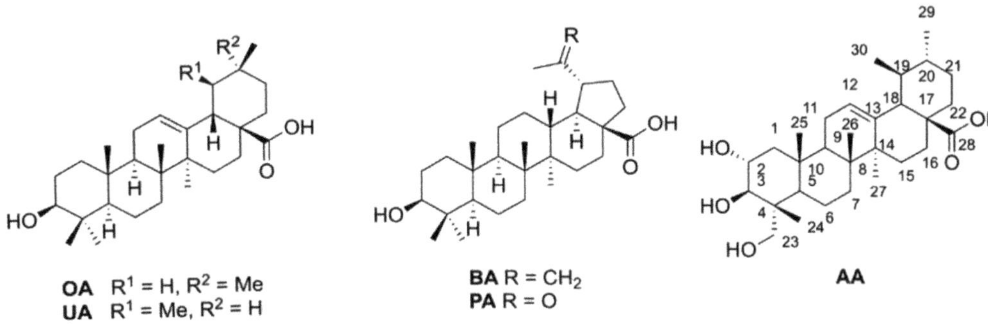

Figure 1. Structure of triterpenoic acid oleanolic acid (OA), ursolic acid (UA), betulinic acid (BA), platanic acid (PA), and asiatic acid (AA); for the latter, a numbering scheme is depicted.

The triterpenoic acids were acetylated to yield the acetates **9–13** (Scheme 2). Rhodamine B and rhodamine 101 were chosen as representative examples of rhodamines. The former compound has been shown in previous studies to be an essential component of mitocan-acting triterpene carboxylic acid amide conjugates; the latter differs from the former in having a somewhat higher lipophilicity (consensus log $P_{o/w}$ 2.21 and 3.96, respectively; from www.swiss.adme.ch, accessed on 2 May 2023), which we consider advantageous for possible interactions with biological membranes. Thus, the reaction of acetates **9–13** with oxalyl chloride followed by the addition of **8** furnished amides **14–18**. Rhodamine B and rhodamine 101 were transformed with oxalyl chloride in situ into their corresponding acid chlorides that were reacted with amides **14–18** to yield rhodamine B-derived conjugates **19–23** and rhodamine 101-derived hybrids **24–28**.

Compounds **14–28** were screened in sulforhodamine B assays employing the breast cancer cell lines MDA-MB-231, HS578T, MCF-7, and T47D (Table 1). Breast cancer could be distinguished into different molecular subtypes: luminal-like (luminal A or B), HER2-enriched, and basal-like, which differ in biology, treatment response, patients' survival, and clinical outcome. These subtypes are also found in cell lines and our investigated breast cancer cell lines have been characterized before. Breast cancer cell lines MDA-MB-231 and HS578T are basal and so-called triple negative, which means neither estrogen receptor (ER) and progesterone receptor (PR) nor human epidermal growth factor receptor 2 (HER2) are expressed. Basal breast cancers are mostly high-grade tumors and no therapeutic targeted therapy can be applied, thus resulting in a poor prognosis for patients although they are relatively sensitive for chemotherapy. MCF-7 and T47D breast cancer cells are luminal A and positive for ER and PR. Breast cancers of this type are often low-grade tumors, which are characterized by chemotherapy resistance, but hold good responses to hormone therapy, resulting in better clinical outcomes compared to basal breast cancers.

As a result, amides of triterpenoic acids 14–18 (Table 1) show cytotoxicity at a low micromolar range for all investigated breast cancer cell lines. IC_{50} values of about 0.5–50 µM were determined. As expected, conjugation of rhodamine B (compounds **19–23**) or rhodamine 101 (compounds **24–28**) led to increased cytotoxicity (in the nanomolar range) in all breast cancer cell lines (Table 1). In the investigated breast cancer cell lines, the IC_{50} values of all homopiperazinyl-spacered rhodamine B derivatives are in a low nano-molar range with rhodamine 101 conjugates being even more cytotoxic. An asiatic acid derivatized rhodamine 101 amide (compound **28**) is the most cytotoxic conjugate in all screened breast cancer cells. The IC_{50} values are in a low nanomolar range (0.6–126 nM). Comparing breast cancer cell lines, the HS578T cell line is the most resistant cell line for rhodamine B or rhodamine 101 conjugates (IC_{50} between 216 nM and 356 nM and between 126 nM and 1.3 µM). Our previous work showed that compounds of this class are also highly able to discriminate between malignant and nonmalignant cells [13,23] and affect mitochondrial ATP synthesis [23]. Future studies will also investigate whether changes in the expression of programmed death ligand-1 (PD-L1) can be observed [50].

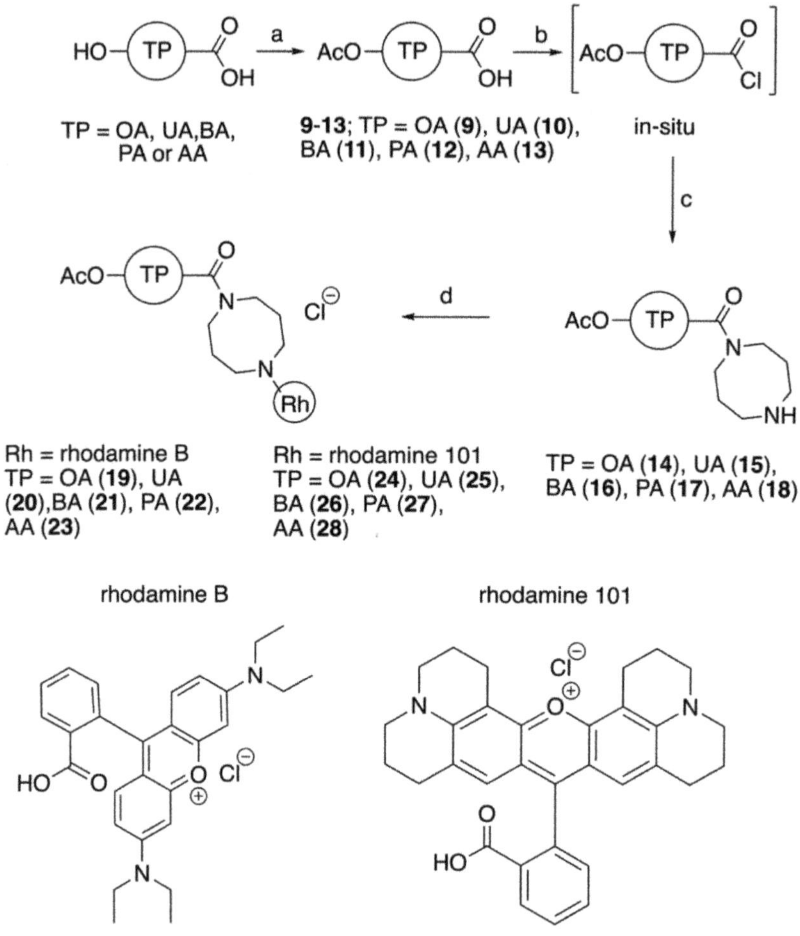

Scheme 2. Synthesis of the rhodamine B and rhodamine 101 conjugates; reactions and conditions: a: Ac_2O, DCM, NEt_3, DMAP (cat.), 21 °C, 24 h; b: $(COCl)_2$, DCM, DMF (cat.), in situ; c: DCM, **8**, NEt_3, DMAP (cat.), 20 °C, 1 h; d: $(COCl)_2$, DCM, DMF (cat.), then rhodamine B or rhodamine 101, 20 °C, 1 h.

In addition to studying the cytotoxicity of **28** in the above-mentioned cell lines, we investigated its ability to overcome resistance. While the IC_{50} of **28** in A2780 cells was 0.72 nM, the resistant A2780cis cells exhibited an IC_{50} of 1.82 nM. Although complete resistance reversal was not achieved, the results highlight the promising potential to partially overcome resistance. We also assessed its selectivity by comparing the cytotoxicity in nonmalignant fibroblasts CCD18Co. The IC_{50} value of **28** in CCD18Co cells was 503.2 nM, which was approximately 800-fold higher than the IC_{50} value observed in the MDA-MB-231 cells.

Table 1. Cytotoxicity of compounds **14–28** determined by SRB assay in four different breast cancer cell lines (MDA-MB-231, HS578T, MCF-7, and T47D). IC_{50} values were calculated after 96 h treatment. The data represent values of at least three independent experiments, which were done each in triplicate.

Compound	MDA-MB-231	HS578T	MCF-7	T47D
14 (μM)	2.88 ± 0.11	3.39 ± 0.92	3.03 ± 0.22	3.86 ± 0.93
15 (μM)	38.91 ± 14.08	15.18 ± 7.18	26.09 ± 10.76	49.67 ± 13.92
16 (μM)	3.36 ± 0.22	4.14 ± 0.13	3.59 ± 0.21	4.39 ± 0.88
17 (μM)	2.58 ± 0.37	2.77 ± 0.41	2.82 ± 0.57	3.78 ± 0.74
18 (μM)	0.46 ± 0.21	2.80 ± 0.16	1.53 ± 0.23	1.97 ± 0.29
19 (nM)	35.87 ± 19.42	280.06 ± 31.25	147.26 ± 68.02	190.96 ± 113.70
20 (nM)	71.76 ± 46.35	215.54 ± 96.53	155.25 ± 64.67	269.61 ± 76.07
21 (nM)	126.46 ± 40.55	351.94 ± 127.31	221.96 ± 90.61	261.83 ± 49.91
22 (nM)	134.05 ± 76.38	356.46 ± 92.90	120.63 ± 43.11	187.07 ± 60.55
23 (nM)	55.99 ± 19.44	275.88 ± 64.62	25.97 ± 21.28	32.71 ± 24.35
24 (nM)	1140.71 ± 255.22	1341.56 ± 74.91	1189.47 ± 325.25	1316.63 ± 713.38
25 (nM)	69.68 ± 8.43	341.79 ± 36.15	138.65 ± 111.56	232.17 ± 65.43
26 (nM)	135.93 ± 71.83	538.92 ± 27.80	239.90 ± 3.63	251.17 ± 56.18
27 (nM)	62.91 ± 22.03	440.34 ± 206.56	103.85 ± 19.75	129.25 ± 38.29
28 (nM)	0.60 ± 0.11	125.79 ± 7.61	3.96 ± 1.95	8.18 ± 6.51

The most cytotoxic compound, **28**, was used for further investigations of proliferation and cell death in sensitive MDA-MB-231 and resistant HS578T breast cancer cells. In MDA-MB-231 cells, compound **28** caused a strong inhibition of proliferation (under 20% compared to the control cells) after treatment with at least 250 nM (Figure 2). However, in HS578T cells, treatment with 250 nM of compound **28** resulted in a less decrease of proliferation by about 50%, but with 500 nM, compound **28** cell number was reduced by up to 20% compared to control cells (Figure 2).

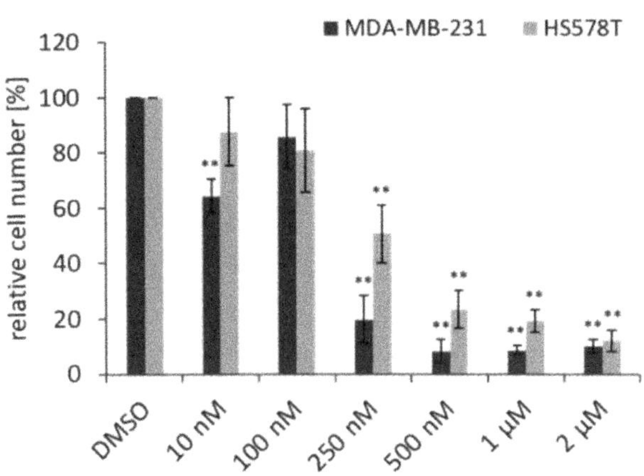

Figure 2. Relative cell number of MDA-MB-231 and HS578T breast cancer cells. Cells were seeded in 6-well plates and treated with different concentrations of compound 28. After 72 h the number of viable cells was counted. Data represent mean values (±SD) of at least three independent experiments. All data were referred to DMSO-treated cells (=100%). Significant p values are highlighted with asterisks (** $p \leq 0.01$).

Cell death analyses were done by use of FITC annexin V-Sytox Deep Red staining in MDA-MB-231 (IC_{50} = 0.6 nM) and HS578T (IC_{50} = 126 nM) breast cancer cell lines to discriminate apoptotic and necrotic cells. An example of the evaluation of cell death via annexin V-Sytox Deep Red staining in the sensitive breast cancer cell line MDA-MB-231 and the resistant breast cancer cell line HS578T is shown in Figure 3A. Cells stained negative for both annexin V and Sytox Deep Red were viable (Q3). Early apoptotic cells stained positive for annexin V but negative for Sytox Deep Red (Q4), whereas late apoptotic or dead cells stained positive for both annexin V and Sytox Deep Red (Q2). Necrotic cells are indicated as negative for annexin V but positive for Sytox Deep Red (Q1).

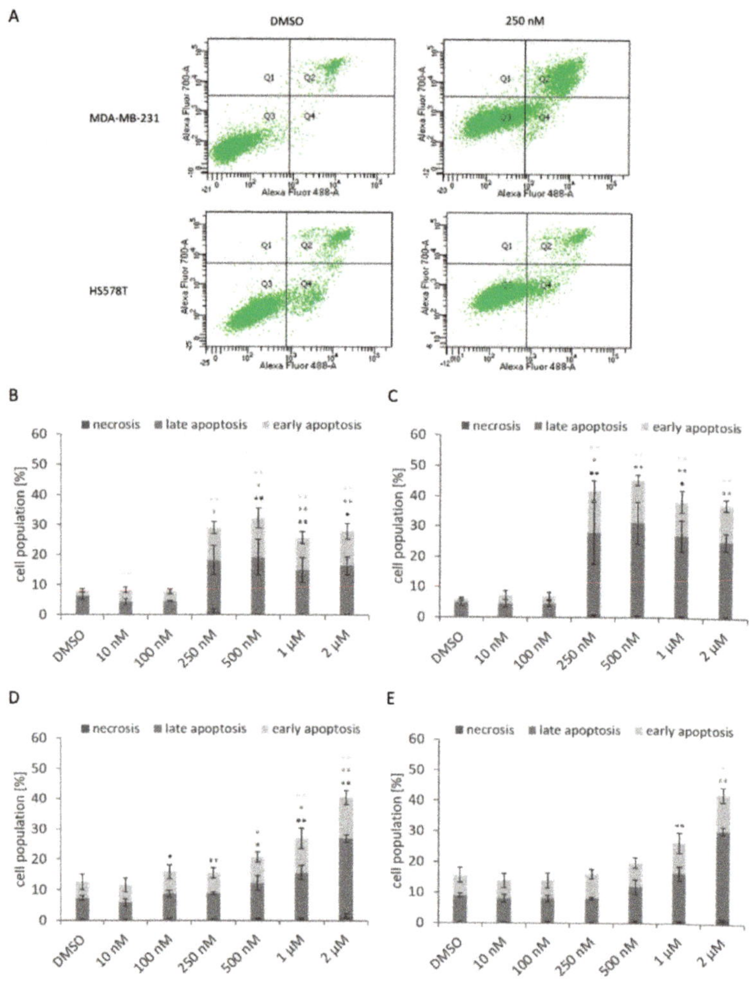

Figure 3. FITC Annexin V (Alexa 488)-Sytox Deep Red (Alexa 700) staining of MDA-MB-231 and HS578T cells. (**A**) Dot Plots of MDA-MB-231 and HS578T cell line after treatment with 250 nM compound 28 (**B–E**). Quantitative analysis of cell death of MDA-MB-231 (**B**,**C**) and HS578T cells (**D**,**E**) after treatment with different concentrations of compound 28 for 48 h (**B**,**D**) and 72 h (**C**,**E**). Data represent mean values (±SD) of at least three independent experiments. Significant p values are highlighted with asterisks (* $p \leq 0.05$; ** $p \leq 0.01$).

Analysis of subcellular localization of compound **28** (Figure 4A) compared to the mitochondrial targeting compound BioTracker™ 488 Green Mitochondria Dye (Figure 4B) in MDA-MB-231 cells shows an identical pattern of accumulation, indicating the mitochondrial targeting of **28**. Using a quantitative analysis of the respective integrated fluorescence intensity, a mitochondrial uptake of about 56% could be determined.

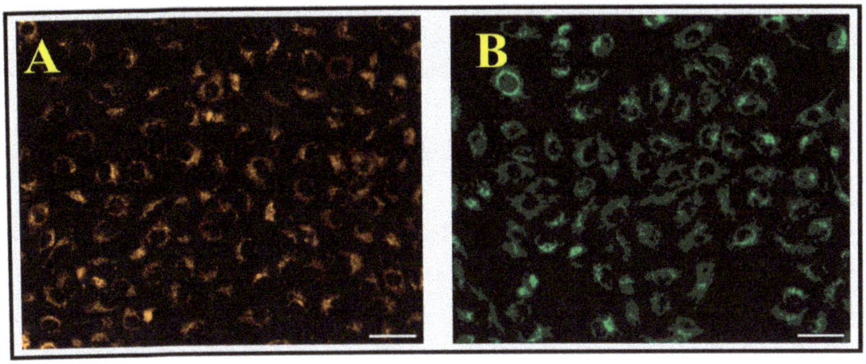

Figure 4. (**A**) Analysis of subcellular localization of compound **28** (**A**) was performed in MDA-MB-231 cells using BioTracker™ 488 Green Mitochondria Dye; (**B**) Cells treated with 100 nM 28 for 6 h or 100 nM BioTracker488 for 30 min, observed: BioTracker (475 nm/514 nm), AS101 (555 nm/592 nm). Scale bar: 50 μm.

In summary, the determination of proliferation and cell death indicates that compound **28** induces inhibition of proliferation or growth arrest at a lower dose, and with increasing dose treatment with compound **28** causes an induction of apoptosis. Furthermore, differential responses to proliferation inhibition and apoptosis induction may explain the differential sensitivity of mammary cell lines to compound **28**.

3. Discussion

1,5-Diazacyclooctane was synthesized through a straightforward synthetic pathway and subsequently linked with pentacyclic triterpenoic acids, namely oleanolic acid, ursolic acid, betulinic acid, platanic acid, and asiatic acid. These resulting amides were activated with oxalyl chloride and reacted with either rhodamine B or rhodamine 101 to form conjugates. These conjugates were then subjected to screening using SRB assays on various breast cancer cell lines, namely MDA-MB-231, HS578T, MCF-7, and T47D. The findings revealed that the conjugates exhibited cytotoxic activity even at low concentrations. Notably, the asiatic acid rhodamine 101 conjugate 28 displayed an IC_{50} = 0.60 nM and demonstrated the ability to induce apoptosis in MDA-MB-231 and HS578T cells. Further investigations demonstrated that the compound acted as a mitocan, resulting in the inhibition of proliferation or growth arrest in MDA-MB-231 cells at lower doses, followed by the induction of apoptosis at higher doses. Moreover, the differential responses observed in terms of proliferation inhibition and apoptosis induction could potentially explain the varying sensitivity of mammary cell lines to compound **28**.

4. Materials and Methods

4.1. General

NMR spectra were recorded using the Varian spectrometers (Darmstadt, Germany) DD2 and VNMRS (400 and 500 MHz, respectively). MS spectra were taken on an Advion expression^{L} CMS mass spectrometer (Ithaca, NY, USA; positive ion polarity mode, solvent: methanol, solvent flow: 0.2 mL/min, spray voltage: 5.17 kV, source voltage: 77 V, APCI corona discharge: 4.2 μA, capillary temperature: 250 °C, capillary voltage: 180 V, sheath gas: N_2). Thin-layer chromatography was performed on precoated silica gel plates supplied by Macherey-Nagel (Düren, Germany). IR spectra were recorded on a Spectrum 1000 FT-IR-spectrometer from Perkin Elmer (Rodgau, Germany). The UV/Vis-spectra were recorded on a Lambda 14 spectrometer from Perkin Elmer (Rodgau, Germany); optical rotations were measured at 20 °C using a JASCO-P2000 instrument (JASCO Germany GmbH, Pfungstadt, Germany). The melting points (m.p.) were determined using the Leica hot-stage microscope Galen III (Leica Biosystems, Nussloch, Germany) and are uncorrected. The solvents were dried according to the usual procedures. Microanalyses were performed with an Elementar Vario EL (CHNS) instrument (Elementar Analysensysteme GmbH, Elementar-Straße 1, D-63505, Langenselbold, Germany).

All dry solvents were distilled over respective drying agents except for DMF which was distilled and stored under argon and a molecular sieve. Reactions using air- or moisture-sensitive reagents were carried out under an argon atmosphere in dried glassware. Triethylamine was stored over potassium hydroxide. Biological assays were performed as previously reported. The parent triterpenoic acids were obtained from local vendors.

4.2. *General Procedure for Acetylation (GP 1)*

To a solution of the parent triterpenoic acid (1 equiv.) in dry DCM, acetic anhydride (3 equiv.), dry triethylamine (3 equiv.), and DMAP (catal. amounts) were added, and the mixture was stirred at 20 °C for one day. The usual aqueous work-up followed by re-crystallization from ethanol furnished the corresponding acetates 9–13. Their respective m.p., $[\alpha]_D^{20}$ values, ^{1}H, and ^{13}C NMR spectra, as well as ESI MS data, correspond to the literature values.

4.3. *General Procedure for the Synthesis of Amides* **14–18** *(GP 2)*

To a solution of acetates 9–13 (1 equiv.) in dry DCM (100 mL), oxalyl chloride (5 equiv.) and DMF (2 drops) were added and the mixture was stirred at 20 °C for 2 h. The volatiles were removed under diminished pressure and the residue was dissolved in dry DCM (100 mL). This solution was slowly added to a solution of the corresponding amine (3 equiv.) in dry acetonitrile (100 mL) in the presence of DMAP (catal. amounts). The mixture was stirred at 20 °C for 1 day, the volatiles were removed under diminished pressure, and the residue was subjected to column chromatography (silica gel) to afford products **14–18**.

4.4. *General Procedure for the Synthesis of the Rhodamine Conjugates* **19–28** *(GP 3)*

To a solution of the rhodamine (rhodamine B or rhodamine 101, 1 equiv.) in dry DCM (100 mL), oxalyl chloride (7 equiv.) and dry DMF (2 drops) were added, and the mixture was stirred at 20 °C for 1 h. The volatiles were removed under diminished pressure and the residue was dissolved in dry DCM (100 mL). A solution of the corresponding amine (1 equiv.) in dry DCM (100 mL) was added, followed by the addition of catal. amounts of triethylamine and DMAP. The mixture was stirred at 20 °C for 1 h (TLC showed completion of the reaction), the solvents were removed in vacuo, and the residue was subjected to column chromatography (silica gel, $CHCl_3$/MeOH) to afford products **19–28**.

4.5. *N,N'-Ditosyl-1,3-propanediamine* (**5**)

Tosyl chloride (40.0 g, 210 mmol) was molten in a beaker at 80 °C and 1,3-propanediamine (3, 8.9 mL, 106 mmol) was added dropwise; to complete the reaction, the mixture was stirred for an additional 30 min at 80 °C. After cooling to 20 °C, aq. HCl (2 M) was added, and the precipitate was washed with water followed by a recrystallization from ethanol to furnish **5** (33.7 g, 83%) as a colorless solid; m.p. 138 °C (lit: [49] 137–140 °C); R_f = 0.75 (silica gel, hexanes/ethyl acetate, 4:6); UV-Vis ($CHCl_3$): λ_{max} (log ε) = 228 nm (4.16); IR (ATR): ν = 3271*w*, 1595*w*, 1431*w*, 1305*s*, 1214*w*, 1154*s*, 1088*m*, 1024*w*, 980*m*, 858*m*, 815*s*, 698*s*, 550*s*, 568*s*, 489*m* cm^{-1}; ^{1}H NMR (400 MHz, $CDCl_3$): δ = 7.73 (*m*, 4H, 4-H, 8-H), 7.32–7.25 (*m*, 4H, 5-H, 7-H), 3.02 (*t*, *J* = 5.8 Hz, 4H, 2-H), 2.42 (*s*, 6H, 9-H), 1.67 (*p*, *J* = 6.2 Hz, 2H, 1-H) ppm; ^{13}C NMR (101 MHz, $CDCl_3$): δ = 143.6 (C-6), 136.8 (C-3), 129.8 (C-5, C-7), 127.0 (C-4, C-8), 39.8 (C-2), 29.9 (C-1), 21.5 (C-9) ppm; MS (ESI, MeOH/$CHCl_3$, 4:1): *m*/*z* = 405.0 (100%, $[M+Na]^+$).

4.6. 1,3-Propanediol Ditosylate (6)

A mixture of 1,3-propanediol (**4**, 16.0 g, 210 mmol) and tosyl chloride (88.0 g, 461 mmol) in dry pyridine (70 mL) was stirred at 0 °C for 1 h. The product was precipitated by adding aq. HCl (2 M), filtered off and dried. Compound **6** (69.9 g, 87%) was obtained as a colorless solid; m.p. 92 °C (lit.: [51] 92–93 °C); R_f = 0.49 (hexanes/ethyl acetate, 6:4); UV-Vis ($CHCl_3$): λ_{max} (log ε) = 225 nm (4.11); IR (ATR): ν = 2978*w*, 1599*m*, 1496*w*, 1470*w*, 1421*w*, 1352*s*, 1293*m*, 1254*w*, 1190*m*, 1172*s*, 1095*m*, 1029*m*, 1021*m*, 941*s*, 892*w*, 852*s*, 810*s*, 739*s*, 660*s*, 580*s*, 568*s*, 549*s*, 488*m* cm^{-1}; ^1H NMR (400 MHz, $CDCl_3$): δ = 7.75–7.23 (*m*, 8H, 4-H, 5-H, 7-H, 8-H), 4.06 (*t*, *J* = 6.0 Hz, 4H, 2-H), 2.46 (s, 6H, 9-H), 1.99 (*p*, *J* = 6.0 Hz, 2H, 1-H) ppm; ^{13}C NMR (101 MHz, $CDCl_3$): δ = 145.1 (C-6), 132.6 (C-3), 130.0 (C-5, C-7), 127.9 (C-4, C-8), 65.9 (C-2), 28.7 (C-1), 21.6 (C-9) ppm; MS (ESI, MeOH/$CHCl_3$, 4:1): *m*/*z* = 407.3 (100%, $[M+Na]^+$).

4.7. 1,5-Bis (p-Toluenesulfonyl)-1,5-diazacyclooctane (7)

To a solution of sodium methanolate (8.0 g, 148 mmol) in dry MeOH (100 mL) **5** (5.0 g, 13 mmol) was added, and the mixture was heated under reflux for 4 h. The solvent was removed, the residue was dissolved in dry DMF (100 mL) and 6 (5.0 g, 13 mmol) was added. The mixture was stirred at 80 °C for 12 h. The product was precipitated by adding aq. HCl (2 M), filtered off, and **7** (4.7 g, 84%) was obtained as a colorless solid; m.p. 214–216 °C (lit. [33]: 214–215 °C); R_f = 0.33 (hexane/ethyl acetate, 7:3); UV-Vis ($CHCl_3$): λ_{max} (log ε) = 232 nm (4.32); IR (ATR): ν = 2953*w*, 1597*w*, 1456*m*, 1378*m*, 1321*s*, 1182*m*, 1150*s*, 1088*s*, 1017*m*, 1059*s*, 987*s*, 927*m*, 837*m*, 812*s*, 723*s*, 644*s*, 627*m*, 543*s*, 487*m*, 462*m*, 408*m* cm^{-1}; ^1H NMR (400 MHz, $CDCl_3$): δ = 7.68 (*d*, *J* = 8.3 Hz, 4H, 5-H, 9-H), 7.33–7.30 (*m*, 4H, 6-H, 8-H), 3.31–3.24 (*m*, 8H, 1-H, 3-H), 2.43 (*s*, 6H, 10-H), 2.04 (*p*, *J* = 5.9 Hz, 4H, 2-H) ppm; ^{13}C NMR (101 MHz, $CDCl_3$): δ = 143.4 (C-7), 135.6 (C-4), 129.8 (C-6, C-8), 127.1 (C-5, C-9), 47.0 (C-1, C-3), 30.2 (C-2), 21.5 (C-10) ppm; MS (ESI, MeOH/$CHCl_3$, 4:1): *m*/*z* = 445.2 (100%, $[M+Na]^+$).

4.8. 1,5-Diazacyclooctane Dihydrobromide (8)

4.8.1. Procedure A

A solution of **7** (2.5 g, 6 mmol) and thioanisole (2.4 mL, 18 mmol) in HBr (33% in glacial acetic acid, 150 mL) was stirred at 80 °C for 3 h. The volatiles were removed under diminished pressure, DCM (30 mL) was added, and the solution was washed with water (3 × 100 mL), followed by decolorization (activated charcoal). The solution was filtered, the solvent removed, and **8** (1.5 g, 5.5 mmol, 92%) was obtained as a colorless solid.

4.8.2. Procedure B

A solution of hydrazine (75 mL, 1.5 mol) in EtOH (200 mL) was heated under reflux, and 1,3-dibromopropane (75 mL, 0.75 mol) was added slowly within 4 h. Stirring was continued for another hour, the solids were filtered off, washed with ethanol (3 × 50 mL), and discarded. The pH of the filtrate [combined with the EtOH washings and additional water (150 mL)] was adjusted to pH =3 by adding aqu. HBr (48% in water). Benzaldehyde (60 mL, 0.6 mol) was added, and the precipitate formed upon addition was filtered off, washed with water (3 × 50 mL), and discarded. The combined filtrates were extracted with ether (1000 mL), and the aq. The layer was concentrated under diminished pressure resulting in the formation of a red solid. Ethanol (250 mL) was added, and shaking of this suspension was continued for another 5 min. The yellowish solid was filtered off, washed with ethanol (250 mL) and ether (5 × 100 mL), and **8** (15.6 g, 7.5%) was obtained as a colorless solid; m.p. = 220–225 °C (lit.: [51,52] >250 °C); R_f = 0.8 ($CHCl_3$:MeOH, 95:5); IR (ATR): ν = 2971*s*, 2728*s*, 2418*m*, 1577*s*, 1461*s*, 1331*m*, 1095*s*, 1027*m*, 890*m*, 696*m*, 547*m*, 491*m*, cm^{-1}; ^1H NMR (400 MHz, D_2O): δ = 3.36–3.31 (*m*, 8H, 1-H, 3-H, 4-H, 6-H), 2.22–2.16 (*m*, 4H, 2-H, 5-H) ppm; ^{13}C NMR (101 MHz, D_2O): δ = 43.8 (C-1, C-3, C-4, C-6), 20.8 (C-2, C-5) ppm; MS (ESI, MeOH/$CHCl_3$, 4:1): *m*/*z* = 115.0 (100%, $[M+H-2 HBr]^+$).

4.9. *(3ß)28-(1,5-Diazocan-1-yl)-28-oxoolean-12-en-3-yl Acetate* (**14**)

Following GP 2 from 3-*O*-acetyl-oleanolic acid (9, 500 mg, 1.0 mmol), followed by chromatography (silica gel, $CHCl_3$/MeOH (2% → 10%), compound **14** (425 mg, 71%) was obtained as a colorless solid; m.p. = 207–210 °C (decomp.); R_f = 0.52 ($CHCl_3$/MeOH, 95:5); $[\alpha]_D^{20}$ = + 3.8° (*c* 0.088, $CHCl_3$); IR (ATR): ν = 2954*m*, 1732*s*, 1626*m*, 1464*m*, 1368*s*, 1245*s*, 1026*s*, 750*s*, 662*w* cm^{-1}; ^1H NMR (400 MHz, $CDCl_3$): δ = 5.25 (*m*, 1H, 12-H), 4.50 (*m*, 1H, 3-H), 3.67–3.11 (*m*, 8H, 33-H, 35-H, 36-H, 38-H), 3.03 (*d*, *J* = 13.8 Hz 1H, 18-H), 2.16–2.12 (m, 1H, 16-H), 2.04 (*s*, 3H, 32-H), 1.87–1.17 (*m*, 23H, 11-H, 34-H, 37-H, 19-H_a, 2-H, 1-H_a, 9-H, 6-H_a, 15-H, 7-H, 21-H, 6 H_b, 22-H, 19-H_b), 1.13 (*s*, 3H, 27-H), 1.01–0.98 (m, 1H, 1-H_b), 0.97-0.93 (*s*, 3H, 25-H), 0.92 (*s*, 3H, 30-H), 0.89 (*s*, 3H, 29-H), 0.85 (*s*, 3H, 23-H), 0.84 (*s*, 3H, 24-H), 0.82-0.81 (*m*, 1H, 5-H), 0.72 (*s*, 3H, 26-H) ppm; ^{13}C NMR (101 MHz, $CDCl_3$): δ = 177.0 (C-28), 171.2 (C-31), 144.7 (C-13), 121.7 (C-12), 81.1 (C-3), 55.5 (C-5), 47.9 (C-33, C-35, C-36, C-38), 47.8 (C-9),47.4 (C-17), 46.6 (C-19), 43.9 (C-18), 42.6 (C-14), 39.2 (C-8), 38.2 (C-1), 37.8 (C-4), 37.1 (C-10), 34.2 (C-21), 33.1 (C-7), 33.0 (C-29), 30.5 (C-34, C-37), 30.4 (C-20),29.8 (C-22), 28.2 (C-23), 27.6 (C-15), 26.0 (C-27), 24.1 (C-30), 23.7 (C-2), 23.5 (C-11), 22.8 (C-16), 21.4 (C-32), 18.3 (C-6), 17.3 (C-26), 16.8 (C-24), 15.6 (C-25) ppm; MS (ESI, MeOH/$CHCl_3$, 4:1): *m*/*z* = 596.3 (100%, $[M+H]^+$); analysis calcd. for $C_{38}H_{62}N_2O_3$ (594.93): C 76.72, H 10.50, N 4.71; found: C 76.47, H 10.74, N 4.50.

4.10. *(3ß) 28-(1,5-Diazocan-1-yl)-28-oxours-12-en-3-yl Acetate* (**15**)

Following GP 2 from 3-*O*-acetyl-ursolic acid (10, 500 mg, 1.0 mmol), followed by chromatography (silica gel, $CHCl_3$/MeOH (2% → 10%), compound **15** (413 mg, 69%) was obtained as an off-white solid; m.p. = 232–235 °C (decomp.); R_f = 0.37 ($CHCl_3$/MeOH, 95:5); $[\alpha]_D^{20}$ = + 0.45° (*c* 0.088, $CHCl_3$); IR (ATR): ν = 2942*m*, 1731*m*, 1627*m*, 1456*m*, 1370*s*, 1245*s*, 1026*s*, 750*s*, 662*m* cm^{-1}; ^1H NMR (400 MHz, $CDCl_3$): δ = 5.18–5.13 (*m*, 1H, 12-H), 4.46–4.39 (*m*, 1H, 3-H), 3.74–3.01 (*m*, 8H, 33-H, 35-H, 36-H, 38-H), 2.39 (*d*, *J* = 11.3 Hz, 1H, 18-H), 1.99 (*s*, 3H, 32-H), 1.88–1.82 (*m*, 2H, 11-H), 1.74–1.67 (*m*, 1H, 20-H), 1.73–1.05 (*m*, 23H, 2-H, 6-H, 15-H, 16-H, 21-H, 7-H, 9-H, 22-H, 1H_a, 19-H, 34-H, 37-H), 1.02 (*s*, 3H, 27-H), 0.99–0.95 (m, 1H, 1H_b), 0.92 (*s*, 3H, 23-H), 0.88 (*s*, 3H, 30-H), 0.86 (*s*, 3H, 25-H), 0.81 (*s*, 3H, 29-H), 0.80 (*s*, 3H, 24-H), 0.77-0.74 (*m*, 1H, 5-H), 0.72 (*s*, 3H, 26-H) ppm; ^{13}C NMR (101 MHz, $CDCl_3$): δ = 174.9 (C-28), 171.0 (C-31), 125.3 (C-12), 80.9 (C-3), 55.2 (C-5), 55.0 (C-18), 48.7 (C-33, C-35, C-36, C-38), 48. 6 (C-17), 47.7 (C-9), 43.4 (C- 8), 43.5 (C-14), 39.4 (C-19), 38.7 (C-20), 38.6 (C-1), 37.6 (C-4), 37.0 (C-10), 33.9 (C-22), 32.9 (C-7), 30.6 (C-21), 28.1 (C-23), 27.3 (C-34, C-37), 27.0 (C-15), 26.4 (C-16), 23,4 (C-27), 23.5 (C-2), 23.3 (C-11), 21.2 (C-32), 21.0 (C-30), 18.3 (C-6), 16.7 (C-29), 16.39 (C-26), 15.62 (C-24), 15.40 (C-25) ppm; MS (ESI, MeOH/$CHCl_3$, 4:1): *m*/*z* = 596.2 (100%, $[M+H]^+$); analysis calcd. for $C_{38}H_{62}N_2O_3$ (594.93): C 76.72, H 10.50, N 4.71; found: C 76.58, H 10.76, N 4.49.

4.11. *(3ß) 28-(1,5-Diazocan-1-yl)-28-oxolup-20(29)-en-3-yl Acetate* (**16**)

Following GP 2 from 3-*O*-acetyl-betulinic acid (11, 500 mg, 1.0 mmol), followed by chromatography (silica gel, ethyl acetate/MeOH (10% → 50%), compound **16** (430 mg, 72%) was obtained as a colorless solid; m.p. 223–234 °C (decomp.); R_f = 0.43 ($CHCl_3$/MeOH, 9:1); $[\alpha]_D^{20}$ = −8.0° (*c* 0.064, $CHCl_3$); IR (ATR): ν = 3408*w*, 2942*m*, 1731*m*, 1632*s*, 1455*m*, 1373*s*, 1246*s*, 1195*m*, 1026*m*, 979*m*, 882*m*, 730*s* cm^{-1}; ^1H NMR (400 MHz, $CDCl_3$): δ = 4.68 (*m*, 1H, 29-H_a), 4.56–4.53 (*m*, 1H, 29-H_b), 4.42 (*dd*, J = 10.1, 6.2 Hz, 1H, 3-H), 4.02–3.19 (*m*, 8H, 33-H, 35-H, 36-H, 38-H), 2.85 (*m*, 2H, 13-H, 19-H), 2.13–2.08 (*m*, 1H, 16-H_a), 2.00 (*s*, 3H, 32-H), 1.96–1.93 (*m*, 1H, 22-H_a), 1.78–1.74 (*m*, 1H, 21-H_a1.65–1.63 (*m*, 5H, 1-H_a, 12-H_a, 30-H), 1.60–1.05 (*m*, 2-H, 16-H_b, 18-H, 6-H_a, 7-H, 21-H, 11-H, 22-H_b,34-H, 37-H, 9-H, 15-H), 0.96–0.94 (*m*, 1H, 1-H_b), 0.92 (*s*, 3H, 27-H), 0.90–0.89 (*m*, 1H, 12-H_b), 0.87 (*s*, 3H, 25-H), 0.80 (*s*, 3H,m 24-H), 0.79 (*s*, 3H, 23-H), 0.76–0.74 (*m*, 1H, 5-H), 0.72 (*s*, 3H, 26-H) ppm; ^{13}C NMR (101 MHz, $CDCl_3$): δ = 175.4 (C-28), 171.0 (C-31), 150.8 (C-20), 109.4 (C-29), 80.9 (C-3), 55.5 (C-5), 55.2 (C-33, C-35, C-36, C-38), 55.0 (C-17), 52.9 (C-18), 50.7 (C-9), 45.6 (C-19), 42.0 (C-14), 40.7 (C-8), 38.8 (C-4), 38.4 (C-1), 37.8 (C-10), 37.1 (C-7), 36.9 (C-13), 36.1 (C-22), 34.3 (C-34, C-37), 32.3 (C-16), 31.4 (C-21), 30.1 (C-15), 25.5 (C-23), 23.7 (C-12), 23.7 (C-2),

21.3 (C-32), 21.1 (C-11), 19.7 (C-30), 18.1 (C-6), 16.4 (C-24), 16.2 (C-25), 16.0 (C-26), 14.6 (C-27) ppm; MS (ESI, MeOH/$CHCl_3$, 4:1): m/z = 596.1 (100%, $[M+H]^+$); analysis calcd. for $C_{38}H_{62}N_2O_3$ (594.93): C 76.72, H 10.50, N 4.71; found: C 76.46, H 10.77, N 4.53.

*4.12. (3ß)28-(1,5-Diazocan-1-yl)-30-nor-20,28-dioxolup-3-yl-acetate (**17**)*

Following GP 2 from 3-*O*-acetyl-platanic acid (12, 500 mg, 1.0 mmol), followed by chromatography (silica gel, ethyl acetate/MeOH (10% → 50%), compound **17** (425 mg, 70%) was obtained as a colorless solid; m.p. = 210–214 °C (decomp.); R_f = 0.44 ($CHCl_3$/MeOH, 9:1); $[\alpha]_D^{20} = -26.6°$ (*c* 0.028, $CHCl_3$); IR (ATR): ν = 3396*w*, 2942*m*, 2866*m*, 1731*m*, 1626*s*, 1466*m*, 1411*m*, 1369*m*, 1197*s*, 1245*m*, 1120*m*, 1025*m*, 978*m* cm^{-1}; ^1H NMR (400 MHz, $CDCl_3$): δ = 4.39 (*dd*, *J* = 10.6, 5.5 Hz, 1H, 3-H), 3.78–3.06 (*m*, 9H, 19-H, 32-H, 34-H, 35-H, 37-H), 2.66–2.56 (*m*, 1H, 13-H), 2.10 (*s*, 3H, 29-H), 2.08–1.98 (*m*, 2H, 16-H_a, 18-H), 1.97 (*s*, 3H, 31-H), 1.94–1.90 (*m*, 1H, 22-H_a), 1.82–1.76 (*m*, 1H, 21-H_a), 1.70–1.05 (*m*, 19H, 1-H_a, 16-H_b, 2-H, 22-H_b, 21-H_b, 6-H_a, 11-H_a, 7-H, 6H_b, 9-H, 15-H, 11-H_b, 33-H, 36-H), 0.98–0.95 (*m*, 2H, 12-H), 0.92 (*s*, 3H, 27-H), 0.91–0.85 (*m*, 1H, 1-H_b), 0.83 (*s*, 3H, 24-H), 0.79–0.77 (*m*, 6H, 23-H, 25-H), 0.76 (*s*, 3H, 26-H), 0.72–0.71 (*m*, 1H, 5-H) ppm; ^{13}C NMR (101 MHz, $CDCl_3$): δ = 212.5 (C-20), 175.3 (C-28), 170.9 (C-30), 80.8 (C-3), 55.4 (C-5), 55.1 (C-32, C-34, C-35, C-37), 52.7 (C-18), 50.6 (C-9), 49.9 (C-19), 46.1 (C-17), 41.8 (C-8), 40.6 (C-14), 38.3 (C-1), 37.7 (C-4), 37.1 (C-10), 35.9 (C-13), 35.8 (C-22), 34.1 (C-7), 31.8 (C-16), 30.3 (C-29), 30.0 (C-15), 28.8 (C-21), 27.9 (C-23), 27.3 (C-12), 23.6 (C-2), 21.3 (C-31), 21.1 (C-11), 18.1 (C-6), 16.4 (C-26), 16.2 (C-25), 15.9 (C-24), 14.6 (C-27) ppm; MS (ESI, MeOH/$CHCl_3$, 4:1): m/z = 597.3 (100%, $[M+H^+)$; analysis calcd. for $C_{37}H_{60}N_2O_4$ (596.90): C 74.45, H 10.13, N 4.69; found: C 74.21, H 10.32, N 4.43.

*4.13. (2α,3ß,4α)28-(1,5-Diazocan-1-yl)-28-oxours-12-ene-2,3,23-triyl Triacetate (**18**)*

Following GP 2 from 2,3,24-tri-*O*-acetyl-asiatic acid (13, 400 mg, 0.8 mmol), followed by chromatography [silica gel, $CHCl_3$/MeOH (2% → 50%)], compound **18** (425 mg, 74%) was obtained as colorless solid; m.p. = 187–190 °C (decomp.); R_f = 0.38 ($CHCl_3$/MeOH, 9:1); $[\alpha]_D^{20} = -30.2°$ (*c* 0.015, $CHCl_3$); IR (ATR): ν = 2925*w*, 1741*s*, 1623*w*, 1368*m*, 1231*s*, 1042*m*, 748*w* cm^{-1}; ^1H NMR (400 MHz, $CDCl_3$): δ = 5.22–5.17 (*m*, 1H, 12-H), 5.14–5.08 (*m*, 1H, 2-H), 5.04–5.01 (*m*, 1H, 3-H), 3.80 (*m*, 1H, 23-H_a), 3.51 (*m*, 1H, 23-H_b), 3.32–2.67 (*m*, 8H, 37-H, 39-H, 40-H, 42-H), 2.40–2.34 (*m*, 1H, 18-H), 2.03 (*s*, 3H, 36-H), 2.02–2.00 (*m*, 1H, 1-H_a), 1.97 (*s*, 3H, 34-H), 1.92 (*s*, 3H, 32-H), 1.88–1.69 (*m*, 5H, 11-H, 16-H 22-H_a), 1.60–1.45 (*m*, 4H, 22-H_b, 9-H, 21-H_a, 7-H_a), 1.53–1.45 (*m*, 2H, 16-H_a, 16-H_b), 1.33–1.14 (*m*, 10H, 19-H, 5-H, 21-H_b, 7-H_b, 15-H, 38-H, 41-H), 1.11–1.09 (*m*, 1H, 1-H_b), 1.05 (*s*, 3H, 27-H), 1.02 (s, 3H, 25-H), 0.99-0.96 (*m*, 1H, 20-H), 0.91 (*s*, 3H, 30-H), 0.84 (*s*, 3H, 24-H), 0.82 (*s*, 3H, 29-H), 0.70 (*s*, 3H, 26-H) ppm; ^{13}C NMR (101 MHz, $CDCl_3$): δ = 176.8 (C-28), 170.8 (C-35), 170.3 (C-33), 170.3 (C-31), 138.7 (C-13), 124.9 (C-12), 74.8 (C-3), 69.8 (C-2), 65.2 (C-23), 55.6 (C-18), 47.6 (C-9), 47.5 (C-5), 46.1 (C-37, C-39, C-40, C-42), 43.7 (C-1), 42.3 (C-14), 41.9 (C-4), 39.5 (C-8), 39.3 (C-19), 38.5 (C-20), 37.8 (C-10), 34.8 (C-22), 34.7 (C-7), 31.9 (C-21), 29.6 (C-15), 23.3 (C-11), 23.2 (C-16), 22.6 (C-38, C-41), 21.2 (C-30), 21.0 (C-36), 20.8 (C-32), 20.7 (C-34), 17.8 (C-6), 17.4 (C-27), 17.3 (C-29), 17.1 (C-25), 13.9 (C-26), 8.7 (C-24) ppm; MS (ESI, MeOH/$CHCl_3$, 4:1): m/z = 711.8 (100%, $[M+H^+)$; analysis calcd. for $C_{42}H_{66}N_2O_7$ (711.00): C 70.95, H 9.36, N 3.94; found: C 70.69, H 9.51, N 3.75.

*4.14. (3ß)-3-Acetyloxy-28-(5-{2-[3,6-bis(diethylamino)xanthen-10-ium-9-yl]benzoyl}-1,5-diazocan-1-yl)-28-oxoolean-12-ene Chloride (**19**)*

Following GP 3 from **14** (150 mg, 0.14 mmol) and rhodamine B (100 mg, 0.2 mmol), followed by chromatography (silica gel, ethyl acetate/MeOH, 10% → 40%), **19** (100 mg, 72%) was obtained as a pink solid; m.p. = 211–216 °C; R_f = 0.44 ($CHCl_3$/MeOH, 9:1); UV-Vis ($CHCl_3$): λ_{max} (log ε) = 562 nm (4.53); IR (ATR): ν = 2926*m*, 2605*w*, 2498*w*, 1729*w*, 1587*s*, 1466*s*, 1412*s*, 1336, 1245*s*, 1180*s*, 1132*m*, 1073*s*, 1009*m*, 921*w*, 748*m*, 683*m* cm^{-1}; ^1H NMR (400 MHz, $CDCl_3$): δ = 7.67–7.57 (*m*, 2H, 43-H, 44-H), 7.53–7.47 (*m*, 1H, 42-H), 7.34–7.26 (*m*,

3H, 45-H, 48-H), 7.14–6.65 (*m*, 4H, 49-H, 51-H), 5.25–5.15 (*m*, 1H, 12-H), 4.51–4.40 (*m*, 1H, 3-H), 3.78–3.20 (*m*, 16H, 33-H, 35-H, 36-H, 38-H, 53-H), 3.05–2.95 (*m*, 1H, 18-H), 2.07–2.02 (*m*, 1H, 16-H_a), 2.01–1.99 (*m*, 3H, 32-H), 1.89–1.81 (*m*, 2H, 11-H), 1.67–1.37 (*m*, 14H, 19-H_a, 1-H_a, 2-H, 9-H, 6-H_a, 15-H_a, 22-H_a, 21-H_a, 6-H_b, 34-H, 37-H), 1.30–1.24 (*m*, 12H, 54-H), 1.23–1.13 (*m*, 6H, 16-H_b, 7-H 22-H_b, 21-Hb, 19-H_b,), 1.08 (*s*, 3H, 27-H), 0.99 (*m*, 2H, 1-H_b, 15-H_b), 0.87 (*s*, 3H, 25-H), 0.86 (*s*, 3H, 29-H), 0.84 (*s*, 3H, 30-H), 0.82 (*s*, 3H, 23-H), 0.80 (*s*, 3H, 24-H), 0.79–0.76 (*m*, 1H, 5-H), 0.68 (*s*, 3H, 26-H) ppm; ^{13}C NMR (101 MHz, $CDCl_3$): δ = 170.9 (C-28, C-31), 168.7 (C-39), 157.7 (C-52), 155.8 (C-46), 155.7 (C-50), 145.4 (C-13), 136.6 (C-41), 132.5 (C-49), 130.4 (C-40), 130.1 (C-42), 130.0 (C-44), 129.4 (C-43), 127.7 (C-45), 121.2 (C-129, 113.9 (C-47), 96.1 (C-48, C-51), 80.9 (C-3), 55.3 (C-5), 48.4 (C-17), 47.6 (C-9), 46.6 (C-19), 46.2 (C-53), 46.1 (C-33, C-35, C-36, C-38), 44.7 (C-18), 42.0 (C-14), 39.1 (C-8), 38.0 (C-1), 37.6 (C-4), 37.0 (C-10), 34.1 (C-21), 32.9 (C-30), 32.8 (C-22), 30.3 (C-20), 29.6 (C-7), 28.0 (C-15), 28.0 (C-23), 25.8 (C-27), 24.0 (C-29), 23.5 (C-2), 23.3 (C-11), 22.6 (C-16), 21.3 (C-32), 18.2 (C-6), 17.2 (C-26), 16.6 (C-24), 15.4 (C-25), 12.7 (C-54) ppm; MS (ESI, MeOH/$CHCl_3$, 4:1): m/z = 1021.4 (98%, $[M\text{-}Cl]^+$); analysis calcd. for $C_{66}H_{91}N_4O_5Cl$ (1055.93): C 75.07, H 8.69, N 5.31; found: C 74.87, H 8.82, N 5.08.

*4.15. (3ß)-3-Acetyloxy-28-(5-{2-[3,6-bis(diethylamino)xanthen-10-ium-9-yl]benzoyl}-1,5-diazocan-1-yl)-28-oxours-12-ene Chloride (**20**)*

Following GP 3 from **15** (150 mg, 0.14 mmol) and rhodamine B (100 mg, 0.2 mmol), followed by chromatography (silica gel, ethyl acetate/MeOH, 10% → 40%), **20** (94 mg, 63%) was obtained as a pink solid; m.p. = 194–197 °C (decomp.); R_f = 0.41 ($CHCl_3$/MeOH, 9:1); UV-Vis ($CHCl_3$): λ_{max} (log ε) = 560 nm (5.54); IR (ATR): ν = 2932*w*, 1726*w*, 1586*s*, 1465*m*, 1411*s*, 1335*s*, 1272*m*, 1245*s*, 1179*s*, 1132*m*, 1073*m*, 1009*m*, 921*m*, 823*w*, 746*m*, 683*m*, 663*m*, 498*m* cm^{-1}; ^{1}H NMR (400 MHz, $CDCl_3$): δ = 7.68–7.56 (*m*, 2H, 43-H, 44-H), 7.53–7.49 (*m*, 1H, 42-H), 7.32–7.25 (*m*, 3H, 45-H, 48-H), 7.18–6.54 (*m*, 4H, 49-H, 51-H), 5.24–5.11 (*m*, 1H, 12-H), 4.50–4.39 (*m*, 1H, 3-H), 4.12–2.76 (*m*, 16H, 33-H, 35-H, 36-H, 38-H,53-H), 2.43–2.33 (*m*, 1H, 18-H), 2.09–2.07 (*m*, 1H, 16-H_a), 2.00 (*s*, 3H, 32-H), 1.91–1.84 (*m*, 2H, 11-H), 1.77–1.36 (*m*, 14H, 1-H_a, 2-H, 21-H_a, 6-H_a, 9-H, 22-H_a, 19-H, 6-H_b, 16-H_b, 34-H, 37-H), 1.29 (*t*, J = 7.1 Hz, 12H, 54-H), 1.23 (*m*, 6H, 7-H, 15-H, 21-H_b, 22-H_b), 1.03 (s, 4H, 1-H_b, 27-H), 0.96–0.93 (*m*, 1H, 20-H), 0.90 (*s*, 3H, 29-H), 0.88 (*s*, 3H, 25-H), 0.83 (*s*, 3H, 30-H), 0.82 (*s*, 3H, 23-H), 0.81 (*s*, 3H, 24-H), 0.77–0.75 (*m*, 1H, 5-H), 0.69 (*s*, 3H, 26-H) ppm; ^{13}C NMR (101 MHz, $CDCl_3$): δ = 170.9 (C-28), 157.7 (C-31), 157.7 (C-39), 155.8 (C-50), 155.7 (C-46) 155.6 (C-52), 136.6 (C-40), 132.9 (C-48), 130.1 (C-44), 130.0 (C-42), 129.4 (C-43), 127.0 (C-45), 125.0 (C-12), 113.9 (C-47), 96.2 (C-49, C-51), 80.9 (C-3), 55.3 (C-18), 55.3 (C-5), 49.4 (C-17), 47.5 (C-9), 46.2 (C-33, C-35, C-36, C-38), 46.1 (C-53), 42.4 (C-14), 39.6 (C-19), 39.3 (C-8), 38.6 (C-20), 38.2 (C-1), 37.6 (C-4), 36.9 (C-10), 32.7 (C-22), 31.9 (C-7), 30.5 (C-21), 29.6 (C-15), 29.3 (C-16), 28.0 (C-23), 23.2 (C-2), 23.1 (C-11), 23.0 (C-27), 18.1 (C-6), 17.4 (C-30), 17.2 (C-26), 16.7 (C-24), 15.5 (C-25), 12.7 (C-54) ppm; MS (ESI, MeOH/$CHCl_3$, 4:1): m/z = 1020.4 (100%, $[M\text{-}Cl]^+$); analysis calcd. For $C_{66}H_{91}N_4O_5Cl$ (1055.93): C 75.07, H 8.69, N 5.31; found: C 74.83, H 8.91, N 5.03.

*4.16. (3ß)-3-Acetyloxy-28-(5-{2-[3,6-bis(diethylamino)xanthen-10-ium-9-yl]benzoyl}-1,5-diazocan-1-yl)-28-oxolup-20(29)-ene Chloride (**21**)*

Following GP 3 from **16** (300 mg, 0.5 mmol) and rhodamine B (200 mg, 0.4 mmol), followed by chromatography (silica gel, $CHCl_3$/MeOH, 9:1), **21** (3536 mg, 69%) was obtained as a pink solid; m.p. = 212–218 °C; R_f = 0.49 ($CHCl_3$/MeOH, 9:1); UV-Vis ($CHCl_3$): λ_{max} (log ε) = 562 nm (4.43); IR (ATR): ν = 2936*w*, 1730*w*, 1587*s*, 1465*m*, 1411*s*, 1335*s*, 1244*s*, 1179*s*, 1132*m*, 1073*m*, 978*w*, 921*w*, 684*m* cm^{-1}; ^{1}H NMR (400 MHz, $CDCl_3$): δ = 7.52–7.47 (*m*, 2H, 43-H, 44-H), 7.43–7.37 (*m*, 1H, 42-H), 7.22–6.99 (*m*, 3H, 45-H, 48-H), 6.97–6.71 (*m*, 2H, 49-H), 6.64–6.57 (*m*, 2H, 51-H), 4.58–4.50 (*m*, 1H, 29-H_a), 4.42–4.37 (*m*, 1H, 29-H_b), 4.30 (*m*, 1H, 3-H), 3.73–2.93 (*m*, 16H, 33-H, 35-H, 36-H, 38-H, 53-H), 2.83–2.68 (*m*, 2H, 19-H, 13-H), 2.00–1.94 (*m*, 1H, 16-H_a), 1.87 (*s*, 3H, 32-H), 1.83–1.54 (*m*, 4H, 22-H_a, 15-H, 21-H_a), 1.53–1.51 (*m*, 2H, 12-H_a, 1-H_a), 1.50 (*s*, 3H, 30-H), 1.47–1.42 (*m*, 2H, 2-H), 1.41–1.36 (*m*, 1H, 18-H), 1.35–1.29 (*m*,

2H, 16-H_a, 6-H_a), 1.28–1.12 (*m*, 21H, 11-H_a, 6-H_b, 7-H, 22-H_b, 54-H, 34-H, 37-H), 1.11–1.09 (*m*, 2H, 11-H_b, 9-H, 21-H_b), 0.83–0.74 (*m*, 8H, 1-H_b, 12-H_b, 23-H, 27-H), 0.69–0.65 (*m*, 9H, 26-H, 25-H, 24-H), 0.63–0.59 (*m*, 1H, 5-H) ppm; ^{13}C NMR (101 MHz, $CDCl_3$): δ = 170.8 (C-28), 168.5 (C-39), 167.6 (C-31), 157.6 (C-50), 155.6 (C-46), 155.5 (C-52), 151.2 (C-20), 136.4 (C-40), 132.3 (C-41), 130.8 (C-48), 130.0 (C-43), 129.4 (C-42), 128.6 (C-45), 127.0 (C-44), 114.6 (C-49), 113.6 (C-47), 108.9 (C-29), 96.0 (C-51), 80.8 (C-3), 55.2 (C-5), 55.1 (C-38, C-36, C-35, C-33), 53.0 (C-18), 50.6 (C-9), 46.1 (C-53), 45.8 (C-19), 41.9 (C-17), 40.6 (C-8), 40.6 (C-14), 38.3 (C-1), 37.7 (C-10), 37.0 (C-4), 36.8 (C-13), 36.0 (C-22), 34.2 (C-7), 32.0 (C-16), 31.3 (C-21), 30.2 (C-34, C-37), 29.8 (C-15), 27.8 (C-24), 25.5 (C-12), 25.4 (C-37, C-34), 23.6 (C-2), 21.2 (C-32), 21.0 (C-11), 19.6 (C-30), 18.1 (C-6), 16.1 (C-25), 15.9 (C-26), 14.6 (C-23), 14.5 (C-27), 12.6 (C-54) ppm; MS (ESI, MeOH/$CHCl_3$, 4:1): *m/z* = 1020.5 (100%, [M-Cl]$^+$); analysis calcd. for $C_{66}H_{91}N_4O_5Cl$ (1055.93): C 75.07, H 8.69, N 5.31; found: C 74.86, H 8.90, N 5.09.

*4.17. (3ß)-3-Acetyloxy-28-(5-{2-[3,6-bis(diethylamino)xanthen-10-ium-9-yl]benzoyl}-1,5-diazocan-1-yl)-28-oxolup-20-oxo Chloride (**22**)*

Following GP 3 from **17** (300 mg, 0.50 mmol) and rhodamine B (300 mg, 0.6 mmol), followed by chromatography (silica gel, ethyl acetate/MeOH, 9:1), **22** (350 mg, 69%) was obtained as a pink solid; m.p. = 198–201 °C; R_f = 0.51 ($CHCl_3$/MeOH, 9:1); UV-Vis ($CHCl_3$): λ_{max} (log ε) = 558 nm (4.73); IR (ATR): *ν* = 2934*w*, 1721*m*, 1585*s*, 1410*m*, 1466*s*, 1334*s*, 1272*s*, 1245*s*, 1131*s*, 1072*s*, 1009*s*, 977*m*, 921*m*, 823*m*, 755*m*, 682*s* cm^{-1}; ^{1}H NMR (400 MHz, $CDCl_3$): δ = 7.67–7.57 (*m*, 2H, 42-H, 43-H), 7.53–7.47 (*m*, 1H, 41-H), 7.35–7.27 (*m*, 3H, 44-H, 47-H), 7.11–6.64 (*m*, 4H, 48-H, 50-H), 4.46–4.36 (*m*, 1H, 3-H), 3.88–3.20 (*m*, 16H, 32-H, 34-H, 35-H, 37-H, 52-H), 3.16–3.05 (*m*, 1H, 18-H), 2.76–2.51 (*m*, 1H, 13-H), 2.11–2.04 (*m*, 4H, 16-H_a, 29-H), 1.98 (*s*, 4H, 19-H, 31-H), 1.78 (*s*, 2H, 21-H_a, 22-H_a), 1.62–1.48 (*m*, 4H, 1-H_a, 2-H, 16-H_a), 1.42 (*m*, 7H, 6-H_a, 22-H_b, 21-H_b, 11-H, 7-H_a, 6-H_b), 1.28 (*t*, *J* = 6.8 Hz, 14H, 7-H_b, 9-H, 53-H), 1.23–1.04 (*m*, 6H, 33-H, 36-H, 15-H), 0.94 (*s*, 2H, 12-H), 0.91 (*s*, 4H, 1-H_b, 24-H), 0.82 (*s*, 3H, 27-H), 0.78 (*m*, 10H, 23-H, 25-H, 26-H, 5-H) ppm; ^{13}C NMR (101 MHz, $CDCl_3$): δ = 212.8 (C-20), 170.9 (C-28, C-30, C- 38), 157.7 (C-49), 155.7 (C-45), 155.6 (C-51), 136.6 (C-39), 136.5 (C-40), 132.4 (C-47), 130.1 (C-42), 129.7 (C-43), 129.4 (C-44), 127.1 (C-41), 114.5 (C-48), 113.7 (C-46), 96.2 (C-50), 80.8 (C-3), 55.4 (C-5), 55.3 (C-32, C-34, C-35, C-37), 53.0 (C-19), 50.6 (C-9), 50.3 (C-18), 49.5 (C-17), 46.2 (C-52), 41.9 (C-14), 40.6 (C-8), 38.3 (C-1), 37.7 (C-4), 37.1 (C-10), 35.8 (C-13), 35.6 (C-22), 34.2 (C-7), 31.6 (C-16), 30.1 (C-29), 29.9 (C-15), 28.8 (C-21), 27.9 (C-23), 27.4 (C-12), 23.6 (C-2), 22.6 (C-33, C-36), 21.1 (C-11), 18.1 (C-6), 16.4 (C-25), 16.2 (C-26), 14.7 (C-24), 14.0 (C-27), 12.7 (C-53) ppm; MS (ESI, MeOH/$CHCl_3$, 4:1): *m/z* = 1022.4 (100%, [M-Cl]$^+$); analysis calcd. for $C_{65}H_{89}N_4O_6Cl$ (1057.90): C 73.80, H 8.48, N 5.30; found: C 73.55, H 8.67, N 5.07.

*4.18. (2α,3ß,4α)2,3,23-Tris (acetyloxy)-28-(5-{2-[3,6-bis(diethylamino)xanthen-10-ium-9-yl]benzoyl}-1,5-diazocan-1-yl)-28-oxours-12-en Chloride (**23**)*

Following GP 3 from **18** (300 mg, 0.4 mmol) and rhodamine B (250 mg, 0.5 mmol), followed by chromatography (silica gel, ethyl acetate/MeOH, 9:1), **23** (184 mg, 60%) was obtained as a pink solid; m.p. = 225 °C; R_f = 0.44 ($CHCl_3$/MeOH, 9:1); UV-Vis ($CHCl_3$): λ_{max} (log ε) = 562 nm (4.50); IR (ATR): *ν* = 2927*w*, 1793*m*, 1587*s*, 1467*m*, 1411*m*, 1336*s*, 1244*s*, 1179*s*, 1042*m*, 921*w*, 684*m*, 436*w* cm^{-1}; ^{1}H NMR (400 MHz, $CDCl_3$): δ = 7.66–7.57 (*m*, 2H, 47-H, 48-H), 7.52–7.47 (*m*, 1H, 46-H), 7.27-7.20 (m, 49-H, 52-H), 7.17–6.63 (*m*, 4H, 53-H, 55-H), 5.20–5.00 (*m*, 3H, 12-H, 2-H, 3-H), 3.82–3.76 (*m*, 1H, 23-H_a), 3.73–2.93 (*m*, 17H, 37-H, 39-H, 40-H, 42-H, 57-H, 23-H_b), 2.44–2.33 (*m*, 1H, 18-H), 2.04 (*s*, 3H, 34-H), 2.02–1.99 (*m*, 1H, 1-H_a), 1.97 (*s*, 3H, 36-H), 1.93 (*s*, 3H, 32-H), 1.90–1.32 (*m*, 15H, 11-H, 9-H, 15-H, 16-Ha, 21-H_a, 22-H_a, 20-H, 38-H, 41-H, 6-H), 1.28 (*t*, *J* = 7.1 Hz, 13H, 5-H, 58-H), 1.25–1.10 (*m*, 5H, 7-H, 16-H_b, 21-H_b, 22-H_b), 1.09–1.07 (*m*, 1H, 1-H_b), 1.04 (*s*, 3H, 30-H), 1.01 (*s*, 3H, 27-H), 0.97–0.92 (*m*, 1H, 19-H), 0.88 (*s*, 3H, 29-H), 0.84 (*s*, 3H, 25-H), 0.81 (*s*, 3H, 26-H), 0.69 (*s*, 3H, 24-H) ppm; ^{13}C NMR (101 MHz, $CDCl_3$): δ = 176.2 (C-43), 170.8 (C-35), 170.4 (C-31, C-33), 170.3 (C-28), 157.7 (C-54), 155.7 (C-56), 155.6 (C-50), 138.6 (C-13), 136.6 (C-45), 132.3 (C-52),

130.1 (C-47), 130.0 (C-49), 129.3 (C-48), 127.2 (C-46), 125.9 (C-12), 113.9 (C-51), 96.2 (C-53, C-55), 74.8 (C-3), 69.9 (C-2), 65.3 (C-23), 55.5 (C-18), 53.4 (C-37, C-39, C-40, C-42), 47.6 (C-5), 47.5 (C-9), 46.2 (C-57), 46.1 (C-17), 43.7 (C-1), 42.5 (C-4), 41.9 (C-14), 38.9 (C-8), 38.7 (C-20), 38.6 (C-19), 37.8 (C-10), 32.6 (C-22), 30.5 (C-21), 29.6 (C-7), 28.4 (C-15), 23.4 (C-27), 23.3 (C-11), 21.2 (C-29), 21.0 (C-32), 20.8 (C-36), 20.7 (C-34), 17.8 (C-6), 17.4 (C-26), 17.2 (C-30), 17.0 (C-24), 13.9 (C-25), 12.6 (C-58) ppm; MS (ESI, MeOH/$CHCl_3$, 4:1): m/z = 1036.5 (100%, $[M-Cl]^+$); analysis calcd. for $C_{70}H_{95}N_4O_9Cl$ (1172.00): C 71.74, H 8.17, N 4.78; found: C 71.49, H 8.35, N 4.47.

*4.19. 3β-Acetyloxy-28-[4-[3-(2,3,6,7,12,13,16,17-octahydro-1H,5H,11H,15H-pyrido [3,2,1-ij]pyrido[1″,2″,3″:1′,8′]quinolino[6′,5′:5,6]pyrano[2,3-f]quinolin-4-ium-9-yl)benzoyl]1,5-diazocan-1-yl]-28-oxo-olean-12-en Chloride (**24**)*

Following GP 3 from **14** (100 mg, 0.14 mmol) and rhodamine 101 (200 mg, 0.4 mmol), followed by chromatography (silica gel, ethyl acetate/MeOH, 10% → 50%), **24** (114 mg, 75%) was obtained as a pink solid; m.p. = 205–210 °C; R_f = 0.41 ($CHCl_3$/MeOH, 9:1); UV-Vis ($CHCl_3$): λ_{max} (log ε) = 580 nm (4.23); IR (ATR): ν = 2942*w*, 1727*m*, 1595*s*, 1493*m*, 1459*m*, 1362*m*, 1295*s*, 1196*s*, 1035*m*, 746*m*, 420*m* cm^{-1}; ^1H NMR (400 MHz, $CDCl_3$): δ = 7.81–7.61 (*m*, 2H, 45-H), 7.54–7.43 (*m*, 1H, 42-H), 7.29 (*s*, 1H, 44-H), 6.86–6.47 (*m*, 2H, 48-H), 5.27–5.21 (*m*, 1H, 12-H), 4.51–4.44 (*m*, 1H, 3-H), 3.79–3.15 (*m*, 16H, 33-H, 35-H, 36-H, 38-H, 52-H, 57-H), 3.09–2.90 (*m*, 5H, 18-H, 55-H,), 2.76–2.47 (*m*, 4H, 50-H), 2.15–2.06 (*m*, 4H, 56-H), 2.03 (*s*, 3H, 32-H), 1.97 (*s*, 5H, 16-H_a, 51-H), 1.85 (*s*, 2H, 11-H), 1.70–1.15 (*m*, 20H, 19-H_a, 21-H, 2-H, 1-H_a, 9-H, 6-H_a, 7-H_a, 6-H_b, 22-H_a, 7-H_b, 15-H, 22-H_b, 19-H_b, 34-H, 37-H), 1.12 (*s*, 3H, 30-H), 1.07–0.97 (*m*, 2H, 1-H_b, 16-H_b), 0.91 (*s*, 3H, 25-H), 0.90 (*s*, 3H, 27-H), 0.88 (*s*, 3H, 29-H), 0.85 (*s*, 3H, 23-H), 0.83 (*s*, 3H, 24-H), 0.81–0.79 (*m*, 1H, 5-H), 0.72 (*s*, 3H, 26-H) ppm; ^{13}C NMR (101 MHz, $CDCl_3$): δ = 171.0 (C-28, C-31, C-39), 164.1 (C-53), 152.0 (C-46), 139.9 (C-58), 134.6 (C-41), 131.0 (C-40), 130.5 (C-44), 129.4 (C-45, C-42), 126.9 (C-43), 125.9 (C-48), 123.5 (C-47), 121.4 (C-12), 113.0 (C-49), 105.3 (C-54), 81.0 (C-3), 55.4 (C-5), 51.1 (C-33, C-35, C-36, C-38), 50.5 (C-52, C-57), 48.2 (C-17), 47.6 (C-9), 46.6 (C-19), 43.7 (C-18), 43.3 (C-14), 39.1 (C-8), 38.1 (C-1), 37.7 (C-4), 37.0 (C-10), 33.9 (C-22), 33.0 (C-29), 32.9 (C-7), 30.5 (C-20), 30.3 (C-21), 29.7 (C-15), 28.0 (C-23), 27.8 (C-16), 27.6 (C-50), 25.8 (C-30), 24.1 (C-27), 23.5 (C-2), 23.4 (C-11), 21.3 (C-32), 20.6 (C-51), 19.9 (C-55), 19.7 (C-56), 18.2 (C-6), 17.2 (C-26), 16.7 (C-24), 15.4 (C-25) ppm; MS (ESI, MeOH/$CHCl_3$, 4:1): m/z = 1068.6 (100%, $[M-Cl]^+$); analysis calcd. For $C_{70}H_{91}N_4O_5Cl$ (1103.97): C 76.16, H 8.31, N 5.08; found: C 75.81, H 8.52, N 4.89.

*4.20. 3β-Acetyloxy-28-[4-[3-(2,3,6,7,12,13,16,17-octahydro-1H,5H,11H,15H-pyrido[3,2,1-ij]pyrido[1″,2″,3″:1′,8′]quinolino[6′,5′:5,6]pyrano[2,3-f]uinoline-4-ium-9-yl)benzoyl]1,5-diazocan-1-yl]-28-oxo-urs-12-en Chloride (**25**)*

Following GP 3 from **15** (150 mg, 0.2 mmol) and rhodamine 101 (150 mg, 0.3 mmol), followed by chromatography (silica gel, ethyl acetate/MeOH, 10% → 50%), **25** (94 mg, 62%) was obtained as a pink solid; m.p. = 199–202 °C; R_f = 0.43 ($CHCl_3$:Methanol, 9:1); UV-Vis ($CHCl_3$): λ_{max} (log ε) = 571 nm (3.94); IR (ATR): ν = 3388*w*, 2925*m*, 1728*m*, 1597*s*, 1495*m*, 1459*m*, 1362*s*, 1297*s*, 1246*s*, 1195*s*, 1100*s*, 1024*s*, 421*s* cm^{-1}; ^1H NMR (400 MHz, $CDCl_3$): δ = 8.36–8.06 (*m*, 1H, 43-H), 7.75–7.63 (*m*, 2H, 42-H, 45-H), 7.24–7.11 (*m*, 1H, 44-H), 6.81–6.50 (*m*, 2H, 48-H), 5.26–5.16 (*m*, 1H, 12-H), 4.49–4.43 (*m*, 1H, 3-H), 3.71–3.21 (*m*, 16H, 33-H, 35-H, 36-H, 38-H, 52-H, 57-H), 3.17–2.90 (*m*, 4H, 55-H), 2.81–2.57 (*m*, 4H, 50-H), 2.23–2.06 (*m*, 4H, 56-H), 2.01 (*s*, 3H, 32-H), 1.98–1.84 (*m*, 6H, 51-H, 11-H_a, 16-H_a), 1.66–1.19 (*m*, 22H, 1-H_a, 11-H_b, 21-H_a, 6-H_a, 22-H_a, 19-H, 6-H_b, 21-H_b, 22-H_b, 2-H, 15-H, 7-H, 16-H_b, 18-H, 34-H, 37-H), 1.13–1.10 (*m*, 3H, 29-H), 1.05 (*s*, 3H, 27-H), 1.04–0.99 (*m*, 2H, 1-H_b, 20-H), 0.92 (*s*, 3H, 24-H), 0.85 (*s*, 3H, 25-H), 0.83 (*s*, 3H, 23-H), 0.82 (*s*, 3H, 30-H), 0.79–0.77 (*m*, 1H, 5-H), 0.72 (*s*, 3H, 26-H) ppm; ^{13}C NMR (101 MHz, $CDCl_3$): δ = 171.0 (C-28), 169.3 (C-31, C-39), 151.2 (C-53), 150.9 (C-46), 135.2 (C-58), 132.3 (C-42), 131.3 (C-43), 130.2 (C-45), 129.1 (C-44), 127.1 (C-48), 125.1 (C-12), 112.6 (C-49), 111.6 (C-47), 105.6 (C-54), 80.9 (C-3), 55.3 (C-5), 47.7 (C-33, C-35, C-36, C-38), 47.5 (C-18), 47.5 (C-9), 45.3 (C-17), 43.3 (C-52, C-57), 41.7 (C-14), 39.6 (C-8),

39.5 (C-19), 38.6 (C-20), 38.2 (C-1), 37.7 (C-4), 36.9 (C-10), 33.1 (C-22), 31.9 (C-7), 30.5 (C-21), 29.7 (C-15), 28.0 (C-16), 27.8 (C-23), 27.5 (C-50), 25.0 (C-34, C-37), 23.5 (C-11), 23.4 (C-27), 23.3 (C-51), 22.6 (C-2), 21.3 (C-32), 19.9 (C-55), 19.7 (C-56), 18.7 (C-29), 18.1 (C-6), 17.3 (C-30), 16.7 (C-26), 15.5 (C-24), 14.1 (C-25) ppm; MS (ESI, MeOH/$CHCl_3$, 4:1): m/z = 1068.4 (100%, $[M-Cl]^+$); analysis calcd. for $C_{70}H_{91}N_4O_5Cl$ (1103.97): C 76.16, H 8.31, N 5.08; found: C 75.87, H 8.59, N 4.83.

4.21. 3β-Acetyloxy-28-[4-[3-(2,3,6,7,12,13,16,17-octahydro-1H,5H,11H,15H-pyrido[3,2,1-ij] pyrido[1″,2″,3″:1′,8′]quinolino[6′,5′:5,6]pyrano[2,3-f]quinolin-4-ium-9-yl)benzoyl] 1,5-diazocan-1-yl]-28-oxo-lup-20(29)-en Chloride (26)

Following GP 3 from **16** (200 mg, 0.14 mmol) and rhodamine 101 (200 mg, 0.4 mmol), followed by chromatography (silica gel, $CHCl_3$/MeOH, 9:1), **26** (103 mg, 68%) was obtained as a pink solid; m.p. = 203–206 °C; R_f = 0.44 ($CHCl_3$/MeOH, 9:1); UV-Vis ($CHCl_3$): λ_{max} (log ε) = 578 nm (4.33); IR (ATR): ν = 2931*w*, 1721*w*, 1595*s*, 1493*s*, 1361*m*, 1294*s*, 1246*s*, 1180*s*, 1035*s*, 746*m*, 622*m*, 421*s* cm^{-1}; ^1H NMR (400 MHz, $CDCl_3$): δ = 7.68–7.53 (*m*, 2H, 43-H, 45-H), 7.52–7.45 (*m*, 1H, 42-H), 7.31–7.26 (*m*, 1H, 44-H), 6.76–6.59 (*m*, 2H, 48-H), 4.70–4.62 (*m*, 1H, 29-H_a), 4.54–4.49 (*m*, 1H, 29-H_b), 4.44–4.38 (*m*, 1H, 3-H), 3.81–3.02 (*m*, 16H, 33-H, 35-H, 36-H, 38-H, 52-H, 57-H), 3.00–2.89 (*m*, 4H, 55-H), 2.88–2.72 (*m*, 2H, 13-H, 18-H), 2.71–2.51 (*m*, 4H, 50-H), 2.16–2.01 (*m*, 5H, 16-H_a, 56-H), 1.99 (*s*, 3H, 32-H), 1.96–1.87 (*m*, 5H, 21-H_a, 51-H), 1.85–1.74 (*m*, 2H, 15-H_a, 22-H_a), 1.70–1.66 (*m*, 1H, 12-H_a), 1.62 (*s*, 4H, 1-H_a, 30-H), 1.60–1.53 (*m*, 2H, 2-H), 1.50–1.47 (*m*, 1H, 9-H), 1.47–1.40 (*m*, 2H, 6-H_a, 16-H_b), 1.36–1.06 (*m*, 13H, 11-H_a, 21-H_b, 6-H_b, 7-H, 15-H_b, 19-H, 22-H_b, 11-H_b, 34-H, 37-H), 0.94 (*s*, 2H, 1-H_b, 12-H_b), 0.90 (*s*, 3H, 24-H), 0.86 (*s*, 3H, 25-H), 0.81 (*s*, 3H, 27-H), 0.79 (*s*, 3H, 23-H), 0.73 (*s*, 3H, 26-H), 0.70–0.59 (*m*, 1H, 5-H) ppm; ^{13}C NMR (101 MHz, $CDCl_3$): δ = 170.9 (C-28), 168.8 (C-31, C-39), 151.9 (C-53), 151.3 (C-46), 151.2 (C-20), 138.4 (C-40, C-41), 136.5 (C-58), 130.4 (C-44), 129.4 (C-45, C-42), 127.1 (C-48), 127.0 (C-43) 123.5 (C-47), 113.1 (C-49), 109.1 (C-29), 105.3 (C-54), 81.0 (C-3), 55.5 (C-5), 53.1 (C-9), 52.9, 50.9 (C-33, C-35, C-36, C-38), 50.7 (C-19), 50.5 (C-52, C-57), 49.4 (C-17), 45.9 (C-13), 42.0 (C-14), 40.7 (C-14), 40.6 (C-8), 38.4 (C-1), 37.8 (C-4), 37.1 (C-10), 36.9 (C-18), 36.1 (C-21), 34.3 (C-7), 32.1 (C-16), 31.4 (C-22), 29.9 (C-15), 27.9 (C-23), 27.5 (C-50), 25.5 (C-12), 23.7 (C-2), 22.6 (C-34, C-37), 21.3 (C-32), 21.1 (C-11), 20.6 (C-51), 19.8 (C-55), 19.6 (C-56), 18.7 (C-30), 18.2 (C-6), 16.5 (C-25), 16.4 (C-26), 14.7 (C-24), 14.6 (C-27) ppm; MS (ESI, MeOH/CHCl3, 4:1): m/z = 1067.2 (100%, $[M-Cl]^+$); analysis calcd. for $C_{70}H_{91}N_4O_5Cl$ (1103.97): C 76.16, H 8.31, N 5.08; found: C 75.98, H 8.52, N 4.83.

4.22. 3β-Acetyloxy-28-[4-[3-(2,3,6,7,12,13,16,17-octahydro-1H,5H,11H,15H-pyrido[3,2,1-ij] pyrido[1″,2″,3″:1′,8′]quinolino[6′,5′:5,6]pyrano[2,3-f]quinolin-4-ium-9-yl)benzoyl] 1,5-diazocan-1-yl]-30-nor-20,28-dioxo-lup-20(29)-en Chloride (27)

Following GP 3 from **17** (200 mg, 0.3 mmol) and rhodamine 101 (100 mg, 0.2 mmol), followed by chromatography (silica gel, $CHCl_3$/MeOH, 9:1), **27** (132 mg, 60%) was obtained as a pink solid; m.p. = 208–210 °C; R_f = 0.49 ($CHCl_3$:MeOH, 9:1); UV-Vis ($CHCl_3$): λ_{max} (log ε) = 577 nm (4.66); IR (ATR): ν = 3350*w*, 1596*s*, 1195*s*, 1298*s*, 1197*s*, 1138*s* cm^{-1}; ^1H NMR (400 MHz, $CDCl_3$): δ = 7.63–7.52 (*m*, 2H, 41-H, 44-H), 7.50–7.43 (*m*, 1H, 42-H), 7.24–7.20 (*m*, 1H, 43-H), 6.72–6.59 (*m*, 2H, 47-H), 4.42–4.33 (*m*, 1H, 3-H), 3.86–3.01 (*m*, 17H, 18-H, 32-H, 34-H, 35-H, 37H, 49-H, 51-H), 2.97–2.85 (*m*, 4H, 54-H), 2.76–2.54 (*m*, 4H, 49-H), 2.52–2.43 (*m*, 1H, 13-H), 2.18–2.06 (*m*, 4H, 21-H_b, 29-H), 2.07–1.99 (*m*, 4H, 55-H), 1.96 (*s*, 4H, 19-H, 31-H), 1.94–1.64 (*m*, 7H, 50-H, 22-H_a, 16-H_a, 15-H_a), 1.60–1.14 (*m*, 18H, 1-H_a, 2-H, 21-H_b, 22-H_b, 6-Ha, 16-H_b, 11-H_a, 7-H, 6-H_b, 11-H_b, 15-H_b), 1.08–0.96 (*m*, 3H, 1-H_b, 12-H), 0.90 (*s*, 3H, 24-H), 0.85 (*s*, 3H, 25-H), 0.80 (*s*, 3H, 27-H), 0.76 (*s*, 3H, 23-H), 0.71 (s, 3H, 26-H), 0.69–0.65 (m, 1H, 5-H) ppm; ^{13}C NMR (101 MHz, $CDCl_3$): δ = 213.2 (C-20), 170.9 (C-28, C-30, C-38), 151.9 (C-52), 151.2 (C-45), 136.6 (C-57), 136.3 (C-39, C-40), 130.4 (C-43), 129.4 (C-41, C-44), 126.8 (C-42), 126.7 (C-47), 123.5 (C-46), 113.0 (C-48), 105.2 (C-53), 80.8 (C-3), 55.4 (C-5), 53.0 (C-19), 50.9 (C-32, C-34, C-35, C-37), 50.6 (C-9), 50.4 (C-51, C-56), 50.3 (C-18), 49.8 (C-17), 44.1 (C-13), 41.8 (C-14), 40.6 (C-8), 38.3 (C-1), 37.7 (C-10), 37.1 (C-4), 35.8 (C-22), 34.2 (C-7), 31.8 (C-21), 30.1 (C-29), 29.9 (C-15), 28.8 (C-16), 27.9 (C-23), 27.5 (C-49), 27.3 (C-12), 23.6 (C-2), 22.6 (C-33, C-36), 21.2 (C-31), 21.1 (C-11), 20.6 (C-50), 19.9 (C-54), 19.6 (C-55), 18.1

(C-6), 16.4 (C-26), 15.9 (C-25), 14.7 (C-24), 14.0 (C-27) ppm; MS (ESI, MeOH/$CHCl_3$, 4:1): m/z = 1070 (100%, $[M-Cl]^+$); analysis calcd. for $C_{69}H_{89}N_4O_6Cl$ (1105.94): C 74.94, H 8.11, N 5.07; found: C 74.73, H 8.35, N 4.81.

*4.23. (2α,3β,4α)2,3,23-Tris(acetoxy)-28-[4-[3-(2,3,6,7,12,13,16,17-octahydro-1H,5H,11H,15H-pyrido[3,2,1-ij]pyrido[1″,2″,3″:1′,8′]quinolino[6′,5′:5,6]pyrano[2,3-f]quinolin-4-ium-9-yl)benzoyl]1,5-diazocan-1-yl]-28-oxo-olean-12-en Chloride (**28**)*

Following GP 3 from **18** (200 mg, 0.3 mmol) and rhodamine 101 (200 mg, 0.4 mmol), followed by chromatography (silica gel, $CHCl_3$/MeOH, 9:1), **28** (232 mg, 64%) was obtained as a pink solid; m.p. = 193–196 °C; R_f = 0.45 ($CHCl_3$:MeOH, 9:1); UV-Vis ($CHCl_3$): λ_{max} (log ε) = 578 nm (4.50); IR (ATR): ν = 2924*w*, 1739*w*, 1594*s*, 1493*s*, 1459*m*, 1361*m*, 1293*s*, 1195*s*, 1180*s*, 1090*s*, 1035*s*, 729*m*, 622*m*, 421*s* cm^{-1}; ^1H NMR (400 MHz, $CDCl_3$): δ =7.67–7.58 (*m*, 2H, 47-H, 49-H), 7.52–7.48 (*m*, 1H, 46-H), 7.29–7.27 (*m*, 1H, 48-H), 6.77–6.65 (*m*, 2H, 52-H), 5.17–5.03 (*m*, 3H, 12-H, 2-H, 3-H), 3.83–3.79 (*m*, 1H, 23-H_a), 3.60–3.16 (*m*, 17H, 23-H_b, 37-H, 39-H, 40-H, 42-H, 56-H, 61-H), 3.00–2.94 (*m*, 4H, 59-H), 2.77–2.63 (*m*, 4H, 54-H), 2.46–2.36 (*m*, 1H, 18-H), 2.07 (*s*, 4H, 60-H), 2.06 (*s*, 3H, 36-H), 2.04–2.01 (*m*, 1H, 1-H_a), 1.99 (*s*, 3H, 34-H), 1.95 (*s*, 7H, 32-H, 55-H), 1.91–1.86 (*m*, 2H, 11-H), 1.60–1.57 (*m*, 1H, 9-H), 1.46–1.42 (*m*, 2H, 21-H_a, 22-H_b), 1.35–1.30 (*m*, 4H, 6-H, 19-H, 5-H), 1.26–1.22 (*m*, 12H, 16-H_a, 38-H, 41-H, 22-H_b, 7-H, 15-H, 21-H_b, 16-H_b), 1.11–1.09 (*m*, 1H, 1-H_b), 1.04 (*s*, 3H, 24-H), 0.98–0.94 (*m*, 1H, 20-H), 0.91 (*s*, 3H, 29-H), 0.85 (*s*, 3H, 25-H), 0.83 (*s*, 3H, 27-H), 0.82 (*s*, 3H, 30-H), 0.72 (*s*, 3H, 26-H) ppm; ^{13}C NMR (101 MHz, $CDCl_3$): δ = 176.3 (C-28), 170.8 (C-35, C-43), 170.4 (C-33), 170.3 (C-31), 152.0 (C-57), 151.3 (C-50), 139.1 (C-62), 136.6 (C-44), 130.3 (C-45), 129.6 (C-48), 129.2 (C-46) 129.1 (C-49), 127.0 (C-47, C-52), 124.5 (C-12), 123.4 (C-51), 113.0 (C-53), 105.2 (C-58), 74.9 (C-3), 69.9 (C-2), 65.3 (C-23), 55.6 (C-18), 51.0 (C-34, C-37, C-40, C-42), 50.5 (C-56, C-61), 47.7 (C-5), 47.5 (C-9), 46.2 (C-17), 43.7 (C-1), 41.9 (C-4, C-14), 39.5 (C-19), 38.6 (C-20), 37.8 (C-10), 32.6 (C-22), 31.9 (C-7), 30.6 (C-21), 29.7 (C-15), 29.6 (C-16), 27.6 (C-54), 23.3 (C-11), 22.6 (C-38, C-41), 22.6 (C-27), 21.2 (C-29), 21.0 (C-32), 20.8 (C-36), 20.7 (C-34), 20.6 (C-55), 19.9 (C-59), 19.7 (C-60), 17.9 (C-6), 17.4 (C-30), 17.1 (C-24), 17.0 (C-26), 14.1 (C-25) ppm; MS (ESI, MeOH/$CHCl_3$, 4:1): m/z = 1084.3 (100%, $[M-Cl]^+$); analysis calcd. for $C_{74}H_{95}N_4O_9Cl$ (1220.04): C 72.85, H 7.85, N 4.59; found: C 72.63, H 8.01, N 4.39.

4.24. Cell Culture

Breast cancer cell lines were obtained from the Department of Radiobiology (MLU Halle-Wittenberg) and previously described. MDA-MB-231, HS578T and MCF-7, and T47D were cultured as a monolayer in RPMI (Thermo Fisher Scientific, Waltham, MA, USA) with 10% fetal bovine serum (Capricorn Scientific, Ebsdorfergrund, Germany), 2% penicillin/streptomycin (Sigma-Aldrich, St. Louis, MO, USA), and 1% sodium pyruvate (Gibco, Thermo Fisher Scientific) at 37 °C and 5% CO_2. All cell lines were regularly tested for mycoplasma contamination.

4.25. SRB Assay

Breast cancer cells were seeded in 96 well plates with different cell numbers depending on the cell line in triplicate and after 24 h treated with different concentrations of compounds **14–28**. Treatment ended after 96 h when cells were fixed with 10% trichloroacetic acid (Carl Roth GmbH, Karlsruhe, Germany) for 1h at 4 °C. Afterwards, cells were washed with ice water four times and stained with 4.4% SRB solution (Sigma–Aldrich) for 10 min at room temperature. After washing cells with 1% acetic acid (Carl Roth GmbH), cells were air-dried overnight and then dissolved with 300 μL 20 mM Tris base solution (Sigma-Aldrich). Excitation was measured at 540 nm with a Spark plate reader (Tecan Treading AG, Männedorf, Switzerland) and IC_{50} values were calculated by dose-response curve fitting using Origin 2019 (OriginLab Corp., Northampton, MA, USA).

4.26. Cell Death

For the determination of apoptotic and necrotic cell death after treatment with compound 28, Annexin V-Sytox Deep Red staining was performed. Therefore, MDA-MB-231 and HS578T cells were seeded in 6-well plates. After 24 h, the cells were treated with different concentrations of compound 28 (10 nM, 100 nM, 250 nM, 500 nM, 1 μM, and 2 μM) for 24 h, 48 h, and 72 h at 37 °C and 5% CO_2. For analysis of cell death, detached cells were collected in tubes and living cells were detached by accutase (Biowest, Nuaillé, France) and collected in the same tube. After several washing steps cells were resuspended in 1x annexin V binding puffer (10 mM HEPES, 140 mM NaCl, 2.5 mM $CaCl_2$) and stained with 5 μL Annexin V-FITC (BioLegend, San Diego, CA, USA) and 1 μL 100 μM Sytox Deep Red Nucleic Acid Stain (Invitrogen, Thermo Fisher Scientific) for 15 min. Afterward, 400 μL 1x annexin V binding puffer were added to each tube. Gating was realized by the use of unstained, single annexin V-FITC or single Sytox Deep Red Nucleic Acid-stained cells, respectively. For quantification of necrotic and apoptotic cells, 10,000 cells were analyzed by LSRFortessa™ flow cytometer (BD Biosciences, Heidelberg, Germany).

4.27. Proliferation

MDA-MB-231 and HS578T cells were seeded in 6-well plates and treated with different concentrations (10 nM, 100 nM, 250 nM, 500 nM, 1 μM, and 2 μM) of compound 28 after 24 h. The number of dead and viable cells was measured by use of a CASY cell counter (OMNI Life Science, Bremen, Germany) after 72 h.

4.28. Staining

Analysis of subcellular localization of compound AS101 was performed in MDA-MB-231 cells using the mitochondrial targeting compound BioTracker™ 488 Green Mitochondria Dye (Sigma-Aldrich Chemie GmbH, Taufkirchen, Germany) for comparison. Cells were seeded in a μ-Plate 96 Well Black plate (ibiTreat: #1.5 polymer coverslip bottom, ibidi GmbH, Gräfelfing, Germany) at a cell density of 50,000 per well. After 24 h, cells were treated with 100 nM AS101 for 6h or 100 nM BioTracker488 for 30 min, followed by rinsing and supplementation with RPMI 1640 w/o Phenol-red (Pan-Biotech GmbH, Aidenbach, Germany). Live-cell imaging was performed on an Axio Observer 7 (Carl Zeiss Microscopy Deutschland GmbH, Oberkochen, Germany) using the settings for Ex/Em as follows: BioTracker (475 nm/514 nm), AS101 (555 nm/592); Scale bar: 50 μm.

Author Contributions: Conceptualization, R.C.; methodology, T.M., M.B. and A.G.; software, N.H.; validation, N.H., T.M., M.B., A.G. and R.C.; formal analysis, N.H.; investigation, N.H., S.B., T.M., M.B. and A.G.; resources, R.C., M.B. and T.M.; data curation, R.C.; writing—original draft preparation, R.C., N.H., M.B., T.M. and A.G.; writing—review and editing, R.C., N.H. and M.B.; visualization, R.C.; supervision, R.C.; project administration, R.C.; funding acquisition, R.C., T.M. and M.B. All authors have read and agreed to the published version of the manuscript.

Funding: This research received no external funding.

Institutional Review Board Statement: Not applicable.

Informed Consent Statement: Not applicable.

Data Availability Statement: The data presented in this study are available on request from the corresponding author.

Acknowledgments: We would like to thank D. Ströhl, Y. Schiller, and S. Ludwig for the NMR spectra and T. Schmidt for the MS measurements. IR, UV/Vis spectra, and optical rotations were recorded by M. Schneider and S. Ludwig; microanalyses were performed by M. Schneider. We would also like to thank J. Block and G. Thomas for their excellent technical assistance. We thank J. Dittmer from the Department of Gynecology (Martin Luther University Halle-Wittenberg) for providing breast cancer cell lines. Additionally, we would like to thank A. Navarette Santos of the Center for Basic Medical Research, who aided in flow cytometry.

Conflicts of Interest: The authors declare no conflict of interest.

References

1. Bai, X.; Ni, J.; Beretov, J.; Graham, P.; Li, Y. Triple-negative breast cancer therapeutic resistance: Where is the Achilles heel. *Cancer Lett.* **2021**, *497*, 100–111. [CrossRef] [PubMed]
2. Borri, F.; Granaglia, A. Pathology of triple negative breast cancer. *Semin. Cancer Biol.* **2021**, *72*, 136–145. [CrossRef]
3. Damaskos, C.; Garmpi, A.; Nikolettos, K.; Vavourakis, M.; Diaman, E.; Patsouras, R.; Farmaki, P.; Nonni, A.; Dimitroulisi, D.; Mantas, D.; et al. Triple-negative breast cancer: The progress of targeted therapies and future tendencies. *Anticancer Res.* **2019**, *39*, 5285–5296. [CrossRef]
4. Garrido-Castro, A.C.; Lin, N.U.; Polyak, K. Insights into molecular classifications of triple-negative breast cancer: Improving patient selection for treatment. *Cancer Discov.* **2019**, *9*, 176–198. [CrossRef]
5. Keenan, T.E.; Tolaney, S.M. Role of immunotherapy in triple-negative breast cancer. *J. Natl. Compr. Cancer Netw.* **2020**, *18*, 479–489. [CrossRef] [PubMed]
6. Liao, M.; Zhang, J.; Wang, G.; Wang, L.; Liu, J.; Ouyang, L.; Liu, B. Small-Molecule Drug Discovery in Triple Negative Breast Cancer: Current Situation and Future Directions. *J. Med. Chem.* **2021**, *64*, 2382–2418. [CrossRef]
7. Waks, A.G.; Winer, E.P. Breast cancer treatment: A review. *JAMA J. Am. Med. Assoc.* **2019**, *321*, 288–300. [CrossRef]
8. Zubair, M.; Wang, S.; Ali, N. Advanced approaches to breast cancer classification and diagnosis. *Front. Pharmacol.* **2020**, *11*, 632079. [CrossRef] [PubMed]
9. Sung, H.; Ferlay, J.; Siegel, R.L.; Laversanne, M.; Soerjomataram, I.; Jemal, A.; Bray, F. Global Cancer Statistics 2020: Globocan Estimates of Incidence and Mortality Worldwide for 36 Cancers in 185 Countries. *CA Cancer J. Clin.* **2021**, *71*, 209–249. [CrossRef]
10. Bache, M.; Muench, C.; Guettler, A.; Wichmann, H.; Theuerkorn, K.; Emmerich, D.; Paschke, R.; Vordermark, D. Betulinyl sulfamates as anticancer agents and radiosensitizers in human breast cancer cells. *Int. J. Mol. Sci.* **2015**, *16*, 26249–26262. [CrossRef]
11. Guettler, A.; Eiselt, Y.; Funtan, A.; Thiel, A.; Petrenko, M.; Kessler, J.; Thondorf, I.; Paschke, R.; Vordermark, D.; Bache, M. Betulin Sulfonamides as Carbonic Anhydrase Inhibitors and Anticancer Agents in Breast Cancer Cells. *Int. J. Mol. Sci.* **2021**, *22*, 8808. [CrossRef] [PubMed]
12. Petrenko, M.; Guettler, A.; Pflueger, E.; Serbian, I.; Kahnt, M.; Eiselt, Y.; Kessler, J.; Funtan, A.; Paschke, R.; Csuk, R.; et al. MSBA-S—A pentacyclic sulfamate as a new option for radiotherapy of human breast cancer cells. *Eur. J. Med. Chem.* **2021**, *224*, 113721. [CrossRef]
13. Sommerwerk, S.; Heller, L.; Kerzig, C.; Kramell, A.E.; Csuk, R. Rhodamine B conjugates of triterpenoic acids are cytotoxic mitocans even at nanomolar concentrations. *Eur. J. Med. Chem.* **2017**, *127*, 1–9. [CrossRef]
14. Heise, N.; Hoenke, S.; Simon, V.; Deigner, H.-P.; Al-Harrasi, A.; Csuk, R. Type and position of linkage govern the cytotoxicity of oleanolic acid rhodamine B hybrids. *Steroids* **2021**, *172*, 108876. [CrossRef]
15. Heise, N.V.; Hoenke, S.; Serbian, I.; Csuk, R. An improved partial synthesis of corosolic acid and its conversion to highly cytotoxic mitocans. *Eur. J. Med. Chem. Rep.* **2022**, *6*, 100073. [CrossRef]
16. Heise, N.V.; Major, D.; Hoenke, S.; Kozubek, M.; Serbian, I.; Csuk, R. Rhodamine 101 Conjugates of Triterpenoic Amides Are of Comparable Cytotoxicity as Their Rhodamine B Analogs. *Molecules* **2022**, *27*, 2220. [CrossRef] [PubMed]
17. Hoenke, S.; Serbian, I.; Deigner, H.-P.; Csuk, R. Mitocanic Di- and triterpenoid rhodamine B conjugates. *Molecules* **2020**, *25*, 5443. [CrossRef]
18. Kahnt, M.; Wiemann, J.; Fischer, L.; Sommerwerk, S.; Csuk, R. Transformation of asiatic acid into a mitocanic, bimodal-acting rhodamine B conjugate of nanomolar cytotoxicity. *Eur. J. Med. Chem.* **2018**, *159*, 143–148. [CrossRef]
19. Kozubek, M.; Denner, T.C.; Eckert, M.; Hoenke, S.; Csuk, R. On the influence of the rhodamine substituents onto the cytotoxicity of mitocanic maslinic acid rhodamine conjugates. *Result. Chem.* **2023**, *5*, 100708. [CrossRef]
20. Kozubek, M.; Hoenke, S.; Deigner, H.-P.; Csuk, R. Betulinic acid and glycyrrhetinic acid derived piperazinyl spacered rhodamine B conjugates are highly cytotoxic and necrotic. *Results Chem.* **2022**, *4*, 100429. [CrossRef]
21. Kraft, O.; Hartmann, A.-K.; Brandt, S.; Hoenke, S.; Heise, N.V.; Csuk, R.; Mueller, T. Asiatic acid as a leading structure for derivatives combining sub-nanomolar cytotoxicity, high selectivity, and the ability to overcome drug resistance in human preclinical tumor models. *Eur. J. Med. Chem.* **2023**, *250*, 115189. [CrossRef]
22. Kraft, O.; Hartmann, A.-K.; Hoenke, S.; Serbian, I.; Csuk, R. Madecassic Acid-A New Scaffold for Highly Cytotoxic Agents. *Int. J. Mol. Sci.* **2022**, *23*, 4362. [CrossRef]
23. Kraft, O.; Hoenke, S.; Csuk, R. A tormentic acid-homopiperazine-rhodamine B conjugate of single-digit nanomolar cytotoxicity and high selectivity for several human tumor cell lines. *Eur. J. Med. Chem. Rep.* **2022**, *5*, 100043. [CrossRef]
24. Serbian, I.; Hoenke, S.; Csuk, R. Synthesis of some steroidal mitocans of nanomolar cytotoxicity acting by apoptosis. *Eur. J. Med. Chem.* **2020**, *199*, 112425. [CrossRef] [PubMed]
25. Serbian, I.; Hoenke, S.; Kraft, O.; Csuk, R. Ester and amide derivatives of rhodamine B exert cytotoxic effects on different human tumor cell lines. *Med. Chem. Res.* **2020**, *29*, 1655–1661. [CrossRef]
26. Wolfram, R.K.; Fischer, L.; Kluge, R.; Stroehl, D.; Al-Harrasi, A.; Csuk, R. Homopiperazine-rhodamine B adducts of triterpenoic acids are strong mitocans. *Eur. J. Med. Chem.* **2018**, *155*, 869–879. [CrossRef]
27. Wolfram, R.K.; Heller, L.; Csuk, R. Targeting mitochondria: Esters of rhodamine B with triterpenoids are mitocanic triggers of apoptosis. *Eur. J. Med. Chem.* **2018**, *152*, 21–30. [CrossRef]

28. Shi, J.; Wang, H.; Wang, Y.; Peng, Y.; Huang, X.; Zhang, Y.; Geng, H.; Wang, Y.; Li, X.; Liu, C.; et al. Mitochondrion-targeting and in situ photocontrolled protein delivery via photocages. *J. Photochem. Photobiol. B* **2023**, *238*, 112624. [CrossRef] [PubMed]
29. Shi, J.; Zhao, D.; Li, X.; Deng, F.; Tang, X.; Liu, N.; Huang, H.; Liu, C. The conjugation of rhodamine B enables carrier-free mitochondrial delivery of functional proteins. *Org. Biomol. Chem.* **2020**, *18*, 6829–6839. [CrossRef]
30. Singh, H.; Sareen, D.; George, J.M.; Bhardwaj, V.; Rha, S.; Lee, S.J.; Sharma, S.; Sharma, A.; Kim, J.S. Mitochondria targeted fluorogenic theranostic agents for cancer therapy. *Coordin. Chem. Rev.* **2022**, *452*, 214283. [CrossRef]
31. Veer, W.L.C. Derivatives of N-bis-phenyl amino propane. *Chem. Zent.* **1939**, *110*, 57–989.
32. Audouze, K.; Oestergaard Nielsen, E.; Olsen, G.M.; Ahring, P.; Jorgensen, T.D.; Peters, D.; Liljefors, T.; Balle, T. New Ligands with Affinity for the α4β2 Subtype of Nicotinic Acetylcholine Receptors. Synthesis, Receptor Binding, and 3D-QSAR Modeling. *J. Med. Chem.* **2006**, *49*, 3159–3171. [CrossRef] [PubMed]
33. Boerjesson, L.; Welch, C.J. An alternative synthesis of cyclic aza compounds. *Acta Chem. Scand.* **1991**, *45*, 621. [CrossRef]
34. Hancock, R.D.; Ngwenya, M.P.; Evers, A.; Wade, P.W.; Boeyens, J.C.A.; Dobson, S.M. Open-chain polyamine ligands with more rigid double connecting bridges. Study of their metal ion selectivities by molecular mechanics calculation, crystallography, and thermodynamics. *Inorg. Chem.* **1990**, *29*, 264. [CrossRef]
35. Majchrzak, M.; Kotelko, A.; Guryn, R. Octahydro-1,5- and octahydro-1,4-diazocine derivatives with expected pharmacological activity. I. Synthesis of N-alkyl derivatives of octahydro-1,5- and octahydro-1,4-diazocine. *Acta Pol. Pharm.* **1975**, *32*, 145.
36. Margaretha, P. Synthesis of alkyl- and cycloalkylamines by reduction of nitrogen-based functional groups. *Sci. Synth.* **2009**, *41*, 19–156.
37. Matveev, S.V.; Matveeva, A.G.; Matrosov, E.I.; Shcherbakov, B.K.; Polikarpov, Y.M.; Kabachnik, M.I. Synthesis and acid-base properties of phosphorylated diazacycloalkanes and their cyclic analogs. *Izv. Akad. Nauk. Ser. Khim.* **1994**, *43*, 1895–1901. [CrossRef]
38. Mikolajewska, H.; Kotelko, A. Hydrogenation of amino nitriles. X. Catalytic hydrogenation of N,N-bis(2-cyanoethyl)amine and its N-alkyl derivatives. *Acta Pol. Pharm.* **1966**, *23*, 425.
39. Mills, D.K.; Font, I.; Farmer, P.J.; Hsiao, Y.-M.; Tuntulani, T.; Buonomo, R.M.; Goodman, D.C.; Musie, G.; Grapperhaus, C.A.; Maguire, M.J.; et al. 1,5-Diazacyclooctane, pendant arm thiolato derivatives and [N,N'-bis(2-mercaptoethyl)-1,5-diazacyclooctanato]nickel(II). *Inorg. Synth.* **1998**, *32*, 89–98.
40. Nagashima, S.; Sasaki, T.; Kamiguchi, S.; Chihara, T. Synthesis of common-sized heterocyclic compounds by intramolecular cyclization over halide cluster catalysts. *Chem. Lett.* **2015**, *44*, 764–766. [CrossRef]
41. Paudler, W.W.; Zeiler, A.G. 3,7-Disubstituted octahydro-1,5-diazocines. Their conversion into tetrahydro-1,5-diazocines and to ring-contracted products. *J. Org. Chem.* **1967**, *32*, 2425. [CrossRef] [PubMed]
42. Stetter, H.; Spangenberger, H. Preparation of cyclic diamines of medium ring size by ring cleavage of bicyclic compounds. *Chem. Ber.* **1958**, *91*, 1982. [CrossRef]
43. Tsutsui, A.; Pradipta, A.R.; Saigitbatalova, E.; Kurbangalieva, A.; Tanaka, K. Exclusive formation of imino[4 + 4]cycloaddition products with biologically relevant amines: Plausible candidates for acrolein biomarkers and biofunctional modulators. *MedChemComm* **2015**, *6*, 431–436. [CrossRef]
44. Baer, T.; Martin, T.; Stadlwieser, J.; Wollin, S.-L.; Zech, K.; Sommerhoff, C.P.; Ulrich, W.-R. Preparation of N,N'-Bis(N-alkanoyl-2-alkoxycarbonyl-4-pyrrolidinyl)-2,6-dioxoperhydro-1,5-diazocine-1,5-diacetamides and Analogs as Tryptase Inhibitors. WO/2002/060895, 8 August 2002. Available online: https://patentscope.wipo.int/search/en/detail.jsf?docId=WO2002060895 (accessed on 2 May 2023).
45. Gawley, R.E. The Beckmann reactions: Rearrangements, elimination-additions, fragmentations, and rearrangement-cyclizations. *Org. React.* **1988**, *35*, 14–24.
46. Ha, K.; Monbaliu, J.-C.M.; Williams, B.C.; Pillai, G.G.; Ocampo, C.E.; Zeller, M.; Stevens, C.V.; Katritzky, A.R. A convenient synthesis of difficult medium-sized cyclic peptides by Staudinger mediated ring-closure. *Org. Biomol. Chem.* **2012**, *10*, 8055–8058. [CrossRef]
47. Rothe, M.; Timler, R. Beckmann and Schmidt rearrangement of alicyclic diketones. Synthesis of cyclodiamides of the medium ring range region. *Chem. Ber.* **1962**, *95*, 783. [CrossRef]
48. Watanab, H.; Kuwat, S.; Koyam, S. Synthesis of cyclic peptide. I. Preparation of cyclodi-β-alanyl from 1,4-cyclohexanedione. *Bull. Chem. Soc. Jpn.* **1963**, *36*, 143. [CrossRef]
49. Norrehed, S.; Karlsson, C.; Light, M.E.; Thapper, A.; Huang, P.; Gogoll, A. Formation of persistent organic diradicals from N,N'-diphenyl-3,7-diazacyclooctanes. *Monatsh. Chem.* **2019**, *150*, 77–84. [CrossRef]
50. Zhou, Z.; Liu, Y.; Jiang, X.; Zheng, C.; Luo, W.; Xiang, X.; Qi, X.; Shen, J. Metformin modified chitosan as a multi-functional adjuvant to enhance cisplatin-based tumor chemotherapy efficacy. *Intern. J. Biol. Macromol.* **2023**, *224*, 797–809. [CrossRef]

51. Dittmer, D.C.; Hertler, W.R.; Winicov, H. Mechanism of trimethylene oxide formation from 3-chloropropyl acetate. *J. Am. Chem. Soc.* **1957**, *79*, 4431. [CrossRef]
52. Halfen, J.A.; Moore, H.L.; Fox, D.C. Synthetic Models of the Reduced Active Site of Superoxide Reductase. *Inorg. Chem.* **2002**, *41*, 3935–3943. [CrossRef] [PubMed]

molecules

MDPI

Article

Phytochemical Analysis and Anticancer Properties of *Drimia maritima* Bulb Extracts on Colorectal Cancer Cells

Khairallah Al-Abdallat [1,2,†], Maher Obeidat [3,†], Nidaa A. Ababneh [3], Suzan Zalloum [4], Sabal Al Hadidi [4], Yahya Al-Abdallat [5], Malek Zihlif [6] and Abdalla Awidi [3,7,*]

1 Bone Marrow Transplantation Unit, Jordan University Hospital, Amman 11942, Jordan
2 Hemostasis and Thrombosis Laboratory, School of Medicine, The University of Jordan, Amman 11942, Jordan
3 Cell Therapy Center, The University of Jordan, Amman 11942, Jordan
4 Department of Medical Laboratory Analysis, Faculty of Science, Al-Balqa Applied University, Al-Salt 19117, Jordan
5 Forensic Laboratory, Department of Public Security, Amman 11942, Jordan
6 Department of Pharmacology, School of Medicine, The University of Jordan, Amman 11942, Jordan
7 Department of Hematology and Oncology, Jordan University Hospital, Amman 11942, Jordan
* Correspondence: aabbadi@ju.edu.jo
† These authors contributed equally to this work.

Abstract: Cancer is a worldwide health problem and is the second leading cause of death after heart disease. Due to the high cost and severe side effects associated with chemotherapy treatments, natural products with anticancer therapeutic potential may play a promising role in anticancer therapy. The purpose of this study was to investigate the cytotoxic and apoptotic characteristics of the aqueous *Drimia maritima* bulb extract on Caco-2 and COLO-205 colorectal cancer cells. In order to reach such a purpose, the chemical composition was examined using the GC-MS method, and the selective antiproliferative effect was determined in colon cancer cell lines in normal gingival fibroblasts. The intracellular ROS, mitochondrial membrane potential, and gene expression changes in selected genes (*CASP8*, *TNF-α*, and *IL-6* genes) were assessed to determine the molecular mechanism of the antitumor effect of the extract. GC-MS results revealed the presence of fifty-seven compounds, and Proscillaridin A was the predominant secondary metabolite in the extract. The IC_{50} of *D. maritima* bulb extract on Caco-2, COLO-205, and the normal human gingival fibroblasts were obtained at 0.9 μg/mL, 2.3 μg/mL, and 13.1 μg/mL, respectively. The apoptotic effect assay indicated that the bulb extract induced apoptosis in both colon cancer cell lines. *D. maritima* bulb extract was only able to induce statistically significant ROS levels in COLO-205 cells in a dose-dependent manner. The mitochondrial membrane potential (MMP) revealed a significant decrease in the MMP of Caco-2 and COLO-205 to various concentrations of the bulb extract. At the molecular level, RT-qPCR was used to assess gene expression of *CASP8*, *TNF-α*, and *IL-6* genes in Caco-2 and COLO-205 cancer cells. The results showed that the expression of pro-inflammatory genes *TNF-α* and *IL-6* were upregulated. The apoptotic initiator gene *CASP8* was also upregulated in the Caco-2 cell line and did not reach significance in COLO-205 cells. These results lead to the conclusion that *D. maritima* extract induced cell death in both cell lines and may have the potential to be used in CRC therapy in the future.

Keywords: colorectal; *Drimia maritima*; anticancer

Citation: Al-Abdallat, K.; Obeidat, M.; Ababneh, N.A.; Zalloum, S.; Al Hadidi, S.; Al-Abdallat, Y.; Zihlif, M.; Awidi, A. Phytochemical Analysis and Anticancer Properties of *Drimia maritima* Bulb Extracts on Colorectal Cancer Cells. *Molecules* **2023**, *28*, 1215. https://doi.org/10.3390/molecules28031215

Academic Editors: Barbara De Filippis, Alessandra Ammazzalorso and Marialuigia Fantacuzzi

Received: 25 October 2022
Revised: 2 January 2023
Accepted: 4 January 2023
Published: 26 January 2023

1. Introduction

Cancer can be defined as a non-communicable disease with progressive uncontrolled cell growth/division with a probability to invade nearby and/or distant tissues and could appear in any part of the body [1–4]. Colorectal cancer, "CRC", is the second most common cancer in both genders [5]. Natural products with anticancer therapeutic potential have earned an increasing interest in recent years. Pharmacological research of plant extracts as a source of secondary metabolites is probably the most important step in the identification of plant-derived compounds with therapeutic promise [6]. Plant extracts are a major source of phenolic compounds and other secondary metabolites, which have shown potential anticancer activities by regulating cell death pathways [7]. Furthermore, most of the anticancer drugs in the market are plant-derived such as taxanes (e.g., paclitaxel (Taxol) and docetaxel (Taxotere)) or synthetic compounds. Therefore, a need for basic and applied research to find novel cancer prevention and treatment options from plants as a source for safe and effective anticancer treatment [8].

To our knowledge, the cytotoxicity of the bulb extract of the medicinal plant *D. maritima* toward CRC cell lines was not previously investigated. Therefore, this research was initiated to study the therapeutic potential of *D. maritima* on CRC via assessment of the cytotoxic activity of *D. maritima* bulb extract on the colorectal Caco-2 and COLO-205 cancer cell lines. In this study, we prepared an aqueous extraction of the medicinal plant *D. maritima* bulb to assess the in vitro antiproliferative effects of *D. maritima* bulb extract against colorectal cancer cells. We also aimed to determine the mechanism of action of active *D. maritima* bulb extract against colorectal cancer cells. Finally, we aimed to examine the gene expression of some cell growth-related genes in bulb extract-treated colorectal cancer cells using quantitative RT-PCR.

2. Results

2.1. *Identification of Chemical Constituents of D. maritima Bulb Extract by GC-MS*

Analysis of the bioactive constituents of the bulb extract of *D. maritima* by GC-MS demonstrated the presence of 57 compounds and their chromatogram, as shown in Figure 1 and Table 1. Major peaks determined in the GC-MS chromatogram and their corresponding components were recognized according to NIST 20 and Willy 19 Libraries. The bulb extract was found to include a variety of essential phytochemicals. The results of GC-MS analysis showed that *D. maritima* bulb extract was rich in the phytosterol "Campesterol" containing ~14%, 2,3-Butanediol (glycol and secondary alcohol) and 5-Hydroxymethylfurfural (furans, an arenecarbaldehyde, and primary alcohol) (~10% each), and ~8% for each of the fatty acid derivatives "Hexadecanoic acid ethyl ester" and "9-Octadecenamide (Z)-". Interestingly, the cardiac glycoside "Proscillaridin" proved to be one of the predominant secondary metabolites in the bulb extract of *D. maritima* with about 5% content which may play an effective role as a pharmaceutical anticancer agent (Table 1).

2.2. *Drimia maritima Bulb Extract and ProA Can Selectively Inhibit the Proliferation of COLO-205 and Caco-2 Cancer Cells*

The MTT assay was performed to evaluate the cell viability and proliferation of COLO-205 and Caco-2 cells upon treatment with different concentrations of *D. maritima* bulb extract, ProA, and Doxorubicin (positive control). The treatment of COLO-205 and Caco-2 with different concentrations of *D. maritima* bulb extract showed cytotoxic effects proportional to the concentration of *D. maritima* bulb extract used. The IC_{50} of *D. maritima* bulb extract on COLO-205 cell lines was ~2.3 μg/mL and for Caco-2 cells was ~0.9 μg/mL (Figure 2). In order to determine whether *D. maritima* bulb extract has cytotoxicity effects on normal human cells, normal HGF cells were treated with the plant extract using the same concentrations used in colon cancer cell lines and incubated for 48 h. The results showed that *D. maritima* bulb extract has minimal cytotoxic effects on normal human cells at low concentrations, and the IC_{50} was achieved at a relatively high concentration of 13.1 μg/mL (Figure 2), indicating that *D. maritima* bulb extract potentially has selective cytotoxic effects on cancer cells but not on normal cells. From the reported IC50s, an estimation for the selectivity index can be found to be approximately 5.7 for the COLO-205 cells and 14.55 for Caco-2 cells.

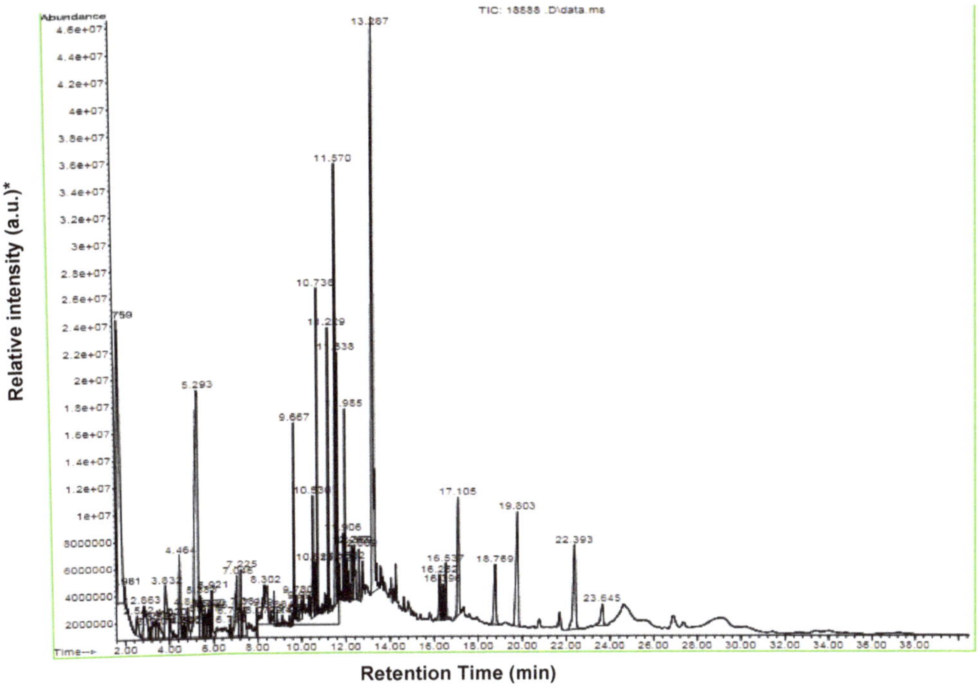

Figure 1. Gas chromatography and mass spectrometry chromatogram showing the major components of the aqueous bulb extract of *Drimia maritima*. * a.u.: arbitrary unit.

Table 1. Gas chromatography and mass spectrometry data of chemical components of *Drimia maritima* bulb extract.

No.	Component	Cas #	Content (%)
1	2,3-Butanediol	513-85-9	10.454
2	Furancarboxaldehyde	98-01-1	0.28
3	Isobutanoic acid	79-31-2	0.544
4	2-Furancarboxaldehyde, 5-methyl	620-02-0	1.389
5	Erythritol	149-32-6	0.267
6	Oxetane, 3,3-dimethyl	6921-35-3	0.626
7	Limonene	138-86-3	0.449
8	Methyl-3-furanthiol	28588-74-1	0.523
9	2H-Pyrazole-3-carbohydrazide	9-64-26275	1.82
10	Butanedioic acid, monomethyl ester	3878-55-5	0.379
11	4H-Pyran-4-one, 2,3-dihydro-3,5-dihydroxy-6-methyl	28564-83-2	1.333
12	(E,5S)-3,5-dimethylhept-3-en-1-yne	997029-22-6	0.219
13	2-Furancarboxaldehyde, 5-(chloromethyl)(	1623-88-7	0.142
14	4H-Pyran-4-one, 3,5-dihydroxy-2-methyl	1073-96-7	0.666
15	5-Hydroxymethylfurfural	67-47-0	9.857

Table 1. *Cont.*

No.	Component	Cas #	Content (%)
16	α-D-Glucopyranoside, O-α-D-glucopyranosyl-(1.fwdarw.3)-β-D-fructofuranosyl	597-12-6	0.843
17	α-D-Glucopyranoside, O-α-D-glucopyranosyl-(1.fwdarw.3)-β-D-fructofuranosyl	597-12-6	0.482
18	3-Methoxybenzyl alcohol	6971-51-3	0.538
19	5-Acetoxymethyl-2-furaldehyde	10551-58-3	0.449
20	5-Hydroxymethylfurfural	67-47-0	0.335
21	Glutaric acid, 2-naphthyl tridecyl ester	998725-55-8	0.56
22	8-Oxabicyclo[5.1.0]oct-5-en-2-ol, 1,4,4-trimethyl	58795-43-0	0.14
23	Cycloheptasiloxane, tetradecamethyl	107-50-6	0.16
24	Ethyl hydrogen succinate	1070-34-4	1.679
25	Phenol, 2,4-bis(1,1-dimethylethyl)	96-76-4	1.029
26	β-D-Glucopyranose, 1,6-anhydro	498-07-7	1.072
27	α-D-Glucopyranoside, O-α-D-glucopyranosyl-(1.fwdarw.3)-β-D-fructofuranosyl	597-12-6	0.217
28	6Methoxy-2-amido-5,6-dihydrothiazolo[2,3-c]-1,2,4-triazole	997204-67-5	3.361
29	Myristic acid	544-63-8	0.155
30	Ethyl hydrogen succinate	1070-34-4	0.339
31	Hexadecanoic acid, 1-(hydroxymethyl)-1,2-ethanediyl ester	761-35-3	0.067
32	Palmitoleic acid	373-49-9	0.063
33	n-Hexadecanoic acid	57-10-3	0.105
34	Hexadecanoic acid, ethyl ester	628-97-7	8.057
35	Heptadecanoic acid	506-12-7	0.159
36	Octadecanoic acid	57-11-4	0.417
37	Octadecenoic acid (Z) 9	112-80-1	1.578
38	Octadecanoic acid	57-11-4	0.73
39	Hexadecanamide	629-54-9	2.309
40	Stearic acid, 2-hydroxy-1-methylpropyl ester	14251-39-9	1.497
41	9-Octadecenamide, (Z)	301-02-0	8.142
42	Octadecanamide	124-26-5	1.513
43	(Z)-(S)-Octadec-9-en-11-olide	997490-85-5	3.409
44	n-Propyl 9-octadecenoate	997641-34-3	0.439
45	Stearic acid, 2-hydroxy-1-methylpropyl ester	14251-39-9	1.569
46	Bis(2-ethylhexyl) phthalate	117-81-7	0.499
47	Elaidamide	301-02-0	0.475
48	Ethyl iso-allocholate	112-84-5	1.244
49	13-Docosenamide, (Z)	112-84-5	0.545
50	Campesterol	474-62-4	13.874
51	6,12-dimethoxy-8-methyl-5,8,9,13-tetrahydro-7H-cyclohept[b]anthracene-5,13-dione	997713-65-8	0.723

Table 1. *Cont.*

No.	Component	Cas #	Content (%)
52	Stigmasterol	83-48-7	0.491
53	β-Sitosterol	83-46-5	0.735
54	Bufa-20,22-dienolide, 14-hydroxy-3-oxo-, (5β)	4029-65-6	2.642
55	Proscillaridin	466-06-8	4.956
56	4-(2,4-Dimethyl-phenyl)-1,7-dimethyl-4-azatricyclo[5.2.1.0(2,6)]decane-3,5,8-trione	997597-94-2	2.78
57	Bufa-20,22-dienolide, 3-(acetyloxy)-14,15-epoxy-5-hydroxy-, (3β,5β,15β)	4029-68-9	0.766

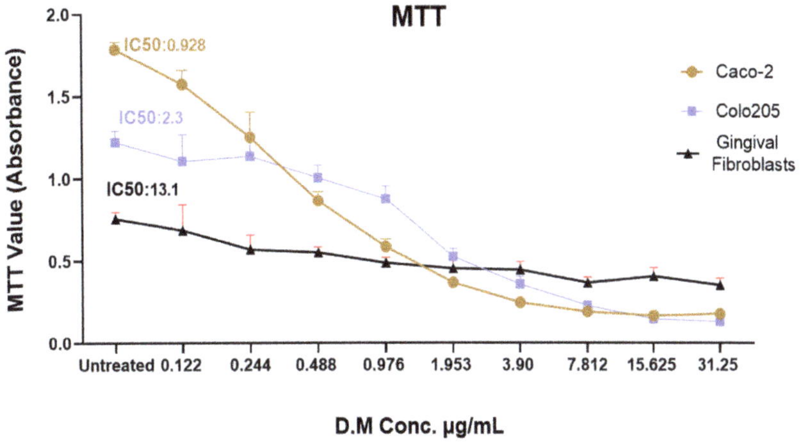

(**A**)

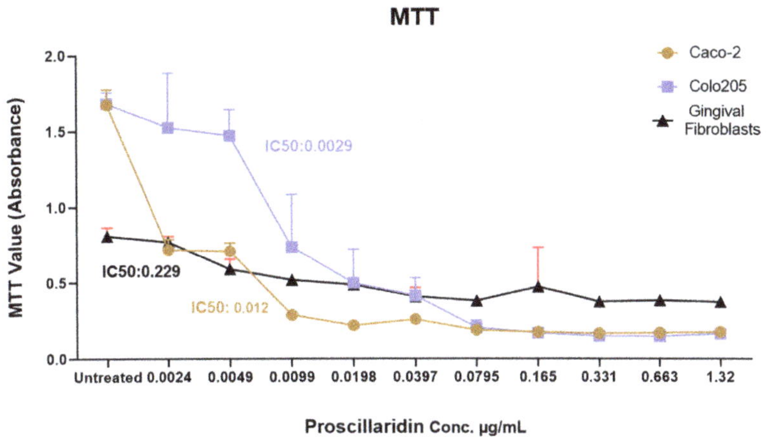

(**B**)

Figure 2. *Cont.*

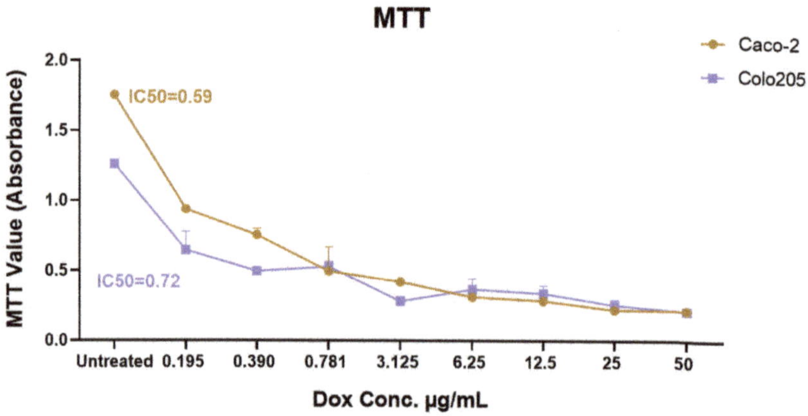

(C)

Figure 2. Cell viability MTT assay of Caco-2 and COLO-205 colon cancer cells and hGFs after treatment with the following: (**A**) increasing concentration of aqueous *Drimia maritima* bulb extract (0.122–31.25 µg/mL); (**B**) Proscillaridin (0.0024–1.32 µg/mL); (**C**) Doxorubicin (from 50 to 0.195 µg/mL). The IC_{50} values were calculated using log-probit analysis. Each value is presented as the mean ± SD of an average of three independent experiments.

On the other hand, to evaluate the cytotoxic effect of ProA, which is one of the major active compounds of *D. maritima* (Table 1), COLO-205 and Caco-2 cells, as well as the normal HGF cells, were treated with different concentrations of ProA ranging from 0.0024 µg/mL to 1.32 µg/mL. The results, as indicated in Figure 2B, showed a significant increase in Caco-2 and COLO-205 cell death, and the IC_{50} was achieved at 0.0029 µg/mL and 0.012 µg/mL, respectively. Moreover, ProA showed a minimal cytotoxic effect on normal HGF, and the IC_{50} was achieved at 0.229 µg/mL.

Doxorubicin was also used to assess the efficacy and the potential of ProA and bulb extract as natural cancer therapeutics. Importantly, ProA showed a more powerful cytotoxic effect than *D. maritima* bulb extract on both Caco-2 and COLO-205 cell lines when compared to Doxorubicin, which was achieved at IC_{50} at 0.78 µg/mL for COLO-205 and 0.59 µg/mL for Caco-2 (Figure 2C).

2.3. *D. maritima Bulb Extract Can Induce Early and Late Apoptosis in Colon Cancer Cell Lines*

In order to clarify whether *D. maritima* bulb extract can induce cell apoptosis in colon cancer cells, *D. maritima*-treated and -untreated Caco-2 and COLO-205 cells were stained with Annexin V and PI to analyze different apoptotic stages using flow cytometry. When compared to untreated cells (control cells), *D. maritima* bulb extract was able to significantly increase both the early and late cell apoptotic percentages in treated colon cancer cells in a concentration-dependent manner. In the COLO-205 cell culture, there was a statistically significant increase in the percentage of early and late apoptotic cells (Figure 3A). These results clearly emphasize that *D. maritima* bulb extract is able to induce cell early and late apoptosis in Caco-2 and COLO-205 cell lines in a concentration-dependent manner (Figure 3B).

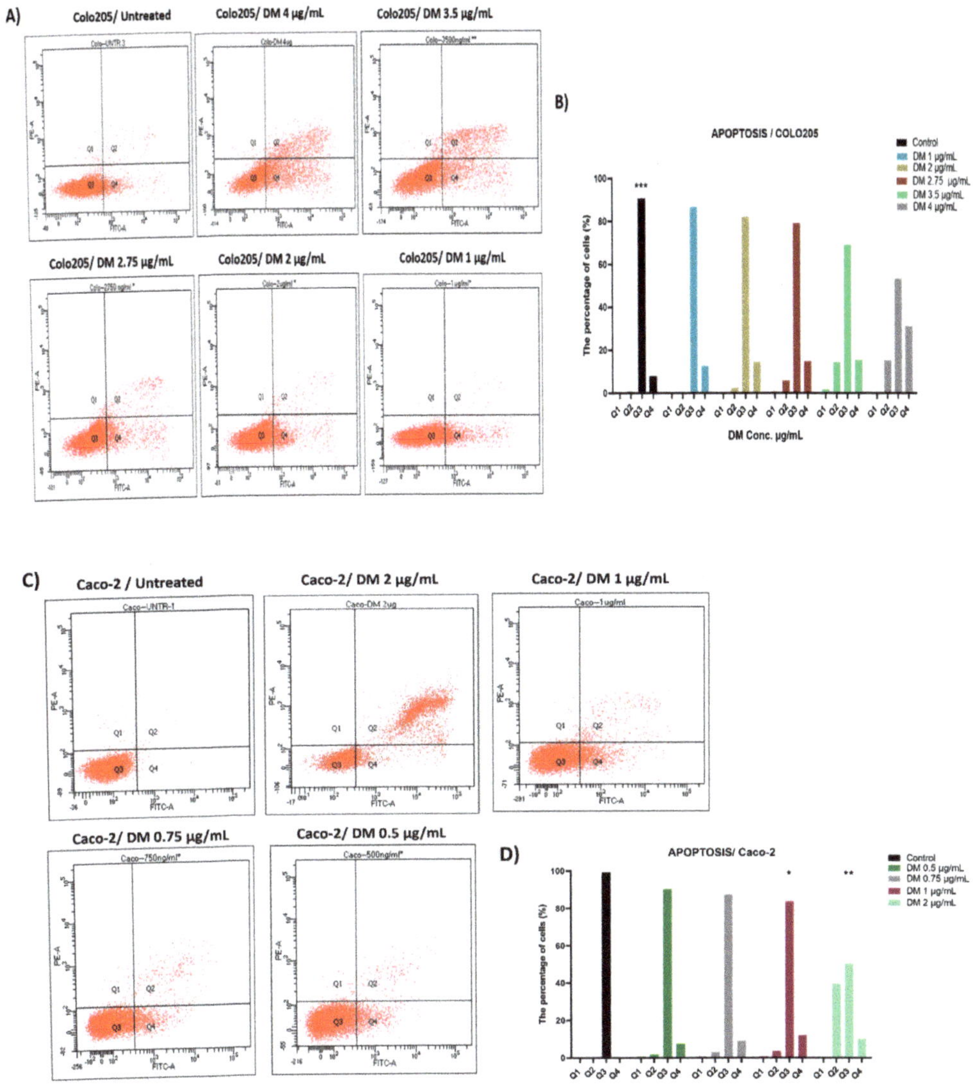

Figure 3. Flow cytometry analysis of D. maritima (DM) bulb extract effect on COLO-205 and Caco-2 cells. (**A**) Representative flow cytometer plots are presented for the untreated group (control) and DM-treated groups (4 µg/Ml, 3.5 µg/mL, 2.75 µg/mL, 2 µg/mL, 1 µg/mL and 0.5 µg/mL) in COLO205 cells. (**B**) The bar graph represents the percentage of early and late apoptotic cells detected by flow cytometer from three separate experiments (mean ± SD, n = 3). (**C**) Representative flow cytometery plots are presented for the control group (Untreated) and DM treated groups (2 µg/mL, 1 µg/mL, 0.75 µg/mL, and 0.5 µg/mL) in Caco-2 cells. (**D**) The bar graph represents the percentage of early and late apoptotic cells detected by flow cytometer from three different individual experiments (mean ± SD, n = 3). ** Significant differences were observed between the DM-treated (2 µg/mL and 1 µg/mL) and untreated control group (*p*-values *** < 0.001, ** < 0.01 and * < 0.05).

2.4. *D. maritima* Bulb Extract Induces the Production of ROS in Colon Cancer Cells

ROS generation was measured after treatment with *D. maritima* bulb extracts in colon cancer cells. *D. maritima* bulb extract was only able to induce statistically significant ROS levels in COLO-205 cells in a dose-dependent manner when treated with concentrations above 2 μg/mL (i.e., 3.5, 2.75, and 2 μg/mL; *p*-value > 0.001) (Figure 4). Although *D. maritima* bulb extract was able to induce ROS in Caco-2 cells at lower plant extract concentrations (0.5 and 1 μg/mL), these results were statistically non-significant (Figure 4). Moreover, *D. maritima* bulb extract was not able to induce a statistically significant level of ROS in Caco-2 cells. Perhaps, this could be referred to the lower concentrations of *D. maritima* bulb extract used to treat Caco-2 cells (1.5, 1, and 0.75 μg/mL) when compared to that used to treat COLO-205.

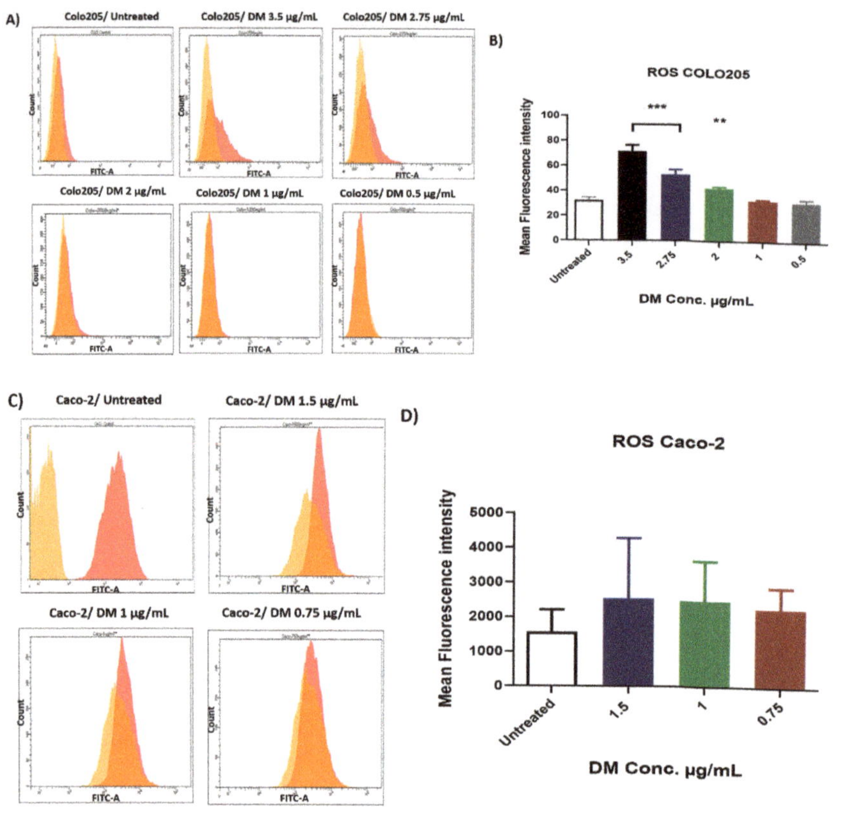

Figure 4. Production of reactive oxygen species (ROS) in COLO-205 and Caco-2 cells incubated for 48 h with *D. maritima* (DM) bulb extract: (**A**,**B**) Histograms and bar graphs of ROS production in COLO-205 cells were obtained by flow cytometer in the FITC channel in different groups. The bar graph shows a remarkable increase in the level of intracellular ROS in the treated group. (**C**,**D**) Representative histograms and bar graphs from Caco-2 cells treated with indicated concentrations of *D. maritima* extract on intracellular ROS levels production in comparison to control (untreated cells) detected by flow cytometer from three separate experiments (mean ± SD, n = 3). *p*-values *** < 0.001, ** < 0.01.

2.5. *D. maritima* Bulb Extract Affects Mitochondrial Membrane Potential (ΔΨm) in Colon Cancer Cells

The effect of *D. maritima* bulb extract on mitochondrial membrane potential (ΔΨm) was assessed in colorectal cancer cells using TMRE cell-permeant red-orange dye to label active mitochondria. FCCP was used as a positive control, which can significantly diminish mitochondrial membrane potential. The results showed that treatment of COLO-205 cells concentrations of *D. maritima* bulb extracts above 2 µg/mL (2.75 and 3.5 µg/mL) resulted in a statistically significant ($p < 0.001$) decrease in ΔΨm of COLO-205 cells (4.569 ± 0.726, and 0.666 ± 0.72, respectively) when compared to control cells (Figure 5). Although the effect of *D. maritima* bulb extracts on ΔΨm in COLO-205 cells at 2 µg/mL concentration was minor, it was statistically significant (15.38 ± 0.72; $p < 0.05$). However, treatment of COLO-205 with 1 µg/mL *D. maritima* bulb extract showed no significant reduction in their ΔΨm.

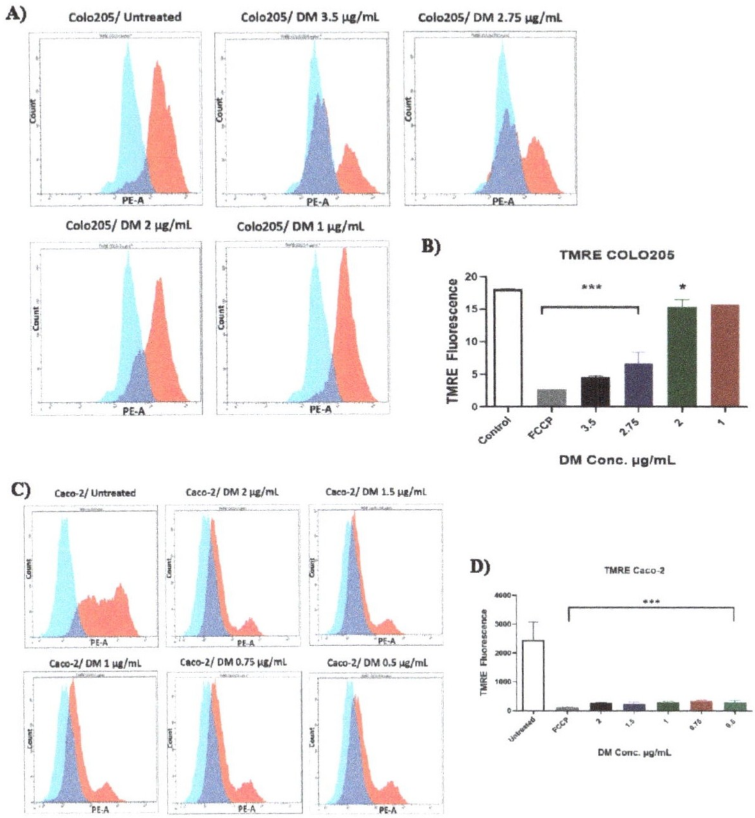

Figure 5. Assessment of the mitochondrial membrane potential (ΔΨm) in COLO-205 and Caco-2 cells after treatment with *D. maritima* (DM) bulb extract for 48 h: (**A**,**B**) Histograms and bar graphs show changes in COLO-205 cells ΔΨm response to various concentrations of DM extract (3.5 µg/mL, 2.75 µg/mL, 2 µg/mL, 1 µg/mL, and 0.5 µg/mL) in comparison to untreated cells. (**C**,**D**) Histogram and bar graphs show loss of ΔΨm following exposure to different concentrations of DM extract (2 µg/mL, 1.5 µg/mL, 1 µg/mL, 0.75 µg/mL, and 0.5 µg/mL) compared to control (untreated cells). All data are expressed as mean ± SD of three separate experiments. All data are expressed as mean ± SD of three separate experiments. (p-values *** < 0.001 ** < 0.01, and * < 0.05).

On the other hand, treatment of Caco-2 cells with different concentrations of *D. maritima* bulb extract of 0.5, 0.75, 1, 1.5, and 2 μg/mL resulted in a statistically significant ($p < 0.001$) reduction in their ΔΨm (260 ± 194.4, 250.3 ± 194.4, 290.3 ± 194.4, 326.0 ± 194.4, and 287.7 ± 194.4, respectively) when compared to the control cells (Figure 5). These results confirmed that *D. maritima* bulb extract could significantly reduce ΔΨm in COLO-205 cells in a dose-dependent manner and also in the Caco-2 cell line.

2.6. The Impact of *D. maritima* Bulb Extract on Gene Expression in Colon Cancer Cell Lines

In order to figure out changes in colon cancer cell lines at the molecular level after the observed growth-inhibitory effect of *D. maritima* bulb extract, RT-qPCR was applied to assess gene expression of multiple genes: *Casp8*, *TNF-α*, and *IL-6* in COLO-205 and Caco-2 cells pre-treated with different concentrations of *D. maritima* bulb extract.

In COLO-205 cells, there was a non-significant upregulation in *Casp8* gene by when the cells were treated with the extract at a concentration of 3.5 μg/mL (Figure 6A). Moreover, treatment with the extract for 48 h at 2.75 and 3.5 μg/mL resulted in statistically significant elevations in the target gene *TNF-α* (5.59-fold and 4.8-fold, respectively). Although there was an elevation in the expression of the *TNF-α* gene when cells were treated with the extract at 2 μg/mL by 1.65-fold, this elevation was statistically non-significant (Figure 6B). Furthermore, there was a non-significant elevation in the expression of the pro-inflammatory cytokine gene *IL-6* when COLO-205 was treated at extract concentrations 2, 2.75, and 3.5 μg/mL (1.2-, 1.6-, and 2.1-fold, respectively) (Figure 6C).

In comparison to the control group (untreated cells), the pro-inflammatory *TNF-α* expression levels in Caco-2 cells were significantly increased by 6.5- and 6.4-fold following treatment with 2 and 1.5 μg/mL of *D. maritima* bulb extracted for 48 h, respectively ($p < 0.0001$), and 5.2-fold when cells were treated with 1 μg/mL ($p < 0.0007$) (Figure 6D). Although the expression levels of *TNF-α* elevated by 3.3- and 3.6-fold when Caco-2 cells were treated with 0.75 and 0.5 μg/mL, respectively, these elevations were not significant. The expression of the *Casp8* gene was significantly upregulated (1.5-fold) following 48 h treatment with 1.5 μg/mL ($p < 0.001$) in Caco-2 cells. Moreover, the expression still elevated significantly by 1.31- and 1.3-fold when decreasing the concentration to 1 and 0.75 μg/mL ($p < 0.041$ and <0.014), respectively (Figure 6E). An elevation also occurred when Caco-2 cells were treated with 0.5 μg/mL, yet, this elevation was statistically non-significant. Furthermore, results showed that *D. maritima* bulb extract could induce the activation of the effector *Casp8* gene in Caco-2 cells (Figure 6E). With respect to the expression of pro-inflammatory cytokine gene *IL-6*, results showed that there was a statistically significant upregulation (6.5-fold increase) when Caco-2 cells were treated with 1.5 μg/mL ($p < 0.0244$) when compared to control cells (Figure 6F). Although there was an increase in the expression of gene *IL-6* (3.4-, 3.2-, and 5.5-fold) upon treatment of Caco-2 cells with 0.5, 0.75, and 1 μg/mL of *D. maritima* bulb extract, respectively, these elevations were statistically non-significant.

In general, the results showed that *D. maritima* bulb extract could affect the expression of cell proliferation-related genes that were examined in this study in both cell lines, i.e., it can upregulate the expression of inflammatory cytokine genes *TNF-α* and *IL-6* and the apoptotic initiator gene *Casp8*.

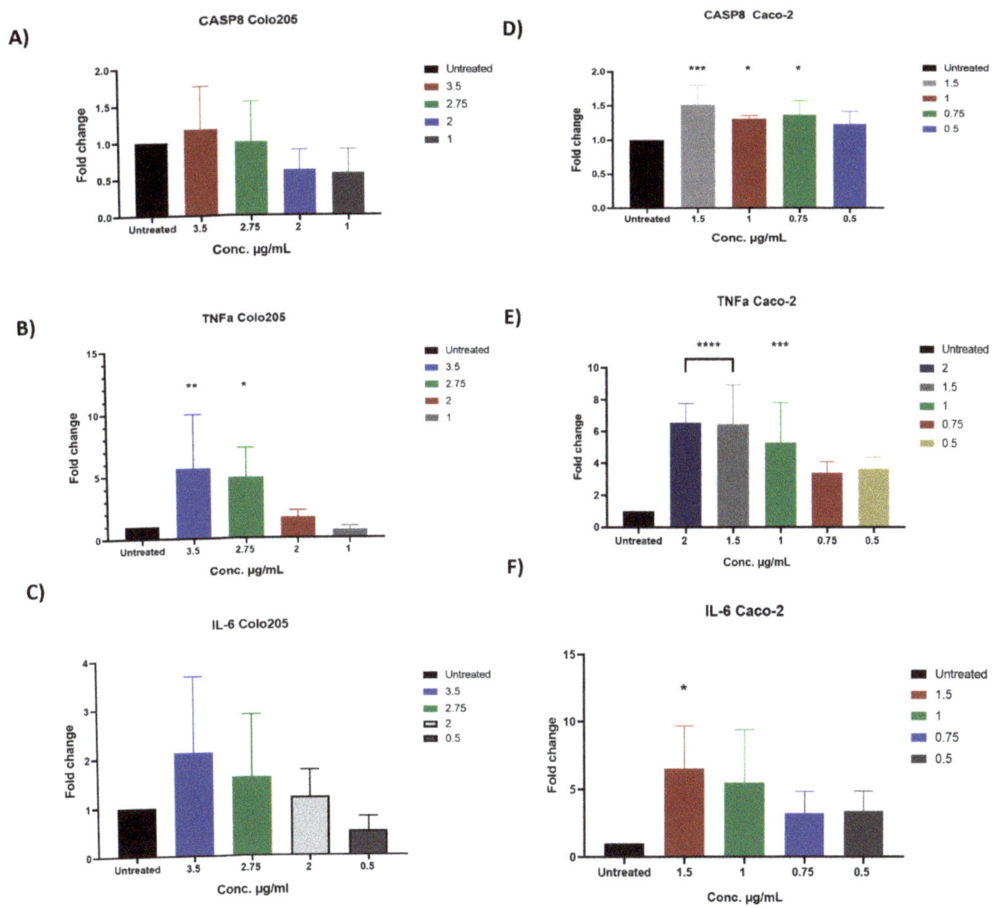

Figure 6. Gene expression analysis of apoptotic initiator gene *CASP8* and two inflammatory cytokine genes *TNF-α* and *IL-6* in COLO-205 and Caco-2 cells after treatment with various concentrations of *D. maritima* (DM) bulb extract for 48 h as examined by quantitative RT–PCR: (**A**,**D**) The graphs reveal fold changes in the expression of *CASP8* in COLO-205 and Caco-2 cells, respectively. (**B**,**E**) *TNF-α* gene in COLO-205 and Caco-2 cells at various extract concentrations (2.0, 1.5, 1.0, 0.75, and 0.5 µg/mL). (**C**,**F**) *IL-6* in COLO-205 and Caco-2 cells treated with different extract concentrations (1.5, 1.0, 0.75, and 0.5 µg/mL). Fold change was calculated using the ΔΔCt method. Untreated cells were used as the control; therefore, the fold change for untreated cells is 1 in all plots. *GAPDH* gene served as an internal reference gene. The error bars indicate the standard deviation from triplicate experiments (* $p < 0.05$; ** $p < 0.01$; *** $p < 0.001$; **** $p < 0.0001$).

3. Discussion

Plants are an interesting and cost-effective natural source of potential therapeutic candidates, and their secondary metabolites, phenols, and extracts have been extensively investigated for a mode of action on cancer cell death and their anticarcinogenic properties [9]. In the current study, the anticancer potential of a novel medicinal plant common in Mediterranean regions, namely *D. maritima* was investigated. *D. maritima* has long been used for the management and treatment of many pathological conditions [10–14]. In cancer settings, several preceding in vitro studies have reported potent anticancerous and selective cytotoxic effects of *D. maritima* on different cancer types, including breast, lung, lymphoma, and prostate cancer [10,11,13,15]. However, [16] the cytotoxic effect of *D. calcarata* bulb extracts against *p53* mutant HT-29 and *p53* wild-type Caco-2 colorectal cancer cells has recently been demonstrated. Herein, to our knowledge, the current study is the first to investigate the anticancerous effect of *D. maritima* bulb extracts on COLO-205 and Caco-2 colorectal cancer cell lines.

In order to evaluate the potential antitumor effect mediated by *D. maritima* bulb extract on the cell proliferation of colon COLO-205 and Caco-2 cancer cell lines, an MTT assay was used to measure mitochondrial activity in viable cells. Interestingly, *D. maritima* bulb extract showed a dose-dependent antiproliferative effect against both colon cancer cell lines (Caco-2 and COLO-205). *D. maritima* bulb extract was able to achieve IC_{50} at 0.92 and 2.3 μg/mL in Caco-2 and COLO-205, respectively. In this study, ProA, which accounts for about 5% of the *D. maritima* bulb extract, was one of the major active phytochemical compounds with potent anticancer activity on different cancer types, including, but not limited to, glioblastoma, lung, and prostate cancers [17,18]. Accordingly, it was assumed that the cytotoxic activity of *D. maritima* bulb extracts on colon COLO-205 and Caco-2 cell lines could be achieved, at least in part, through ProA as an active compound. Interestingly, ProA was highly effective in inhibiting COLO-205 and Caco-2 cell lines and achieved IC_{50} at concentrations of 0.0029 μg/mL and 0.012μg/mL, respectively. Additionally, both *D. maritima* bulb extract and ProA express minimal cytotoxic effects against normal HGF when compared to cancer cells (IC_{50} equals 13.1 μg/mL and 0.229 μg/mL, respectively), indicating that their cytotoxic activities are selective to colon cancer cells, with a very attractive selectivity index of 14.6 for Caco-2 and 5.6 for COLO-205. Interestingly, the obtained IC50 values in this study are relatively lower than the previously reported IC50 against different breast cancer cell lines. For example, Hamzeloo-Moghadam reported that the IC50 values for the non-hemolytic ethanol extract of U. maritima against breast cancer MCF7 cells were 11.01 μg/mL. Additionally, IC50 values for the non-hemolytic acetone extract of U. maritima against breast cancer MCF7 cells was 6.01 μg/mL, while the Doxorubicin drug (positive control) exhibited a cytotoxic effect with a higher IC50 value (52.35 μg/mL) [19]. Another example is the study conducted by Obeidat and Sharan, which found that the effective doses of *D. maritima* that inhibited 50% of growth (IC50) of MCF-7 and MDA-MB-468 cells were 20.48 ± 1.17 μg/mL and 25.74 ± 2.05 μg/mL, respectively. Interestingly, Obeidat and Sharab's study revealed that *D. maritima* displays significantly lower cytotoxicity against AGO1522, a normal human fibroblast cell, with IC_{50} values of 43.5 ± 1.73 μg/mL [13].

Under normal physiological conditions, apoptosis "programmed cell death" is considered a mechanism to eliminate aged or abnormal cells; however, in cancer settings, cancer cells are, in general, resistant to apoptosis and induce apoptosis "therapeutically", which is considered an effective way to eliminate cancer cells [20]. The findings of this study showed that when compared to untreated cells (control), *D. maritima* bulb extract was able to induce early and late cell apoptosis in a concentration-dependent manner.

D. maritima bulb extract was able to significantly ($p < 0.0001$) induce ROS production in both Caco-2 and COLO-205 cancer cell lines after 48 h of treatment in a dose-dependent manner. As aforementioned, intracellular ROS generation in large amounts is considered a mechanism to trigger cell apoptosis, in part, through triggering the endoplasmic reticulum stress [21], and thus, colon cancer cells apoptosis investigated in this study could be a result of excessive intracellular ROS generation mediated by *D. maritima* bulb extract. On the other hand, excessive ROS generation can cause cell cycle arrest as described previously [22], but still, our results did not confirm the finding; at the same time, this possibility cannot be excluded.

In order to further understand the mechanisms that promoted apoptosis in colon cancer cells upon treatment with *D. maritima* bulb extract, studying the mitochondrial membrane potential, ΔΨm, is of significant value in this context. In particular, ΔΨm has considered one of the key markers of apoptosis [23]. Accordingly, the changes in the ΔΨm were evaluated by tracking TMRE fluorescent signal in colon cancer cells (Caco-2 and COLO-205 cell lines) after treatment with different concentrations of *D. maritima* bulb extract for 48 h. Importantly, when compared to untreated cells (control), a significant reduction in ΔΨm was observed in colon cancer cells ($p < 0.0001$), and this effect was dose-dependent. Notably, the Colo-205 represents a metastatic colorectal cancer, as this cell was isolated from the ascitic fluid of a 70-year-old Caucasian male with carcinoma of the colon. The patient had been treated with 5-fluorouracil for 4–6 weeks before the removal of the fluid specimen. Additionally, Caco-2 cells represent relatively sensitive cells toward the 5-fluorouracil. Interestingly, the extract used in this study shows a relatively higher activity toward the colorectal Caco-2 cells. Interestingly, the apoptosis assay has also shown less apoptosis percentage than those seen in the case of the Caco-2 cells. These results inversely correlate with the ROS results, indicating that there is a negative correlation between ROS generation and ΔΨm, which is consistent with the results of [24], and showed that curcumin is able to induce apoptosis in melanoma cancer cells by increasing the production of ROS and reducing ΔΨm

Finally, in order to track the molecular pathway through which *D. maritima* bulb extract was able to induce apoptosis in colon cancer cell lines, RT-qPCR was used to quantify the following target genes: genes encoding for pro-inflammatory cytokines, including TNF-α and IL-6, as well as the gene encoding for caspase-8. TNF-α is an important pleiotropic pro-inflammatory cytokine that, once produced at the site of inflammation, can mediate a wide range of cellular responses that include but are not limited to stimulating the production of pro-inflammatory cytokines, affecting the survival and proliferation of cells and/or inducing cell death under certain circumstances [25]. In fact, TNF-α can positively regulate the survival and proliferation of cells if it activates certain NF-kB-dependent genes involved in cell survival and proliferation [26,27]. The latter can be achieved through the activation of distinct caspase-8 activation pathways [27]. Furthermore, it has been reported that upregulating the gene expression of *TNF-α* and *IL-6* can participate in inducing Caco-cell death [28]. This explains why the above-mentioned three gene targets are examined in this study. Importantly, the results showed that upon treatment of both colon cancer cell lines with the *D. maritima* bulb extract, there was a statistically significant increase in the expression of all three gene targets tested in this study. This may indicate that *D. maritima* bulb extract induces apoptosis in colon cancer cells through the *TNF-α*, *IL-6*, and caspase-8 activation pathways [29]. The results of this study are in agreement with [13], which showed that the expression levels of *TNF-α* and *IL-6* gene were induced in MCF7 cells treated with fruit extracts of *D. maritima*.

4. Materials and Methods

4.1. Plant Collection, Classification, and Extraction

The plant *D. maritima* was collected in March 2021 from Princess Tasneem bint Ghazi Technological Research Station in Al-Salt (Jordan), with coordinates: 32°05′ N 35°40′ E. The collected plant was identified by a taxonomist specialist Mr. Refad Khawaldeh at Jordan Royal Botanical Garden, where a voucher specimen (073/2021) is conserved for future reference. Then, a powder of *D. maritima* bulbs was prepared after the bulbs were cleaned with water. The grinding process was achieved manually by mortar and pestle. In the next step, the crude powdered plant (30 g) was macerated in 100 mL water for two weeks with continuous shaking at 150 rpm at RT. At the end of this period, the mixture was filtered using a clean white canvas and filter papers to yield the aqueous *D. maritima* bulb extract. Then, the aqueous part of the solution was dried out (evaporated) using a lyophilizer to obtain the desired *D. maritima* bulbs to extract in a lyophilized form. Finally, 100 mg of the *D. maritima* bulb extract was dissolved in 1 mL of DMSO to make a 100 mg/mL stock solution for the treatment experiments.

4.2. *Identification and Characterization of D. maritima Bulb Extract by Gas Chromatography-Mass Spectrometry (GC-MS)*

Gas chromatography–mass spectrometry (GC-MS) analysis of the extracted sample was performed using an Agilent 5977B GC/MSD (Agilent, Santa Clara, CA, USA). Gas Chromatograph was equipped and coupled to a mass detector Turbo Mass Gold, PerkinElmer Turbo Mass 5.1 spectrometer with an Elite-1 (100% dimethylpolysiloxane), DB-5MS, 30 m × 0.25 mm i.d., 0.25 µm film thickness of capillary column. The instrument was set to an initial temperature of 80 °C and maintained at this temperature for 1 min. At the end of this duration, the oven temperature was raised to 300 °C, at the rate of an increase of 15 °C/min, and maintained for 9 min. The injection port temperature was ensured at 290 °C, and the helium flow rate was one mL/min. The ionization voltage was 70 eV. Samples were injected in split mode as 10:1. Mass spectral scan range was set at 30–600 (m/z) [30].

4.3. *Drugs Preparation*

Proscillaridin A (Sigma-Aldrich, St. Louis, MO, USA) and Doxorubicin (EBEWE Pharma, Rome, Italy) were completely dissolved in DMSO and then prepared in 20 mM and 100 mM stock solutions, respectively. Then serial dilutions for both were prepared in DMEM medium and stored at −20 °C until use.

4.4. *Cell Culture*

Two human colorectal carcinoma cell lines from the American Type Culture Collection (ATCC), namely COLO-205 (ATCC® CCL-222™) and Caco-2 (ATCC® HTB-37™), were used in this study. Additionally, normal human gingival fibroblasts (hGFs) samples prepared at the Cell Therapy Center (CTC) were used to assess the cytotoxic effects of the plant extract and drugs/treatments. All cells were cultured under the same conditions in 75 cm^2 tissue culture flasks and maintained in cell culture media (CCM) consisting of DMEM (Euroclone, Pero, Italy) high-glucose supplemented with 10% (*v*/*v*) heat-inactivated FBS, 1X penicillin/streptomycin, 1X non-essential amino acid, sodium pyruvate, and 1X L-Glutamine and incubated in a humidified incubator at 37 °C and 5% CO_2. When the confluence of cells reached 70–80 percent, cells were passaged with 1X trypsin/EDTA (Euroclone, Italy) and centrifuged at 1400 rpm, 25 °C for five min. Different characteristics for the used cell line is listed in Table 2.

Table 2. Type of cells used in the study.

Cell Line	Organism	Tissue	Morphology	Culture Properties	Mutant Gene	Chemoresistance
COLO-205 (ATCC® CCL-222™) *	*Homo sapiens*, human	Colon	Epithelial	Mixed; adherent and suspension	APC, BRAF SMAD4, TP53	Cisplatin
Caco-2 (ATCC® HTB-37™) *	*Homo sapiens*, human	Colon	Epithelial	Adherent	APC, SMAD4 TP53	5-fluorouracil

*; https://www.atcc.org (accessed on 20 December 2022).

4.5. *Cell Viability and Proliferation Assay*

The antiproliferative effect and the median inhibitory concentration (IC_{50}) of *D. maritima* bulb extract and ProA was assessed on COLO-205, Caco-2, and hGF cells using an MTT assay. In brief, cells were seeded in 96-well plates at a concentration of 8 × 10^3 cells/well and incubated for 24 h at 37 °C. The next day, cells were treated with *D. maritima* bulb extract and ProA at concentrations ranging from 0.122 µg to 500 to /mL and 2.46 to 5307 µg/mL, respectively, in a quadruplicate manner. The plates were incubated at 37 °C for 48 h. COLO-205, Caco-2, and hGF cells were also treated with a 2-fold serial dilution of Doxorubicin at concentrations ranging from 0.024 to 50 µg/mL under the same conditions.

DMSO was used as a drug solvent in minimal concentrations. Furthermore, each cell line used in this study was treated with 1% DMSO as a control. Additionally, untreated cells were used as a negative control. At the end of the incubation period, DMEM media were aspirated, and 10 μL of MTT dye solution (Promega, USA) was added to each well. After 4 h of incubation at 37 °C, the dye solution was removed, 100 μL of DMSO was added to each well, and the absorbance was measured using a 96-well plate reader at 560 and 750 nm wavelength. The IC_{50} values were determined using the logarithmic trend line of the cytotoxicity graph using the GraphPad PRISM® 8.0 software (GraphPad Software, Inc., San Diego, CA, USA).

4.6. Apoptosis Assay

Cell apoptosis was determined using the Annexin V-FITC/Propidium Iodide (PI) apoptosis detection assay Kit (Invitrogen, Waltham, MA, USA). In brief, Caco-2 and COLO-205 cells were seeded in 6-well plates at a concentration of 3×10^5 cells/well, treated with different concentrations of the *D. maritima* bulb extract, and incubated for 24 h at 37 °C, 5% CO_2. According to the IC_{50}, Caco-2 cells were treated with different concentrations ranging from 0.5 to 2 μg/mL, COLO-205 cells were treated with different concentrations ranging from 0.5 to 3.5 μg/mL, and then both cells were incubated for 48 h at 37 °C, 5% CO_2. The cells were harvested using 1X TrypLE Express, washed twice with PBS, and suspended in equal volumes of Annexin V and PI reagents (2 μL each) diluted in 100 μL of 1X binding buffer. All cells were incubated in a dark place at room temperature for 15–20 min. After that, cells were analyzed by flow cytometry BD FACSCanto software (BD FACSCanto, Wokingham, UK)

4.7. Total Reactive Oxygen Species Measurement

Seeding and treatment conditions and cell preparation were similar to apoptosis analyses. Cells were incubated with 1X ROS stain (Invitrogen, USA) (100 μL/sample) and incubated for 60 min at 37 °C, with 5% CO_2. Then the stained cells were analyzed by flow cytometer by measuring the fluorescence emission at 520 nm.

4.8. Mitochondrial Membrane Potential ($\Delta\Psi m$)

Mitochondrial membrane potential ($\Delta\Psi$m) was assessed in colon cancer cell lines using a Tetramethylrhodamine ethyl ester (TMRE) mitochondrial membrane potential assay kit (Abcam, Boston, MA, USA). Colon cancer cells were treated as described above, and then 0.8 μL of trifluoromethoxy carbonylcyanide phenylhydrazone (FCCP) was added to the untreated cells only (control) and incubated for 15 min at 37 °C, 5% CO_2. Treated cells were stained with TMRE by adding 0.8 μL of TMRE/well to the cell suspensions, and then cells were re-incubated for an additional 30 min. Next, cells were harvested, centrifuged, and resuspended in PBS and then analyzed by flow cytometer and measured at 549/575 nm.

4.9. Real-Time Quantitative Polymerase Chain Reaction (RT-qPCR) Amplification

Total RNA was extracted from cell pellets using Qiagen RNeasy Mini Kit (Qiagen, Germany), according to the manufacturer's instructions. Complementary DNA (cDNA) was prepared using 1 μg RNA and PrimeScript RT Master Mix Kit (TaKaRa, Kusatsu, Japan) according to the manufacturer's instructions. The cDNA synthesis reaction was performed using veriti 96 well Thermal Cycler (Thermo Fisher Scientific, Waltham, MA, USA), under the following conditions: "37 °C" (reverse-transcription) for 15 min, "85 °C" (heat inactivation for reverse-transcription) for 5 s, and "4 °C" holds. Finally, the samples were stored at −20 °C until use.

cDNA samples were diluted in 1:10 using nuclease-free water. Samples were performed in replicate. qPCR *assay* was performed *in* a 10 μL total reaction using specific primers to amplify *CASP8*, *TNF-α*, *IL-6*, and *GADPH* genes, which are responsible for the expression of caspase-8, tumor necrosis factor-alpha, interleukin-6, and glyceraldehyde-3-phosphate dehydrogenase, as the following: "95 °C" for 2 min as initial denaturation cycle, then 40 cycles of 95 °C for 15 s (denaturation), "58 °C" for 60 s (annealing), and "72 °C" for 30 s (extension). The primers sequences are listed in Table 3. The PCR data analysis was performed using the ΔΔCt method (delta delta cycle threshold); the analysis was performed automatically according to CFX Maestro Software of Bio-Rad Company (Hercules, CA, USA). The data were normalized, across all plates, to the housekeeping gene *GAPDH*.

Table 3. List of primers for qPCR amplification.

Gene	Forward Primer Sequence (5′-3′)	Reverse Primer Sequence (5′-3′)
CASP8	CTG CTG GGG ATG GCC ACT GTG	TCG CCT CGA GGA CAT CGC TCT C
TNF-a	GTC AAC CTC CTC TCT GCC AT	CCA AAG TAG ACC TGC CCA GA
IL-6	TTC CAA AGA TGT AGC CGC CC	ACC AGG CAA GTC TCC TCA TT
GAPDH	CCT GTT CGA CAG TCA GCC G	CGA CCA AAT CCG TTG ACT CC

4.10. Statistical Analysis

All statistical analyses were performed using GraphPad Prism software version 8.0 (GraphPad Software, San Diego, CA, USA). The comparison between different groups of numerical variables was performed using one-way or two-way ANOVA. Homogeneity of variances was tested using Dunnett's and Bonferroni's multiple comparisons tests, and a p-value less than 0.05 ($p < 0.05$) was considered statistically significant.

The IC_{50} values were determined by using log–probit analysis; log (concentration) plotted on the x-axis and inhibition percentage plotted on the y-axis; percent of inhibition was calculated, after correction of the absorbance (A) measurements for the background (blank) absorbance, according to the equation; Inhibition% = $((A_{control} - A_{treatment})/A_{control}) \times 100\%$.

5. Conclusions

In summary, *D. maritima* bulb extract and ProA showed a selective inhibitory activity on the proliferation of colorectal cancer cell lines. Such a finding was supported by the results of the apoptosis, intracellular ROS, and mitochondrial membrane potential assays. On the molecular level, the expression of pro-inflammatory genes *TNF-α* and *IL-6* and the apoptotic initiator gene *CASP8* was also confirmative for the antiproliferative effect of the *D. maritima* bulb extract. Taken together, the findings of this study elect *D. maritima* for further investigation and validation on CRC animal cancer xenograft models.

Author Contributions: Conceptualization, M.Z., K.A.-A., N.A.A. and M.O.; methodology, N.A.A., S.A.H., Y.A.-A. and S.Z.; software, K.A.-A.; formal analysis, M.Z, K.A.-A.; investigation, K.A.-A., N.A.A.; supervision, A.A, N.A.A. and M.O.; project administration, M.Z., N.A.A. and A.A; funding acquisition, M.O. and A.A. All authors have read and agreed to the published version of the manuscript.

Funding: This study was supported by the Deanship of Scientific Research and Innovation, Al-Balqa Applied University (Grant number: 497/2020/2021).

Institutional Review Board Statement: Not applicable.

Informed Consent Statement: Not applicable.

Data Availability Statement: All data are available upon request from the corresponding author.

Conflicts of Interest: The authors declare no conflict of interest.

Sample Availability: Samples of the compounds are available from the corresponding author upon request.

References

1. Blackburn, E.H.; Collins, K. Telomerase: An RNP enzyme synthesizes DNA. *Cold Spring Harb. Perspect. Biol.* **2011**, *3*, a003558. [CrossRef]
2. Adjiri, A. DNA Mutations May Not Be the Cause of Cancer. *Oncol. Ther.* **2017**, *5*, 85–101. [CrossRef]

3. Donnem, T.; Reynolds, A.R.; Kuczynski, E.A.; Gatter, K.; Vermeulen, P.B.; Kerbel, R.S.; Harris, A.L.; Pezzella, F. Non-angiogenic tumours and their influence on cancer biology. *Nat. Rev. Cancer* **2018**, *18*, 323–336. [CrossRef] [PubMed]
4. van Zijl, F.; Krupitza, G.; Mikulits, W. Initial steps of metastasis: Cell invasion and endothelial transmigration. *Mutat. Res.* **2011**, *728*, 23–34. [CrossRef]
5. Alzaghal, M. Epidemiology of Colorectal Cancer in Jordan, From 2003 to 2012. *J. Glob. Oncol.* **2018**, *4*, 32s. [CrossRef]
6. Nobili, S.; Lippi, D.; Witort, E.; Donnini, M.; Bausi, L.; Mini, E.; Capaccioli, S. Natural compounds for cancer treatment and prevention. *Pharmacol. Res.* **2009**, *59*, 365–378. [CrossRef] [PubMed]
7. Anantharaju, P.G.; Gowda, P.C.; Vimalambike, M.G.; Madhunapantula, S.V. An overview on the role of dietary phenolics for the treatment of cancers. *Nutr. J.* **2016**, *15*, 99. [CrossRef]
8. Habtemariam, S.; Lentini, G. Plant-derived anticancer agents: Lessons from the pharmacology of geniposide and its aglycone, genipin. *Biomedicines* **2018**, *6*, 39. [CrossRef] [PubMed]
9. Brglez Mojzer, E.; Hrncic, M.K.; Skerget, M.; Knez, Z.; Bren, U. Polyphenols: Extraction Methods, Antioxidative Action, Bioavailability and Anticarcinogenic Effects. *Molecules* **2016**, *21*, 901. [CrossRef]
10. Naghibi, F.; Khalaj, A.; Mosaddegh, M.; Malekmohamadi, M.; Hamzeloo-Moghadam, M. Cytotoxic activity evaluation of some medicinal plants, selected from Iranian traditional medicine Pharmacopoeia to treat cancer and related disorders. *J. Ethnopharmacol.* **2014**, *155*, 230–239. [CrossRef] [PubMed]
11. Mohamed, G.A.; Ibrahim, S.R.; Shaala, L.A.; Alshali, K.Z.; Youssef, D.T. Urgineaglyceride A: A new monoacylglycerol from the Egyptian Drimia maritima bulbs. *Nat. Prod. Res.* **2014**, *28*, 1583–1590. [CrossRef] [PubMed]
12. Nejatbakhsh, F.; Karegar-Borzi, H.; Amin, G.; Eslaminejad, A.; Hosseini, M.; Bozorgi, M.; Gharabaghi, M.A. Squill Oxymel, a traditional formulation from Drimia Maritima (L.) Stearn, as an add-on treatment in patients with moderate to severe persistent asthma: A pilot, triple-blind, randomized clinical trial. *J. Ethnopharmacol.* **2017**, *196*, 186–192. [CrossRef]
13. Obeidat, M.; Sharab, A. Antimicrobial and anticancer activities of extracts from *Urginea maritima* fruits. *Afr. J. Tradit. Complement. Altern. Med.* **2018**, *15*, 74–84. [CrossRef]
14. Rhimi, W.; Salem, I.B.; Camarda, A.; Saidi, M.; Boulila, A.; Otranto, D.; Cafarchia, C. Chemical characterization and acaricidal activity of Drimia maritima (L) bulbs and Dittrichia viscosa leaves against Dermanyssus gallinae. *Vet. Parasitol.* **2019**, *268*, 61–66. [CrossRef]
15. El-Seedi, H.R.; Burman, R.; Mansour, A.; Turki, Z.; Boulos, L.; Gullbo, J.; Goransson, U. The traditional medical uses and cytotoxic activities of sixty-one Egyptian plants: Discovery of an active cardiac glycoside from Urginea maritima. *J. Ethnopharmacol.* **2013**, *145*, 746–757. [CrossRef]
16. Laka, K.; Mapheto, K.B.F.; Mbita, Z. Selective in vitro cytotoxicity effect of Drimia calcarata bulb extracts against p53 mutant HT-29 and p53 wild-type Caco-2 colorectal cancer cells through STAT5B regulation. *Toxicol. Rep.* **2021**, *8*, 1265–1279. [CrossRef] [PubMed]
17. Berges, R.; Denicolai, E.; Tchoghandjian, A.; Baeza-Kallee, N.; Honore, S.; Figarella-Branger, D.; Braguer, D. Proscillaridin A exerts anti-tumor effects through GSK3beta activation and alteration of microtubule dynamics in glioblastoma. *Cell Death Dis.* **2018**, *9*, 984. [CrossRef] [PubMed]
18. Li, R.Z.; Fan, X.; Duan, F.; Jiang, Z.; Pan, H.; Luo, L.; Zhou, Y.; Li, Y.; Yao, Y.J.; Yao, X.J.; et al. Proscillaridin A induces apoptosis and suppresses non-small-cell lung cancer tumor growth via calcium-induced DR4 upregulation. *Cell Death Dis.* **2018**, *9*, 696. [CrossRef] [PubMed]
19. Hamzeloo-Moghadam, M.; Aghaei, M.; Abdolmohammadi, M.H.; Khalaj, A.; Fallahian, F. Cytotoxic effect of *Drimia maritima* bulb extract and induction of mitochondrial apoptotic signaling in human breast cancer cells, MCF-7 and MDA-MB-468. *OncoTargets Ther.* **2018**, *11*, 7669–7677. [CrossRef]
20. Kaczanowski, S. Apoptosis: Its origin, history, maintenance and the medical implications for cancer and aging. *Phys. Biol.* **2016**, *13*, 031001. [CrossRef] [PubMed]
21. Banerjee, A.; Banerjee, V.; Czinn, S.; Blanchard, T. Increased reactive oxygen species levels cause ER stress and cytotoxicity in andrographolide treated colon cancer cells. *Oncotarget* **2017**, *8*, 26142–26153. [CrossRef]
22. Kuczler, M.D.; Olseen, A.M.; Pienta, K.J.; Amend, S.R. ROS-induced cell cycle arrest as a mechanism of resistance in polyaneuploid cancer cells (PACCs). *Prog. Biophys. Mol. Biol.* **2021**, *165*, 3–7. [CrossRef] [PubMed]
23. Elmore, S. Apoptosis: A review of programmed cell death. *Toxicol. Pathol.* **2007**, *35*, 495–516. [CrossRef] [PubMed]
24. Kocyigit, A.; Guler, E.M. Curcumin induce DNA damage and apoptosis through generation of reactive oxygen species and reducing mitochondrial membrane potential in melanoma cancer cells. *Cell. Mol. Biol.* **2017**, *63*, 97–105. [CrossRef] [PubMed]
25. Wang, P.; Qiu, W.; Dudgeon, C.; Liu, H.; Huang, C.; Zambetti, G.P.; Yu, J.; Zhang, L. PUMA is directly activated by NF-kappaB and contributes to TNF-alpha-induced apoptosis. *Cell Death Differ.* **2009**, *16*, 1192–1202. [CrossRef]
26. Rath, P.C.; Aggarwal, B.B. TNF-induced signaling in apoptosis. *J. Clin. Immunol.* **1999**, *19*, 350–364. [CrossRef] [PubMed]
27. Wang, L.; Du, F.; Wang, X. TNF-alpha induces two distinct caspase-8 activation pathways. *Cell* **2008**, *133*, 693–703. [CrossRef] [PubMed]
28. Machado, A.R.T.; Aissa, A.F.; Ribeiro, D.L.; Hernandes, L.C.; Machado, C.S.; Bianchi, M.L.P.; Sampaio, S.V.; Antunes, L.M.G. The toxin BjussuLAAO-II induces oxidative stress and DNA damage, upregulates the inflammatory cytokine genes TNF and IL6, and downregulates the apoptotic-related genes BAX, BCL2 and RELA in human Caco-2 cells. *Int. J. Biol. Macromol.* **2018**, *109*, 212–219. [CrossRef]

29. Yaseen, M.M.; Abuharfeil, N.M.; Darmani, H. The impact of MDSCs on the efficacy of preventive and therapeutic HIV vaccines. *Cell. Immunol.* **2021**, *369*, 104440. [CrossRef]
30. Knittel, D.N.; Stintzing, F.C.; Kammerer, D.R. Simultaneous determination of bufadienolides and phenolic compounds in sea squill (*Drimia maritima* (L.) Stearn) by HPLC-DAD-MS n as a means to differentiate individual plant parts and developmental stages. *Anal. Bioanal. Chem.* **2014**, *406*, 6035–6050. [CrossRef]

molecules

MDPI

Article

Synthesis of Oleanolic Acid-Dithiocarbamate Conjugates and Evaluation of Their Broad-Spectrum Antitumor Activities

Liyao Tang [1,†], Yan Zhang [1,†], Jinrun Xu [1,†], Qingfan Yang [2], Fukuan Du [1,3], Xu Wu [1,3], Mingxing Li [1,3], Jing Shen [1,3], Shuai Deng [1,3], Yueshui Zhao [1,3], Zhangang Xiao [2,3,*] and Yu Chen [1,3,*]

1 Laboratory of Molecular Pharmacology, Department of Pharmacology, School of Pharmacy, Southwest Medical University, Luzhou 646000, China
2 Department of Oncology, The Affiliated Hospital of Southwest Medical University, Southwest Medical University, Luzhou 646000, China
3 Cell Therapy & Cell Drugs of Luzhou Key Laboratory, Southwest Medical University, Luzhou 646000, China
* Correspondence: zhangangxiao@swmu.edu.cn (Z.X.); chenyu2021@swmu.edu.cn (Y.C.)
† These authors contributed equally to this work.

Abstract: Efficient and mild synthetic routes for bioactive natural product derivatives are of current interest for drug discovery. Herein, on the basis of the pharmacophore hybrid strategy, we report a two-step protocol to obtain a series of structurally novel oleanolic acid (OA)-dithiocarbamate conjugates in mild conditions with high yields. Moreover, biological evaluations indicated that representative compound **3e** exhibited the most potent and broad-spectrum antiproliferative effects against Panc1, A549, Hep3B, Huh-7, HT-29, and Hela cells with low cytotoxicity on normal cells. In terms of the IC_{50} values, these OA-dithiocarbamate conjugates were up to 30-fold more potent than the natural product OA. These compounds may be promising hit compounds for the development of novel anti-cancer drugs.

Keywords: structural modification; oleanolic acid; natural product derivative; dithiocarbamate; hybrid strategy; antitumor activity

Citation: Tang, L.; Zhang, Y.; Xu, J.; Yang, Q.; Du, F.; Wu, X.; Li, M.; Shen, J.; Deng, S.; Zhao, Y.; et al. Synthesis of Oleanolic Acid-Dithiocarbamate Conjugates and Evaluation of Their Broad-Spectrum Antitumor Activities. *Molecules* **2023**, *28*, 1414. https://doi.org/10.3390/molecules28031414

Academic Editors: Barbara De Filippis, Alessandra Ammazzalorso and Marialuigia Fantacuzzi

Received: 4 January 2023
Revised: 27 January 2023
Accepted: 30 January 2023
Published: 2 February 2023

1. Introduction

Natural products and their derivatives have a long history in cancer therapy and are important for drug development. Efficient and mild synthetic routes for bioactive natural product derivatives are of current interest for drug discovery [1–4]. Recently, pentacyclic triterpenes have been identified as the main biologically active components in many traditional Chinese medicines [5,6]. Among them, oleanolic acid (OA) is the most abundant and cheap; thus, OA and its derivatives have been widely investigated for their diverse biological activities, including their anti-cancer, anti-inflammatory, anti-HIV, anti-bacterial, anti-diabetic, and anti-hepatotoxic effects, among others [7–11]. Derivatization of OA has yielded a wide variety of novel compounds for anti-cancer investigations (Scheme 1) [11–15]; however, poor pharmacokinetic properties, low cell selectivities, limited bioavailabilities, and synthetic complexity have hindered further clinical application [7]. Therefore, methods for readily accessible modification of OA to enhance its polarity and anti-proliferative activity are urgently required.

Dithiocarbamates are an important class of sulfur-containing organic compounds with a wide range of applications in both academia and industry [16–27]. They serve as fungicides and pesticides in agriculture [17–19], vulcanization agents in the rubber industry [20], radical chain transfer agents in polymerization [21], effective ligands in coordination chemistry [22], and, last but not least, as biologically important structural motifs in medicinal chemistry (Scheme 2) [23–27].

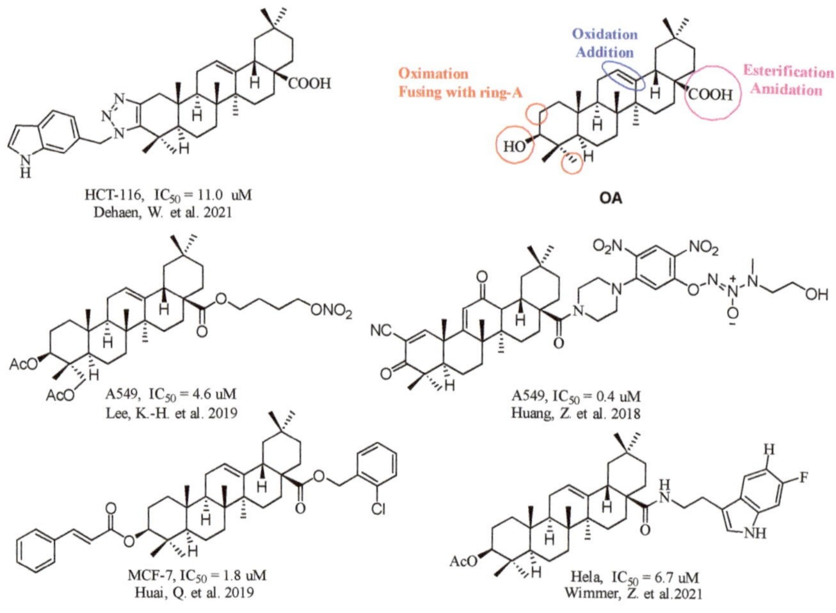

Scheme 1. Oleanolic Acid and Its Derivatization for Antitumor Medicinal Chemistry [11–15].

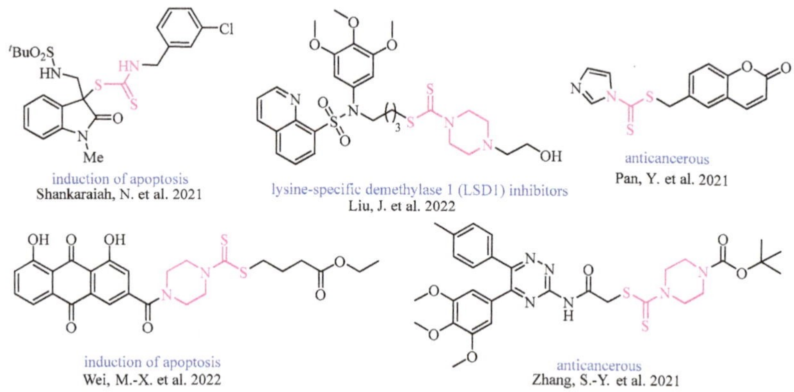

Scheme 2. Pharmaceutically Important Dithiocarbamates [23–27].

In recent years, the pharmacophore hybrid strategy has emerged as an essential method for the discovery and modification of lead compounds [28–31]. Covalently combining two known pharmacophores yields a novel hybrid molecule, which can possess integrated advantages for optimizing certain biological activities and overcoming the deficiencies of a single drug [32–35]. In view of the high performance of dithiocarbamate derivatives in structural modification, the synthesis of OA-dithiocarbamate conjugates may enhance the polarities and antitumor properties of the reaction products in a readily accessible manner [7,23–27]. The structural modifications of OA have mainly focused on the C-3 hydroxyl and C-28 carboxyl groups (Scheme 1) [7]. The C-28 carboxyl group can easily be esterified by alcohols or amidated by amines; however, the preparation of OA-dithiocarbamate conjugates has not yet been documented in the literature [7–11]. In order to simplify the synthetic route and control the polarity of target molecules, ethylidene was chosen as a linker between OA and dithiocarbamates.

2. Results and Discussion

To establish the optimal reaction conditions, we prepared key intermediate **2**, as previously described [36,37]. Under the "standard" conditions, the reaction of **2** with CS_2 and pyrrolidine in a one-pot manner afforded the target product **3a** in an 80% isolated yield. In the "standard" conditions, 2 equiv. of K_3PO_4 was shown to be essential to yield the desired product **3a** (Entries 1–4, Table 1). Lowering the loading of K_3PO_4 to 1.5 equiv. led to a decreased yield of **3a** (Entry 1, Table 1), while replacement of it by K_2HPO_4 or Li_2CO_3 resulted in no desired product (Entries 2–3, Table 1). On the other hand, in the presence of 2 equiv. of K_2CO_3, product **3a** could be isolated with a 62% yield (Entry 4, Table 1). Changing the reaction temperature or using other solvents, such as DMF, CH_3CN, and EtOH, did not offer better results (Entries 5–8, Table 1). Lower amounts of CS_2 or pyrrolidine resulted in a decreased yield of **3a** (Entries 9–10, Table 1).

Table 1. Optimization of Reaction Conditions.

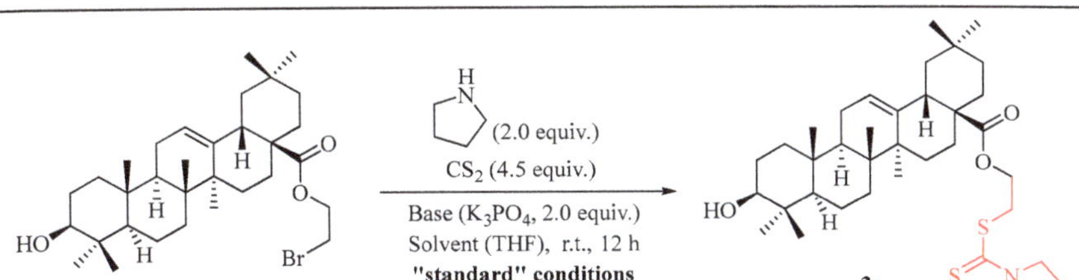

2 (0.4 mmol)

3a
80% isolated yield

Entry	Base (equiv.)	Solvent	Isolated Yield of 3a (%)
1	K_3PO_4 (1.5)	THF	72
2	K_2HPO_4 (2.0)	THF	0
3	Li_2CO_3 (2.0)	THF	0
4	K_2CO_3 (2.0)	THF	62
5	K_3PO_4 (2.0)	DMF	23
6	K_3PO_4 (2.0)	CH_3CN	19
7	K_3PO_4 (2.0)	EtOH	34
8 [a]	K_3PO_4 (2.0)	THF	78
9 [b]	K_3PO_4 (2.0)	THF	64
10 [c]	K_3PO_4 (2.0)	THF	70

Variations from the "standard" conditions. [a] Reaction temperature was raised to 60 °C. [b] CS_2 was used in 3.0 equiv. instead of 4.5 equiv. [c] Pyrrolidine was used in 1.5 equiv. instead of 2.0 equiv.

With the optimal reaction conditions in hand, the substrate scope was subsequently investigated, and the results are compiled in Figure 1. The replacement of the H-atom of the pyrrolidine ring with other substituents, such as methyl, dimethyl, hydroxy, and hydroxymethyl, worked well, affording the corresponding products **3b**–**3e** in 69–85% yields. Among them, hydroxyl containing products were obtained at slightly lower yields. This reaction was also tolerant of fused-ring substrates, such as hexahydroisoindoline and isoindoline, resulting in **3f** and **3g** with 77% and 90% yields, respectively.

To further enhance the structural diversity of products, various types of piperidine-derived substrates were also examined, and all of them were compatible with the established reaction conditions. First, methyl-, hydroxy-, hydroxymethyl-, hydroxyethyl-, and phenyl-substituted piperidines reacted smoothly to give **3h**–**3m** in 70–88% yields. Then, methyl-, hydroxyethyl-, phenyl-, and aryl-substituted piperazines were also viable substrates, affording **3n**–**3s** in 71–89% yields. Moreover, thiomorpholine was also compatible, leading to the formation of **3t** in 72% yield. Gratifyingly, the mild reaction conditions, high yields of products, and good functional group tolerances clearly demonstrated the advantages of our pharmacophore hybrid strategy for the structural modification of OA. The isolated compounds **3a–3t** were fully characterized by ^{1}H and ^{13}C NMR spectroscopy as well as high-resolution mass spectrometry (see the Supplementary Information for details).

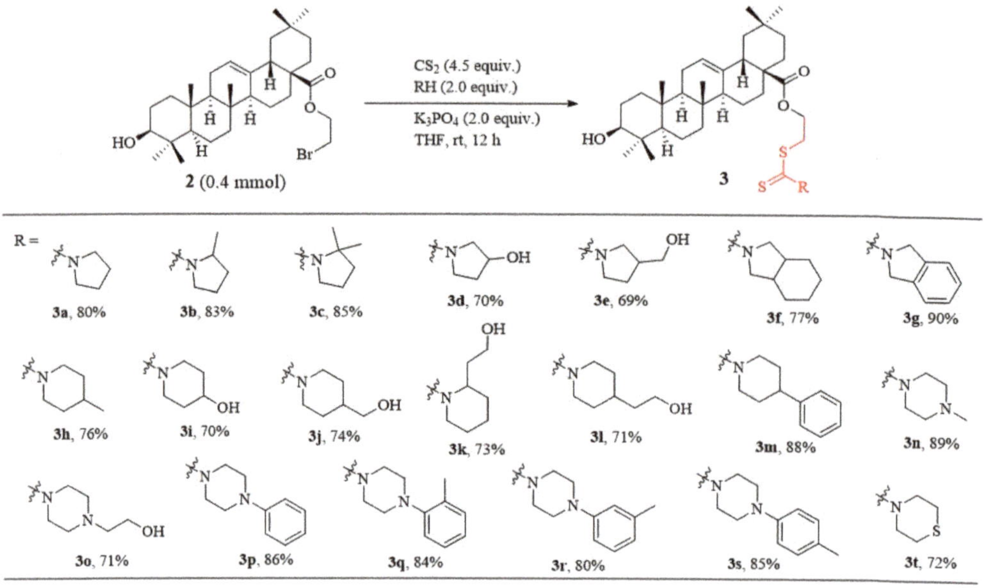

Figure 1. Synthesis of OA-Dithiocarbamate Derivatives.

Having obtained a series of structurally diverse OA-dithiocarbamates, we next performed a systematic biological evaluation to examine whether introducing an extra dithiocarbamate group could improve antitumor activities. These compounds were evaluated by MTT assay against human pancreatic cancer (Panc1), human lung cancer (A549), human hepatoma cell (Hep3B), human hepatoma cell (Huh-7), human colon cancer (HT-29), and human cervical cancer (Hela) cells, with the widely used anticancer drugs fluorouracil, docetaxel, and cisplatin as positive controls (Table 2). Most of the compounds exhibited remarkable antiproliferative activities, and the IC_{50} values of ten selected compounds were less than 50 μM on certain tumor cell lines. Among them, compounds **3e, 3i, 3j,** and **3l** were shown to be excellent, with broad-spectrum antitumor activities as well as being up to 30-fold more potent than the natural product OA and the positive controls; this might be ascribed to the introduction of hydroxyl groups. Particularly, compound **3p** was also found to be a promising hit compound that was 20-fold more potent than the natural product OA against HT-29 cells. Moreover, the cytotoxicities of compounds **3a-3t** were also evaluated in human normal hepatocytes (LO2) to determine whether these compounds preferred killing tumor cells over normal cells. Excitingly, the IC_{50} value of compound **3e** in LO2 cells was 62.8 μM, which was several times higher than that in the tumor cells.

Table 2. In Vitro Cytotoxicity Data of OA and Its Derivatives.

Compound	IC_{50} ^{a} (μM)						
	Panc1	A549	Hep3B	Huh-7	HT-29	Hela	LO2
OA	>200	>200	>200	>200	>200	>200	140.1
5-fluorouracil	160.0	125.3	152.2	140.0	93.3	130.4	108.9
Docetaxel	>200	>200	172.2	104.1	>200	135.0	139.7
Cisplatin	>200	>200	>200	>200	>200	142.5	>200

Table 2. *Cont.*

Compound	IC_{50} [a] (μM)						
	Panc1	A549	Hep3B	Huh-7	HT-29	Hela	LO2
3a	>200	92.1	>200	144.9	ND [b]	89.4	113.4
3b	130.0	135.8	>200	>200	100.3	77.1	136.0
3c	>200	64.3	ND	>200	>200	133.7	ND
3d	15.7	42.5	26.3	64.6	~18.3	11.9	34.1
3e	13.1	28.8	15.2	29.9	~17.6	7.0	62.8
3f	ND	ND	ND	ND	ND	ND	ND
3g	185.2	>200	>200	>200	121.3	>200	>200
3h	>200	ND	176.5	96.9	106.7	106.2	>200
3i	16.9	24.4	~18.7	70.6	~18.4	7.8	30.3
3j	13.5	33.6	16.9	49.4	7.6	10.9	25.2
3k	59.0	>200	>200	106.7	>200	49.8	>200
3l	13.4	34.3	14.7	39.9	8.3	ND	ND
3m	>200	>200	160.1	>200	81.8	131.2	>200
3n	39.5	34.5	124.3	132.8	62.2	48.6	76.9
3o	31.1	32.6	35.8	22.9	27.5	36.4	24.1
3p	14.6	25.2	13.9	59.1	10.3	ND	20.6
3q	>200	ND	ND	183.1	187.4	>200	ND
3r	>200	>200	161.2	>200	>200	192.0	>200
3s	>200	ND	>200	102.1	ND	115.4	ND
3t	>200	40.3	64.5	72.9	ND	175.4	114.7

[a] Concentration inhibiting 50% of cell growth for 48 h exposure period of tested samples. [b] ND, not determined.

3. Materials and Methods

3.1. General Information

All organic solvents were dried and distilled by standard methods prior to use. ^1H and ^{13}C NMR spectra were recorded on a Bruker AV II-400 spectrometer (BURKERT, Ingelfingen, Germany) at 400 and 100 MHz, respectively. All chemical shifts were reported in δ units with references to the residual solvent resonances of the deuterated solvents for proton and carbon chemical shifts. High Resolution Mass Spectra (HRMS) were obtained on a Thermo Q Exactive™ Focus Hybrid Quadrupole-Orbitrap™ Mass Spectrometer (SCIEX, Framingham, Massachusetts, USA). All other chemicals were purchased from either Aldrich (Sigma-Aldrich, Shanghai, China) or Aladdin Chemical Co. (Aladdin Holdings Group Co., Ltd, Shanghai, China) and used as received, unless otherwise specified.

The optical density at 490 nm of each well was measured using a microplate reader (Molecular devices corporation, Sunnyvale, CA. USA) to calculate the percent of cell viability. The inhibition rates were calculated using GraphPad Prism 7.0 software. The seven tested cell lines were obtained from the laboratory of Molecular Pharmacology, Department of Pharmacology, School of Pharmacy, Southwest Medical University.

3.2. Experimental Section of Synthesis

[2-bromoethyl] 3-hydroxy-12-en-28-oic acid (**2**) [36–38] To a mixture of oleanolic acid (913.4 mg, 2.0 mmol), K_2CO_3 (552.8 mg, 4.0 mmol), and DMF (40 mL), 1, 2-dibromoethane (513 μL, 6.0 mmol) was slowly added at room temperature, and the mixture was then stirred at 40 °C for 4 h. The resulting mixture was cooled to room temperature, then quenched with ice water (50.0 mL), and the insoluble material was removed by a Buchner funnel. The organic layer was separated, and the aqueous layer was extracted with ethyl acetate (50 mL × 3). The organic solutions were combined and dried over anhydrous $MgSO_4$. After removal of the solvent, the residue was submitted to column chromatography on silica gel (200-300 mesh) using petroleum ether and ethyl acetate (15/1 in v/v) as eluents to give **2** (957.6 mg, 85% yield) as a white solid. ^1H NMR (400 MHz, $CDCl_3$): δ 5.30 (s, 1H, H-12), 4.35 (m, 2H, -OCH_2C-), 3.49 (t, J = 5.5 Hz, 2H, BrCH_2C-), 3.20 (d, J = 6.9 Hz, 1H, H-3), 2.87 (d, J = 12.2 Hz, 1H, H-18), 1.99 (m, 1H, -*OH*), 1.87 (m, 2H, -CH_2), 1.72 (m, 3H, H-22, -*CH*, -CH_2,), 1.62 (m, 6H, 3 × -CH_2), 1.54

(m, 3H, H-22, -*CH*, -*CH*$_2$), 1.33 (m, 6H, 3 × -*CH*$_2$), 1.18 (s, 1H, H-9), 1.13 (s, 3H, -*CH*$_3$), 1.06 (s, 1H, H-5), 0.98 (s, 3H, -*CH*$_3$), 0.93 (s, 3H, -*CH*$_3$), 0.90 (s, 6H, 2 × -*CH*$_3$), 0.77 (s, 3H, -*CH*$_3$), 0.73 (s, 3H, -*CH*$_3$). ^{13}C NMR (100 MHz, CDCl$_3$): δ 177.2 (C-28), 143.4 (C-13), 122.6 (C-12), 78.8 (C-3), 63.6 (-CO-), 55.2 (C-5), 47.6 (C-9), 46.8 (C-17), 45.7 (C-19), 41.6 (C-14), 41.2 (C-18), 39.3 (C-8), 38.7 (C-1), 38.4 (C-4), 37.0 (C-10), 33.8 (C-29), 33.1 (C-22), 32.7 (C-21), 32.4 (C-7), 30.7 (C-20), 29.1 (-CBr), 28.2 (C-15), 27.7 (C-23), 27.1 (C-27), 25.9 (C-30), 23.6 (C-2), 23.4 (C-11), 22.9 (C-16), 18.3 (C-6), 17.0 (C-26), 15.6 (C-24), 15.3 (C-25). HRMS (ESI): m/z calculated for $C_{32}H_{51}BrO_3$ [M+H]$^+$: 563.3100. Found: 563.3054.

[2-((pyrrolidine-1-carbonothioyl)thio)ethyl] 3-hydroxy-12-en-28-oic acid (**3a**). To a mixture of CS_2 (1.8 mmol, 108 μL), anhydrous K_3PO_4 (0.8 mmol, 169.1 mg), and THF (8.0 mL), pyrrolidine (1.0 mmol, 82 μL) was slowly added at 0 °C, and the reaction mixture was then stirred at 0 °C for 0.5 h. To the resulting mixture another THF solution (4.0 mL) of **2** (0.4 mmol, 225.4 mg) was added dropwise. The reaction mixture was stirred for 12 h at room temperature, then quenched with ice water (15.0 mL), and the insoluble material was removed by a Buchner funnel. After removal of the solvent, the residue was dissolved in ethyl acetate (15.0 mL). Water (15.0 mL) was added to the resulting solution, the organic layer was separated, and the aqueous layer was extracted with ethyl acetate (15.0 mL × 2). The organic solutions were combined and dried over anhydrous Na_2SO_4. After removal of the solvent, the residue was submitted to column chromatography on silica gel (200–300 mesh) using petroleum ether and ethyl acetate (2/1 in v/v) as eluents to give **3a** (201.3 mg, 80% yield) as a white solid. ^{1}H NMR (400 MHz, CDCl$_3$): δ 5.29 (s, 1H, H-12), 4.27 (m, 2H, -O*CH*$_2$C-), 3.92 (t, *J* = 6.9 Hz, 2H, -S*CH*$_2$), 3.66 (t, *J* = 6.8 Hz, 2H, -N*CH*$_2$), 3.59 (m, 2H, -N*CH*$_2$), 3.20 (m, 1H, H-3), 2.87 (dd, *J* = 13.5, 3.4 Hz, 1H, H-18), 2.10 (m, 1H, -*OH*), 1.97 (m, 5H, H-22, -*CH*, 2 × -*CH*$_2$), 1.87 (m, 2H, -*CH*$_2$), 1.66 (d, *J* = 8.4 Hz, 3H, -NCH$_2$***CH***$_2$***CH***), 1.59 (m, 5H, -NCH$_2$CH$_2$***CH***, 2 × -*CH*$_2$), 1.53 (m, 3H, H-22, -*CH*, -*CH*$_2$), 1.35 (m, 6H, 3 × -*CH*$_2$), 1.16 (d, *J* = 4.0 Hz, 1H, H-9), 1.13 (s, 3H, -*CH*$_3$), 1.04 (s, 1H, H-5), 0.98 (s, 3H, -*CH*$_3$), 0.93 (s, 3H, -*CH*$_3$), 0.90 (s, 6H, 2 × -*CH*$_3$), 0.77 (s, 3H, -*CH*$_3$), 0.73 (s, 3H, -*CH*$_3$). ^{13}C NMR (100 MHz, CDCl$_3$): δ 191.7 (-CS$_2$), 177.4 (C-28), 143.6 (C-13), 122.5 (C-12), 78.8 (C-3), 62.5 (-CO-), 55.2 (-NCH$_2$), 55.1 (-NCH$_2$), 50.6 (C-5), 47.6 (C-9), 46.7 (C-17), 45.8 (C-19), 41.6 (C-14), 41.2 (C-18), 39.3 (C-8), 38.7 (C-1), 38.5 (C-4), 37.0 (C-10), 35.0 (-CS), 33.8 (C-29), 33.1 (C-22), 32.7 (C-21), 32.4 (C-7), 30.7 (C-20), 28.1 (C-15), 27.7 (C-23), 27.2 (C-27), 26.1 (-CH$_2$), 25.9 (C-30), 24.3 (-CH$_2$), 23.7 (C-2), 23.4 (C-11), 22.9 (C-16), 18.3 (C-6), 17.1 (C-26), 15.7 (C-24), 15.3 (C-25). HRMS (ESI): m/z calculated for $C_{37}H_{59}NO_3S_2$ [M+H]$^+$: 630.4015. Found: 630.3961.

[2-((2-methylpyrrolidine-1-carbonothioyl)thio)ethyl] 3-hydroxy-12-en-28-oic acid (**3b**). To a mixture of CS_2 (1.8 mmol, 108 μL), anhydrous K_3PO_4 (0.8 mmol, 169.1 mg), and THF (8.0 mL), 2-methylpyrrolidine (1.0 mmol, 101 μL) was slowly added at 0 °C, and the reaction mixture was then stirred at 0 °C for 0.5 h. Another THF solution (4.0 mL) of **2** (0.4 mmol, 225.2 mg) was added dropwise to the resulting mixture. The reaction mixture was stirred for 12 h at room temperature, then quenched with ice water (15.0 mL), and the insoluble material was removed by a Buchner funnel. After removal of the solvent, the residue was dissolved in ethyl acetate (15.0 mL). Water (15.0 mL) was added to the resulting solution, the organic layer was separated, and the aqueous layer was extracted with ethyl acetate (15.0 mL × 2). The organic solutions were combined and dried over anhydrous Na_2SO_4. After removal of the solvent, the residue was submitted to column chromatography on silica gel (200–300 mesh) using petroleum ether and ethyl acetate (10/1 in v/v) as eluents to give **3b** (213.6 mg, 83% yield) as a white solid. ^{1}H NMR (400 MHz, CDCl$_3$): δ 5.30 (s, 1H, H-12), 4.52 (m, 1H, -*OH*), 4.26 (m, 2H, -O*CH*$_2$C-), 3.93 (m, 1H, -N*CH*), 3.73 (m, 1H, -N*CH*), 3.44 (m, 2H, -S*CH*$_2$), 3.21 (m, 1H, H-3), 2.87 (dd, *J* = 13.7, 3.8 Hz, 1H, H-18), 2.25 (m, 1H, -N*CH*), 2.02 (m, 4H, 2 × -*CH*$_2$), 1.81 (m, 3H, H-11, -*CH*, -*CH*$_2$), 1.63 (m, 7H,-NCH$_2$*CH*$_2$, -NCH$_2$***CH***$_2$, H-22, -*CH*, -*CH*$_2$), 1.53 (m, 3H, H-22, -*CH*, -*CH*$_2$), 1.42 (m, 2H, -*CH*$_2$), 1.35 (m, 4H, 2 × -*CH*$_2$), 1.28 (m, 3H, -*CH*$_3$), 1.16 (t, *J* = 4.2 Hz, 1H, H-9), 1.13 (s, 3H, -*CH*$_3$), 1.04 (s, 1H, H-5), 0.98 (s, 3H, -*CH*$_3$), 0.93 (s, 3H, -*CH*$_3$), 0.90 (s, 6H, 2 × -*CH*$_3$), 0.77 (s, 3H, -*CH*$_3$), 0.74 (s, 3H, -*CH*$_3$). ^{13}C NMR (100 MHz, CDCl$_3$): δ 191.7 (-CS$_2$), 177.5 (C-28), 143.6 (C-13), 122.5 (C-12), 78.9 (C-3), 62.6 (-CO-), 61.3 (-NCH$_2$CH$_3$), 58.0(-CH$_3$), 55.2 (C-5), 50.4 (-NCH$_2$), 47.6 (C-9), 46.7 (C-17), 45.8 (C-19), 41.7 (C-14), 41.3 (C-18),

39.4 (C-8), 38.8 (C-1), 38.5 (C-4), 37.0 (C-10), 34.8 (-CS), 33.9 (C-29), 33.1 (C-22), 32.4 (C-21), 31.3 (C-7), 30.7 (C-20), 28.1 (C-15), 27.7 (C-23), 27.2 (C-27), 25.9 (C-30), 23.7 (C-2), 22.9 (C-11), 21.6 (C-16), 18.6 (-CH_2), 18.3 (C-6), 17.5 (-CH_2), 17.1 (C-26), 15.6 (C-24), 15.4 (C-25). HRMS (ESI): m/z calculated for $C_{38}H_{61}NO_3S_2$ $[M+H]^+$: 644.4171. Found: 644.4116.

[2-((2,2-dimethylpyrrolidine-1-carbonothioyl)thio)ethyl] 3-hydroxy-12-en-28-oic acid (**3c**). To a mixture of CS_2 (1.8 mmol, 108 μL), anhydrous K_3PO_4 (0.8 mmol, 169.1 mg), and THF (8.0 mL), 2,2-dimethylpyrrolidine (1.0 mmol, 120 μL) was slowly added at 0 °C, and the reaction mixture was then stirred at 0 °C for 0.5 h. Another THF solution (4.0 mL) of **2** (0.4 mmol, 225.9 mg) was added dropwise to the resulting mixture. The reaction mixture was stirred for 12 h at room temperature, then quenched with ice water (15.0 mL), and the insoluble material was removed by a Buchner funnel. After removal of the solvent, the residue was dissolved in ethyl acetate (15.0 mL). To the resulting solution was added water (15.0 mL), the organic layer was separated, and the aqueous layer was extracted with ethyl acetate (15.0 mL × 2). The organic solutions were combined and dried over anhydrous Na_2SO_4. After removal of the solvent, the residue was submitted to column chromatography on silica gel (200–300 mesh) using petroleum ether and ethyl acetate (10/1 in v/v) as eluents to give **3c** (223.5 mg, 85% yield) as a white solid. ^{1}H NMR (400 MHz, $CDCl_3$): δ 5.30 (s, 1H, H-12), 4.26 (m, 2H, -OCH_2C-), 3.83 (t, J = 6.8 Hz, 1H, -NCH), 3.56 (m, 2H, -SCH_2), 3.21 (m, 1H, -NCH), 2.87 (dd, J = 13.6, 3.7 Hz, 1H, H-18), 2.01 (m, 1H, -OH), 1.96 (m, 2H, -CH_2), 1.88 (m, 3H, H-22, -CH, -CH_2), 1.73 (s, 6H, 3 × -CH_2), 1.63 (m, 8H, 4 × -CH_2), 1.55 (m, 3H, -CH_3), 1.46 (m, 3H, -CH_3), 1.31 (m, 6H, 3 × -CH_2), 1.16 (t, J = 5.6 Hz, 1H, H-9), 1.13 (s, 3H, -CH_3), 1.04 (s, 1H, H-5), 0.98 (s, 3H, -CH_3), 0.93 (s, 3H, -CH_3), 0.90 (s, 6H, 2 × -CH_3), 0.78 (s, 3H, -CH_3), 0.73 (s, 3H, -CH_3). ^{13}C NMR (100 MHz, $CDCl_3$): δ 191.4 (-CS_2), 177.5 (C-28), 143.7 (C-13), 122.5 (C-12), 79.0 (C-3), 69.2 (-N$C$$CH_3$$CH_3$), 62.7 (-CO-), 55.2 (-N$CH_2$), 53.8 (C-5), 47.6 (C-9), 46.7 (C-17), 45.8 (C-19), 43.3 (-CH_2), 41.7 (C-14), 41.3 (C-18), 39.4 (C-8), 38.8 (C-1), 38.5 (C-4), 37.0 (C-10), 34.7 (-CS), 33.9 (C-29), 33.2 (C-22), 32.8 (C-21), 32.4 (C-7), 30.7 (C-20), 28.2 (C-15), 27.7 (C-23), 27.2 (C-27), 26.1 (-CH_2), 25.9 (C-30), 24.8 (-CH_2), 23.7 (C-2), 23.5 (C-11), 22.9 (C-16), 22.1 (-CH_2), 18.4 (C-6), 17.1 (C-26), 15.7 (C-24), 15.4 (C-25). HRMS (ESI): m/z calculated for $C_{39}H_{63}NO_3S_2$ $[M+H]^+$: 658.4328. Found: 658.4303.

[2-((3-hydroxypyrrolidine-1-carbonothioyl)thio)ethyl] 3-hydroxy-12-en-28-oic acid (**3d**). To a mixture of CS_2 (1.8 mmol, 108 μL), anhydrous K_3PO_4 (0.8 mmol, 169.1 mg), and THF (8.0 mL), 3-hydroxypyrrolidine (1.0 mmol, 81 μL) was slowly added at 0 °C, and the reaction mixture was then stirred at 0 °C for 0.5 h. Another THF solution (4.0 mL) of **2** (0.4 mmol, 224.7 mg) was added dropwise to the resulting mixture. The reaction mixture was stirred for 12 h at room temperature, then quenched with ice water (15.0 mL), and the insoluble material was removed by a Buchner funnel. After removal of the solvent, the residue was dissolved in ethyl acetate (15.0 mL). Water (15.0 mL) was added to the resulting solution, the organic layer was separated, and the aqueous layer was extracted with ethyl acetate (15.0 mL × 2). The organic solutions were combined and dried over anhydrous Na_2SO_4. After removal of the solvent, the residue was submitted to column chromatography on silica gel (200–300 mesh) using petroleum ether and ethyl acetate (2/1 in v/v) as eluents to give **3d** (180.7 mg, 70% yield) as a yellowish gel. ^{1}H NMR (400 MHz, $CDCl_3$): δ 5.31 (s, 1H, H-12), 4.57 (m, 1H, -OH), 4.21 (m, 2H, -OCH_2C-), 4.03 (m, 2H, -SCH_2), 3.82 (m, 2H, -NCH_2), 3.55 (m, 2H, -NCH_2), 3.20 (m, 1H, H-3), 2.86 (d, J = 12.2 Hz, 1H, H-18), 2.15 (m, 1H, -OH), 2.05 (m, 2H, -CH_2), 1.89 (m, 4H, 2 × -CH_2), 1.67 (m, 6H, 3 × -CH_2), 1.53 (m, 4H, 2 × -CH_2), 1.33 (m, 7H, -CHOH, 3 × -CH_2), 1.16 (t, J = 3.8 Hz, 1H, H-9), 1.13 (s, 3H, -CH_3), 1.05 (s, 1H, H-5), 0.97 (s, 3H, -CH_3), 0.93 (s, 3H, -CH_3), 0.90 (d, J = 2.3 Hz, 6H, 2 × -CH_3), 0.77 (s, 3H, -CH_3), 0.73 (s, 3H, -CH_3). ^{13}C NMR (100 MHz, $CDCl_3$): δ 192.5 (-CS_2), 177.7 (C-28), 143.5 (C-13), 122.5 (C-12), 79.0 (C-3), 70.7 (-COH), 68.8 (-NCH$_2$CH), 63.2 (-NCH_2), 62.5 (-CO-), 55.2 (C-5), 52.9 (-CH_2), 48.6 (C-7), 47.6 (C-9), 46.8 (C-17), 45.8 (C-19), 41.7 (C-14), 41.3 (C-18), 39.3 (C-8), 38.7 (C-1), 38.5 (C-4), 37.0 (C-10), 35.0 (-CS), 33.8 (C-29), 32.9 (C-22), 32.4 (C-21), 30.7 (C-20), 28.1 (C-15), 27.7 (C-23), 27.1 (C-27), 25.9 (C-30), 23.7 (C-2), 23.4 (C-11), 22.9 (C-16), 18.3 (C-6), 17.1 (C-26), 15.7 (C-24), 15.4 (C-25). HRMS (ESI): m/z calculated for $C_{37}H_{59}NO_4S_2$ $[M+H]^+$: 646.3964. Found: 646.3917.

[2-((3-(hydroxymethyl)pyrrolidine-1-carbonothioyl)thio)ethyl] 3-hydroxy-12-en-28-oic acid (**3e**). To a mixture of CS_2 (1.8 mmol, 108 μL), anhydrous K_3PO_4 (0.8 mmol, 169.1 mg), and THF (8.0 mL), 3-(hydroxymethyl)pyrrolidine (1.0 mmol, 103 μL) was slowly added at 0 °C, and the reaction mixture was then stirred at 0 °C for 0.5 h. Another THF solution (4.0 mL) of **2** (0.4 mmol, 225.8 mg) was added dropwise to the resulting mixture. The reaction mixture was stirred for 12 h at room temperature, then quenched with ice water (15.0 mL), and the insoluble material was removed by a Buchner funnel. After removal of the solvent, the residue was dissolved in ethyl acetate (15.0 mL). Water (15.0 mL) was added to the resulting solution, the organic layer was separated, and the aqueous layer was extracted with ethyl acetate (15.0 mL × 2). The organic solutions were combined and dried over anhydrous Na_2SO_4. After removal of the solvent, the residue was submitted to column chromatography on silica gel (200–300 mesh) using petroleum ether and ethyl acetate (1/1 in *v*/*v*) as eluents to give **3e** (181.9 mg, 69% yield) as a yellowish gel. ^{1}H NMR (400 MHz, $CDCl_3$): δ 5.30 (t, *J* = 3.2 Hz, 1H, H-12), 4.25 (m, 2H, -O*CH*$_2$C-), 3.85 (m, 1H, -*OH*), 3.68 (m, 2H, -S*CH*$_2$), 3.54 (m, 3H, -***CH***$_2$OH, -N*CH*), 3.21 (m, 1H, H-3), 2.86 (dd, *J* = 13.7, 3.9 Hz, 1H, H-18), 2.55 (m, 1H, -N*CH*), 2.22 (m, 1H, -N*CH*), 2.08 (m, 1H, -N*CH*), 1.95 (m, 2H, -*CH*$_2$), 1.84 (m, 3H, -NCH$_2$C***H***, -*CH*$_2$), 1.70 (m, 1H, -*OH*), 1.63 (m, 6H, 2 × -*CH*$_3$), 1.53 (m, 3H, -NCH$_2$C***H***, -*CH*$_2$), 1.42 (m, 3H, H-22, -*CH*, -*CH*$_2$), 1.28 (m, 5H, H-22, -*CH*, 2 × -*CH*$_2$), 1.21 (s, 1H, -C***H***CH$_2$OH), 1.17 (t, *J* = 3.2 Hz, 1H, H-9), 1.13 (s, 3H, -*CH*$_3$), 1.05 (s, 1H, H-5), 0.98 (s, 3H, -*CH*$_3$), 0.93 (s, 3H, -*CH*$_3$), 0.90 (s, 6H, 2 × -*CH*$_3$), 0.77 (s, 3H, -*CH*$_3$), 0.73 (s, 3H, -*CH*$_3$). ^{13}C NMR (100 MHz, $CDCl_3$): δ 192.0 (-CS$_2$), 177.6 (C-28), 143.6 (C-13), 122.5 (C-12), 79.0 (C-3), 63.6 (-COH), 62.4 (-CO-), 57.5 (-N*C*H$_2$CH), 55.2 (-*C*'OH), 54.5 (-N*C*'H$_2$CH), 53.1 (-N*C*H$_2$CH$_2$), 50.1 (C-5), 47.6 (C-9), 46.8 (C-17), 45.8 (C-19), 41.7 (C-14), 41.3 (C-18), 39.5 (-*C*CH$_2$OH), 39.3 (C-8), 38.7 (C-1), 38.5 (C-4), 37.0 (C-10), 35.0 (-CS), 33.8 (C-29), 33.1 (C-22), 32.7 (C-21), 32.4 (C-7), 31.5 (-N*C*'H$_2$CH$_2$), 30.7 (C-20), 30.2 (-NCH$_2$*C*H$_2$), 28.4 (-***C***'CH$_2$OH), 28.1 (C-15), 27.7 (C-23), 27.1 (C-27), 26.6 (-*C*'CH$_2$OH), 25.9 (C-30), 23.7 (C-2), 23.4 (C-11), 22.9 (C-16), 18.3 (C-6), 17.1 (C-26), 15.7 (C-24), 15.4 (C-25). HRMS (ESI): *m*/*z* calculated for $C_{38}H_{61}NO_4S_2$ [M+H]$^+$: 660.4120. Found: 660.4069.

[2-((octahydro-1H-isoindole-2-carbonothioyl)thio)ethyl] 3-hydroxy-12-en-28-oic acid (**3f**). To a mixture of CS_2 (1.8 mmol, 108 μL), anhydrous K_3PO_4 (0.8 mmol, 169.1 mg), and THF (8.0 mL), octahydro-1H-isoindole (1.0 mmol, 115 μL) was slowly added at 0 °C, and the reaction mixture was then stirred at 0 °C for 0.5 h. Another THF solution (4.0 mL) of **2** (0.4 mmol, 225.5 mg) was added dropwise to the resulting mixture. The reaction mixture was stirred for 12 h at room temperature, then quenched with ice water (15.0 mL), and the insoluble material was removed by a Buchner funnel. After removal of the solvent, the residue was dissolved in ethyl acetate (15.0 mL). Water (15.0 mL) was added to the resulting solution, the organic layer was separated, and the aqueous layer was extracted with ethyl acetate (15.0 mL × 2). The organic solutions were combined and dried over anhydrous Na_2SO_4. After removal of the solvent, the residue was submitted to column chromatography on silica gel (200–300 mesh) using petroleum ether and ethyl acetate (10/1 in *v*/*v*) as eluents to give **3f** (210.4 mg, 77% yield) as a yellowish gel. ^{1}H NMR (400 MHz, $CDCl_3$): δ 5.20 (s, 1H, H-12), 4.18 (m, 2H, -O*CH*$_2$C-), 3.76 (m, 2H, -S*CH*$_2$), 3.52 (m, 4H, 2 × -N*CH*$_2$), 3.10 (m, 1H, H-3), 2.77 (d, *J* = 11.0 Hz, 1H, H-18), 2.26 (m, 2H, -*CH*$_2$), 2.09 (m, 1H, -*OH*), 1.84 (m, 3H, H-22, -*CH*, -*CH*$_2$), 1.52 (m, 8H, 4 × -*CH*$_2$), 1.44 (m, 5H, H-22, -*CH*, 2 × -*CH*$_2$), 1.30 (m, 8H, 4 × -*CH*$_2$), 1.18 (m, 4H, 2 × -*CH*$_2$), 1.07 (s, 1H, H-9), 1.04 (s, 3H, -*CH*$_3$), 0.95 (s, 1H, H-5), 0.88 (s, 3H, -*CH*$_3$), 0.83 (s, 3H, -*CH*$_3$), 0.80 (s, 6H, 2 × -*CH*$_3$), 0.67 (s, 3H, -*CH*$_3$), 0.64 (s, 3H, -*CH*$_3$). ^{13}C NMR (100 MHz, $CDCl_3$): δ 192.3 (-CS$_2$), 177.3 (C-28), 143.5 (C-13), 122.5 (C-12), 78.6 (C-3), 62.5 (-CO-), 58.9 (2 × -CH$_2$), 55.2 (C-5), 54.5 (2 × -CH$_2$), 47.5 (C-9), 46.6 (C-17), 45.7 (C-19), 41.6 (C-14), 41.2 (C-18), 39.3 (C-8), 38.7 (C-1), 37.6 (C-4), 36.9 (C-10), 35.8 (-CS), 34.9 (2 × -CH$_2$), 33.8 (C-29), 33.1 (C-22), 32.7 (C-21), 32.3 (C-7), 30.6 (C-20), 28.1 (C-15), 27.7 (C-23), 27.1 (C-27), 26.9 (C-30), 25.9 (C-2), 25.6 (2 × -CH$_2$), 23.6 (C-11), 22.6 (C-16), 18.3 (C-6), 17.1 (C-26), 15.7 (C-24), 15.3 (C-25). HRMS (ESI): *m*/*z* calculated for $C_{41}H_{65}NO_3S_2$ [M+H]$^+$: 684.4484. Found: 684.4430.

[2-((isoindoline-2-carbonothioyl)thio)ethyl] 3-hydroxy-12-en-28-oic acid (**3g**). To a mixture of CS_2 (1.8 mmol, 108 μL), anhydrous K_3PO_4 (0.8 mmol, 169.1 mg), and THF (8.0 mL), isoindoline (1.0 mmol, 113 μL) was slowly added at 0 °C, and the reaction mixture was then stirred at 0 °C for 0.5 h. Another THF solution (4.0 mL) of **2** (0.4 mmol, 226.4 mg) was added dropwise to the resulting mixture. The reaction mixture was stirred for 12 h at room temperature, then quenched with ice water (15.0 mL), and the insoluble material was removed by a Buchner funnel. After removal of the solvent, the residue was dissolved in ethyl acetate (15.0 mL). Water (15.0 mL) was added to the resulting solution, the organic layer was separated, and the aqueous layer was extracted with ethyl acetate (15.0 mL × 2). The organic solutions were combined and dried over anhydrous Na_2SO_4. After removal of the solvent, the residue was submitted to column chromatography on silica gel (200–300 mesh) using petroleum ether and ethyl acetate (10/1 in *v*/*v*) as eluents to give **3g** (243.9 mg, 90% yield) as a yellowish solid. ^{1}H NMR (400 MHz, $CDCl_3$): δ 7.31 (m, 4H, Ar-*H*), 5.30 (t, *J* = 3.3 Hz, 1H, H-12), 5.20 (s, 2H, -OCH_2C-), 4.99 (s, 2H, -NCH_2), 4.32 (m, 2H, -NCH_2), 3.66 (m, 2H, -SCH_2), 3.19 (m, 1H, H-3), 2.95 (m, 1H, -O*H*), 2.88 (dd, *J* = 13.7, 4.0 Hz, 1H, H-18), 1.85 (m, 2H, -CH_2), 1.69 (m, 3H, H-22, -C*H*, -CH_2), 1.54 (m, 6H, 3 × -CH_2), 1.42 (m, 3H, H-22, -C*H*, -CH_2), 1.23 (m, 6H, 3 × -CH_2), 1.17 (t, *J* = 4.4 Hz, 1H, H-9), 1.12 (s, 3H, -CH_3), 1.04 (s, 1H, H-5), 0.95 (s, 3H, -CH_3), 0.93 (s, 3H, -CH_3), 0.90 (s, 3H, -CH_3), 0.86 (s, 3H, -CH_3), 0.74 (s, 3H, -CH_3), 0.72 (s, 3H, -CH_3). ^{13}C NMR (100 MHz, $CDCl_3$): δ 192.7 (-CS_2), 177.5 (C-28), 143.6 (C-13), 135.2 (*Ph*), 134.9 (*Ph*), 128.1 (*Ph*), 127.9 (*Ph*), 122.8 (*Ph*), 122.7 (*Ph*), 122.5 (C-12), 78.9 (C-3), 62.3 (-CO-), 60.5 (-NCH_2), 55.7 (-NCH_2), 55.1 (C-5), 47.5 (C-9), 46.7 (C-17), 45.8 (C-19), 41.6 (C-14), 41.3 (C-18), 39.3 (C-8), 38.7 (C-1), 38.4 (C-4), 37.0 (C-10), 35.3 (-CS), 33.8 (C-29), 33.1 (C-22), 32.7 (C-21), 32.4 (C-7), 30.7 (C-20), 28.1 (C-15), 27.7 (C-23), 27.1 (C-27), 25.9 (C-30), 23.6 (C-2), 23.4 (C-11), 22.9 (C-16), 18.2 (C-6), 17.1 (C-26), 15.5 (C-24), 15.3 (C-25). HRMS (ESI): *m*/*z* calculated for C41H59NO3S2 [M+H]+: 678.4015. Found: 678.3996.

[2-((4-methylpiperidine-1-carbonothioyl)thio)ethyl] 3-hydroxy-12-en-28-oic acid (**3h**). To a mixture of CS_2 (1.8 mmol, 108 μL), anhydrous K_3PO_4 (0.8 mmol, 169.1 mg), and THF (8.0 mL), 4-methylpiperidine (1.0 mmol, 100 μL) was slowly added at 0 °C, and the reaction mixture was then stirred at 0 °C for 0.5 h. Another THF solution (4.0 mL) of **2** (0.4 mmol, 224.6 mg) was added dropwise to the resulting mixture. The reaction mixture was stirred for 12 h at room temperature, then quenched with ice water (15.0 mL), and the insoluble material was removed by a Buchner funnel. After removal of the solvent, the residue was dissolved in ethyl acetate (15.0 mL). Water (15.0 mL) was added to the resulting solution, the organic layer was separated, and the aqueous layer was extracted with ethyl acetate (15.0 mL × 2). The organic solutions were combined and dried over anhydrous Na_2SO_4. After removal of the solvent, the residue was submitted to column chromatography on silica gel (200–300 mesh) using petroleum ether and ethyl acetate (10/1 in *v*/*v*) as eluents to give **3h** (199.8 mg, 76% yield) as a white solid. ^{1}H NMR (400 MHz, $CDCl_3$): δ 5.23 (s, 1H, H-12), 4.21 (m, 2H, -OCH_2C-), 3.54 (m, 2H, -SCH_2), 3.10 (m, 3H, -NCH_2, H-3), 2.80 (d, *J* = 12.2 Hz, 1H, H-18), 1.89 (m, 1H, -O*H*), 1.80 (m, 2H, -NCH_2), 1.70 (m, 3H, H-22, -C*H*, -CH_2), 1.58 (m, 7H, -**C*H***CH_3, 3 × -CH_2), 1.46 (m, 4H, 2 × -CH_2), 1.33 (m, 5H, H-22, -C*H*, 2 × -CH_2), 1.20 (m, 6H, 3 × -CH_2), 1.10 (s, 1H, H-9), 1.06 (s, 3H, -CH_3), 0.98 (s, 1H, H-5), 0.92 (s, 6H, 2 × -CH_3), 0.86 (s, 3H, -CH_3), 0.83 (s, 6H, 2 × -CH_3), 0.71 (s, 3H, -CH_3), 0.67 (s, 3H, -CH_3). ^{13}C NMR (100 MHz, $CDCl_3$): δ 194.8 (-CS_2), 177.5 (C-28), 143.7 (C-13), 122.6 (C-12), 79.1 (C-3), 62.5 (-CO-), 55.3 (C-5), 53.6 (-NCH_2, -NCH_2), 47.7 (C-9), 46.8 (C-17), 45.9 (C-19), 41.8 (C-14), 41.4 (C-18), 39.4 (C-8), 38.8 (C-1), 38.5 (C-4), 37.1 (C-10), 35.8 (-CS), 34.0 (C-29), 33.2 (-NCH_2*C*H_2, -NCH_2*C*H_2), 33.1 (C-22), 32.8 (C-21), 32.5 (C-7), 31.0 (-*C*CH_3), 30.8 (C-20), 28.2 (C-15), 27.8 (C-23), 27.3 (C-27), 26.0 (C-30), 23.7 (C-2), 23.5 (C-11), 23.0 (C-16), 21.4 (-CH_3), 18.4 (C-6), 17.2 (C-26), 15.7 (C-24), 15.4 (C-25). HRMS (ESI): *m*/*z* calculated for $C_{39}H_{63}NO_3S_2$ $[M+H]^+$: 658.4328. Found: 658.4275.

[2-((4-hydroxypiperidine-1-carbonothioyl)thio)ethyl] 3-hydroxy-12-en-28-oic acid (**3i**). To a mixture of CS_2 (1.8 mmol, 108 μL), anhydrous K_3PO_4 (0.8 mmol, 169.1 mg), and THF (8.0 mL), 4-hydroxypiperidine (1.0 mmol, 103.5 mg) was slowly added at 0 °C, and the reaction mixture was then stirred at 0 °C for 0.5 h. Another THF solution (4.0 mL) of **2**

(0.4 mmol, 225.4 mg) was added dropwise to the resulting mixture. The reaction mixture was stirred for 12 h at room temperature, then quenched with ice water (15.0 mL), and the insoluble material was removed by a Buchner funnel. After removal of the solvent, the residue was dissolved in ethyl acetate (15.0 mL). Water (15.0 mL) was added to the resulting solution, the organic layer was separated, and the aqueous layer was extracted with ethyl acetate (15.0 mL × 2). The organic solutions were combined and dried over anhydrous Na_2SO_4. After removal of the solvent, the residue was submitted to column chromatography on silica gel (200–300 mesh) using petroleum ether and ethyl acetate (1/1 in v/v) as eluents to give **3i** (184.6 mg, 70% yield) as a yellow gel. ^{1}H NMR (400 MHz, $CDCl_3$): δ 5.50 (s, 1H, -*OH*), 5.30 (s, 1H, H-12), 4.60 (s, 1H, -C*H*OH), 4.28 (m, 2H, -SC*H*$_2$), 3.61 (m, 2H, -NC*H*$_2$), 3.21 (m, 1H, H-3), 3.08 (s, 2H, -NC*H*$_2$), 2.87 (d, *J* = 11.0 Hz, 1H, H-18), 2.00 (m, 1H, -*OH*), 1.87 (s, 2H, -C*H*$_2$), 1.76 (m, 3H, H-22, -C*H*, -C*H*$_2$), 1.62 (m, 6H, 3 × -C*H*$_2$), 1.53 (m, 5H, H-22, -C*H*, 2 × -C*H*$_2$), 1.42 (m, 4H, 2 × -C*H*$_2$), 1.27 (m, 6H, 3 × -C*H*$_2$), 1.16 (t, *J* = 3.7 Hz, 1H, H-9), 1.13 (s, 3H, -C*H*$_3$), 1.04 (s, 1H, H-5), 0.98 (s, 3H, -C*H*$_3$), 0.93 (s, 3H, -C*H*$_3$), 0.90 (s, 6H, 2 × -C*H*$_3$), 0.77 (s, 3H, -C*H*$_3$), 0.74 (s, 3H, -C*H*$_3$). ^{13}C NMR (100 MHz, $CDCl_3$): δ 194.6 (-CS_2), 177.4 (C-28), 143.6 (C-13), 122.5 (C-12), 78.9 (C-3), 62.4 (-CO-), 55.2 (C-5), 47.6 (C-9), 46.7 (C-17), 45.8 (C-19), 41.7 (C-14), 41.3 (C-18), 39.4 (C-8), 38.8 (C-1), 38.5 (C-4), 37.0 (C-10), 35.7 (-CS), 33.9 (C-29), 33.1 (C-22), 32.8 (C-21), 32.4 (C-7), 31.0 (-COH), 30.7 (C-20), 28.1 (C-15), 27.7 (C-23), 27.2 (C-27), 26.9 (-NCH$_2$, -NCH$_2$), 25.9 (C-30), 23.7 (C-2), 23.4 (C-11), 22.9 (C-16), 21.3 (-NCH$_2$CH$_2$, -NCH$_2$CH$_2$), 18.4 (C-6), 17.1 (C-26), 15.6 (C-24), 15.4 (C-25). HRMS (ESI): m/z calculated for $C_{38}H_{61}NO_4S_2$ [M+H]$^+$: 660.4120. Found: 660.4080.

[2-((4-(hydroxymethyl)piperidine-1-carbonothioyl)thio)-ethyl] 3-hydroxy-12-en-28-oic acid (**3j**). To a mixture of CS_2 (1.8 mmol, 108 µL), anhydrous K_3PO_4 (0.8 mmol, 169.1 mg), and THF (8.0 mL), 4-(hydroxymethyl)piperidine (1.0 mmol, 115.3 mg) was slowly added at 0 °C, and the reaction mixture was then stirred at 0 °C for 0.5 h. Another THF solution (4.0 mL) of **2** (0.4 mmol, 225.9 mg) was added dropwise to the resulting mixture. The reaction mixture was stirred for 12 h at room temperature, then quenched with ice water (15.0 mL), and the insoluble material was removed by a Buchner funnel. After removal of the solvent, the residue was dissolved in ethyl acetate (15.0 mL). Water (15.0 mL) was added to the resulting solution, the organic layer was separated, and the aqueous layer was extracted with ethyl acetate (15.0 mL × 2). The organic solutions were combined and dried over anhydrous Na_2SO_4. After removal of the solvent, the residue was submitted to column chromatography on silica gel (200–300 mesh) using petroleum ether and ethyl acetate (2/1 in v/v) as eluents to give **3j** (199.3 mg, 74% yield) as a yellow gel. ^{1}H NMR (400 MHz, $CDCl_3$): δ 5.57 (s, 1H, -C*H*CH$_2$OH), 5.31 (s, 1H, H-12), 4.64 (s, 1H, -C*H*OH), 4.26 (m, 2H, -OC*H*$_2$C-), 3.60 (m, 2H, -SC*H*$_2$), 3.51 (m, 2H, -NC*H*$_2$), 3.21 (m, 2H, -NC*H*$_2$), 3.13 (m, 1H, H-3), 2.86 (dd, *J* = 13.5, 3.7 Hz, 1H, H-18), 1.96 (m, 1H, -*OH*), 1.91 (m, 2H, -C*H*$_2$), 1.87 (m, 3H, -*OH*, -C*H*$_2$), 1.63 (m, 6H, 3 × -C*H*$_2$), 1.52 (m, 5H, -C*H*OH, 2 × -C*H*$_2$), 1.38 (m, 6H, 3 × -C*H*$_2$), 1.27 (m, 4H, 2 × -C*H*$_2$), 1.16 (t, *J* = 4.4 Hz, 1H, H-9), 1.13 (s, 3H, -C*H*$_3$), 1.05 (s, 1H, H-5), 0.98 (s, 3H, -C*H*$_3$), 0.93 (s, 3H, -C*H*$_3$), 0.90 (s, 6H, 2 × -C*H*$_3$), 0.77 (s, 3H, -C*H*$_3$), 0.73 (s, 3H, -C*H*$_3$). ^{13}C NMR (100 MHz, $CDCl_3$): δ 194.8 (-CS_2), 177.5 (C-28), 143.6 (C-13), 122.5 (C-12), 78.9 (C-3), 66.5 (-CH$_2$OH), 62.4 (-CO-), 55.2 (C-5), 47.6 (C-9), 46.7 (C-17), 45.8 (C-19), 41.6 (C-14), 41.3 (C-18), 39.3 (C-8), 38.7 (C-1), 38.5 (C-4), 38.4 (-NCH$_2$, -NCH$_2$), 37.0 (C-10), 36.6 (-NCH$_2$CH$_2$, -NCH$_2$CH$_2$), 35.6 (-CS), 33.8 (C-29), 33.1 (C-22), 32.7 (C-21), 32.4 (C-7), 31.5 (-CCH$_2$OH), 30.7 (C-20), 28.1 (C-15), 27.7 (C-23), 27.1 (C-27), 25.9 (C-30), 23.6 (C-2), 23.4 (C-11), 22.9 (C-16), 18.3 (C-6), 17.1 (C-26), 15.6 (C-24), 15.3 (C-25). HRMS (ESI): m/z calculated for $C_{39}H_{63}NO_4S_2$ [M+H]$^+$: 674.4277. Found: 674.4230.

[2-((2-(2-hydroxyethyl)piperidine-1-carbonothioyl)thio)ethyl] 3-hydroxy-12-en-28-oic acid (**3k**). To a mixture of CS_2 (1.8 mmol, 108 µL), anhydrous K_3PO_4 (0.8 mmol, 169.1 mg), and THF (8.0 mL), 2-(2-hydroxyethyl)piperidine (1.0 mmol, 128.1 mg) was slowly added at 0 °C, and the reaction mixture was then stirred at 0 °C for 0.5 h. Another THF solution (4.0 mL) of **2** (0.4 mmol, 225.6 mg) was added dropwise to the resulting mixture. The reaction mixture was stirred for 12 h at room temperature, then quenched with ice water (15.0 mL), and the insoluble material was removed by a Buchner funnel. After removal of the solvent, the residue was dissolved in ethyl acetate (15.0 mL). Water (15.0 mL) was added to the resulting solution, the organic layer was separated, and the aqueous layer was extracted with ethyl acetate (15.0 mL × 2). The organic solutions were combined and dried over anhydrous Na_2SO_4. After removal of the solvent, the residue was submitted to column chromatography on silica gel (200–300 mesh) using petroleum ether and ethyl acetate (2/1 in v/v) as eluents to give **3k** (200.7 mg, 73% yield) as a yellowish gel. ^{1}H NMR (400 MHz, $CDCl_3$): δ 5.93 (m, 1H, -O*H*), 5.30 (t, *J* = 3.3 Hz, 1H, H-12), 4.55 (m, 1H, -C*H*OH), 4.28 (m, 2H, -OCH_2C-), 3.62 (m, 3H, -C*H*OH, -SCH_2), 3.39 (m, 1H, H-3), 3.16 (m, 3H, -NCH_2, -NC*H*), 2.87 (dd, *J* = 13.7, 3.9 Hz, 1H, H-18), 2.14 (m, 1H, -O*H*), 1.95 (m, 2H, -CH_2), 1.87 (m, 3H, -CHCH_2CH$_2$OH, H-22, -C*H*), 1.79 (m, 1H, H-22, -C*H*), 1.70 (m, 6H, 3 × -CH_2), 1.59 (m, 6H, 3 × -CH_2), 1.53 (m, 4H, 2 × -CH_2), 1.38 (m, 6H, 3 × -CH_2), 1.17 (t, *J* = 4.3 Hz, 1H, H-9), 1.13 (s, 3H, -CH_3), 1.05 (s, 1H, H-5), 0.98 (s, 3H, -CH_3), 0.93 (s, 3H, -CH_3), 0.90 (s, 6H, 2 × -CH_3), 0.77 (s, 3H, -CH_3), 0.74 (s, 3H, -CH_3). ^{13}C NMR (100 MHz, $CDCl_3$): δ 196.4 (-CS_2), 177.4 (C-28), 143.5 (C-13), 122.5 (C-12), 78.8 (C-3), 58.1 (-CO-), 56.0 (-NCH), 55.2 (C-5), 47.6 (C-9), 46.7 (C-17), 46.0 (C-19), 45.8 (-CH_2OH), 41.6 (C-14), 41.3 (C-18), 39.3 (C-8), 38.7 (C-1), 38.5 (C-4), 37.0 (C-10), 35.6 (-CS), 33.8 (C-29), 33.1 (C-22), 32.9 (C-21), 32.7 (C-7), 32.4 (-NCH_2), 30.7 (C-20), 29.3 (-CH_2CH$_2$OH), 28.1 (C-15), 27.7 (C-23), 27.1 (C-27), 25.9 (C-30), 25.8 (-NCHCH_2), 23.6 (C-2), 23.4 (C-11), 22.9 (C-16), 19.2 (-NCH$_2$CH$_2$$CH_2$), 18.3 (C-6), 17.1 (C-26), 17.1 (-NCH$_2$$CH_2$), 15.6 (C-24), 15.3 (C-25). HRMS (ESI): m/z calculated for $C_{40}H_{65}NO_4S_2$ $[M+H]^+$: 688.4433. Found: 688.4418.

[2-((4-(2-hydroxyethyl)piperidine-1-carbonothioyl)thio)ethyl] 3-hydroxy-12-en-28-oic acid (**3l**). To a mixture of CS_2 (1.8 mmol, 108 μL), anhydrous K_3PO_4 (0.8 mmol, 169.1 mg), and THF (8.0 mL), 4-(2-hydroxyethyl)piperidine (1.0 mmol, 130.8 mg) was slowly added at 0 °C, and the reaction mixture was then stirred at 0 °C for 0.5 h. Another THF solution (4.0 mL) of **2** (0.4 mmol, 226.4 mg) was added dropwise to the resulting mixture. The reaction mixture was stirred for 12 h at room temperature, then quenched with ice water (15.0 mL), and the insoluble material was removed by a Buchner funnel. After removal of the solvent, the residue was dissolved in ethyl acetate (15.0 mL). Water (15.0 mL) was added to the resulting solution, the organic layer was separated, and the aqueous layer was extracted with ethyl acetate (15.0 mL × 2). The organic solutions were combined and dried over anhydrous Na_2SO_4. After removal of the solvent, the residue was submitted to column chromatography on silica gel (200–300 mesh) using petroleum ether and ethyl acetate (2/1 in v/v) as eluents to give **3l** (195.2 mg, 71% yield) as a yellowish gel. ^{1}H NMR (400 MHz, $CDCl_3$): δ 5.23 (t, *J* = 3.3 Hz, 1H, H-12), 4.53 (m, 1H, -O*H*), 4.21 (m, 2H, -OCH_2C-), 3.95 (m, 2H, -SCH_2), 3.75 (m, 2H, -NCH_2), 3.53 (m, 2H, -NCH_2), 3.14 (m, 1H, H-3), 2.79 (dd, *J* = 13.6, 3.7 Hz, 1H, H-18), 2.07 (m, 2H, -CH_2), 1.90 (m, 1H, -O*H*), 1.81 (m, 3H, -CH_2, -NCH$_2$CH$_2$C*H*), 1.61 (m, 2H, -CH_2), 1.56 (m, 6H, 3 × -CH_2), 1.45 (m, 4H, 2 × -CH_2), 1.25 (m, 6H, 3 × -CH_2), 1.10 (t, *J* = 4.6 Hz, 1H, H-9), 1.06 (s, 3H, -CH_3), 0.98 (s, 1H, H-5), 0.91 (s, 3H, -CH_3), 0.86 (s, 3H, -CH_3), 0.83 (s, 6H, 2 × -CH_3), 0.70 (s, 3H, -CH_3), 0.67 (s, 3H, -CH_3). ^{13}C NMR (100 MHz, $CDCl_3$): δ 194.5 (-CS_2), 177.5 (C-28), 143.5 (C-13), 122.5 (C-12), 77.0 (C-3), 62.4 (-CO-), 60.4 (-CH_2OH), 59.6 (-NCH_2), 55.2 (C-5), 52.3 (-NCH_2), 50.4 (-CH_2CH$_2$OH), 47.5 (C-9), 46.7 (C-17), 45.7 (C-19), 41.6 (C-14), 41.2 (C-18), 39.3 (C-8), 38.7 (C-1), 38.5 (C-4), 36.9 (C-10), 35.6 (-CS), 33.8 (C-29), 33.1 (C-22), 32.7 (C-21), 32.4 (C-7), 31.6 (-NCH$_2$$CH_2$), 30.7 (C-20), 28.1 (C-15), 27.6 (C-23), 27.1 (C-27), 25.9 (C-30), 23.6 (C-2), 23.4 (C-11), 22.9 (C-16), 21.1 (-*C*HCH$_2$CH$_2$OH), 18.3 (C-6), 17.1 (C-26), 15.7 (C-24), 15.3 (C-25). HRMS (ESI): m/z calculated for $C_{40}H_{65}NO_4S_2$ $[M+H]^+$: 688.4433. Found: 688.4366.

[2-((4-phenylpiperidine-1-carbonothioyl)thio)ethyl] 3-hydroxy-12-en-28-oic acid (**3m**). To a mixture of CS_2 (1.8 mmol, 108 μL), anhydrous K_3PO_4 (0.8 mmol, 169.1 mg), and THF (8.0 mL), 4-phenylpiperidine (1.0 mmol, 164.7 mg) was slowly added at 0 °C, and the reaction mixture was then stirred at 0 °C for 0.5 h. Another THF solution (4.0 mL) of **2** (0.4 mmol, 225.2 mg) was added dropwise to the resulting mixture. The reaction mixture was stirred for 12 h at room temperature, then quenched with ice water (15.0 mL), and the insoluble material was removed by a Buchner funnel. After removal of the solvent, the residue was dissolved in ethyl acetate (15.0 mL). Water (15.0 mL) was added to the resulting solution, the organic layer was separated, and the aqueous layer was extracted with ethyl acetate (15.0 mL × 2). The organic solutions were combined and dried over anhydrous Na_2SO_4. After removal of the solvent, the residue was submitted to column chromatography on silica gel (200–300 mesh) using petroleum ether and ethyl acetate (10/1 in *v*/*v*) as eluents to give **3m** (253.2 mg, 88% yield) as a yellowish gel. ^1H NMR (400 MHz, $CDCl_3$): δ 7.31 (m, 2H, Ar-*H*), 7.21 (m, 3H, Ar-*H*), 5.30 (t, *J* = 3.3 Hz, 1H, H-12), 4.32 (m, 2H, -OCH_2C-), 3.63 (m, 2H, -SCH_2), 3.20 (m, 3H, H-3, -NCH_2), 2.88 (m, 2H, H-18, -NCH_2CH_2*CH*), 1.99 (m, 1H, -*OH*), 1.96 (m, 2H, -CH_2), 1.88 (m, 3H, H-22, -*CH*, -CH_2), 1.64 (m, 8H, 2 × -NCH_2, 2 × -CH_2), 1.51 (m, 3H, H-22, -*CH*, -CH_2), 1.44 (m, 4H, 2 × -NCH_2), 1.28 (m, 6H, 3 × -CH_2), 1.17 (t, *J* = 3.6 Hz, 1H, H-9), 1.13 (s, 3H, -CH_3), 1.05 (s, 1H, H-5), 0.97 (s, 3H, -CH_3), 0.93 (s, 3H, -CH_3), 0.90 (s, 3H, -CH_3), 0.89 (s, 3H, -CH_3), 0.76 (s, 3H, -CH_3), 0.75 (s, 3H, -CH_3). ^{13}C NMR (100 MHz, $CDCl_3$): δ 195.1 (-CS_2), 177.5 (C-28), 144.3 (*Ph*), 143.6 (C-13), 128.7 (*Ph*), 126.8 (*Ph*), 122.6 (C-12), 78.9 (C-3), 62.4 (-CO-), 55.2 (C-5), 47.6 (C-9), 46.8 (C-17), 45.8 (C-19), 42.6 (-NCH_2), 41.7 (C-14), 41.3 (C-18), 39.4 (C-8), 38.8 (C-1), 38.5 (C-4), 37.0 (C-10), 35.9 (-CS), 34.7 (-NCH_2CH_2CH), 33.9 (C-29), 33.2 (C-22), 32.8 (C-21), 32.4 (C-7), 30.7 (C-20), 28.2 (C-15), 27.7 (C-23), 27.2 (C-27), 27.0 (-NCH_2CH_2), 25.9 (C-30), 25.3 (-NCH_2CH_2), 23.7 (C-2), 23.5 (C-11), 23.0 (C-16), 18.4 (C-6), 17.2 (C-26), 15.7 (C-24), 15.4 (C-25). HRMS (ESI): *m*/*z* calculated for $C_{44}H_{65}NO_3S_2$ $[M+H]^+$: 720.4484. Found: 720.4450.

[2-((4-methylpiperazine-1-carbonothioyl)thio)ethyl] 3-hydroxy-12-en-28-oic acid (**3n**). To a mixture of CS_2 (1.8 mmol, 108 μL), anhydrous K_3PO_4 (0.8 mmol, 169.1 mg), and THF (8.0 mL), 4-methylpiperazine (1.0 mmol, 112 μL) was slowly added at 0 °C, and the reaction mixture was then stirred at 0 °C for 0.5 h. Another THF solution (4.0 mL) of **2** (0.4 mmol, 225.0 mg) was added dropwise to the resulting mixture. The reaction mixture was stirred for 12 h at room temperature, then quenched with ice water (15.0 mL), and the insoluble material was removed by a Buchner funnel. After removal of the solvent, the residue was dissolved in ethyl acetate (15.0 mL). Water (15.0 mL) was added to the resulting solution, the organic layer was separated, and the aqueous layer was extracted with ethyl acetate (15.0 mL × 2). The organic solutions were combined and dried over anhydrous Na_2SO_4. After removal of the solvent, the residue was submitted to column chromatography on silica gel (200–300 mesh) using petroleum ether and ethyl acetate (1/4 in *v*/*v*) as eluents to give **3n** (234.3 mg, 89% yield) as a yellowish gel. ^1H NMR (400 MHz, $CDCl_3$): 5.30 (t, *J* = 3.3 Hz, 1H, H-12), 4.36 (s, 2H, -OCH_2C-), 4.28 (m, 2H, -NCH_2), 3.96 (s, 2H, -NCH_2), 3.61 (m, 2H, -SCH_2), 3.21 (m, 1H, H-3), 2.87 (dd, *J* = 13.6, 4.0 Hz, 1H, H-18), 2.50 (s, 4H, 2 × -NCH_2), 2.34 (s, 3H, -CH_3), 1.97 (m, 1H, -*OH*), 1.87 (m, 2H, -CH_2), 1.64 (m, 6H, 3 × -CH_2), 1.53 (m, 3H, H-22, -*CH*, -CH_2), 1.40 (m, 3H, H-22, -*CH*, -CH_2), 1.27 (m, 6H, 3 × -CH_2), 1.16 (t, *J* = 4.3 Hz, 1H, H-9), 1.13 (s, 3H, -CH_3), 1.05 (s, 1H, H-5), 0.98 (s, 3H, -CH_3), 0.93 (s, 3H, -CH_3), 0.90 (s, 6H, 2 × -CH_3), 0.78 (s, 3H, -CH_3), 0.73 (s, 3H, -CH_3). ^{13}C NMR (100 MHz, $CDCl_3$): δ 195.9 (-CS_2), 177.4 (C-28), 143.6 (C-13), 122.5 (C-12), 78.9 (C-3), 62.3 (-CO-), 55.2 (C-5), 54.4 (-NCH_2), 47.6 (C-9), 46.7 (C-17), 46.4 (-CH_2CH_2), 45.8 (C-19), 45.6 (-NCH_3), 41.7 (C-14), 41.3 (C-18), 39.3 (C-8), 38.7 (C-1), 38.4 (C-4), 37.0 (C-10), 35.6 (-CS), 33.8 (C-29), 33.1 (C-22), 32.7 (C-21), 32.4 (C-7), 30.7 (C-20), 28.1 (C-15), 27.7 (C-23), 27.2 (C-27), 25.9 (C-30), 23.6 (C-2), 23.4 (C-11), 22.9 (C-16), 18.3 (C-6), 17.1 (C-26), 15.6 (C-24), 15.3 (C-25). HRMS (ESI): *m*/*z* calculated for $C_{38}H_{62}N_2O_3S_2$ $[M+H]^+$: 659.4280. Found: 659.4239.

[2-((4-(2-hydroxyethyl)piperazine-1-carbonothioyl)thio)ethyl] 3-hydroxy-12-en-28-oic acid (**3o**). To a mixture of CS_2 (1.8 mmol, 108 μL), anhydrous K_3PO_4 (0.8 mmol, 169.1 mg), and THF (8.0 mL), 4-(2-hydroxyethyl)piperazine (1.0 mmol, 123 μL) was slowly added at 0 °C, and the reaction mixture was then stirred at 0 °C for 0.5 h. Another THF solution (4.0 mL) of **2** (0.4 mmol, 224.9 mg) was added dropwise to the resulting mixture. The reaction mixture was stirred for 12 h at room temperature, then quenched with ice water (15.0 mL), and the insoluble material was removed by a Buchner funnel. After removal of the solvent, the residue was dissolved in ethyl acetate (15.0 mL). Water (15.0 mL) was added to the resulting solution, the organic layer was separated, and the aqueous layer was extracted with ethyl acetate (15.0 mL × 2). The organic solutions were combined and dried over anhydrous Na_2SO_4. After removal of the solvent, the residue was submitted to column chromatography on silica gel (200–300 mesh) using petroleum ether and ethyl acetate (1/5 in *v*/*v*) as eluents to give **3o** (195.5 mg, 71% yield) as a yellowish gel. ^{1}H NMR (400 MHz, $CDCl_3$): δ 5.30 (t, *J* = 3.1 Hz, 1H, H-12), 4.33 (s, 1H, -NC*H*), 4.28 (m, 2H, -OC*H*$_2$C-), 3.99 (s, 1H, -NC*H*), 3.69 (m, 2H, -NC*H*$_2$), 3.61 (m, 2H, -SC*H*$_2$), 3.21 (m, 1H, H-3), 2.86 (dd, *J* = 13.7, 4.1 Hz, 1H, H-18), 2.63 (t, *J* = 5.2 Hz, 4H, 2 × -NC*H*$_2$), 2.61 (s, 1H, -O*H*), 1.97 (m, 1H, -O*H*), 1.88 (m, 2H, -C*H*$_2$), 1.66 (m, 2H, -C*H*$_2$), 1.60 (m, 5H, H-22, -C*H*, 2 × -C*H*$_2$), 1.53 (m, 4H, 2 × -C*H*$_2$), 1.43 (m, 3H, H-22, -C*H*, -C*H*$_2$), 1.33 (m, 4H, 2 × -C*H*$_2$), 1.27 (m, 4H, 2 × -C*H*$_2$), 1.16 (t, *J* = 4.4 Hz, 1H, H-9), 1.13 (s, 3H, -C*H*$_3$), 1.05 (s, 1H, H-5), 0.98 (s, 3H, -C*H*$_3$), 0.93 (s, 3H, -C*H*$_3$), 0.90 (s, 6H, 2 × -C*H*$_3$), 0.77 (s, 3H, -C*H*$_3$), 0.73 (s, 3H, -C*H*$_3$). ^{13}C NMR (100 MHz, $CDCl_3$): δ 196.1 (-CS_2), 177.5 (C-28), 143.6 (C-13), 122.5 (C-12), 79.0 (C-3), 62.3 (-CO-), 59.1 (-N*C*H$_2$CH$_2$OH), 57.9 (-NCH$_2$*C*H$_2$OH), 55.2 (C-5), 52.3 (-N*C*H$_2$CH$_2$), 47.6 (C-9), 46.8 (C-17), 45.8 (C-19), 41.7 (C-14), 41.3 (C-18), 39.4 (C-8), 38.8 (C-1), 38.5 (C-4), 37.0 (C-10), 35.7 (-CS), 33.9 (C-29), 33.1 (C-22), 32.4 (C-21), 31.5 (C-7), 30.7(-NCH$_2$*C*H$_2$), 30.2 (C-20), 28.1 (C-15), 27.7 (C-23), 27.2 (C-27), 25.9 (C-30), 23.7 (C-2), 23.4 (C-11), 22.9 (C-16), 18.4 (C-6), 17.1 (C-26), 15.6 (C-24), 15.4 (C-25). HRMS (ESI): *m*/*z* calculated for $C_{39}H_{64}N_2O_4S_2$ [M+H]$^+$: 689.4386. Found: 689.4336.

[2-((4-phenylpiperazine-1-carbonothioyl)thio)ethyl] 3-hydroxy-12-en-28-oic acid (**3p**). To a mixture of CS_2 (1.8 mmol, 108 μL), anhydrous K_3PO_4 (0.8 mmol, 169.1 mg), and THF (8.0 mL), 4-phenylpiperazine (1.0 mmol, 150 μL) was slowly added at 0 °C, and the reaction mixture was then stirred at 0 °C for 0.5 h. Another THF solution (4.0 mL) of **2** (0.4 mmol, 226.7 mg) was added dropwise to the resulting mixture. The reaction mixture was stirred for 12 h at room temperature, then quenched with ice water (15.0 mL), and the insoluble material was removed by a Buchner funnel. After removal of the solvent, the residue was dissolved in ethyl acetate (15.0 mL). Water (15.0 mL) was added to the resulting solution, the organic layer was separated, and the aqueous layer was extracted with ethyl acetate (15.0 mL × 2). The organic solutions were combined and dried over anhydrous Na_2SO_4. After removal of the solvent, the residue was submitted to column chromatography on silica gel (200–300 mesh) using petroleum ether and ethyl acetate (1/5 in *v*/*v*) as eluents to give **3p** (247.8 mg, 86% yield) as a yellowish solid. ^{1}H NMR (400 MHz, $CDCl_3$): δ 7.30 (m, 2H, Ar-*H*), 6.93 (m, 3H, Ar-*H*), 5.30 (t, *J* = 3.2 Hz, 1H, H-12), 4.49 (s, 2H, -OC*H*$_2$C-), 4.29 (m, 2H, -NC*H*$_2$), 4.10 (m, 2H, -NC*H*$_2$), 3.64 (m, 2H, -SC*H*$_2$), 3.30 (t, *J* = 4.9 Hz, 4H, 2 × -NC*H*$_2$), 3.20 (m, 1H, H-3), 2.87 (dd, *J* = 13.6, 3.9 Hz, 1H, H-18), 1.97 (m, 1H, -O*H*), 1.88 (m, 2H, -C*H*$_2$), 1.67 (m, 4H, 2 × -C*H*$_2$), 1.58 (m, 4H, 2 × -C*H*$_2$), 1.51 (m, 3H, H-22, -C*H*, -C*H*$_2$), 1.35 (m, 7H, H-22, -C*H*, 3 × -C*H*$_2$), 1.17 (t, *J* = 4.0 Hz, 1H, H-9), 1.13 (s, 3H, -C*H*$_3$), 1.05 (s, 1H, H-5), 0.97 (s, 3H, -C*H*$_3$), 0.93 (s, 3H, -C*H*$_3$), 0.90 (s, 3H, -C*H*$_3$), 0.89 (s, 3H, -C*H*$_3$), 0.76 (s, 3H, -C*H*$_3$), 0.74 (s, 3H, -C*H*$_3$). ^{13}C NMR (100 MHz, $CDCl_3$): δ 196.1 (-CS_2), 177.4 (*Ph*), 150.2 (*Ph*), 143.6 (C-13), 129.3 (*Ph*), 122.5 (C-12), 120.6 (*Ph*), 116.3 (*Ph*), 78.9 (C-3), 62.2 (-CO-), 55.2 (C-5), 48.7 (-NCH$_2$), 48.2 (-NCH$_2$), 47.6 (C-9), 46.7 (C-17), 45.8 (C-19), 41.6 (C-14), 41.3 (C-18), 39.3 (C-8), 38.7 (C-1), 38.4 (C-4), 37.0 (C-10), 35.6 (-CS), 33.8 (C-29), 33.1 (C-22), 32.7 (C-21), 32.4 (C-7), 30.7 (C-20), 28.1 (C-15), 27.7 (C-23), 27.1 (C-27), 25.9 (C-30), 23.6 (C-2), 23.4 (C-11), 22.9 (C-16), 18.3 (C-6), 17.1 (C-26), 15.6 (C-24), 15.3 (C-25). HRMS (ESI): *m*/*z* calculated for $C_{43}H_{64}N_2O_3S_2$ [M+H]$^+$: 721.4437. Found: 721.4411.

[2-((4-(o-tolyl)piperazine-1-carbonothioyl)thio)ethyl] 3-hydroxy-12-en-28-oic acid (**3q**). To a mixture of CS_2 (1.8 mmol, 108 μL), anhydrous K_3PO_4 (0.8 mmol, 169.1 mg), and THF (8.0 mL), 4-(o-tolyl)piperazine (1.0 mmol, 177.9 mg) was slowly added at 0 °C, and the reaction mixture was then stirred at 0 °C for 0.5 h. Another THF solution (4.0 mL) of **2** (0.4 mmol, 225.9 mg) was added dropwise to the resulting mixture. The reaction mixture was stirred for 12 h at room temperature, then quenched with ice water (15.0 mL), and the insoluble material was removed by a Buchner funnel. After removal of the solvent, the residue was dissolved in ethyl acetate (15.0 mL). Water (15.0 mL) was added to the resulting solution, the organic layer was separated, and the aqueous layer was extracted with ethyl acetate (15.0 mL × 2). The organic solutions were combined and dried over anhydrous Na_2SO_4. After removal of the solvent, the residue was submitted to column chromatography on silica gel (200–300 mesh) using petroleum ether and ethyl acetate (10/1 in *v*/*v*) as eluents to give **3q** (246.7 mg, 84% yield) as a yellowish gel. ^{1}H NMR (400 MHz,

$CDCl_3$): δ 7.17 (t, *J* = 7.9 Hz, 1H, Ar-*H*), 6.73 (m, 3H, Ar-*H*), 5.30 (t, *J* = 3.1 Hz, 1H, H-12), 4.46 (s, 2H, -O*CH*$_2$C-), 4.27 (m, 2H, -N*CH*$_2$), 4.10 (s, 2H, -N*CH*$_2$), 3.64 (m, 2H, -S*CH*$_2$), 3.28 (t, *J* = 5.0 Hz, 4H, 2 × -N*CH*$_2$), 3.18 (m, 1H, H-3), 2.87 (dd, *J* = 13.6, 3.8 Hz, 1H, H-18), 2.32 (s, 3H, -*CH*$_3$), 1.97 (m, 1H, -*OH*), 1.87 (m, 2H, -*CH*$_2$), 1.69 (m, 4H, 2 × -*CH*$_2$), 1.58 (m, 5H, H-22, -*CH*, 2 × -*CH*$_2$), 1.51 (m, 3H, H-22, -*CH*, -*CH*$_2$), 1.35 (m, 6H, 3 × -*CH*$_2$), 1.17 (t, *J* = 3.8 Hz, 1H, H-9), 1.13 (s, 3H, -*CH*$_3$), 1.05 (s, 1H, H-5), 0.97 (s, 3H, -*CH*$_3$), 0.93 (s, 3H, -*CH*$_3$), 0.90 (s, 3H, -*CH*$_3$), 0.89 (s, 3H, -*CH*$_3$), 0.76 (s, 3H, -*CH*$_3$), 0.74 (s, 3H, -*CH*$_3$). ^{13}C NMR (100 MHz, $CDCl_3$): δ 195.9 (-CS_2), 177.4 (C-28), 150.2 (*Ph*), 143.5 (C-13), 139.0 (*Ph*), 129.1 (*Ph*), 122.5 (C-12), 121.5 (*Ph*), 117.1 (*Ph*), 113.4 (*Ph*), 78.8 (C-3), 62.3 (-CO-), 55.2 (C-5), 48.8 (-NCH_2), 47.6 (C-9), 46.7 (C-17), 45.8 (C-19), 41.6 (C-14), 41.3 (C-18), 39.3 (C-8), 38.7 (C-1), 38.4 (C-4), 37.0 (C-10), 35.6 (-CS), 33.8 (C-29), 33.1 (C-22), 32.7 (C-21), 32.4 (C-7), 30.7 (C-20), 28.1 (C-15), 27.7 (C-23), 27.1 (C-27), 26.9 (-NCH_2CH_2), 25.9 (C-30), 23.6 (C-2), 23.4 (C-11), 22.9 (C-16), 21.8 (-CH_3), 18.3 (C-6), 17.1 (C-26), 15.6 (C-24), 15.4 (C-25). HRMS (ESI): *m*/*z* calculated for $C_{44}H_{66}N_2O_3S_2$ [M+H]$^+$: 735.4593. Found: 735.4540.

[2-((4-(m-tolyl)piperazine-1-carbonothioyl)thio)ethyl] 3-hydroxy-12-en-28-oic acid (**3r**). To a mixture of CS_2 (1.8 mmol, 108 μL), anhydrous K_3PO_4 (0.8 mmol, 169.1 mg), and THF (8.0 mL), 4-(m-tolyl)piperazine (1.0 mmol, 174 μL) was slowly added at 0 °C, and the reaction mixture was then stirred at 0 °C for 0.5 h. Another THF solution (4.0 mL) of **2** (0.4 mmol, 226.1 mg) was added dropwise to the resulting mixture. The reaction mixture was stirred for 12 h at room temperature, then quenched with ice water (15.0 mL), and the insoluble material was removed by a Buchner funnel. After removal of the solvent, the residue was dissolved in ethyl acetate (15.0 mL). Water (15.0 mL) was added to the resulting solution, the organic layer was separated, and the aqueous layer was extracted with ethyl acetate (15.0 mL × 2). The organic solutions were combined and dried over anhydrous Na_2SO_4. After removal of the solvent, the residue was submitted to column chromatography on silica gel (200–300 mesh) using petroleum ether and ethyl acetate (10/1 in *v*/*v*) as eluents to give **3r** (235.0 mg, 80% yield) as a white solid. ^{1}H NMR (400 MHz, $CDCl_3$): δ 7.16 (t, *J* = 7.9 Hz, 1H, Ar-*H*), 6.72 (m, 3H, Ar-*H*), 5.30 (s, 1H, H-12), 4.40 (s, 2H, -O*CH*$_2$C-), 4.28 (m, 2H, -N*CH*$_2$), 4.11 (m, 2H, -N*CH*$_2$), 3.60 (m, 2H, -S*CH*$_2$), 3.27 (m, 4H, 2 × -N*CH*$_2$), 3.18 (m, 1H, H-3), 2.87 (dd, *J* = 13.5, 3.5 Hz, 1H, H-18), 2.32 (s, 3H, -*CH*$_3$), 1.95 (m, 1H, -*OH*), 1.86 (m, 2H, -*CH*$_2$), 1.62 (m, 7H, H-22, -*CH*, 3 × -*CH*$_2$), 1.51 (m, 3H, H-22, -*CH*, -*CH*$_2$), 1.42 (m, 2H, -*CH*$_2$), 1.32 (m, 6H, 3 × -*CH*$_2$), 1.17 (t, *J* = 3.1 Hz, 1H, H-9), 1.13 (s, 3H, -*CH*$_3$), 1.04 (s, 1H, H-5), 0.96 (s, 3H, -*CH*$_3$), 0.93 (s, 3H, -*CH*$_3$), 0.90 (s, 3H, -*CH*$_3$), 0.89 (s, 3H, -*CH*$_3$), 0.75 (s, 3H, -*CH*$_3$), 0.74 (s, 3H, -*CH*$_3$). ^{13}C NMR (100 MHz, $CDCl_3$): δ 195.9 (-CS_2), 177.4 (C-28), 150.2 (*Ph*), 143.5 (C-13), 139.0 (*Ph*), 129.1 (*Ph*), 122.5 (C-12), 121.5 (*Ph*), 117.1 (*Ph*), 113.4 (*Ph*), 78.8 (C-3), 62.3 (-CO-), 55.2 (C-5), 48.8 (-NCH_2), 47.6 (C-9), 46.7 (C-17), 45.8 (C-19), 41.6 (C-14), 41.3 (C-18), 39.3 (C-8), 38.7 (C-1), 38.4 (C-4), 37.0 (C-10), 35.6 (-CS), 33.8 (C-29), 33.1 (C-22), 32.7 (C-21), 32.4 (C-7), 30.7 (C-20), 28.1 (C-15), 27.7 (C-23), 27.1 (C-27), 26.9 (-NCH_2CH_2), 25.9 (C-30), 23.6 (C-2), 23.4 (C-11), 22.9 (C-16), 21.8 (-CH_3), 18.3 (C-6), 17.1 (C-26), 15.6 (C-24), 15.4 (C-25). HRMS (ESI): *m*/*z* calculated for $C_{44}H_{66}N_2O_3S_2$ [M+H]$^+$: 735.4593. Found: 735.4537.

[2-((4-(p-tolyl)piperazine-1-carbonothioyl)thio)ethyl] 3-hydroxy-12-en-28-oic acid (**3s**). To a mixture of CS_2 (1.8 mmol, 108 μL), anhydrous K_3PO_4 (0.8 mmol, 169.1 mg), and THF (8.0 mL), 4-(p-tolyl)piperazine (1.0 mmol, 177.1 mg) was slowly added at 0 °C, and the reaction mixture was then stirred at 0 °C for 0.5 h. Another THF solution (4.0 mL) of **2** (0.4 mmol, 225.8 mg) was added dropwise to the resulting mixture. The reaction mixture was stirred for 12 h at room temperature, then quenched with ice water (15.0 mL), and the insoluble material was removed by a Buchner funnel. After removal of the solvent, the residue was dissolved in ethyl acetate (15.0 mL). Water (15.0 mL) was added to the resulting solution, the organic layer was separated, and the aqueous layer was extracted with ethyl acetate (15.0 mL × 2). The organic solutions were combined and dried over anhydrous Na_2SO_4. After removal of the solvent, the residue was submitted to column chromatography on silica gel (200–300 mesh) using petroleum ether and ethyl acetate (10/1 in *v*/*v*) as eluents to give **3s** (249.6 mg, 85% yield) as a white solid. ^{1}H NMR (400 MHz, $CDCl_3$): δ 7.10 (d, *J* = 8.3 Hz, 2H, Ar-*H*), 6.84 (d, *J* = 8.5 Hz, 2H, Ar-*H*), 5.30 (t, *J* = 3.3 Hz, 1H, H-12), 4.48 (s, 2H, -N*CH*$_2$), 4.30 (m, 2H, -O*CH*$_2$C-), 4.10 (s, 2H, -N*CH*$_2$), 3.64 (m, 2H,

-SCH_2), 3.23 (m, 4H, 2× -NCH_2), 3.19 (d, *J* = 4.8 Hz, 1H, H-3), 2.87 (dd, *J* = 13.7, 4.0 Hz, 1H, H-18), 2.28 (s, 3H, -CH_3), 1.97 (m, 1H, -*OH*), 1.87 (m, 2H, 2× -CH_2), 1.65 (m, 6H, 3× -CH_2), 1.50 (m, 4H, 2× -CH_2), 1.40 (m, 4H, 2× -CH_2), 1.29 (m, 4H, 2× -CH_2) 1.17 (t, *J* = 4.1 Hz, 1H, H-9), 1.13 (s, 3H, -CH_3), 1.05 (s, 1H, H-5), 0.97 (s, 3H, -CH_3), 0.93 (s, 3H, -CH_3), 0.90 (s, 3H, -CH_3), 0.89 (s, 3H, -CH_3), 0.76 (s, 3H, -CH_3), 0.74 (s, 3H, -CH_3). ^{13}C NMR (100 MHz, $CDCl_3$): δ 196.0 (-CS_2), 177.4 (C-28), 148.1 (*Ph*), 143.6 (C-13), 130.3 (*Ph*), 129.8 (*Ph*), 122.5 (C-12), 116.8 (*Ph*), 78.9 (C-3), 62.3 (-CO-), 55.2 (C-5), 49.4 (-NCH_2), 47.6 (C-9), 46.7 (C-17), 45.8 (C-19), 41.7 (C-14), 41.5 (C-18), 41.3 (-NCH_2CH_2), 39.3 (C-8), 38.7 (C-1), 38.4 (C-4), 37.0 (C-10), 35.6 (-CS), 33.8 (C-29), 33.1 (C-22), 32.7 (C-21), 32.4 (C-7), 30.7 (C-20), 28.1 (C-15), 27.7 (C-23), 27.1 (C-27), 25.9 (C-30), 23.6 (C-2), 23.4 (C-11), 22.9 (C-16), 20.5 (-CH_3), 18.3 (C-6), 17.1 (C-26), 15.6 (C-24), 15.3 (C-25). HRMS (ESI): *m*/*z* calculated for $C_{44}H_{66}N_2O_3S_2$ $[M+H]^+$: 735.4593. Found: 735.4562.

[2-((thiomorpholine-4-carbonothioyl)thio)ethyl] 3-hydroxy-12-en-28-oic acid (**3t**). To a mixture of CS_2 (1.8 mmol, 108 μL), anhydrous K_3PO_4 (0.8 mmol, 169.1 mg), and THF (8.0 mL), thiomorpholine (1.0 mmol, 94 μL) was slowly added at 0 °C, and the reaction mixture was then stirred at 0 °C for 0.5 h. Another THF solution (4.0 mL) of **2** (0.4 mmol, 225.1 mg) was added dropwise to the resulting mixture. The reaction mixture was stirred for 12 h at room temperature, then quenched with ice water (15.0 mL), and the insoluble material was removed by a Buchner funnel. After removal of the solvent, the residue was dissolved in ethyl acetate (15.0 mL). Water (15.0 mL) was added to the resulting solution, the organic layer was separated, and the aqueous layer was extracted with ethyl acetate (15.0 mL × 2). The organic solutions were combined and dried over anhydrous Na_2SO_4. After removal of the solvent, the residue was submitted to column chromatography on silica gel (200–300 mesh) using petroleum ether and ethyl acetate (10/1 in *v*/*v*) as eluents to give **3t** (190.4 mg, 72% yield) as a white gel. ^{1}H NMR (400 MHz, $CDCl_3$): δ 5.29 (s, 1H, H-12), 4.61 (s, 2H, -OCH_2C-), 4.26 (m, 2H, -NCH_2), 3.61 (m, 2H, -SCH_2), 3.21 (m, 1H, H-3), 2.86 (dd, *J* = 13.5, 3.6 Hz, 1H, H-18), 2.75 (m, 4H, 2 × -SCH_2), 1.97 (m, 1H, -*OH*), 1.88 (m, 2H, -CH_2), 1.63 (m, 6H, 3 × -CH_2), 1.53 (m, 3H, H-22, -*CH*, -CH_2), 1.42 (m, 4H, 2 × -CH_2), 1.35 (m, 3H, H-22, -*CH*, -CH_2), 1.27 (m, 4H, 2 × -CH_2), 1.16 (t, *J* = 3.6 Hz, 1H, H-9), 1.13 (s, 3H, -CH_3), 1.04 (s, 1H, H-5), 0.98 (s, 3H, -CH_3), 0.93 (s, 3H, -CH_3), 0.90 (s, 6H, 2 × -CH_3), 0.78 (s, 3H, -CH_3), 0.73 (s, 3H, -CH_3). ^{13}C NMR (100 MHz, $CDCl_3$): δ 195.9 (-CS_2), 177.5 (C-28), 143.6 (C-13), 122.6 (C-12), 79.0 (C-3), 62.2 (-CO-), 55.3 (C-5), 47.7 (C-9), 46.8 (C-17), 45.8 (C-19), 41.7 (C-14), 41.3 (C-18), 39.4 (C-8), 38.8 (C-1), 38.5 (C-4), 37.1 (C-10), 35.8 (-CS), 33.9 (C-29), 33.2 (C-22), 32.8 (C-21), 32.5 (C-7), 30.8 (C-20), 28.2 (C-15), 27.8 (C-23), 27.2 (C-27), 27.0 (-NCH_2), 25.9 (C-30), 23.7 (C-2), 23.5 (C-11), 23.0 (C-16), 18.4 (C-6), 17.2 (C-26), 15.7 (C-24), 15.4 (C-25), 14.2 (-SCH_2). HRMS (ESI): *m*/*z* calculated for $C_{37}H_{59}NO_3S_3$ $[M+H]^+$: 662.3735. Found: 662.3673.

3.3. Preliminary Biological Study

The in vitro cytotoxic activities of the compounds were evaluated by MTT assay against Pancl, A549, Hep3B, Huh-7, HT-29, Hela, LO2. Cell lines were obtained from the Laboratory of Molecular Pharmacology, Southwest Medical University. Briefly, different tumor cells grew in DMEM medium except for A549, which used 1640 medium. Cells ((3–5) × 10^3 cells/well) were harvested at the log phase of growth and seeded in 96-well plates. After 24 h incubation at 37 °C in 5% CO_2 to allow cell attachment, cultures were exposed to various concentrations of the isolated compounds for 48 h. Finally, the MTT solution was added. Plates were further incubated for 4 h at 37 °C after adding 150 μL/well of DMSO and shaking for 10 min on the shaker platform. The plates were read in a 96-well plate reader at 490 nm wavelength. The results were expressed as IC_{50} values, and were defined as the concentration at which 50% survival of cells was obtained. Fluorouracil, docetaxel, and cisplatin were co-assayed as positive controls.

4. Conclusions

In summary, we have synthesized a series of OA-dithiocarbamate derivatives in a two-step protocol at room temperature, offering a readily accessible synthetic route to obtain novel OA derivatives in high yields. Moreover, some of the compounds were shown to be promising hit compounds, with remarkably improved broad-spectrum antiproliferative activities compared to the natural product OA. Mechanistic insights of their activities on certain tumor cell lines are currently underway in our laboratory.

Supplementary Materials: The following supporting information can be downloaded at: https://www.mdpi.com/article/10.3390/molecules28031414/s1. Figures S1–S42: ^{1}H and ^{13}C NMR spectrum of **2**, **3a–t**; Figures S43–S63: HRMS spectrum of **2**, **3a–t**.

Author Contributions: Y.C., Z.X. and Y.Z. (Yueshui Zhao). conceptualized and designed this article. L.T., Y.Z. (Yan Zhang) and J.X. conducted the experiments and wrote the manuscript. Q.Y., F.D., X.W., M.L., J.S. and S.D. provided critical comments and edited the manuscript. All authors have read and agreed to the published version of the manuscript.

Funding: This work was supported by the National Natural Science Foundation of China (Grant No. 81972643), SCU-Luzhou Platform Construction of Scientific and Technological Innovation (Grant No. 2022CDLZ-20), and the Research Fund of Southwest Medical University (Grant No. 2021ZKQN106).

Institutional Review Board Statement: Not applicable.

Informed Consent Statement: Not applicable.

Data Availability Statement: Not applicable.

Conflicts of Interest: The authors declare no conflict of interest.

References

1. Li, J.; Cai, Z.; Li, X.-W.; Zhuang, C. Natural Product-Inspired Targeted Protein Degraders: Advances and Perspectives. *J. Med. Chem.* **2022**, *65*, 13533–13560. [CrossRef] [PubMed]
2. Liu, M.; Martyn, A.P.; Quinn, R.J. Natural product-based PROteolysis TArgeting Chimeras (PROTACs). *Nat. Prod. Rep.* **2022**, *39*, 2292. [CrossRef] [PubMed]
3. Rahman, M.M.; Sarker, M.T.; Alam Tumpa, M.A.; Yamin, M.; Islam, T.; Park, M.N.; Islam, M.R.; Rauf, A.; Sharma, R.; Cavalu, S.; et al. Exploring the recent trends in perturbing the cellular signaling pathways in cancer by natural products. *Front. Pharmacol.* **2022**, *13*, 950109. [CrossRef]
4. Man, S.; Luo, C.; Yan, M.; Zhao, G.; Ma, L.; Gao, W. Treatment for liver cancer: From sorafenib to natural products. *Eur. J. Med. Chem.* **2021**, *224*, 113690. [CrossRef] [PubMed]
5. Li, H.; Li, M.; Xu, R.; Wang, S.; Zhang, Y.; Zhang, L.; Zhou, D.; Xiao, S. Synthesis, structure activity relationship and in vitro anti-influenza virus activity of novel polyphenol-pentacyclic triterpene conjugates. *Eur. J. Med. Chem.* **2019**, *163*, 560–568. [CrossRef] [PubMed]
6. Zhang, B.-W.; Xing, Y.; Wen, C.; Yu, X.-X.; Sun, W.-L.; Xiu, Z.-L.; Dong, Y.-S. Pentacyclic triterpenes as α-glucosidase and α-amylase inhibitors: Structure-activity relationships and the synergism with acarbose. *Bioorg. Med. Chem. Lett.* **2017**, *27*, 5065–5070. [CrossRef]
7. Wang, W.; Li, Y.; Li, Y.; Sun, D.; Li, H.; Chen, L. Recent Progress in Oleanolic Acid: Structural Modification and Biologi-cal Activity. *Curr. Top. Med. Chem.* **2022**, *22*, 3–23. [CrossRef]
8. Gou, W.; Luo, N.; Yu, B.; Wu, H.; Wu, S.; Tian, C.; Guo, J.; Ning, H.; Bi, C.; Wei, H.; et al. Ursolic Acid Deriva-tive UA232 Promotes Tumor Cell Apoptosis by Inducing Endo-plasmic Reticulum Stress and Lysosomal Dysfunction. *Int. J. Biol. Sci.* **2022**, *18*, 2639–2651. [CrossRef]
9. Gou, W.; Luo, N.; Wei, H.; Wu, H.; Yu, X.; Duan, Y.; Bi, C.; Ning, H.; Hou, W.; Li, Y. Ursolic acid derivative UA232 evokes apoptosis of lung cancer cells induced by endoplasmic reticulum stress. *Pharm. Biol.* **2020**, *58*, 707–715. [CrossRef] [PubMed]
10. Cheng, K.-G.; Su, C.-H.; Yang, L.-D.; Liu, J.; Chen, Z.-F. Synthesis of oleanolic acid dimers linked at C-28 and evaluation of anti-tumor activity. *Eur. J. Med. Chem.* **2015**, *89*, 480–489. [CrossRef]
11. Chen, Z.; Huang, K.-Y.; Ling, Y.; Goto, M.; Duan, H.-Q.; Tong, X.-H.; Liu, Y.-L.; Cheng, Y.-Y.; Morris-Natschke, S.L.; Yang, P.-C.; et al. Discovery of an Oleanolic Acid/Hederagenin-Nitric Oxide Donor Hybrid as an EGFR Tyrosine Kinase Inhibitor for Non-Small-Cell Lung Cancer. *J. Nat. Prod.* **2019**, *82*, 3065–3073. [CrossRef] [PubMed]
12. Wang, R.; Li, Y.; Hu, H.; Persoons, L.; Daelemans, D.; De Jonghe, S.; Luyten, W.; Krasniqi, B.; Dehaen, W. Antibacterial and antitumoral properties of 1,2,3-triazolo fused triterpenes and their mechanism of inhibiting the proliferation of HL-60 cells. *Eur. J. Med. Chem.* **2021**, *224*, 113727. [CrossRef] [PubMed]

13. Kang, F.; Ai, Y.; Zhang, Y.; Huang, Z. Design and synthesis of new hybrids from 2-cyano-3,12-dioxooleana- 9-dien-28-oic acid and O2-(2,4-dinitrophenyl) diazeniumdiolate for intervention of drug-resistant lung cancer. *Eur. J. Med. Chem.* **2018**, *149*, 269–280. [CrossRef] [PubMed]
14. Wang, R.; Yang, W.; Fan, Y.; Dehaen, W.; Li, Y.; Li, H.; Wang, W.; Zheng, Q.; Huai, Q. Design and synthesis of the novel oleanolic acid-cinnamic acid ester derivatives and glycyrrhetinic acid-cinnamic acid ester derivatives with cytotoxic properties. *Bioorg. Chem.* **2019**, *88*, 102951. [CrossRef]
15. Bildziukevich, U.; Kvasnicová, M.; Šaman, D.; Rárová, L.; Wimmer, Z. Novel Oleanolic Acid-Tryptamine and -Fluorotryptamine Amides: From Adaptogens to Agents Targeting In Vitro Cell Apoptosis. *Plants* **2021**, *10*, 2082. [CrossRef] [PubMed]
16. Martins, F.C.O.L.; Batista, A.D.; Melchert, W.R. Current overview and perspectives in environmentally friendly microextractions of carbamates and dithiocarbamates. *Compr. Rev. Food Sci. Food Saf.* **2021**, *20*, 6116–6145. [CrossRef]
17. Ajiboye, T.O.; Ajiboye, T.T.; Marzouki, R.; Onwudiwe, D.C. The Versatility in the Applications of Dithiocarbamates. *Int. J. Mol. Sci.* **2022**, *23*, 1317. [CrossRef]
18. Arslan, S.; Güler, A.; Güngör, N.; Dağaşan, Ö.; Yiğitkaya, S.; Kale, L.Y.; Numanoğlu, E.; Balaban, B.; Özaltın, K.E.; Merken, Ö.; et al. False positive effect of sulfur sources used in growing and processing of vine (*Vitis Vinifera* L.) leaves on the results of dithiocarbamate analysis based on carbon di-sulfide measurement. *Food Addit. Contam. Part A Chem. Anal. Control Expo. Risk Assess* **2022**, *39*, 1565–1575. [CrossRef]
19. Wu, Z.; Su, R. Pesticide thiram exposure alters the gut microbial diversity of chickens. *Front. Microbiol.* **2022**, *13*, 966224. [CrossRef]
20. Hansen, A.; Brans, R.; Sonsmann, F. Allergic contact dermatitis to rubber accelerators in protective gloves: Problems, challenges, and solutions for occupational skin protection. *Allergol. Select.* **2021**, *5*, 335–344. [CrossRef]
21. Guan, Z.; Guo, Y.; Mo, Z.; Chen, S.; Liang, J.; Liao, X.; Zhang, Y.; Huang, Z.; Song, W.; Xu, Y.; et al. High-efficiency treatment of electroless nickel plating effluent using core-shell $MnFe_2O_4$-C@Al_2O_3 combined with ozonation: Performance and mechanism. *J. Hazard. Mater.* **2022**, *433*, 128768. [CrossRef] [PubMed]
22. Wang, Y.; Shen, H.; Qiu, J.; Chen, M.; Song, W.; Zhao, M.; Wang, L.; Bai, F.; Wang, H.; Wu, Z. Copper-Promoted Hiyama Cross-Coupling of Arylsilanes With Thiuram Reagents: A Facile Synthesis of Aryl Dithiocarbamates. *Front. Chem.* **2022**, *10*, 867806. [CrossRef] [PubMed]
23. Liu, J.; Zhu, X.; Yu, L.; Mao, M. Discovery of novel sul-phonamide hybrids that inhibit LSD1 against bladder cancer cells. *J. Enzyme Inhib. Chem.* **2022**, *37*, 866–875. [CrossRef] [PubMed]
24. Wei, M.-X.; Zhou, Y.-X.; Lin, M.; Zhang, J.; Sun, X. De-sign, synthesis and biological evaluation of rhein-piperazine-dithiocarbamate hybrids as potential anticancer agents. *Eur. J. Med. Chem.* **2022**, *241*, 114651. [CrossRef]
25. Sakla, A.P.; Panda, B.; Laxmikeshav, K.; Soni, J.P.; Bhandari, S.; Godugu, C.; Shankaraiah, N. Dithiocarbamation of spiro-aziridine oxindoles: A facile access to C3-functionalised 3-thiooxindoles as apoptosis inducing agents. *Org. Biomol. Chem.* **2021**, *19*, 10622–10634. [CrossRef]
26. Song, J.; Liu, Y.; Yuan, X.-Y.; Liu, W.-B.; Li, Y.-R.; Yu, G.-X.; Tian, X.-Y.; Zhang, Y.-B.; Fu, X.-J.; Zhang, S.-Y. Discovery of 1,2,4-triazine dithiocarbamate derivatives as NEDDylation ago-nists to inhibit gastric cancers. *Eur. J. Med. Chem.* **2021**, *225*, 113801. [CrossRef]
27. Zhu, H.; Ying, S.; Zhou, B.; Hu, X.; Liang, X.; Li, W.; Wang, D.; Jin, H.; Pan, Y. Design, synthesis, and evaluation of novel coumarin-dithiocarbamate derivatives (IDs) as anti-colorectal cancer agents. *J. Enzyme. Inhib. Med. Chem.* **2021**, *36*, 593–604. [CrossRef]
28. Sflakidou, E.; Leonidis, G.; Foroglou, E.; Siokatas, C.; Sarli, V. Recent Advances in Natural Product-Based Hybrids as Anti-Cancer Agents. *Molecules* **2022**, *27*, 6632. [CrossRef]
29. Singh, A.K.; Kumar, A.; Singh, H.; Sonawane, P.; Paliwal, H.; Thareja, S.; Pathak, P.; Grishina, M.; Jaremko, M.; Emwas, A.-H.; et al. Khalilullah, H.; Kumar, P. Con-cept of Hybrid Drugs and Recent Advancements in Anticancer Hybrids. *Pharmaceuticals* **2022**, *15*, 1071. [CrossRef]
30. Padhi, D.; Govindaraju, T. Mechanistic Insights for Drug Repurposing and the Design of Hybrid Drugs for Alzheimer's Disease. *J. Med. Chem.* **2022**, *65*, 7088–7105. [CrossRef]
31. Hosseini-Zare, M.S.; Sarhadi, M.; Zarei, M.; Thilagavathi, R.; Selvam, C. Synergistic effects of curcumin and its analogs with other bioactive compounds: A comprehensive review. *Eur. J. Med. Chem.* **2021**, *210*, 113072. [CrossRef] [PubMed]
32. Wang, C.; Wang, X.; Wang, H.; Pu, J.; Li, Q.; Li, J.; Liu, Y.; Lu, L.; Jiang, S. A "Two-Birds-One-Stone" Approach toward the Design of Bifunctional Human Immunodeficiency Virus Type 1 Entry Inhibitors Targeting the CCR5 Coreceptor and gp41 N-Terminal Heptad Repeat Region. *J. Med. Chem.* **2021**, *64*, 11460–11471. [CrossRef] [PubMed]
33. Yilmaz-Goler, A.M.; Jannuzzi, A.T.; Bayrak, N.; Yıldız, M.; Yıldırım, H.; Otsuka, M.; Fujita, M.; Radwan, M.O.; TuYuN, A.F. In Vitro and In Silico Study to Assess Toxic Mechanisms of Hybrid Molecules of Quinone-Benzocaine as Plastoquinone Analogues in Breast Cancer Cells. *ACS Omega* **2022**, *7*, 30250–30264. [CrossRef] [PubMed]
34. Bonifazi, A.; Newman, A.H.; Keck, T.M.; Gervasoni, S.; Vistoli, G.; Del Bello, F.; Giorgioni, G.; Pavletić, P.; Quaglia, W.; Piergentili, A. Scaffold Hybridization Strategy Leads to the Dis-covery of Dopamine D3 Receptor-Selective or Multitarget Bitop-ic Ligands Potentially Useful for Central Nervous System Disor-ders. *ACS Chem. Neurosci.* **2021**, *12*, 3638–3649. [CrossRef]
35. Channar, P.A.; Aziz, M.; Ejaz, S.A.; Chaudhry, G.-E.; Saeed, A.; Ujan, R.; Hasan, A.; Ejaz, S.R.; Saeed, A. Structural and functional insight into thiazolidinone derivatives as novel candidates for anticancer drug design: In vitro biological and in-silico strategies. *J. Biomol. Struct. Dyn.* **2023**, *41*, 942–953. [CrossRef]

36. Chi, K.-Q.; Wei, Z.-Y.; Wang, K.-S.; Wu, J.; Chen, W.-Q.; Jin, X.-J.; Piao, H.-R. Design, synthesis, and evaluation of novel ursolic acid derivatives as HIF-1α inhibitors with anticancer po-tential. *Bioorg. Chem.* **2017**, *75*, 157–169. [CrossRef] [PubMed]
37. Liu, C.-M.; Huang, J.-Y.; Sheng, L.-X.; Wen, X.-A.; Cheng, K.-G. Synthesis and antitumor activity of fluorouracil—Oleanolic acid/ursolic acid/glycyrrhetinic acid conjugates. *Medchemcomm.* **2019**, *10*, 1370–1378. [CrossRef]
38. Sheng, L.-X.; Huang, J.-Y.; Liu, C.-M.; Zhang, J.-Z.; Cheng, K.-G. Synthesis of oleanolic acid/ursolic acid/glycyrrhetinic acid-hydrogen sulfide donor hybrids and their antitumor activity. *Med. Chem. Res.* **2019**, *28*, 1212–1222. [CrossRef]

molecules

MDPI

Article

Genistein Inhibits Proliferation and Metastasis in Human Cervical Cancer Cells through the Focal Adhesion Kinase Signaling Pathway: A Network Pharmacology-Based In Vitro Study in HeLa Cells

Tingting Chen [1,†], Juan Wang [1,†], Min Li [1], Qingqing Wu [1] and Shuna Cui [1,2,3,*]

1 Jiangsu Key Laboratory of Integrated Traditional Chinese and Western Medicine for Prevention and Treatment of Senile Diseases, Medical College of Yangzhou University, Jiangyang Middle Road 136, Yangzhou 225001, China
2 Department of Gynecology and Obstetrics, Affiliated Hospital of Yangzhou University, Yangzhou 225009, China
3 Jiangsu Co-Innovation Center for Prevention and Control of Important Animal Infectious Diseases and Zoonoses, College of Veterinary Medicine, Yangzhou 225001, China
* Correspondence: sncui@yzu.edu.cn
† These authors contributed equally to this work.

Abstract: Previous studies have provided evidence that genistein exerts a therapeutic effect on different tumor cells. However, the mechanism of action of genistein against cervical cancer cells remains largely unknown. The aim of this study was to comprehensively decipher the anti-metastatic effect and molecular mechanism of genistein action on cervical cancer cells. We developed an integrated strategy from genotype to phenotype, combining network pharmacology and a transcriptome screening approach, to elucidate the underlying mechanism of action of genistein against human cervical cancer cells. In silico studies predicted that the focal adhesion pathway may be an important signaling cascade targeted by genistein treatment. Using RNA sequencing analysis, representative genes of the focal adhesion pathway were demonstrated to be significantly downregulated. Phenotypic studies revealed that genistein demonstrated strong anti-proliferative and anti-metastatic activity in HeLa cells. Moreover, genistein modulated this activity in a concentration-dependent manner. Genistein also inhibited both the activation and gene expression of FAK (Focal Adhesion Kinase) and paxillin. In addition, vimentin and β-catenin protein expression, and Snail and Twist gene expression, were strongly inhibited by genistein. Our findings provide strong evidence for a pleiotropic effect of genistein on cervical cancer cells, mediated through the focal adhesion pathway.

Keywords: genistein; cervical cancer; metastasis; network pharmacology; RNA expression profiling

Citation: Chen, T.; Wang, J.; Li, M.; Wu, Q.; Cui, S. Genistein Inhibits Proliferation and Metastasis in Human Cervical Cancer Cells through the Focal Adhesion Kinase Signaling Pathway: A Network Pharmacology-Based In Vitro Study in HeLa Cells. *Molecules* **2023**, *28*, 1919. https://doi.org/10.3390/molecules28041919

Academic Editors: Barbara De Filippis, Alessandra Ammazzalorso and Marialuigia Fantacuzzi

Received: 4 January 2023
Revised: 7 February 2023
Accepted: 7 February 2023
Published: 17 February 2023

1. Introduction

Cervical cancer is known to be the fourth most common malignancy, leading to a substantial burden and threatening women's health worldwide [1]. A persistent infection by human papilloma virus (HPV), especially HPV16 and 18, is critical for cervical cancer initiation and progression [2,3]. The implementation of HPV vaccines, HPV testing, and cervical cytology has notably decreased the incidence of early-stage cervical cancer [2,4,5]. However, patients with advanced cervical cancer still have unfavorable outcomes due to the high incidence of metastasis, which is still one of the main factors influencing the prognosis of patients. Moreover, the clinical application of immunotherapy or adjuvant chemotherapy approaches in advanced cervical cancer has not been as effective as once expected [6,7]. Therefore, there is an urgent need for novel therapeutic approaches.

Cervical cancer is a complicated disease involving the disruption of normal complex biological networks in the human body [8]. Upon HPV infection, several key molecular events are involved in the initiation and progression of cervical cancer, including the

Toll-like receptor (TLR) pathway, the nuclear factor-kappa B (NF-κB) pathway, the Notch signal pathway, the Hippo-Yes-associated protein (YAP1) pathway [9–11], and the focal adhesion pathway [12]. However, drugs that act on single-molecular targets usually exert an unsuccessful effect or show strong toxic side effects in clinical practice. Considering the complexity of the pathogenesis of cancers, attention has switched from focusing on single drug targets towards a more systemic view of drug targets [13]. Network pharmacology is considered a powerful tool in deciphering the complexity of biological systems and provides a new concept for understanding the interplay of molecular networks of compounds [14]. This approach is now widely used in the study of the pharmacological effects of compounds, where it promotes new directions for efficient drug discovery.

Genistein is a well-studied natural flavone compound with a wide range of biological effects, including tyrosine kinase inhibitory, anti-inflammatory, phytoestrogen, and anticancer effects [15–20]. Several studies have already been published concerning genistein treatment during cervical cancer development, and the reported activities of genistein include inducing cell cycle G2-M phase arrest and apoptosis, inhibiting the action of histone deacetylases and DNA methyltransferases, and synergizing the radiation effect by cell cycle G2-M phase arrest and AKT (Protein Kinase B) activation [21–26]. Considering the range of activities identified in the above-mentioned studies, the precise molecular action of genistein against cervical cancer remains largely unknown. Therefore, in order to investigate the molecular action of genistein against cervical cancer more comprehensively, this study employed an integrated strategy that combined the network pharmacology approach and RNA-seq analysis to identify critical targets related to the genistein treatment of cervical cancer.

2. Results

2.1. Identification of Potential Genistein Targets against Human Cervical Cancer

The targets of genistein and human cervical cancer were downloaded from the Comparative Toxicogenomics Database (CTD). In total, 28,150 protein-coding genes were related to the progression of human cervical cancer, and 2647 protein-coding genes were confirmed as the effective targets of genistein. A total of 2647 genes were identified in a Venn plot (Figure 1). Since a large number of genes were identified, we performed secondary screening using an Interaction Count (human cervical cancer target > 50; genistein target > 2). Finally, 371 genes were selected as the core targets involved in the action of genistein (data not shown), and the following analysis is based on these genes.

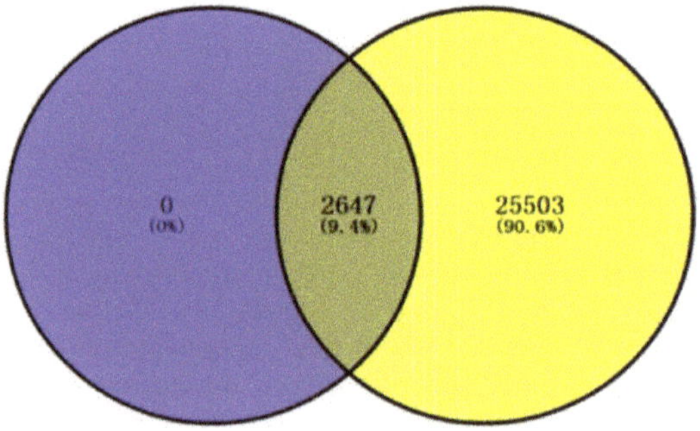

Figure 1. Venn plot of genes potentially involved in genistein's action against human cervical cancer. The purple color represents the targets of genistein, and the yellow color represents the genes related to the progression of human cervical cancer.

2.2. PPI Network Construction and Identification of Hub Genes

The 371 core targets were introduced into the STRING database to build the PPI (Protein-Protein Interaction) network of genistein's action against human cervical cancer. A confidence score of protein and protein interaction of >0.9 was set, and data were collected and visualized using Cytoscape. As shown in Figure 2, the network contained 317 nodes and 1754 edges; the cluster coefficient was 0.33, and the network centralization value was 0.170. The top 10 hub genes in this network were subsequently identified by MCC (Maximal Clique Centrality) algometrical analysis: FN1, TIMP1, GAS6, IL6, C3, IGFBP3, IGFBP4, IGFBP1, CST3 and SPP1. The increasing significance of genes in the network is represented by the color change (yellow to red) (Figure 3).

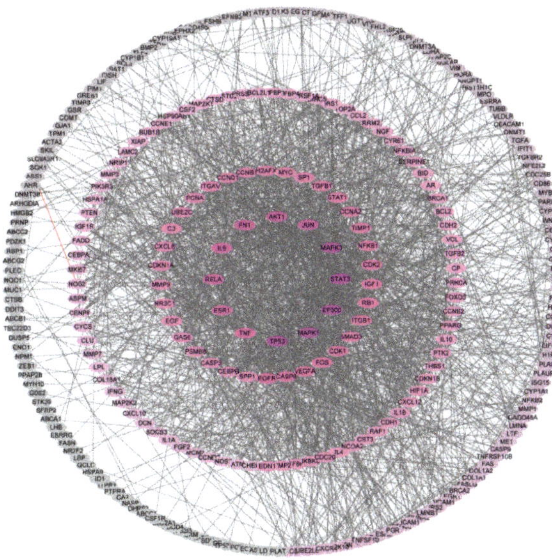

Figure 2. PPI network of the core genes in genistein's action against human cervical cancer (dark purple color indicates high degree; grey color indicates low degree).

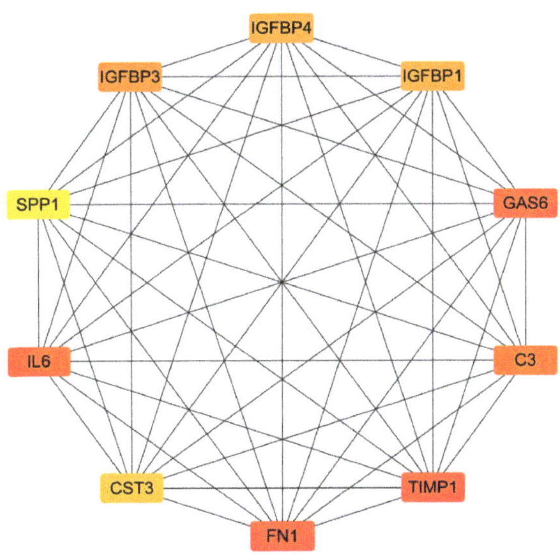

Figure 3. Hub gene analysis of the PPI network. The color change from yellow to red indicates the increasing importance of related genes in the network. The red color indicates the highest significance.

2.3. GO Enrichment Analyses of Core Targets

The predicted core targets were further analyzed by GO (Gene Ontology) and KEGG (Kyoto Encyclopedia of Genes and Genomes) pathway enrichment in the DAVID database. The top 20 biological processes of predicted core targets were identified (Figure 4A); the core targets are mainly involved in the response to organic substances, regulation of programmed cell death, regulation of cell death, regulation of apoptosis, response to endogenous stimulus, regulation of cell proliferation, response to hormone stimulus, and response to extracellular stimulus. The enriched KEGG pathways (Figure 4B) included the following: pathways in cancer; the p53 signaling pathway; the cell cycle; apoptosis; the MAPK (Mitogen Activated Protein Kinase) signaling pathway; the TLR (Toll Like Recepter) signaling pathway; and focal adhesion. From the hub gene analysis, FN1 was selected as the most significant hub gene in genistein's action against the cervical cancer network. Therefore, we predicted that the focal adhesion pathway is a novel pathway targeted by genistein in the treatment of cervical cancer. To gain a deeper insight, all the predicted genes in this pathway potentially regulated by genistein are highlighted in red (Figure 5).

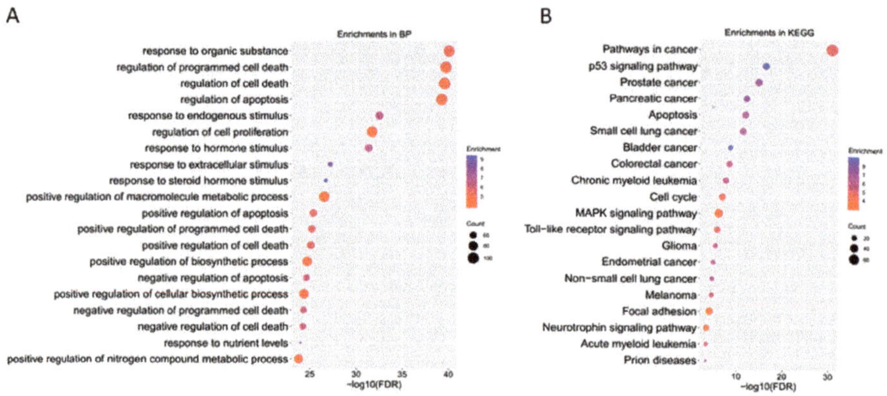

Figure 4. GO ontology and KEGG pathway enrichment of the core targets. (**A**) Biological processes and (**B**) KEGG pathways involved in genistein's action against human cervical cancer.

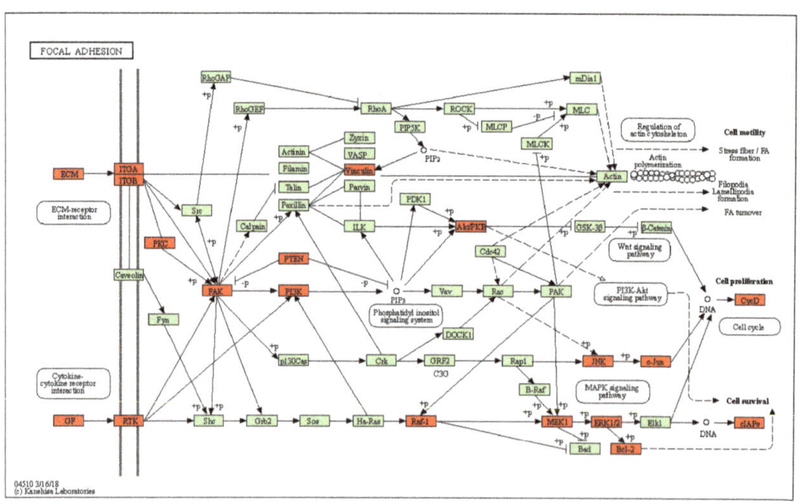

Figure 5. Predicted targets of genistein's action in the focal adhesion pathway. Proteins highlighted in red indicate potential targets of genistein's action against human cervical cancer.

2.4. Genistein Attenuates Cell Viability and Growth in HeLa Cells

According to in silico studies, genistein showed multiple effects on cervical cancer. Next, we experimentally validated these effects using human cervical cancer cells in vitro. The high−risk HPV 16 and 18 are highly associated with the pathogenesis of cervical cancer. Moreover, according to the literature, HeLa cells are more sensitive to genistein treatment. Therefore, in this study, we used HeLa cells for the following experiments [27]. As shown in Figure 6A, genistein significantly inhibited cell growth in a time- and dose-dependent manner after 24 h and 48 h of treatment by CCK−8 (Cell Counting Kit−8) assay. Moreover, 5-fluorouracil (5−FU), clinically used as an anti-tumor drug, was used as a positive control. The concentration of 5−FU was chosen based on the literature [28]. The result showed that 80 μM of 5−FU inhibited the viability of HeLa cells compared with the DMSO (Dimethyl sulfoxide) control. The results indicate that genistein exerted the same inhibitory effect on the human cervical cancer cells as the anti-cancer drug 5−FU. Moreover, we further tested the effects of genistein on cell growth by using cell number counting. The results indicate a prominent effect of genistein on cell growth; the cell number was significantly decreased after genistein (12.5–100 μM) treatment for 24–48 h (Figure 6B). Furthermore, genistein strongly inhibited the colony formation ability of cervical cells (Figure 6C). While cervical cells formed large colonies in the control group, this colony-forming ability was significantly decreased after genistein treatment, indicating that genistein (12.5–100 μM) strongly inhibited HeLa cells' proliferation. Overall, these results demonstrate that 12.5–100 μM genistein strongly inhibited HeLa cells' viability and proliferation.

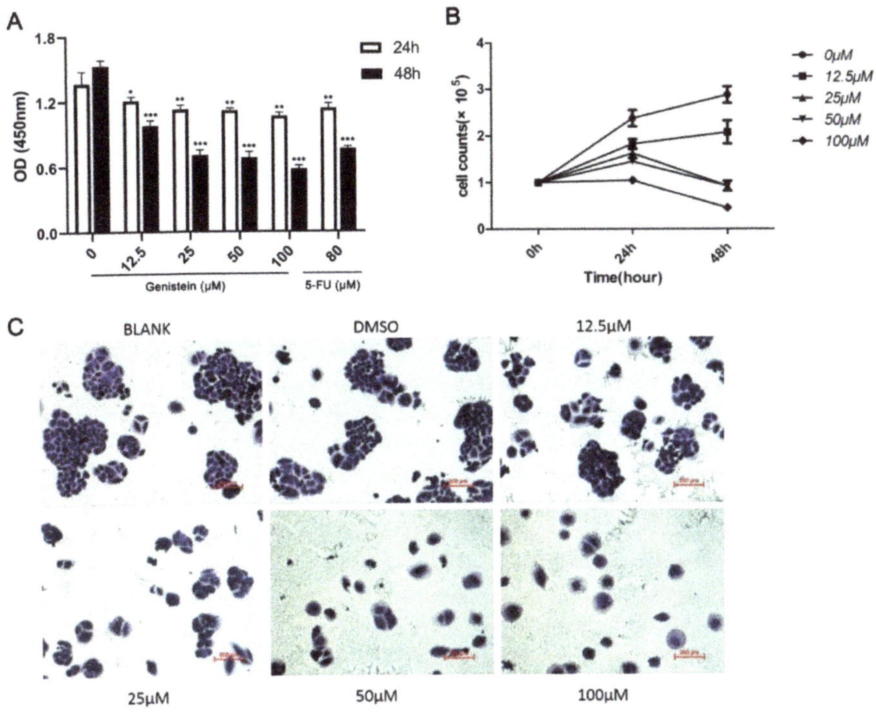

Figure 6. (**A**). Effects of genistein treatment on the proliferation of HeLa cells for 24–48 h were detected by CCK−8 assay. (**B**). Effects of genistein treatment on cell growth were counted by hemocytometer after 24–48 h. (**C**). Representative images of HeLa cell colony formation after genistein treatment (0–100 μM). The data shown are the average of three replicates; the experiments were performed three times independently. *** $p < 0.001$, ** $p < 0.01$, * $p < 0.05$ compared with solvent control. Scale bar: 200 μm.

2.5. Genistein Inhibits HeLa Cell Adhesion

Since adhesion is the first critical step in cancer metastasis, we initially investigated the influence of genistein on HeLa cells' adhesion. The data demonstrate that genistein dose-dependently inhibited cell adhesion in cervical cancer cells (Figure 7A,B). Compared to the control, 92%, 82%, 81%, and 71% inhibition of adhesion was observed with 12.5 μM, 25 μM, 50 μM, and 100 μM of genistein, respectively. Thus, HeLa cell adhesion was significantly inhibited after genistein (25–100 μM) treatment ($p < 0.01$; $p < 0.05$) (Figure 7A).

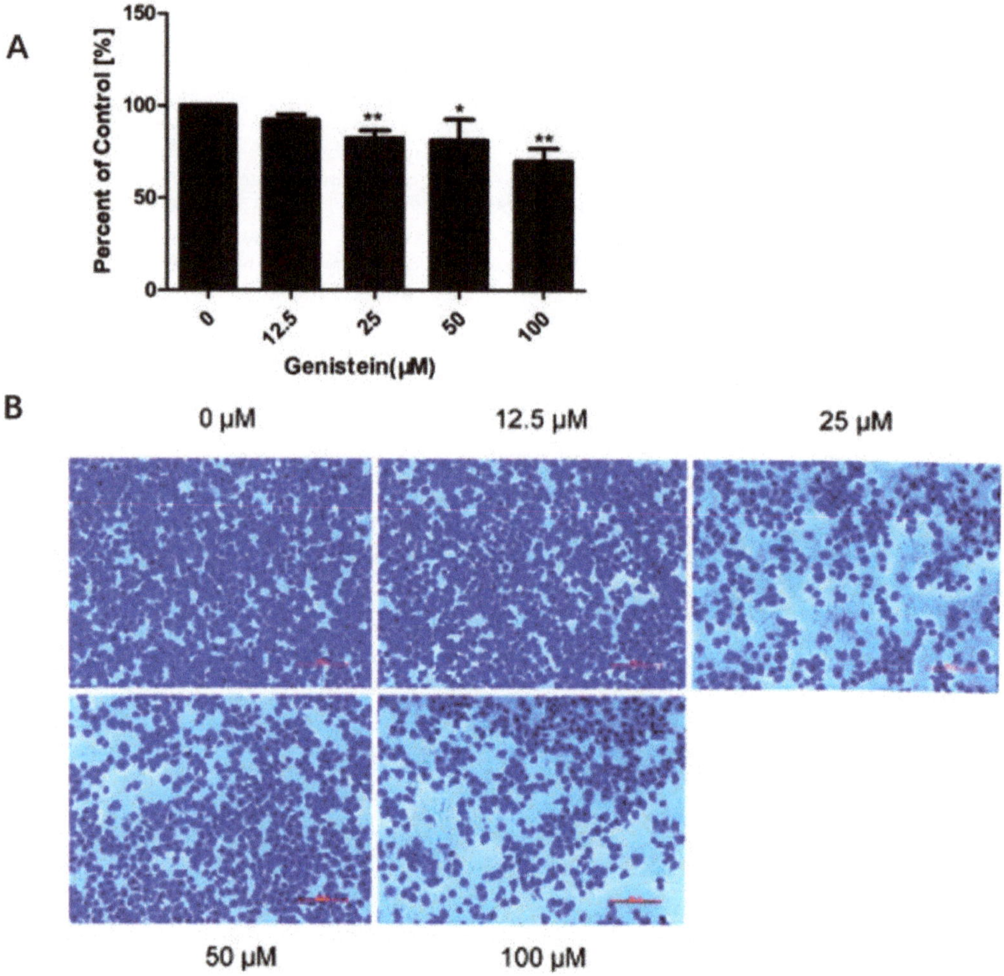

Figure 7. Effects of genistein on HeLa cell adhesion. Cells were grown in the presence of different doses of genistein for 24 h, and reseeded for 3 h. Adherent cells were then fixed by PFA (Paraformaldehyde) and stained with crystal violet solution. Absorbance readings were detected at OD570 nm by microplate reader. (**A**). Percentage of adhesion was then calculated based on the OD value of the adhered cells in the genistein-treated group (compared to control values (100%)). The experiment was performed three times independently, and data shown are the average of all three replicates. (**B**). Representative images from the three independent experiments. ** $p < 0.01$ vs. DMSO control; * $p < 0.05$ vs. DMSO control. Scale bar: 200 μm.

2.6. Genistein's Inhibition of Cell Migration in the Wound—Healing Assay

We also assessed cell migration activities using a wound-healing assay. As shown in Figure 8A,B, the continuous migration of HeLa cells was observed in the control group after 8 h and 24 h. HeLa cell migration was significantly reduced in the presence of 12.5–100 μM genistein. The results indicate that genistein strongly inhibits cell migration in a concentration-dependent manner ($p < 0.01$; $p < 0.05$).

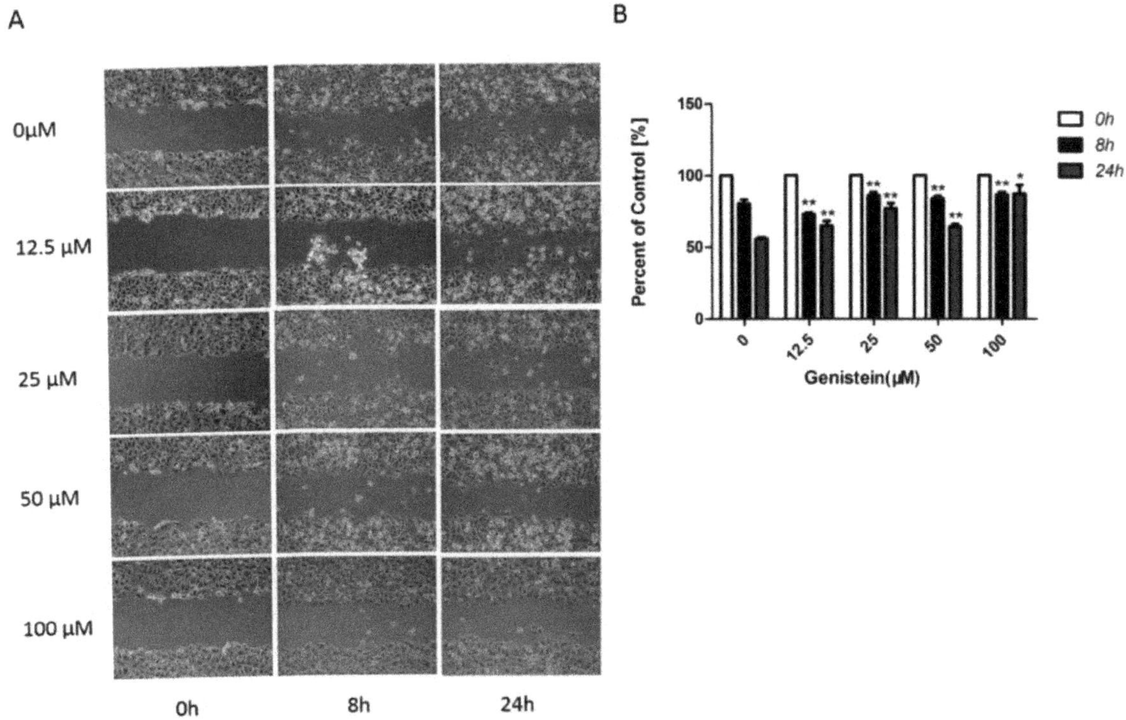

Figure 8. Effect of genistein on the mobility of HeLa cells. (**A**) Representative images of wound-healing assay. (**B**) Cell migration was calculated by measuring the distances from the wound edges in each treatment group using Image J software. Cell migration activity (as a percentage) was calculated from the migration distances in the genistein treatment group (compared to the control (100%)). The experiment was repeated three times. ** $p < 0.01$ vs. DMSO control. * $p < 0.05$ vs. DMSO control; Scale bar: 200 μm.

2.7. Genistein Inhibited Cell Migration and Invasion of HeLa Cells in Transwell® Assays

The inhibition of cell migration by genistein was verified using the Transwell assay. A remarkable decrease in cell migration activity was observed with increasing concentrations of genistein; 12.5 μM–100 μM of genistein decreased cell migration activity by 81%, 85%, 50%, and 36% compared with the solvent control, respectively (Figure 9A–C). As shown in Figure 9B–D, genistein (12.5–100 μM) also significantly inhibited cell-invasive activity; 12.5 μM, 25 μM, 50 μM, and 100 μM of genistein decreased cell invasion activity compared with the solvent control by 36%, 39%, 30%, and 27%, respectively. Compared with the inhibition of cell migration activity, genistein exerted a stronger inhibitory effect on cell invasion activity. Moreover, compared with the cell viability results, the inhibition of cell migration and invasion was not entirely due to the inhibition of cell viability.

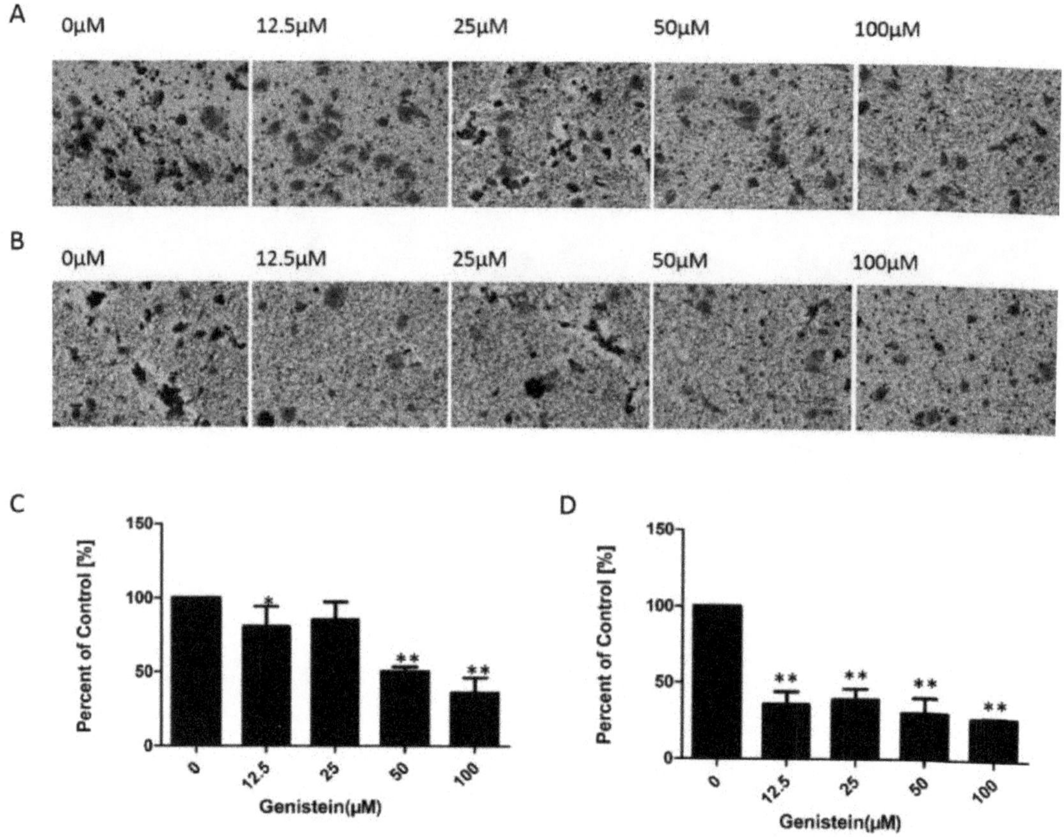

Figure 9. Effect of genistein on the migration and invasion activities of HeLa cells. Cells were seeded on membranes and co-cultured with different doses of genistein for 24 h. (**A**) Cells that migrated to the lower surface of the filter were fixed and stained with crystal violet, and then photographed by an inverted microscope at ×100. (**B**) Cell invasion was assessed by following cell movement through the Matrigel to the lower surface of the filter. Invading cells were fixed, stained with crystal violet, and photographed under an inverted microscope at ×100. (**C**) Cell migration was quantified from at least three images randomly using Image J software. (**D**) Cell invasion was quantified from at least three images randomly using the Image J software. The experiment was repeated three times. ** $p < 0.01$ vs. DMSO control. * $p < 0.05$ vs. DMSO control; scale bar: 200 μm.

2.8. Identification of Differentially Expressed Genes (DEGs) Associated with Genistein Treatment

To further decipher the mechanism of genistein's action on cervical cancer cells, we analyzed global gene expression profiles in genistein- and DMSO-treated cells by using RNA sequencing. Approximately 59–67 million (M) clean reads from six samples (three for genistein treatment; three for control) were obtained after deletion of the low-quality and adaptor sequences; Q30 bases ranged from 92.72% to 93.32% (data not shown). These results demonstrate that the samples were of good quality, and that the coverage of the cervical cancer cell genome was high.

We previously observed significant changes in the proliferation and metastasis of cervical cancer cells after genistein treatment. The transcriptome screening results provide strong evidence that these changes were accompanied by significant differences in gene expression. A total list of expressed genes was determined using RNA-Seq data (Figure 10).

Among these, genes that were upregulated (orange) and downregulated (blue) following genistein treatment (compared with control) were identified ($p < 0.05$; $|\log_2\text{FoldChange}| > 1$).

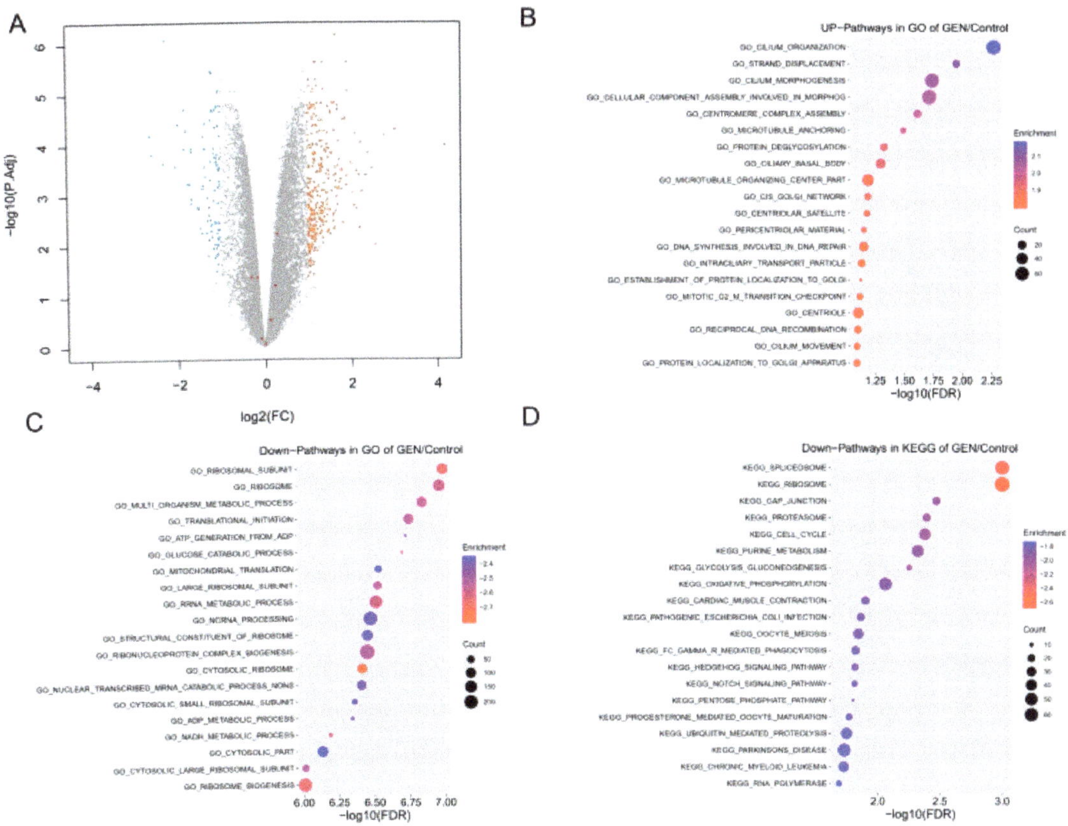

Figure 10. (**A**) Volcano plot of DEGs identified following genistein treatment (compared with control). Grey dots, genes with no significant difference in expression; blue dots, downregulated genes; and orange dots, upregulated genes. Fold-change was calculated using gene-normalized expression of the genistein group/gene-normalized expression of the control group. Differences in expression with a p value < 0.05 and a Log_2 (fold change) > 1 were considered statistically significant. (**B**,**C**) Gene ontology enrichment of up- and downregulated DEGs after genistein treatment. (**D**) KEGG enrichment of upregulated DEGs after genistein treatment.

Gene ontology of the DEGs was analyzed by GESA (Gene Set Enrichment Analysis), and the upregulated and downregulated DEGs were enriched for biological process analysis. The upregulated DEGs are involved in morphological processes, including cilium organization, strand displacement, and cilium morphogenesis. In contrast, the downregulated DEGs are associated with ribosomal subunits, the ribosome, the multi-organism metabolic process, and mitochondrial translation. GESA analysis revealed that the gene clusters involved in the regulation of mitochondrion organization, substrate adhesion-dependent cell spreading, and focal adhesion were significantly downregulated (Figures 10B,C and 11A,B,E,F). Moreover, the top KEGG pathways are listed in Figure 10D. The downregulated DEGs are involved in the spliceosome, ribosome, GAP junction, proteasome, cell cycle, purine metabolism, glycolysis metabolism, and oxidative phosphorylation. Previously, we predicted that the focal adhesion pathway was a promising target for genistein treatment in silico (Figures 3 and 4). The RNA sequencing results validated these predictions, and numerous genes in the focal adhesion pathway were downregulated after genistein treatment, including FAK, PAK, Src, Shc, Actinin, Talin, and ILK. Moreover, mitochondrion function was also significantly inhibited by genistein, while adhesion-related pathways involving adherent junctions were also downregulated (Figure 11C,D,G,H). Interestingly, our data provide evidence that genistein mainly exerted a downregulation effect on cervical cancer cells.

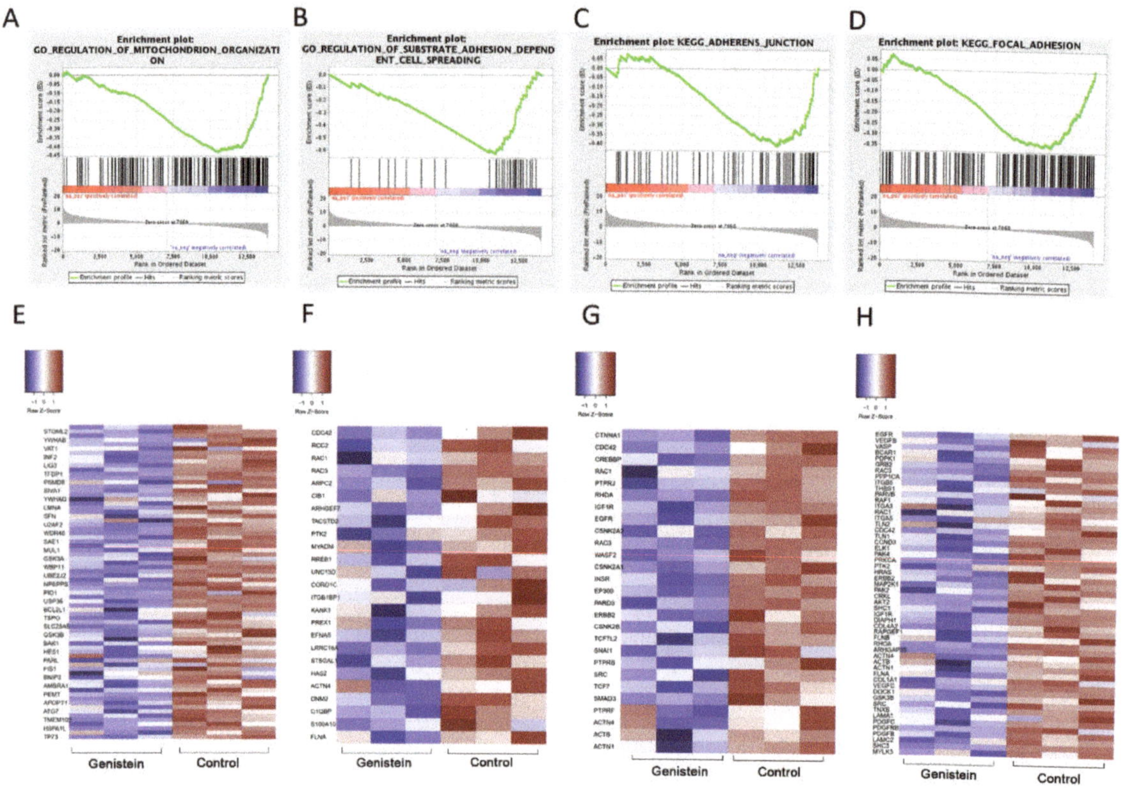

Figure 11. (**A**–**D**) Representative enrichment of gene signatures in genistein and control group by gene set enrichment analysis (GESA). Representative enriched gene sets are shown (FDR q value < 0.05). (**E**–**H**). Heatmap of the representative DEGs between genistein and control group in parallel with GESA analysis.

2.9. Genistein Inhibits Activation of the FAK–Paxillin Pathway

To investigate whether genistein inhibited cell migration and invasion through inhibition of the FAK–paxillin pathway, we performed Western blot analyses to detect the expression of the relevant proteins. As shown in Figure 12, genistein treatment strongly decreased the phosphorylation of paxillin and FAK. In addition, the expression of β-catenin and vimentin was inhibited by genistein. The results suggest that the molecular mechanism of genistein on cell proliferation and metastasis involves inactivation of the FAK–paxillin pathway.

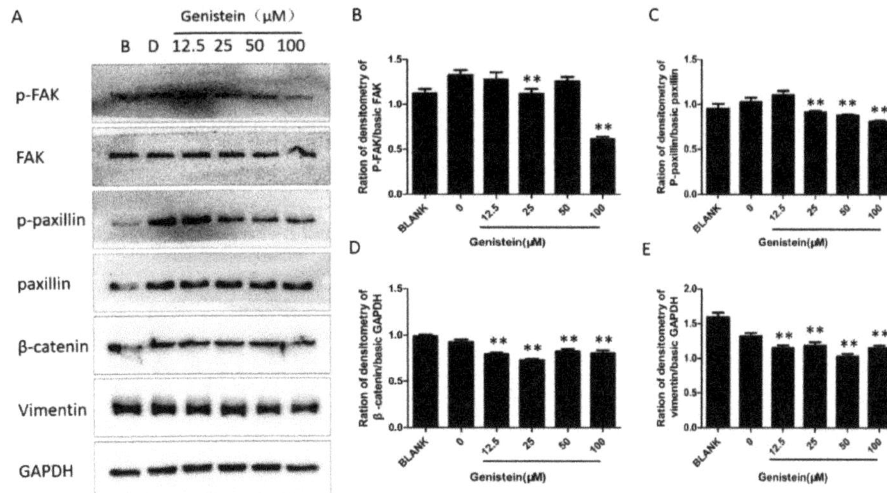

Figure 12. Effect of genistein on the focal adhesion protein expression in HeLa cells. (**A**) Cells were grown with or without different doses of genistein for 30 min. The expression levels of specific proteins were detected by Western blot analysis. GAPDH was used as a control. All first antibodies were used at a dilution of 1:1000. Secondary antibodies were used at a concentration of 1:3000. (**B–E**) Integrated optical intensity of the bands was determined by Image J software (https://imagej.net, accessed on 3 January 2023). The experiment was repeated three times. ** $p < 0.01$ vs. DMSO control.

2.10. Genistein Inhibits Gene Expression of FAK, Paxillin, Snail, and Twist

After confirming that genistein inhibits the activation of the focal adhesion pathway, we next investigated whether genistein inhibits FAK and paxillin gene expression levels. qRT-PCR results indicated that 50–100 μM genistein strongly downregulated paxillin and FAK mRNA expression. In addition, we analyzed the expression of other genes of interest. Snail is a transcription factor that regulates the expression of E-cadherin. Twist is closely associated with cervical cancer progression [29–31]. Our results showed that high doses of genistein (50–100 μM) inhibited Snail and Twist expression ($p < 0.01$; $p < 0.05$) (Figure 13). These results confirmed that genistein inhibits migration and invasion via Snail- and Twist-mediated EMT (Epithelial Mesenchymal Transition).

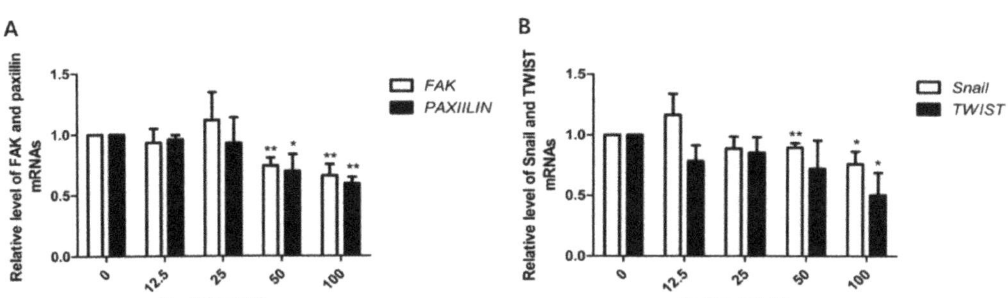

Figure 13. Effect of genistein on specific gene expression in HeLa cells. (**A**) Genistein inhibited FAK and paxillin, and (**B**) Snail and Twist mRNA expression in HeLa cells. Gene expression was analyzed by qRT-PCR. mRNA relative expression levels were evaluated using the $2^{-\triangle\triangle Ct}$ method. GAPDH was used as an internal control. The experiment was repeated three times. ** $p < 0.01$ vs. DMSO control; * $p < 0.05$ vs. DMSO control.

3. Discussion

The effects of genistein (alone or in combination with anti-cancer drugs) on growth regulation, angiogenesis, and metastasis have been extensively investigated in several different tumors [32–34]. Multiple molecular mechanisms have been implicated in its actions, including inhibition of the NF-κB, Wingless, and integration 1 beta-catenin (Wnt/beta-catenin); mitogen-activated protein kinase (MAPK); and phosphoinositide 3 kinase/Akt (PI3K/Akt) signaling pathways [35]. However, evidence regarding the effects of genistein on cervical cancer is limited. Therefore, the underlying mechanism of genistein's action against human cervical cancer, especially its anti-metastatic potential, remains unknown. The present study was designed to elucidate the mechanism of genistein's action against cervical cancer.

We first used a network pharmacological approach to predict potential targets of genistein's action against human cervical cancer in silico. We identified 10 hub targets of genistein treatment: FN1; TIMP1, GAS6, IL6, C3, IGFBP3, IGFBP4, IGFBP1, CST3, and SPP1. FN1 encodes fibronectin, which monitors proliferation and metastasis by regulating the FAK signaling pathway in cervical cancer cells [12]. Previous in silico studies have identified the focal adhesion pathway as a key pathway in cervical cancer [36]. Moreover, the focal adhesion pathway is already considered a potential target in the treatment of highly invasive cancers [37–39]. Focal adhesion kinase (FAK) is an intracellular tyrosine kinase and plays an important role in the regulation of ECM integrin signaling [40–43]. Evidence is accumulating that demonstrates that FAK promotes tumorigenesis through a wide range of cellular processes, including proliferation, survival, metastasis, angiogenesis, epithelial–mesenchymal transition (EMT), cancer stem cell activities, and the metabolism of glucose, lipids, and glutamine [12,44,45]. In our in silico study, focal adhesion was identified using KEGG pathway enrichment analysis as one of the targeted pathways that regulate the anti-cancer effects of genistein (Figures 4 and 11). Considering all the evidence, the FAK pathway was selected as the main pathway for experimental validation.

Phenotypic studies revealed that genistein decreased the proliferation of HeLa cells. This observation is consistent with a previous study indicating that genistein demonstrates cytotoxic properties in numerous different cell types [17,20]. Moreover, genistein is reported to inhibit the proliferation of HeLa, CaSki, and C33 cell lines, and HeLa cells are more sensitive to genistein [27]; therefore, we used the HeLa cell line for our mechanism study. According to our results, genistein also dose-dependently inhibited the HeLa cells' adhesion and metastasis. The inhibition of adhesion is consistent with genistein's inhibition of focal adhesion pathway activation and genistein's inhibition of vimentin and β-catenin expression. Thus, our results provide evidence that genistein suppresses cervical cancer cell metastasis by regulating the FAK/paxillin pathway. Genistein has previously been shown to influence cervical cancer by altering epigenetic modulatory signatures and inducing apoptosis [21,23]. Our results provide strong evidence that genistein inhibits both the activation of the FAK/paxillin pathway and FAK and paxillin gene expression in cervical cancer cells. These results are consistent with the published data and our previously obtained data [17]. We showed that genistein inhibited p-FAK after only 10 min treatment and had a stable inhibitory effect after 24 h treatment in melanoma cells. In human cervical cells, genistein exerts the same behavior. Furthermore, we have previously reported that high concentrations of genistein strongly decrease Snail expression in melanoma cells [17]. Snail is an important transcription factor regulating the process of EMT; the overexpression of Snail in several tumor tissues is associated with metastasis and recurrence [46]. Here, we show that genistein also inhibits Snail expression in human cervical cancer cells.

The role of genistein in cervical cancer was also explored by RNA expression profiling. Thus, the influence of genistein on the regulation of RNA transcription, processing, and splicing in cervical cancer cells was elucidated. The top KEGG pathways enriched using the downregulated DEGs included the spliceosome, ribosome, cell cycle, RNA transport, ribosome biogenesis in eukaryotes, ubiquitin-mediated proteolysis, RNA polymerase, steroid biosynthesis, viral carcinogenesis, central carbon metabolism in cancer, microRNAs in cancer, focal adhesion, cellular senescence, and thyroid hormone signaling pathways. Using RNA sequencing analysis, we were able to confirm our in silico predictions that focal adhesion was a target pathway. In addition to inhibiting focal adhesion, genistein downregulated the expression of PKC, Src, Shc, Pak, Actinin, Talin, and ILK (Figure 11). Protein kinase C (PKC) is a serine-threonine kinase found in most cell types, where it exerts a strong influence on signal transduction events. Elevated expression of PKC has been highly associated with several human cancers, and inhibition of PKC signaling retards the growth and invasion of cervical cells [47]. The proto-oncogene tyrosine-protein kinase Src (Src) is involved in cell growth, differentiation, migration, and survival. FAK and Src are recruited upon integrin activation to form the FAK–Src complex, and this complex phosphorylates downstream adaptor proteins such as paxillin. The activated FAK–Src complex has an essential role in controlling cell shape and cell motility [48,49].

Our RNA profiling analysis revealed that the downregulated DEGs are involved in the regulation of the cell cycle. This result is consistent with our earlier published data. We previously found that genistein could block the cell cycle arrest of macrophages in the G2/M phase [50]. In addition, genistein strongly downregulated mitochondrial organization and disrupted several metabolic pathways, including the glucose catabolic process, ATP (Adenosinetriphosphate) generation from ADP (Adenosinediphosphate), and multi-organism metabolic processes. According to previous reports, genistein can trigger anti-cancer activity against several cancer cells involved in mitochondrial apoptosis [51–53]. However, in cervical cancer, genistein's action on mitochondrial function has not yet been reported. Therefore, this result may herald a new direction in cervical cancer research.

In conclusion, our study provides evidence that the mode of action of genistein against cervical cancer is comprehensive, from genotype to phenotype. Our results reveal that genistein exerts its anti-proliferation and anti-metastatic activities against cervical cancer by interacting with several key pathways. Genistein inhibits the FAK/paxillin pathway and strongly regulates Twist/Snail-mediated EMT, two pathways related to the progression of cervical cancer. Differing from the dual function of genistein in regulating the metastasis of melanoma cells [17], the predominant inhibitory effects of genistein on cervical cancer cells were identified based on RNA expression profiling and phenotypic studies. The novel mechanisms of action of genistein against cervical cancer identified in this study should prove useful in future research and in clinical applications. Overall, our study provides strong evidence that genistein is a promising chemotherapeutic agent against cervical cancer.

4. Materials and Methods

4.1. Prediction of Genistein's Anti-Human Cervical Cancer Targets

All verified targets of genistein and human cervical cancer were screened in the Comparative Toxicogenomics Database (CTD) (http://ctdbase.org/) (accessed on 13 June 2018) [54–57]. CTD is a unique tool in which three types of core data can be obtained, including chemical–gene (and protein) interactions, chemical–disease relationships, and gene–disease relationships. It offers the basis for testable hypotheses about the mechanisms underlying the etiology of environmental diseases [54]. The selected genes were further selected according to the interaction count value, compound targets ≥ 2, disease targets ≥ 50. Finally, potential targets of genistein against human cervical carcinomas were obtained by overlapping the compound targets and disease targets.

4.2. PPI Network Analysis and Identification of Hub Genes

The STRING database [58] was applied to build the PPI network. The confidence score for protein–protein interactions was selected as >0.9. The PPI network for genistein against human cervical carcinoma was visualized using Cytoscape (v3.7.1). The hub genes in the PPI network were calculated using the CytoHubba plugin based on the MCC algorithm [59].

4.3. GO and KEGG Pathway Enrichment Analyses of Core Targets

The Database for Annotation, Visualization, and Integrated Discovery (DAVID) (https://david.ncifcrf.gov/) (accessed on 17 September 2018) was used for Gene Ontology and KEGG pathway enrichment analysis of core targets. Bubble charts of BP and KEGG pathways were produced by ggplot2, implemented in the R platform.

4.4. Experimental Verification

4.4.1. Reagent Source

Fetal bovine serum (FBS), 100× penicillin, streptomycin, and Dulbecco's modified Eagle's medium (DMEM) were purchased from Lonza (Verviers, Belgium). Genistein was obtained from Selleck (Shanghai, China). Genistein was dissolved in DMSO with a stock solution of 100 mM and diluted in culture medium to final concentrations (12.5–100 μM). Phosphatase and protease inhibitor cocktail set I and WST-8 buffer were purchased from Biotool (Shanghai, China). Enhanced chemiluminescence (ECL) detection buffer was purchased from Beyotime Biotechnology (Shanghai, China). Antibodies used in this study were purchased from Cell Signaling Technology (Danvers, MA, USA), and are listed in Table 1.

Table 1. List of antibodies used in the experiments.

	Name	Source	ID
1	Paxillin	Rabbit, pAb	#2542 Cell signaling
2	Anti-rabbit IgG, HRP-linked antibody	Goat	#7074 Cell signaling
3	Phospho-Paxillin (Tyr118)	Rabbit, pAb	#2541 Cell signaling
4	FAK	Rabbit, pAb	#13430 Cell signaling
5	Phospho-FAK (Tyr925)	Rabbit, pAb	#9330 Cell signaling
6	Vimentin (D21H3)	Rabbit, mAb	#9782 Cell signaling
7	β-Catenin (D10A8)	Rabbit, mAb	#9782 Cell signaling
8	GAPDH-HRP	Mouse mAb	#: ab011 Multi Science

4.4.2. Cell Culture and CCK-8 Cell Viability Test

The human cervical cancer cell line HeLa (HPV 18 positive) was purchased from the Type Culture Collection of the Chinese Academy of Sciences (Shanghai, China). Cells were cultured in DMEM with 10% FBS, penicillin (100 units/mL), and streptomycin (100 μg/mL), in an incubator at 37 °C with 5% CO_2. The CCK-8 test was performed as previously described [17,41]. Briefly, HeLa cells (1×10^5 cells/mL) were cultured in DMEM with different doses of genistein and solvent control for 24–48 h. CCK-8 was then added to the culture medium and was incubated for 1 h. The absorbance was measured at a wavelength of 450 nm (OD450 nm) in a microtiter plate reader (BioRad, Hercules, CA, USA).

4.4.3. Colony Formation Assay

Cells (1×10^3 cells/well) were initially grown in DMEM with or without different concentrations of genistein and solvent control. After 7–10 days, the cells were fixed with PFA and stained with crystal violet. Images of five randomly selected fields were captured under an inverted microscope (Nikon, Tochigi, Japan).

4.4.4. Adhesion Assay

This assay was performed according to previous protocols [60,61]. Cells (1×10^5 cells/mL) were grown for 2 h and then cultured with or without genistein (0–100 μM) for another 24 h in a 12-well plate. Cells were collected and reseeded with the concentration of 1×10^5 cells/mL in a 96-well plate for 3 h. Afterwards, cells were washed, fixed with PFA, and finally stained with crystal violet. Adhesion was assessed at OD570 nm using a microplate reader. Images of five randomly selected fields were captured under an inverted microscope. The percentage of adherent cells was calculated from the OD values of the genistein-treated group (relative to the OD values of the control group).

4.4.5. Wound-Healing Mobility Assay

This assay was performed according to previous protocols [17]. Briefly, cells (1×10^5 cells/well) were grown in a 6-well plate for 24 h to achieve 90% confluency. The medium was discarded and cell monolayers were scratched with a sterile P200 micropipette tip. After the debris was washed away, cells were allowed to grow in serum-free medium with different doses of genistein and solvent control for 24 h. Images of the wound areas were captured at 0 h, 8 h, and 24 h. Cell migration was calculated by measuring cell distances from the wound edges in each treatment group. Cell migration (as a percentage) was calculated based on the migration distances in the genistein-treated group (relative to those of the control group).

4.4.6. Transwell Assay

The assay was performed according to previous protocols [17]. Cells were cultured in a Transwell® cell culture chamber (8 mm pore size; Corning, Lowell, MA, USA) at a density of 2×10^4/well. For a 24-h invasion assay, the chambers were first coated with Matrigel™. A cell suspension in serum-free DMEM was cultured in the upper chamber of the Transwell® insert with or without different doses of genistein and solvent control. The lower part was filled with DMEM containing 20% FBS as a chemoattractant. After 24 h, cells that migrated or invaded into the lower surface of the membrane were fixed with 4% PFA and stained with crystal violet solution. Images of five random fields were captured by an inverted microscope. Cell migration/invasion was subsequently assessed using Image J software. Cell migration/invasion was calculated (as a percentage) from the relative numbers of cells in the genistein-treated and control groups.

4.4.7. Western Blotting Assay

The assay was carried out according to previous protocols [17]. Briefly, cells were grown with or without different concentrations of genistein (12.5–100 μM) and solvent control for 30 min. Cells were then harvested and lysed in ice-cold cell lysis buffer. After protein extraction, the total protein concentration was quantified using standard protocols. Total protein (20 μg of protein/lane) was then separated on a 10% SDS-PAGE gel by electrophoresis. Separated proteins were transferred onto PVDF (Polyvinylidene Fluoride) membranes (BioRad, USA) and subsequently probed with the respective primary antibody followed by an HRP (Horse Radish peroxidase) -conjugated secondary antibody. Finally, the blots were developed by ECL (Electrochemiluminescence).

4.4.8. RNA Sequencing

RNA sequencing was carried out as previously reported [62,63]. Cells were grown with DMSO and genistein (50 μM) for 5 h. Total RNA was isolated using the RNeasy Plus Mini Kit, following the manufacturer's instructions (Qiagen, Germantown, MD, USA). The quality of the RNA was first confirmed, and then the RNA was sequenced using the Illumina Hiseq X ten platform in GeneChem. Data from the sequencer were first subjected to quality control using FastQC and trimmed using trimgalore. Data processing included (i) trimming the Illumina adapter sequence and low-quality bases (phred score < 20) at the 3′ end; (ii) discarding the reads with a length shorter than 20 (the paired reads were removed if any of the two reads did not meet the minimum length). Duplicates were then removed using Picard. For each sample, we counted the reads of individual transcripts using htseq-count. Differential analysis between treatments (genistein) and the control was performed using a count-based method, limma, implemented in R, and voom for normalization [64,65]. Significantly expressed genes were first screened for BH-adjusted p values less than 0.05 [66] and further filtered using a 2-fold-change minimum boundary (up- and downregulated genes labeled in the volcano plot). In parallel, we used GSEA v3.0 (Broad Institute, PreRanked mode) for enrichment analysis. To ensure consistency in our method for identifying significant genes, we used the t-statistic output from the limma as a metric for ranking. Here, 1000 gene set permutations were set as default, and gene sets were obtained by collecting pathways from KEGG and biological processes from GO. A gene set with an FDR q value less than 0.05 was considered significantly enriched. For the heatmap, log_2 transformed FPKM values (fragments per kilobase of transcript per million mapped reads) of the significant genes were used as input for heatmap generation.

4.4.9. Quantitative Real-Time RT-PCR

Cells were grown with or without different doses of genistein and solvent control for 5 h. Total RNA was isolated using the RNeasy Plus Mini Kit. The cDNA was synthesized using a reverse transcription reagent kit (Selleck, Shanghai, China). Target genes were amplified with the following specific primers in the Light Cycler® 96 Real-Time PCR System (Roche, Indianapolis, IN, USA):

GAPDH: 5′-GGAGCGAGATCCCTCCAAAAT-3′ (forward) and
5′-GGCTGTTGTCATACTTCTCATGG-3′ (reverse);
FAK: 5′-TGGTGCAATGGAGCGAGTATT-3′(forward) and
5′-CAGTGAACCTCCTCTGACCG-3′(reverse);
Paxillin: 5′-CTGCTGGAACTGAACGCTGTA-3′ (forward) and
5′-GGGGCTGTTAGTCTCTGGGA-3′ (reverse);
Snail: 5′-TCGGAAGCCTAACTACAGCGA-3′ (forward) and
5′-AGATGAGCATTGGCAGCGAG-3′ (reverse);
Twist: 5′-GTCCGCAGTCTTACGAGGAG-3′ (forward) and
5′-GCTTGAGGGTCTGAATCTTGCT-3′ (reverse).

GAPDH was used as a normalization control. Each treatment was tested in triplicate. The relative expression levels of genes were normalized using the $2^{-\Delta\Delta Ct}$ method.

4.5. *Statistical Analyses*

Data are reported as the mean ± S.D. from at least three independent experiments. A $p < 0.05$ was used to measure statistical significance. Student's *t*-tests were used to compare statistical significance between the treated groups.

Author Contributions: T.C.: Data curation; Writing—Original draft preparation. J.W.: Data curation; Writing—Original draft preparation. M.L.: Data curation. Q.W.: Data curation; Reviewing and Editing. S.C.: Conceptualization; Supervision; Writing—Original draft preparation; Reviewing and Editing. All authors have read and agreed to the published version of the manuscript.

Funding: This research was funded by the National Natural Science Foundation of China (NSFC) (81703969), Scientific Research Foundation of Jiangsu Province, China (BK20211327), The Natural Science Foundation of Jiangsu Higher Education Institutions of China (21KJA360004) Jiangsu Province "Qinglan" project (2022), and Yangzhou University "Qinglan" project (2018).

Institutional Review Board Statement: Not applicable.

Informed Consent Statement: Not applicable.

Data Availability Statement: The data presented in this study are available on request from the corresponding author.

Acknowledgments: We acknowledge the National Natural Science Foundation of China, Scientific Research Foundation of Jiangsu Province, The Natural Science Foundation of Jiangsu Higher Education Institutions of China, Yangzhou University "Qinglan" project, and Jiangsu Province "Qinglan" project for the financial support.

Conflicts of Interest: The authors declare no conflict of interest.

Sample Availability: Samples of the compounds are not available from the authors.

References

1. Bray, F.; Ferlay, J.; Soerjomataram, I.; Siegel, R.L.; Torre, L.A.; Jemal, A. Global cancer statistics 2018: GLOBOCAN estimates of incidence and mortality worldwide for 36 cancers in 185 countries. *CA Cancer J. Clin.* **2018**, *68*, 394–424. [CrossRef] [PubMed]
2. Chan, C.K.; Aimagambetova, G.; Ukybassova, T.; Kongrtay, K.; Azizan, A. Human Papillomavirus Infection and Cervical Cancer: Epidemiology, Screening, and Vaccination-Review of Current Perspectives. *J. Oncol.* **2019**, *2019*, 3257939. [CrossRef]

3. Curty, G.; de Carvalho, P.S.; Soares, M.A. The Role of the Cervicovaginal Microbiome on the Genesis and as a Biomarker of Premalignant Cervical Intraepithelial Neoplasia and Invasive Cervical Cancer. *Int. J. Mol. Sci.* **2019**, *21*, 222. [CrossRef] [PubMed]
4. Latsuzbaia, A.; Hebette, G.; Fischer, M.; Arbyn, M.; Weyers, S.; Vielh, P.; Schmitt, F.; Mossong, J. Introduction of liquid-based cytology and human papillomavirus testing in cervical cancer screening in Luxembourg. *Diagn. Cytopathol.* **2017**, *45*, 384–390. [CrossRef] [PubMed]
5. Sasaki, Y.; Iwanari, O.; Arakawa, I.; Moriya, T.; Mikami, Y.; Iihara, K.; Konoro, R. Cervical Cancer Screening With Human Papillomavirus DNA and Cytology in Japan. *Int. J. Gynecol. Cancer* **2017**, *27*, 523–529. [CrossRef]
6. Gupta, S. Adjuvant chemotherapy in locally advanced cervical cancer: The ceiling remains unbroken. *J. Gynecol. Oncol.* **2019**, *30*, e97. [CrossRef]
7. Liontos, M.; Kyriazoglou, A.; Dimitriadis, I.; Dimopoulos, M.A.; Bamias, A. Systemic therapy in cervical cancer: 30 years in review. *Crit. Rev. Oncol. Hematol.* **2019**, *137*, 9–17. [CrossRef]
8. Azmi, A.S. Adopting network pharmacology for cancer drug discovery. *Curr. Drug Discov. Technol.* **2013**, *10*, 95–105. [CrossRef]
9. Balasubramaniam, S.D.; Balakrishnan, V.; Oon, C.E.; Kaur, G. Key Molecular Events in Cervical Cancer Development. *Medicina* **2019**, *55*, 384. [CrossRef]
10. He, C.; Lv, X.; Huang, C.; Angeletti, P.C.; Hua, G.; Dong, J.; Zhouu, J.; Wang, Z.; Ma, B.; Chen, X.; et al. A Human Papillomavirus-Independent Cervical Cancer Animal Model Reveals Unconventional Mechanisms of Cervical Carcinogenesis. *Cell Rep.* **2019**, *26*, 2636–2650.e5. [CrossRef]
11. Wang, C.; Davis, J.S. At the center of cervical carcinogenesis: Synergism between high-risk HPV and the hyperactivated YAP1. *Mol. Cell Oncol.* **2019**, *6*, e1612677. [CrossRef] [PubMed]
12. Zhou, Y.; Shu, C.; Huang, Y. Fibronectin promotes cervical cancer tumorigenesis through activating FAK signaling pathway. *J. Cell Biochem.* **2019**, *120*, 10988–10997. [CrossRef] [PubMed]
13. Zhang, R.; Zhu, X.; Bai, H.; Ning, K. Network Pharmacology Databases for Traditional Chinese Medicine: Review and Assessment. *Front. Pharmacol.* **2019**, *10*, 123. [CrossRef] [PubMed]
14. Muhammad, J.; Khan, A.; Ali, A.; Fang, L.; Yanjing, W.; Xu, Q.; Wei, D.Q. Network Pharmacology: Exploring the Resources and Methodologies. *Curr. Top. Med. Chem.* **2018**, *18*, 949–964. [CrossRef] [PubMed]
15. Cepeda, S.B.; Sandoval, M.J.; Rauschemberger, M.B.; Massheimer, V.L. Beneficial role of the phytoestrogen genistein on vascular calcification. *J. Nutr. Biochem.* **2017**, *50*, 26–37. [CrossRef]
16. Cui, S.; Bilitewski, U. Effect of genistein on the TLR and MAPK transduction cascades in lipopolysaccharide-stimulated macrophages. *Xi Bao Yu Fen Zi Mian Yi Xue Za Zhi* **2014**, *30*, 233–236.
17. Cui, S.N.; Wang, J.; Wu, Q.Q.; Qian, J.; Yang, C.S.; Bo, P. Genistein inhibits the growth and regulates the migration and invasion abilities of melanoma cells via the FAK/paxillin and MAPK pathways. *Oncotarget* **2017**, *8*, 21674–21691. [CrossRef]
18. Jaiswal, N.; Akhtar, J.; Singh, S.P.; Badruddeen; Ahsan, F. An Overview on Genistein and its Various Formulations. *Drug Res.* **2019**, *69*, 305–313. [CrossRef]
19. Mukund, V.; Mukund, D.; Sharma, V.; Mannarapu, M.; Alam, A. Genistein: Its role in metabolic diseases and cancer. *Crit. Rev. Oncol. Hematol.* **2017**, *119*, 13–22. [CrossRef]
20. Tuli, H.S.; Tuorkey, M.J.; Thakral, F.; Sak, K.; Kumar, M.; Sharma, A.K.; Sharma, U.; Jain, A.; Aggarwal, V.; Bishayee, A. Molecular Mechanisms of Action of Genistein in Cancer: Recent Advances. *Front. Pharmacol.* **2019**, *10*, 1336. [CrossRef]
21. Sundaram, M.K.; Ansari, M.Z.; Al Mutery, A.; Ashraf, M.; Nasab, R.; Rai, S.; Rais, N.; Hussain, A. Genistein Induces Alterations of Epigenetic Modulatory Signatures in Human Cervical Cancer Cells. *Anticancer Agents Med. Chem.* **2018**, *18*, 412–421. [CrossRef] [PubMed]
22. Wang, S.Y.; Yang, K.W.; Hsu, Y.T.; Chang, C.L.; Yang, Y.C. The differential inhibitory effects of genistein on the growth of cervical cancer cells in vitro. *Neoplasma* **2001**, *48*, 227–233. [PubMed]
23. Yang, Y.M.; Yang, Y.; Dai, W.W.; Li, X.M.; Ma, J.Q.; Tang, L.P. Genistein-induced apoptosis is mediated by endoplasmic reticulum stress in cervical cancer cells. *Eur. Rev. Med. Pharmacol. Sci.* **2016**, *20*, 3292–3296. [PubMed]
24. Yashar, C.M.; Spanos, W.J.; Taylor, D.D.; Gercel-Taylor, C. Potentiation of the radiation effect with genistein in cervical cancer cells. *Gynecol. Oncol.* **2005**, *99*, 199–205. [CrossRef]
25. Zhang, B.; Liu, J.Y.; Pan, J.S.; Han, S.P.; Yin, X.X.; Wang, B.; Hu, G. Combined treatment of ionizing radiation with genistein on cervical cancer HeLa cells. *J. Pharmacol. Sci.* **2006**, *102*, 129–135. [CrossRef]
26. Zhang, H.; Liu, G.; Zeng, X.; Wu, Y.; Yang, C.; Mei, L.; Wang, Z.; Huang, L. Fabrication of genistein-loaded biodegradable TPGS-b-PCL nanoparticles for improved therapeutic effects in cervical cancer cells. *Int. J. Nanomed.* **2015**, *10*, 2461–2473. [CrossRef]
27. Kim, S.H.; Kim, S.H.; Lee, S.C.; Song, Y.S. Involvement of Both Extrinsic and Intrinsic Apoptotic Pathways in Apoptosis Induced by Genistein in Human Cervical Cancer Cells. *Nat. Compd. Role Apoptotic Cell Signal. Pathw.* **2009**, *1171*, 196–201. [CrossRef]
28. Lin, Y.J.; Zhen, Y.Z.; Zhao, Y.F.; Wei, J.; Hu, G. Rhein Lysinate Induced S-Phase Arrest and Increased the Anti-Tumor Activity of 5-FU in HeLa Cells. *Am. J. Chin. Med.* **2011**, *39*, 817–825. [CrossRef]
29. Lee, M.Y.; Chou, C.Y.; Tang, M.J.; Shen, M.R. Epithelial-mesenchymal transition in cervical cancer: Correlation with tumor progression, epidermal growth factor receptor overexpression, and snail up-regulation. *Clin. Cancer Res.* **2008**, *14*, 4743–4750. [CrossRef]

30. Li, C.; Ao, H.; Chen, G.; Wang, F.; Li, F. The Interaction of CDH20 With beta-Catenin Inhibits Cervical Cancer Cell Migration and Invasion via TGF-beta/Smad/SNAIL Mediated EMT. *Front. Oncol.* **2019**, *9*, 1481. [CrossRef]
31. Ou, J.; Guan, D.; Yang, Y. Non-contact co-culture with human vascular endothelial cells promotes epithelial-to-mesenchymal transition of cervical cancer SiHa cells by activating the NOTCH1/LOX/SNAIL pathway. *Cell Mol. Biol. Lett.* **2019**, *24*, 39. [CrossRef] [PubMed]
32. Park, S.J.; Kim, M.J.; Kim, Y.K.; Kim, S.M.; Park, J.Y.; Myoung, H. Combined cetuximab and genistein treatment shows additive anti-cancer effect on oral squamous cell carcinoma. *Cancer Lett.* **2010**, *292*, 54–63. [CrossRef] [PubMed]
33. Sarkar, F.H.; Adsule, S.; Padhye, S.; Kulkarni, S.; Li, Y. The role of genistein and synthetic derivatives of isoflavone in cancer prevention and therapy. *Mini Rev. Med. Chem.* **2006**, *6*, 401–407. [CrossRef]
34. Davis, D.A.; Sarkar, S.H.; Hussain, M.; Li, Y.W.; Sarkar, F.H. Increased therapeutic potential of an experimental anti-mitotic inhibitor SB715992 by genistein in PC-3 human prostate cancer cell line. *BMC Cancer* **2006**, *6*, 22. [CrossRef] [PubMed]
35. Spagnuolo, C.; Russo, G.L.; Orhan, I.E.; Habtemariam, S.; Daglia, M.; Sureda, A.; Nabavi, S.M. Genistein and cancer: Current status, challenges, and future directions. *Adv. Nutr.* **2015**, *6*, 408–419. [CrossRef] [PubMed]
36. Wu, K.; Yi, Y.; Liu, F.; Wu, W.; Chen, Y.; Zhang, W. Identification of key pathways and genes in the progression of cervical cancer using bioinformatics analysis. *Oncol. Lett.* **2018**, *16*, 1003–1009. [CrossRef]
37. Cao, F.Y.; Zhou, X.P.; Su, J.; Yang, X.H.; Mu, F.H.; Shen, J.Y.; Sun, W. Chemical Structure Characteristics and Bioactivity of Small Molecule FAK Inhibitors. *Anticancer Agents Med. Chem.* **2015**, *16*, 934–941. [CrossRef]
38. Lv, P.C.; Jiang, A.Q.; Zhang, W.M.; Zhu, H.L. FAK inhibitors in Cancer, a patent review. *Expert Opin. Ther. Pat.* **2018**, *28*, 139–145. [CrossRef]
39. Roy-Luzarraga, M.; Hodivala-Dilke, K. Molecular Pathways: Endothelial Cell FAK-A Target for Cancer Treatment. *Clin. Cancer Res.* **2016**, *22*, 3718–3724. [CrossRef]
40. Alanko, J.; Ivaska, J. Endosomes: Emerging Platforms for Integrin-Mediated FAK Signalling. *Trends Cell Biol.* **2016**, *26*, 391–398. [CrossRef]
41. Cui, S.; Wu, Q.; Wang, J.; Li, M.; Qian, J.; Li, S. Quercetin inhibits LPS-induced macrophage migration by suppressing the iNOS/FAK/paxillin pathway and modulating the cytoskeleton. *Cell Adh. Migr.* **2019**, *13*, 1–12. [CrossRef] [PubMed]
42. Kanteti, R.; Batra, S.K.; Lennon, F.E.; Salgia, R. FAK and paxillin, two potential targets in pancreatic cancer. *Oncotarget* **2016**, *7*, 31586. [CrossRef] [PubMed]
43. Yoon, H.; Dehart, J.P.; Murphy, J.M.; Lim, S.T. Understanding the roles of FAK in cancer: Inhibitors, genetic models, and new insights. *J. Histochem. Cytochem.* **2015**, *63*, 114–128. [CrossRef] [PubMed]
44. Lee, B.Y.; Timpson, P.; Horvath, L.G.; Daly, R.J. FAK signaling in human cancer as a target for therapeutics. *Pharmacol. Ther.* **2015**, *146*, 132–149. [CrossRef] [PubMed]
45. Yeh, C.M.; Hsieh, M.J.; Yang, J.S.; Yang, S.F.; Chuang, Y.T.; Su, S.C.; Liang, M.-Y.; Chen, M.-K.; Lin, C.-W. Geraniin inhibits oral cancer cell migration by suppressing matrix metalloproteinase-2 activation through the FAK/Src and ERK pathways. *Environ. Toxicol.* **2019**, *34*, 1085–1093. [CrossRef]
46. Herzinger, T.; Wolf, D.A. Snail puts melanoma on the fast track. *Pigment. Cell Melanoma Res.* **2009**, *22*, 150–151. [CrossRef]
47. Wang, Q.; Xu, H.; Zhao, X. Baicalin Inhibits Human Cervical Cancer Cells by Suppressing Protein Kinase C/Signal Transducer and Activator of Transcription (PKC/STAT3) Signaling Pathway. *Med. Sci. Monit.* **2018**, *24*, 1955–1961. [CrossRef]
48. Bolos, V.; Gasent, J.M.; Lopez-Tarruella, S.; Grande, E. The dual kinase complex FAK-Src as a promising therapeutic target in cancer. *OncoTargets Ther.* **2010**, *3*, 83–97. [CrossRef]
49. Mitra, S.K.; Schlaepfer, D.D. Integrin-regulated FAK-Src signaling in normal and cancer cells. *Curr. Opin. Cell Biol.* **2006**, *18*, 516–523. [CrossRef]
50. Cui, S.; Wienhoefer, N.; Bilitewski, U. Genistein induces morphology change and G2/M cell cycle arrest by inducing p38 MAPK activation in macrophages. *Int. Immunopharmacol.* **2014**, *18*, 142–150. [CrossRef]
51. Farruggio, S.; Cocomazzi, G.; Marotta, P.; Romito, R.; Surico, D.; Calamita, G.; Bellan, M.; Pirisi, M.; Grossini, E. Genistein and 17beta-Estradiol Protect Hepatocytes from Fatty Degeneration by Mechanisms Involving Mitochondria, Inflammasome and Kinases Activation. *Cell Physiol. Biochem.* **2020**, *54*, 401–416. [CrossRef] [PubMed]
52. Qin, J.; Teng, J.; Zhu, Z.; Chen, J.; Huang, W.J. Genistein induces activation of the mitochondrial apoptosis pathway by inhibiting phosphorylation of Akt in colorectal cancer cells. *Pharm. Biol.* **2016**, *54*, 74–79. [CrossRef]
53. Zhang, Q.; Bao, J.; Yang, J. Genistein-triggered anticancer activity against liver cancer cell line HepG2 involves ROS generation, mitochondrial apoptosis, G2/M cell cycle arrest and inhibition of cell migration. *Arch. Med. Sci.* **2019**, *15*, 1001–1009. [CrossRef] [PubMed]
54. Davis, A.P.; Murphy, C.G.; Saraceni-Richards, C.A.; Rosenstein, M.C.; Wiegers, T.C.; Mattingly, C.J. Comparative Toxicogenomics Database: A knowledgebase and discovery tool for chemical-gene-disease networks. *Nucleic Acids Res.* **2009**, *37*, D786–D792. [CrossRef] [PubMed]
55. Mattingly, C.J.; Rosenstein, M.C.; Davis, A.P.; Colby, G.T.; Forrest, J.N.; Boyer, J.L. The Comparative Toxicogenomics Database: A cross-species resource for building chemical-gene interaction networks. *Toxicol. Sci.* **2006**, *92*, 587–595. [CrossRef]
56. Mattingly, C.J.; Colby, G.T.; Rosenstein, M.C.; Forrest, J.N.; Boyer, J.L. Promoting comparative molecular studies in environmental health research: An overview of the comparative toxicogenomics database (CTD). *Pharm. J.* **2004**, *4*, 5–8. [CrossRef]

57. Mattingly, C.J.; Rosenstein, M.C.; Colby, G.T.; Forrest, J.N.; Boyer, J.L. The Comparative Toxicogenomics Database (CTD): A resource for comparative toxicological studies. *J. Exp. Zool. Part A Ecol. Integr. Physiol.* **2006**, *305a*, 689–692. [CrossRef]
58. von Mering, C.; Huynen, M.; Jaeggi, D.; Schmidt, S.; Bork, P.; Snel, B. STRING: A database of predicted functional associations between proteins. *Nucleic Acids Res.* **2003**, *31*, 258–261. [CrossRef]
59. Chin, C.H.; Chen, S.H.; Wu, H.H.; Ho, C.W.; Ko, M.T.; Lin, C.Y. CytoHubba: Identifying hub objects and sub-networks from complex interactome. *BMC Syst. Biol.* **2014**, *8*, S11. [CrossRef]
60. Wu, Z.Y.; Lien, J.C.; Huang, Y.P.; Liao, C.L.; Lin, J.J.; Fan, M.J.; Ko, Y.-C.; Hsiao, Y.-P.; Lu, H.-F.; Chung, J.-G. Casticin Inhibits A375.S2 Human Melanoma Cell Migration/Invasion through Downregulating NF-kappaB and Matrix Metalloproteinase-2 and -1. *Molecules* **2016**, *21*, 384. [CrossRef]
61. Wu, S.H.; Hsiao, Y.T.; Kuo, C.L.; Yu, F.S.; Hsu, S.C.; Wu, P.P.; Chen, J.C.; Hsia, T.C.; Liu, H.C.; Hsu, W.H.; et al. Bufalin Inhibits NCI-H460 Human Lung Cancer Cell Metastasis In Vitro by Inhibiting MAPKs, MMPs, and NF-kappa B Pathways. *Am. J. Chin. Med.* **2015**, *43*, 1247–1264. [CrossRef] [PubMed]
62. Lv, Z.; Hu, C.; Jiang, J.; Jin, S.; Wei, Q.; Wei, X.; Yu, D.; Shi, F. Effects of High-Dose Genistein on the Hypothalamic RNA Profile and Intestinal Health of Female Chicks. *J. Agric. Food Chem.* **2019**, *67*, 13737–13750. [CrossRef] [PubMed]
63. Wang, Q.; Liu, X.; Zhou, J.; Yang, C.; Wang, G.; Tan, Y.; Wu, Y.; Zhang, S.; Yi, K.; Kang, C. The CRISPR-Cas13a Gene-Editing System Induces Collateral Cleavage of RNA in Glioma Cells. *Adv. Sci.* **2019**, *6*, 1901299. [CrossRef] [PubMed]
64. Law, C.W.; Chen, Y.; Shi, W.; Smyth, G.K. Voom: Precision weights unlock linear model analysis tools for RNA-seq read counts. *Genome Biol.* **2014**, *15*, R29. [CrossRef]
65. Liu, R.; Holik, A.Z.; Su, S.; Jansz, N.; Chen, K.; Leong, H.S.; Blewitt, M.E.; Asselin-Labat, M.-L.; Smyth, G.K.; Ritchie, M.E. Why weight? Modelling sample and observational level variability improves power in RNA-seq analyses. *Nucleic Acids Res.* **2015**, *43*, e97. [CrossRef]
66. Benjamini, Y.; Hochberg, Y. Controlling the false discovery rate—A practical and powerful approach to multiple testing. *J. R. Statist. Soc. Ser. B* **1995**, *57*, 289–300. [CrossRef]

marine drugs

MDPI

Article

Anti-Proliferative and Pro-Apoptotic vLMW Fucoidan Formulas Decrease PD-L1 Surface Expression in EBV Latency III and DLBCL Tumoral B-Cells by Decreasing Actin Network

Jennifer Saliba [1], Chanez Manseur [2], Hugo Groult [2], Hussein Akil [1], Mona Tannoury [3], Danielle Troutaud [1], Thierry Maugard [2], Jean Feuillard [1,4], Ingrid Arnaudin [2] and Chantal Jayat-Vignoles [1,*]

1 UMR CNRS 7276, INSERM 1262, CRIBL Laboratory, Faculty of Medecine, Limoges University, 87000 Limoges, France
2 UMR CNRS 7266, LIENSs Laboratory, La Rochelle University, 17000 La Rochelle, France
3 Faculty of Sciences II, Lebanese University, Beirut RGHC+4PR, Lebanon
4 Hematology Laboratory, CHU Dupuytren, 2 Avenue Martin Luther King, CEDEX 87042 Limoges, France
* Correspondence: chantal.vignoles@unilim.fr; Tel.: +33-(0)-5-19-564-221; Fax: +33-(0)-555-435-897

Abstract: Epstein–Barr virus (EBV) infects 95% of the world's population and persists latently in the body. It immortalizes B-cells and is associated with lymphomas. LCLs (lymphoblastoid cell lines, EBV latency III B-cells) inhibit anti-tumoral T-cell response following PD-L1 overexpression (programmed death-ligand 1 immune checkpoint). Many cancer cells, including some DLBCLs (diffuse large B-cell lymphomas), also overexpress PD-L1. Immunotherapies are based on inhibition of PD-L1/PD-1 interactions but present some dose-dependent toxicities. We aim to find new strategies to improve their efficiency by decreasing PD-L1 expression. Fucoidan, a polysaccharide extracted from brown seaweed, exhibits immunomodulatory and anti-tumor activities depending on its polymerization degree, but data are scarce on lymphoma cells or immune checkpoints. LCLs and DLBCLs cells were treated with native fucoidan (*Fucus vesiculosus*) or original very-low-molecular-weight fucoidan formulas (vLMW-F). We observed cell proliferation decrease and apoptosis induction increase with vLMW-F and no toxicity on normal B- and T-cells. We highlighted a decrease in transcriptional and PD-L1 surface expression, even more efficient for vLMW than native fucoidan. This can be explained by actin network alteration, suggesting lower fusion of secretory vesicles carrying PD-L1 with the plasma membrane. We propose vLMW-F as potential adjuvants to immunotherapy due to their anti-proliferative and proapoptotic effects and ability to decrease PD-L1 membrane expression.

Keywords: fucoidan; very-low-molecular-weight fucoidan; PD-L1; EBV latency III B-cells; DLBCLs; actin network

Citation: Saliba, J.; Manseur, C.; Groult, H.; Akil, H.; Tannoury, M.; Troutaud, D.; Maugard, T.; Feuillard, J.; Arnaudin, I.; Jayat-Vignoles, C. Anti-Proliferative and Pro-Apoptotic vLMW Fucoidan Formulas Decrease PD-L1 Surface Expression in EBV Latency III and DLBCL Tumoral B-Cells by Decreasing Actin Network. *Mar. Drugs* **2023**, *21*, 132. https://doi.org/10.3390/md21020132

Academic Editors: Barbara De Filippis, Alessandra Ammazzalorso and Marialuigia Fantacuzzi

Received: 26 January 2023
Revised: 13 February 2023
Accepted: 15 February 2023
Published: 18 February 2023

1. Introduction

EBV is an oncogenic virus that infects about 95% of the worldwide adult population. After primo-infection, it remains hidden in nuclei of memory B-cells, resulting in life-long persistent infection. During infection, including transient reactivation, some infected B-cells enter the lytic cycle or EBV latency III program (also called proliferation program), with transcription of the full range of latent genes [1]. In an immunocompetent host, the balance established between the immune system and the virus avoids development of cancers. However, a rupture in equilibrium can occur, causing EBV lymphoproliferative disorders, such as Hodgkin lymphomas (HL), Burkitt lymphomas (BL) or DLBCLs [2], which is the most common non-Hodgkin lymphoma. This aggressive tumor affects B-lymphocytes and has two major biologically distinct subtypes: germinal center B-cell (GCB) and activated B-cell (ABC) [3]. ABC-DLBCL is associated with worse outcomes when treated with chemo-immunotherapy, the standard clinical care for this pathology.

Inhibitory immune checkpoints exert inhibitory effects on adaptive and innate immune systems. They are crucial for self-tolerance but also mediate immune evasion of cancer cells, contributing to tumor emergence and development [4]. PD-L1 (also known as B7-H1 or CD274) is expressed on a sizeable fraction of tumor types and is one of the most critical [5]. It can interact with its receptor, PD-1, which is expressed on numerous cells involved in anti-tumor response (such as activated T-cells, dendritic cells or NK cells) and leads to inhibitory signals [6]. We have previously shown that PD-L1 is also overexpressed on EBV latency III B-cells and strongly inhibits anti-tumoral T-cell response in an autologous B/T model; expansion of anergic conventional and unconventional $CD4^+$ Tregs (regulatory T-cells) leads to inhibition of $CD4^+$ and $CD8^+$ effector T-cells proliferation [7]. The PD-L1/PD-1 axis is also critical for numerous B-cell lymphomas, such as HL and non-Hodgkin lymphomas, among them follicular lymphoma and DLBCL (which variably express PD-L1) [8,9]. PD-L1 overexpression in many cancer types and strong immune response inhibition following interaction with PD-1 have led to development of anti-PD-L1 and anti-PD-1 immunotherapies to block the PD-L1/PD-1 axis and restore immune response [10,11]. However, immune checkpoint inhibitors have some limitations since tolerance breakdown is not limited to tumors; related adverse events can affect multiple organ systems (gut, skin, endocrine glands, liver or lung) [12–14]. While keeping the advantage of immunotherapy, new therapeutic strategies can be considered, such as use of adjuvants capable of decreasing PD-L1 membrane expression and consequently lowering antibody doses [15].

Fucoidans are non-allergenic, non-irritating, biodegradable and biocompatible sulfated fucose-based polysaccharides constituents of brown seaweeds [16,17]. Extracts from *Fucus vesiculosus* algae are approved by the FDA (Food and Drug Administration) as GRAS (generally recognized as safe). In Europe, preparations that contain fucoidans are registered by the EMA (European Medicines Agency) for use as ingredients in food categories [17,18]. Numerous studies report bioactive properties with health benefits, predominantly dependent on the natural source extraction method, sulfate groups content and molecular weight of polysaccharide. For instance, fucoidans possess antioxidant, anticoagulant, anti-pathogenic and anti-inflammatory activities [19–21]. They also exhibit *in vitro* and *in vivo* anticancer properties, almost exclusively studied on solid tumor cells (colon, breast, lung, bladder, hepatoma or melanoma). The mechanisms of action described are generally cell cycle arrest, apoptosis, anti-metastatic effects and stimulation of macrophages, T-cells and NK cells. Nevertheless, scarce studies indicate decrease in PD-L1 checkpoint [22,23], which can be consistent with the fact that fucoidan impairs pathways responsible for PD-L1 expression: PI3k/AKT, NF-κB or RAS/ERK1/2 [24–29]. Fucoidan extracts can also protect against side effects associated with chemotherapeutic drugs and radiation-induced damages [16,30]. As suggested by some authors who evaluated pre-clinical safety of fucoidan extracts [31], they may become an appropriate and natural anticancer therapeutic as an adjunctive antitumor drug. However, more information is needed, particularly in the field of hematological malignancies and immune checkpoints, such as PD-L1, which is the overall objective in this study. We evaluated opportunity to use vLMW-F to decrease PD-L1 membrane expression and associated molecular mechanisms.

2. Results

2.1. Proliferation Inhibition and Apoptosis Induction of Tumoral B-Cells

Anti-cancer properties of fucoidan (mainly with extracted fucoidan of high molecular weight) were almost exclusively studied on solid tumors and emphasized anti-proliferative and pro-apoptotic events [32]. In order to confirm this role on lymphoma B-cells, we performed cell cycle analysis by flow cytometry on EBV latency III B-cells (three LCLs) and DLBCL cells (two ABCs: U2932 and OCILy10 and two GCBs: SUDHL4 and SUDHL6 cell lines) treated with native or vLMW-F F1 and F2. Estimation of cell population percentage in the different phases of the cell cycle highlighted significant decrease in S phase after treatment with vLMW-F in contrast to the native form (Figure 1A, B). This was consistent with inhibition of cell proliferation. A significant increase in subG1 peak on DNA content histograms (subsequent to fragmentation of nuclear DNA in late apoptosis) was also sometimes observed, depending on cell types, for treatment by vLMW-F, especially F2 (Figure 1C).

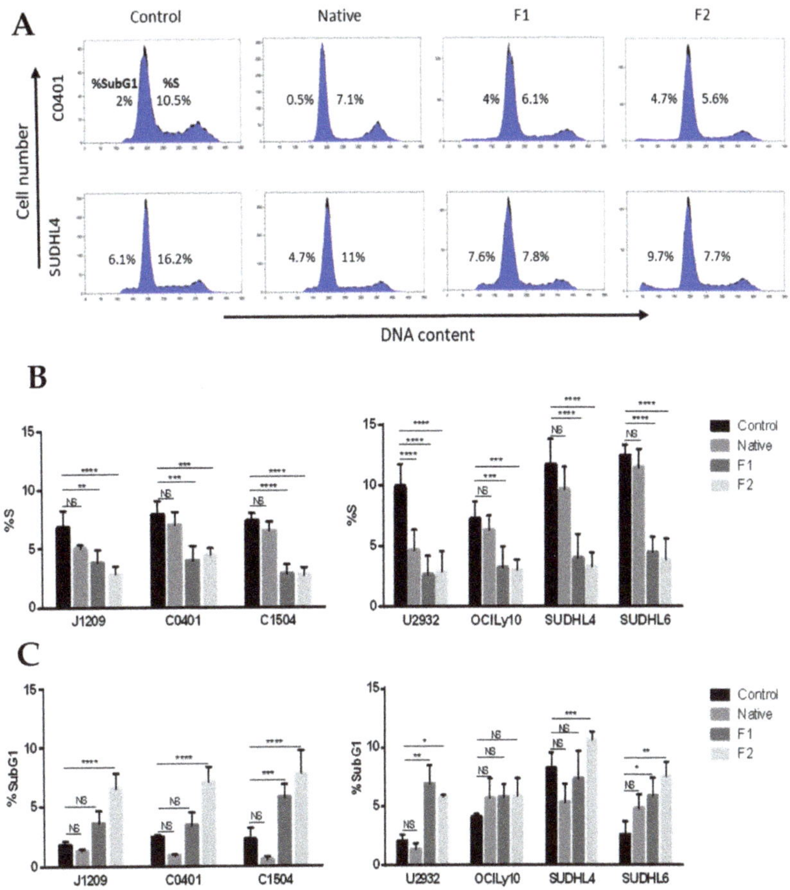

Figure 1. vLMW-F decrease the percentage of LCLs and DLBCLs cells in S-phase. LCLs (J1209, C0401, C1504) and DLBCLs (U2932, OCILy10, SUDHL4, SUDHL6) cells were treated or not (control) with 100µg/mL of native fucoidan or vLMW-F (F1 and F2) for 48 h. Flow cytometry analysis was performed to determine cell-cycle distribution in all tested conditions. Results were obtained from three independent experiments. (**A**) Examples of cell cycle profiles for C0401 (LCL) and SUDHL4 (DLBCL). (**B**) Percentage of LCLs or DLBCLs cells in S-phase: fewer cells are in S-phase after 48 h treatment of 100 µg/mL vLMW-F in contrast with the native form and compared to the control. (**C**) Percentage of LCLs or DLBCLs cells in SubG1 phase: the increase in cell percentage in SubG1 phase occasionally observed suggests apoptosis induction. NS: not significant; * $p < 0.05$; ** $p < 0.01$; *** $p < 0.001$; **** $p < 0.0001$.

To refine the apoptotic response, we evaluated percentage of apoptotic cells, from early to late stages, for the same cell lines and in the same treatment conditions. Annexin-V binding to externalized phosphatidylserine revealed apoptosis induction only with the two vLMW-F (Figure 2). The importance of the process depended on the cell lines (up to 50% for J1209 and SUDHL6) and was similar for the two fractions. Our results emphasized that, unlike the native form, vLMW-F possess anti-proliferative and pro-apoptotic properties for EBV latency III and DLBCL tumoral cells at the tested dose. This suggests a better cytotoxic effect for vLMW-F. We verified that toxicity (viability and apoptosis) was due to the formulas and not L-Fucose since it is the smallest subunit of fucoidan skeleton (Figure S2).

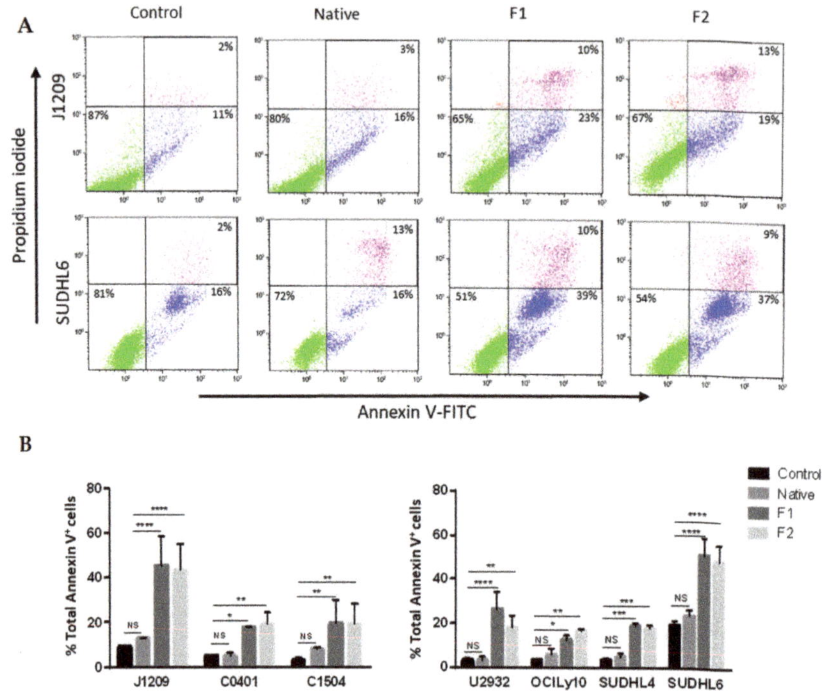

Figure 2. vLMW-F induce apoptosis in LCLs and DLBCLs. LCLs (J1209, C0401, C1504) and DLBCLs (U2932, OCILy10, SUDHL4, SUDHL6) cells were treated or not (control) with 100µg/mL of native fucoidan or vLMW-F (F1 and F2) for 48 h, followed by apoptosis analysis (Annexin V/PI staining) by flow cytometry. Results were obtained from three independent experiments. (**A**) Examples of cell apoptosis for J1209 (LCL) and SUDHL6 (DLBCL) are shown (intact cells: green events–early apoptotic cells: blue events–late apoptotic cells: purple events). (**B**) Percentage of LCLs or DLBCLs total Annexin V+ cells. vLMW-F fractions induce similar apoptosis. NS: not significant; * $p < 0.05$; ** $p < 0.01$; *** $p < 0.001$; **** $p < 0.0001$.

2.2. *Absence of Toxicity for Normal B- and T-Cells*

Potential use of native fucoidan or vLMW-F for biomedical application and specificity of the treatment require that they do not display toxicity for normal cells. We chose to focus on peripheral blood mononuclear cells and particularly on normal B-cells (for comparison with tumoral B-cells), T-cells and activated T-cells (frequently implicated in anti-tumor responses via the PD-L1/PD-1 axis). We performed an Annexin V-based flow cytometry test that enables assessing simultaneously apoptosis and viability. No cytotoxic effect was observed for either the native form or the two vLMW-F (Figure 3).

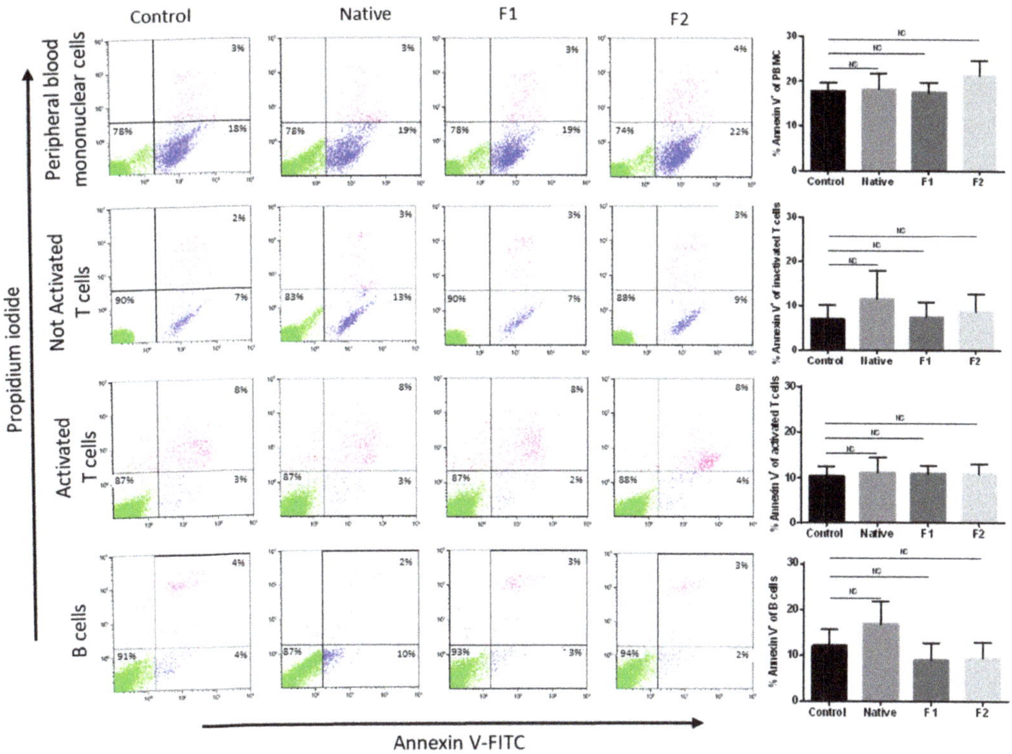

Figure 3. Native fucoidan or vLMW-F are not toxic for normal lymphocyte cells. Normal cells (mononuclear cells, B-cells, T-cells activated or not) were treated or not (control) with 100µg/mL of native fucoidan or vLMW-F (F1 and F2) for 48 h. Apoptosis analysis (Annexin V/PI staining) was realized by flow cytometry. Results were obtained from three independent experiments. An example of each population is shown (intact cells: green events–early apoptotic cells: blue events–late apoptotic cells: purple events) as well as the percentage of total Annexin V^+ cells for each condition. No apoptosis induction was observed. NS: not significant.

2.3. *Decrease in PD-L1 Transcriptional Expression*

PD-L1 transcriptional expression involves signaling pathways that can be inhibited by fucoidan, such as PI3k/AKT, NF-κB or RAS/ERK1/2 [33–36]. Therefore, we studied the effect of native and vLMW-F (F1 and F2) on mRNA expression of *PD-L1* for the three LCLs and four DLBCLs cell lines. We showed that it was strongly decreased in LCLs regardless of treatment and to a lesser extent in DLBCLs (Figure 4). Our results emphasized that transcriptional expression of *PD-L1* can be strongly impaired by native fucoidan or vLMW-F.

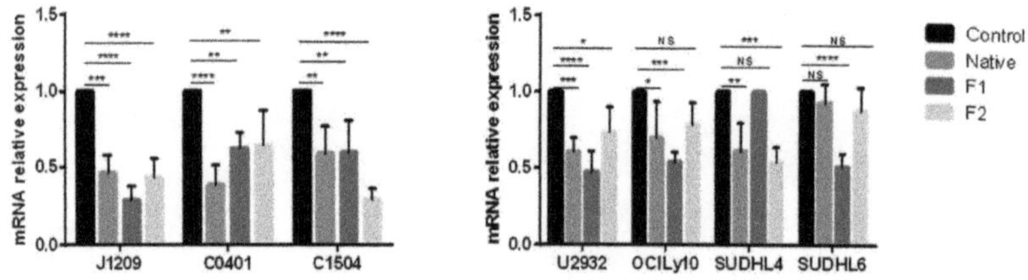

Figure 4. Fucoidan downregulates transcriptional expression of *PD-L1* in LCLs and DLBCLs cells. LCLs (J1209, C0401, C1504) and DLBCLs (U2932, OCILy10, SUDHL4, SUDHL6) were treated with 100µg/mL of native fucoidan or vLMW-F (F1 and F2) for 48 h followed by RNA extraction and RT-qPCR. Results were obtained from three independent experiments. mRNA relative expression of *PD-L1* was decreased either for the native form or the fractions. NS: not significant; * $p< 0.05$; ** $p < 0.01$; *** $p < 0.001$; **** $p < 0.0001$.

2.4. Decrease of membrane, but Not of total, PD-L1 protein expression

Since mRNA expression can differ from protein expression, especially due to translational regulation, we studied the total protein expression of PD-L1 for the same cell lines and in the same treatment conditions. All the cell lines strongly expressed PD-L1 and, surprisingly, despite inhibition of transcriptional regulation, total PD-L1 expression remained unchanged or occasionally slightly modified whatever the cell line and treatment, as observed by Western blot (Figure 5) or flow cytometry (Figure S3). This could be explained by the fact that PD-L1 is stored in secretory lysosomes before their migration *via* the actin network and their fusion with the plasma membrane, which could mask transcriptional regulation.

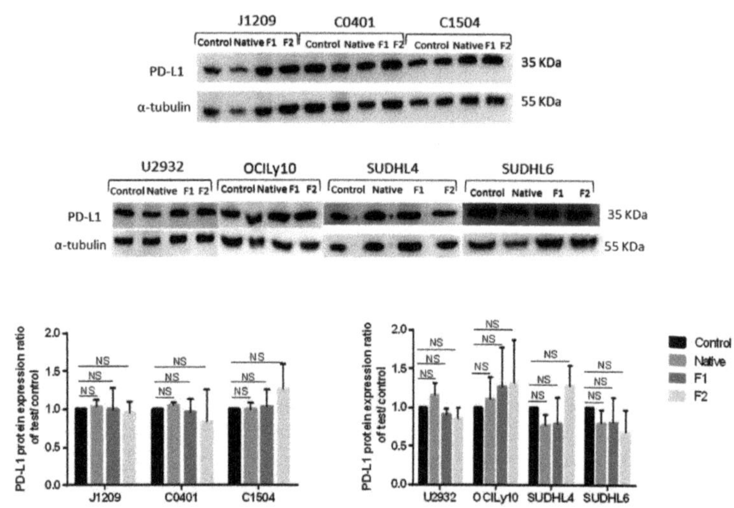

Figure 5. Native fucoidan or vLMW-F do not modify PD-L1 total expression. PD-L1 total expression analysis for LCLs (J1209, C0401, C1504) and DLBCLs (U2932, OCILy10, SUDHL4, SUDHL6) by Western blot after 48 h of 100 µg/mL native fucoidan or vLMW-F (F1 and F2) treatment. No significant change was observed for PD-L1 total expression. Results were obtained from three independent experiments. NS: not significant.

Since the active fraction of PD-L1 responsible for interaction with PD-1 is that at the cell surface, we have also studied its specific expression. Cytometry analysis was carried out on viable cells populations in order not to consider possible degradation of the protein on dead cells. As expected, cytometry analysis showed overexpression of surface PD-L1, which was much higher for LCLs [37] than for DLBCLs cells [8] (Figure 6A). However, unlike for total expression, fucoidan treatments significantly decreased PD-L1 membrane expression for the three LCLs and four DLBCLs, with generally better results for vLMW-F (Figure 6B). Otherwise, PD-L1 decrease was more important for LCLs than DLBCLs that have, however, lower baseline expression. Our results emphasized a specific decrease in PD-L1 membrane expression in the presence of fucoidan species, especially effective on LCLs when treated with vLMW-F. Since total expression remained unchanged, this could be due to regulation of membrane traffic. We verified that a decrease in membrane PD-L1 expression was due to the fractions of vLMW-F and not L-Fucose since it is the smallest subunit of fucoidan skeleton (Figure S4).

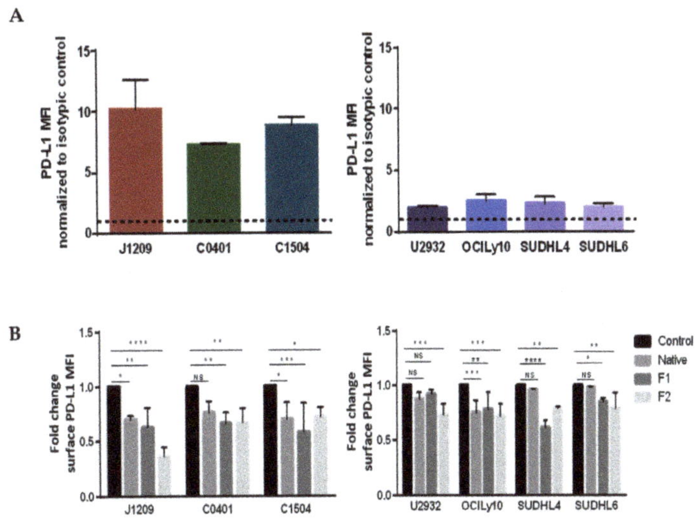

Figure 6. vLMW-F decrease PD-L1 surface expression in LCLs and DLBCLs cells. LCLs (J1209, C0401, C1504) and DLBCLs (U2932, OCILy10, SUDHL4, SUDHL6) cells were treated with 100µg/mL of native fucoidan or vLMW-F (F1 and F2) for 48 h followed by immunofluorescent staining for PD-L1 analyzed by flow cytometry. Results were obtained from three independent experiments. (**A**) PD-L1 is overexpressed by LCLs compared to DLBCLs. (**B**) Fold change (ratio of MFI test/MFI control, both normalized to isotypic control. MFI: mean fluorescence intensity) of PD-L1 surface expression for LCLs and DLBCLs. vLMW-F generally decreased more efficiently than the native form, PD-L1 surface expression for LCLs and DLBCLs. NS: not significant; * $p< 0.05$; ** $p < 0.01$; *** $p < 0.001$; **** $p < 0.0001$.

2.5. Disruption of Actin Network and Decrease in Secretory Activity

We have already shown for LCLs that PD-L1 membrane expression involved migration of LAMP2$^+$/PD-L1$^+$ secretory lysosome via the densified actin network and vesicular membrane traffic [37]. Therefore, we studied the impact of native and vLMW-F fractions F1 and F2 on actin network. F-actin was stained by fluorescent phalloidin. We emphasized a marked decrease in actin polymerization, especially for LCLs and to a lesser extent for DLBCLs cells, as visualized by confocal microscopy (Figure 7A) and quantified by flow cytometry (Figure 7B). Furthermore, we showed, by quantifying the F-actin, that, for normal B-cells, neither native fucoidan nor vLMW-F modify actin network (Figure 7C). To assess vesicular membrane traffic, we focused on LCLs, for which PD-L1 membrane expression and actin network were more affected. We studied native fucoidan and vLMW-F effects on two specific reporter molecules, which are constitutive of intracellular vesicles and expressed at the plasma membrane following their fusion: CD63 and LAMP2. Moreover, LAMP2 is otherwise a lysosomal-associated protein expressed by secretory lysosomes (storage location of PD-L1). Analysis by flow cytometry showed a decrease in the two secretory vesicle markers at the plasma membrane for the native fucoidan and even more for vLMW-F F1 and F2 (Figure 7D). Our results suggest that fucoidan impedes secretory activity through the actin network and vesicle fusion with plasma membrane, which leads to decrease in PD-L1 membrane expression.

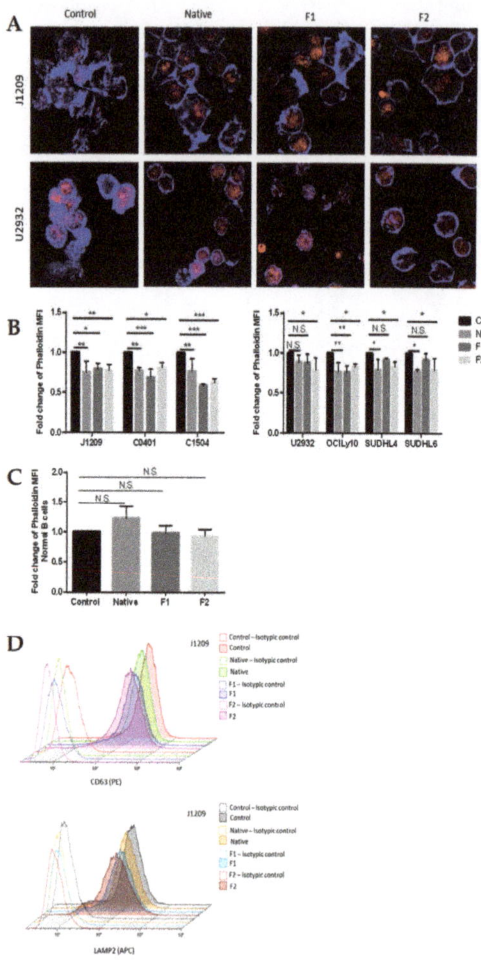

Figure 7. vLMW-F decrease actin polymerization and vesicle markers expression at plasma membrane. (**A**) LCLs (J1209, C0401, C1504) and DLBCLs (U2932, OCILy10, SUDHL4, SUDHL6) cells were treated or not (control) with 100µg/mL of native fucoidan or vLMW-F (F1 and F2) for 48 h, followed by phalloidin staining (F-actin, blue) and TOPRO-3 (nuclei, red) before confocal microscopy observations. (**B, C**) Quantification of F-actin in the same conditions analyzed by flow cytometry for (**B**) LCLs and DLBCLs or (**C**) normal B-cells. vLMW-F significantly decreased content of actin polymerization strongly in LCLs and to a lesser extent in DLBCLs but not in normal B-cells. Results were obtained for three independent experiments. (**D**) Flow cytometry fluorescence histograms of surface CD63 and LAMP2 (secretory vesicle markers) for J1209 (obtained for three independent experiments). The decrease is more efficient with vLMW-F than with the native form. NS: not significant; * $p < 0.05$; ** $p < 0.01$; *** $p < 0.001$.

3. Discussion

Our results show that vLMW-F decrease cell proliferation and induce apoptosis of LCLs and DLBCLs tumoral B-cells without being toxic for normal B- and T-cells. Furthermore, these formulas decreased PD-L1 expression at transcriptional and cell surface levels. These results may be explained by actin network alteration that could be associated with deregulation of cells secretory activity, reducing thereby PD-L1 externalization.

Numerous studies report *in vitro* and *in vivo* anti-cancer effects (such as anti-proliferative, pro-apoptotic, anti-angiogenic and anti-metastatic) of fucoidan extracts or their low-molecular-weight derivatives against multiple types of solid tumors, such as colon, breast, hepatocarcinoma, lung or bladder [16,32,38]. On the contrary, scarce data are reported regarding their effects on liquid tumors, especially concerning LMW derivatives of fucoidan. Few studies have shown that native fucoidan extracted from *Fucus vesiculosus* can inhibit proliferation of myeloid and monocytic leukemia cell lines by inducing their apoptosis [24,30,39] or arrest ABC- or GCB-DLBCL cell cycle [40]. Therefore, we first confirmed these effects previously reported on lymphocytic B lineage and demonstrated for the first time that these anti-proliferative and pro-apoptotic activities are also extended to LCLs. We also highlighted that extremely depolymerized formulas (< 600 Da) maintain specific anti-tumor activity with more efficiency than native form while being non-toxic for normal B- and T-cells. This is consistent with the fact that depolymerized forms are generally more potent [21,23] and in agreement with non-toxicity of fucoidans [16,32,41]. Use of depolymerized form enables being more specific with fewer unwanted effects.

We wanted to confirm the role of fucoidans since they, or derivatives, cover a wide range of immunomodulatory effects and can participate in immune response against several cancers and infectious diseases [42,43], sulfate and acetyl groups mainly contributing to the activity [44]. For instance, they have been shown to enhance dendritic cell maturation, cytotoxic T-cell activation, antibody production or memory T-cells production [45,46]. They can also increase production of TNFα by neutrophils *in vitro* and *in vivo*, delaying their apoptosis [45,46], or induce NO synthesis [47] and activate *in vitro* and *in vivo* NK cells [45,48]. However, scarce data exist either for solid or liquid tumors in regard to their effects on the inhibitory immune checkpoints responsible for tumor cells escape from immune surveillance, especially regarding the PD1/PD-L1 axis. Yet, other data have shown that fucoidan impairs pathways responsible for PD-L1 expression, such as PI3k/AKT, NF-κB or RAS/ERK1/2 [33–36], making them very promising candidates for immune checkpoint modulation. To date, only two articles have reported a native fucoidan that can decrease PD-L1 expression in tumor tissues of experimental-induced mammary cancer [22] and a LMW one that can decrease transcriptional expression of *PD-L1* and *PD-L2* and PD-L1 protein level in fibrosarcoma cells [23]. Thus, it is particularly interesting to better understand effects on PD-L1 since it is particularly critical in immune escape and now of great interest in clinical care/immunotherapy approaches. The decrease in transcriptional expression that we found is in agreement with other studies that have demonstrated that signaling pathways involved in PD-L1 expression (PI3k/AKT, NF-κB or RAS/ERK1/2) can be inhibited by fucoidan [33–36]. Especially, our results confirm such effect for the first time in B-lymphoma cells, whether with the native form or vLMW-F.

In tumor cells, transcriptional expression of *PD-L1* is often not directly related to protein expression due to stabilizing post-translational modifications, such as N-glycosylation and phosphorylation [49,50]. Moreover, it can be accumulated in vesicles, such as exosomes [5] or secretory lysosomes, as demonstrated for LCLs [37], where we observed cytoplasmic accumulation. The relevant fraction of PD-L1 is that expressed at cell surface and able to interact with inhibitor receptor PD-1 expressed on anti-tumor immune cells. As expected, we observed overexpression for LCLs [37] compared with DLBCLs cells [8]. Interestingly, we next showed a PD-L1 decrease on lymphoma B-cells after treatment by native and our two fucoidan fractions, with little more efficiency for vLMW-F than the native form. It is of importance to note that PD-L1 decrease occurs on viable cells since it reduces their inhibition towards anti-tumor immune cells, while some of them die by apoptosis.

The same tests realized with L-fucose monomer showed no effect, clearly demonstrating the real added value for these original vLMW-F.

Maintenance of high intracellular level of PD-L1 and decrease on cell surface emphasized that native fucoidan, as well as vLMW-F, can regulate membrane secretory traffic of this immune checkpoint. A prerequisite for vesicle secretion is their migration close to the plasma membrane *via* the actin network [51,52]. Remodeling and molecular modification of actin network occur in tumor cells [53,54] and constitute a specific and original therapeutic target [55,56]. We previously showed that actin network is increased in LCLs by EBV latency III program and responsible for fusion of secretory lysosome with plasma membrane, leading to PD-L1 overexpression at the cell surface [37]. Presently, we show that native fucoidan, as well as vLMW-F, decrease actin polymerization for LCLs and to a lesser extent for DLBCLs cells, which can be associated with reduction in PD-L1 membrane expression. This is also supported by decrease in LAMP2 membrane expression, particularly after treatment with vLMW-F, which has been correlated with vesicles secretory activity of cells. Data in the literature confirm some links between fucoidan and actin pathway, such as decrease in expression of genes implicated in polymerization, organization and stabilization [57] or disruption of F-actin stress fibers [58,59]. In this context and as a first hypothesis, the difference between native and vLMW forms might be explained by variation in the internalized amount of the different species, especially for their molecular weight differences. No effect on normal cells, associated with lack of toxicity, suggests very interesting specific sensitivity for tumoral actin network. Our results also suggest that expression of other inhibitory immune checkpoints could be decreased insofar as they pass through secretory vesicles [4], secretory lysosomes [37,60] or exosomes [61,62].

As native fucoidan is mainly composed of fucose and because the F1 and F2 fractions present very low DP, such formulas may comprise mono-, di- or tri-saccharides of fucose that are imputable of the effects observed on our cellular models. Results obtained with the single L-fucose monosaccharide did not show any effect. This suggests that F1 and F2 present other original fucoidan-derived compounds of vLMW responsible for these bioactivities, perhaps including glucuronic acid, galactose and xylose (the other principal sugar found in fucoidan) [63], or backbone modifications because of the depolymerization method (opening or creation of insaturation because of H_2O_2-based hydrolysis) [64].

Altogether, our results suggest that efficiency of vLMW-F is correlated to their low molecular weight (by comparison with the native form), which is consistent with the literature [23,65]. It will be interesting to study if this can be associated with different capacities of internalization. However, no noteworthy differences were observed between the two fractions, F1 and F2, that differ mainly by their sulfation degree. These slight differences in sulfation percentage could explain the different effects observed with the two vLMW-F in some experiments. Negatively charged sulfate groups are responsible for interaction with numerous molecules and involved in various biological process. They contribute to fucoidan activity. However, at a very low fraction size, this parameter does not seem to be a key factor in the bioactivities observed. Considering their very small size, high internalization of vLMW-F could explain that a lower degree of sulfation is sufficient for optimal activity. Establishing a complete picture of the structure (Mn and % S)/bioactivity relationship of such a complex fucoidan molecular structure is tedious as both parameters can differently influence the outcome of the effect according to the bioactivity sought and the experimental model used. However, in perspective, it could be interesting to compare the results obtained in this work with ones of desulfated native fucoidan and/or oversulfated vLMW-F.

In translational medicine, fucoidan extracts are considered of great interest as adjuvants for cancer therapy [66,67]; benefits are also observed with anti-PD-L1 or anti-PD-1 immunotherapies in mice models. Fucoidan extracted from *Fucus vesiculosus* promoted activation of tumor-infiltrating $CD8^+$ T-cells and strongly inhibited growth of melanoma cells when co-administrated with anti-PD-1, particularly when applied before immunotherapy [35]. Fucoidan extracted from three species of algae, among them *Fucus vesiculosus*, promoted proliferation and activity of *ex vivo* PBMCs and potentiated anti-PD-1 effects [68]. Intranasal administration of *Ecklonia-cava*-extracted fucoidan enhanced anti-PD-L1 mediated anti-cancer activities against melanoma and carcinoma tumor growth in lungs [69]. Fucoidan of *Luminaria japonica* enhanced anticancer efficacy of anti-PD-L1 antibodies against Lewis lung carcinoma [70].

Algal polysaccharides, such as fucoidan, could provide novel therapeutic alternatives and promising supplements, especially for cancer treatments. Clinical trials are actually in course for hepatocellular carcinoma (NCT04066660) and rectal cancer (NCT04342949). It could be useful combined with immune checkpoint blockade therapies to treat lymphoproliferative malignancies.

Our results suggest that vLMW-F (<600 Da) could be effective potential adjuvants of anti-PD-L1 or anti-PD-1 immunotherapy thanks to their favorable anti-proliferative and pro-apoptotic effects associated with their ability to decrease membrane PD-L1 *via* actin depolymerization. Since fucoidan possesses anti-inflammatory properties, which could interfere with antitumoral functions (reduction in recruitment of antitumoral killing cells and increase in cancer cell apoptosis and chemo-sensitivity), it will be important to further investigate this activity for vLMW-F. Otherwise, the PD-L1/PD-1 axis plays a crucial role in the tumor microenvironment and interactions between antitumor and cancerous cells. Therefore, functional *in vitro* studies on co-culture models with autologous T-cells or NK cells and *in vivo* studies on mice models are the next steps. Treatments with anti-PD-L1 or anti-PD-1 antibodies and fucoidan (native and vLMW-F) remain to be evaluated, independently and in combination.

4. Materials and Methods

4.1. Fucoidan Samples

Native fucoidan of *Fucus vesiculosus* was obtained from Sigma-Aldrich. Original formulas were depolymerized by our collaborators from LIENSs laboratory (UMR CNRS 7266, La Rochelle University, France) from the native fucoidan using a radical H_2O_2-based hydrolysis method previously published with other types of polysaccharides [71]. Briefly, native fucoidan was dissolved in Milli-Q water (25 mg/mL), and then the solution was purged with argon and heated until 60°C. Addition of H_2O_2 30% (Sigma-Aldrich) at a weight/weight ratio of 0.5 and 1.5 resulted in production of two different vLMW-F fractions, named F1 and F2, respectively, after 96 h and 72 h of depolymerization. The chromatographic profile shows that F1 and F2 fractions are practically eluted at the same time and after the native fucoidan, which attests that the H_2O_2-based hydrolysis reaction worked well (Figure S1). Number-average molecular weights (Mn), degree of polymerization (DP) and polydispersity index (I) were estimated by SEC-HPLC according procedures already published [71] using calibrant curves made of pullulans standards (Polymer Standards Service GmbH, Mainz, Germany) for native fucoidan and heparin standards (Iduron, UK) for F1 and F2 fractions. Degree of sulfation (DS) was calculated by an Azure-A-based-colorimetric assay (Sigma-Aldrich) according to a state-of-the-art technique. Results of these characterizations are summarized in Table 1.

Table 1. Characteristics of native fucoidan and vLMW-F (F1 and F2). Number-average molecular weights (Mn), degree of polymerization (DP), polydispersity index (I) and degree of sulfation (DS). *: calculated with pullulans standards. **: calculated with heparin standards.

Sample	H_2O_2 (*w*/*w*)	Time (h)	Mn (Da)	DP	I	DS (% SO_3^-)
Native fucoidan	0	0	66744 *	240.5 *	1.4 *	41.5 ± 0.7
F1 fraction	0.5	96	604 **	3.5 **	1.3 **	6.0 ± 1.0
F2 fraction	1.5	72	562 **	3.4 **	1.1 **	2.1 ± 0.4

As shown in Table 1, the F1 and F2 fractions contain a mixture of different fucoidan-derived compounds with similar very-low-mean DPs between 3.4 and 3.5 but are distinct by their mean sulfation degree, 6% against 2.1%, respectively. Further, LC–MS (data not shown) confirmed that these fractions contain predominantly di- and tri-oligofucoidan with, interestingly, several unsaturated species.

4.2. Cell Culture Conditions

Lymphoblastoid cell lines (LCLs–J1209, C0401, C1504) were established and characterized by the Genethon (Evry, France). They were cultured in RPMI 1640 medium (Eurobio Scientific) supplemented with 10% decomplemented FBS (PAN^{TM} Biotech). Amino acids, vitamins, sodium pyruvate, penicillin/streptomycin and 2 mM L-glutamine were added at 1× concentrations from 100× stock solutions (all from Gibco, ThermoFisher). Four cell lines of DLBCLs, two ABC subtypes (U2932 and OCILy10) and two GCB subtypes (SUDHL4 and SUDHL6), were cultured in RPMI 1640 medium supplemented with 10% decomplemented FBS, pyruvate (1×), Penicillin/Streptomycin (1×), L-glutamine (1X) and 10 mM of HEPES buffer solution (Gibco ThermoFisher). All cell lines were maintained at 37 °C in a humified 5% CO_2 atmosphere and were mycoplasma-free (MycoAlert Mycoplasma Detection Kit). Samples from healthy subjects were obtained from the University Hospital Center of Limoges after their informed consent.

4.3. Cell Cycle Analysis

LCLs and DLBCLs cells were seeded in plates (5×10^5 cells/well) for 24 h and then treated with 100 μg/mL of native fucoidan or F1/F2 fractions. After 48 h, cells were collected, washed twice in Dulbecco's Phosphate Buffered Saline (DPBS–Eurobio Scientific) and fixed with ice-cold 70% ethanol overnight. For Propidium Iodide (PI–Sigma Life Sciences) staining, fixed cells were washed twice with cold DPBS and incubated in 30μL of RNase working solution (10 mg/mL) and 1 mL cold DPBS for 20 min at room temperature (RT). Then, samples were stained with PI and analyzed using a BD FACSCalibur flow cytometer and Kaluza Analysis 2.1 Software (Beckman Coulter).

4.4. Apoptosis Analysis

We followed the same protocol of seeding and treatments as described above for cell cycle analysis. LCLs and DLBCLs (5×10^5 cells/well) cells were collected and washed with DPBS containing Ca^{2+}. Then, they were stained with Annexin V-FITC (Biolegend) and PI (5μg/mL) for 15 min, in the dark, at RT. Stained cells were analyzed using a BD FACSCalibur flow cytometer and Kaluza Analysis 2.1 Software.

4.5. Isolation of Healthy PBMC and Cell Subtypes (B- and T-Cells) for Apoptosis Assay

Isolated peripheral blood mononuclear cells (PBMCs) from all healthy donors were obtained after written consent and were issued from the cell biological collection of the Tissue and Cell Bank CRBioLim of the Limoges Hospital University Center, this cell collection being declared to and authorized by the French Health Ministry with session n° "AC-2021-4790" according to French law. PBMCs were isolated from leukocyte buffy coats by lymphocyte medium separation (MSL, Eurobio Scientific) density gradient centrifugation. T-cells were purified from PBMC by CD3/CD4 EasySep^{TM} human T-cell isolation kit (STEMCELL Technologies) according to the manufacturer's instructions. Activated T lymphocytes were obtained using T-cell activation/expansion kit (Anti-Biotin MACSiBead Particles and biotinylated antibodies against human CD2, CD3 and CD28) according to the manufacturer's protocol (Miltenyi Biotec). All cell subtypes were seeded in plates (5×10^5 cells/well) and, after 24 h, were treated or not with 100μg/mL of native fucoidan or vLMW-F. After 48 h, Annexin V/PI staining was performed for cell apoptosis analysis as described above for all cells groups. For flow cytometry analysis, B-cells were identified from mononuclear cells by staining with anti-CD19 (APC) conjugated antibody (Biolegend).

The different antibodies and conjugated fluorochromes, as well as final dilutions, are listed in Table S1.

4.6. RNA Extraction, Reverse Transcriptase and Real-Time Quantitative PCR

Total RNA was extracted using TRIzol reagent (Life Technologies) from 10^6 LCLs and DLBCLs cells treated or not. Total RNA (1 µg) was reverse transcribed using the high capacity cDNA Reverse Transcription Kit (Applied Biosystems) according to the manufacturer's instructions, with 20µL of final reaction volume. Quantitative mRNA relative expression of PD-L1 was performed in triplicate, with 50 ng cDNA, using the Taqman Assay Gene Expression system of PD-L1 (Hs01125296_m1) or GAPDH–internal control–(Hs02758991_g1) (both from ThermoFisher Scientific) with SensiFast Probe HiRox Mix (Bioline), on a Quant Studio3 cycler. Each quantitative PCR was performed in triplicate. The expression level of each gene was normalized to the GAPDH expression level. The calculated relative mRNA expression level was equal to $2^{-\Delta\Delta Ct}$ with untreated cells (control) as reference.

4.7. Western Blot Analysis

Control or treated groups were dry pelleted after 48 h of treatment and lysed with equal volumes of 1× lysis buffer (1 mM PMSF and 1 X protease Inhibitor Cocktail) on ice for 30 min. Then, they were sonicated and centrifuged at 18000 G for 20 min at 4 °C. Protein concentrations were determined by Bradford protein assay. Equal amounts of proteins (30 µg) were separated by 12% SDS PAGE gel electrophoresis and then transferred to PVDF membranes that were blocked in PBS 5% BSA containing 0.1% Tween 20 at room temperature for 1 h. Afterward, the membranes were incubated with primary antibodies against PD-L1 (1:200) (Santa Cruz: Biotechnology) or α-tubulin (1:5000) (Cell Signaling) overnight at 4 °C. The next day, membranes were washed (PBS-0.1% Tween) and incubated with HRP-secondary antibody (1:5000) at room temperature for 1 h. After washing, the protein bands were detected with a chemiluminescence detection system (ChemiDoc^{TM} Touch Gel Imaging System—Bio-Rad Laboratories), which were quantified and numerated using Fiji software (Rasband, W.S., ImageJ). A ratio was calculated for PD-L1 expression/α-tubulin expression, and then a second ratio was calculated for test/control to compare expression of treated to untreated cells.

4.8. PD-L1 Expression Analysis: Immunofluorescent Staining and Flow Cytometry

For surface labeling, the same protocol of seeding and treatment as described above for cell cycle analysis was followed. LCLs and DLBCLs cells were collected and washed with DPBS. Then, they were labeled for 15 min in the dark at RT with anti-PD-L1-PE (Biolegend) (Table S1). Intracellular PD-L1 staining was performed on LCLs and DLBCLs cells treated with native fucoidan or F1/F2 fractions using the IntraPrep Permeabilization Reagent kit (Beckman Coulter) according to the protocol recommended by the supplier. Acquisitions were performed on FACSCalibur. Results were analyzed with Kaluza Analysis 2.1 Software. Fold change was calculated based on the mean fluorescence intensity ratio of PD-L1 on its isotypic control, and then normalized to the control (untreated cells).

4.9. F-Actin Cytoskeleton Immunofluorescence

Following the same experimental protocol of treatment as described above, LCLs and DLBCLs cells were collected and washed with DPBS. After washing, they were fixed with 4% paraformaldehyde for 10 min at RT and washed with DPBS. Actin fibers were revealed using 405-Phalloidin-iFluor reagent (Abcam) as per the manufacturer's instructions.

Finally, after 30 min of phalloidin incubation, nuclei were stained with TOPRO-3 (1:1000—Fisher scientific) for 15 min at RT. Cells were visualized using a ZEISS LSM 900 confocal microscope (40 × oil lens). Images were constructed using the Fiji software. For actin quantification by flow cytometry, the same experimental protocol was followed. Intracellular actin fibers labeling (45 min of phalloidin staining) was performed after permeabilization (IntraPrep Permeabilization Reagent kit–Beckman Coulter) according to the protocol recommended by the supplier. Acquisitions were performed on the Cytoflex cytometer (Beckman Coulter). Results were analyzed with Kaluza Analysis 2.1 Software. Fold change was calculated based on the mean fluorescence intensity ratio of phalloidin of the test normalized to the control.

4.10. Statistical Analysis

One-way or two-way analysis of variance (ANOVA) and *t*-test were performed to identify significant differences between the control and experimental groups. All experimental data were acquired from at least three independent experiments. All statistical analyses were performed with GraphPad Prism 6.05 for Windows. A probability (p) value of <0.05 was considered statistically significant.

Supplementary Materials: The following supporting information can be downloaded at: https://www.mdpi.com/article/10.3390/md21020132/s1, Table S1: Antibodies used for flow cytometry; Figure S1: SEC-HPLC analysis with refractive detector of native fucoidan with F1- and F2-produced fractions; Figure S2: L-fucose does not induce apoptosis in LCLs and DLBCLs; Figure S3: Native fucoidan or vLMW-F do not (or slightly) change PD-L1 total expression; Figure S4: L-fucose does not decrease PD-L1 surface expression in LCLs and DLBCLs cells.

Author Contributions: Conceptualization, J.S., C.M., H.G., H.A., M.T., D.T., T.M., J.F., I.A. and C.J.-V.; methodology, J.S.; validation, J.S. and C.J.-V.; formal analysis, J.S.; investigation, J.S. and C.M.; resources, H.G., I.A., J.F. and C.J.-V.; data curation, J.S.; writing—original draft preparation, C.J.-V. and J.S.; writing—review and editing, J.S., C.M., H.G., H.A., M.T., D.T., T.M., J.F., I.A. and C.J.-V.; visualization, J.S. and C.J.-V.; supervision, C.J.-V., J.F., I.A. and M.T.; project administration, J.S. and C.J.-V.; funding acquisition, C.J.-V. All authors have read and agreed to the published version of the manuscript.

Funding: This work was supported by the Ligue Nationale Contre le Cancer and Ligue Régionale Contre le Cancer (Limousin – MM/CF n°8 & 22, Charente, Charente-Maritime). Author S.J. has received research support from Hariri Foundation for Sustainable Human Development.

Institutional Review Board Statement: The cell biological collection issued from Tissue and Cell Bank CRBioLim of the Limoges Hospital University Center was declared to and authorized by the French Health Ministry with session n° "AC-2021-4790" according to French law.

Informed Consent Statement: Informed consent was obtained from all subjects involved in the study.

Data Availability Statement: The datasets generated and analyzed during the current study are available from the corresponding author on reasonable request.

Acknowledgments: We thank the flow cytometry and microscopy facilities of the BISCEm US 042 INSERM/UMS 2015 CNRS technological platform of the University of Limoges for their technical assistance as well as the immunology laboratory of the Limoges University Hospital Center. All individuals included in the section acknowledgment have consented.

Conflicts of Interest: The authors declare no conflict of interest.

References

1. Rowe, M.; Raithatha, S.; Shannon-Lowe, C. Counteracting Effects of Cellular Notch and Epstein-Barr Virus EBNA2: Implications for Stromal Effects on Virus-Host Interactions. *J. Virol.* **2014**, *88*, 12065–12076. [CrossRef]
2. Shannon-Lowe, C.; Rickinson, A. The Global Landscape of EBV-Associated Tumors. *Front. Oncol.* **2019**, *9*, 713. [CrossRef]
3. Susanibar-Adaniya, S.; Barta, S.K. 2021 Update on Diffuse large B cell lymphoma: A review of current data and potential applications on risk stratification and management. *Am. J. Hematol.* **2021**, *96*, 617–629. [CrossRef] [PubMed]
4. He, X.; Xu, C. Immune checkpoint signaling and cancer immunotherapy. *Cell Res.* **2020**, *30*, 660–669. [CrossRef]
5. Cha, J.-H.; Chan, L.-C.; Li, C.-W.; Hsu, J.L.; Hung, M.-C. Mechanisms Controlling PD-L1 Expression in Cancer. *Mol. Cell* **2019**, *76*, 359–370. [CrossRef]
6. Wu, Y.; Chen, W.; Xu, Z.P.; Gu, W. PD-L1 Distribution and Perspective for Cancer Immunotherapy—Blockade, Knockdown, or Inhibition. *Front. Immunol.* **2019**, *10*, 2022. [CrossRef]

7. Auclair, H.; Ouk-Martin, C.; Roland, L.; Santa, P.; Mohamad, H.A.; Faumont, N.; Feuillard, J.; Jayat-Vignoles, C. EBV Latency III–Transformed B Cells Are Inducers of Conventional and Unconventional Regulatory T Cells in a PD-L1–Dependent Manner. *J. Immunol.* **2019**, *203*, 1665–1674. [CrossRef] [PubMed]
8. Boussiotis, V.A. Cell-specific PD-L1 expression in DLBCL. *Blood* **2015**, *126*, 2171–2172. [CrossRef]
9. Yamamoto, R.; Nishikori, M.; Kitawaki, T.; Sakai, T.; Hishizawa, M.; Tashima, M.; Kondo, T.; Ohmori, K.; Kurata, M.; Hayashi, T.; et al. PD-1-PD-1 ligand interaction contributes to immunosuppressive microenvironment of Hodgkin lymphoma. *Blood* **2008**, *111*, 3220–3224. [CrossRef] [PubMed]
10. Gu, D.; Ao, X.; Yang, Y.; Chen, Z.; Xu, X. Soluble immune checkpoints in cancer: Production, function and biological significance. *J. Immunother. Cancer* **2018**, *6*, 132. [CrossRef]
11. Khan, M.; Arooj, S.; Wang, H. Soluble B7-CD28 Family Inhibitory Immune Checkpoint Proteins and Anti-Cancer Immunotherapy. *Front. Immunol.* **2021**, *12*, 651634. [CrossRef]
12. Conroy, M.; Naidoo, J. Immune-related adverse events and the balancing act of immunotherapy. *Nat. Commun.* **2022**, *13*, 392. [CrossRef]
13. Michot, J.M.; Bigenwald, C.; Champiat, S.; Collins, M.; Carbonnel, F.; Postel-Vinay, S.; Berdelou, A.; Varga, A.; Bahleda, R.; Hollebecque, A.; et al. Immune-related adverse events with immune checkpoint blockade: A comprehensive review. *Eur. J. Cancer* **2016**, *54*, 139–148. [CrossRef]
14. Palmieri, D.J.; Carlino, M.S. Immune Checkpoint Inhibitor Toxicity. *Curr. Oncol. Rep.* **2018**, *20*, 72. [CrossRef] [PubMed]
15. Wu, M.; Huang, Q.; Xie, Y.; Wu, X.; Ma, H.; Zhang, Y.; Xia, Y. Improvement of the anticancer efficacy of PD-1/PD-L1 blockade via combination therapy and PD-L1 regulation. *J. Hematol. Oncol.* **2022**, *15*, 24. [CrossRef] [PubMed]
16. Jin, J.-O.; Chauhan, P.S.; Arukha, A.P.; Chavda, V.; Dubey, A.; Yadav, D. The Therapeutic Potential of the Anticancer Activity of Fucoidan: Current Advances and Hurdles. *Mar. Drugs* **2021**, *19*, 265. [CrossRef]
17. Citkowska, A.; Szekalska, M.; Winnicka, K. Possibilities of Fucoidan Utilization in the Development of Pharmaceutical Dosage Forms. *Mar. Drugs* **2019**, *17*, 458. [CrossRef]
18. Committee on Herbal Medicinal Products. In *Assessment Report on Fucus vesiculosus L., Thallus*; European Medecine Agency: Amsterdam, The Netherlands, 2014; p. 55.
19. Cumashi, A.; Ushakova, N.A.; Preobrazhenskaya, M.E.; D'Incecco, A.; Piccoli, A.; Totani, L.; Tinari, N.; Morozevich, G.E.; Berman, A.E.; Bilan, M.I.; et al. A comparative study of the anti-inflammatory, anticoagulant, antiangiogenic, and antiadhesive activities of nine different fucoidans from brown seaweeds. *Glycobiology* **2007**, *17*, 541–552. [CrossRef] [PubMed]
20. Fitton, J.H.; Stringer, D.N.; Karpiniec, S.S. Therapies from Fucoidan: An Update. *Mar. Drugs* **2015**, *13*, 5920–5946. [CrossRef]
21. Wang, Y.; Xing, M.; Cao, Q.; Ji, A.; Liang, H.; Song, S. Biological Activities of Fucoidan and the Factors Mediating Its Therapeutic Effects: A Review of Recent Studies. *Mar. Drugs* **2019**, *17*, 183. [CrossRef]
22. Xue, M.; Liang, H.; Tang, Q.; Xue, C.; He, X.; Zhang, L.; Zhang, Z.; Liang, Z.; Bian, K.; Zhang, L.; et al. The Protective and Immunomodulatory Effects of Fucoidan Against 7,12-Dimethyl benz[a]anthracene-Induced Experimental Mammary Carcinogenesis Through the PD1/PDL1 Signaling Pathway in Rats. *Nutr. Cancer* **2017**, *69*, 1234–1244. [CrossRef] [PubMed]
23. Teruya, K.; Kusumoto, Y.; Eto, H.; Nakamichi, N.; Shirahata, S. Selective Suppression of Cell Growth and Programmed Cell Death-Ligand 1 Expression in HT1080 Fibrosarcoma Cells by Low Molecular Weight Fucoidan Extract. *Mar. Drugs* **2019**, *17*, 421. [CrossRef]
24. Jin, J.-O.; Song, M.-G.; Kim, Y.-N.; Park, J.-I.; Kwak, J.-Y. The mechanism of fucoidan-induced apoptosis in leukemic cells: Involvement of ERK1/2, JNK, glutathione, and nitric oxide. *Mol. Carcinog.* **2010**, *49*, 771–782. [CrossRef]
25. Lee, H.; Kim, J.-S.; Kim, E. Fucoidan from Seaweed Fucus vesiculosus Inhibits Migration and Invasion of Human Lung Cancer Cell via PI3K-Akt-mTOR Pathways. *PLoS ONE* **2012**, *7*, e50624. [CrossRef] [PubMed]
26. Boo, H.-J.; Hong, J.-Y.; Kim, S.-C.; Kang, J.-I.; Kim, M.-K.; Kim, E.-J.; Hyun, J.-W.; Koh, Y.-S.; Yoo, E.-S.; Kwon, J.-M.; et al. The Anticancer Effect of Fucoidan in PC-3 Prostate Cancer Cells. *Mar. Drugs* **2013**, *11*, 2982–2999. [CrossRef] [PubMed]
27. Liu, S.; Yang, J.; Peng, X.; Li, J.; Zhu, C. The Natural Product Fucoidan Inhibits Proliferation and Induces Apoptosis of Human Ovarian Cancer Cells: Focus on the PI3K/Akt Signaling Pathway. *Cancer Manag. Res.* **2020**, *12*, 6195–6207. [CrossRef]
28. Han, Y.; Lee, J.H.; Lee, S.H. Antitumor Effects of Fucoidan on Human Colon Cancer Cells via Activation of Akt Signaling. *Biomol. Ther.* **2015**, *23*, 225–232. [CrossRef]
29. Chen, J.; Jiang, C.C.; Jin, L.; Zhang, X.D. Regulation of PD-L1: A novel role of pro-survival signalling in cancer. *Ann. Oncol.* **2016**, *27*, 409–416. [CrossRef]
30. Atashrazm, F.; Lowenthal, R.M.; Woods, G.M.; Holloway, A.F.; Dickinson, J.L. Fucoidan and Cancer: A Multifunctional Molecule with Anti-Tumor Potential. *Mar. Drugs* **2015**, *13*, 2327–2346. [CrossRef]
31. Mathew, L.; Burney, M.; Gaikwad, A.; Nyshadham, P.; Nugent, E.K.; Gonzalez, A.; Smith, J.A. Preclinical Evaluation of Safety of Fucoidan Extracts from *Undaria pinnatifida* and Fucus vesiculosus for Use in Cancer Treatment. *Integr. Cancer Ther.* **2017**, *16*, 572–584. [CrossRef]
32. Lin, Y.; Qi, X.; Liu, H.; Xue, K.; Xu, S.; Tian, Z. The anti-cancer effects of fucoidan: A review of both in vivo and in vitro investigations. *Cancer Cell Int.* **2020**, *20*, 154. [CrossRef] [PubMed]
33. Reyes, M.E.; Riquelme, I.; Salvo, T.; Zanella, L.; Letelier, P.; Brebi, P. Brown Seaweed Fucoidan in Cancer: Implications in Metastasis and Drug Resistance. *Mar. Drugs* **2020**, *18*, 232. [CrossRef] [PubMed]

34. Vincent-Fabert, C.; Roland, L.; Zimber-Strobl, U.; Feuillard, J.; Faumont, N. Pre-clinical blocking of PD-L1 molecule, which expression is down regulated by NF-κB, JAK1/JAK2 and BTK inhibitors, induces regression of activated B-cell lymphoma. *Cell Commun. Signal.* **2019**, *17*, 89. [CrossRef] [PubMed]
35. Yang, J.; Yang, X.; Pan, W.; Wang, M.; Lu, Y.; Zhang, J.; Fang, Z.; Zhang, X.; Ji, Y.; Bei, J.-X.; et al. Fucoidan-Supplemented Diet Potentiates Immune Checkpoint Blockage by Enhancing Antitumor Immunity. *Front. Cell Dev. Biol.* **2021**, *9*, 733246. [CrossRef] [PubMed]
36. Ye, J.; Chen, D.; Ye, Z.; Huang, Y.; Zhang, N.; Lui, E.M.K.; Xue, C.; Xiao, M. Fucoidan Isolated from Saccharina japonica Inhibits LPS-Induced Inflammation in Macrophages via Blocking NF-κB, MAPK and JAK-STAT Pathways. *Mar. Drugs* **2020**, *18*, 328. [CrossRef] [PubMed]
37. Durand-Panteix, S.; Farhat, M.; Youlyouz-Marfak, I.; Rouaud, P.; Ouk-Martin, C.; David, A.; Faumont, N.; Feuillard, J.; Jayat-Vignoles, C. B7-H1, which represses EBV-immortalized B cell killing by autologous T and NK cells, is oppositely regulated by c-Myc and EBV latency III program at both mRNA and secretory lysosome levels. *J. Immunol.* **2012**, *189*, 181–190. [CrossRef]
38. Tsai, H.-L.; Tai, C.-J.; Huang, C.-W.; Chang, F.-R.; Wang, J.-Y. Efficacy of Low-Molecular-Weight Fucoidan as a Supplemental Therapy in Metastatic Colorectal Cancer Patients: A Double-Blind Randomized Controlled Trial. *Mar. Drugs* **2017**, *15*, 122. [CrossRef]
39. Park, H.S.; Hwang, H.J.; Kim, G.-Y.; Cha, H.-J.; Kim, W.-J.; Kim, N.D.; Yoo, Y.H.; Choi, Y.H. Induction of apoptosis by fucoidan in human leukemia U937 cells through activation of p38 MAPK and modulation of Bcl-2 family. *Mar. Drugs* **2013**, *11*, 2347–2364. [CrossRef]
40. Yang, G.; Zhang, Q.; Kong, Y.; Xie, B.; Gao, M.; Tao, Y.; Xu, H.; Zhan, F.; Dai, B.; Shi, J.; et al. Antitumor activity of fucoidan against diffuse large B cell lymphoma in vitro and in vivo. *Acta Biochim. Biophys. Sin.* **2015**, *47*, 925–931. [CrossRef]
41. Hwang, P.-A.; Yan, M.-D.; Lin, H.-T.V.; Li, K.-L.; Lin, Y.-C. Toxicological Evaluation of Low Molecular Weight Fucoidan In Vitro and In Vivo. *Mar. Drugs* **2016**, *14*, 121. [CrossRef]
42. Apostolova, E.; Lukova, P.; Baldzhieva, A.; Katsarov, P.; Nikolova, M.; Iliev, I.; Peychev, L.; Trica, B.; Oancea, F.; Delattre, C.; et al. Immunomodulatory and Anti-Inflammatory Effects of Fucoidan: A Review. *Polymers* **2020**, *12*, 2338. [CrossRef]
43. Hwang, J.; Yadav, D.; Lee, P.C.; Jin, J.-O. Immunomodulatory effects of polysaccharides from marine algae for treating cancer, infectious disease, and inflammation. *Phytother. Res.* **2022**, *36*, 761–777. [CrossRef] [PubMed]
44. Ferreira, S.S.; Passos, C.P.; Madureira, P.; Vilanova, M.; Coimbra, M.A. Structure-function relationships of immunostimulatory polysaccharides: A review. *Carbohydr. Polym.* **2015**, *132*, 378–396. [CrossRef] [PubMed]
45. Jin, J.-O.; Zhang, W.; Du, J.-Y.; Wong, K.-W.; Oda, T.; Yu, Q. Fucoidan can function as an adjuvant in vivo to enhance dendritic cell maturation and function and promote antigen-specific T cell immune responses. *PLoS ONE* **2014**, *9*, e99396. [CrossRef] [PubMed]
46. Zhang, W.; Oda, T.; Yu, Q.; Jin, J.-O. Fucoidan from Macrocystis pyrifera has powerful immune-modulatory effects compared to three other fucoidans. *Mar. Drugs* **2015**, *13*, 1084–1104. [CrossRef]
47. Jiang, Z.; Okimura, T.; Yamaguchi, K.; Oda, T. The potent activity of sulfated polysaccharide, ascophyllan, isolated from Ascophyllum nodosum to induce nitric oxide and cytokine production from mouse macrophage RAW264.7 cells: Comparison between ascophyllan and fucoidan. *Nitric Oxide Biol. Chem.* **2011**, *25*, 407–415. [CrossRef]
48. Ale, M.T.; Maruyama, H.; Tamauchi, H.; Mikkelsen, J.D.; Meyer, A.S. Fucoidan from Sargassum sp. and Fucus vesiculosus reduces cell viability of lung carcinoma and melanoma cells in vitro and activates natural killer cells in mice in vivo. *Int. J. Biol. Macromol.* **2011**, *49*, 331–336. [CrossRef]
49. Fan, Z.; Wu, C.; Chen, M.; Jiang, Y.; Wu, Y.; Mao, R.; Fan, Y. The generation of PD-L1 and PD-L2 in cancer cells: From nuclear chromatin reorganization to extracellular presentation. *Acta Pharm. Sin. B* **2022**, *12*, 1041–1053. [CrossRef]
50. Yu, X.; Li, W.; Young, K.H.; Li, Y. Posttranslational Modifications in PD-L1 Turnover and Function: From Cradle to Grave. *Biomedicines* **2021**, *9*, 1702. [CrossRef]
51. Li, P.; Bademosi, A.T.; Luo, J.; Meunier, F.A. Actin Remodeling in Regulated Exocytosis: Toward a Mesoscopic View. *Trends Cell Biol.* **2018**, *28*, 685–697. [CrossRef]
52. Porat-Shliom, N.; Milberg, O.; Masedunskas, A.; Weigert, R. Multiple roles for the actin cytoskeleton during regulated exocytosis. *Cell. Mol. Life Sci.* **2013**, *70*, 2099–2121. [CrossRef] [PubMed]
53. Aseervatham, J. Cytoskeletal Remodeling in Cancer. *Biology* **2020**, *9*, 385. [CrossRef] [PubMed]
54. Suresh, R.; Diaz, R.J. The remodelling of actin composition as a hallmark of cancer. *Transl. Oncol.* **2021**, *14*, 101051. [CrossRef]
55. Datta, A.; Deng, S.; Gopal, V.; Yap, K.C.-H.; Halim, C.E.; Lye, M.L.; Ong, M.S.; Tan, T.Z.; Sethi, G.; Hooi, S.C.; et al. Cytoskeletal Dynamics in Epithelial-Mesenchymal Transition: Insights into Therapeutic Targets for Cancer Metastasis. *Cancers* **2021**, *13*, 1882. [CrossRef] [PubMed]
56. Ong, M.S.; Deng, S.; Halim, C.E.; Cai, W.; Tan, T.Z.; Huang, R.Y.-J.; Sethi, G.; Hooi, S.C.; Kumar, A.P.; Yap, C.T. Cytoskeletal Proteins in Cancer and Intracellular Stress: A Therapeutic Perspective. *Cancers* **2020**, *12*, 238. [CrossRef]
57. Kwack, K.H.; Ji, J.Y.; Park, B.; Heo, J.S. Fucoidan (*Undaria pinnatifida*)/Polydopamine Composite-Modified Surface Promotes Osteogenic Potential of Periodontal Ligament Stem Cells. *Mar. Drugs* **2022**, *20*, 181. [CrossRef]
58. Wu, S.-Y.; Chen, Y.-T.; Tsai, G.-Y.; Hsu, F.-Y.; Hwang, P.-A. Protective Effect of Low-Molecular-Weight Fucoidan on Radiation-Induced Fibrosis through TGF-β1/Smad Pathway-Mediated Inhibition of Collagen I Accumulation. *Mar. Drugs* **2020**, *18*, 136. [CrossRef]

59. Mustafa, S.; Pawar, J.S.; Ghosh, I. Fucoidan induces ROS-dependent epigenetic modulation in cervical cancer HeLa cell. *Int. J. Biol. Macromol.* **2021**, *181*, 180–192. [CrossRef]
60. Wang, H.; Han, X.; Xu, J. Lysosome as the Black Hole for Checkpoint Molecules. *Adv. Exp. Med. Biol.* **2020**, *1248*, 325–346. [CrossRef]
61. Hu, Y.; Zhang, R.; Chen, G. Exosome and Secretion: Action On? *Adv. Exp. Med. Biol.* **2020**, *1248*, 455–483. [CrossRef]
62. Xing, C.; Li, H.; Li, R.-J.; Yin, L.; Zhang, H.-F.; Huang, Z.-N.; Cheng, Z.; Li, J.; Wang, Z.-H.; Peng, H.-L. The roles of exosomal immune checkpoint proteins in tumors. *Mil. Med. Res.* **2021**, *8*, 56. [CrossRef]
63. Oliveira, R.M.; Câmara, R.B.G.; Monte, J.F.S.; Viana, R.L.S.; Melo, K.R.T.; Queiroz, M.F.; Filgueira, L.G.A.; Oyama, L.M.; Rocha, H.A.O. Commercial Fucoidans from Fucus vesiculosus Can Be Grouped into Antiadipogenic and Adipogenic Agents. *Mar. Drugs* **2018**, *16*, 193. [CrossRef] [PubMed]
64. Courtois, J. Oligosaccharides from land plants and algae: Production and applications in therapeutics and biotechnology. *Curr. Opin. Microbiol.* **2009**, *12*, 261–273. [CrossRef]
65. Gupta, D.; Silva, M.; Radziun, K.; Martinez, D.C.; Hill, C.J.; Marshall, J.; Hearnden, V.; Puertas-Mejia, M.A.; Reilly, G.C. Fucoidan Inhibition of Osteosarcoma Cells is Species and Molecular Weight Dependent. *Mar. Drugs* **2020**, *18*, 104. [CrossRef] [PubMed]
66. Hsu, H.-Y.; Hwang, P.-A. Clinical applications of fucoidan in translational medicine for adjuvant cancer therapy. *Clin. Transl. Med.* **2019**, *8*, e15. [CrossRef] [PubMed]
67. Kwak, J.-Y. Fucoidan as a marine anticancer agent in preclinical development. *Mar. Drugs* **2014**, *12*, 851–870. [CrossRef]
68. Park, A.Y.; Nafia, I.; Stringer, D.N.; Karpiniec, S.S.; Fitton, J.H. Fucoidan Independently Enhances Activity in Human Immune Cells and Has a Cytostatic Effect on Prostate Cancer Cells in the Presence of Nivolumab. *Mar. Drugs* **2021**, *20*, 12. [CrossRef]
69. Zhang, W.; Hwang, J.; Yadav, D.; An, E.-K.; Kwak, M.; Lee, P.C.-W.; Jin, J.-O. Enhancement of Immune Checkpoint Inhibitor-Mediated Anti-Cancer Immunity by Intranasal Treatment of Ecklonia cava Fucoidan against Metastatic Lung Cancer. *Int. J. Mol. Sci.* **2021**, *22*, 9125. [CrossRef]
70. An, E.-K.; Hwang, J.; Kim, S.-J.; Park, H.-B.; Zhang, W.; Ryu, J.-H.; You, S.; Jin, J.-O. Comparison of the immune activation capacities of fucoidan and laminarin extracted from Laminaria japonica. *Int. J. Biol. Macromol.* **2022**, *208*, 230–242. [CrossRef]
71. Groult, H.; Cousin, R.; Chot-Plassot, C.; Maura, M.; Bridiau, N.; Piot, J.-M.; Maugard, T.; Fruitier-Arnaudin, I. λ-Carrageenan Oligosaccharides of Distinct Anti-Heparanase and Anticoagulant Activities Inhibit MDA-MB-231 Breast Cancer Cell Migration. *Mar. Drugs* **2019**, *17*, 140. [CrossRef]

marine drugs

MDPI

Article

A Novel Aldisine Derivative Exhibits Potential Antitumor Effects by Targeting JAK/STAT3 Signaling

Dong-Ping Wang [1,2,†], Li-Hong Wu [1,3,†], Rui Li [1,3,†], Na He [1,3], Qian-Yue Zhang [1,3], Chen-Yang Zhao [1,4,*] and Tao Jiang [1,2,*]

1 Key Laboratory of Marine Drugs, Ministry of Education, School of Medicine and Pharmacy, Ocean University of China, Qingdao 266003, China
2 Laboratory for Marine Drugs and Bioproducts, Qingdao National Laboratory for Marine Science and Technology, Qingdao 266237, China
3 Innovation Platform of Marine Drug Screening & Evaluation, Qingdao National Laboratory for Marine Science and Technology, Qingdao 266100, China
4 Department of Cancer Biology, Cleveland Clinic, 9500 Euclid Ave, Cleveland, OH 44195, USA
* Correspondence: zhaoc2@ccf.org (C.-Y.Z.); jiangtao@ouc.edu.cn (T.J.)
† These authors contributed equally to this work.

Abstract: The JAK/STAT3 signaling pathway is aberrantly hyperactivated in many cancers, promoting cell proliferation, survival, invasiveness, and metastasis. Thus, inhibitors targeting JAK/STAT3 have enormous potential for cancer treatment. Herein, we modified **aldisine** derivatives by introducing the isothiouronium group, which can improve the antitumor activity of the compounds. We performed a high-throughput screen of 3157 compounds and identified compounds **11a**, **11b**, and **11c**, which contain a pyrrole [2,3-c] azepine structure linked to an isothiouronium group through different lengths of carbon alkyl chains and significantly inhibited JAK/STAT3 activities. Further results showed that compound **11c** exhibited the optimal antiproliferative activity and was a pan-JAKs inhibitor capable of inhibiting constitutive and IL-6-induced STAT3 activation. In addition, compound **11c** influenced STAT3 downstream gene expression (Bcl-xl, C-Myc, and Cyclin D1) and induced the apoptosis of A549 and DU145 cells in a dose-dependent manner. The antitumor effects of **11c** were further demonstrated in an in vivo subcutaneous tumor xenograft experiment with DU145 cells. Taken together, we designed and synthesized a novel small molecule JAKs inhibitor targeting the JAK/STAT3 signaling pathway, which has predicted therapeutic potential for JAK/STAT3 overactivated cancer treatment.

Keywords: JAK/STAT3 signaling pathway; aldisine derivatives; isothiouronium; antitumor activity; JAK inhibitor; high-throughput screening

Citation: Wang, D.-P.; Wu, L.-H.; Li, R.; He, N.; Zhang, Q.-Y.; Zhao, C.-Y.; Jiang, T. A Novel Aldisine Derivative Exhibits Potential Antitumor Effects by Targeting JAK/STAT3 Signaling. *Mar. Drugs* **2023**, *21*, 218. https://doi.org/10.3390/md21040218

Academic Editors: Barbara De Filippis, Alessandra Ammazzalorso and Marialuigia Fantacuzzi

Received: 26 February 2023
Revised: 24 March 2023
Accepted: 27 March 2023
Published: 29 March 2023

1. Introduction

Cancer presenting as an incurable advanced or metastatic disease is common, and the development of new targeted antitumor drugs is of great significance to human health [1]. The Janus kinase (JAK) and signal transducer and activator of transcription 3 (STAT3) signaling pathway is aberrantly hyperactivated in many types of cancer, and such hyperactivation is generally associated with a poor clinical prognosis [2,3]. It plays a central role in immune response, cell proliferation, differentiation, and survival [4,5]. In the tumor microenvironment, numerous cytokines, such as IL-6 and IFNα/β, can activate JAKs by phosphorylating tyrosine residues, which in turn phosphorylate and activate STAT3 to regulate the transcription of downstream target genes [6,7]. Examples of these genes include those which drive cell proliferation (cyclin D1), promote tumor survival BCL2-like protein 1 (BCL-xL), and regulate immune response (IFN-γ) [2,8]. There are 11 JAK inhibitors approved for the treatment of various diseases that exert inhibitory effects through competitive and non-competitive reactions with the amino acid residues in JAKs [9]. An example of a JAK inhibitor used in treatment is ruxolitinib, which has been approved by the U.S. Food and Drug Administration (FDA) for the treatment of myelofibrosis and polycythemia vera [10]. In addition, dozens of potential JAK inhibitors are under clinical trials to further evaluate their antitumor activity; for example, DZD4205 in the treatment of T-cell lymphoma [11]. Therefore, the JAK/STAT pathway is a potential therapeutic target with great value for cancer treatment; among these, small molecules to inhibit JAK activity have attracted much attention.

Marine sponges are an important source of potential natural bioactive ingredients that have formed natural secondary metabolites with complex and unique structures to adapt to the harsh marine survival conditions [12,13]. **Aldisine** (Figure 1) and its derivatives are the secondary metabolites from sponges with unique pyrrolo [2,3-c] azepine skeleton structural features that exhibit antitumor activity by inhibiting protein kinase [14,15]. It was reported that the oximes, oxime ethers, and hydrazones groups in **aldisine** can provide numerous hydrogen bond donor and acceptor moieties, which showed antiviral, larvicidal, and anti-phytopathogenic-fungus activities [16]. Modified **aldisine** at N-1 and C-4 positions obtained compounds **1** to **3** (Figure 1), which could enhance its antiproliferative activity [17–20]. The extensive antiproliferative properties of **aldisine** have made it a significant drug for cancer therapy. Due to its promising biological activities and multi-site modification, **aldisine** has become a focus of pharmaceutical chemistry as a lead compound, especially in antitumor aspects.

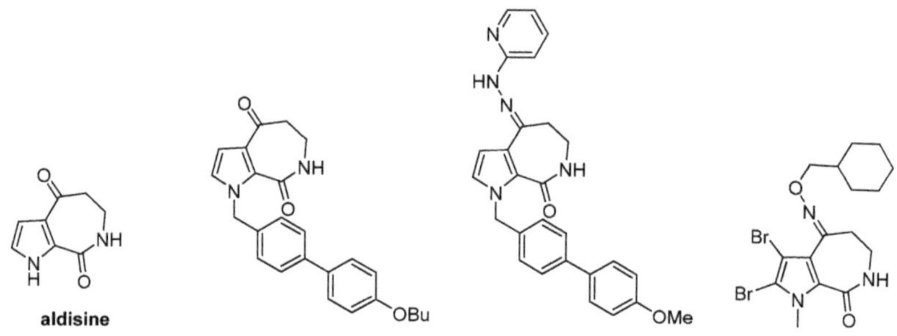

Figure 1. The structures of **aldisine** and its derivatives.

These previous results guide us to put our efforts into designing and modifying **aldisine**. Isothiouronium is a positively charged group that induces G2/M cell cycle arrest and promotes cell apoptosis [21,22]. Previous studies have shown that isothiouronium-modified analogs may be promising anticancer agents, novel Golgi staining reagents, and useful research tools for studying Golgi functions in normal or cancer cells [23]. Therefore, compounds **10a**, **10b**, **10c**, **11a**, **11b**, and **11c** were obtained by introducing the isothiouronium groups to **aldisine** at the N-1 and N-7 positions with different lengths of carbon alkyl chains. The carbon alkyl chains increase their flexibility and liposolubility, and the introduction of isothiouronium makes it easier to enter cells to enhance antitumor activity.

Therefore, we first tested the antitumor activities of **aldisine** and its derivatives and found that compounds **11a**, **11b**, and **11c** significantly reduced cell viability in the treatment of cancer cells. In parallel, we screened tens of thousands of collected compounds in a STAT3 binding promoter driving luciferase reporter system according to the method reported in references [20,21], in which compounds **11a**, **11b**, and **11c** showed remarkable STAT3 inhibitory activity, with compound **11c** showing the optimal activity. Further experiments focused on compound **11c** revealed its inhibitory efficacy against JAKs. In addition, inhibition of JAK/STAT3 signaling by compound **11c** induced substantial tumor cell apoptosis and influenced cell proliferation. Notably, compound **11c** significantly reduced tumor growth by induced apoptosis in a mouse subcutaneous tumor implantation model in vivo, suggesting a potential for compound **11c** to be further developed as a JAK/STAT3 signaling inhibitor for the treatment of cancer.

2. Results

2.1. Chemistry

Design and Synthesis of Aldisine Derivatives

Considering the rotatability of different lengths of carboxyalkyl chains (n = 4,5,6) and the positive charge of the isothiouronium group, which can easily approach the cell membrane, we first designed and synthesized isothiouronium-modified **aldisine** derivatives at N1 positions in two steps as outlined in Scheme 1. Compound **7** was prepared from the 2-(trichloroacetyl) pyrrole according to the synthesis procedure of marine natural products **Stevensine** [24]. Subsequently, compound **7** reacts with excessive dibromoalkanes (n = 4,5,6) in DMSO for 1.5 h under the basic condition of KOH to obtain bromoalkyl derivatives **8a, 8b, 8c, 9a, 9b**, and **9c**, which were separated by silica gel chromatography with a 39~56% yield. Then **8a, 8b, 8c, 9a, 9b**, and **9c** were reacted with thiourea reflux for 12 h in ethanol to produce the target compounds **10a, 10b, 10c, 11a, 11b**, and **11c** with a yield of 57~67%.

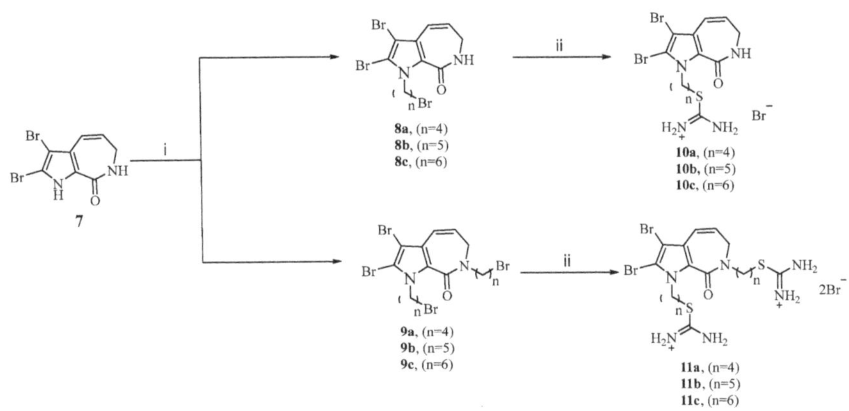

Scheme 1. Synthesis of the isothiouronium-modified **aldisine** derivatives. Reagents and conditions: (i) Br-$(CH_2)_n$-Br, KOH, DMSO, 25 °C, 1.5 h, 39–56%; (ii) Thiourea, EtOH, 80 °C, 12 h, 57–67%.

The general synthesized procedures for compounds **8a, 8b, 8c, 9a, 9b, 9c** and **10a, 10b, 10c, 11a, 11b, 11c** are in the Supplementary Materials.

2.2. Biological Activity Assessment of Compound 11c

2.2.1. Compound 11c Exhibited Antiproliferative Activity and was Identified as a JAK-STAT3 Signaling Inhibitor

After a series of **aldisine** derivatives were synthesized with similar structures and chemical properties, as shown in the chemistry section, we conducted high-throughput screening on them and found that the compound **11c**, containing two six-carbon chain lengths of alkyl isothiourea groups at the N1 and N7 positions significantly inhibit JAK/STAT3 activity. Whereas compounds **10a, 10b**, and **10c**, containing only one different length of alkyl isothiourea at the N1 position, demonstrated lower inhibition of JAK/STAT 3 activity than **11c** (Table S1; Figure S1).

Next, for further understanding of the structure-activity relationship between **aldisine** derivatives, the inhibitory activities of **11a, 11b**, and **11c** were tested. The results showed that compounds **11a, 11b**, and **11c** exhibited significant antiproliferative activity against four human cancer cell lines: prostate cancer (DU145), non-small cell lung cancer (A549), breast cancer (MDA-MB-231), and cervical cancer (HeLa) (Table 1), with **11c** being the most potent. Compound **11c** inhibited the growth of DU145 cells with an IC_{50} value of

2.37 μM (Figure 2A) and HeLa cells with an IC_{50} value of 5.12 μM (Figure 2B). STAT3 can be activated in cancer cells in a constitutive or IL-6-induced manner [25,26]. In both DU145 and A549 cells, STAT3 is constitutively activated, whereas in Hela and MDA-MB231 cells, IL-6 can induce significant STAT3 activation [27–29]. Therefore, we next evaluated whether **aldisine** derivatives can inhibit STAT3 signaling. A STAT3 transcriptional activity-based high-throughput luciferase reporter was applied [23]. Interestingly, STAT3 luciferase inhibitory activities as well as the antiproliferative effects were indeed observed for **11a, 11b**, and **11c** (Figure S1; Figure 2C,D). The IC_{50} value of **11a**, **11b**, and **11c** was generally lower and exhibited greater inhibitory activity as the length of alkyl carbon groups increased. Compound **11c** with two six-carbon chain lengths showed the highest activity, which inhibited cancer cell growth in a dose-dependent manner and could be a potential JAK/STAT3 pathway inhibitor at a relatively low concentration.

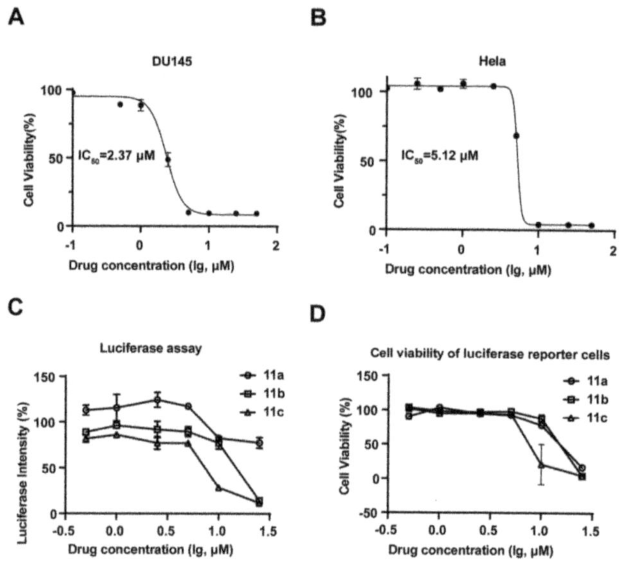

Figure 2. Compound **11c** was indicated as a JAK/STAT3 pathway inhibitor and exhibited antiproliferative activity. (**A**,**B**) Cell viability assay was determined by resazurin on DU145 (**A**) and Hela (**B**) cells after being treated with **11c** for 72 h at the indicated concentrations ($n = 3$). (**C**) SKA cells (8000 cells/well) were seeded in 96-well plates and cultured overnight. Cells were then treated with **11a**, **11b**, and **11c** at the indicated concentrations for 24 h before the STAT3-driven luciferase activity was measured. (**D**) Cell viability assay was determined by resazurin on SKA cells after being treated with **11c** for 72 h at the indicated concentrations ($n = 3$).

Table 1. Antiproliferative activity of **aldisine** derivatives against human cancer cell lines.

Compounds	IC_{50} value (μM) [1]			
	DU145	A549	Hela	MDA-MB231
11a	29.09 ± 4.21	8.48 ± 0.31	8.10 ± 1.27	12.59 ± 0.17
11b	7.28 ± 0.13	7.60 ± 0.08	12.14 ± 0.01	4.46 ± 0.22
11c	2.37 ± 0.09	3.62 ± 0.00	5.12 ± 0.37	3.49 ± 0.09

[1] Four cancer cell lines were used to measure the antiproliferative activity of compounds **11a**, **11b**, and **11c** by the resazurin cell viability assay. All experiments were performed independently at least three times and the IC_{50} values are expressed as means ± SD.

2.2.2. **11c** Inhibits Constitutive and IL-6-induced STAT3 Activation

To further determine whether **11c** can inhibit the activation of STAT3, we first treated DU145 and A549 cells with **11c** at the indicated concentrations for 2 h and then analyzed the phosphorylation of STAT3 by Western blot (Figure 3A,B). Compound **11c** inhibited constitutively activated STAT3 at the concentration of 5 μM both in DU145 and A549 cell lines. In consideration of IL-6 as the major cytokine participant in STAT3 activation and its significance in cancer formation and suppressing the antitumor immune response [4,30], we further examined the effect of **11c** on IL-6-induced STAT3 activation cell lines such as Hela and MB231 cells (Figure 3C,D). The results indicated that **11c** inhibited non-constitutive STAT3 activation at the concentration of 7 μM in a dose-dependent manner. Taken together, the Western blot analysis results suggested that **11c** treatment inhibits the constitutive and IL-6-induced STAT3 phosphorylation in cancer cells.

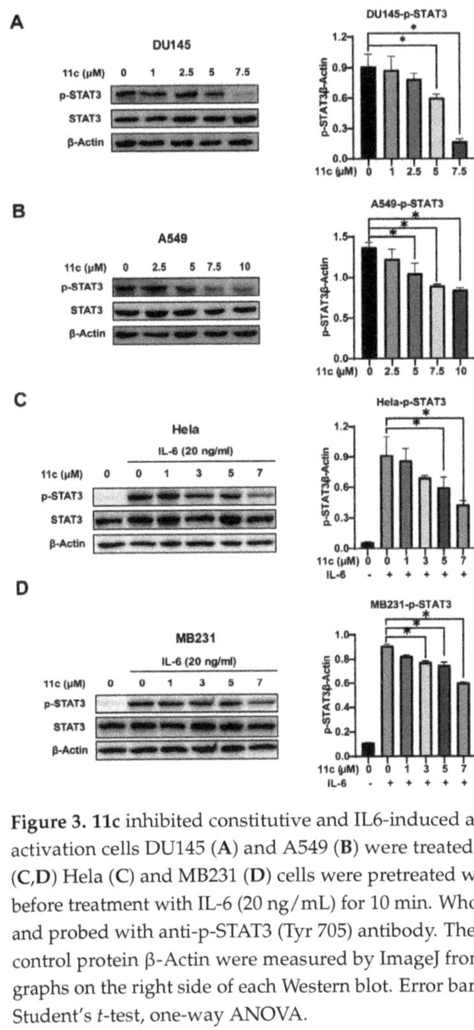

Figure 3. **11c** inhibited constitutive and IL6-induced activation of STAT3. (**A**,**B**) Constitutive STAT3 activation cells DU145 (**A**) and A549 (**B**) were treated with **11c** at the specific concentration for 2 h. (**C**,**D**) Hela (**C**) and MB231 (**D**) cells were pretreated with **11c** at the indicated concentrations for 2 h before treatment with IL-6 (20 ng/mL) for 10 min. Whole cell lysates were processed for Western blot and probed with anti-p-STAT3 (Tyr 705) antibody. The relative expressions compared to the loading control protein β-Actin were measured by ImageJ from 3 individual experiments and shown as bar graphs on the right side of each Western blot. Error bars indicate means ± SD. $p < 0.05$ (*), significant, Student's *t*-test, one-way ANOVA.

2.2.3. **11c** Inhibits the Phosphorylation of JAK Family Members

The activation of STAT3 is usually regulated by its upstream JAK kinases phosphorylation [31]. To further explore whether **11c** inhibits STAT3 phosphorylation by influencing JAK kinases, DU145 and A549 cells were treated with **11c** for 1 h and JAK kinase phosphorylation was determined (Figure 4A,B). Phosphorylation of JAK1, JAK2, JAK3, and TYK2 were decreased after **11c** treatment at 5 μM in DU145 and 7.5 μM in A549 cells. These data suggest that **11c** is a pan-JAK inhibitor and has a higher affinity. Then, to determine whether **11c** specifically inhibited the JAK/STAT3 pathway or not, we analyzed other signaling kinases including IKK, AKT, NF-κB, p38, p-JNK, and GSK-3β (Figure 4C,D). The results indicated that **11c** had no substantial inhibitory effect on the phosphorylation of IKK, AKT, and GSK-3β, with slight inhibitory activities on NF-κB at the higher concentration and stimulatory effects on the phosphorylation of p38 and JNK. In conclusion, the above data demonstrate that **11c** inhibits the activation of JAK kinases in constitutively activated STAT3 cancer cells.

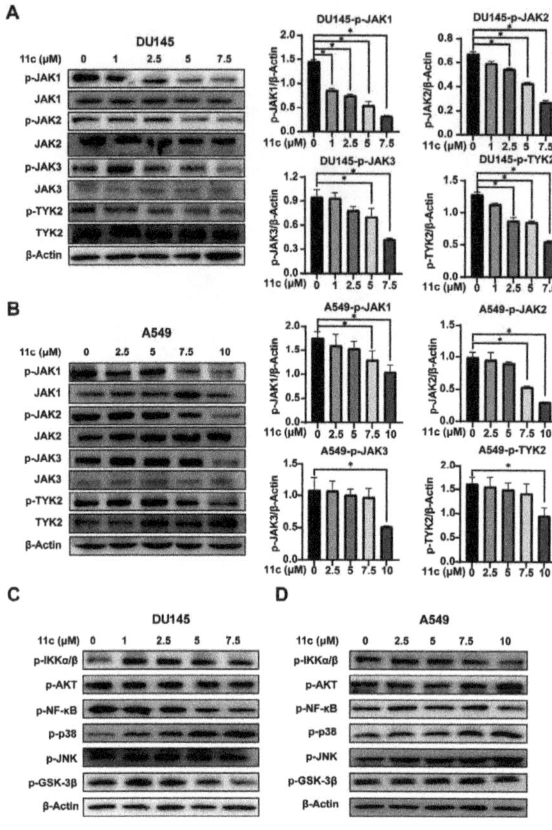

Figure 4. 11c was indicated as a pan-JAK inhibitor. Constitutive STAT3 activation cells DU145 and A549 were treated with **11c** at the indicated concentration for 1 h and then total protein was analyzed by Western blot. (**A**,**B**) Phosphorylation and total expression of four JAK members were detected. (**C**,**D**) Phosphorylation of IKKα/β, AKT, NF-κB, p38, JNK, and GSK-3β were detected. The relative expressions compared to the loading control protein β-Actin were measured by ImageJ from 3 individual experiments and shown as bar graphs on the right side of each Western blot. Error bars indicate means ± SD. $p < 0.05$ (*), significant, Student's *t*-test, one-way ANOVA.

2.2.4. Molecular Docking Revealed That Hydrogen Bonding Is the Major Interaction between **11c** and JAKs

JAKs, with a total length of 120–140 kD, are essential for many biological outcomes of cytokine signaling. The JAK family contains four members (JAK1, JAK2, JAK3, and TYK2), with the end being a catalytic or kinase domain at the carboxyl end, and the front is a pseudokinase (PK) or kinase-like domain. JAK binds to the Box1 and Box2 domains of cytokine receptors through the amino-terminal ezrin-radixin- moesin (FERM) domain and Src Homology 2 (SH2) domain [32–34]. Molecular docking software provides a good platform for the interaction between molecules (ligands) and target proteins (receptors) [32]. In our research, molecular docking was conducted to examine the interaction between compound **11c** and JAK1 (PDB number: 4EHZ), JAK2 (PDB number: 7Q7W), JAK3 (PDB number: 4Z16), and TYK2 (PDB number: 4GJ2). The data indicated that the hydrophobic fatty chain was surrounded by a hydrophobic pocket. In addition, the isothiouronium and hydrogen interact with amino acid residues through hydrogen bonding, forming six hydrogen bonds with Glu-957, Met-956, Gly-1020, and Asp-1039 in JAK1 (Figure 5A). Similarly, in JAK2, it forms four hydrogen bonds with Lys-857, Met-865, and Gln-853 residues (Figure 5B), while in TYK2, it forms two hydrogen bonds with Asp-988 and Tyr-989 (Figure 5D). Specifically, in JAK3, in addition to four hydrogen bonds with Asp-912 and Asp-967, a π–π interaction is also formed with the indole ring of compound **11c** (Figure 5C). Overall, molecular docking revealed that the hydrogen bond is the main interaction between **11c** and JAK members; furthermore, the interaction intensity differences in the four JAK members were related to the inhibition effect of **11c**.

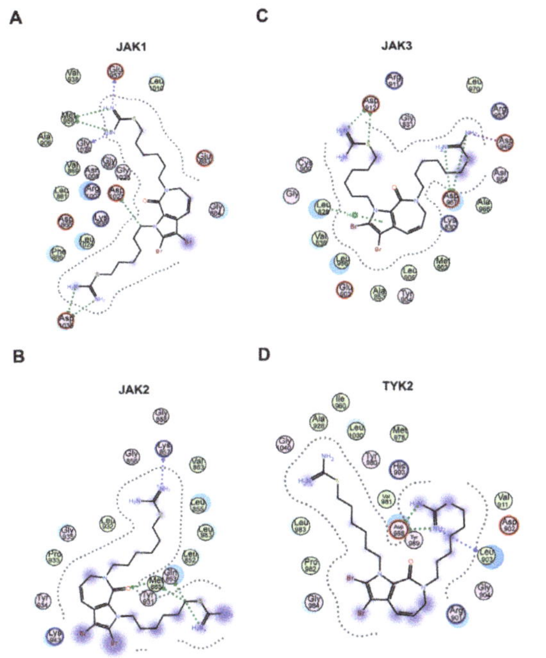

Figure 5. Molecular docking revealed that hydrogen bonding is the main interaction between **11c** and JAKs. (**A–D**) Molecular docking analysis 2D results of JAK1 (**A**), JAK2 (**B**), JAK3 (**C**), and TYK2 (**D**) with compound **11c** by MOE software. The centered chemical structure is compound **11c**. Each circle represents the amino acid residue of JAK proteins. The interaction forces between the amino acid site and the compound structure are represented by a dashed line with an arrow.

2.2.5. **11c** Downregulates Anti-apoptosis Gene Expression and Induces Cancer Cell Apoptosis In Vitro

Since JAK/STAT3 signaling plays an essential role in cell proliferation and survival by reducing the expression of cell-cycle-related genes (Cyclin D) and anti-apoptotic genes (Bcl-xl) [35,36], we analyzed the effect of **11c** on cell-cycle-related gene expression. As shown in Figure 6A,B, the downstream genes C-Myc, Bcl-xL, and cyclin D1 were significantly downregulated at the **11c** concentration of 7.5 μM and both DU145 and A549. Furthermore, we investigated whether **11c** induced apoptosis in vitro by flow cytometry. As the results show, in DU145 cells, the ratio of cells in early (Annexin V^+/PI^-) and late apoptosis (Annexin V^+/PI^+) was a total of 19.16% in the 7.5 μM **11c** treatment groups and reached 52.35% in the 10 μM **11c** treatment groups (Figure 6C). Similarly, in A549 cells, the ratio of cells in early and late apoptosis was a total of 20.49% in the 7.5 μM **11c** treatment groups and reached 52.4% in the 10 μM **11c** treatment groups (Figure 6D). Therefore, we demonstrated that **11c** downregulated anti-apoptosis gene expression and induced apoptosis activities in vitro.

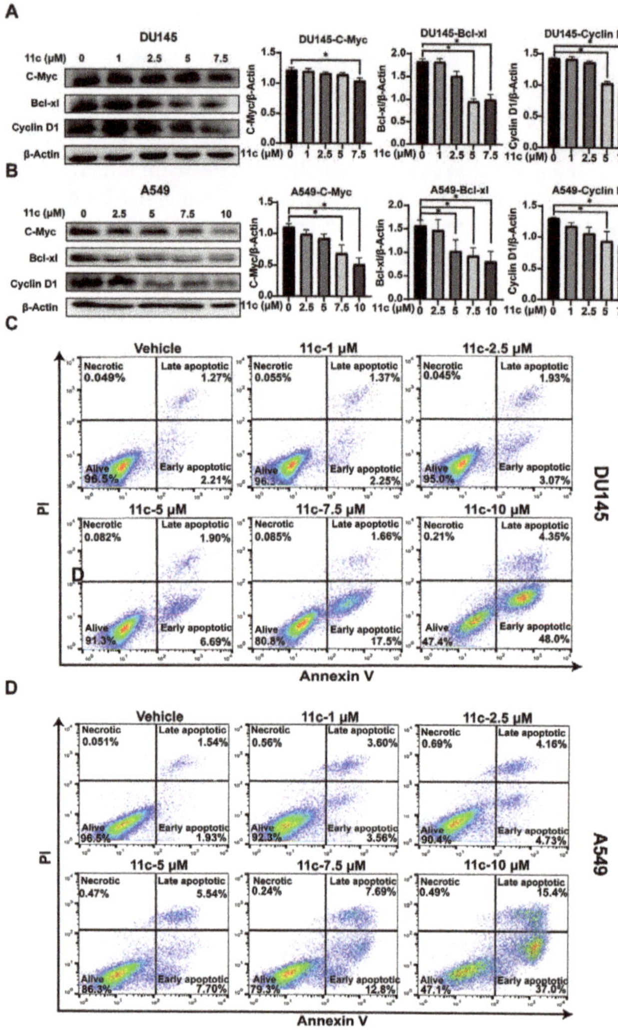

Figure 6. 11c downregulates anti-apoptosis gene expression and induces cancer cell apoptosis in vitro. (**A**,**B**) DU145 (**A**) and A549 (**B**) cells were treated with **11c** at the specific concentrations for 2 h. The levels of C-Myc, Bcl-xl, and Cyclin D1 were detected by Western blot. The relative expressions compared to the loading control protein β-Actin were measured by ImageJ from 3 individual experiments and shown as bar graphs on the right side of each Western blot. Error bars indicate means ± SD. $p < 0.05$ (*), significant, Student's *t*-test, one-way ANOVA. (**C**,**D**) DU145 (**A**) and A549 (**B**) cells were treated with **11c** at specific concentrations for 24 h. After that, cell apoptosis was measured by Annexin V-FITC/PI detection assay.

2.2.6. **11c** Inhibits the Growth of DU145 Cells by Inducing Apoptosis In Vivo

To further investigate the effects of **11c** on cancer cell growth in vivo, we examined the effect of compound **11c** in the DU145 xenograft tumors nude model. Tumor xenograft animal models, especially subcutaneous tumor xenograft model in mice, is a widely used tool to bridge basic and clinical cancer research [37,38]. After establishing the model and drug treatment for 21 days, as shown in Figure 7A,B, 10 mg/kg **11c** potently inhibited DU145 cell growth compared to the controlled vehicle group. The tumor inhibitory effects at the 10 mg/kg **11c** (i.p.) dose reached more than 40% efficiency. The solid tumor images after treatment are shown in Figure 7C. In addition, we investigated whether the inhibition of **11c** on tumor growth in vivo also functions via induction of cell-cycle arrest and apoptosis, which is similar to the observation obtained in the in vitro experiments (Figure 6). Ki67, Tunel, and p-STAT3 staining were performed, as shown in Figure 7D, and the Ki67 positive area decreased after **11c** treatment, indicating inhibited tumor proliferation. Meanwhile, an increased Tunel positive area indicated that **11c** treatment caused tumor cell apoptosis in vivo. Consistent with these observations, **11c** inhibited the phosphorylation of STAT3 in vivo. The body weight of the mice (Figure 7E) suggests that all treatments exhibited high efficacy without toxicity.

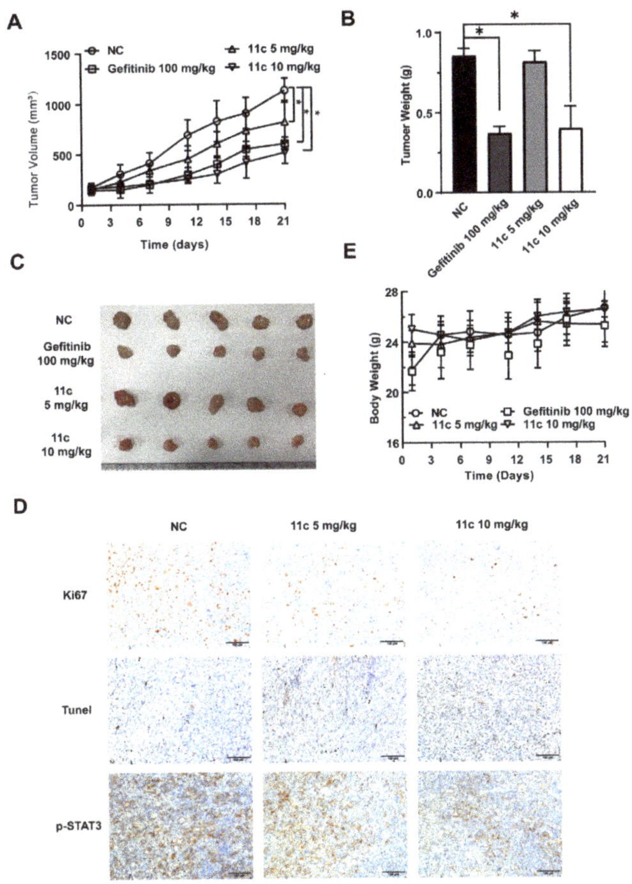

Figure 7. 11c inhibits the growth of DU145 cells in vivo. Nude mice with DU145 xenograft tumors were treated with vehicle, Gefitinib (100 mg/kg, p.o., q.2d.) or **11c** (5 or 10 mg/kg, i.p., q.2d.) for 21 days. On the last day, nude mice were sacrificed. (**A**) The tumor volumes before excision were calculated every three days. (**B**) The tumor weights were measured on the day before the nude mice sacrifice. (**C**) Tumors were excised and photographed. (**D**) Immunohistochemical (IHC) analysis of tumor slices by Ki67, Tunel, and p-STAT3 staining. (**E**) The body weights were recorded every three days. Error bars indicate means ± SEM. $p < 0.05$ (*), significant, Student's *t*-test, two-way ANOVA.

3. Discussion

The JAK/STAT3 is a classical intracellular signaling pathway in the regulation of tumor cell proliferation, survival, invasiveness, and metastasis [2,4,39]. Therefore, the JAK/STAT3 signaling pathway was considered as an effective therapeutic target for numerous cancers [40]. In the current study, we synthesized **aldisine** derivatives named compounds **11a**, **11b**, and **11c**, and their inhibitory effect on JAK/STAT3 signaling was explored in a STAT3 transcriptional activity driven luciferase reporter cell line. In particular, compound **11c** with the longest carbon atom links exhibited the highest biological activity. The Western blot analysis results elucidated that **11c** inhibits the phosphorylation of STAT3 and its upstream JAKs. Compound **11c** was identified as a new pan-JAK kinase inhibitor. Moreover, the introduction of two isothiouronium groups contains a stronger film-breaking property with a positive charge that is superior to a single group. In addition, compound **11c** induced the apoptosis of A549 and DU145 cancer cells by decreasing cell cycle and anti-apoptosis gene expression. Further in vivo antitumor studies showed that apoptosis also plays an important role in **11c** suppressed xenograft tumor growth. Taken together, we have identified a novel compound **11c** that inhibits the phosphorylation of JAKs that induce cell apoptosis to decrease cell proliferation based on the JAK/STAT3 signaling pathway.

The improved understanding of the JAK/STAT3 signaling participation in cancer treatment has led to the increasing discovery of therapeutic intervention with JAK inhibitors [41]. Previous reports have indicated that JAK inhibitors can be used to treat rheumatoid arthritis, cancer, hemophagocytic lymphohistiocytosis, atopic dermatitis, and so on [42–44]. Nowadays, several JAK inhibitors have been developed, but the clinical use of pan-JAK inhibitors in cancer therapy is still limited, perhaps due to the selectivity of JAK inhibitors [45,46]. Recent research has focused on more selective JAK inhibitors because specific JAK inhibitors may reduce side effects while increasing safety and efficacy [47,48]. Our molecular docking data showed that the hydrogen bond is the major interaction route between **11c** and the JAK's amino acid residues. In addition, the hydrogen bond interaction intensity, which was different in the four JAK members, was related to the inhibitory effect of **11c**. This discovery may provide evidence for the further modification of compound **11c** to improve its selectivity of JAK members. At the same time, there are some therapeutic interests in the future; for example, which JAK structural motif the **11c** is targeting and how it works concretely.

In conclusion, our research identified compound **11c** as a novel antitumor drug by specifically targeting the JAK/STAT3 signaling pathway. Compound **11c** exhibited inhibitory activity on JAKs activation, and efficiently inhibited cancer cell growth in vitro and in vivo. The synthesis and modification route of compound **11c** provides the potential for marine drug development in cancer treatment. In the future, compound **11c** may serve as a new skeleton molecule for further development into a JAKs' inhibitor, which has great potential for cancer treatment in clinical applications.

4. Materials and Methods

4.1. Chemical Design and Synthesis Materials

All raw materials required in this article were purchased from commercial channels. All reactions were tracked by thin-layer chromatography (TLC) and observed under 254 nm ultraviolet light using precoated silica gel plates. The specification of silica gel used for column chromatography is 200–300 mesh. ^{1}H NMR and ^{13}C NMR spectra were recorded with a Jeol JNM-ECP 600 MHz spectrometer (Celes Automation Technology Co., Ltd., Tianjin, China), using TMS as an internal standard. Chemical shifts were reported on the δ scale and *J* values were given in Hz. High resolution mass spectra (HRMS) were recorded on a Q-TOF Global Mass Spectrum (Agilent, Beijing, China). The following abbreviations are used: s = singlet, d = doublet, t = triplet, q = quartet, m = multiplet, dd = double-doublet.

4.2. Antibodies and Reagents

Antibodies against STAT3, p-STAT3 (Tyr705), JAK1, JAK2, JAK3, TYK2, Bcl-xl, C-Myc, CyclinD1, p-JAK1 (Tyr1022/1023), p-JAK2 (Tyr1007/1008), p-TYK2 (Tyr1054/1055), p-JAK(Tyr980/981), p-IKK-α/β(Ser176/180), p-NF-κB p65(Ser536)(93H1), p-Akt (Ser473) (D9E) XP®, p-GSK-3β(Ser9)(D85E12), p-p38 (Thr180/Tyr182), p-JNK (Thr183/Tyr185), and β-Actin were all obtained from Cell Signaling Technology (Danvers, MA, USA). Obtained recombinant human IL6 (Cat. 216-16) was from PeproTech. Protease and phosphatase inhibitors A and B were purchased from Millipore (Billerica, MA, USA). Bioactive drugs and compounds used for high-throughput screening were provided by TargetMol (Shanghai, China). **Aldisine** derivatives were obtained as mentioned in the chemical part.

4.3. Cell Culture

A549, DU145, MDA-MB231, and Hela were purchased from the American Type Culture Collection (Manassas, VA, USA). SKA cells were established by transfected A549 cells with a vector containing STAT3-based luciferase reporter gene as in previously reported methods [49]. The DU145 cells were cultured in RPMI 1640 complete medium (Gibco, Grand Island, NY, USA), the others were cultured in DMEM complete medium (Gibco, Grand Island, NY, USA). Prepared complete medium with added 1% streptomycin, 1% penicillin, and 10% fetal bovine serum (FBS, Gibco, Grand Island, NY, USA). Cells were incubated in a 37 °C temperature incubator with 5% CO_2.

4.4. Animals

Nude mice (male, six-week-old, weight 17–20 g) were purchased from Beijing Vital River Laboratory Animal Technology (Beijing, China). Mice were bred in a specific pathogen-free environment with controlled temperature and humidity and 12 h light and dark alternate. The Committee of Experimental Animals of the Ocean University of China (OUC-SMP-2020-11-01) has approved the animal experiments.

4.5. Luciferase Reporter Assay

SKA cells (8000 cells/well) were bedded into white 96-well plates (Corning, NY, USA) and incubated in an incubator at 37 °C containing 5% CO_2 overnight and then treated with the vehicle or indicated concentrations of compounds. Twenty-four hours later, luciferase activity was detected by adding a luciferase substrate (Cat. E2510, Promega, Beijing, China) and read by a SpectraMax® L microplate reader (Molecular Devices, Shanghai, China) [49,50].

4.6. Western Blot Analysis

After stimulating with compounds, we washed the cells twice with phosphate-buffered saline (PBS) and lysed the cells with the RIPA buffer including 1% phosphatase and 1% protease inhibitors. Protein lysis was quantified by a BCA kit (Solarbio, Beijing, China) and separated by 10% SDS-PAGE. Later they were transferred onto nitrocellulose membranes (GE Healthcare) at 90v for 2 h and incubated with primary antibodies at 4 °C overnight. After that, they were incubated with anti-rabbit horseradish peroxidase (HRP)-conjugated secondary antibodies at room temperature for 1 h, detected with chemiluminescence HRP substrate (Millipore, Billerica, MA, USA) and photographed by Chemiluminescence Imaging System (Tanon 5200, Shanghai, China).

4.7. Cell Viability and Antiproliferation Activity Assay

Cell viability and antiproliferation activity was evaluated by the resazurin indicator [51]. Cells (3500 cells/well) were seeded into 96-well plates overnight and treated with the vehicle or indicated drug concentrations for 72 h. An amount of 10 μL of 1 mg/mL resazurin solution was added per well and, after incubating for 3 h, relative cell viability was detected using a SpectraMax Mode Plate Reader (Molecular Devices, Shanghai, China) at a 595-nm emission wavelength and a 549-nm excitation wavelength. The half-maximal inhibitory concentration value (IC_{50}) of **11c** was determined using GraphPad Prism 8 software.

4.8. Molecular Docking

The docking results of compound **11c** (ligand) and JAK proteins (receptor) were calculated by the MOE (version 2020) molecular docking program. Crystal structures of all JAK proteins were obtained from the RCSB Protein Data Bank (RCSB PDB). Firstly, compound **11c** was subjected to an energy minimization processing through Chemdraw 3D software (version, 14.0.0.17). Secondly, the water molecules of the receptor protein and the existing small molecule ligands in the crystal were removed. Finally, compound **11c** was introduced into the protein structure and docked in the pocket of the original ligand. Based on the scores calculated by GBVI/WSA combined with free energy, the top 5 results were analyzed using MOE.

4.9. Flow cytometry Analysis of Apoptosis

A549 and DU145 cells (5×10^5 cells/well) were bedded into 6-well plates and treated with **11c** at the indicated concentrations. After 24 h incubation, the cells were washed with phosphate-buffered saline (PBS) twice followed by incubating with the eBioscience™ Annexin VFITC Apoptosis Kit (Invitrogen, City, Carlsbad, California, USA) according to the manufacturer's instructions. Finally, cell apoptosis was analyzed by flow cytometry and the results were processed by flowjo software(version 10.6.2).

4.10. Subcutaneous Tumor Xenograft Model and Antitumor Assay In Vivo

Nude mice were randomly divided into 4 treatment groups (n = 5/group) before being implanted with subcutaneous tumor xenograft cells. DU145 cells were harvested, counted, and reserved on ice. About 15×10^6 cells were injected to establish a tumor transplantation nude mouse model. The four groups were treated as follows: vehicle group, Gefitinib (100 mg/kg) group, and **11c** (5 mg/kg or 10 mg/kg) group. Tumor size ($1/2 \times$ length $\times$ width^2) and body weight were measured every 3 days for 21 days. On the last day the mice were sacrificed, and the tumor weight was determined [6].

4.11. Immunohistochemical (IHC) Analysis

The xenograft model tumor of mice was collected and fixed with 4% paraformaldehyde (PFA) for 72 h at 4 °C and then embedded in paraffin and cut into slices. After, the slices were baked, dewaxed in xylene, gradients ethanol, and boiled in a microwave to repair antigen [31]. The inactivation of endogenous peroxidase was blocked by incubating with fresh 3% H_2O_2. The slices were blocked with fat free milk and incubated with the primary antibody (1:3000) at 4 °C overnight. After that, they were washed with PBS followed by incubation with the HRP-conjugated secondary antibody at room temperature (Boster, Wuhan, China). Finally, slices were dyed by DAB/H_2O_2 reaction, brown color in the cell membrane indicated positive staining. Images were captured using an upright fluorescence microscope (Olympus BX53, Tokyo, Japan) [6,52].

4.12. Statistical Analysis

The data were presented as mean ± SD. GraphPad prism (version 8.0.2) was used for statistical analysis. p-value < 0.05 (*) was considered a significant difference, which was calculated by t-test, one and two-way ANOVA (analysis of variance).

Supplementary Materials: The following supporting information can be downloaded at: https://www.mdpi.com/article/10.3390/md21040218/s1, The general procedures for compounds **8a, 8b, 8c, 9a, 9b, 9c, 10a, 10b, 10c, 11a, 11b**, and **11c**. The data of ^1H and ^{13}C NMR of all the compounds are shown in Supplementary Materials. Table S1: The high-throughput-screen result of **aldisine** derivatives. Figure S1: The high-throughput screen of compounds graph.

Author Contributions: Conceptualization, C.-Y.Z. and T.J.; experimental studies performed by, D.-P.W., L.-H.W., R.L., N.H. and Q.-Y.Z.; writing–original draft preparation, L.-H.W., D.-P.W. and R.L.; writing–review and editing, C.-Y.Z. and T.J.; Our manuscript is original content and has not been submitted to other journals. All authors have read and agreed to the published version of the manuscript.

Funding: This research was funded by Natural Science Foundation of China: Grant No. 82073759; Shandong Provincial Key Laboratory Platform Project No. 2021ZDSYS11; Shandong Province Major Scientific and Technological Innovation Project: No. 2020CXGC010503; National Natural Science Foundation of China Major Project: No. 81991525.

Institutional Review Board Statement: The animal study protocol was approved by Committee of Experimental Animals of the Ocean University of China (protocol code: OUC-SMP-2020-11-01 and date of approval: 2 November 2020).

Informed Consent Statement: Not applicable.

Data Availability Statement: The authors declare that supporting data of this study are available within the article and the Supplementary Materials.

Conflicts of Interest: Authors have no conflict of interest.

References

1. Sung, H.; Ferlay, J.; Siegel, R.L.; Laversanne, M.; Soerjomataram, I.; Jemal, A.; Bray, F. Global Cancer Statistics 2020: GLOBOCAN Estimates of Incidence and Mortality Worldwide for 36 Cancers in 185 Countries. *CA Cancer J. Clin.* **2021**, *71*, 209–249. [CrossRef] [PubMed]
2. Johnson, D.E.; O'Keefe, R.A.; Grandis, J.R. Targeting the IL-6/JAK/STAT3 signalling axis in cancer. *Nat. Rev. Clin. Oncol.* **2018**, *15*, 234–248. [CrossRef] [PubMed]
3. Calautti, E.; Avalle, L.; Poli, V. Psoriasis: A STAT3-Centric View. *Int. J. Mol. Sci.* **2018**, *19*, 171. [CrossRef] [PubMed]
4. Manore, S.G.; Doheny, D.L.; Wong, G.L.; Lo, H.-W. IL-6/JAK/STAT3 Signaling in Breast Cancer Metastasis: Biology and Treatment. *Front. Oncol.* **2022**, *12*, 866014. [CrossRef]
5. Xu, J.; Zhang, J.; Mao, Q.-F.; Wu, J.; Wang, Y. The Interaction Between Autophagy and JAK/STAT3 Signaling Pathway in Tumors. *Front. Genet.* **2022**, *13*, 880359. [CrossRef]
6. Zhang, J.-Q.; Li, R.; Dong, X.-Y.; He, N.; Yin, R.-J.; Yang, M.-K.; Liu, J.-Y.; Yu, R.-L.; Zhao, C.-Y.; Jiang, T. Design, Synthesis and Structure-Activity Relationship Studies of Meridianin Derivatives as Novel JAK/STAT3 Signaling Inhibitors. *Int. J. Mol. Sci.* **2022**, *23*, 2199. [CrossRef]
7. E Fragoulis, G.; McInnes, I.B.; Siebert, S. JAK-inhibitors. New players in the field of immune-mediated diseases, beyond rheumatoid arthritis. *Rheumatology* **2019**, *58*, i43–i54. [CrossRef]
8. Owen, K.L.; Brockwell, N.K.; Parker, B.S. JAK-STAT Signaling: A Double-Edged Sword of Immune Regulation and Cancer Progression. *Cancers* **2019**, *11*, 2002. [CrossRef]
9. Shawky, A.M.; Almalki, F.A.; Abdalla, A.N.; Abdelazeem, A.H.; Gouda, A.M. A Comprehensive Overview of Globally Approved JAK Inhibitors. *Pharmaceutics* **2022**, *14*, 1001. [CrossRef]
10. Bryan, J.C.; Verstovsek, S. Overcoming treatment challenges in myelofibrosis and polycythemia vera: The role of ruxolitinib. *Cancer Chemother. Pharmacol.* **2016**, *77*, 1125–1142. [CrossRef]
11. Kim, W.; Yoon, D.; Song, Y.; Koh, Y.; Cao, J.; Ji, D.; Yang, H.; Eom, H.; Jing, H.; Kwak, J.; et al. Early Safety and Efficacy Data from a Phase I/II Trial of DZD4205, a Selective Jak1 Inhibitor, in Relapsed/Refractory Peripheral T-Cell Lymphoma. *Hematol. Oncol.* **2021**, *39*, 101–102. [CrossRef]
12. Rigogliuso, S.; Campora, S.; Notarbartolo, M.; Ghersi, G. Recovery of Bioactive Compounds from Marine Organisms: Focus on the Future Perspectives for Pharmacological, Biomedical and Regenerative Medicine Applications of Marine Collagen. *Molecules* **2023**, *28*, 1152. [CrossRef]
13. Bai, X.; Liu, Y.; Wang, H.; Zhang, H. Natural Products from the Marine Sponge Subgenus *Reniera*. *Molecules* **2021**, *26*, 1097. [CrossRef] [PubMed]
14. Ebada, S.S.; Linh, M.H.; Longeon, A.; de Voogd, N.J.; Durieu, E.; Meijer, L.; Bourguet-Kondracki, M.L.; Singab, A.N.B.; Müller, W.E.; Proksch, P. Dispacamide E and other bioactive bromopyrrole alkaloids from two Indonesian marine sponges of the genus Stylissa. *Nat. Prod. Res.* **2015**, *29*, 231–238. [CrossRef]
15. Tasdemir, D.; Mallon, R.; Greenstein, M.; Feldberg, L.R.; Kim, S.C.; Collins, K.; Wojciechowicz, D.; Mangalindan, G.C.; Concepción, G.P.; Harper, M.K.; et al. Aldisine Alkaloids from the Philippine Sponge *Stylissa massa* Are Potent Inhibitors of Mitogen-Activated Protein Kinase Kinase-1 (MEK-1). *J. Med. Chem.* **2001**, *45*, 529–532. [CrossRef]
16. Xu, W.; Yang, R.; Hao, Y.; Song, H.; Liu, Y.; Zhang, J.; Li, Y.; Wang, Q. Discovery of Aldisine and Its Derivatives as Novel Antiviral, Larvicidal, and Antiphytopathogenic-Fungus Agents. *J. Agric. Food Chem.* **2022**, *70*, 12355–12363. [CrossRef]

17. Xie, J.; Tian, J.; Su, L.; Huang, M.; Zhu, X.; Ye, F.; Wan, Y. Pyrrolo[2,3-c]azepine derivatives: A new class of potent protein tyrosine phosphatase 1B inhibitors. *Bioorganic Med. Chem. Lett.* **2011**, *21*, 4306–4309. [CrossRef]
18. White, A.W.; Carpenter, N.; Lottin, J.R.; McClelland, R.A.; Nicholson, R.I. Synthesis and evaluation of novel anti-proliferative pyrroloazepinone and indoloazepinone oximes derived from the marine natural product hymenialdisine. *Eur. J. Med. Chem.* **2012**, *56*, 246–253. [CrossRef]
19. Cimino, G.; De Rosa, S.; De Stefano, S.; Mazzarella, L.; Puliti, R.; Sodano, G. Isolation and X-ray crystal structure of a novel bromo-compound from two marine sponges. *Tetrahedron Lett.* **1982**, *23*, 247–259. [CrossRef]
20. Wan, Y.; Hur, W.; Cho, C.Y.; Liu, Y.; Adrian, F.J.; Lozach, O.; Bach, S.; Mayer, T.; Fabbro, D.; Meijer, L.; et al. Synthesis and target identification of hymenialdisine analogs. *Chem. Biol.* **2004**, *11*, 247–259. [CrossRef]
21. Bhuyan, B.K.; Scheidt, L.G.; Fraser, T.J. Cell cycle phase specificity of antitumor agents. *Cancer Res* **1972**, *32*, 398–407.
22. Ferreira, M.; Assunção, L.S.; Silva, A.H.; Filippin-Monteiro, F.B.; Creczynski-Pasa, T.B.; Sá, M.M. Allylic isothiouronium salts: The discovery of a novel class of thiourea analogues with antitumor activity. *Eur. J. Med. Chem.* **2017**, *129*, 151–158. [CrossRef]
23. Tong, S.; Zhang, M.; Wang, S.; Yin, R.; Yu, R.; Wan, S.; Jiang, T.; Zhang, L. Isothiouronium modification empowers pyrimidine-substituted curcumin analogs potent cytotoxicity and Golgi localization. *Eur. J. Med. Chem.* **2016**, *123*, 849–857. [CrossRef]
24. Xu, Y.Z.; Yakushijin, K.; Horne, D.A. Synthesis of C11N5 marine sponge alkaloids:(±)-Hymenin, stevensine, hymenialdisine, and debromohymenialdisine. *J. Org. Chem.* **1997**, *62*, 456–464. [CrossRef]
25. Suter, M.A.; Tan, N.Y.; Thiam, C.H.; Khatoo, M.; MacAry, P.A.; Angeli, V.; Gasser, S.; Zhang, Y.L. cGAS-STING cytosolic DNA sensing pathway is suppressed by JAK2-STAT3 in tumor cells. *Sci. Rep.* **2021**, *11*, 7243. [CrossRef]
26. Yeh, H.-H.; Lai, W.-W.; Chen, H.H.W.; Liu, H.-S.; Su, W.-C. Autocrine IL-6-induced Stat3 activation contributes to the pathogenesis of lung adenocarcinoma and malignant pleural effusion. *Oncogene* **2006**, *25*, 4300–4309. [CrossRef]
27. Schabath, M.B.; Cote, M.L. Cancer Progress and Priorities: Lung Cancer. *Cancer Epidemiol. Biomark. Prev. A Publ. Am. Assoc. Cancer Res. Cosponsored Am. Soc. Prev. Oncol.* **2019**, *28*, 1563–1579. [CrossRef]
28. Nagpal, J.K.; Mishra, R.; Das, B.R. Activation of Stat-3 as one of the early events in tobacco chewing-mediated oral carcinogene-sis. *Cancer* **2002**, *94*, 2393–2400. [CrossRef]
29. Suradej, B.; Sookkhee, S.; Panyakaew, J.; Mungkornasawakul, P.; Wikan, N.; Smith, D.R.; Potikanond, S.; Nimlamool, W. Kaempferia parviflora Extract Inhibits STAT3 Activation and Interleukin-6 Production in HeLa Cervical Cancer Cells. *Int. J. Mol. Sci.* **2019**, *20*, 4226. [CrossRef]
30. Zhang, L.; Song, Q.; Zhang, X.; Li, L.; Xu, X.; Xu, X.; Li, X.; Wang, Z.; Lin, Y.; Li, X.; et al. Zelnorm, an agonist of 5-Hydroxytryptamine 4-receptor, acts as a potential antitumor drug by targeting JAK/STAT3 signaling. *Investig. New Drugs* **2019**, *38*, 311–320. [CrossRef]
31. Aaronson, D.S.; Horvath, C.M. A Road Map for Those Who Don't Know JAK-STAT. *Science* **2002**, *296*, 1653–1655. [CrossRef]
32. Pellegrini, S.; Dusanter-Fourt, I. The Structure, Regulation and Function of the Janus Kinases (JAKs) and the Signal Transducers and Activators of Transcription (STATs). *JBIC J. Biol. Inorg. Chem.* **1997**, *248*, 615–633. [CrossRef]
33. Glassman, C.R.; Tsutsumi, N.; Saxton, R.A.; Lupardus, P.J.; Jude, K.M.; Garcia, K.C. Structure of a Janus kinase cytokine receptor complex reveals the basis for dimeric activation. *Science* **2022**, *376*, 163–169. [CrossRef]
34. Xin, P.; Xu, X.; Deng, C.; Liu, S.; Wang, Y.; Zhou, X.; Ma, H.; Wei, D.; Sun, S. The role of JAK/STAT signaling pathway and its inhibitors in diseases. *Int. Immunopharmacol.* **2020**, *80*, 106210. [CrossRef]
35. de Araujo, E.D.; Orlova, A.; Neubauer, H.A.; Bajusz, D.; Seo, H.-S.; Dhe-Paganon, S.; Keserű, G.M.; Moriggl, R.; Gunning, P.T. Structural Implications of STAT3 and STAT5 SH2 Domain Mutations. *Cancers* **2019**, *11*, 1757. [CrossRef]
36. Fukada, T.; Ohtani, T.; Yoshida, Y.; Shirogane, T.; Nishida, K.; Nakajima, K.; Hibi, M.; Hirano, T. STAT3 orchestrates contradictory signals in cytokine-induced G1 to S cell-cycle transition. *EMBO J.* **1998**, *17*, 6670–6677. [CrossRef]
37. Lee, N.P.; Chan, C.M.; Tung, L.N.; Wang, H.K.; Law, S. Tumor xenograft animal models for esophageal squamous cell carcinoma. *J. Biomed. Sci.* **2018**, *25*, 66. [CrossRef]
38. Bürtin, F.; Mullins, C.S.; Linnebacher, M. Mouse models of colorectal cancer: Past, present and future perspectives. *World J. Gastroenterol.* **2020**, *26*, 1394–1426. [CrossRef]
39. Yu, H.; Lee, H.; Herrmann, A.; Buettner, R.; Jove, R. Revisiting STAT3 signalling in cancer: New and unexpected biological functions. *Nat. Rev. Cancer* **2014**, *14*, 736–746. [CrossRef]
40. Zou, S.; Tong, Q.; Liu, B.; Huang, W.; Tian, Y.; Fu, X. Targeting STAT3 in Cancer Immunotherapy. *Mol. Cancer* **2020**, *19*, 145. [CrossRef]
41. McLornan, D.P.; E Pope, J.; Gotlib, J.; Harrison, C.N. Current and future status of JAK inhibitors. *Lancet* **2021**, *398*, 803–816. [CrossRef]
42. Taylor, P.C.; Keystone, E.C.; Van Der Heijde, D.; Weinblatt, M.E.; Del Carmen Morales, L.; Gonzaga, J.R.; Yakushin, S.; Ishii, T.; Emoto, K.; Beattie, S.; et al. Baricitinib versus Placebo or Adalimumab in Rheumatoid Arthritis. *N. Engl. J. Med.* **2017**, *376*, 652–662. [CrossRef]
43. Chovatiya, R.; Paller, A.S. JAK inhibitors in the treatment of atopic dermatitis. *J. Allergy Clin. Immunol.* **2021**, *148*, 927–940. [CrossRef]
44. Keenan, C.; Nichols, K.E.; Albeituni, S. Use of the JAK Inhibitor Ruxolitinib in the Treatment of Hemophagocytic Lymphohistiocytosis. *Front. Immunol.* **2021**, *12*, 614704. [CrossRef]

45. Clarke, B.; Yates, M.; Adas, M.; Bechman, K.; Galloway, J. The safety of JAK-1 inhibitors. *Rheumatology* **2021**, *60*, ii24–ii30. [CrossRef]
46. Traves, P.G.; Murray, B.; Campigotto, F.; Galien, R.; Meng, A.; A Di Paolo, J. JAK selectivity and the implications for clinical inhibition of pharmacodynamic cytokine signalling by filgotinib, upadacitinib, tofacitinib and baricitinib. *Ann. Rheum. Dis.* **2021**, *80*, 865–875. [CrossRef]
47. Virtanen, A.T.; Haikarainen, T.; Raivola, J.; Silvennoinen, O. Selective JAKinibs: Prospects in Inflammatory and Autoimmune Diseases. *BioDrugs Clin. Immuno-Ther. Biopharm. Gene Ther.* **2019**, *33*, 15–32. [CrossRef]
48. Smyth, L.A.; Collins, I. Measuring and interpreting the selectivity of protein kinase inhibitors. *J. Chem. Biol.* **2009**, *2*, 131–151. [CrossRef]
49. Chen, X.; Du, Y.; Nan, J.; Zhang, X.; Qin, X.; Wang, Y.; Hou, J.; Wang, Q.; Yang, J. Brevilin A, a Novel Natural Product, Inhibits Janus Kinase Activity and Blocks STAT3 Signaling in Cancer Cells. *PLoS ONE* **2013**, *8*, e63697. [CrossRef]
50. Li, M.; Yan, Y.; Zhang, X.; Zhang, Y.; Xu, X.; Zhang, L.; Lu, L.; Wang, J.; Zhang, Y.; Song, Q.; et al. Scaffold compound L971 exhibits anti-inflammatory activities through inhibition of JAK/STAT and NFκB signalling pathways. *J. Cell. Mol. Med.* **2021**, *25*, 6333–6347. [CrossRef]
51. Kumar, P.; Nagarajan, A.; Uchil, P. Analysis of Cell Viability by the alamarBlue Assay. *Cold Spring Harb. Protoc.* **2018**, *2018*, pdb.prot095489. [CrossRef] [PubMed]
52. Tan, W.C.C.; Nerurkar, S.N.; Cai, H.Y.; Ng, H.H.M.; Wu, D.; Wee, Y.T.F.; Lim, J.C.T.; Yeong, J.; Lim, T.K.H. Overview of multiplex immunohistochemistry/immunofluorescence techniques in the era of cancer immunotherapy. *Cancer Commun.* **2020**, *40*, 135–153. [CrossRef] [PubMed]

marine drugs

MDPI

Article

Light-Mediated Transformation of Renieramycins and Semisynthesis of 4′-Pyridinecarbonyl-Substituted Renieramycin-Type Derivatives as Potential Cytotoxic Agents against Non-Small-Cell Lung Cancer Cells

Suwimon Sinsook [1,2], Koonchira Buaban [1,3], Iksen Iksen [4], Korrakod Petsri [4,5], Bhurichaya Innets [4,5], Chaisak Chansriniyom [1,3], Khanit Suwanborirux [1,3], Masashi Yokoya [6], Naoki Saito [6], Varisa Pongrakhananon [4,7], Pithi Chanvorachote [4,5] and Supakarn Chamni [1,3,*]

1 Department of Pharmacognosy and Pharmaceutical Botany, Faculty of Pharmaceutical Sciences, Chulalongkorn University, Bangkok 10330, Thailand; nhamsuwimon1997@gmail.com (S.S.); koonchira.buaban@gmail.com (K.B.); chaisak.c@pharm.chula.ac.th (C.C.); khanit.s@chula.ac.th (K.S.)
2 Pharmaceutical Sciences and Technology Program, Faculty of Pharmaceutical Sciences, Chulalongkorn University, Bangkok 10330, Thailand
3 Natural Products and Nanoparticles Research Unit (NP2), Chulalongkorn University, Bangkok 10330, Thailand
4 Department of Pharmacology and Physiology, Faculty of Pharmaceutical Sciences, Chulalongkorn University, Bangkok 10330, Thailand; ikseniksen08@gmail.com (I.I.); korrakod.petsri@gmail.com (K.P.); 6481004120@student.chula.ac.th (B.I.); varisa.p@pharm.chula.ac.th (V.P.); pithi.c@chula.ac.th (P.C.)
5 Center of Excellence in Cancer Cell and Molecular Biology, Faculty of Pharmaceutical Sciences, Chulalongkorn University, Bangkok 10330, Thailand
6 Graduate School of Pharmaceutical Sciences, Meiji Pharmaceutical University, 2-522-1 Noshio, Tokyo 204-8588, Japan; yokoya@my-pharm.ac.jp (M.Y.); naoki@my-pharm.ac.jp (N.S.)
7 Preclinical Toxicity and Efficacy, Assessment of Medicines and Chemicals Research Unit, Chulalongkorn University, Bangkok 10330, Thailand
* Correspondence: supakarn.c@pharm.chula.ac.th; Tel.: +66-2-218-8357

Citation: Sinsook, S.; Buaban, K.; Iksen, I.; Petsri, K.; Innets, B.; Chansriniyom, C.; Suwanborirux, K.; Yokoya, M.; Saito, N.; Pongrakhananon, V.; et al. Light-Mediated Transformation of Renieramycins and Semisynthesis of 4′-Pyridinecarbonyl-Substituted Renieramycin-Type Derivatives as Potential Cytotoxic Agents against Non-Small-Cell Lung Cancer Cells. *Mar. Drugs* **2023**, *21*, 400. https://doi.org/10.3390/md21070400

Academic Editors: Barbara De Filippis, Alessandra Ammazzalorso and Marialuigia Fantacuzzi

Received: 24 June 2023
Revised: 9 July 2023
Accepted: 10 July 2023
Published: 13 July 2023

Abstract: The semisynthesis of renieramycin-type derivatives was achieved under mild and facile conditions by attaching a 1,3-dioxole-bridged phenolic moiety onto ring A of the renieramycin structure and adding a 4′-pyridinecarbonyl ester substituent at its C-5 or C-22 position. These were accomplished through a light-induced intramolecular photoredox reaction using blue light (4 W) and Steglich esterification, respectively. Renieramycin M (**4**), a bis-tetrahydroisoquinolinequinone compound isolated from the Thai blue sponge (*Xestospongia* sp.), served as the starting material. The cytotoxicity of the 10 natural and semisynthesized renieramycins against non-small-cell lung cancer (NSCLC) cell lines was evaluated. The 5-*O*-(4′-pyridinecarbonyl) renieramycin T (**11**) compound exhibited high cytotoxicity with half-maximal inhibitory concentration (IC_{50}) values of 35.27 ± 1.09 and 34.77 ± 2.19 nM against H290 and H460 cells, respectively. Notably, the potency of compound **11** was 2-fold more than that of renieramycin T (**7**) and equal to those of **4** and doxorubicin. Interestingly, the renieramycin-type derivatives with a hydroxyl group at C-5 and C-22 exhibited weak cytotoxicity. In silico molecular docking and dynamics studies confirmed that the mitogen-activated proteins, kinase 1 and 3 (MAPK1 and MAPK3), are suitable targets for **11**. Thus, the structure–cytotoxicity study of renieramycins was extended to facilitate the development of potential anticancer agents for NSCLC cells.

Keywords: *Xestospongia* sp.; cytotoxicity; renieramycins; semisynthesis; light-induced intramolecular photoredox reaction; non-small-cell lung cancer; bis-tetrahydroisoquinoline; molecular docking; molecular dynamics

1. Introduction

Renieramycins, bis-tetrahydroisoquinolinequinone marine alkaloids, along with ecteinascidins and jorunnamycins, have been reported to exhibit significant anticancer activity (Figure 1) [1,2]. Trabectedin (also known as ecteinascidin 743, **1**), which was isolated from the Caribbean tunicate (*Ecteinascidia turbinate*), was approved by the United States Food and Drug Administration in 2015 for the treatment of advanced soft tissue sarcoma and ovarian carcinoma [3–5]. Lurbinectedin (PM01183, **2**), a bis-tetrahydroisoquinoline analog of **1**, was approved for the second-line treatment of metastatic small-cell lung cancer in 2020 [6,7]. Compounds **1** and **2** are chemotherapeutic drugs that covalently bind specifically to the N2 position of guanine in the DNA minor groove, leading to double-strand breaks and apoptosis in cancer cells [3,6].

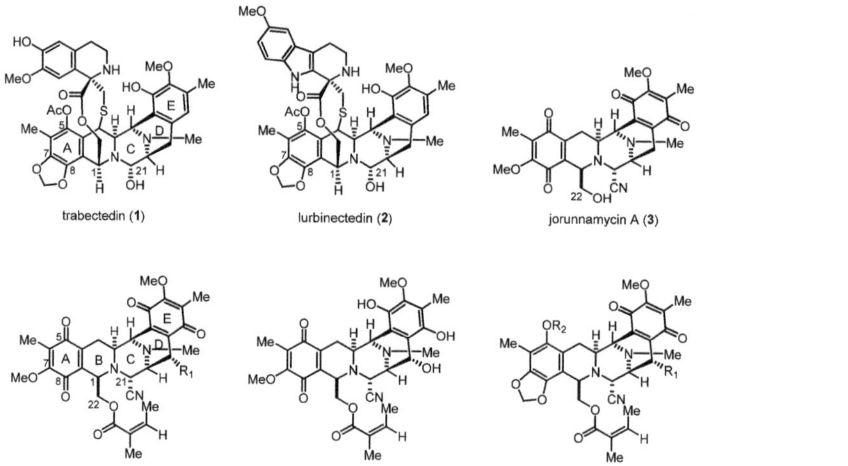

Figure 1. Structures of the bis-tetrahydroisoquinoline alkaloids as anticancer drugs and promising drug leads.

Renieramycins are isolated from marine sponges, such as genera *Reniera* [8,9], *Cribrochalina* [10], and *Xestospongia* [11,12], and they possess a pentacyclic bis-tetrahydroisoquinolinequinone moiety as the core scaffold (Figure 1). Several renieramycins containing an angelate ester at the C-22 position display potent bioactivities, including antimicrobial [8], antileishmanial [13], and anticancer [11,12,14,15] activities. Interestingly, renieramycins M (**4**) and N (**5**) have been successfully isolated in the gram scale of the Thai blue sponge (*Xestospongia* sp.) [11]. Renieramycins M, N, and O (**4**–**6**) have been demonstrated to exhibit potent cytotoxicity against colon (HCT116) and lung carcinoma (QG56) [11,12]. Additionally, compound **4** has been reported to display strong cytotoxicity against various human cancer cell lines, including colon (DLD1), lung (NCI-H460), pancreatic adenocarcinoma (AsPC1), and ductal breast epithelial (T47D) cells [11,12,14]. Renieramycins T (**7**) and U (**8**), renieramycin–ecteinascidin hybrid marine natural alkaloids containing a 1,3-dioxole ring that is similar to the left-side carbon framework of trabectedin, exhibit strong in vitro anticancer activity against non-small-cell lung cancer (NSCLC) cells [14]. Furthermore, the cytotoxicity mechanisms of the renieramycin–ecteinascidin hybrid derivatives against NSCLC cells have been revealed. Compound **7** was discovered to enhance apoptosis induction via the degradation of the myeloid cell leukemia 1 (Mcl-1) protein in NSCLC [16,17]. Further, it suppressed mouse melanoma (B16F10) cell metastasis and migration through the downregulation of

NF-E2-related factor 2 [18]. Moreover, the 5-*O*-ester derivatives of **7**, which possess acetyl and *N*-Boc-L-alaninoyl substituents, induced apoptosis and suppressed cancer stem cell markers via protein kinase B (AKT) inhibition in NSCLC cells [19,20].

According to the structure–activity relationship (SAR) study, nitrogen-containing heterocyclic ester substituents, particularly 4′-pyridinecarbonyl ester derivatives, as side chains on the renieramycin framework have a remarkable effect on the cytotoxicity of renieramycin against various cancer cells (Figure 2). The 22-*O*-(4′-pyridinecarbonyl) jorunnamycin A compound (**9**) exhibited significantly better cytotoxicity than jorunnamycin A (**3**), its parent compound, against human colon (HCT116), breast (MDA-MB-435), and NSCLC (H292 and H460) cell lines [21,22]. Furthermore, hydroquinone 5-*O*-(4′-pyridinecarbonyl) renieramycin M (**10**) was prepared from **4** by a two-step process, including hydrogenation and Steglich esterification. The resulting derivative (**10**) exhibited cytotoxicity against the highly metastatic H292 and H460 NSCLC cell lines at inhibitory concentration (IC_{50}) values in the nanomolar range [15].

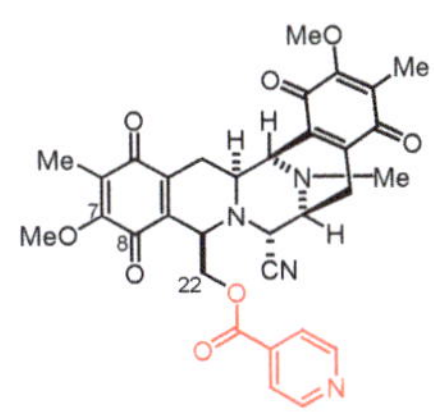

22-*O*-(4′-pyridinecarbonyl) jorunnamycin A (**9**)

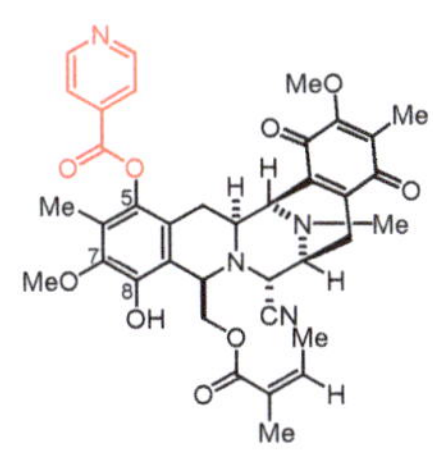

hydroquinone 5-*O*-(4′-pyridinecarbonyl) renieramycin M (**10**)

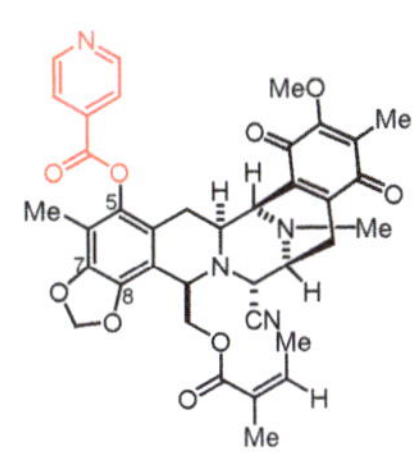

5-*O*-(4′-pyridinecarbonyl) renieramycin T (**11**)

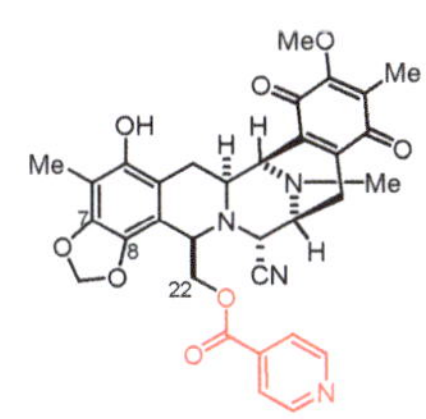

22-*O*-(4′-pyridinecarbonyl) renieramycin T (**12**)

Figure 2. Semisynthetic derivatives of the renieramycin-type derivatives containing a 4′-pyridinecarbonyl ester substituent.

Regarding the continuous structure–cytotoxicity relationship study of the renieramycin-type derivatives, the semisynthesis of the renieramycin–ecteinascidin hybrid derivatives of natural bis-tetrahydroisoquinolinequinones (**4**–**6**) was conducted via a facile, light-induced intramolecular photoredox reaction to transform quinone ring A into the 1,3-dioxole-bridged phenolic moiety. The mild photoredox reaction enables the selective one-step modification of the methoxy-substituted quinone unit located on ring A of renieramycins, resulting in the formation of 5-hydroxy-tetrahydroisoquinol-1,3-dioxoles with excellent yields [23]. This transformation yields a series of renieramycin–ecteinascidin derivatives that closely resemble the structure of ring A found in Trabectedin and Lurbinectedin, well-known tetrahydroisoquinoline-based chemotherapeutic drugs. Next, a series of 4′-pyridinecarbonyl esters for the renieramycin-type derivatives were prepared by mild and selective Steglich esterification. The new 4′-pyridinecarbonyl esters, **11** and **12**, were obtained (Figure 2). The in vitro cytotoxicity of the compounds against human H292 and H460 NSCLC cell lines was evaluated using the 3-(4,5-dimethylthiazol-2-yl)-2,5-diphenyltetrazolium bromide (MTT) assay. Additionally, the in silico prediction of the target genes and molecular pathways associated with the activity of the compounds was achieved by virtual network pharmacology study, including molecular docking and molecular dynamics studies.

2. Results and Discussion

2.1. Light-Induced Intramolecular Photoredox Reaction of Renieramycins

Renieramycins **4**–**6** were isolated from the Thai blue sponge (*Xestospongia* sp.) by pretreatment with 10% potassium cyanide following a previously reported protocol [11,12]. The photoredox reactions occurring through the light-induced radical formation and intramolecular cyclization of the natural bis-tetrahydroisoquinolinequinone alkaloids (**4**–**6**) were investigated (Scheme 1 and Table 1) [23]. To determine the optimal reaction conditions, we experimented with compound **4**, along with various solvents and light sources. Through irradiation by an 18-W fluorescent lamp (white light) in dichloromethane (CH_2Cl_2) for 24 h, compound **4** was smoothly transformed into compound **7** in 64% yield (Table 1, entry 1). The application of chloroform ($CHCl_3$) and tetrahydrofuran (THF) as solvents for the photoredox reaction of compound **4** furnished compound **7** in 46% and 47% yields, respectively (Table 1, entries 2 and 3). Further improvement in the yield was achieved when the reaction solution was exposed to irradiation by a 4-W light-emitting diode (LED) lamp (blue light) in CH_2Cl_2, affording **7** in excellent yield (81% yield, entry 4). However, using $CHCl_3$ and THF with blue light irradiation decreased the yields of **7** to 51% and 54%, respectively (Table 1, entries 5 and 6). Thus, optimized photoredox reactions using blue light and CH_2Cl_2 were further performed with natural alkaloids **5** and **6** (Table 1, entries 7 and 8).

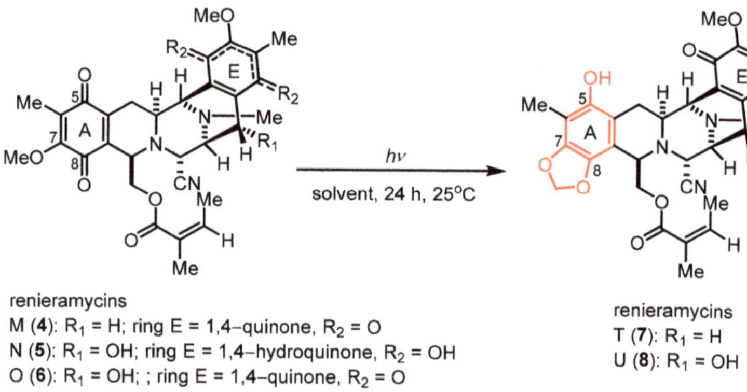

Scheme 1. Photoredox reaction of the natural renieramycins.

Table 1. Optimization of the conditions for the photoredox of natural renieramycins.

Entry	Starting Material	Light Source [a]	Solvent	Renieramycin Product	Isolated Yield (%)
1	4	18 W	CH_2Cl_2	7	64
2	4	18 W	$CHCl_3$	7	46
3	4	18 W	THF	7	47
4	4	4 W	CH_2Cl_2	7	81
5	4	4 W	$CHCl_3$	7	51
6	4	4 W	THF	7	54
7	5	4 W	CH_2Cl_2	6:8 = 1:2 [b]	18:37 [c]
8	6	4 W	CH_2Cl_2	8	48

[a] 18 W refers to the white light fluorescent lamp, and 4 W refers to the blue LED lamp. [b] Ratio was determined based on the proton signal of H-3 by nuclear magnetic resonance (NMR) spectroscopy analysis. [c] The yield of the major product was determined after column chromatographic purification.

Unexpectedly, the photoredox reaction of compound **5** yielded a mixture of bis-tetrahydroisoquinolinequinones **6** and **8** (Table 1, entry 7). Compound **8** was obtained as the major product in 37% yield, two times higher than the yield of compound **6** (18% yield). Meanwhile, the photoredox reaction of compound **6** under the optimized condition yielded compound **8** in 48% yield (Table 1, entry 8). Therefore, the light-induced radical formation and intramolecular cyclization of compound **5** to yield compounds **6** and **8** were proposed to occur via stepwise transformations. The mechanism involved air oxidation to convert the unstable 1,4-hydroquinone into the 1,4-quinone moiety, followed by the photoredox reaction [24] (Scheme 2). The results of the light-mediated transformation highlight the chemical diversity of the natural renieramycins found around the blue *Xestospongia* sponge habitat.

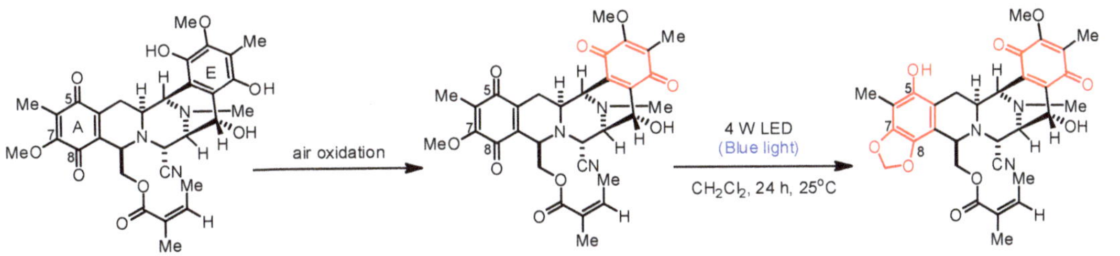

Scheme 2. Proposed transformation mechanism of **5** into **6** and **8**.

2.2. Semisynthesis of 4′-Pyridinecarbonyl-Substituted Renieramycin-Type Derivatives

The semisynthesis of the 4′-pyridinecarbonyl-substituted renieramycin–ecteinascidin hybrid derivative (**11**) started with the photoredox transformation and esterification (Scheme 3). The irradiation of **4** under the 4-W LED light in CH_2Cl_2 furnished **7**. Subsequently, a 4′-pyridinecarbonyl motif of **7** was installed by Steglich esterification using isonicotinoyl chloride as an acylating agent, 1-ethyl-3-(3-dimethylaminopropyl) carbodiimide (EDCI) as a coupling reagent, and 4-dimethylaminopyridine (DMAP) as a nucleophilic base catalyst to obtain the desired product (**11**) in acceptable yield. The semisynthesis protocol of the renieramycin-type derivative (**12**) was envisioned. Compound **3** was prepared from compound **4** by hydrogenation, hydride reduction, and air oxidation [21,24]. Ester compound **12** was obtained in excellent yield by attaching the 4′-pyridinecarbonyl substituent to the C-22 position of renieramycin by Steglich esterification, followed by the formation of the 1,3-dioxole-bridged phenolic moiety via light-induced radical formation and intramolecular cyclization.

The chemical structures of all semisynthetic renieramycin-type derivatives were characterized by spectroscopic techniques (see Supporting Information for the spectra, Figures S1–S15). The spectral data of compounds **7**–**9** were consistent with previous reports [14,22]. Regarding the 4′-pyridinecarbonyl-substituted renieramycin–ecteinascidin hybrid derivatives (**11** and **12**), the characteristic chemical shift of the methylene moiety (–CH_2–) at the newly constructed 1,3-dioxole ring showed a proton signal as a pair of doublets at 5.95 ± 0.07 ppm and a carbon signal at 101.6 ± 0.3 ppm. Moreover, the C-7 and C-8 quaternary carbon signals of both compounds **11** and **12** shifted upfield, compared with the signals of the parent compound **4**. The carbonyl carbon signals of the resulting 4′-pyridinecarbonyl ester were confirmed at 167.0 and 164.2 ppm for **11** and **12**, respectively. Moreover, the chemical shifts of the carbonyl carbon at C-15 and C-18 for both **11** and **12** are located at 186.0 ± 0.2 ppm and 182.5 ± 0.1 ppm, respectively, indicating the presence of the quinone group on ring E.

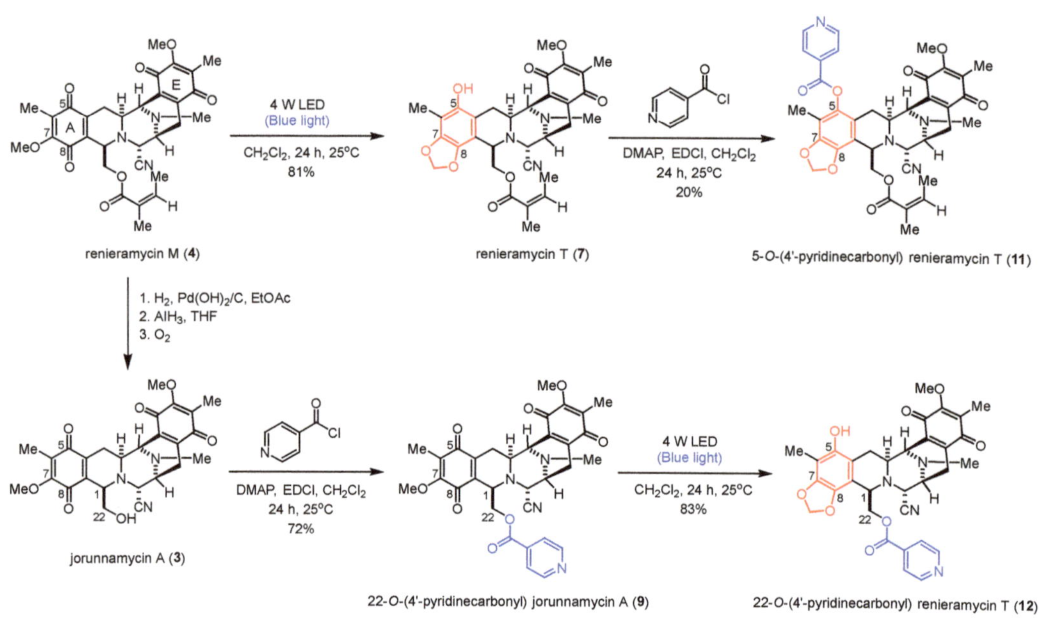

Scheme 3. Semisynthesis of the 4′-pyridinecarbonyl-substituted renieramycin-type derivatives.

The heteronuclear multiple bond correlations (HMBCs) between the methylene proton at the 1,3-dioxole ring and the quaternary aromatic carbons at C-7 and C-8 clearly confirmed the fused ring structure at ring A in compounds **11** and **12** (Figure 3). The key HMBCs of compound **11** included the correlations between the C-5 quaternary carbon and both the C-4 methylene protons and the C-6 methyl protons, along with those of the C-1′ pyridine carbon, all the protons at the C-2′ and C-3′ position of pyridine, and C-6 methyl motifs. Compound **12** exhibited significant HMBCs between the C-24 carbonyl carbon and both the C-22 methylene protons and the C-2′ pyridine proton.

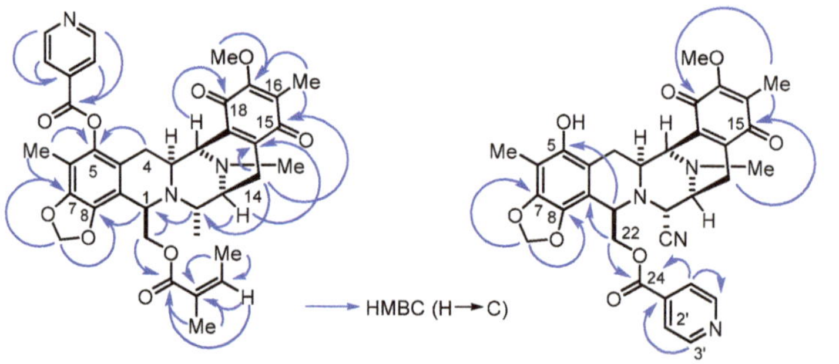

Figure 3. HMBCs (blue arrows) for the 4′-pyridinecarbonyl-substituted derivatives (**11** and **12**).

2.3. *Cytotoxicity of Compounds* **3–12** *against NSCLC Cell Lines*

The in vitro cytotoxic activities of the series of semisynthesized renieramycin-type derivatives and the natural renieramycins analogs were analyzed by MTT assay against the human H292 and H460 NSCLC cell lines (Table 2). The positive controls were cisplatin and doxorubicin, which were the first-line chemotherapeutic drugs. The results showed that compound **3**, which has a primary alcohol at the C-22 position, and renieramycins **5–8**, which possess unique structures (1,4-quinone or 1,3-dioxole-bridged phenol at ring A, methylene or secondary alcohol at C-14 of ring D, and 1,4-quinone or 1,4-hydroquinone at ring E), exhibited weak cytotoxicity against both H292 and H460 NSCLC cell lines at the IC_{50} values of 72.64–183.37 nM (Table 2, entries 1 and 3–6). However, compound **4** exhibited the strongest cytotoxicity among the series of natural renieramycins at the IC_{50} values of 35.36 and 33.86 nM against H292 and H460 cells, respectively (Table 2, entry 2). The semisynthesized renieramycin-type derivatives (**9**–**11**) exhibited substantially high cytotoxic activity at nanomolar concentrations against both cell lines (Table 2, entries 7–9). The known semisynthesized alkaloid (**9**), which possesses bis-tetrahydroisoquinolinequinone and 4′-pyridinecarbonyl moieties, exhibited the strongest cytotoxicity among all the renieramycin derivatives in this study. The compound **9** was approximately 10-fold and 9-fold more potent than the parent compound (**4**) against H292 and H460 NSCLC cell lines, respectively [22]. Both compound **10**, the known 8-hydroquinone, and compound **11**, the renieramycin–ecteinascidin hybrid derivative, contained the 5-*O*-(4′-pyridinecarbonyl) ester. They exhibited significant cytotoxicity, similar to those of **4** and docxorubicin, at the same IC_{50} level. Moreover, compound **11** was 3-fold and 2-fold more potent than **7**, the parent compound, against the H292 and H460 cell lines. Interestingly, compound **12**, a renieramycin-type derivative with a hydroxyl group at C-5, lost its cytotoxic activity and inhibited both the H292 and H460 cell lines at micromolar IC_{50} values (Table 2, entry 10). However, compound **12** exhibited 3-fold and 2-fold stronger potency than cisplatin against the H292 and H460 NSCLC cell lines, respectively. Therefore, the presence of the 4′-pyridinecarbonyl ester and the chemical structure of ring A constitute the essential pharmacophore controlling the cytotoxic potency [15,22,25]. The cytotoxicity of the renieramycin-type derivatives having a hydroxyl group at either the C-5 or C-22 position was weak.

Table 2. Cytotoxicity of the natural renieramycins and semisynthesized renieramycin derivatives against non-small-cell lung cancer cell lines.

Entry	Compound	5-*O*-Substituents	22-*O*-Substituents	$IC_{50} \pm$ S.D. (nM)	
				H292	H460
1	**3**	carbonyl	OH	97.85 ± 6.75	157.53 ± 6.65
2	**4**	carbonyl	angeloyl	35.36 ± 4.51	33.86 ± 2.16
3	**5**	carbonyl	angeloyl	170.03 ± 10.07	104.36 ± 22.02
4	**6**	carbonyl	angeloyl	111.74 ± 12.94	99.74 ± 0.13
5	**7**	OH	angeloyl	72.64 ± 2.55	83.32 ± 4.72
6	**8**	OH	angeloyl	183.37 ± 37.04	167.97 ± 3.53
7	**9**	carbonyl	4′-pyridinecarbonyl	3.52 ± 0.62	3.98 ± 0.38
8	**10**	4′-pyridinecarbonyl	angeloyl	33.79 ± 0.40	35.77 ± 2.11
9	**11**	4′-pyridinecarbonyl	angeloyl	35.27 ± 1.09	34.77 ± 2.19
10	**12**	OH	4′-pyridinecarbonyl	1.27 ± 0.20 μM	1.83 ± 0.83 μM
11	Cisplatin			4.23 ± 0.40 μM	3.86 ± 0.46 μM
12	Doxorubicin			37.54 ± 4.41	43.37 ± 5.60

2.4. *In Silico Prediction of the Target Genes and Molecular Pathways*

The series of the 4′-pyridinecarbonyl ester of the renieramycin-type derivatives (**10** and **11**) exhibited significant cytotoxicity against NSCLC cells. The anticancer mechanisms of compounds **10** and **11** were not investigated because of their limited quantity. Regarding data mining from several databases, pharmaco-mapping, and computational strategies, network pharmacology has recently emerged as a comprehensive tool for elucidating the putative biomolecular targets, signaling pathway complexities, and protein–protein interactions (PPIs) of potential leads [26,27]. Therefore, the inhibition mechanism and molecular pathways of both **10** and **11** against NSCLC were investigated by molecular docking and molecular dynamics studies, enabling the identification of the primary target genes.

2.4.1. Investigation of the Potential Targets against NSCLC

The Swiss Target Prediction online tool was employed to compare the renieramycin-type derivatives (**10** and **11**) to a massive internal pharmacophore model database to identify prospective drug targets using reverse pharmacophore alignment (Figure 4) [28]. One hundred and sixteen potential targets related to **10** and **11** were found. From the following four databases: GeneCards, Therapeutic Targets Database (TTD), Online Mendelian Inheritance in Man (OMIM), and DisGeNET, 6431 genes were found in association with NSCLC. Overlapping the corresponding genes using a Venn diagram, 94 prospective targets of **10** and **11** against NSCLC were generated (Figure 4C).

A

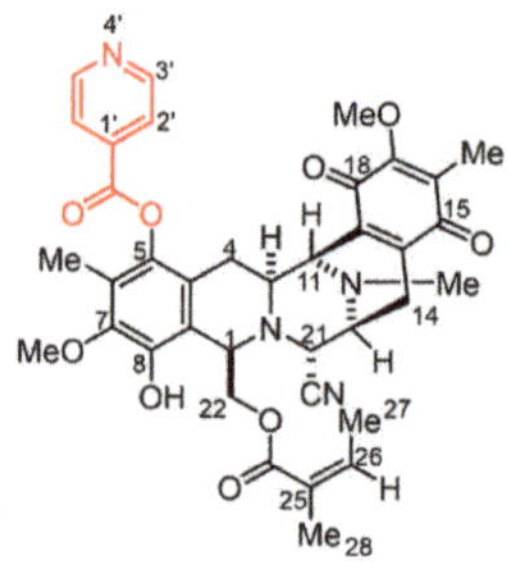

10

B

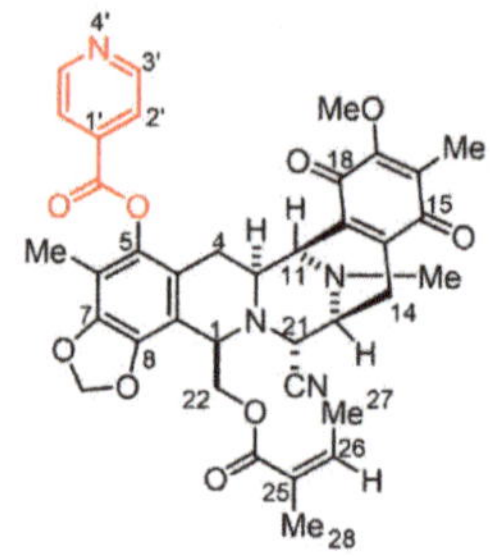

11

C

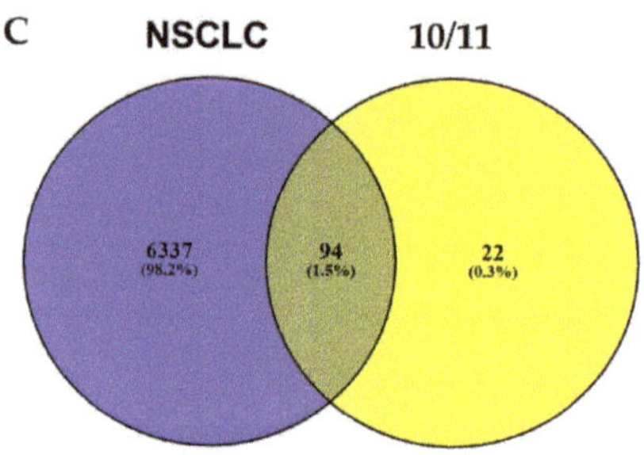

Figure 4. Structure and putative analysis of **10** and **11** against NSCLC. (**A**) Structure of **10**. (**B**) Structure of **11**. (**C**) Venn diagram analysis showing both **10** and **11** associated with 116 targets, whereas the NSCLC cells are associated with 6431 targets. The interception analysis showing 94 overlapping targets between **10**/**11** and NSCLC.

2.4.2. Protein–Protein Interaction Network Construction and Core Target Identification

To envision the relationship between the 94 prospective targets matched with **10** and **11** against NSCLC, a PPI network was retrieved and visualized using Cytoscape v3.9.1 after the resulting putative targets were loaded into the STRING platform (Figure 5A). The PPI network illustrates the interactions between the targets, with highly linked proteins in the network having a comparatively high number of interactions. CytoHubba, a plugin for Cytoscape, was employed to perform a topological analysis, which revealed the top 10 proteins linked to the number of degrees (Figure 5B). The colors from yellow to red represent small to large degrees. The results revealed several proteins, including signal transducer and activator of transcription 3 (STAT3), mitogen-activated protein kinase 1 (MAPK1), mitogen-activated protein kinase 3 (MAPK3), cyclin-dependent kinase 4 (CDK4), cyclin-dependent kinase 1 (CDK1), cyclin-dependent kinase 2 (CDK2), 90 kDa heat shock protein (HSP90AA1), phosphatidylinositol-4,5-bisphosphate 3-kinase catalytic subunit alpha (PIK3CA), cyclin D1 (CCND1), and cyclin E1 (CCNE1), as the 10 core hub proteins serving as potential therapeutic targets against NSCLC. Regarding the previous virtual study, gene ontology and KEGG pathway enrichment analyses depicted that MAPKs were potential targets of **9** toward the induction of NSCLC apoptosis [29]. Thus, we focused on MAPK1 and MAPK3 for further analysis due to the structural similarities between **9** and **11**, which are the 4′-pyridinecarbonyl esters of the tetrahydroisoquinolinequinone alkaloids.

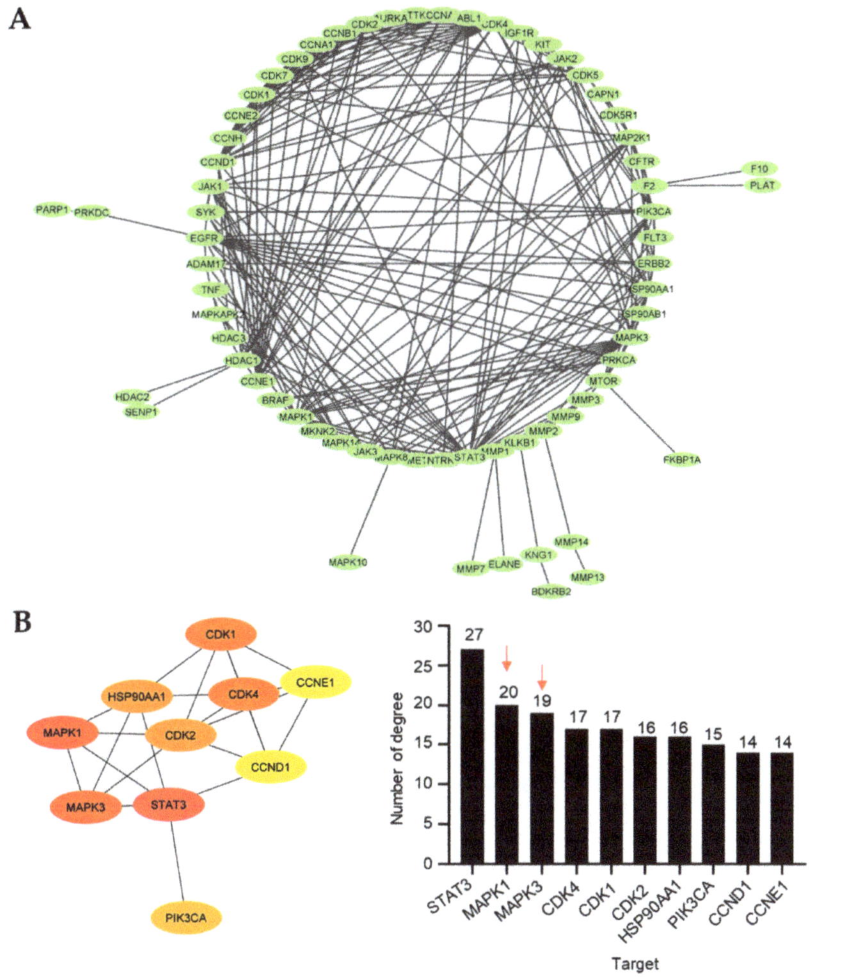

Figure 5. Protein–protein interaction (PPI). (**A**) The main cluster of the PPI obtained from the 94 overlapping targets and visualized using Cytoscape 3.9.1. (**B**) Top 10 targets based on the number of degrees visualized by the CytoHubba plugin. More than 10 degrees are displayed for all the main targets. The intensity of the colors represents the degree values, where red, orange, and yellow correspond to large, medium, and small values, respectively. Red arrow indicates the MAPK family.

2.4.3. Molecular Docking of MAPK1 and MAPK3

To explore the binding relationships between the MAPK1 and MAPK3 proteins, compounds **10** and **11** were docked in comparison with Ravoxertinib, a known inhibitor of both MAPK1 and MAPK3 (see Supporting Information, Figure S16). From the binding energy calculations, **11** exhibited the lowest binding energies of −9.8 kcal/mol and −9.9 kcal/mol, respectively, for MAPK1 and MAPK3, which was better than those of **10** and Ravoxertinib (Figure 6A). Furthermore, docking studies were conducted for the protonated forms of compounds **10** and **11**, specifically protonated at the nitrogen at position 12, as shown in the Supporting Information (Figure S17). Both the neutral and protonated forms of compounds **10** and **11** exhibited similar binding energy values. Docking with MAPK-1 revealed that both the neutral and protonated forms of compounds **10** and **11** predominantly displayed comparable binding interactions with amino acid residues. Interestingly, the protonated forms of compounds **10** and **11** exhibited hydrogen bonding interactions rather than hydrophobic interactions. Docking with MAPK-3 demonstrated that the protonated forms of compounds **10** and **11** could engage in additional interactions at the enzyme site. However, these additional interactions primarily resulted from hydrophobic interactions, which are generally weaker compared to hydrogen bonding interactions. Upon considering the binding interactions of amino acid residues at the enzyme active site, the neutral forms of compounds **10** and **11** exhibited a closer match with the known ligand, Ravoxertinib, compared to the protonated forms. Specifically, for MAPK-1, the neutral forms of compounds **10** and **11** demonstrated interactions with amino acid residues, including ASP111, ILE31, ILE103, and LEU156. For MAPK-3, the neutral forms of compounds 10 and 11 displayed interactions with LEU173 and VAL56. The number of interacting bonds involving hydrogen, hydrophobic interactions, and electrostatic interactions demonstrated the stability of both **10** and **11** in the binding pocket of both MAPK1 and MAPK3. However, compound **11** interacted with both MAPK1 and MAPK3 with stronger hydrogen binding than that of **10** (Figure 6B,C). Regarding the amino acid residues of MAPK1 that interacted with **11**, the key binding site of MAPK1 comprised ALA52, ASN154, ASP111, CYS166, GLU71, and ILE103. The interactions between **11** and MAPK3 at the specific amino acid residues involved ASN171, GLN122, ILE48, LEU173, LYS71, and TYR130. Interestingly, compounds **10** and **11**, along with compound **9**, had similar binding sites, which confirmed that MAPK1 and MAPK3 are the biomolecular targets. The docking conformations of **11** with MAPK1 and MAPK3 demonstrated stable ligand–receptor binding and increased interaction, thereby affirming the necessity of validating the interaction stability through molecular dynamics simulation.

2.4.4. Molecular Dynamics Analysis of MAPK1 and MAPK3 with **11**

To gain an in-depth understanding of the protein–ligand interaction of **11**, a molecular dynamics study was conducted on the core proteins of MAPK1 and MAPK3, utilizing the protein–ligand complexes obtained from the results of the molecular docking simulations. When the trajectory exhibits steep changes, it indicates that the system has undergone a significant transition, whereas a smooth trajectory signifies that the system has reached equilibrium. One crucial parameter in molecular dynamics simulations is the root mean square deviation (RMSD), which serves as a measure of the stability of the trajectory. In this simulation, the conformation and movement of the ligand were analyzed using the RMSD value. The RMSD (Å) values of the ligand conformations for MAPK1 and MAPK3 were found to be 2.38 ± 0.15 and 1.79 ± 0.19, respectively, as depicted in Figure 7A. The ligand conformation analysis revealed that both MAPK1 and MAPK3 maintained consistent proximity throughout the entire 15 ns duration of the experiment. However, when comparing the RMSD values, the interaction between **11** and MAPK3 exhibited greater stability in the ligand conformation, and both protein targets did not show significant differences in terms of their interactions. Additionally, the RMSD (Å) of the ligand movement between **11** and these targets was assessed. The results indicated that the average RMSD values for MAPK1 and MAPK3 were 5.68 ± 0.52 and 5.63 ± 2.04, respectively (Figure 7B). A relatively small RMSD of the ligand movement indicates good proximity between the ligand and the targets. The stability of the interaction between compound **11** and MAPK3 showed a greater tendency to fluctuate at 5, 7.5, and 13.2 ns compared to the interaction with MAPK1, particularly at 5 ns intervals.

A

Target	Binding energy (Kcal/mol)		
	Compounds		
	10	11	Ravoxertinib
MAPK1	−9.7	−9.8	−8.5
MAPK3	−9.6	−9.9	−9.2

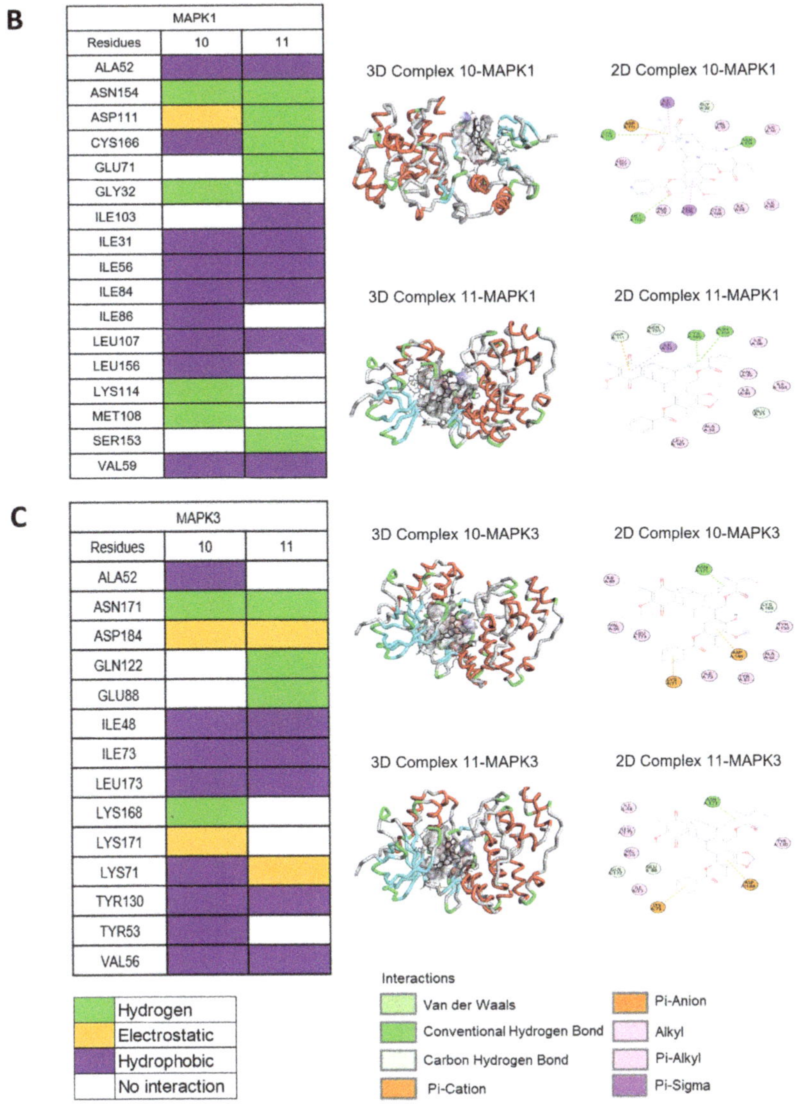

Figure 6. Molecular docking of **10** and **11** with both MAPK1 (ERK2) and MAPK3 (ERK1). (**A**) Binding energies indicate that the interactions of **10** and **11** with both MAPK1 and MAPK3, compared to Ravoxertinib, a known inhibitor. (**B**) Interactions between the amino acid residues of MAPK1 and both **10** and **11**. (**C**) Interactions between the amino acid residues of MAPK3 and both **10** and **11**.

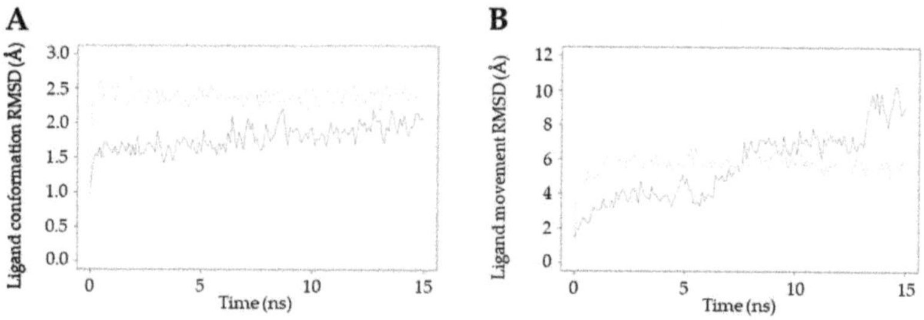

Figure 7. Molecular dynamics study of the interactions between **11** and MAPK1 and MAPK3. Green line shows the interaction with MAPK1, whereas the red line shows the interaction with MAPK3. (**A**) The ligand conformation and (**B**) ligand movement interaction of **11** with MAPK1 and MAPK3.

Considering all these findings, we hypothesized that **11** interacts with multiple targets in the MAPK family. Among these targets, MAPK1 demonstrated the highest potential and consistently engaged in strong interactions with **11**, aligning with our previous investigation. According to previous studies investigating the structure-cytotoxicity relationship, which employed both in vitro and in silico approaches, the mechanistic pathways underlying the anti-lung cancer effects of marine alkaloids from the tetrahydroisoquinolinequinone family have been elucidated. Specifically, compounds such as 5-*O*-(*N*-Boc-L-alanine)-renieramycin T, a renieramycin-ecteinascidin derivative [20], (1R,4R,5S)-10-(benzyloxy)-9-methoxy-8,11-dimethyl-3-(thiazol-5-ylmethyl)-1,2,3,4,5,6-hexahydro-1,5-epimi- nobenzo [d]azocine-4-carbonitrile (DH_25), a right-half C–E ring analog of renieramycins [30], and 22-*O*-(4′-pyridinecarbonyl) jorunnamycin A, a 4′-pyridinecarbonyl substituted renieramycin-type derivative [29], have demonstrated efficacy against non-small cell lung cancer (NSCLC) cells through modulation of the protein kinase B (Akt), myeloid cell leukemia-1 (MCL-1), and mitogen-activated protein kinase (MAPK) signaling pathways, leading to the induction of apoptosis. The proteins Akt, MCL-1, and MAPK are interconnected targets of cellular signaling networks involved in the regulation of apoptosis. While the MAPK pathway exerts pro-apoptotic effects, Akt signaling generally promotes cell survival. Furthermore, MCL-1, functioning as an anti-apoptotic protein, is influenced by both the MAPK and Akt pathways, thereby contributing to the delicate balance between cell survival and apoptosis in cancer cells [31,32]. Therefore, targeting these signaling pathways and their interactions holds promise for therapeutic interventions aimed at inducing apoptosis in cancer therapy.

3. Materials and Methods

3.1. General Experimental Procedures

All commercial reagents were purchased from Tokyo Chemical Industry, Tokyo, Japan. The glassware was dried in an oven (105 °C) before the experiment. Photochemical reactions were carried out using a commercially supplied LED (4W LED Filament GLS Blue, 220–240 V, EVE) and 18-W fluorescent light (100 V, HATAYA, Tokyo, Japan). All reactions were monitored by thin-layer chromatography (TLC) using aluminum silica gel 60 F254 (Merck, Darmstadt, Germany), and the TLC chromatogram was recorded under UV light at 254 and 365 nm. Flash column chromatographic purification was performed with silica gel (230–400 mesh) using a mixture of ethyl acetate and hexane as the mobile phase. Moreover, ^{1}H and ^{13}C NMR spectra were recorded on a Bruker ADVANCE NEO NMR spectrometer (Bruker, Massachusetts, MA, USA) at 400 and 100 MHz, respectively. Deuterated chloroform ($CDCl_3$) was used as the internal standard for the ^{13}C (77.0 ppm) and ^{1}H (7.27 ppm) spectroscopic analyses. Infrared spectra were measured using a Perkin Frontier Fourier-Transform Infrared Spectrometer (PerkinElmer, Massachusetts, MA, USA). High-resolution mass spectrometry was conducted using a microTOF Bruker Daltonics mass spectrometer. Optical rotations were measured with a JASCO P-2000 polarimeter using a 1-mL cell with a cell path length of 1 dm. The spectra of electronic circular dichroism were obtained using a JASCO J-815 CD spectrometer (JASCO, Maryland, MD, USA).

3.2. Extraction and Isolation

With assistance from the Aquatic Resources Research Institute, Chulalongkorn University and approval from the Department of Fisheries, Ministry of Agriculture and Cooperatives, Thailand (0510.2/8234, Date: 28 October 2019), a Thai blue sponge (*Xestospongia* sp.) was collected during a SCUBA diving mission at a depth of 3–5 m at Sichang Island, the Gulf of Thailand. The fresh blue sponge was mashed and subsequently pre-treated with 10% potassium cyanide solution in a phosphate-buffered solution at pH 7. Next, the suspension was macerated with methanol. The extraction process was repeated three times. The methanolic extracts were filtered, combined, and concentrated at reduced pressure. The condensed aqueous-methanolic extract was partitioned with hexane and ethyl acetate. The ethyl acetate extract was further concentrated and purified by silica gel column chromatography using hexane and ethyl acetate as the eluent. Natural renieramycins, including renieramycin M (**4**), renieramycin N (**5**) [11], and renieramycin O (**6**) [12], were obtained. Thereafter, compound **4** was transformed into Jorunnamycin A (**3**) under a three-step semisynthesis including hydrogenation, hydride reduction, and air oxidation [21,24].

3.3. Screening of the Photoredox Reaction Conditions with the Renieramycins

Natural renieramycins **4–6** were employed as the starting material for the light-induced intramolecular photoredox reaction. A solution of the renieramycin alkaloid (15 mg) with 20 mL of the selected solvent (CH_2Cl_2, $CHCl_3$, and THF) was stirred vigorously under a light source comprising white light (18 W fluorescent) and blue light (4 W LED) for 24 h at room temperature under a nitrogen atmosphere. The reaction was monitored by TLC using a solution of ethyl acetate and hexane (1:1 v/v) as the mobile phase. After the completion of the reaction, the solvent was evaporated under reduced pressure. The resultant crude product was purified by flash column chromatography using silica gel as the stationary phase and the mixed solvents of ethyl acetate and hexane as the mobile phase to afford the corresponding products, **7** and **8**.

3.4. Procedure for the Semisynthesis of Compound 11

Compound **4** (15 mg, 0.03 mmol) in dry CH_2Cl_2 (20 mL) was irradiated by a 4 W LED lamp (blue light) at room temperature under a nitrogen atmosphere for 24 h. The reaction was monitored by TLC using a hexane and ethyl acetate solution (1:1 v/v) as the mobile phase. After the completion of the reaction, the solvent was removed under reduced pressure. The crude product was precipitated using hexane, affording **7** as a yellow amorphous solid. Compound **7** was employed in the next step without further purification. Next, compound **7** (21 mg, 0.04 mmol), 4-dimethylaminopyridine (DMAP) (5 mg, 0.04 mmol), 1-(3-dimethylaminopropyl)-3-ethylcarbodiimide hydrochloride (EDCI) (8 mg, 0.04 mmol), and isonicotinoyl chloride hydrochloride (32 mg, 0.18 mmol) were dissolved in CH_2Cl_2 (20 mL). The mixture was stirred for 24 h at room temperature under a nitrogen atmosphere. After the completion of the reaction, as determined by TLC, the reaction mixture was quenched by adding distilled H_2O (20 mL) and extracted with CH_2Cl_2 (20 mL, three times). The organic layers were combined and dried over anhydrous magnesium sulfate ($MgSO_4$), filtered, and concentrated under reduced pressure. After purification by silica gel flash chromatography using the hexane and ethyl acetate solution as the eluent, 5-*O*-(4′-pyridinecarbonyl) renieramycin T (**11**) was obtained in 20% yield as a yellow amorphous powder.

3.5. Procedure for the Semisynthesis of Compound 12

Jorunnamycin A (**3**) (25 mg, 0.05 mmol) was placed into an oven-dried, round-bottomed flask and dissolved in dry CH_2Cl_2 (10 mL). Thereafter, DMAP (31 mg, 0.25 mmol), EDCI (49 mg, 0.25 mmol), and isonicotinoyl chloride hydrochloride (45 mg, 0.25 mmol) were added. The mixture was stirred for 24 h at room temperature under a nitrogen atmosphere and monitored by TLC using a mixture solvent of ethyl acetate and hexane (1:1 *v*/*v*) as the mobile phase. After completion, the solution was concentrated under reduced pressure. Next, the resultant crude product was purified by flash column chromatography using silica gel as the stationary phase and the mixed solvent of ethyl acetate and hexane as the mobile phase to yield a yellow product (**9**) in 72% yield. Subsequently, compound **9** (6 mg, 0.01 mmol) was dissolved in CH_2Cl_2 (15 mL) and irradiated by a 4 W LED lamp (blue light) at room temperature under a nitrogen atmosphere for 24 h. The reaction mixture was monitored by TLC and further purified following the procedure described above to obtain 22-*O*-(4′-pyridinecarbonyl) renieramycin T (**12**) as an amorphous yellow powder in 83% yield.

3.6. Cytotoxic Evaluations against NSCLC Cell Lines

The in vitro cytotoxicity of compounds **3**–**12** against H292 and H460 NSCLC cell lines was determined by MTT colorimetric assay. The H292 and H460 cultured cell lines were obtained from the American Type Culture Collection (Manassas, VA, USA). The Roswell Park Memorial Institute (RPMI) medium 1640, fetal bovine serum (FBS), L-glutamine, a penicillin/streptomycin solution, and Albumax I were purchased from Gibco (Gaithersburg, MA, USA). Dimethyl sulfoxide (DMSO) was acquired from Merck Millipore (Billerica, MA, USA) or Sigma-Aldrich. All cell lines were cultured in the RPMI 1640 medium, supplemented with 10% FBS, 2 mM L-glutamine, and 100 units/mL of penicillin/streptomycin, and the temperature was maintained at 37 °C under 5% CO_2. Cells were trypsinized and seeded at a density of 5000 cells/well with the RPMI media for 24 h in a 96-well plate. A 10 mm stock solution of each test compound in DMSO was prepared and diluted into the serial concentrations at 1–250 nM, with a DMSO concentration of less than 0.2% *v*/*v*. The cells were treated with various concentrations of each derivative for 72 h. Next, the cells were incubated with 0.5 mg/mL of MTT for 2 h. After solubilizing the resulting formazan salt with 100 µL of DMSO, the absorbance of the formed formazan was measured by a spectrophotometric microtiter plate reader (Perkin Elmer Victor 3 1420 Multilabel Plate Counter, Massachusetts, MA, USA) at 570 nm. The experiment was performed in three replicate wells with at least five concentrations of the tested compounds. The cell viability was determined using the GraphPad Prism software (version 5), calculated as a percentage of non-treated control cells and the mean of the half-maximal inhibitory concentration (IC_{50}) values. Cisplatin and doxorubicin were used as the positive controls, and 0.2% DMSO was used as the negative control.

3.7. Network Pharmacology Study

3.7.1. Database Mining and Identification of **10**, **11**, and NSCLC-Related Targets

The Swiss Target Prediction database (http://www.swisstargetprediction.ch), which was accessed on 14 January 2023, was utilized to gather information on the probable targets of **10** and **11**. To identify potential targets associated with NSCLC cells, various human genetic databases, such as GeneCards, TTD, OMIM, and DisGeNET, were screened. A Venn diagram illustrating the overlapping targets between **10** and **11** with respect to NSCLC can be viewed at this link (https://bioinfogp.cnb.csic.es/tools/venny/, accessed on 15 March 2023). The Venn diagram was generated using Venny 2.1.0 (Centro Nacional de Biotecnología, Madrid, Spain), https://bioinfogp.cnb.csic.es/tools/venny/, accessed on 15 March 2020.

3.7.2. Construction of Protein–Protein Interaction Network and Identification of Potential Core Targets

The overlapping targets derived from the Venn diagram were inputted into the STRING database. For STRING analysis, the organism parameter was set to Homo sapiens with the highest confidence level of 0.900. The obtained results were gathered and imported into Cytoscape v3.9.1 (The Cytoscape Consortium, San Diego, CA, USA) for visualization and further analysis. To examine the top 10 core targets, the CytoHubba plugin was employed, using the number of degrees as the primary parameter.

3.8. Molecular Docking Study

The ligand structures (**10**, **11**, and Ravoxertinib) were prepared using ChemDraw Ultra 15.0 (Perkin Elmer, MA, USA). The protonation state of **10** and **11** were prepared using Open Babel GUI and Command Prompt with pH 7.4. To predict the potential binding interactions between the compounds and the core targets, an in silico assay was conducted using PyRx Virtual Screening Tools v0.8. The X-ray crystal structures of the proteins were obtained from the Protein Data Bank (https://www.rcsb.org/, accessed on 16 March 2023), e.g., 6GES for MAPK3 (ERK1) and 1WZY for MAPK1 (ERK2). Prior to the analysis, the proteins were prepared by removing water molecules and any other ligands attached to the main protein using Pymol v2.5 (https://pymol.org/2/, accessed on 16 March 2023). The free binding energies (ΔG), interaction types, and amino acid residues were calculated and analyzed using BIOVIA Discovery Studio Visualizer 2022 (Biovia, CA, USA).

3.9. Molecular Dynamics Study

The stability of the interactions between ligand **11** and the proteins was assessed using Yasara Dynamic, following the previously described methodology [29]. In summary, the optimal binding between ligand **11** and the proteins was selected for further analysis, incorporating the AMBER14 force field with standard parameters. The simulation was conducted at a temperature of 298 K and a pH of 7.4 for 15 ns. Two RMSD parameters were employed: RMSD ligand conformation and RMSD ligand movement. The evaluation utilized the default scripts: md_run.mcr and md_analyse.mcr. The RMSD plots were generated using the Rstudio program (https://posit.co/products/open-source/rstudio/, accessed on 17 March 2023).

4. Conclusions

Here, 4′-pyridinecarbonyl-substituted renieramycin-type derivatives were prepared from compound **4** using light-induced intramolecular photoredox reactions and Steglich esterification. The optimal conditions for the photoredox reaction were achieved by employing 4 W blue light and dichloromethane. The natural renieramycins (**4**–**6**) were successfully transformed into their corresponding derivatives (**7** and **8**, which contained a 1,3-dioxole-bridged phenolic moiety on ring A) in excellent–moderate yields (yields: 81%–37%). The attachment of the 4′-pyridinecarbonyl ester at the C-5 and C-22 positions was accomplished smoothly. Cytotoxicity study revealed that compounds **4** and **9** exhibited the most potent cytotoxicity against the human H292 and H460 NSCLC cell lines among the natural renieramycins and semisynthesized renieramycin-type derivatives, respectively. Interestingly, compound **11**, which contained both the 4′-pyridinecarbonyl ester at C-5 and the 1,3-dioxole-bridged phenolic motifs on ring A, showed better cytotoxicity than its parent compound (**7**). In addition, the renieramycin-type derivatives with a hydroxyl group at C-5 and C-22 lost their cytotoxicity against the NSCLC cells. Thus, the conformation of ring A featuring the 4′-pyridinecarbonyl ester at C-5 is crucial for the cytotoxic activity of renieramycins. Due to the limited quantity of the compound, a virtual network pharmacology study was conducted to simulate the target genes and molecular pathways. Molecular docking and dynamics studies predicted that the target proteins of compound **11** were MAPK1 and MAPK3. In future studies, the renieramycin-type derivatives will be further explored for their potential as anti-lung cancer agents.

Supplementary Materials: The following supporting information can be downloaded at: https://www.mdpi.com/article/10.3390/md21070400/s1, Figures S1–S15: ^{1}H NMR, ^{13}C NMR and 2D NMR spectra of compounds **7**–**9** and **11**–**12**, Figures S16 and S17: Molecular docking of Ravoxertinib and the protonated **10** and **11** with both MAPK1 (ERK2) and MAPK3 (ERK1), Tables S1 and S2: Theoretical level of minimization of the 3D structures of **10** and **11**.

Author Contributions: Conceptualization, S.C.; methodology, S.S., K.B., K.P., B.I., K.S., M.Y., N.S., P.C. and S.C.; software, V.P., I.I. and S.C.; validation, K.S., M.Y., N.S. and S.C.; formal analysis, S.S., K.B., I.I., K.P., B.I., C.C. and S.C.; investigation, S.S., K.B., I.I., K.P., B.I. and S.C.; resources, P.C. and S.C.; data curation, S.C.; writing—original draft preparation, S.S., I.I. and K.B.; writing—review and editing, S.C.; visualization, S.C.; supervision, S.C.; project administration, S.C.; funding acquisition, S.C. All authors have read and agreed to the published version of the manuscript.

Funding: This research was funded by the Thai Research Fund, Thailand (RSA 6280009) to S.C.

Data Availability Statement: The data described and analyzed in this study are available from the corresponding author upon reasonable request.

Acknowledgments: This research is supported by the 90th anniversary of Chulalongkorn university fund No. GCUGR1125661018M (Ratchadaphiseksomphot Endowment Fund) for S.S. and the Second Century Fund (C2F), Chulalongkorn University for postdoctoral research fellowship to K.B. We gratefully acknowledge the Natural Products and Nanoparticles Research Unit (NP2) and the Department of Pharmacognosy and Pharmaceutical Botany and the Department of Pharmacology and Physiology, Faculty of Pharmaceutical Sciences, Chulalongkorn University for their scientific support.

Conflicts of Interest: The authors declare no conflict of interest.

References

1. Fang, Y.; Li, H.; Ji, B.; Cheng, K.; Wu, B.; Li, Z.; Zheng, C.; Hua, H.; Li, D. Renieramycin-type alkaloids from marine-derived organisms: Synthetic chemistry, biological activity and structural modification. *Eur. J. Med. Chem.* **2021**, *210*, 113092. [CrossRef] [PubMed]
2. Saito, N. Chemical Research on Antitumor Isoquinoline Marine Natural Products and Related Compounds. *Chem. Pharm. Bull.* **2021**, *69*, 155–177. [CrossRef] [PubMed]
3. D'Incalci, M.; Galmarini, C.M. A Review of Trabectedin (ET-743): A Unique Mechanism of Action. *Mol. Cancer Ther.* **2010**, *9*, 2157–2163. [CrossRef] [PubMed]
4. Gordon, E.M.; Sankhala, K.K.; Chawla, N.; Chawla, S.P. Trabectedin for Soft Tissue Sarcoma: Current Status and Future Perspectives. *Adv. Ther.* **2016**, *33*, 1055–1071. [CrossRef]
5. Cesne, A.L.; Martín-Broto, J.; Grignani, G. A review of the efficacy of trabectedin as second-line treatment of advanced soft tissue sarcoma. *Future Oncol.* **2022**, *18*, 5–11. [CrossRef]
6. Patel, S.; Petty, W.J.; Sands, J.M. An overview of lurbinectedin as a new second-line treatment option for small cell lung cancer. *Ther. Adv. Med. Oncol.* **2021**, *13*, 17588359211020529. [CrossRef]
7. Manzo, A.; Sforza, V.; Carillio, G.; Palumbo, G.; Montanino, A.; Sandomenico, C.; Costanzo, R.; Esposito, G.; Laudato, F.; Mercadante, E.; et al. Lurbinectedin in small cell lung cancer. *Front. Oncol.* **2022**, *12*, 932105. [CrossRef]
8. Frincke, J.M.; Faulkner, D.J. Antimicrobial metabolites of the sponge *Reniera* sp. *J. Am. Chem. Soc.* **1982**, *104*, 265–269. [CrossRef]
9. He, H.Y.; Faulkner, D.J. Renieramycins E and F from the sponge *Reniera* sp.: Reassignment of the stereochemistry of the renieramycins. *J. Org. Chem.* **1989**, *54*, 5822–5824. [CrossRef]
10. Pettit, G.R.; Knight, J.C.; Collins, J.C.; Herald, D.L.; Pettit, R.K.; Boyd, M.R.; Young, V.G. Antineoplastic Agents 430. Isolation and Structure of Cribrostatins 3, 4, and 5 from the Republic of Maldives *Cribrochalina* Species. *J. Nat. Prod.* **2000**, *63*, 793–798. [CrossRef]
11. Suwanborirux, K.; Amnuoypol, S.; Plubrukarn, A.; Pummangura, S.; Kubo, A.; Tanaka, C.; Saito, N. Chemistry of Renieramycins. Part 3. Isolation and Structure of Stabilized Renieramycin Type Derivatives Possessing Antitumor Activity from Thai Sponge *Xestospongia* Species, Pretreated with Potassium Cyanide. *J. Nat. Prod.* **2003**, *66*, 1441–1446. [CrossRef]
12. Amnuoypol, S.; Suwanborirux, K.; Pummangura, S.; Kubo, A.; Tanaka, C.; Saito, N. Chemistry of Renieramycins. Part 5. Structure Elucidation of Renieramycin-Type Derivatives O, Q, R, and S from Thai Marine Sponge *Xestospongia* Species Pretreated with Potassium Cyanide. *J. Nat. Prod.* **2004**, *67*, 1023–1028. [CrossRef]
13. Nakao, Y.; Shiroiwa, T.; Murayama, S.; Matsunaga, S.; Goto, Y.; Matsumoto, Y.; Fusetani, N. Identification of Renieramycin A as an Antileishmanial Substance in a Marine Sponge *Neopetrosia* sp. *Mar. Drugs* **2004**, *2*, 55–62. [CrossRef]
14. Daikuhara, N.; Tada, Y.; Yamaki, S.; Charupant, K.; Amnuoypol, S.; Suwanborirux, K.; Saito, N. Chemistry of renieramycins. Part 7: Renieramycins T and U, novel renieramycin–ecteinascidin hybrid marine natural products from Thai sponge Xestospongia sp. *Tetrahedron Lett.* **2009**, *50*, 4276–4278. [CrossRef]
15. Chamni, S.; Sirimangkalakitti, N.; Chanvorachote, P.; Saito, N.; Suwanborirux, K. Chemistry of Renieramycins. 17. A New Generation of Renieramycins: Hydroquinone 5-*O*-Monoester Analogues of Renieramycin M as Potential Cytotoxic Agents against Non-Small-Cell Lung Cancer Cells. *J. Nat. Prod.* **2017**, *80*, 1541–1547. [CrossRef] [PubMed]
16. Petsri, K.; Chamni, S.; Suwanborirux, K.; Saito, N.; Chanvorachote, P. Renieramycin T Induces Lung Cancer Cell Apoptosis by Targeting Mcl-1 Degradation: A New Insight in the Mechanism of Action. *Mar. Drugs* **2019**, *17*, 301. [CrossRef] [PubMed]

17. Petsri, K.; Yokoya, M.; Tungsukruthai, S.; Rungrotmongkol, T.; Nutho, B.; Vinayanuwattikun, C.; Saito, N.; Matsubara, T.; Sato, R.; Chanvorachote, P. Structure–Activity Relationships and Molecular Docking Analysis of Mcl-1 Targeting Renieramycin T Analogues in Patient-derived Lung Cancer Cells. *Cancers* **2020**, *12*, 875. [CrossRef] [PubMed]
18. Yu, B.; Liang, J.; Li, X.; Liu, L.; Yao, J.; Chen, X.; Chen, R. Renieramycin T Inhibits Melanoma B16F10 Cell Metastasis and Invasion via Regulating Nrf2 and STAT3 Signaling Pathways. *Molecules* **2022**, *27*, 5337. [CrossRef]
19. Chantarawong, W.; Chamni, S.; Suwanborirux, K.; Saito, N.; Chanvorachote, P. 5-*O*-Acetyl-Renieramycin T from Blue Sponge *Xestospongia* sp. Induces Lung Cancer Stem Cell Apoptosis. *Mar. Drugs* **2019**, *17*, 109. [CrossRef]
20. Suksamai, D.; Racha, S.; Sriratanasak, N.; Chaotham, C.; Aphicho, K.; Lin, A.C.K.; Chansriniyom, C.; Suwanborirux, K.; Chamni, S.; Chanvorachote, P. 5-*O*-(*N*-Boc-l-Alanine)-Renieramycin T Induces Cancer Stem Cell Apoptosis via Targeting Akt Signaling. *Mar. Drugs* **2022**, *20*, 235. [CrossRef]
21. Charupant, K.; Daikuhara, N.; Saito, E.; Amnuoypol, S.; Suwanborirux, K.; Owa, T.; Saito, N. Chemistry of renieramycins. Part 8: Synthesis and cytotoxicity evaluation of renieramycin M–jorunnamycin A analogues. *Bioorg. Med. Chem.* **2009**, *17*, 4548–4558. [CrossRef] [PubMed]
22. Sirimangkalakitti, N.; Chamni, S.; Charupant, K.; Chanvorachote, P.; Mori, N.; Saito, N.; Suwanborirux, K. Chemistry of Renieramycins. 15. Synthesis of 22-*O*-Ester Derivatives of Jorunnamycin A and Their Cytotoxicity against Non-Small-Cell Lung Cancer Cells. *J. Nat. Prod.* **2016**, *79*, 2089–2093. [CrossRef]
23. Yokoya, M.; Yamazaki-Nakai, M.; Nakai, K.; Sirimangkalakitti, N.; Chamni, S.; Suwanborirux, K.; Saito, N. Transformation of Renieramycin M into Renieramycins T and S by Intramolecular Photoredox Reaction of 7-Methoxy-6-methyl-1,2,3,4-tetrahydroisoquinoline-5,8-dione Derivatives. *J. Nat. Prod.* **2023**, *86*, 222–231. [CrossRef]
24. Saito, N.; Tanaka, C.; Koizumi, Y.-I.; Suwanborirux, K.; Amnuoypol, S.; Pummangura, S.; Kubo, A. Chemistry of renieramycins. Part 6: Transformation of renieramycin M into jorumycin and renieramycin J including oxidative degradation products, mimosamycin, renierone, and renierol acetate. *Tetrahedron* **2004**, *60*, 3873–3881. [CrossRef]
25. Chamni, S.; Sirimangkalakitti, N.; Chanvorachote, P.; Suwanborirux, K.; Saito, N. Chemistry of Renieramycins. Part 19: Semi-Syntheses of 22-*O*-Amino Ester and Hydroquinone 5-*O*-Amino Ester Derivatives of Renieramycin M and Their Cytotoxicity against Non-Small-Cell Lung Cancer Cell Lines. *Mar. Drugs* **2020**, *18*, 418. [CrossRef] [PubMed]
26. Xi, P.; Niu, Y.; Zhang, Y.; Li, W.; Gao, F.; Gu, W.; Kui, F.; Liu, Z.; Lu, L.; Du, G. The mechanism of dioscin preventing lung cancer based on network pharmacology and experimental validation. *J. Ethnopharmacol.* **2022**, *292*, 115138. [CrossRef]
27. Iksen, I.; Witayateeraporn, W.; Wirojwongchai, T.; Suraphan, C.; Pornputtapong, N.; Singharajkomron, N.; Nguyen, H.M.; Pongrakhananon, V. Identifying molecular targets of Aspiletrein-derived steroidal saponins in lung cancer using network pharmacology and molecular docking-based assessments. *Sci. Rep.* **2023**, *13*, 1545. [CrossRef]
28. Gfeller, D.; Grosdidier, A.; Wirth, M.; Daina, A.; Michielin, O.; Zoete, V. SwissTargetPrediction: A web server for target prediction of bioactive small molecules. *Nucleic Acids Res.* **2014**, *42*, W32–W38. [CrossRef] [PubMed]
29. Iksen, I.; Sinsook, S.; Wattanathamsan, O.; Buaban, K.; Chamni, S.; Pongrakhananon, V. Target Identification of 22-(4-Pyridinecarbonyl) Jorunnamycin A, a Tetrahydroisoquinoline Derivative from the Sponge *Xestospongia* sp., in Mediating Non-Small-Cell Lung Cancer Cell Apoptosis. *Molecules* **2022**, *27*, 8948. [CrossRef]
30. Petsri, K.; Yokoya, M.; Racha, S.; Thongsom, S.; Thepthanee, C.; Innets, B.; Ei, Z.Z.; Hotta, D.; Zou, H.; Chanvorachote, P. Novel Synthetic Derivative of Renieramycin T Right-Half Analog Induces Apoptosis and Inhibits Cancer Stem Cells via Targeting the Akt Signal in Lung Cancer Cells. *Int. J. Mol. Sci.* **2023**, *24*, 5345. [CrossRef]
31. Kitazumi, I.; Tsukahara, M. Regulation of DNA fragmentation: The role of caspases and phosphorylation. *FEBS J.* **2011**, *278*, 427–441. [CrossRef] [PubMed]
32. Pithi, C.; Supakarn, C.; Chuanpit, N.; Preeyaporn Plaimee, P. Potential Anti-metastasis Natural Compounds for Lung Cancer. *Anticancer Res.* **2016**, *36*, 5707.

Scientia Pharmaceutica

ÖSTERREICHISCHE PHARMAZEUTISCHE GESELLSCHAFT MDPI

Article

Immuno-Modulatory Effects of Korean Mistletoe in MDA-MB-231 Breast Cancer Cells and THP-1 Macrophages

Wan-Taek Lim †, Chang-Eui Hong † and Su-Yun Lyu *

Department of Pharmacy, College of Pharmacy, Sunchon National University, Suncheon 57922, Republic of Korea; top951324@naver.com (W.-T.L.); gruni80@naver.com (C.-E.H.)

* Correspondence: suyun96@yahoo.com; Tel.: +82-61-750-3750

† These authors contributed equally to this work.

Abstract: Korean mistletoe (*Viscum album* var. *coloratum*) has been traditionally used as a remedy for cancer, diabetes, and hypertension. This study investigated the immuno-modulatory effects of Korean mistletoe water extract, specifically on MDA-MB-231 cells, a highly metastatic breast cancer cell line, when co-cultured with THP-1 human macrophage cells. When compared to MDA-MB-231 cells cultured alone, the co-culture of MDA-MB-231/THP-1 cells treated with mistletoe extract showed a significant reduction in IL-6 secretion. Additionally, these co-cultures exhibited elevated levels of IL-4, TGF-β, and IFN-y. These results suggest that water extracts from mistletoe have the potential to induce mitochondria-targeted apoptosis in MDA-MB 231 cells stimulated by THP macrophages. Regarding apoptosis, in MDA-MB-231 cells co-cultured with THP-1 macrophages, mistletoe water extract treatment triggered a significant increase in Bax/Bcl-2 ratio, caspase-3 activation, and PARP inactivation. In addition, there was a significant increase in E-cadherin and a decrease in N-cadherin. Treatment of Korean mistletoe also led to significant reductions in both MMP-2 and -9. Furthermore, inhibition of cell migration in MDA-MB-231/THP-1 co-cultured cells was observed. In summary, this study highlights the potential of Korean mistletoe as a prospective drug for the treatment of triple-negative breast cancer, particularly through its ability to regulate human immunity.

Keywords: MDA-MD-231; breast cancer; THP-1; macrophage; mistletoe

Citation: Lim, W.-T.; Hong, C.-E.; Lyu, S.-Y. Immuno-Modulatory Effects of Korean Mistletoe in MDA-MB-231 Breast Cancer Cells and THP-1 Macrophages. *Sci. Pharm.* **2023**, *91*, 48. https://doi.org/10.3390/scipharm91040048

Academic Editor: Barbara De Filippis

Received: 30 August 2023
Revised: 23 September 2023
Accepted: 4 October 2023
Published: 18 October 2023

1. Introduction

European mistletoe (Loranthaceae) grows parasitically on trees, including oaks and apples, across Europe and Asia [1]. This semi-parasite has been used for generations as a medicinal plant in Germany and Switzerland to treat hypertension, arterial sclerosis, and cancer [2,3]. Several studies are proving its pharmacological effects. Various active components isolated from mistletoe have been demonstrated to possess anti-cancer effects in extensive detail [4,5]. The active ingredients responsible for these effects are lectin (a glycoprotein), viscotoxin (a protein component), and oleanolic acid (a triterpenoid). Scientific evidence suggests that these components not only possess anti-cancer properties but also play a vital role in enhancing the immune system's activity [2,6–9]. For example, among the pharmacological components of mistletoe, polysaccharides, oligosaccharides, amines, and alkaloids have a lesser direct killing effect on cancer cells than lectin, but they can activate macrophages to induce cell-mediated immunity [10]. In particular, a variant of European mistletoe, Korean mistletoe (*Viscum album* L. var. *coloratum*), has been reported to have superior immune cell stimulation activity compared to European mistletoe [11]. Korean mistletoe is a domestically native plant distinct from European mistletoe, and it has been used as a medicine for back pain, high blood pressure, and toothache in private and oriental medicine [12,13]. Recently, researchers have actively investigated the anti-cancer activity of Korean mistletoe extract. Most studies on chemotherapy with mistletoe use mistletoe water extract [14]. The anti-cancer activity of mistletoe extract is produced not only by the direct cytotoxic effects of its constituents but also by inducing tumor-specific cell-mediated immune enhancement. This occurs due to the activation of immune cells (such as macrophages) against tumor cells [15].

Clinically diverse phenotypes characterize breast cancer, with different subtypes classified into progesterone receptor (PR), estrogen receptor (ER), and human epithelial growth factor receptor 2 (HER2) based on immunohistochemical staining expression [16]. Triple-negative breast cancer, a subtype in which PR, ER, and HER2 are not expressed, represents 10–20% of all breast cancer patients [17–19]. Therapeutic effects are noticeably lower in triple-negative breast cancers compared to other hormone receptors or treatments targeting HER2-positive subtypes. Consequently, treatment for triple-negative breast cancer still relies heavily on non-specific measures such as surgery, radiation therapy, and chemotherapy, despite their associated side effects [19,20]. Furthermore, triple-negative breast cancer aggressively metastasizes to major organs such as the bone, liver, lung, and brain throughout the course of the tumor. Doctors identify metastasis as a significant obstacle in effectively treating triple-negative breast cancer, which consequently results in a clinically poor prognosis [21–26].

Breast cancer encompasses an intricate microenvironment within the tumor, involving blood vessels, immune cells, fibroblasts, cytokines, and extracellular matrices. These components interact with each other, playing significant roles at every stage of metastasis [27]. Macrophages, integral to innate immunity, function differently within the tumor microenvironment compared to general macrophages. Specifically, in breast cancer microenvironments, they transform into tumor-associated macrophages (TAMs) upon activation [28]. TAMs constitute around 50% of the total cell population in this microenvironment, making them the most abundant component. They secrete stimulatory or inhibitory signaling molecules that manipulate growth during solid tumor progression [29–31].

The human immune response and inflammation lead to the secretion of inflammatory mediators from cells to protect against external stimuli like infections or tissue damage. However, this process can also promote chronic cancer cell death by inhibiting inflammatory mediators like interleukin (IL)-4, IL-6, interferon (IFN)-γ, and transforming growth factor (TGF)-β [13,32]. Tumor cells secrete matrix metalloproteases (MMPs) and proteolytic enzymes, along with inflammatory cytokines, that degrade the extracellular matrix forming the cellular scaffold and modulate the intra-tumoral environment [33,34].

Moreover, an inflamed microenvironment leads to the persistent activation of signal transducer and transcription (STAT) proteins within cells, triggering further inflammation along with metastasis and neovascular synthesis in cancerous cells, exacerbating the tumor [35]. Under normal conditions, STAT proteins play crucial roles in cell development, differentiation, and survival. However, excessive activation of these same proteins often underlies cancer development. An illustrative case of this phenomenon is the active pathway of STAT3, extensively studied due to its overexpression across various cancer cell types [36]. In an inflammatory microenvironment, tumor cells interact with IL-6 via IL-6 receptors, leading to their conversion into phospho-STAT3 (p-STAT3), an activated form [37]. P-STAT3 infiltrates the nucleus of tumor cells, upregulating metastasis and neovascularization-related genes [38]. While advancements in early diagnosis technology and anti-cancer drugs have led to a decrease in cancer mortality rates [39], cancer cell metastasis remains the primary cause of death in cancer patients [40]. Thus, the development of anti-cancer drugs inhibiting STAT3 activation is anticipated to offer therapeutic benefits by curbing cancer cell metastasis and new blood vessel synthesis.

In addition, the activation of Bcl-2 family proteins such as Bax and Bcl-2 triggers the direct apoptosis of tumor cells [41]. These activated Bax protein oligomers bind to the mitochondrial outer membrane, inducing mitochondrial outer membrane permeabilization (MOMP) [42,43]. This process allows apoptosome leakage from the mitochondria, subsequently activating cysteine-aspartic proteases (caspases) [44]. Among these, caspase-3 acts as an effector caspase, inducing apoptosis by deactivating poly ADP-ribose polymerase (PARP) in the nucleus of tumor cells, thereby hindering DNA repair [45]. Apoptosis is genetically regulated by infection and DNA damage, setting it apart from necrosis. In the study of anti-cancer drugs, inducing apoptosis is crucial; unlike necrosis, it avoids triggering additional inflammatory reactions. Consequently, only tumor cells are selectively eliminated without causing harm to normal tissues [46].

Furthermore, cancer cell metastasis is a sequential process, progressing from primary tumors to the development of new tumors in distant organs. Epithelial–mesenchymal transition (EMT) is a theory closely associated with the early stages of this metastasis process [47]. The initiation phase occurs when MMP-2 and MMP-9 are secreted by the primary tumor, enabling the infiltration of local tissues and blood vessels [48]. Consequently, these infiltrated cancer cells gradually undergo a phenotypic change from epithelial to mesenchymal cells, characterized by a decrease in the expression of the cell adhesion molecule E-cadherin and an increase in the expression of N-cadherin, which weakens cell adhesion [49,50]. EMT transforms solid tumor cells into mesenchymal cells, endowing these newly transformed cells with enhanced mobility. This mobility allows detached cancerous epithelial cells to enter circulatory systems like blood vessels and metastasize to other organs. A notable feature of EMT is the conversion of cadherins, in particular an increase in N-cadherin accompanied by a loss of E-cadherin [51].

Recent studies have actively pursued immuno-cancer research, with a focus on investigating anti-cancer activity by meticulously examining and enhancing tumor microenvironments. However, no research has reported on how mistletoe water extract activates macrophages to improve the tumor microenvironment. Therefore, in this experiment, we aimed to explore the potential of Korean mistletoe extract as an immune enhancer. We sought to compare and investigate whether activated macrophages induce apoptosis more effectively in triple-negative breast cancer cells while concurrently inhibiting EMT and neovascular synthesis.

2. Materials and Methods

2.1. Reagents and Antibodies

The antibodies used in this study were obtained from multiple providers: Cell Signaling Technology (CST, Danvers, MA, USA), Thermo Fisher Scientific (Waltham, MA, USA), and BD Biosciences (Franklin Lakes, NJ, USA). The biotin anti-human IL-6 detection antibody used for the enzyme-linked immunosorbent assay (ELISA) was procured from BD Biosciences. For Western blot experiments, primary antibodies were supplied by CST, including anti-mouse Bcl-2 (1:1000, Cat#15071), anti-rabbit Bax (1:1000, Cat#5023), anti-rabbit caspase-3 (1:1000, Cat#9664), anti-rabbit cleaved caspase-3 (1:1000, Cat#9664), anti-rabbit PARP (poly ADP-ribose polymerase, Cat#9532) (1:1000), anti-rabbit cleaved PARP (1:1000, Cat#5625), anti-mouse STAT3 (Tyr705, 1:1000, Cat#9138), anti-mouse p-STAT3 (1:1000, Cat#9145), anti-rabbit MMP-2 (1:1000, Cat#40994), anti-rabbit MMP-9 (1:1000, Cat#13667), anti-rabbit E-cadherin (1:1000, Cat#3195), and anti-rabbit N-cadherin (1:1000, Cat#13116). Cleaved caspase-3 (1:1000, Cat#700182) and β-actin antibodies (Cat#MA1-744) were obtained from Thermo Fisher Scientific. For Western blot experiments, secondary antibodies including anti-mouse IgG and horseradish peroxidase (HRP)-linked antibodies (Cat#7056) as well as anti-rabbit IgG and HRP-linked antibodies (Cat#7074), were procured from CST. In the immunofluorescence experiment, Alexa Fluor™ 488 goat anti-rabbit IgG (H+L) served as the secondary antibody and was acquired from Thermo Fisher Scientific.

2.2. Manufacturing Mistletoe Water Extract

Korean mistletoe was harvested from oak trees in Kangwon-do, Korea. The botanical verification was conducted by Professor Jon-Suk Lee from Seoul Women's University, Korea, and a voucher specimen (VCA101) was deposited at the College of Pharmacy, Sunchon National University, Korea. Initially, 100 g of crushed samples containing dried mistletoe leaves, stems, and branches (EV-MC6000, Everyhome Co., Busan, Republic of Korea) were combined with distilled water in a proportion of four times the weight of the dried sample. This mixture was gently agitated for a day within a shaking incubator operating at

120 rpm and maintained at a temperature of 4 °C. Subsequently, the resulting supernatant was separated via filtration using cotton material. The remaining residue underwent two additional extraction cycles using the same quantity of distilled water, followed by shaking. The obtained supernatant was then subjected to centrifugation at 4 °C for 20 min at 4500 rpm utilizing a centrifuge (VS-550, Vision Co., Daejeon, Republic of Korea), and then filtered using filter paper (No. 2, Advantec Toyo Roshi Kaisha, Ltd., Tokyo, Japan). The filtered supernatant was freeze-dried and stored at −20 °C until it was ready for use.

2.3. Cell Culture

Human breast cancer cells (MDA-MB-231) and human mononuclear cells (THP-1) were procured from the Korean Cell Line Bank (Seoul, Republic of Korea). Both cell lines were cultivated in a RPMI 1640 medium supplemented with 10% fetal bovine serum (FBS, Gibco Co., Grand Island, NY, USA), 2.05 mM L-glutamine, and 1% antibiotics (100 U/mL penicillin-100 µg/mL streptomycin). The cells were maintained in a controlled environment at 37 °C in a 5% CO_2 incubator (Sanyo, Osaka, Japan).

2.4. Cell Viability

The MTT (3-(4,5-dimethylthiazol-2-yl) assay was employed to evaluate the effect of mistletoe extract on the viability of MDA-MB-231 cells and THP-1 cells. The MTT reagent used for this assay was procured from Duchefa Biochemie (Haarlem, Netherlands). For the MDA-MB-231 cells, a concentration of 1×10^4 cells/well was added to 96-well plates (SPL Life Sciences Co., Ltd., Pocheon-si, Republic of Korea) and subsequently cultured at 37 °C for 24 h within a humidified 5% CO_2 incubator (Sanyo) without mistletoe extract. After removing the supernatant, mistletoe water extract was introduced, and the cells were further cultured for either 24 h or 48 h. In the case of THP-1 cells, differentiation into macrophages was achieved by treating the cells with phorbol 12-myristate 13-acetate (PMA, Sigma-Aldrich, St. Louis, MO, USA). The differentiated macrophages were then distributed into a 100 mm cell culture dish and incubated at 37 °C for 48 h within a humidified 5% CO_2 incubator (Sanyo). Afterward, the differentiated macrophages were washed with phosphate-buffered saline (PBS, VWR Life Science, Radnor, PA, USA), followed by an additional 48 h incubation with the same medium. The cells were subsequently seeded into a 96-well plate at a concentration of 1×10^4 cells/well and exposed to various concentrations (0.1–500 µg/mL) of mistletoe extract. To measure cell viability, 50 µL of MTT solution (5 mg/mL) prepared in PBS was added to each well and allowed to incubate at 37 °C for 4 h. After the supernatant was removed and the formazan crystals were dissolved using with 200 µL of dimethyl sulfoxide (DMSO), absorbance was assessed at 570 nm using a microplate reader (Sunrise Technologies, Männedorf, Zürich, Switzerland).

2.5. MDA-MB-231/THP-1 Co-Culture Model

The co-culture of MDA-MB-231 cells and THP-1 macrophages was performed using a Transwell system (Corning, NY, USA), utilizing both 6-well and 24-well plates. THP-1 cells, previously differentiated into macrophages, were introduced into the upper chamber of the Transwell insert, which had a pore size of 0.4 µm. On the other hand, MDA-MB-231 cells were added to the lower chamber of the Transwell system. The cells added to their respective compartments were cultured and allowed to attach for a period of 24 h at 37 °C within a humidified 5% CO_2 incubator (Sanyo). Following the attachment phase, mistletoe water extract at various concentrations was introduced, and the co-culture was continued for an additional 24 and 48 h. Subsequently, the MDA-MB-231 cells that were attached to the lower chamber were recovered, and the supernatants were collected for use in the subsequent experimental procedures. A schematic representation of the co-culture of MDA-MB-231 and M0 macrophages is provided in Figure 1.

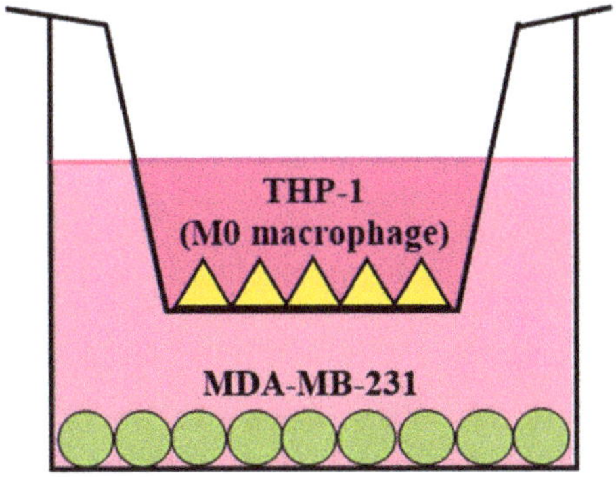

Figure 1. MDA-MB-231/THP-1 M0 macrophage co-culture model using Transwell system. THP-1 monocytes were differentiated with PMA (10 ng/mL) for 48 h before being plated in the upper insert. MDA-MB-231 cells were plated in the bottom chamber. Subsequently, both cell types were incubated in the presence or absence of mistletoe water extracts.

2.6. Wound Healing Assay

MDA-MB-231 cells were plated in a 24-well plate at a concentration of 2×10^5 cells/mL. They were then allowed to culture for 24 h, reaching a cell density of approximately 90%. Following this incubation period, a gap of a certain size was created by gently scratching the central portion of the cell monolayer on the plate using a sterile 200 μL pipette tip. The scratched monolayer was subsequently washed twice with phosphate-buffered saline (PBS). After the creation of the scratch, various concentrations of mistletoe water extract were added to the wells, and the cells were further cultured for 24 and 48 h. During this time, the extent of cell movement into the scratched area was observed and documented using an optical microscope (Nikon, Tokyo, Japan). The resulting gaps caused by the migration of cells were then quantified using Image J software (version 1.53e, National Institutes of Health, Bethesda, MD, USA).

2.7. Migration Assay

To assess the migration of MDA-MB-231 cells, a 24-Transwell plate with an 8.0 μm pore size was employed. Initially, M0 macrophages or RPMI with 10% FBS were introduced into the Transwell chamber and incubated for 24 h at 37 °C in a 5% CO_2 incubator (Sanyo). The mistletoe water extract was diluted with serum-free RPMI, and 100 μL of the diluted extract was added to the Transwell insert. MDA-MB-231 cells were suspended in the serum-free RPMI 1640 medium and placed in the Transwell insert, where they were incubated for either 24 or 48 h. For the visualization of cells that migrated through the filter and reached the bottom surface of the insert, Giemsa staining was employed. Briefly, the residual medium within the insert was removed, and the insert was washed twice with PBS (pH 7.4). The cells were fixed at room temperature for 2 min using 3.7% formaldehyde. After two washes with PBS to remove the formaldehyde, 100% methanol was added and incubated for 20 min at room temperature. Following this, the insert was washed twice with PBS, and a 0.4% Giemsa solution (Sigma-Aldrich) was added. The insert was further incubated for 15 min at room temperature. After removing excess reagents with PBS, the cells on the top surface of the insert were gently wiped away using a cotton swab. The insert was then dried, and an optical microscope (Nikon) was used to count the number of cells that had migrated.

2.8. ELISA

The quantification of secreted IL-6 from MDA-MB-231 cells and THP-1 M0 macrophages was performed using an ELISA kit (BD Biosciences), following the provided instructions. Initially, 100 μL of the capture antibody diluted in a coating buffer

(0.1 M sodium carbonate, pH 9.0) was added to each well of a 96-well EIA/RIA plate (Corning), and the plate was incubated at 4 °C for 24 h. Subsequently, the plate was washed three times with a washing buffer containing PBS and 0.05% Tween-20. Then, a blocking buffer consisting of PBS with 1% bovine serum albumin (BSA) was added to the wells and allowed to incubate at room temperature for 1 h. After another three washes, the cell supernatant and the standard solutions were added to the wells and incubated at room temperature for 2 h. After an additional five washes with the washing buffer, the detection antibody was added to the wells, and the plate was incubated in darkness for 1 h. Following this, equal volumes of 3,3′,5,5′-Tetramethylbiphenyl-4,4′-diamine (TMB) Solution (0.4 g/L, Thermo Scientific, Cat#34021) and Peroxide Solution (0.02% hydrogen peroxide in citric acid buffer, Thermo Scientific, Cat#34021) were mixed, and 100 μL was added to each well; the plate was once again placed in darkness for an incubation of 30 min. After this incubation, 100 μL of 2 M sulfuric acid was introduced into the wells to stop the reaction, and the absorbance was measured at a wavelength of 450 nm.

2.9. Cytokine Array

The qualitative analysis of human inflammatory cytokines was carried out following the provided instructions using the Multi-analyte ELISArray kit (MEH-003A, QIAGEN, Hilden, Germany). In this assay, each well of the ELISArray plate was loaded with the assay buffer and 50 μL of the cell supernatant. The plate was then allowed to incubate at room temperature for a period of 2 h. Following the incubation, the plate was subjected to a series of washing steps, performed three times using a washing buffer to remove any residual contents from the wells. Subsequently, 100 μL of the detection antibody was added to each well, and the plate was once again incubated at room temperature for 1 h. After this incubation, the plate was washed three times to ensure proper removal of excess detection antibody. Next, 100 μL of avidin-HRP conjugate antibody was introduced to the wells, and the plate was incubated in darkness for 30 min. Following this incubation, the plate underwent four additional washing steps. Subsequently, 100 μL of the developing solution was added to each well, and the plate was placed in darkness for an additional incubation of 15 min. To stop the reaction, an equal volume of stop solution was added to each well. The absorbance of the samples was measured at a wavelength of 450 nm using a microplate reader (Sunrise Technologies).

2.10. Western Blotting

Cells were washed twice with PBS. To each well, 180 μL of radio-immuno preservation assay (RIPA) buffer (Thermo Scientific) and 1.8 μL of protease and phosphatase inhibitor cocktail (×100) (Thermo Scientific) were added. Centrifugation was performed at 4 °C for 20 min at 14,000 rpm. The total protein content was determined using the bicinchoninic acid (BCA) Protein Assay Kit (Thermo Scientific) following the manufacturer's protocol. The sample was mixed with sample loading dye (×5) (Chembio, Medford, NY, USA) and heated at 100 °C for 5 min. The mixture was loaded into the wells of a 12% sodium dodecyl sulfate-polyacrylamide gel electrophoresis (SDS-PAGE) setup. The protein was transferred from the gel to a polyvinylidene fluoride (PVDF) membrane filter (Merck Millipore Ltd., Middlesex, MA, USA). The membrane was washed with tris-buffered saline (TBS) containing 50 mM tris-Cl and 150 mM NaCl (pH 7.5) for 5 min. The membrane was blocked with a solution of 5% (w/v) bovine serum albumin (BSA) (VWR Life Science) at room temperature. The membrane was washed three times with TBS-T (TBS with 0.1% Tween-20), and 10 μL of the primary antibody was diluted in 10 mL of blocking buffer, added to the membrane, and incubated at 4 °C for 24 h. The membrane was washed three times with TBS-T. The membrane was exposed to a horseradish peroxidase (HRP)-conjugated secondary antibody at room temperature for 1 h. The membrane was washed three times with TBS-T and the expressed protein was visualized using the Western Bright ECL kit (Advansta Inc., San Jose, CA, USA).

2.11. Immunofluorescence

MDA-MB-231 cells were attached to a 24-well plate containing a coverslip (12 mm, SPL Life Sciences), and various concentrations of mistletoe water extract were added and incubated for 48 h at 37 °C in a humidified 5% CO_2 incubator (Sanyo). After washing three times with PBS, 500 µL of 4% formaldehyde (pH 7.4) was added and incubated at 37 °C for 10 min to fix the cells. After washing three times, 0.1% Triton X-100 was added and incubated for 15 min at room temperature. After washing three times, 500 µL of 2% (*w/v*) BSA (VWR Life Science) was added and incubated at room temperature for 1 h. The primary antibody was added and incubated at 4 °C for 24 h. After washing three times, the secondary antibody was added and incubated for 45 min at room temperature. After washing three times, DNA was stained with 4,6-diamidino-2-phenylindole (DAPI) for 20 min in the dark and observed with a fluorescence microscope (Nikon).

2.12. Statistical Analysis

All experiments were conducted in triplicate, and the results are presented as means ± standard deviation (S.D.). Statistical analysis of the data was performed using GraphPad software (version 7.00). Significant differences between groups were determined using a one-way analysis of variance (ANOVA), followed by Tukey's multiple comparison tests for post hoc analysis. Statistical significance was defined as $p < 0.05$, $p < 0.01$, and $p < 0.001$, indicating the level of significance for the observed differences between groups.

3. Results

3.1. Cell Viability

Different concentrations of mistletoe extract were introduced to the MDA-MB-231 human triple-negative breast cancer cell line and THP-1 human mononuclear cells that had been differentiated into macrophages. Subsequently, the cells were incubated for either 24 h or 48 h, and their viability was assessed using the MTT assay (Figure 2). Through this analysis, we determined that THP-1 macrophages exhibited a survival rate of over 80% when treated with concentrations of 2 µg/mL or lower for both the 24 and 48 h groups. As a result, we selected two specific doses for further experimentation.

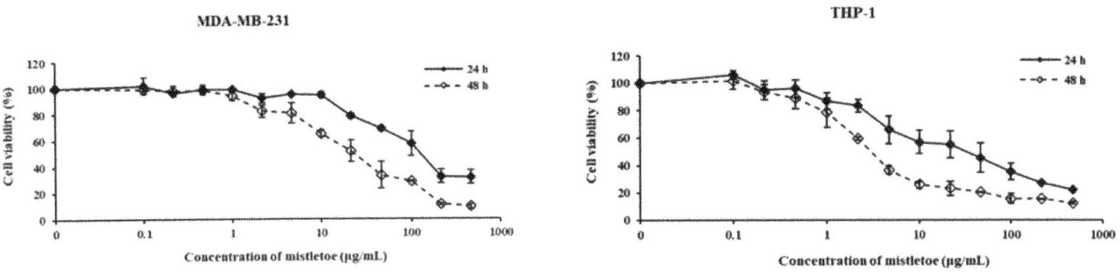

(**a**) (**b**)

Figure 2. Cytotoxic effect of mistletoe water extracts in (**a**) MDA-MB-231 and (**b**) THP-1 cells for 24 and 48 h. Both cell lines were exposed to various concentrations of mistletoe water extracts. Cell viability was assessed using the MTT assay. Untreated control cell viability was set at 100%. Results represent the means ± standard deviation (S.D.) of triplicate experiments.

3.2. Wound Healing and Migration Assay

For the wound healing assay, we first cut an arbitrary wound into the plate, treated it with mistletoe water extract, then monitored cell movement towards the wounded area over time (Figure 3). As a result, 61.1 ± 3.4% and 74.8 ± 3.8% of the wound area were moved in the MDA-MB-231 cells treated with mistletoe at 0.1 µg/mL concentrations for 24 and 48 h, respectively, whereas the MDA-MB-231/THP-1 co-culture group was significantly inhibited by 38.2 ± 3.4% and 57.9 ± 4.4% at 24 and 48 h, respectively. In addition,

57.6 ± 3.3% and 68.9 ± 2.9% of the wound area were moved in the MDA-MB-231 group treated with 2 μg/mL mistletoe for 24 and 48 h, respectively, whereas the MDA-MB-231/THP-1 co-culture group was significantly inhibited by 36.7 ± 1.6% and 45.9 ± 4.8% at 24 and 48 h, respectively (Figure 3d). Using the Transwell migration assay method, the MDA-MB-231 or MDA-MB-231/THP-1 groups were added into the insert membranes with pore sizes that cells can penetrate, and the number of breast cancer cells moving through the membranes under mistletoe extract treatment was observed (Figure 4). As a result, when mistletoe at a concentration of 0.1 μg/mL was treated for 48 h, 71.5 ± 5.3% of cells migrated through the membrane in the MDA-MB-231 group compared to the control, whereas 60.0 ± 3.2% of cells migrated through the membrane in the MDA-MB-231/THP-1 co-culture group compared to the control. When 2 μg/mL mistletoe was added for 48 h, 64.4 ± 2.8% of cells migrated through the membrane in the MDA-MB-231 group compared to the control, whereas 48.3 ± 2.4% of cells migrated through the membrane in the MDA-MB-231/THP-1 co-culture group.

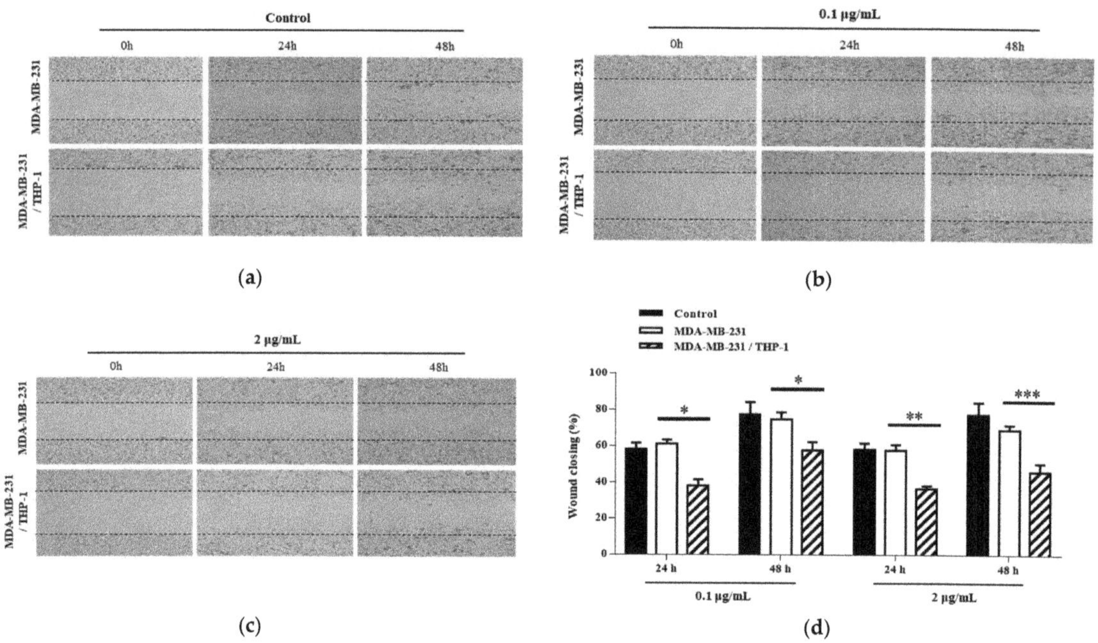

Figure 3. Effects of Korean mistletoe water extracts on wound healing assay in MDA-MB-231 and MDA-MB-231/THP-1 co-cultured cells. Following the creation of scratches on both cell groups, various concentrations of Korean mistletoe water extracts (**a**) 0, (**b**) 0.1, and (**c**) 2 μg/mL were applied immediately. Representative images from the wound healing assay were captured at 0, 24, and 48 h post-treatment. The closure of the wound area was observed under a light microscope (×40). Additionally, (**d**) a quantitative bar graph of the closed wound area was generated using an image analysis software (Image J). The results are represented as the mean ± standard deviation (S.D.). The *p*-value indicates significant differences between MDA-MB-231 and MDA-MB-231/THP-1 co-cultured cells (*** $p < 0.001$, ** $p < 0.01$, * $p < 0.001$).

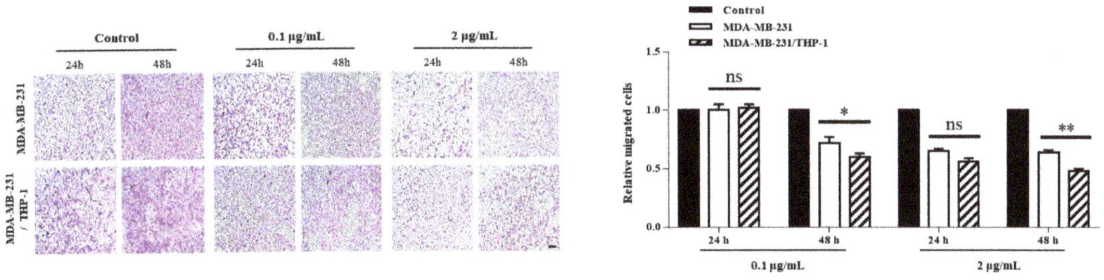

(**a**) (**b**)

Figure 4. Effect of Korean mistletoe water extracts on Transwell migration assay in (**a**) MDA-MB-231 and (**b**) MDA-MB-231/THP-1 co-cultured cells. Mistletoe water extracts were applied at various concentrations (0, 0.1, and 2 μg/mL) for 24 and 48 h. Migrated cells were observed using a light microscope (magnification, ×100; scale bar, 100 μm). The number of migrated cells was quantified using Image J software. Scale bars: 20 μm. The results are represented as the mean ± standard deviation (S.D.). The *p*-value indicates significant differences between MDA-MB-231 and MDA-MB-231/THP-1 co-cultured cells (** $p < 0.01$, * $p < 0.001$, ns: not significant).

3.3. Secretion of Inflammatory Cytokines

A quantitative and qualitative study was conducted by ELISA and cytokines array to investigate if Korean mistletoe water extract may modulate the release of inflammation-related cytokines produced by triple-negative breast cancer cells by activating macrophages. Initially, MDA-MB-231 cells and MDA-MB-231/THP-1 co-cultured cells underwent treatment with or without 100 ng/mL lipopolysaccharides (LPS); this process served to induce the expression of inflammatory cytokines in MDA-MD-231 cells. Following treatment with 0.1 and 2 μg/mL concentrations of Korean mistletoe water extracts for a period of 48 h, MDA-MB-231 cells, THP-1 macrophages, and MDA-MB-231/THP-1 co-cultured cells underwent testing to quantify IL-6 expression through ELISA. Consequently, when cells were not stimulated with LPS, MDA-MB-231 cells secreted 1501.5 ± 110.6 pg/mL and MDA-MB231/THP-1 co-cultured cells secreted 1418.5 ± 80.4 pg/mL of IL-6. However, after exposure to 100 ng/mL LPS, MDA-MB-231 cells and MDA-MB-231/THP-1 co-cultured cells showed an elevated IL-6 expression of to1987.6 ± 65.7 pg/mL and 1847.9 ± 120.5 pg/mL, respectively. There was no significant difference in IL-6 expression between the MDA-MB-231 cells and MDA-MB-231/THP-1 co-cultured cells. Following this, when 0.1 μg/mL mistletoe water extract was administered to MDA-MB-231 cells, we confirmed an IL-6 secretion level of 2053.1 ± 77.9 pg/mL, whereas MBA-MB-231/THP-1 co-cultured cells showed an IL-6 secretion level of 1503.2 ± 89.8 pg/mL. Additionally, treatment of MDA-MB-231 cells with 2 μg/mL mistletoe water extract resulted in an IL-6 secretion of 1993.1 ± 71.6 pg/mL. However, in MDA-MB-231/THP-1 co-cultured cells, the expression of IL-6 was significantly inhibited to 1447.6 ± 74.5 pg/mL (Figure 5). Moreover, through qualitative analysis aimed at determining the regulation of cytokine expression, it was observed that there was an increase in the expression levels of IL-4, TGF-β, and IFN-γ in MDA-MB-231/THP -1 co-cultured cells compared to the MDA-MB-231 group (Figure 6).

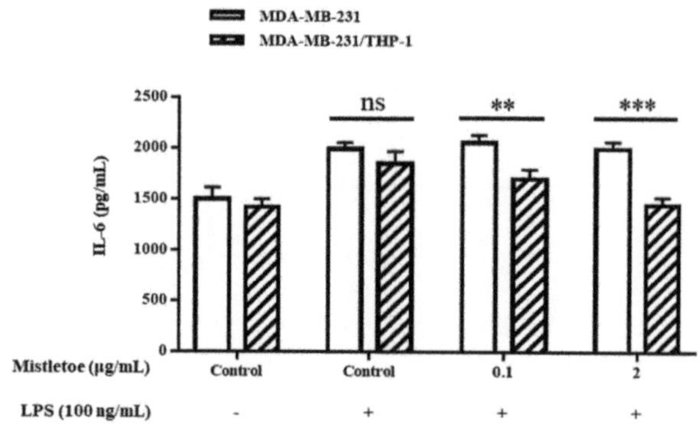

Figure 5. Effects of mistletoe water extracts on pro-inflammatory cytokine (IL-6) production in LPS-stimulated MDA-MB-231 and MDA-MDA-MB-231/THP-1 co-cultured cells. Cells were treated with or without various concentrations of mistletoe water extracts (0, 0.1, and 2 µg/mL) and LPS (100 ng/mL) for 48 h. Cell supernatant was collected and assessed using an ELISA kit. The results are represented as the mean ± standard deviation (S.D.). The *p*-value indicates significant differences between MDA-MB-231 and MDA-MB-231/THP-1 co-cultured cells (*** $p < 0.001$, ** $p < 0.01$, ns: not significant).

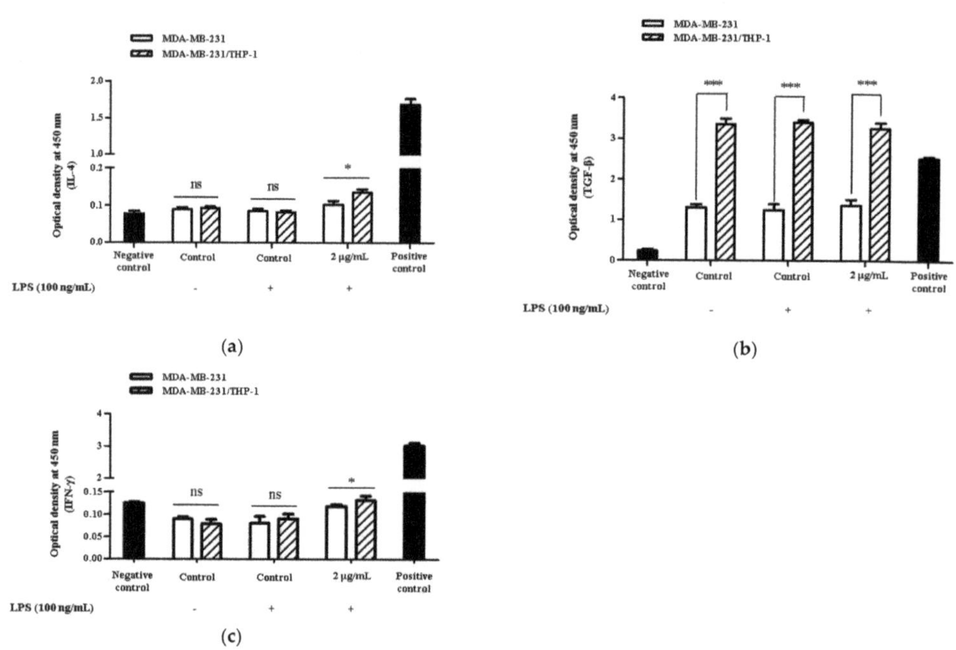

Figure 6. Effects of Korean mistletoe water extracts on (**a**) IL-4, (**b**) TGF-β, and (**c**) IFN-γ secretion in MDA-MB-231 and MDA-MB-231/THP-1 co-cultured cells. Both cell groups were treated with or without mistletoe water extracts (0 or 2 µg/mL) and LPS (100 ng/mL) for 48 h. Cell supernatants were then collected and qualitative relative profiling of cytokine levels was measured using the Multi-Analyte ELISArray kit according to the manufacturer's protocol. The results are represented as the mean ± standard deviation (S.D.). The *p*-value indicates significant differences between MDA-MB-231 and MDA-MB-231/THP-1 co-cultured cells (*** $p < 0.001$, * $p < 0.001$, ns: not significant).

3.4. Expression of Apoptosis-Related Proteins

The apoptosis-related protein expressions were assessed in triple-negative breast cancer cells upon administration of Korean mistletoe extract. Mistletoe water extract was administered to MDA-MB-231 cells and MDA-MB-231 cells co-cultured with THP-1 cells for a duration of 48 h, followed by conducting Western blot and immunofluorescence assays. Western blot analysis measured the ratio of Bax and Bcl-2 proteins, which are proteins that induce MOMP in mitochondrial outer membranes. When treated with 0.1 μg/mL mistletoe extract, MBA-MB-231 cells and MBA-MB-231/THP-1 co-cultured cells showed no significant difference in Bax/Bcl-2 protein ratio, compared to the controls. However, when treated with 2 μg/mL mistletoe extract, the MDA-MB-231/THP-1 co-culture group showed a protein ratio of 2.1 ± 0.1 times (Figure 7c). To determine if MOMP induced the activation of caspase-3 protein to cleaved caspase-3, we measured the ratio of cleaved caspase-3 and caspase-3 proteins via Western blot. Upon treatment with 0.1 μg/mL Korean mistletoe water extract, no significant differences were shown in either group when compared to the control. However, when treated with 2 μg/mL mistletoe extract, MDA-MB-231 cells and MDA-MB-231/THP-1 co-cultured cells showed a cleaved caspase-3/caspase-3 protein ratio of 1.6 ± 0.1 and 2.7 ± 0.1 times, respectively (Figure 7d). Therefore, the ratio of cleaved caspase-3/caspase-3 protein was significantly increased in MDA-MB-231 cells co-cultured with THP-1 cells compared to single-cultured MDA-MB-231 cells. We also assessed the influence of cleaved caspase-3 on PARP protein deactivation through its transformation into cleaved PARP. As a result, when treated with 0.1 μg/mL mistletoe extract, the expression of cleaved PARP protein was 0.9 ± 0.1 times and 1.2 ± 0.1 times that of the control in MDA-MB-231 cells and MDA-MB-231/THP-1 co-cultured cells, respectively. In addition, when treated with 2 μg/mL mistletoe extract, the expression of cleaved PARP protein was 0.9 ± 0.2 times and 1.4 ± 0.2 times that of the control in MDA-MB-231 cells and MDA-MB-231/THP-1 co-cultured cells, respectively (Figure 7e). The immunofluorescence staining confirmed the expression level of apoptosis proteins Bax, cleaved caspase-3, and cleaved PARP; interestingly, the protein expression of Bax and cleaved-caspase-3 increased dose-dependently in MDA-MB-231/THP-1 co-cultured cells (Figure 8a,b). However, there were no significant differences in cleaved PARP expression in both MDA-MB-231 cells and MDA-MB-231/THP-1 co-cultured cells, compared to the controls (Figure 8c).

3.5. Inhibition of STAT3 Activation

Unregulated STAT3 protein activation is frequently seen in cancer cells, and it is involved in cell proliferation and differentiation, which leads to tumor malignancy [52]. Therefore, to confirm whether Korean mistletoe extract can inhibit STAT3 protein activation in triple-negative breast cancer cells in the breast cancer microenvironment, Western blot assay was performed by treating MDA-MB-231 cells and MDA-MB-231/THP-1 co-cultured cells for 48 h with 0.1 and 2 μg/mL of Korean mistletoe extract (Figure 9a,b). The ratio of the expression of the total STAT3 protein and the phosphorylated and activated p-STAT3 protein was calculated and compared. When 0.1 μg/mL mistletoe was treated, p-STAT3/STAT3 protein was expressed 0.9 ± 0.1 times and 1.13 ± 0.1 times more than the control in the MDA-MB-231 and MDA-MB-231/THP-1 co-culture group, respectively, and no significant difference was observed between the two groups. However, when 2 μg/mL mistletoe was treated, p-STAT3/STAT3 protein was expressed 1.2 ± 0.1 times and 0.7 ± 0.1 times in the MDA-MB-231 and MDA-MB-231/THP-1 co-culture group, respectively, showing a significant difference in inhibiting the activation of the STAT3 protein (Figure 9c).

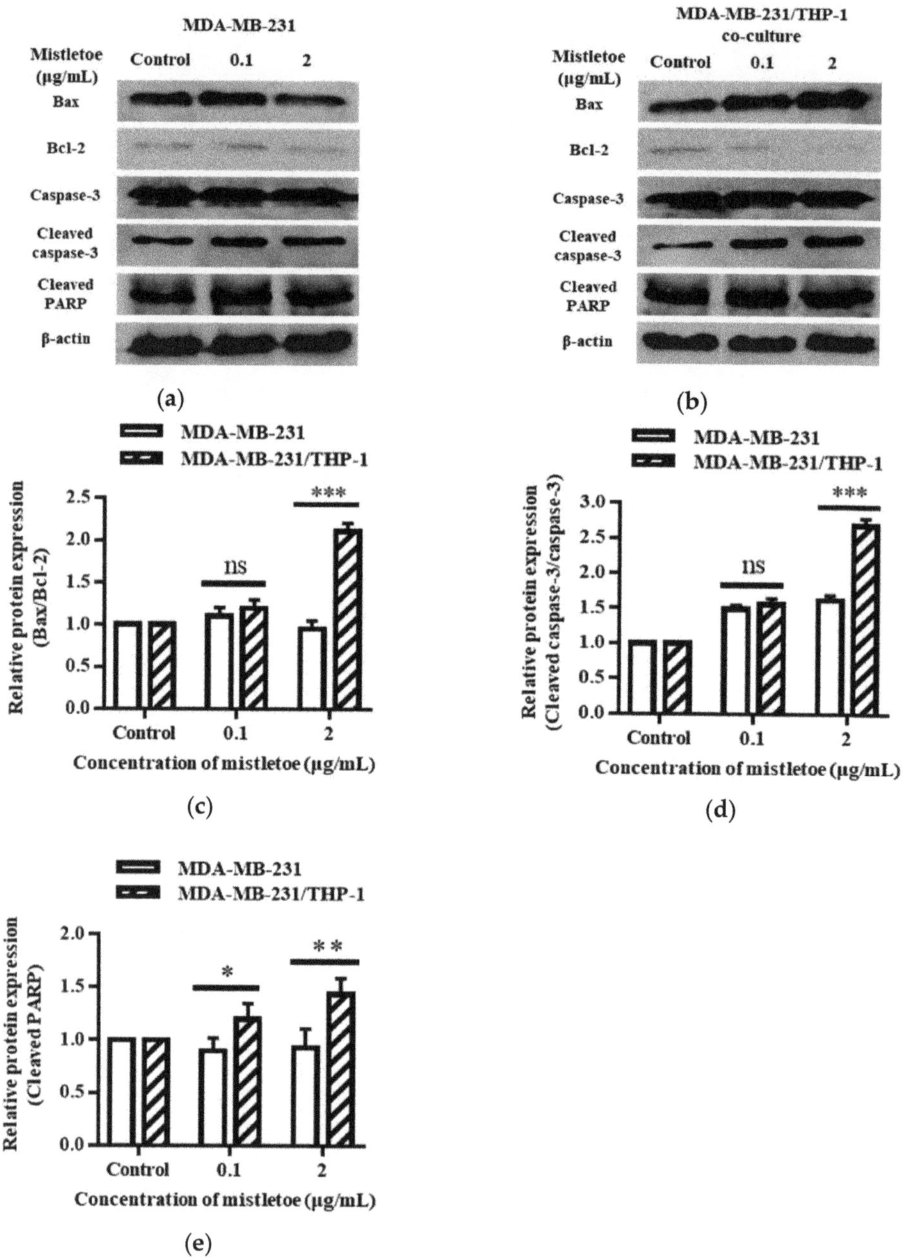

Figure 7. Effects of Korean mistletoe water extracts on apoptosis-related protein expression in (**a**) MDA-MDA-231 and (**b**) MDA-MB-231/THP-1 co-cultured cells using Western blot analysis. Both cell groups were treated with mistletoe water extracts (0, 0.1 and 2 μg/mL) for 48 h, and their relative protein expression levels (**c**) Bax/Bcl-2, (**d**) cleaved caspase-3/caspase-3, and (**e**) cleaved PARP were quantified and presented using a bar graph. The results are represented as the mean ± standard deviation (S.D.). The p-value indicates significant differences between MDA-MB-231 and MDA-MB-231/THP-1 co-cultured cells (*** $p < 0.001$, ** $p < 0.01$, * $p < 0.001$, ns: not significant).

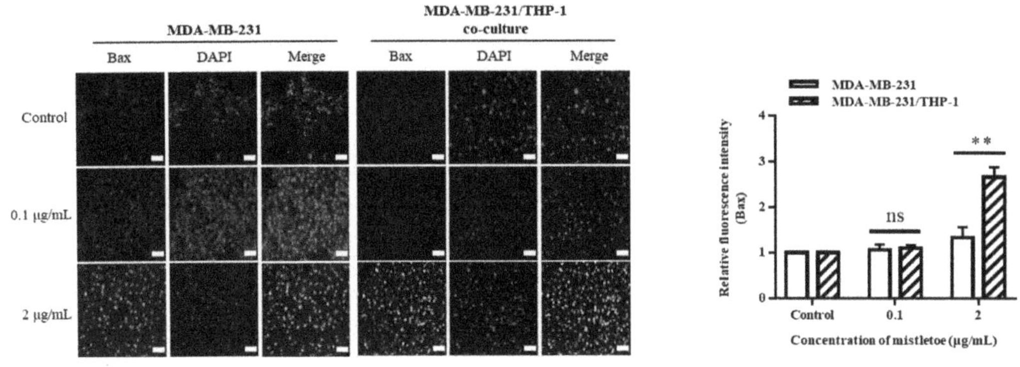

(a)

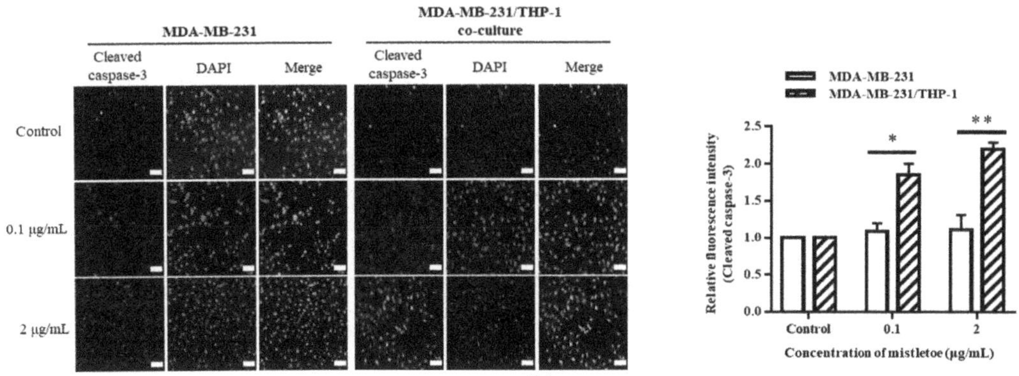

(b)

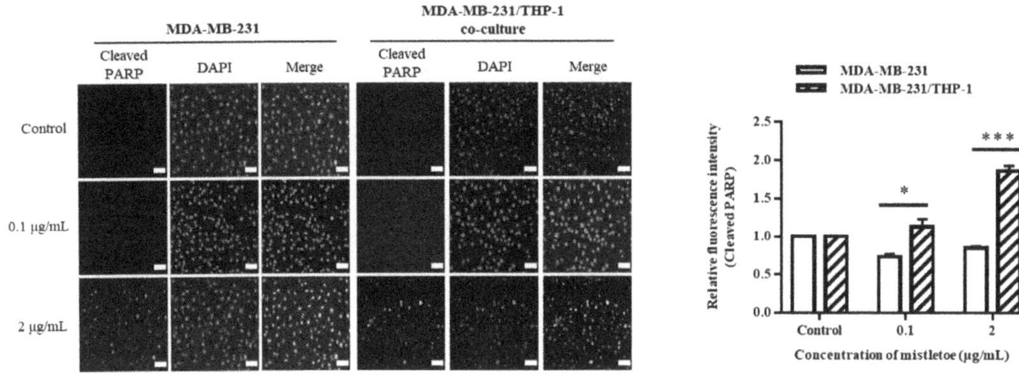

(c)

Figure 8. Representative images and quantitative bar graph of pro-apoptosis proteins using immunofluorescence staining. MDA-MB-231 and MDA-MB-231/THP-1 co-cultured cells were treated with various concentrations of Korean mistletoe water extracts (0, 0.1, and 2 μg/mL) for 48 h. The expressed proteins (**a**) Bax, (**b**) cleaved caspase-3, and (**c**) cleaved PARP were labeled with Alexa Fluor™ 488 (green), while nuclear DNA was counterstained with DAPI (blue) then observed using fluorescence microscope (magnification ×200). Fluorescence intensity was quantified using Image J software. Scale bars: 20 μm. The results are represented as the mean ± standard deviation (S.D.). The p-value indicates significant differences between MDA-MB-231 and MDA-MB-231/THP-1 co-cultured cells (*** $p < 0.001$, ** $p < 0.01$, * $p < 0.001$, ns: not significant).

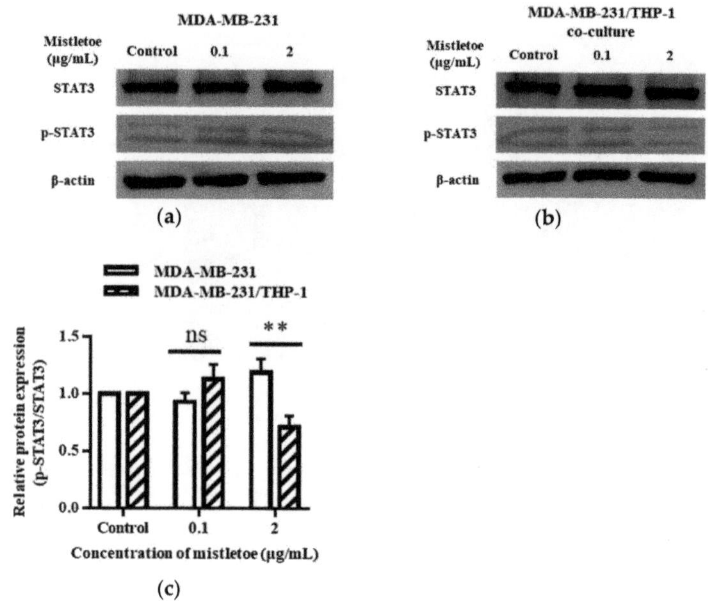

Figure 9. Inhibitory effects of Korean mistletoe water extract on STAT3 activation in (**a**) MDA-MB-231 and (**b**) MDA-MB-231/THP-1 co-cultured cells. After treatment with Korean mistletoe water extracts at concentrations of 0, 0.1, and 2 μg/mL for 48 h, Western blot analysis was conducted. (**c**) The quantification bar graph represents the ratio of p-STAT3/STAT3 protein expression. Each bar represents the mean ± standard deviation (S.D.) of experiments performed in triplicates. The *p*-value indicates significant differences between MDA-MB-231 and MDA-MB-231/THP-1 co-cultured cells (** $p < 0.01$, ns: not significant).

3.6. Inhibition of MMP-2 and -9 Expression

MMP-2 and MMP-9 are enzymes released by the metastatic cancer cell line MDA-MB-231 that tear down the extracellular matrix, a barrier surrounding the cell that allows tumor cells to migrate to neighboring organs [53]. We confirmed the suppression of MMP-2 or MMP-9 expression through Western blot and immunofluorescence assays after treating MDA-MB-231 cells and MDA-MB-231/THP-1 co-cultured cells for 48 h with 0.1 and 2 μg/mL of mistletoe extract (Figure 10a,b). As a result, when MDA-MB-231 and MDA-MB-231/THP-1 co-culture groups were treated with 0.1 g/mL mistletoe extract, no significant difference in MMP-2 protein expression was found. However, when 2 μg/mL mistletoe was treated, MMP-1 protein was expressed 0.9 ± 0.1 times and 0.4 ± 0.2 times less in the MDA-MB-231 and MDA-MB-231/THP-1 co-culture group, respectively, showing a significant difference in inhibiting the MMP-1 protein expression (Figure 10a). Similarly, when MDA-MB-231 and MDA-MB-231/THP-1 co-culture groups were treated with 0.1 g/mL mistletoe extract, no significant difference in MMP-9 protein expression was found. On the other hand, when 2 μg/mL mistletoe was treated, MMP-1 protein was expressed 0.7 ± 0.1 times and 0.4 ± 0.1 times less in the MDA-MB-231 and MDA-MB-231/THP-1 co-culture group, respectively, showing a significant difference in inhibiting the MMP-9 protein expression (Figure 10b). In addition, immunofluorescence revealed a significant inhibition of expression in the MBA-MB-231/THP-1 co-culture group upon treatment with 2 μg/mL mistletoe water extract (Figure 11).

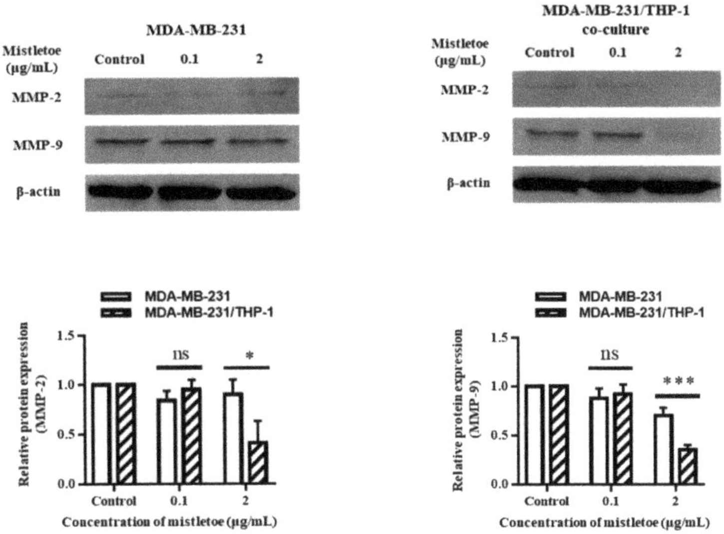

(a) (b)

Figure 10. Inhibitory effects of mistletoe water extract on MMP-2 and MMP-9 expression in (**a**) MDA-MB-231 and (**b**) MDA-MB-231/THP-1 co-cultured cells. Both groups were treated with mistletoe water extracts (0, 0.1, and 2 μg/mL) for 48 h, and their relative protein expression levels were quantified and presented using a bar graph. Each bar represents the mean ± standard deviation (S.D.) of experiments performed in triplicates. The p-value indicates significant differences between MDA-MB-231 and MDA-MB-231/THP-1 co-cultured cells (*** $p < 0.001$, * $p < 0.001$, ns: not significant).

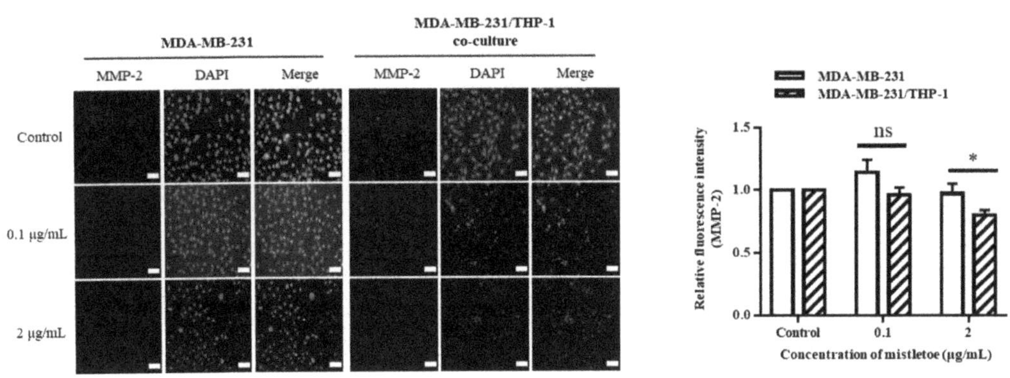

(a) (b)

Figure 11. Representative images from immunofluorescence staining of (**a**) MMP-2 and (**b**) their quantitative bar graph. MDA-MB-231 and MDA-MB-231/THP-1 co-cultured cells were treated with various concentrations of Korean mistletoe water extracts (0, 0.1, and 2 μg/mL) for 48 h. The expressed proteins were labeled with Alexa Fluor™ 488 (green), while nuclear DNA was counterstained with DAPI (blue) then observed using a fluorescence microscope (magnification ×200). Fluorescence intensity was quantified using Image J software. Scale bars: 20 μm. The results are represented as the mean ± standard deviation (S.D.). The p-value indicates significant differences between MDA-MB-231 and MDA-MB-231/THP-1 co-cultured cells (* $p < 0.001$, ns: not significant).

3.7. Effect on EMT Marker Expression

Through the regulation of related proteins, epithelial–mesenchymal transition (EMT) converts epithelial cells into an invasive and metastatic state. E-cadherin and N-cadherin are recognized as the markers for this transformation, where E-cadherin is a suppressor and N-cadherin an activator [54]. To evaluate whether mistletoe could inhibit the metastasis of breast cancer cells by modulating the expression of cadherin protein, 0.1 and 2 μg/mL of mistletoe extract was added to MDA-MB-231 cells and MDA-MB-231/THP-1 co-cultured cells and incubated for 48 h. As a result, E-cadherin, an EMT-inhibiting protein, was expressed 1.7 ± 0.2 times more than the control in MDA-MB-231/THP-1 co-cultured cell when treated with 0.1 μg/mL mistletoe extract; however, there was no significant difference in MDA-MB-231 cells. When 2 μg/mL of mistletoe was treated, E-cadherin protein was expressed 1.4 ± 0.1 times and 2.5 ± 0.3 times more than the control in the MDA-MB-231 and MDA-MB-231/THP-1 co-culture group, respectively, showing a significant difference between the two groups (Figure 12).

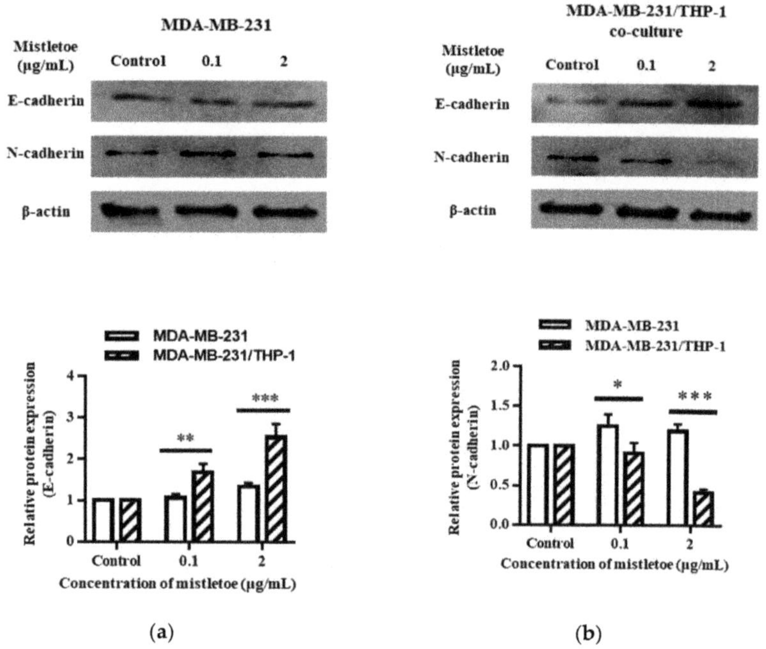

Figure 12. Effects of Korean mistletoe water extracts on regulating EMT markers in (**a**) MDA-MB-231 and (**b**) MDA-MB-231/THP-1 co-cultured cells using Western blot analysis. Both cell groups were treated with mistletoe water extracts (0, 0.1, and 2 μg/mL) for 48 h, and their relative protein expression levels were quantified and presented using a bar graph. The results are represented as the mean ± standard deviation (S.D.). The p-value indicates significant differences between MDA-MB-231 and MDA-MB-231/THP-1 co-cultured cells (*** $p < 0.001$, ** $p < 0.01$, * $p < 0.001$).

In addition, the expression of N-cadherin, a protein that induces EMT, was confirmed via Western blot. When 0.1 μg/mL of mistletoe was treated, N-cadherin protein was expressed 1.3 ± 0.2 times and 0.9 ± 0.1 times more compared to the control in the MDA-MB-231 and MDA-MB-231/THP-1 co-culture group, respectively, showing a significant difference between the two groups. In the case of 2 μg/mL mistletoe treatment, N-cadherin protein was expressed 1.2 ± 0.1 times and 0.4 ± 0.1 times more compared to the control in the MDA-MB-231 and MDA-MB-231/THP-1 co-culture group, respectively, showing a significant difference between the two groups (Figure 12).

4. Discussion

Breast cancer is a major problem for women worldwide, accounting for around one-quarter of all female cancer cases [39,55,56]. Breast cancer treatment often entails targeting particular receptors such as ER, PR, and HER2, inducing pharmacological reactions that result in cell death. Developing medications that successfully attack triple-negative breast cancer, on the other hand, provides a distinct difficulty. This subtype, which affects around 10% to 20% of patients, lacks the typical receptors ER, PR, and HER2 [16]. The only therapy presently approved by the Food and Medication Administration (FDA) in the United States is a medication that inhibits the expression of programmed death-ligand 1 (PD-L1) in triple-negative breast cancer [48]. To make things worse, triple-negative breast cancer is notorious for its high recurrence rates and disease spread to distant organs, both of which contribute considerably to death rates [40]. To prevent any further complications, the primary treatment for triple-negative breast cancer involves surgical surgery, radiation therapy, and non-specific chemotherapy [20]; however, these chemotherapeutic procedures—utilizing highly cytotoxic drugs—are associated with a wide range of side effects. These adverse reactions in turn diminish the quality of life among patients suffering from triple-negative breast cancer [18]. Therefore, discovering medications that precisely suppress triple-negative breast cancer without causing adverse effects is emerging.

Mistletoe, a medicinal plant widely distributed throughout Europe and Asia, serves as a complementary agent for anti-cancer drugs that increase apoptosis in cancer cells, decrease cancer mortality, and lessen drug adverse effects [1,3]. Recent studies have shown that mistletoe water extract promotes cell-mediated immunity to tumor cells by protecting monocytes DNA and stimulating immune cells such as macrophages as well as direct cytotoxicity to cancer cells [57]. The bone marrow produces monocytes, which then differentiate into macrophages; these macrophages undergo further differentiation, dependent on various environmental factors, which enable them to perform dual functions within the tumor microenvironment. In general, macrophages use cell-mediated immune responses to kill cancer cells, mediate phagocytosis, and cause vascular damage and necrosis of tumors; however, in a malignly established tumor microenvironment, cancer cells survive, proliferate angiogenesis, and their immune avoidance contributes to cancer progression and metastasis [58]. In recent immuno-cancer studies using macrophages, methods of manipulating macrophages to enhance anti-cancer activity or blocking the access of macrophages to tumors have been mainly proposed. This study confirms that mistletoe water extract holds potential as an immuno-cancer drug for treating triple-negative breast cancer by manipulating the function of macrophages.

When we treated mistletoe extract on MDA-MB-231 cells, a triple-negative breast cancer cell, for 48 h, the 50% inhibitory concentration (IC50) was 20 μg/mL. According to the plant screening system of the National Cancer Institute (NCI) in the United States, the crude extract of plants is considered to be cytotoxic in vitro when IC50 is less than 20 μg/mL after 24–72 h culture [59]. Our results are similar to those of Goda et al., who conducted prior studies on the cytotoxicity of mistletoe extracts in MDA-MB-231 cells [60]. Therefore, we considered mistletoe water extract as a potential cytotoxic drug for triple-negative breast cancer. Furthermore, when mistletoe extracts were treated on THP-1 cells (human mononuclear cell lines), our findings revealed a survival rate of more than 80% at dosages less than 2 μg/mL. Mishra et al. confirmed that the mistletoe water extract for THP-1 cells showed a survival rate of about 60% at 2 g/mL [61], which differed slightly from our findings. However, this might be because Mishra et al. employed *Viscum articulatum* and did not differentiate THP-1 cells into macrophages, which differs from our work.

Cancer cells secrete inflammatory mediators; these are a significant factor in tumor progression [32]. For instance, in the case of triple-negative breast cancer-secreting cytokines such as IL-4, IL-6, IFN-, and TGF-β, it is these that cause chronic inflammation within this specific microenvironment. The over-expression of such inflammatory cytokines results in accelerated metastasis, alongside neovascularization and cancer cell infiltration [62]. The inflammatory cytokine, IL-6, which plays a pivotal role in cancer progression through the activation of the JAK2/STAT3 signaling pathway [48], has been found to associate STAT3-activated cancer cells with survival and differentiation, metastasis, and infiltration, as well as an increase in EMT [18]. This study's results revealed that when THP-1 cells (differentiated into macrophages) and MDA-MB-231/THP-1 co-cultured cells were treated with 0.1 and 2 μg/mL Korean mistletoe water extract, there was a significant reduction in IL-6 secretion compared to that seen in MDA-MB-231 cells. Additionally, we studied the JAK2/STAT3 signaling pathway using Western blotting. When we treated the MDA-MB-231/THP-1 co-cultured cells with mistletoe extract at a concentration of 2 μg/mL, it significantly reduced p-STAT3 protein expression. Choi et al. reported through their studies on complex plant extracts that they inhibit STAT3 activation within MDA-MB-231 cells; such inhibition further suppresses IL-6 production in cancer cells [17]. Based on this report, we can assume that Korean mistletoe extract actively reduces the secretion of IL-6 in MDA-MB231 cells by inhibiting the activation of STAT3 between tumor cells and macrophages. Faggioli et al. [63] observed an increase in IL-6 expression within MDA-MB231 cells via nuclear factor kappa (NF-kB)-light-chain enhancer pathway in parallel studies [63], and Suarez-Crevo et al. [64] suggested that the increase in p38, which is a mitogen-activated protein kinase (MAPK) signaling subgroup, and extracellular signal-regulated kinases (ERK1/2) mediated IL-6 expression in MDA-MB-231 cells [64]. However, since this study cannot confirm whether mistletoe water extract affects IL-6 expression in MDA-MB-231 cells by targeting molecules other than STAT3 in MDA-MB-231 cells, it is necessary to study other signaling proteins closely related to inflammatory cytokines. In addition, expressions of IL-4, TGF-β, and IFN-γ were qualitatively analyzed using the Multi-Analyte ELISArray kit (Qiagen) to find out what immune regulation Korean mistletoe extract is involved in between MDA-MB-231 and macrophages. As a result, the expression of the anti-inflammatory cytokines IL-4 and TGF-β increased in the MDA-MB-231/THP-1 co-culture group compared to the MBA-MB-231 cell culture group. It was reported that TGF-β reacts with TGF-β receptor 1 to activate the formation of reactive oxygen specifications (ROS) in cells through the TGF-β/Smad pathway, which activates the suppressor of mothers again (Smad) protein, resulting in the activation of mitochondria, cytochrome c, caspase-9, and finally caspase-3 [65,66]. Since ELISArray confirmed that TGF-β increased expression in the MDA-MB-231/THP-1 co-culture group compared to the MDA-MB-231 cell culture group, we expected that apoptosis targeting mitochondria in triple-negative breast cancer cells would increase in the co-culture group. Also, it was reported that IFN-γ is involved when M0 macrophages are differentiated into M1 macrophages [67]. Based on these facts, we can assume that Korean mistletoe extract can differentiate M0 macrophages into M1 via initiating IFN-γ expression. However, a follow-up study is needed.

Aside from direct apoptosis, the mechanism of tumor cell death produced by the component of mistletoe water extract is linked to immune cell activation, namely natural killer cells (NK cells), lymphocytes, and macrophages [67–69]. Clinical investigations have indicated that immune cells triggered by mistletoe water extracts react directly or indirectly to tumor cells, inhibiting tumor cell proliferation and improving patient survival rates [12,70]. Therefore, we investigated whether the activation of human macrophage THP-1 by Korean mistletoe water extract could induce apoptosis in MDA-MB-231 cells through cell-mediated immunity. MDA-MB-231 cells and the MDA-MB-231/THP-1 co-culture group were each exposed to Korean mistletoe water extracts at concentrations of 0.1 and 2 μg/mL for a duration of 48 h. It was observed that in the MDA-MB-231/THP-1 co-culture group at a concentration of 2 μg/mL, there was a significant augmentation in the Bax/Bcl-2 protein expression ratio compared to the MDA-MB-231 cell culture group, indicating a significant increase in the initiation of apoptosis.

Additionally, we hypothesized that mistletoe could release apoptosomes into the mitochondria's cytoplasm, through Bcl-2 family regulation, which leads to caspase-3 activation. Typically, caspase-3 exists in the cytoplasm in an inactive form, and when cleaved by caspase-9 or other proteases, it is activated when the active site is exposed [71]. To compare and analyze the degree of activation of caspase-3 in this study, the ratio of cleaved caspase-3 was confirmed. When 2 μg/mL mistletoe extract was treated, the expression of cleaved caspase-3 increased significantly in the MDA-MB-231/THP-1 co-culture group. From this result, it can be said that mistletoe can regulate Bax and Bcl-2 proteins leading to an increase in MOMP, resulting in caspase-3 activation.

Apoptosis is caused when cleaved caspase-3 cuts and inactivates PARP, which aids in the repair of damaged DNA in tumor cells' nuclei. Therefore, increasing cleaved PARP induces apoptosis in tumor cells [72].

In this study, cleaved PARP expression increased in both the 0.1 and 2 μg/mL mistletoe-treated MDA-MB-231/THP co-culture group. However, the expression of cleaved caspase-3 increased only in the 2 μg/mL mistletoe-treated MDA-MB-231/THP-1 co-culture group. There was a correlation between the increase in cleaved caspase-3 and cleaved PARP, but it was not proportional. This could be explained by a previous study indicating that cleaved caspase-3 enters the nucleus through active transport in the nuclear pore complex rather than through simple diffusion. Furthermore, active nuclear transport of cleaved caspase-3 is dependent on morphological changes in the nucleus caused by various apoptotic triggers and transport proteins that carry out active nuclear transport [73]. Also, Cui et al. reported that the cutting of PARP during apoptosis was performed by calpain, a calcium-dependent protease, rather than caspase-3, by inducing p53 genes and caspase-9 in breast cancer cell lines [74]. Based on the findings, it is possible to explain why there was an increase in cleaved PARP expression even though there was no significant rise in cleaved caspase-3 when mistletoe water extract at 0.1 g/mL was treated. The mechanism by which mistletoe extract induces apoptosis in MDA-MB-231 cells is likely to cleave PARP and trigger apoptosis through pathways other than caspase-3.

At each stage of metastasis, breast cancer epithelial cells are polarized into endothelial cell phenotypes through the progress of EMT, increasing mobility, and a loss of E-cadherin and an increase in N-cadherin are observed at the molecular level [75,76]. In addition, MMPs are involved in the process of cancer cells breaking down and invading the extra-cellular matrix. Among various types of MMPs, MMP-2 and MMP-9, with the activity of breaking down gelatin, are secreted to the cell surface and locally decompose the extra-cellular matrix that binds to the cell membrane, making the cell motile [77]. Because the findings imply that the mobility of cancer cells is connected to the level of MMP expression, investigations on cancer metastasis inhibition targeting MMPs are being conducted [78–80]. Therefore, in this study, when mistletoe water extract was treated on MDA-MB-231 cells and MDA-MB-231/THP-1 co-cultured cells, the difference in mobility inhibition between the two groups was compared via wound healing and Transwell migration assay. Also, to validate the suppression of metastasis of triple-negative breast cancer cells, the regulation of E-cadherin and N-cadherin, and the inhibition of MMP-2 and MMP-9 expression, were confirmed. Firstly, the MDA-MB-231 cell culture group and the MDA-MB-231/THP-1 co-culture group were attached to a plate or membrane insert, and then the mobility inhibition of MDA-MB-231 cells was observed after they were treated with mistletoe extract. It was confirmed that the co-culture group significantly inhibited the movement to the wound area compared to the MDA-MB-231 cell culture group. The mobility of MDA-MB-231 attached to the insert membrane was inhibited by mistletoe extract, dose-dependently.

To compare the inhibition of metastasis between the two groups due to the regulation of cell movement-related protein expression at the molecular level, an EMT marker that regulates the mobility of cancer cells within the tumor microenvironment was observed through Western blot analysis. First, when the expression of E-cadherin, an EMT inhibitor, was observed, there was a significant increase in expression in the MDA-MB-231/THP-1 co-culture group compared to the MDA-MB-231 cell culture group. In addition, expression of the EMT product, N-cadherin, was considerably reduced in the co-culture group compared to the single culture group. Therefore, it was confirmed that mistletoe water extract can inhibit the EMT of MDA-MB-231 cells at the molecular level by activating THP-1 macrophages. Furthermore, the comparison of Western blot results between the two groups revealed a significant inhibition in the expression of MMP-2 and MMP-9. Following 48 h of treatment with mistletoe water extract at a dosage of 2 μg/mL, both MMP-2 and MMP-9 were considerably suppressed in the MDA-MB-231/THP-1 co-culture group. Therefore, it was confirmed at the molecular level that mistletoe water extract can inhibit metastasis by inhibiting the stage of local infiltration of tissue by activating THP-1 macrophages and inhibiting the expression of MMP-2 and MMP-9 in MDA-MB-231 cells through cell-mediated immunity. The observed effects on EMT markers and MMPs provide valuable insights into the potential mechanisms underlying mistletoe water extract's anti-metastatic properties. These findings align with previous research indicating the anti-cancer properties of mistletoe extracts and highlight its potential as a therapeutic agent in the field of metastatic breast cancer [81].

According to the findings of this research, Korean mistletoe water extract inhibits triple-negative breast cancer cells by enhancing the human immune system via activating macrophages. In particular, we could confirm apoptosis which induced MOMP in triple-negative breast cancer cells through cell-mediated immunity of activated macrophages. In addition, we looked into the STAT3 pathway and also the regulation of cancer cell mobility by controlling numerous inflammation-related cytokines. However, further studies are needed to determine whether mistletoe can influence the immunity of breast cancer subtypes other than triple-negative breast cancer cells. We also need to determine how macrophages were activated and which component in mistletoe extract contributes to this activation. Lastly, the subject of whether mistletoe influences other immune cells in the human body, such as natural killer (NK) cells, remains unanswered, thus further study is needed.

Author Contributions: Conceptualization: C.-E.H. and S.-Y.L.; funding acquisition: S.-Y.L.; investigation: W.-T.L., C.-E.H. and S.-Y.L.; methodology: W.-T.L. and C.-E.H.; resources: W.-T.L. and C.-E.H.; supervision: S.-Y.L.; writing—original draft: W.-T.L.; writing—review and editing: S.-Y.L. All authors have read and agreed to the published version of the manuscript.

Funding: This research received no external funding.

Institutional Review Board Statement: Not applicable.

Informed Consent Statement: Not applicable.

Data Availability Statement: Not applicable.

Conflicts of Interest: The authors declare no conflict of interest.

References

1. Orhan, D.D.; Küpeli, E.; Yesilada, E.; Ergun, F. Anti-inflammatory and antinociceptive activity of flavonoids isolated from Viscum album ssp. album. *Z. Naturforsch. C, J. Biosci.* **2006**, *61*, 26–30. [CrossRef] [PubMed]
2. Kuttan, G.; Vasudevan, D.M.; Kuttan, R. Effect of a preparation from Viscum album on tumor development in vitro and in mice. *J. Ethnopharmacol.* **1990**, *29*, 35–41. [CrossRef] [PubMed]
3. Kienle, G.S.; Kiene, H. Review article: Influence of Viscum album L (European mistletoe) extracts on quality of life in cancer patients: A systematic review of controlled clinical studies. *Integr. Cancer Ther.* **2010**, *9*, 142–157. [CrossRef]
4. Onay-Uçar, E.; Karagöz, A.; Arda, N. Antioxidant activity of Viscum album ssp. album. *Fitoterapia* **2006**, *77*, 556–560. [CrossRef] [PubMed]
5. Attar, R.; Tabassum, S.; Fayyaz, S.; Ahmad, M.S.; Nogueira, D.R.; Yaylim, I.; Timirci-Kahraman, O.; Kucukhuseyin, O.; Cacina, C.; Farooqi, A.A.; et al. Natural products are the future of anticancer therapy: Preclinical and clinical advancements of Viscum album phytometabolites. *Cell. Mol. Biol. (Noisy-le-grand)* **2015**, *61*, 62–68.
6. Park, J.H.; Hyun, C.K.; Shin, H.K. Cytotoxic effects of the components in heat-treated mistletoe (Viscum album). *Cancer Lett.* **1999**, *139*, 207–213. [CrossRef]
7. Zarkovic, N.; Vukovic, T.; Loncaric, I.; Miletic, M.; Zarkovic, K.; Borovic, S.; Cipak, A.; Sabolovic, S.; Konitzer, M.; Mang, S. An overview on anticancer activities of the Viscum album extract Isorel. *Cancer Biother. Radiopharm.* **2001**, *16*, 55–62. [CrossRef] [PubMed]
8. Enesel, M.B.; Acalovschi, I.; Grosu, V.; Sbarcea, A.; Rusu, C.; Dobre, A.; Weiss, T.; Zarkovic, N. Perioperative application of the Viscum album extract Isorel in digestive tract cancer patients. *Anticancer Res.* **2005**, *25*, 4583–4590.
9. Jurin, M.; Zarkovic, N.; Borovic, S.; Kissel, D. Viscum album L. preparation Isorel modifies the immune response in normal and in tumour-bearing mice. *Anti-Cancer Drugs* **1997**, *8* (Suppl. S1), S27–S31. [CrossRef]

10. Mueller, E.A.; Anderer, F.A. AViscum album oligosaccharide activating human natural cytotoxicity is an interferon γ inducer. *Cancer Immunol. Immunother.* **1990**, *32*, 221–227. [CrossRef]
11. Kim, J.C.; Yoon, T.J.; Song, T.; Kim, Y.H.; An, H.S.; Kim, J.B. ucosal Immunoadjuvant Activity of Korean Mistletoe Lectin-C. *Korean J. Food Sci. Technol.* **2011**, *43*, 72–76. [CrossRef]
12. Lee, J.L.; Jeon, Y.H.; Yang, H.S.; Lee, K.B.; Song, K.S.; Kang, T.B.; Kim, J.B.; Yoo, Y.C. The immunostimulatory activity of the water-extract of Korean mistletoe fruit to activate murine peritoneal macrophages. *Kor. J. Pharmacogn.* **2010**, *41*, 122–129.
13. Lee, S.-j.; Lee, M.K.; Choi, G.-P.; Yu, C.Y.; Roh, S.-K.; Kim, J.-D.; Lee, H.Y.; Lee, J.-H. Growth enhancement and cytotoxicity of Korean mistletoe fractions on human cell lines. *Korean J. Med. Crop Sci.* **2003**, *11*, 62–70.
14. Melo, M.N.O.; Oliveira, A.P.; Wiecikowski, A.F.; Carvalho, R.S.; Castro, J.L.; de Oliveira, F.A.G.; Pereira, H.M.G.; da Veiga, V.F.; Capella, M.M.A.; Rocha, L.; et al. Phenolic compounds from Viscum album tinctures enhanced antitumor activity in melanoma murine cancer cells. *Saudi Pharm. J.* **2018**, *26*, 311–322. [CrossRef] [PubMed]
15. Yoon, T.J.; Yoo, Y.C.; Kang, T.B.; Song, S.K.; Lee, K.B.; Her, E.; Song, K.S.; Kim, J.B. Antitumor activity of the Korean mistletoe lectin is attributed to activation of macrophages and NK cells. *Arch. Pharm. Res.* **2003**, *26*, 861–867. [CrossRef] [PubMed]
16. Nielsen, T.O.; Hsu, F.D.; Jensen, K.; Cheang, M.; Karaca, G.; Hu, Z.; Hernandez-Boussard, T.; Livasy, C.; Cowan, D.; Dressler, L.; et al. Immunohistochemical and clinical characterization of the basal-like subtype of invasive breast carcinoma. *Clin. Cancer Res.* **2004**, *10*, 5367–5374. [CrossRef]
17. Choi, Y.K.; Cho, S.G.; Woo, S.M.; Yun, Y.J.; Park, S.; Shin, Y.C.; Ko, S.G. Herbal extract SH003 suppresses tumor growth and metastasis of MDA-MB-231 breast cancer cells by inhibiting STAT3-IL-6 signaling. *Mediators Inflamm.* **2014**, *2014*, 492173. [CrossRef]
18. Noori, S.; Rezaei Tavirani, M.; Deravi, N.; Mahboobi Rabbani, M.I.; Zarghi, A. Naringenin Enhances the Anti-Cancer Effect of Cyclophosphamide against MDA-MB-231 Breast Cancer Cells Via Targeting the STAT3 Signaling Pathway. *Iran J. Pharm. Res.* **2020**, *19*, 122–133. [CrossRef]
19. Adams, L.S.; Phung, S.; Yee, N.; Seeram, N.P.; Li, L.; Chen, S. Blueberry phytochemicals inhibit growth and metastatic potential of MDA-MB-231 breast cancer cells through modulation of the phosphatidylinositol 3-kinase pathway. *Cancer Res.* **2010**, *70*, 3594–3605. [CrossRef]
20. Gurunathan, S.; Han, J.W.; Eppakayala, V.; Jeyaraj, M.; Kim, J.H. Cytotoxicity of biologically synthesized silver nanoparticles in MDA-MB-231 human breast cancer cells. *Biomed Res. Int.* **2013**, *2013*, 535796. [CrossRef] [PubMed]
21. Bäuerle, T.; Adwan, H.; Kiessling, F.; Hilbig, H.; Armbruster, F.P.; Berger, M.R. Characterization of a rat model with site-specific bone metastasis induced by MDA-MB-231 breast cancer cells and its application to the effects of an antibody against bone sialoprotein. *Int. J. Cancer* **2005**, *115*, 177–186. [CrossRef] [PubMed]
22. Adams, L.S.; Kanaya, N.; Phung, S.; Liu, Z.; Chen, S. Whole blueberry powder modulates the growth and metastasis of MDA-MB-231 triple negative breast tumors in nude mice. *J. Nutr.* **2011**, *141*, 1805–1812. [CrossRef]
23. Lee, Y.J.; Lin, W.L.; Chen, N.F.; Chuang, S.K.; Tseng, T.H. Demethylwedelolactone derivatives inhibit invasive growth in vitro and lung metastasis of MDA-MB-231 breast cancer cells in nude mice. *Eur. J. Med. Chem.* **2012**, *56*, 361–367. [CrossRef]
24. An, J.; Wang, L.; Zhao, Y.; Hao, Q.; Zhang, Y.; Zhang, J.; Yang, C.; Liu, L.; Wang, W.; Fang, D.; et al. Effects of FSTL1 on cell proliferation in breast cancer cell line MDA-MB-231 and its brain metastatic variant MDA-MB-231-BR. *Oncol. Rep.* **2017**, *38*, 3001–3010. [CrossRef] [PubMed]
25. Dent, R.; Hanna, W.M.; Trudeau, M.; Rawlinson, E.; Sun, P.; Narod, S.A. Pattern of metastatic spread in triple-negative breast cancer. *Breast Cancer Res. Treat.* **2009**, *115*, 423–428. [CrossRef] [PubMed]
26. Wang, S.J.; Saadi, W.; Lin, F.; Minh-Canh Nguyen, C.; Li Jeon, N. Differential effects of EGF gradient profiles on MDA-MB-231 breast cancer cell chemotaxis. *Exp. Cell Res.* **2004**, *300*, 180–189. [CrossRef]
27. Place, A.E.; Jin Huh, S.; Polyak, K. The microenvironment in breast cancer progression: Biology and implications for treatment. *Breast Cancer Res.* **2011**, *13*, 227. [CrossRef]
28. Lu, X.; Yang, R.; Zhang, L.; Xi, Y.; Zhao, J.; Wang, F.; Zhang, H.; Li, Z. Macrophage Colony-stimulating Factor Mediates the Recruitment of Macrophages in Triple negative Breast Cancer. *Int. J. Biol. Sci.* **2019**, *15*, 2859–2871. [CrossRef]
29. Lopez-Yrigoyen, M.; Cassetta, L.; Pollard, J.W. Macrophage targeting in cancer. *Ann. N. Y. Acad. Sci.* **2021**, *1499*, 18–41. [CrossRef]
30. Park, H.J.; Chi, G.Y.; Choi, Y.H.; Park, S.H. The root bark of Morus alba L. regulates tumor-associated macrophages by blocking recruitment and M2 polarization of macrophages. *Phytother. Res.* **2020**, *34*, 3333–3344. [CrossRef]
31. Thabet, N.A.; El-Guendy, N.; Mohamed, M.M.; Shouman, S.A. Suppression of macrophages- Induced inflammation via targeting RAS and PAR-4 signaling in breast cancer cell lines. *Toxicol. Appl. Pharmacol.* **2019**, *385*, 114773. [CrossRef] [PubMed]
32. Multhoff, G.; Molls, M.; Radons, J. Chronic inflammation in cancer development. *Front. Immunol.* **2011**, *2*, 98. [CrossRef]
33. Zhao, L.; Zhang, C. Berberine Inhibits MDA-MB-231 Cells by Attenuating Their Inflammatory Responses. *Biomed Res. Int.* **2020**, *2020*, 3617514. [CrossRef]
34. Lee, H.S.; Seo, E.Y.; Kang, N.E.; Kim, W.K. [6]-Gingerol inhibits metastasis of MDA-MB-231 human breast cancer cells. *J. Nutr. Biochem.* **2008**, *19*, 313–319. [CrossRef]
35. Huynh, J.; Chand, A.; Gough, D.; Ernst, M. Therapeutically exploiting STAT3 activity in cancer—Using tissue repair as a road map. *Nat. Rev. Cancer* **2019**, *19*, 82–96. [CrossRef]
36. Santoni, M.; Conti, A.; Piva, F.; Massari, F.; Ciccarese, C.; Burattini, L.; Cheng, L.; Lopez-Beltran, A.; Scarpelli, M.; Santini, D.; et al. Role of STAT3 pathway in genitourinary tumors. *Future Sci. OA* **2015**, *1*, Fso15. [CrossRef]

37. Siveen, K.S.; Sikka, S.; Surana, R.; Dai, X.; Zhang, J.; Kumar, A.P.; Tan, B.K.; Sethi, G.; Bishayee, A. Targeting the STAT3 signaling pathway in cancer: Role of synthetic and natural inhibitors. *Biochim. Biophys. Acta* **2014**, *1845*, 136–154. [CrossRef] [PubMed]
38. Byun, H.J.; Darvin, P.; Kang, D.Y.; Sp, N.; Joung, Y.H.; Park, J.H.; Kim, S.J.; Yang, Y.M. Silibinin downregulates MMP2 expression via Jak2/STAT3 pathway and inhibits the migration and invasive potential in MDA-MB-231 cells. *Oncol. Rep.* **2017**, *37*, 3270–3278. [CrossRef]
39. Sun, Y.S.; Zhao, Z.; Yang, Z.N.; Xu, F.; Lu, H.J.; Zhu, Z.Y.; Shi, W.; Jiang, J.; Yao, P.P.; Zhu, H.P. Risk Factors and Preventions of Breast Cancer. *Int. J. Biol. Sci.* **2017**, *13*, 1387–1397. [CrossRef] [PubMed]
40. O'Shaughnessy, J. Extending survival with chemotherapy in metastatic breast cancer. *Oncologist* **2005**, *10* (Suppl. S3), 20–29. [CrossRef]
41. Beberok, A.; Wrześniok, D.; Rok, J.; Rzepka, Z.; Respondek, M.; Buszman, E. Ciprofloxacin triggers the apoptosis of human triple-negative breast cancer MDA-MB-231 cells via the p53/Bax/Bcl-2 signaling pathway. *Int. J. Oncol.* **2018**, *52*, 1727–1737. [CrossRef]
42. Czabotar, P.E.; Westphal, D.; Dewson, G.; Ma, S.; Hockings, C.; Fairlie, W.D.; Lee, E.F.; Yao, S.; Robin, A.Y.; Smith, B.J.; et al. Bax crystal structures reveal how BH3 domains activate Bax and nucleate its oligomerization to induce apoptosis. *Cell* **2013**, *152*, 519–531. [CrossRef] [PubMed]
43. Gillies, L.A.; Kuwana, T. Apoptosis regulation at the mitochondrial outer membrane. *J. Cell. Biochem.* **2014**, *115*, 632–640. [CrossRef]
44. Lindholm, D.; Eriksson, O.; Korhonen, L. Mitochondrial proteins in neuronal degeneration. *Biochem. Biophys. Res. Commun.* **2004**, *321*, 753–758. [CrossRef] [PubMed]
45. Jeong, J.W.; Baek, J.Y.; Kim, K.D.; Choi, Y.H.; Lee, J.D. Induction of apoptosis by pachymic acid in T24 human bladder cancer cells. *J. Life Sci. (Calicut)* **2015**, *1*, 93–100. [CrossRef]
46. McConkey, D.J. Biochemical determinants of apoptosis and necrosis. *Toxicol. Lett.* **1998**, *99*, 157–168. [CrossRef]
47. Lambert, A.W.; Pattabiraman, D.R.; Weinberg, R.A. Emerging Biological Principles of Metastasis. *Cell* **2017**, *168*, 670–691. [CrossRef] [PubMed]
48. Nordin, F.J.; Pearanpan, L.; Chan, K.M.; Kumolosasi, E.; Yong, Y.K.; Shaari, K.; Rajab, N.F. Immunomodulatory potential of Clinacanthus nutans extracts in the co-culture of triple-negative breast cancer cells, MDA-MB-231, and THP-1 macrophages. *PLoS ONE* **2021**, *16*, e0256012. [CrossRef]
49. Ko, Y.S.; Lee, W.S.; Panchanathan, R.; Joo, Y.N.; Choi, Y.H.; Kim, G.S.; Jung, J.M.; Ryu, C.H.; Shin, S.C.; Kim, H.J. Polyphenols from Artemisia annua L Inhibit Adhesion and EMT of Highly Metastatic Breast Cancer Cells MDA-MB-231. *Phytother. Res.* **2016**, *30*, 1180–1188. [CrossRef]
50. Olmeda, D.; Moreno-Bueno, G.; Flores, J.M.; Fabra, A.; Portillo, F.; Cano, A. SNAI1 is required for tumor growth and lymph node metastasis of human breast carcinoma MDA-MB-231 cells. *Cancer Res.* **2007**, *67*, 11721–11731. [CrossRef]
51. Ameri, K.; Luong, R.; Zhang, H.; Powell, A.A.; Montgomery, K.D.; Espinosa, I.; Bouley, D.M.; Harris, A.L.; Jeffrey, S.S. Circulating tumour cells demonstrate an altered response to hypoxia and an aggressive phenotype. *Br. J. Cancer* **2010**, *102*, 561–569. [CrossRef] [PubMed]
52. Kamran, M.Z.; Patil, P.; Gude, R.P. Role of STAT3 in cancer metastasis and translational advances. *Biomed Res. Int.* **2013**, *2013*, 421821. [CrossRef]
53. Parsons, S.L.; Watson, S.A.; Brown, P.D.; Collins, H.M.; Steele, R.J. Matrix metalloproteinases. *Br. J. Surg.* **1997**, *84*, 160–166. [PubMed]
54. De Craene, B.; Berx, G. Regulatory networks defining EMT during cancer initiation and progression. *Nat. Rev. Cancer* **2013**, *13*, 97–110. [CrossRef] [PubMed]
55. Akram, M.; Iqbal, M.; Daniyal, M.; Khan, A.U. Awareness and current knowledge of breast cancer. *Biol. Res.* **2017**, *50*, 33. [CrossRef]
56. Cheng, M.; Liu, P.; Xu, L.X. Iron promotes breast cancer cell migration via IL-6/JAK2/STAT3 signaling pathways in a paracrine or autocrine IL-6-rich inflammatory environment. *J. Inorg. Biochem.* **2020**, *210*, 111159. [CrossRef]
57. Büssing, A.; Raak, C.; Ostermann, T. Quality of life and related dimensions in cancer patients treated with mistletoe extract (iscador): A meta-analysis. *Evid. Based Complement. Alternat. Med.* **2012**, *2012*, 219402. [CrossRef]
58. Mantovani, A.; Allavena, P.; Marchesi, F.; Garlanda, C. Macrophages as tools and targets in cancer therapy. *Nat. Rev. Drug Discov.* **2022**, *21*, 799–820. [CrossRef]
59. Marvibaigi, M.; Amini, N.; Supriyanto, E.; Abdul Majid, F.A.; Kumar Jaganathan, S.; Jamil, S.; Hamzehalipour Almaki, J.; Nasiri, R. Antioxidant Activity and ROS-Dependent Apoptotic Effect of Scurrula ferruginea (Jack) Danser Methanol Extract in Human Breast Cancer Cell MDA-MB-231. *PLoS ONE* **2016**, *11*, e0158942. [CrossRef]
60. Goda, M.S.; Elhady, S.S.; Nafie, M.S.; Bogari, H.A.; Malatani, R.T.; Hareeri, R.H.; Badr, J.M.; Donia, M.S. Phragmanthera austroarabica A.G.Mill. and J.A.Nyberg Triggers Apoptosis in MDA-MB-231 Cells In Vitro and In Vivo Assays: Simultaneous Determination of Selected Constituents. *Metabolites* **2022**, *12*, 921. [CrossRef]
61. Mishra, R.; Sharma, S.; Sharma, R.S.; Singh, S.; Sardesai, M.M.; Sharma, S.; Mishra, V. Viscum articulatum Burm. f. aqueous extract exerts antiproliferative effect and induces cell cycle arrest and apoptosis in leukemia cells. *J. Ethnopharmacol.* **2018**, *219*, 91–102. [CrossRef] [PubMed]

62. Iwashima, T.; Kudome, Y.; Kishimoto, Y.; Saita, E.; Tanaka, M.; Taguchi, C.; Hirakawa, S.; Mitani, N.; Kondo, K.; Iida, K. Aronia berry extract inhibits TNF-α-induced vascular endothelial inflammation through the regulation of STAT3. *Food Nutr. Res.* **2019**, *63*. [CrossRef] [PubMed]
63. Faggioli, L.; Costanzo, C.; Merola, M.; Bianchini, E.; Furia, A.; Carsana, A.; Palmieri, M. Nuclear factor kappa B (NF-kappa B), nuclear factor interleukin-6 (NFIL-6 or C/EBP beta) and nuclear factor interleukin-6 beta (NFIL6-beta or C/EBP delta) are not sufficient to activate the endogenous interleukin-6 gene in the human breast carcinoma cell line MCF-7. Comparative analysis with MDA-MB-231 cells, an interleukin-6-expressing human breast carcinoma cell line. *Eur. J. Biochem.* **1996**, *239*, 624–631. [CrossRef] [PubMed]
64. Suarez-Cuervo, C.; Harris, K.W.; Kallman, L.; Väänänen, H.K.; Selander, K.S. Tumor necrosis factor-alpha induces interleukin-6 production via extracellular-regulated kinase 1 activation in breast cancer cells. *Breast Cancer Res. Treat.* **2003**, *80*, 71–78. [CrossRef] [PubMed]
65. Moriguchi, M.; Yamada, M.; Miake, Y.; Yanagisawa, T. Transforming growth factor β inducible apoptotic cascade in epithelial cells during rat molar tooth eruptions. *Anat. Sci. Int.* **2010**, *85*, 92–101. [CrossRef]
66. Tewari, D.; Priya, A.; Bishayee, A.; Bishayee, A. Targeting transforming growth factor-β signalling for cancer prevention and intervention: Recent advances in developing small molecules of natural origin. *Clin. Transl. Med.* **2022**, *12*, e795. [CrossRef]
67. Chen, S.; Yang, J.; Wei, Y.; Wei, X. Epigenetic regulation of macrophages: From homeostasis maintenance to host defense. *Cell. Mol. Immunol.* **2020**, *17*, 36–49. [CrossRef]
68. Coeugniet, E.G.; Elek, E. Immunomodulation with Viscum album and Echinacea purpurea extracts. *Onkologie* **1987**, *10*, 27–33. [CrossRef]
69. Elluru, S.; Duong Van Huyen, J.P.; Delignat, S.; Prost, F.; Bayry, J.; Kazatchkine, M.D.; Kaveri, S.V. Molecular mechanisms underlying the immunomodulatory effects of mistletoe (Viscum album L.) extracts Iscador. *Arzneimittelforschung* **2006**, *56*, 461–466. [CrossRef]
70. Heiny, B.M.; Beuth, J. Mistletoe extract standardized for the galactoside-specific lectin (ML-1) induces beta-endorphin release and immunopotentiation in breast cancer patients. *Anticancer Res.* **1994**, *14*, 1339–1342.
71. Boatright, K.M.; Salvesen, G.S. Mechanisms of caspase activation. *Curr. Opin. Cell Biol.* **2003**, *15*, 725–731. [CrossRef] [PubMed]
72. Park, S.-Y.; Kim, E.-J.; Lim, D.; Kim, J.-S.; Lim, S.; Shin, H.-K.; Park, J.-H. Inhibitory Effect of the Hexane Extract of Saussurea lappa on the Growth of LNCaP Human Prostate Cancer Cells. *J. Korean Soc. Food Sci. Nutr.* **2008**, *37*, 8–15. [CrossRef]
73. Kamada, S.; Kikkawa, U.; Tsujimoto, Y.; Hunter, T. Nuclear translocation of caspase-3 is dependent on its proteolytic activation and recognition of a substrate-like protein(s). *J. Biol. Chem.* **2005**, *280*, 857–860. [CrossRef] [PubMed]
74. Cui, Q.; Yu, J.H.; Wu, J.N.; Tashiro, S.; Onodera, S.; Minami, M.; Ikejima, T. P53-mediated cell cycle arrest and apoptosis through a caspase-3- independent, but caspase-9-dependent pathway in oridonin-treated MCF-7 human breast cancer cells. *Acta Pharmacol. Sin.* **2007**, *28*, 1057–1066. [CrossRef] [PubMed]
75. Khan, N.; Mukhtar, H. Cancer and metastasis: Prevention and treatment by green tea. *Cancer Metastasis Rev.* **2010**, *29*, 435–445. [CrossRef] [PubMed]
76. Yang, Z.; Garcia, A.; Xu, S.; Powell, D.R.; Vertino, P.M.; Singh, S.; Marcus, A.I. Withania somnifera root extract inhibits mammary cancer metastasis and epithelial to mesenchymal transition. *PLoS ONE* **2013**, *8*, e75069. [CrossRef] [PubMed]
77. VanSaun, M.N.; Matrisian, L.M. Matrix metalloproteinases and cellular motility in development and disease. *Birth Defects Res. C Embryo Today* **2006**, *78*, 69–79. [CrossRef]
78. Chambers, A.F.; Matrisian, L.M. Changing views of the role of matrix metalloproteinases in metastasis. *J. Natl. Cancer Inst.* **1997**, *89*, 1260–1270. [CrossRef]
79. Itoh, T.; Tanioka, M.; Matsuda, H.; Nishimoto, H.; Yoshioka, T.; Suzuki, R.; Uehira, M. Experimental metastasis is suppressed in MMP-9-deficient mice. *Clin. Exp. Metastasis* **1999**, *17*, 177–181. [CrossRef]
80. Shay, G.; Lynch, C.C.; Fingleton, B. Moving targets: Emerging roles for MMPs in cancer progression and metastasis. *Matrix Biol.* **2015**, *44–46*, 200–206. [CrossRef]
81. Kienle, G.S.; Kiene, H. Complementary cancer therapy: A systematic review of prospective clinical trials on anthroposophic mistletoe extracts. *Eur. J. Med. Res.* **2007**, *12*, 103–119. [PubMed]

molecules

MDPI

Review

Molecular Mechanism of Tanshinone against Prostate Cancer

Wei Li †, Tao Huang †, Shenghan Xu †, Bangwei Che, Ying Yu, Wenjun Zhang and Kaifa Tang *

Department of Urology, The Affiliated Hospital of Guizhou Medical University, Guiyang 550004, China
* Correspondence: tangkaifa@gmc.edu.cn
† These authors contributed equally to this work.

Abstract: Prostate cancer (PCa) is the most common malignant tumor of the male urinary system in Europe and America. According to the data in the World Cancer Report 2020, the incidence rate of PCa ranks second in the prevalence of male malignant tumors and varies worldwide between regions and population groups. Although early PCa can achieve good therapeutic results after surgical treatment, due to advanced PCa, it can adapt and tolerate androgen castration-related drugs through a variety of mechanisms. For this reason, it is often difficult to achieve effective therapeutic results in the treatment of advanced PCa. Tanshinone is a new fat-soluble phenanthraquinone compound derived from Salvia miltiorrhiza that can play a therapeutic role in different cancers, including PCa. Several studies have shown that Tanshinone can target various molecular pathways of PCa, including the signal transducer and activator of transcription 3 (STAT3) pathway, androgen receptor (AR) pathway, phosphatidylinositol-3-kinase (PI3K)/protein kinase B (Akt)/mammalian target of rapamycin (mTOR) pathway, and mitogen-activated protein kinase (MAPK) pathway, which will affect the release of pro-inflammatory cytokines and affect cell proliferation, apoptosis, tumor metabolism, genomic stability, and tumor drug resistance. Thus, the occurrence and development of PCa cells are inhibited. In this review, we summarized the in vivo and in vitro evidence of Tanshinone against prostate cancer and discussed the effect of Tanshinone on nuclear factor kappa-B (NF-κB), AR, and mTOR. At the same time, we conducted a network pharmacology analysis on the four main components of Tanshinone to further screen the possible targets of Tanshinone against prostate cancer and provide ideas for future research.

Keywords: prostate cancer; Tanshinone; mTOR; Apoptosis; NF-κB

Citation: Li, W.; Huang, T.; Xu, S.; Che, B.; Yu, Y.; Zhang, W.; Tang, K. Molecular Mechanism of Tanshinone against Prostate Cancer. *Molecules* **2022**, 27, 5597. https://doi.org/10.3390/molecules27175594

Academic Editor: Saverio Bettuzzi

Received: 18 July 2022
Accepted: 22 August 2022
Published: 30 August 2022

1. Introduction

1.1. Current Status of PCa

PCa is the most common malignant tumor in the urinary system of men in Europe and the United States. According to the data of the World Cancer Report 2020, the number of new cases of PCa registered globally was 1,414,259, ranking second in the prevalence of male malignant tumors [1], with the highest incidence in Oceania and North America, followed by Europe. Rates in Africa and Asia are lower than in developed countries. In PCa, the incubation period is very long and is usually diagnosed in older men. At the time of diagnosis, about 90% of PCa is organ-confined or locally advanced [2,3]. Localized PCa is treated with active monitoring and local radiotherapy or resection of the prostate to achieve good treatment effects, but with the progression of the disease, advanced PCa can only be treated with surgery or chemical castration of androgen deprivation therapy (ADT), but most patients develop ADT resistance and progress to castration-resistant PCa (CRPC) in about 18 to 36 months, and once progress to CRPC is made, existing drugs and methods are often difficult to obtain effective results [4]. At the same time, the treatment of advanced PCa is still troubled by the highly toxic side effects of synthetic drugs [5]. Therefore, there is an urgent need to develop a new drug that is safe, effective, affordable, and easy to manufacture to treat androgen-independent PCa (AIPC). In recent years, natural products from fungi, plants, and animals for medical trends are emerging. Medicinal plants used for the purpose of health care in the world have increased dramatically. This is mainly because they have definite efficacy and low toxicity. In fact, more than half of the currently available drugs come from natural products [6].

1.2. The Basic Introduction of Tanshinone

Tanshinone is the fat-soluble component of the active ingredient of Salvia miltiorrhiza. Since the Japanese scholar Nakao first isolated Tanshinone IIA from salvia miltiorrhiza and identified its chemical structure in 1934, with the development of clinical application of salvia miltiorrhiza and the progress of extraction and separation technology in traditional Chinese medicine, the specific composition of Tanshinone has gradually become clear. So far, more than 40 Tanshinones have been isolated from salvia miltiorrhizae, among which the most important ones are Tanshinone I (TsI), Tanshinone II A (Ts II A), Dihydrotanshinone I (DHTI) and Cryptotanshinone (CYT) (Figure 1) [7,8]. The main precursor of Tanshinone biosynthesis is geraniyldiphosphate (GPP), which is derived from mevalproic acid and the 2-c-methyl-d-erythritol 4-phosphate pathway. GPP is eventually converted into Tanshinone through a series of downstream enzymes involved in various steps of catalytic biosynthesis [9,10]. Tanshinone has powerful pharmacological effects with anti-inflammatory, antioxidant stress, and anti-metabolic syndrome, and its water-soluble derivative, Tanshinone SODIUM IIA sulfonate, has been widely used in the clinical treatment of cardiovascular diseases [11]. Interestingly, more and more studies have reported the anti-tumor potential of Tanshinone, and previous studies have shown that Tanshinone can inhibit the proliferation, metastasis, and progression of various cancer cells (including PCa) by regulating transcription and growth factors, inflammatory cytokines, and intracellular signaling pathways [12,13]. Interestingly, a growing number of studies report the effects of Tanshinone on PCa cells. These studies shed light on their mechanisms of action and their potential as anti-PCa drugs. Here, we review the available evidence for Tanshinone against PCa and the molecular targets of its action.

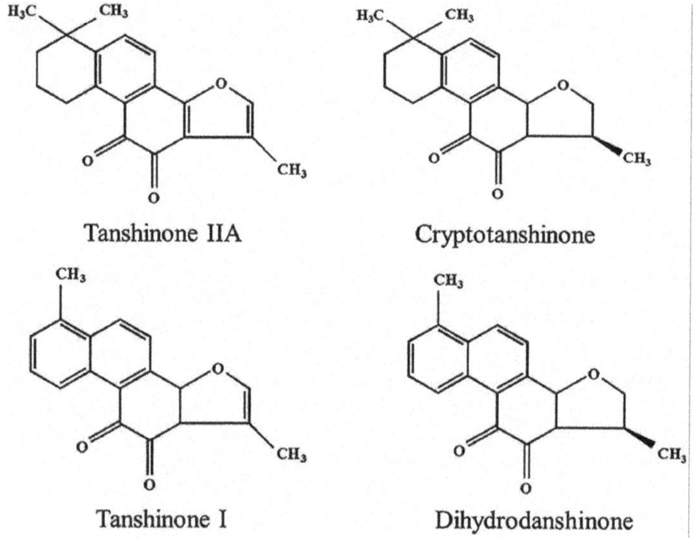

Figure 1. Chemical structures of four Tanshinone monomers.

1.3. Comparison of Main Components of Tanshinone

Tanshinones are uniquely characterized by the presence of 14,16-ether D rings, such as CYT and DHTI, but this heterocycle is usually further converted to furan, as in TsI and TsIIA [14,15]. Tanshinone generally consists of four rings, including naphthalene or tetrahydronaphthalene rings A and B, a normal or paraquinone or lactone ring C, and a furan or dihydrofuran ring D [15,16]. Just as A, B, C, and D rings as shown in the above figure (Figure 1). Obviously, although the molecular skeleton of the four main components of Tanshinone is similar, the groups, group positions, and double bond positions are slightly different.

Secondly, there are some differences in the pharmacokinetics of Tanshinone in vivo, but generally speaking, all Tanshinones, whether oral administration, intravenous administration, subcutaneous injection, or conventional delivery, all have the characteristics of short half-life and low bioavailability [17,18]. Interestingly, there seems to be a certain synergistic effect among the components of Tanshinone. Multiple components of Tanshinone given together can improve the bioavailability of some components, such as Tanshinone IIA and Tanshinone I, which indicates that drug interactions occur among the components of Tanshinone [19]. Tanshinone pharmacokinetics have been well summarized in previous work [20,21]. In addition, the metabolism of different types of Tanshinone in vivo is also different. It is reported that the metabolism of Tanshinones mainly depends on their saturation and substituents in their skeletons. For example, the main metabolic pathway of CYT with saturated A and D rings is dehydrogenation; DHTI with saturated D rings is mainly metabolized by D ring hydrolysis; and hydroxylation is the main metabolic pathway of TsIIA with saturated A rings [22].

In addition, there are differences among Tanshinone components in terms of antitumor pharmacological characteristics, and the conformational relationships show that the pharmacological effects of Tanshinone depend mainly on its D-ring (furan/dihydrofuran) and steroidal structure [14,23], and it has been reported that during the antitumor response, DNA molecules bind to the phenanthrene ring structure of Tanshinone, which in turn affects the synthesis of tumor DNA, while the furan ring and steroidal structure also generate free radicals, which in turn impede DNA synthesis in tumor cells [24,25]. In addition, the antioxidant effect of Tanshinone is also dependent on the D-ring, and changes in the structure of the D-ring can often affect the antioxidant capacity of Tanshinone. For example, Tanshinone containing the dihydrofuran D-ring has a stronger antioxidant capacity than those containing the furan D-ring [26], which is also reflected in the antitumor pharmacological effect. TsIIA's tumor suppressive effect, for example, is primarily dependent on the PI3K/AKT/mTOR signaling pathway and the JNK pathway, whereas CYT is more dependent on State3-mediated anti-tumor effects and has stronger immunomodulatory effects than the other three components [27–29].

In addition, the antitumor potency of Tanshinone components differed among them, and the potency (either induction of apoptosis, inhibition of invasion, or inhibition of proliferation) among the components of Tanshinone was reported to be TsI > TsIIA > CYT in all three prostate cancer cell lines, whether DU145, PC3, or LNCaP [30], which may be partly due to the stronger anti-vascular activity of TsI. In addition, CYT appears to have a stronger anti-androgenic effect, but interestingly, the toxic effect of CYT on DU145 is more enhanced than that of LNCaP [31], suggesting that CYT may be more dependent on other pathways in prostate cancer.

1.4. Tanshinone and PCa

In a recent population-based retrospective study of 40,692 men diagnosed with PCa, the protective effect of salvia miltiorrhiza on PCa was confirmed by a 5–10% increase in survival rates among men who took salvia miltiorrhiza compared with those who did not. This protective effect is positively correlated with the dose and time of salvia miltiorrhiza use [32]. However, unfortunately, there is only one study on clinical evidence of salvia miltiorrhiza and PCa at present, and in this study, the experimenters also did not further verify whether the intake of salvia miltiorrhiza could inhibit the occurrence of castration-resistant PCa, the occurrence of biochemical recurrence of PCa after radical prostatectomy, and the increase in the aggressivity of PCa.

However, there are many in vitro studies on Tanshinone and PCa cell lines. Human PCa cells: LNCaP, PC3, DU145, and 22RV1, which are commonly used as cell models for PCa in vitro experiments, have different characteristics, respectively. For example, LNCaP has functional ARs, so it is sensitive to androgen and secretes prostate-specific antigen (PSA). 22RV1 cells were androgen-sensitive but not androgen-dependent and showed low aggressiveness.PC3 cells do not depend on androgens, are highly invasive, and have a strong potential for metastasis.DU145 cells are also androgen-independent cells with strong proliferation ability but only moderate metastasis ability [33]. In these in vitro experiments, the researchers pretreated PCa cell lines with varying biological characteristics with a specific concentration of Tanshinone and then used various modern molecular biological methods to identify proteins involved in the cell cycle, apoptosis, growth, and metastasis. Finally, they confirmed that Tanshinone in vitro by adjusting the related protein expression and signaling pathway in PCa cells induced the stagnation of the cell cycle and apoptosis, inhibiting metastasis and invasion of tumor cells (Figure 2). We put the current relevant Tanshinone in vitro effect on Pca-related research summarized in Table 1.

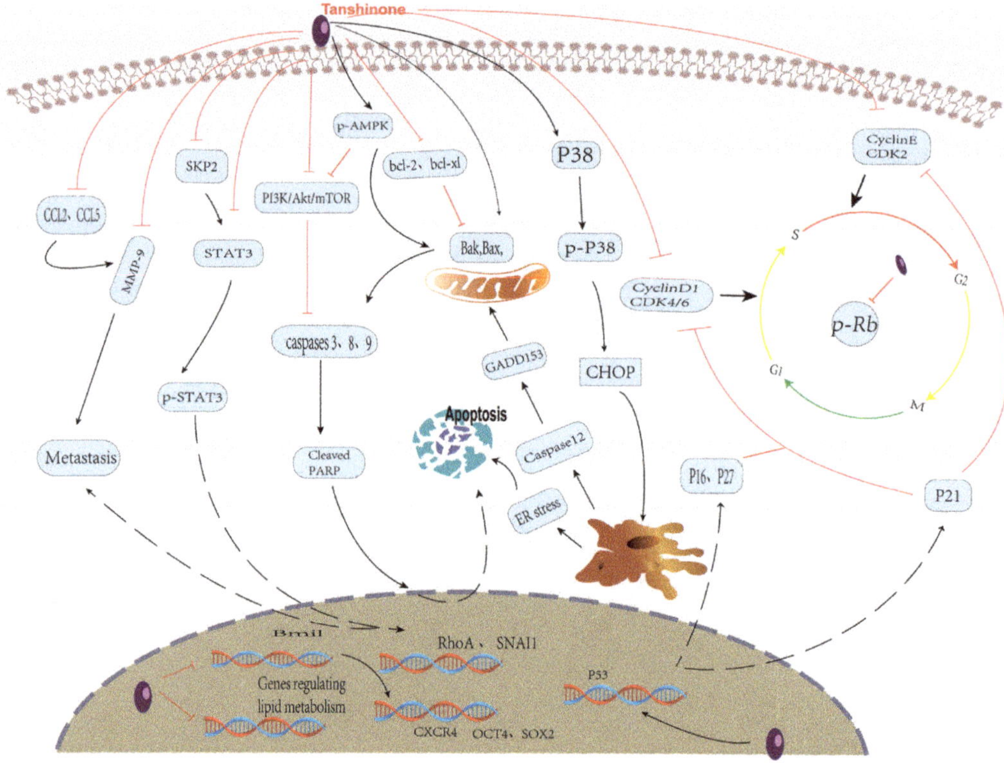

Figure 2. Effect of Tanshinone on prostate cancer. induced by Tanshinone are noted by using →, while the inhibition represented by ⊣ symbol.

Similarly, in vivo experiments with Tanshinone against PCa are also under way. In the experiments, the researchers transplanted human PCa cells (LNCaP, PC3, and 22Rv1) subcutaneously or in situ into immunodeficient mice that did not reject human cells to establish animal models. Finally, it was confirmed that Tanshinone could effectively inhibit the growth of tumors in vivo, whether injected orally or subcutaneously/intraperitoneally. It is worth noting that in the current animal experiment, it has not been observed that the activity of Tanshinone on other organs and tissues, except tumor tissues, has toxic effects. Table 2 summarizes the current state of Tanshinone and PCa in vivo research.

Table 1. Tanshinone and PCa in vitro.

Compound	Dose	Cell	Mechanism	Reference
TsIIA	0, 1.25, 2.5, 5, 10 uM	LNCaP	Cell cycle arrest and apoptosis are induced by the activation of P53 (dose-dependent).	[34]
TsIIA	5 μM	PC-3	Induced autophagy and apoptosis	[35]
TsIIA	20 umol/L	LNCaP, PC3	enhancing the effect of the anti-tumor activity of cisplatin.	[36]
TsIIA	0, 40, 80 μM	PC-3	Inducing autophagy by up-regulated expression of microtubule-associated protein light chain 3 (LC3) II	[37]
TsIIA	10, 25, 50 uM	LNCaP, PC-3	inducing mitochondrial-dependent cell apoptosis by inhibiting PIK3/AKT	[38]
TsIIA	2.5, 5 μg/ml	LNCaP	Induced apoptosis and induced cell cycle arrest by endoplasmic reticulum stress	[39]
TsIIA	—	LNCaP	Cell proliferation was inhibited by inhibiting the AR signal.	[40]
TsIIA	—	—	Maspin expression was induced, AR expression was inhibited, and apoptosis was induced.	[41]
TsIIAD	2.5 μM	PC3	Binding NQO1 protein causes cell cycle arrest and apoptosis.	[42]
CYT	10 umol/L	DU145	Apoptosis was induced and the expression of isomucin was inhibited by inhibiting the PI3K/AKT signaling pathway.	[43]
CYT	10 μM	LNCaP, 22Rv1, and PC3	The activity and expression of AR were inhibited by inhibiting LSD1-mediated H3K9 demethylation.	[44]
CYT	1.0 ug/ml	DU145	To activate Fas-mediated apoptosis	[45]
CYT	0.5 μM	LNCaP, 22Rv1	Cell proliferation was inhibited by inhibiting AR expression and activity.	[46]
CYT	1.5 μM	LNCaP	Tumor-initiating cells are influenced by down-regulating dry gene expression.	[47]
CYT	5, 10 μM	DU145, LNCaP, and PC-3	Inhibiting HIF-1 and AEG-1 inhibits angiogenesis and induces cell cycle arrest and apoptosis.	[31]
CYT	10 μM	PC3	Cell proliferation is inhibited by decreasing the stability and expression of DNA topoisomerase 2.	[48]
CYT	5 uM	22Rv1 and PC-3	AR expression and activity were reduced, and MMP9 secretion was also reduced.	[49]
CYT	0–40 μM	DU145	Apoptosis was induced by inhibiting phosphorylation of mTOR and Rb.	[50]
CYT	7 μmol/L	DU145	Inhibition of STAT3Tyr705 and its upstream tyrosine kinase induces cell cycle arrest and apoptosis.	[51]
TsI	20, 40, 80 μM	PC-3, DU145	Apoptosis is induced by upregulation of microRNA135A-3p and death receptor 5.	[52]
TsI	3–6 μM	PC-3, LNCaP, and DU-145	inhibiting angiogenesis and inducing apoptosis by down-regulating AuroraA expression.	[30]
DHT	5–10 μM	PC-3, DU145, and 22Rv1	inhibiting EMT by inhibition of the CCL2/STAT3 axis	[34]
DHT	0.1 ug/mL and 1.5 ug/mL	DU145	Inducing cell cycle arrest by activating the ER pathway	[53]
TsD	3, 6, 12 μM	PC3, LNCAP	Inducing cell cycle arrest and apoptosis	[54]
TsD	2 μM	LNCaP, C4-2	AR expression and activity were reduced, and cell proliferation was slowed.	[55]
SME	3.125, 12.5, 25 and 50 μg/mL	DU-145	Cell cycle arrest and apoptosis are mediated by P53	[56]
SME	20 μg/ml	PC-3, LNCaP, and DU-145	Inducing cell cycle arrest and apoptosis	[57]
TsIIAN	—	PC-3 and DU145	Induction of apoptosis	[58]
SMEN	—	LNCap	Inducing apoptosis and up-regulating ROS in cells	[59]
NCDT	—	LNCaP	Enhancing toxicity of doxorubicin	[60]

Table 2. In animal study of Tanshinone and PCa.

Animal Models	Dose	Delivery Way	Result	Reference
22Rv1 allograft mouse model	CYT (5 mg/Kg) and CYT (25 mg/Kg)	Intraperitoneal injections were given every two days for four weeks.	Tumor growth was inhibited in both the low-dose and high-dose groups.	[46]
PC-3 allograft mouse model	TsI (150 mg/kg)	Tube feeding, once a day, for 2 weeks	Tumor weight (67%) and intratumor blood vessels (80%) were reduced.	[30]
PC-3 allograft mouse model	SME (100 mg/kg)	Oral and tube feeding, once a day, for 6 weeks	The incidence and weight of tumors were reduced.	[57]
LNCaP allograft mouse model	TsIIA (25 mg/kg)	Orally, once daily for 6 weeks	Tumor growth and the expression of AR were inhibited.	[40]
PC-3 allograft mouse model	CYT (10 mg/kg)	Intraperitoneal injection, once a day	Tumor weight (46.4%) and intratumor blood vessels were reduced.	[31]
DU-145 allograft mouse model	SME (500 mg/kg)	Orally, once daily for 2 weeks	Tumor growth was inhibited	[56]
PC-3 allograft mouse model	TsD (60 mg/kg)	Subcutaneous injections were given every two days for 18 days	Tumor growth was inhibited	[54]
LNCaP allograft mouse model	TsIIA (60 or 90 mg/kg)	Subcutaneous injections were given every two days for 13 days	Tumor weight (86.4%) was reduced.	[39]
CWR22Rv1 allograft mouse model	CYT (25 mg/kg)	Intraperitoneal injections were given 3 times per week for 4 weeks	Tumor metastasis is inhibited.	[49]
LNCaP allograft mouse model	NCDT (5 mg/Kg)	It was injected once every two days for 18 days.	To enhance the toxicity of Doxorubicin	[60]

Note: *Tanshinone I (TsI), Tanshinone II A (TsIIA), Tanshinone II B (TsIIB), Dihydrotanshinone I (DHT), Cryptotanshinone (CYT), Tanshinone derivatives (TsD), Tanshinone IIA derivatives (TIIAD), TsIIA nanoparticles (TsIIAD), Nanoparticles containing doxorubicin and Tanshinone (NCDT), Nanoparticles synthesized from salvia miltiorrhiza extract (SMED).*

2. Tanshinone as a Potential Anti-Cancer Agent for PCa

2.1. Tanshinone-Induced Stagnation of the PCa Cell Cycle

A normal cell cycle is essential for homeostasis and normal development of an organism, and dysregulation of this system often leads to uncontrolled cell proliferation, leading to the occurrence of tumors [61]. The progress of the cell cycle depends on the regulation of various cyclins, cell cycle-dependent protein kinases (CDK), and CDK inhibitors. In mammals, the normal progress of the cell cycle is carefully edited with the expression of different cyclin proteins in characteristic cell cycle stages as the center of the molecular mechanism, and they are assembled with specific CDKs to promote the phosphorylation of the retinoblastoma tumor suppressor (Rb) so as to promote the cell cycle to the next stage [62,63]. Therefore, in order to maintain their own biological characteristics (uncontrolled proliferation), tumor cells induce protein expression of cell cycle progression and the genes encoding the cell cycle inhibitors are missing, or there is inactivation of cell cycle regulators such as Rb and P53 [64,65]. Interestingly, current publications suggest that Tanshinone can significantly inhibit PCa proliferation by inducing PCa cell cycle arrest. The mechanism is that Tanshinone can significantly reduce cyclinD1, A, and E (cyclinD1, A, and E) in PCa cells [34,51,54,56], which seems to be partly due to Tanshinone's ability to directly inhibit the phosphorylation of the pro-proliferative signaling pathway STAT3Tyr705 in PCa cells [51]. Tanshinone also has a significant ability to relate to CDK family-relative proteins in PCa cells. Previous studies have shown that Tanshinone can not only inhibit the expression of CDK in PCa cells but also increase the activation and expression of CDK inhibition (P21, P27, p16) by promoting the phosphorylation of Ser15 residues of p53 [34,59]. It can also significantly inhibit the hyperphosphorylation of Rb in PCa cells [54], which seems to be caused to some extent by Tanshinone increasing ROS in PCa cells [35,66]. In addition, the normal of the cell cycle also depends on other factors of the adjustment.

These factors are not only for genomic stability and integrity maintenance, which is very important, but they also participate in the spindle and maintain normal mitosis of the structure of the adjustment. It is interesting to note that, according to the existing literature, Tanshinone and its derivatives in PCa cells also show the effect on the regulation of these factors. including: stasis and DNA damage-inducing protein (GADD45A), polo-like kinase 1 (PLK1), and checkpoint-related protein [54].

2.2. *Tanshinone-Induced Apoptosis of PCa Cells*

According to reports, tumor progression frequently means apoptosis and proliferation imbalances, which are related to apoptosis signaling molecules and proteins that scientists are concerned about [67,68]. Interestingly, previous studies have shown that Tanshinone induces apoptosis in PCa cells by altering the balance between the expression of pro-apoptotic and anti-apoptotic proteins in the b-cell lymphoma-2 (bcl-2) family [34,35,38,50,51,55–58]. Secondly, caspase containing cysteine is a key enzyme for performing apoptosis, and caspase-3 is a key executor of apoptosis in mammalian cells [68]. Studies have shown that Tanshinone can significantly induce its expression and phosphorylation in PCa. It also significantly increases the activation and expression of caspase-8 or-9 upstream promoters [34,35,38,50,51,55–58]. The regulation of these proteins by Tanshinone is partly due to the inhibition of the pi3k/akt pathway and MAPK pathway and the expression of hypoxia stress factor 1 (HIF-1) in PCa cells [38,45]. In fact, Tanshinone also has a significant effect on the regulation of ROS and LC3II in PCa cells for the process [36]. In addition, Tanshinone induces apoptosis of PCa cells by other mechanisms. As the report goes, Tanshinone activates mitochondrial-dependent apoptosis of PCa cells by inhibiting the expression of mitochondrial protective Bcl-2 family protein Mcl-1 by inducing the cleavage of ADP ribose polymerase (PARP), promoting the release of cytochrome c from the mitochondria to the cytoplasm and reducing mitochondrial membrane potential. which seems to be partly due to the inhibition of pik3/Akt in PCa cells [38]. Similarly, Tanshinone derivatives also have the same pharmacological effects. In the experiments conducted by Wang et al., they found that Tanshinone derivatives induce PCa cell apoptosis by regulating p53, ERK1, BAX, P38, Bcl-2, caspase-8, cleavedcaspase-8, and PARP1, and significantly affect the phosphorylation of ERK1 and P38 in P38 [54]. Second, Tanshinone has been shown to induce ER stress pathway apoptosis in PCa cells by increasing the expression of key proteins of ER stress pathway apoptosis, such as glucose regulatory protein 78 (BIP/GRP78), ER stress sensor (IRE1-) and its downstream target CAAT/enhancer binding protein homologous protein/growth arrest and DNA-damage-inducing gene 153 (gadd153/cho) [48,53]. In addition, Tanshinone has been reported to up-regulate Fas sensitivity of PCa cells and promote Fas (APO1/CD95) mediated apoptosis of PCa cells by inhibiting phosphorylation of Janus kinase (JAK) and p38MAPK [45]. In addition, Tanshinone has been shown to be an effective sensitizer of tumor necrosis factor-associated apoptosis-inducing ligand (TRAIL) to enhance TRAIL-mediated apoptosis, which seems to be related to Tanshinone activation of mir135A-3p mediated up-regulation of death receptor 5 (DR5) in PCa cells [52].

2.3. *Tanshinone-Induced Motility Inhibition of PCa Cells*

Metastasis of tumor cells is often one of the main causes of death in patients. Previous studies have shown that prostate cancer can metastasize through a variety of mechanisms. Among these are the secretion of matrix metalloproteinases (MMPs) to dissolve the extracellular matrix, the promotion of angiogenesis, the recruitment of some cytokines and chemokines, and so on [69,70], which pose significant challenges to clinicians' diagnosis and treatment. Fortunately, existing literature shows that Tanshinone can act as an effective inhibitor of the metastasis and invasion of PCa cells. In the experiment of WuCY et al., Tanshinone inhibits the translocation of phosphorylated STAT3 and protein expression of P-STAT3 and Skp2 in PCa cells in a dose-dependent manner, resulting in inhibition of the translation and transcription of RhoA and SNAI1 genes in PCa cells, which results in reduced invasiveness of PCa cells [35]. Interestingly, inhibition of this pathway also has a significant impact on the ability of PCa cells to recruit macrophages. Inhibition of this pathway will lead to reduced secretion of related cytokines in PCa cells [32], including CCL2, CCL5, interleukin-1 receptor antagonists (il-1ra) and intercellular adhesion molecule-1, which are significantly associated not only with PCa metastasis but also with the ability to recruit macrophages of Pca [71,72]. In addition, literature has shown that Tanshinone has a significant pharmacological effect of inhibiting angiogenesis in PCa cells, which seems to be related to the inhibition of hif-1 expression induction of vascular endothelial growth factor and its receptor in PCa cells by Tanshinone intervention [30,31]. Similarly, Tanshinone derivatives also have significant inhibitory effects on the metastasis and invasion of PCa cells. In the experiment of Wang et al., they found that Tanshinone derivatives can reduce the expression of protein molecules related to metastasis and invasion in PCa cells, including MMP-1, MMP-9, and VEGF-1 [54].

2.4. *Tanshinone Maintains Gene Stability of PCa Cells*

Tanshinone also regulates the expression of epigenetic-modification-related genes in PCa cells. Among 84 epigenetic-modification-related genes in PCa cells treated with Tanshinone (mainly TsI), the expression of 32 genes was down-regulated [30], including AuroraA kinase, DNA methyltransferase, histone acetyltransferase, histone deacetylase, Lysine (K)-specific demethylase, and protein arginine methyltransferase. The PCa cells treated with CYT and TsIIA only had the expression of AuroraA kinase inhibited. However, previous studies have shown that epigenetic disorders such as histone modification and DNA methylation contribute to the initiation and progression of PCa. AuroraA kinase is a key mitotic regulator required to maintain chromosome stability [73], and its overexpression often indicates a higher degree of malignancy in tumors. In addition, Tanshinone has been reported to be significantly associated with the down-regulation of astrocyte elevating gene 1 (AEG-1) in PCa cells [31], which is involved in the regulation of multiple signaling pathways in cancer cells, including PI3K/Akt, NF-κB, Wnt/-catenin, and MAPK. They synergistically promote the oncogenic and metastatic potential of transformed cells [74]. In addition, Tanshinone can reduce the transcription and translation of topoisomerase 2A in PCa cells [52], which is critical for genomic stability and replication. Interestingly, Tanshinone has been reported to regulate the activity and elongation of the RNA-binding protein HuR and telomerase. This coordinates mRNA stabilization and translation [75–78], which is critical for inflammation and tumor progression.

In fact, the antioxidant capacity of Tanshinone also plays a significant role in maintaining the genetic stability of prostate cancer cells. Although this has not been confirmed, studies have shown that oxidative stress can often damage DNA molecules, leading to the occurrence of tumors [79]. However, the specific antioxidant activity of Tanshinone is that it can effectively inhibit the interaction between DNA and intracellular lipid peroxidation products, thereby stabilizing DNA molecules [80]. However, the current research does not pay attention to the influence of Tanshinone on the factors and pathways related to oxidative stress in prostate cancer cells. Secondly, the special skeleton structure of Tanshinone also has an effect on the stability of DNA. It is reported that the Tanshinone D ring can bind to the small grooves in DNA molecules, thereby stabilizing DNA molecules [23,25]. In addition, the regulatory effect of Tanshinone on microRNAs in prostate cancer cells seems to be involved in this process. After all, microRNAs are closely related to gene expression and synthesis, and mutations of microRNAs often lead to cancer [81,82]. Unfortunately, although Tanshinone has been proven to be able to regulate microRNAs in other cancer cells [27,83], the current study has not confirmed the regulatory effect of Tanshinone on microRNAs in prostate cancer cells. Based on the fact that microRNA not only plays a key role in the process of gene expression and synthesis but also has significant significance in maintaining the malignant behavior of cancer cells, future research should also pay attention to the regulatory effect of Tanshinone on microRNA in prostate cancer cells. In conclusion, the current research is limited. Although laboratory data have confirmed that

Tanshinone has the ability to stabilize the genetic stability of prostate cancer cells, there is no exact evidence and the corresponding mechanism is not clear.

2.5. Tanshinone Reverses Multidrug Resistance in PCa

Tanshinone also has a regulatory effect on multidrug resistance (MDR) of tumor cells, and MDR is the main factor for clinical chemotherapy failure. Although chemotherapy is not recommended as a first-line treatment for PCa in the early stages of the disease, it is often recommended as a first-line treatment for PCa in the advanced stages [84,85]. Existing literature shows that Tanshinone can adjust the genes associated with MDR (P glycoprotein, topoisomerase, lung resistance protein expression) to reverse the drug resistance of tumor cells to chemotherapy drugs [86]. Although this has not been confirmed in PCa, it is interesting to note that after Tanshinone pretreatment, the toxic effects of cisplatin and azithromycin on PCa increased [36,60]. In addition, tumor stem cells are also considered to be one of the key factors in the occurrence of MDR [87]. It is noteworthy that Tanshinone has also shown a regulatory effect on tumor-initiating cells in PCa. In an experiment, YingZhang et al. found that Tanshinone can regulate the expression of prostatic cancer cell globogenesis and stem cell genes (Nanog, OCT4, SOX2, -catenin, CXCR4) and simultaneously change the cell proliferation, cell cycle state, migration, and colony formation of prostate tumor-initiating cells (CD44 + CD24-population) [57]. This could be because Tanshinone significantly reduced Bmi1 gene expression and protein levels (key regulators of stem cell self-renewal and malignant transformation) [88].

Tanshinone can prevent the occurrence of MDR in prostate cancer cells by down-regulating the genes related to the occurrence of MDR and inhibiting the tumor-initiating cells closely related to the occurrence of MDR. It is worth noting that Tanshinone can also greatly improve the adverse reactions caused by radiotherapy and chemotherapy [89]. Research shows that Tanshinone can significantly improve the organ nerve loss caused by radiotherapy and chemotherapy [89,90]. Therefore, based on the current research, we believe that Tanshinone combined with radiotherapy and chemotherapy in the treatment of drug-resistant prostate cancer will become a possibility. However, the current research is limited, and the specific mechanism of Tanshinone enhancing the toxic reaction of chemotherapy drugs to prostate cancer is still unclear, so further research is needed.

2.6. Tanshinone Changes the Metabolic Process of PCa

Tanshinone has also been reported to regulate the metabolic process of PCa. Existing publications show that the expression of some genes related to steroid and cholesterol biosynthesis in PCa cells treated with Tanshinone (mainly Tanshinone IIA) is significantly reduced [91], including methylsterol monooxygenase 1 (MSMO1/SC4MOL), squalene monooxygenase (SQLE), ATP-binding box subfamily G member 1 (ABCG1) and preprotein invertase subtilin kexin9 (PCSK9s). Although this has not been proven to be associated with tanshoneinhibition of PCa, it is worth mentioning that Tanshinontong changes the way tumor cell metabolism works, including down-regulating the enzymes involved in glucose uptake and metabolism in cancer cells (especially those related to glycolysis), affecting the energy metabolism of tumor cells, and then inducing apoptosis of cancer cells [92,93].

It is reported that in the process of progression, tumors often change their metabolism to quickly obtain energy or synthesize substances they need [94]. This process is critical for prostate cancer. Previous studies have shown that advanced prostate cancer may be more dependent on lipid metabolism. The expression of genes related to lipid synthesis in advanced prostate cancer cells is significantly higher than that in early prostate cancer cells [95,96]. Prostate cancer increases the synthesis of its own lipids in this way, thereby providing more abundant raw materials for androgen synthesis so as to tolerate the low level of androgen brought on by castration treatment [96,97]. Therefore, regulating the metabolism of prostate cancer has significant significance for the treatment of prostate cancer. As evidenced based on appeal, the metabolic rearrangement of Tanshinone on prostate cancer cells should also be paid attention to in future research. The molecular mechanism involved should also be further explored.

3. Molecular Targets of Tanshinone Action

3.1. Tanshinone and NF-κB

NF-κB is a multipotent transcription factor responsible for regulating cell signaling and various biological processes, such as immune response, inflammation, cell transformation, cell proliferation, angiogenesis, cancer invasion, and metastasis [98]. This factor can be activated by a variety of signals, including growth factors, protein kinases, oxidative stress inducers, mitogens, pro-inflammatory cytokines, and chemokines (TNF-, Il-1, Il-8, Il-6, CXCL12), and environmental stress factors [98,99]. In addition, NF-κB has been proven to be significantly related to the occurrence and progression of PCa. During the development of PCa, NF-κB can promote the survival, invasion, angiogenesis, metastasis, and chemical resistance of cancer cells by inducing pro-survival genes (such as bcl-2 and bcl-xl), pro-inflammatory cytokines, and vascular growth factors [100,101]. Second, IκB kinase -α (IKKα) and IκB kinase -β (IKKβ) signaling molecules upstream of the NF-κB signaling pathway can directly affect AR activity via phosphorylation and induce the expression of the constitutive active AR splicing form (AR-v7), which is one of the key factors in PCa castration resistance and drug resistance [102,103]. Interestingly, available laboratory data have long shown that Tanshinone inhibits cancer cell growth and progression by inhibiting the overactivation of NF-κB in cancer cells [104,105], although this has not yet been demonstrated in PCa cells. Tanshinone has been shown to inhibit the secretion of NF-κB activating factors such as interleukins, vascular cell adhesion molecule-1 (VCMM-1), and intercellular adhesion molecule-1 (ICAM-1) as well as monocyte chemoattractant protein 1 (MCP-1) and tumor necrosis factor (TNF-α). It can also directly inhibit the phosphorylation of upstream molecules by IB kinase-IKK and IKK and simultaneously induce degradation of IKK and IKK. It can also inhibit the NF-κB pathway by decreasing the expression levels of toll-like receptor (TLR), myeloid differentiation factor 88 (MyD88), transferrin 6 (TRF6), and other proteins involved in the NF-κB signaling pathway and directly inhibiting the activation and expression of NF-κB [106–108]. It is noteworthy that Tanshinone can inhibit the activity of COX2 and play a significant inhibitory role in the transcription and expression of COX2 by acting similarly to non-steroidal anti-inflammatory drugs [108–110], while the prostaglandins generated by COX2-mediated production not only have a direct nourishing effect on PCa cells [111]. It also acts as an effective activator of NF-κB

Inflammation is essential for the occurrence and development of all kinds of cancers, including prostate cancer. The signal pathway most closely associated with the inflammatory response is NF-κB. It not only promotes the onset and progression of prostate cancer but also has a clear crosstalk relationship with androgen receptor signals. In fact, it has crosstalk with most signal molecules in the cell. Therefore, based on the current laboratory data, targeting NF-κB is probably a promising treatment [112]. Tanshinone can inhibit the occurrence and progression of prostate cancer by virtue of its excellent ability to regulate inflammation and NF-κB. Unfortunately, current studies have not confirmed the effects of Tanshinone on inflammatory cytokines and the NF-κB pathway in prostate cancer cells. Therefore, future studies should pay attention to the regulation of inflammation-related molecules and signaling pathways in prostate cancer.

3.2. Tanshinone and AR

Androgen is very important for PCa. It is reported that testosterone, after binding to hormone ligands, is transferred to the nucleus and combined with androgen response elements (ARE) located in the promoter region of genes involved in cell proliferation and escape from apoptosis to promote the growth and development of PCa cells. It can also promote the growth and development of PCa by activating other extracellular signaling pathways that crosstalk with androgen signaling pathways [113,114]. Androgen deprivation therapy (ADT) is widely used as a first-line treatment method for metastatic androgen-dependent PCa. However, accept the ADT after treatment of PCa, often in about two years into a more aggressive PCa (CRPC) [4]. Previous views that CRPC does not depend on the nourishment effect of androgens; however, recent laboratory evidence suggests that CRPC still relies on androgen to nourish them either by synthesizing more bioactive androgen through themselves and the adrenal cortex or by increasing the expression of ARs and inducing them to mutate into a more active form to tolerate low androgen levels induced by castration therapy [115–117]. Therefore, inhibition of androgen nourishing effects is of great significance for the treatment of PCa.

Interestingly, Tanshinone inhibits androgen signaling through a variety of mechanisms. Cryptotanshinone has been reported to have a chemical structure similar to dihydrotestosterone (DHT), the most effective androgen for AR activation, and can bind to AR receptors as a competitive antagonist of DHT, thereby inhibiting DHT-mediated AR trans-activation [46]. Tanshinone also has a significant regulatory effect on the expression and activity of AR. According to current published reports, Tanshinone can not only directly inhibit the expression of AR [34,40], but also increase the monomethyl and dimethylation of lysine 9 (H3K9) of histone H3 by targeting the lysine-specific demethylase 1 (LSD1) complex. In addition, AR activity and expression can be inhibited by inhibiting AR N and C terminal dimerization and the formation of an AR-regulator complex [46,55], and reducing the availability of AR by overexpressing heat shock protein (Hsp90) can be changed [30], and it also has a regulatory effect on ARE [46]. Tanshinone, by regulating ARE, can inhibit the transcriptional regulation of AR signaling to its target genes. In addition, Tanshinone also regulates AR receptor mutations. In a study by Liu et al., Tanshinone IIA and its derivatives not only significantly inhibited AR expression but also acted as effective inhibitors of AR receptor mutations, thereby inhibiting AR receptor mutations [41]. Furthermore, it also has a certain regulatory effect on androgen secretion. Previous studies have shown that Tanshinone can not only regulate the expression of key enzymes related to androgen biosynthesis but also regulate extracellular signal-regulated kinase (ERK)/C-FOS/17, 20-lyase (CYP17), leading to androgen biosynthesis levels being down [118,119]. However, it is worth noting that, in addition to having similar pharmacological effects, Tanshinone has other advantages over existing anti-male drugs. As reported, Tanshinone derivatives can significantly inhibit AR trans-activation mediated by 17-estradiol (E2) and androgen-5–Δene-3, 7-diol (Δ5-androstenediol or Adiol) [55]. E2 and Adiol are natural hormones in PCa cells. Because current adt-related drugs do not target these two natural hormones, and because they have the characteristics of converting to testosterone and even acting as effective activators of the AR signaling pathway, they are significantly associated with drug resistance and castration resistance in PCa [120,121]. Secondly, in a clinical trial, LinTH et al. found that although the use of enzaluamide and bicaluamide could lead to the reduction of the primary tumor and PSA, the invasion of PCa cells was significantly enhanced, while the use of Tanshinone could not only achieve the reduction of the primary tumor and PSA but also inhibit PCa cell invasion to a certain extent [53]. Similarly, for other steroid receptors present in PCa, Tanshinone has been reported to inhibit prostatic stromal and epithelial proliferation by down-regulating estrogen receptorα (ERα) [122]. Interestingly, ER is limited to basal cells and stromal cells of the prostate epithelium [123]. It is associated with mitogen-activated protein kinase (MAPK) activity and maintenance of the phosphoinositol 3-kinase (PI3K) signaling pathway in PCa [124].

In short, the occurrence and progression of prostate cancer are inextricably linked to the nourishing effect of androgens. Even if it is CCRP, inhibiting the nourishing effect of androgen in prostate cancer is still the primary purpose of endocrine therapy for prostate cancer. Therefore, as previously described, Tanshinone has a significant inhibitory effect not only on androgen biosynthesis but also on the expression and synthesis of various proteins and genes related to the androgen pathway. Tanshinone has been shown to be more effective than some anti-androgenic drugs because, when compared to these anti-androgenic drugs, Tanshinone not only achieves the same effect but also inhibits prostate cancer cell metastasis. In fact, compared with traditional antiandrogenic drugs, the inhibition of the androgen-mediated signaling pathway by Tanshinone is multi-pathway and multi-target. These data once again confirm the possibility of Tanshinone as an anti-prostate drug.

3.3. *Tanshinone and mTOR*

mTOR is a conserved and universally expressed serine-threonine kinase. In mammals, it is usually assembled with Raptor, rictor, lst8, and msin1 to form two catalytic subunits of different protein complexes (mTORC1 sensitive to rapamycin and mTORC2 insensitive to rapamycin) and participates in a variety of signal pathways in vivo to regulate cell proliferation, autophagy, and apoptosis. Among them, mTORC1 is the most important. mTORC1 not only consists of three core components: mTOR, regulatory-associated protein of mTOR (raptor), and mammalian lethal with SEC13 protein 8 (mlst8), but also contains two inhibitory subunits: 40 kDa proline-rich Akt substrate (PRAS40) and regulatory-associated protein of mTOR (deptor) [125,126]. Here, we mainly review the regulatory effect of Tanshinone on mTORC1.

In terms of assembly, Tanshinone can not only directly inhibit the expression and phosphorylation of mTOR so that it interferes with the assembly of the mTORC1 subunit [23], but also inhibit the promotion of mTORC1 assembled catalyst and stabilizer (heat shock protein 90) [30,127,128]. In terms of activity, the activity of mTORC1 is regulated by growth factors, cell energy, stress, and nucleotides, and the lysosome is the main site of its activation [126,129]. In fact, the activity of mTORC1 is mainly related to the tuberous sclerosis complex (TSC), which can inactivate Ras homolog enriched in the brain (rheb) (an important activator of mTORC1), thereby inhibiting mTORC1 [130]. Interestingly, the existing literature shows that Tanshinone can inhibit not only the expression of growth factors and their receptors [131] but also the expression of rheb [132]. In addition, the activity of mTORC1 is also regulated by the energy sensor AMP-dependent kinase (AMPK). AMPK can promote the inhibition of rheb by TSC by stimulating the gap activity of TSC, resulting in the down-regulation of mTORC1 [133,134], which means that activating AMPK in cancer cells can affect mTORC1 to a certain extent. Interestingly, Tanshinone has been shown to inhibit the mTORC1-mediated signal pathway by activating the AMPK-TSC2 axis [135]. Sestrins negatively regulate mTORC1 signaling through GATOR2/Rag and its components, SESN1 and SESN2, can directly bind to complex and AMPK, resulting in AMPK activation and autophosphorylation in a p53-dependent manner. This stimulates AMPK-mediated TSC2 phosphorylation to negatively regulate mTORC1 signaling [136,137]. Previous literature shows that Tanshinone induces the expression of BECN1 and SESN2 proteins in a dose-dependent manner and then induces autophagy in osteosarcoma cells [138]. It also regulates the upstream gene p53 of the SESN2 protein. Secondly, the down-regulation of pyruvate dehydrogenase kinase 4 (PDK4) has also been reported to lead to the inactivation of mTORC1 [139], and Tanshinone is known as an inhibitor of PDK4, which means that the inhibition of mTORC1 activity by Tanshinone may be partly due to the inhibition of PDK4 [140]. In addition, mitogen-activated protein kinase (MAPK) downstream of the growth factor receptor can also up-regulate mTORC1 activity. MAPK-related signal molecules can promote the activation of mTORC1 through the phosphorylation of Raptor. For example, MEK1/2 can not only phosphorylate Raptor but also promote Raptor phosphorylation through ERK1/2 and P90 ribosomal S6 kinase (RSK1/2). This increases mTORC1 activity [141,142]. Secondly, RAS and RAF kinases, key molecules in the MAPK-mediated signal pathway, also regulate the activation of its upstream signal molecule, PI3K [143,144]. In fact, MAPK and mTOR-mediated signaling pathways have mutual crosstalk in many aspects. They not only receive the activation of various growth factors but also have the same downstream molecules, such as Src kinase, FOXO (forkhead box o), c-myc transcription factor, and various metabolism-related enzymes [143]. This means that inhibition of this pathway can inhibit the activation of mTORC1 and its related pathways to a certain extent. Tanshinone not only directly inhibits the expression and phosphorylation of MAPK but also inhibits the activation and expression of related molecules of its mediated signal pathway, including ERK, JNK, p38 MAPK, Ras, etc. [45,54,145,146]. It can also indirectly affect MAPK by up-regulating ROS in cancer cells [66].

PI3K is a large class of lipid kinases and one of the most important upstream molecules of mTORC1-mediated related pathways. At present, it is mainly divided into three categories: class I (subdivided into classes IA and IB), class II, and class III, of which class I is the most important [142], and class IA PI3K is a heterodimer that consists of a catalytic subunit (P110α, p110β or P110δ) and a regulatory subunit (p85α/p55α/p50α, p85β, or p55γ). It is activated by various growth factors. After being activated, class IA PI3Ks synthesize lipid secondary messenger phosphatidylinositol 3,4,5 triphosphate (PIP3) from phosphatidylinositol 4,5 diphosphate (PIP2), which recruits protein kinase Akt to the plasma membrane, where it is activated by 3-phosphoinositide dependent kinase 1 (PDK1), Subsequently, activated Akt phosphorylates TSC2 and inhibits the TSC complex, eventually leading to the activation of mTORC1 [142,147]. However, as described above, Tanshinone can inhibit the expression of various growth factors and their receptors. In fact, Tanshinone can weaken or even inhibit the induction of PI3K protein expression and phosphorylation by these factors, which is partly because Tanshinone directly inhibits PI3K protein expression and phosphorylation [148–150]. Secondly, Tanshinone also showed the pharmacological action of inhibiting the phosphorylation and expression of catalytic subunit P110α/γ and subunit p85 (down-regulating the expression of its gene) [38,151–153]. In addition, Tanshinone has the pharmacological effect of promoting the expression of phosphatase and tensin homologue (PTEN), a negative regulatory gene of PI3K [133,154,155], which negatively regulates PI3K Akt mTOR signal transduction by transforming PIP3 back to PIP2 [156] and the deletion of this gene usually occurs with the progression of prostate cancer [157,158]. In addition, the expression and phosphorylation of PDK1 and Akt downstream of PI3K were also inhibited by Tanshinone [148–150,159].

The two most important molecules in mTORC1-mediated cell activity are P70S6 kinase 1 (S6K1) and eIF4E binding protein (4E-BP) 1 [160]. The phosphorylation of S6K1 by mTORC1 leads to increased protein and nucleotide synthesis [125,126,160]. 4ebp is a negative regulator of 5′cap dependent mRNA translation, and mTORC1 induces the separation of 4E-BP1 from eIF4E so as to reduce its inhibition of protein synthesis [125,126,160]. By targeting these two molecules, mTORC1 synthesizes proteins required for cell growth, cell cycle process, and cell metabolism, and then induces tumor growth and progression. Tanshinone also has a regulatory effect on these two molecules. As shown in previous literature, Tanshinone can not only prevent the binding of S6K1 to mTORC1 [161] but also significantly inhibit the expression and phosphorylation of S6K1 and 4E-BP1 [159,162]. It is worth mentioning that Tanshinone also regulates the key downstream molecule PKC of mtorc2 [128]. Protein kinase C (PKC) is considered to be the main downstream molecule of mtorc2. Mtorc2 completes various cell activities by targeting the special type of this molecule [126].

This laboratory evidence shows that Tanshinone can inhibit mTOR-mediated tumor malignant behavior in prostate cancer cells by regulating the expression and phosphorylation of upstream and downstream protein molecules of the mTOR-mediated signaling pathway or by regulating other molecular pathways with obvious crosstalk with mTOR. It is worth noting that although Tanshinone is similar to rapamycin in structure, the regulation of mTOR does not directly inhibit the synthesis of mTOR like rapamycin, which means that Tanshinone has fewer side effects on normal tissue and is safer [163,164]. In short, Tanshinone has a significant inhibitory effect on prostate cancer. its pharmacological mechanism. As previously described, it depends on the regulation of the mTOR-mediated signaling pathway, but the current research is still limited, The regulatory mechanism of some Tanshinones on mTOR has only been confirmed in other tumor cells. Therefore, a large number of studies are still needed to further clarify the effect of Tanshinone on the mTOR-mediated signaling pathway in prostate cancer cells. Furthermore, State3 [27] is another key molecule of Tanshinone that exerts an anti-tumor effect. Although it has been confirmed to be involved in the inhibitory effect of Tanshinone on prostate cancer, the current research is very lacking and should be given enough attention in the future. We plotted the relevant regulation of Tanshinone on the mTOR pathway in Figure 3

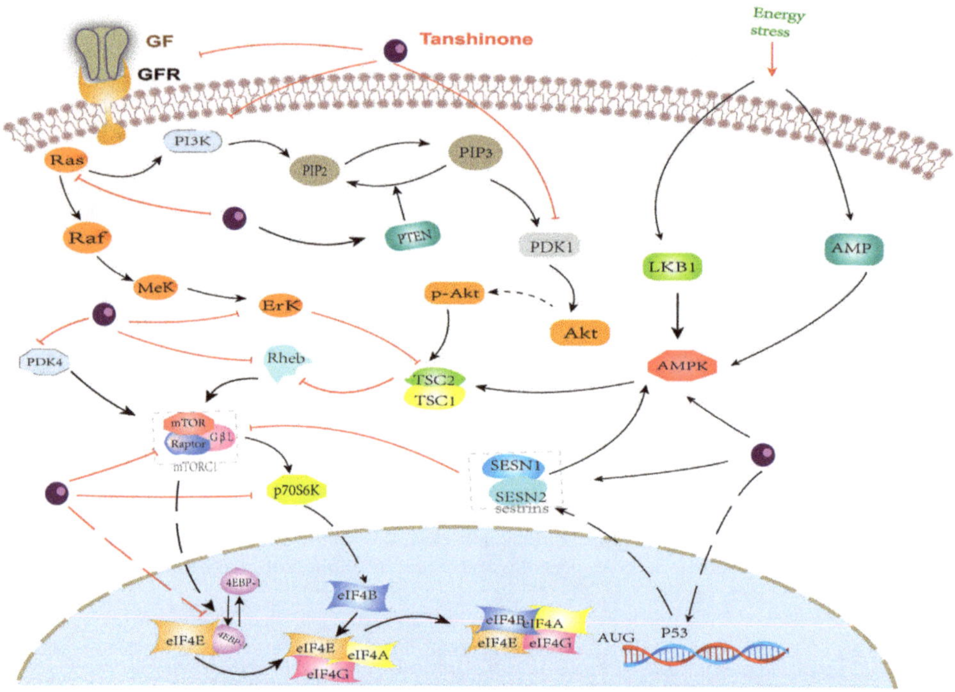

Figure 3. Effect of Tanshinone on mTOR. induced by Tanshinone are noted by using →, while the inhibition represented by ⊣ symbol.

4. Dilemma of Clinical Application of Tanshinone

Tanshinone, as a secondary metabolite, accumulates mainly in the roots of Salvia miltiorrhiza, but in very low yields. Currently, Tanshinone relies on traditional chemical isolation and purification from Salvia divinorum roots [8]. However, traditional methods are characterized by low efficiency, high energy consumption, and unfriendliness to the environment and plant resources [8,165], and secondly, due to the increasing demand for Tanshinone in the market, wild salvia has been over-harvested and the resources are on the verge of extinction [8,165]. Although artificial domestication of salvia has been cultivated since the 1970s, due to the low yield of secondary metabolites and the long growth period of cultivated plants, the production of Tanshinone from cultivated salvia cannot meet the rapidly growing market demand [17]. Therefore, both the reform of the purification process of Tanshinone and the improvement of yield through modern biotechnology have received great attention. Various in vitro culture systems of Salvia divinorum, including suspension cells, guard tissues, adventitious roots, hairy roots, and new techniques such as the use of endophytic fungi and transgenic plants, have been reported to significantly increase the yield of Tanshinone [18,166]. However, these efforts are still insufficient for the increased demand for Tanshinone in the market, and therefore a new technique with a higher yield is urgently needed to provide the supply.

In recent years, the discovery of key genes for the biosynthesis of pharmaceutical active ingredients and the use of synthetic biology strategies to design and modify microbial strains to produce natural products are considered to be promising resource acquisition methods [167]. It is reported that at present, with Saccharomyces cerevisiae as the chassis cell, a high-yield engineering strain of miltiradiene, an important intermediate of Tanshinone, with a yield of up to 488 mg/L has been constructed through functional module design, and cloned the modifying enzyme gene CYP76AH1 of the Tanshinone biosynthesis pathway, which successfully converted miltiradiene into ferruginol [17,168]. However, due to the limited understanding of the transcription genes of Salvia miltiorrhiza, the further elucidation of Tanshinone biosynthesis has been hindered [167,169]. It is worth mentioning that the formation of the furan ring, which has puzzled scientists for a long time, has been gradually decoded [170]. However, there is still a long way to go. It is still necessary to pay more attention to and explore genes and enzymes related to Tanshinone biosynthesis in the future.

Second, like most natural drugs, Tanshinone also has the characteristics of low water solubility, poor stability, large first-pass elimination, and low bioavailability [17,171], which greatly limits the clinical application of Tanshinone. It is reported that when Cryptotanshinone is administered at a body weight of 100 mg/kg (mg/kg), the bioavailability of oral and intraperitoneal injection in rats is 2.1% and 10.6%, respectively. In fact, most of the studies on Tanshinone have pointed out the nanomolar to lower micromolar after oral administration. The maximum/peak concentration (Cmax) value within the range [17,18] greatly limits the clinical application of Tanshinone. Although the currently prepared new formulations of Tanshinone for injection, such as microemulsion, microspheres, solid dispersion, liposomes, and nanoparticles, can significantly improve the bioavailability of Tanshinone, the complexity of the process, high cost, and low tissue specificity still limit the clinical application of these formulations [166,171]. However, it is worth noting that in previous studies, researchers greatly enhanced the specificity of Tanshinone nanoparticles for prostate cancer tissue by combining them with prostate-specific membrane antigen [60], which provides a way for the development of Tanshinone anti-prostate cancer-related nanoparticles in the future. However, the clinical trials of Tanshinone nanoparticles are still lacking, and the clinical application of Tanshinone nanoparticles is still making little progress. In addition, Tanshinone derivatives by changing the Tanshinone skeleton group also seem to be a promising solution, but in most cases, the anti-tumor effect of Tanshinone derivatives will be reduced or even lost, for example, sodium Tanshinone sulfonate [172,173]. Although previous studies have found some Tanshinone derivatives with significantly increased bioavailability and anti-tumor efficacy [42,54,55], due to the lack of in vivo experiments and related toxicological experiments, the safety of these Tanshinone derivatives is also a worrying problem and is also limited by the lack of raw materials. Therefore, future research should not only explore new Tanshinone derivatives but also focus on the safety of Tanshinone derivatives.

In addition, the safety of Tanshinone is also an aspect of concern for scientists. Although the experiments of Wang et al. confirmed that in both acute and subchronic toxicity studies, no abnormalities of other organs were observed in Sprague Dawley rats treated with Tanshinone injection, except that it caused focal inflammation at the injection site [174], which is consistent with the conclusions drawn from the in vivo experiments of Tanshinone and prostate cancer. In fact, limited studies pointed out that high concentrations of TsIIA and CYT showed serious growth inhibition, developmental malformation, and cardiotoxicity to zebrafish embryos [175,176]. Similarly, high concentrations of TsIIA were also toxic to normal human endothelial cells. It was reported that high concentrations of (25 uM) TsIIA could kill endothelial cells within 24 h [177]. Therefore, future research should focus on the toxic reaction of Tanshinone to normal tissues to confirm the safety and stability of Tanshinone, which is crucial for the development of clinical drugs.

5. Conclusions and Prospects

It is well understood that blocking the products of a single signal pathway or gene is frequently insufficient to prevent or treat malignant tumors. Tanshinone is expected to be a candidate drug for the treatment of prostate cancer because it can regulate the proliferation, survival, migration, and metabolism of prostate cancer through multiple targets, links, and pathways. Although the current experiments have confirmed the significant anti-prostate cancer effect of Tanshinone, there are still some problems with the current research. First, the current research on the anti-prostate cancer effect of Tanshinone is still limited, and most of the studies remain to verify the expression of proteins and genes related to apoptosis, cell cycle, and invasion in prostate cancer cells. In order to further explore the specific molecular mechanism that causes these changes, more research is still needed to explore the specific mechanism of Tanshinone against prostate cancer in the future. In addition, as described above, TsI and DHT have stronger anti-prostate cancer effects. However, current research is mostly focused on TsIIA and CYT. TsI and TsIIA should be given sufficient attention in the future. In addition, Tanshinone can significantly regulate the tumor immune microenvironment, which is more important for prostate cancer with poor immunotherapeutic efficacy. In the future, we should also pay attention to the effect of Tanshinone on the immune microenvironment of prostate cancer.

Although Tanshinone has been widely reported to be beneficial to health, its clinical application is still subject to many restrictions. First, as a secondary metabolite, Tanshinone mainly comes from the root of Salvia miltiorrhiza. Due to the characteristics of the long growth cycle and low yield of cultivated plants, the supply of Tanshinone is difficult to meet the market demand, although the current research on Tanshinone biosynthesis has made good progress. However, there are many key conversion processes that we are not clear about. Hence, it is still necessary to further explore the genes and enzymes related to Tanshinone biosynthesis. Secondly, like most natural drugs, Tanshinone also has the characteristics of low water solubility and low bioavailability. Fortunately, the currently prepared Tanshinone injection microemulsions, microspheres, solid dispersions, liposomes, nanoparticles, and other new dosage forms can greatly improve the bioavailability of Tanshinone. However, it is still subject to the limitations of complex processes, high costs, and low tissue specificity. Therefore, further preclinical and clinical studies are needed to explore new preparations with low cost, simple processes, and high tissue specificity. It was previously reported that Tanshinone nanoparticles developed in combination with prostate-cancer-specific membrane antigen can significantly enhance the tissue specificity of Tanshinone nanoparticles for prostate cancer. Therefore, future research will continue to consider the development of drug nanoparticles in combination with tumor-specific antigens. Secondly, Tanshinone derivatives synthesized by the Tanshinone skeleton should also be a focus of future research. Although the anti-tumor effect of these derivatives is significantly lower than that of Tanshinone in most cases, some Tanshinone derivatives with increased bioavailability and anti-tumor effects have been found in the current research. Secondly, the current research on the toxic reaction of Tanshinone and Tanshinone derivatives to normal tissues is limited and cannot confirm the safety and stability of Tanshinone and its derivatives. Therefore, more attention should be paid to the study on the toxic reaction of Tanshinone and its derivatives to normal tissues in the future to further clarify the safety of Tanshinone and its derivatives. Finally, in order to better guide future research and verify the possibility of Tanshinone as an anti-prostate cancer drug, we conducted a bioinformatics analysis on the four components of Tanshinone to further determine the possible anti-prostate cancer targets of Tanshinone.

First, after determining the structural formulas of four Tanshinone components (TsI, TsIIA, DHTI, and CYT) through Pubchem (https://pubchem.ncbi.nlm.nih.gov (accessed on 10 July 2022)), we screened drug targets using the Swiss target prediction database (http://www.swisstargetprediction.ch/ (accessed on 10 July 2022)) and the traditional Chinese Medicine System Pharmacology database (https://www.tcmsp-e.com/ (accessed on 10 July 2022)), and submitted the collected targets to the UniProt database (https://www.uniprot.org/ (accessed on 10 July 2022)), limiting the species to "Homo sapiens", converting the protein targets into official gene names, select gene targets with probability greater than 0 in the Swiss target prediction database, and obtain drug target genes: TsI (53), TsIIA (145), DHTI (80), CYT (94) after excluding duplicate genes. Secondly, we searched the Genecards (https://www.genecards.org/ (accessed on 10 July 2022)) and Disgenet databases (https://www.disgenet.org/ (accessed on 10 July 2022)) by using the keyword "prostate cancer" to obtain disease targets, and obtained 12,555 disease target genes after excluding duplicate targets in the two databases. Then, we input the drug target genes and disease target genes obtained by the above methods into the online Venny 2.1 mapping platform (https://www.bioinformatics.com.cn/ (accessed on 10 July 2022)) to obtain the cross-target genes of "prostate cancer" and "four Tanshinone components" (Figure 3), TsI (49), TsIIA (126), DHTI (68) and CYT (85) were obtained (Figure 4).

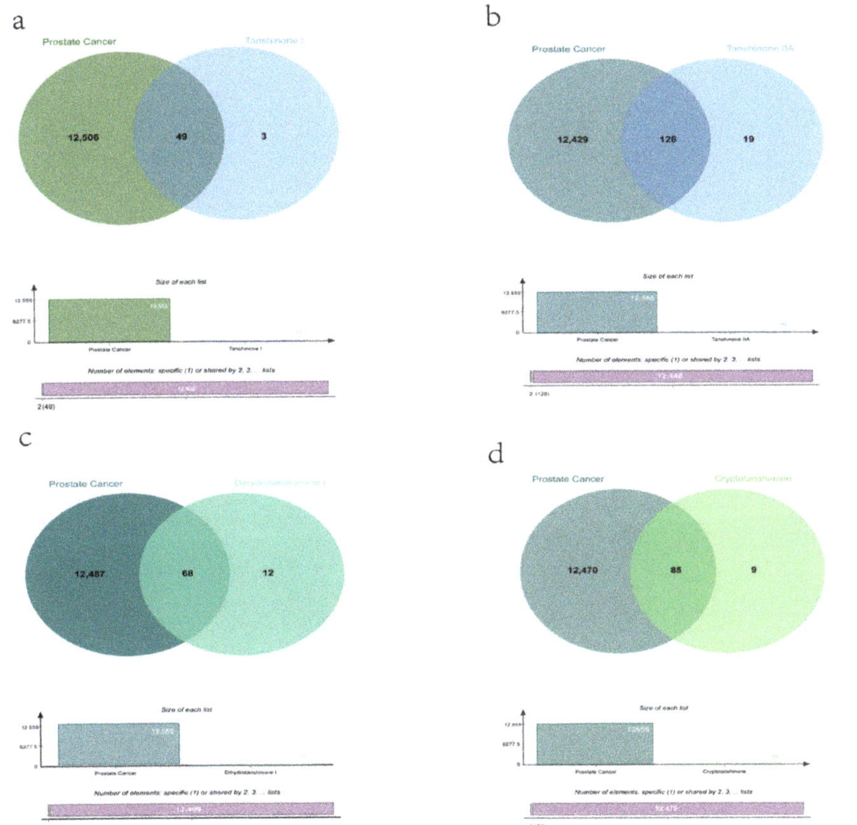

Figure 4. Venny of four components of Tanshinone ((**a**): Tanshinone I and Prostate Cancer; (**b**): Tanshinone IIA and Prostate Cancer; (**c**): Dihydrotanshinone I and Prostate Cancer; (**d**): Cryptotanshinone and Prostate Cancer).

These cross genes are considered possible targets of Tanshinone against prostate cancer, and we analyzed them through a range of methods. First, we uploaded these genes to the String online database (https://string-db.org/ (accessed on 10 July 2022)) to form a protein-protein interaction map. The species is "human" and the comprehensive score > 0.4 is the critical value for inclusion in the network. We further visualized these results with the help of Cytoscape 3.9.1 (Figure 5), To find the key targets of four Tanshinone components. At the same time, we also carried out the Gene Ontology (GO) function and Kyoto Encyclopedia of Genes and Genomes (KEGG) pathway analysis. After inputting these gene data into the David data platform (https://david.ncifcrf.gov/tools.jsp (accessed on 10 July 2022)) and setting the species as "Homo species", we further analyzed the enrichment analysis of four Tanshinone components on prostate cancer-related biological processes (BP), cellular components (CC), molecular functions (MF) and signal pathways. For the obtained information, we met the p-value < 0.05; sorted according to the number of genes; selected the top 10 enrichment information of BP, CC, and MF, and the top 20 enrichment information of KEGG; and used the bioinformatics online platform (https://www.bioinformatics.com.cn/ (accessed on 10 July 2022)) to visualize the analysis results (Figures 6 and 7).

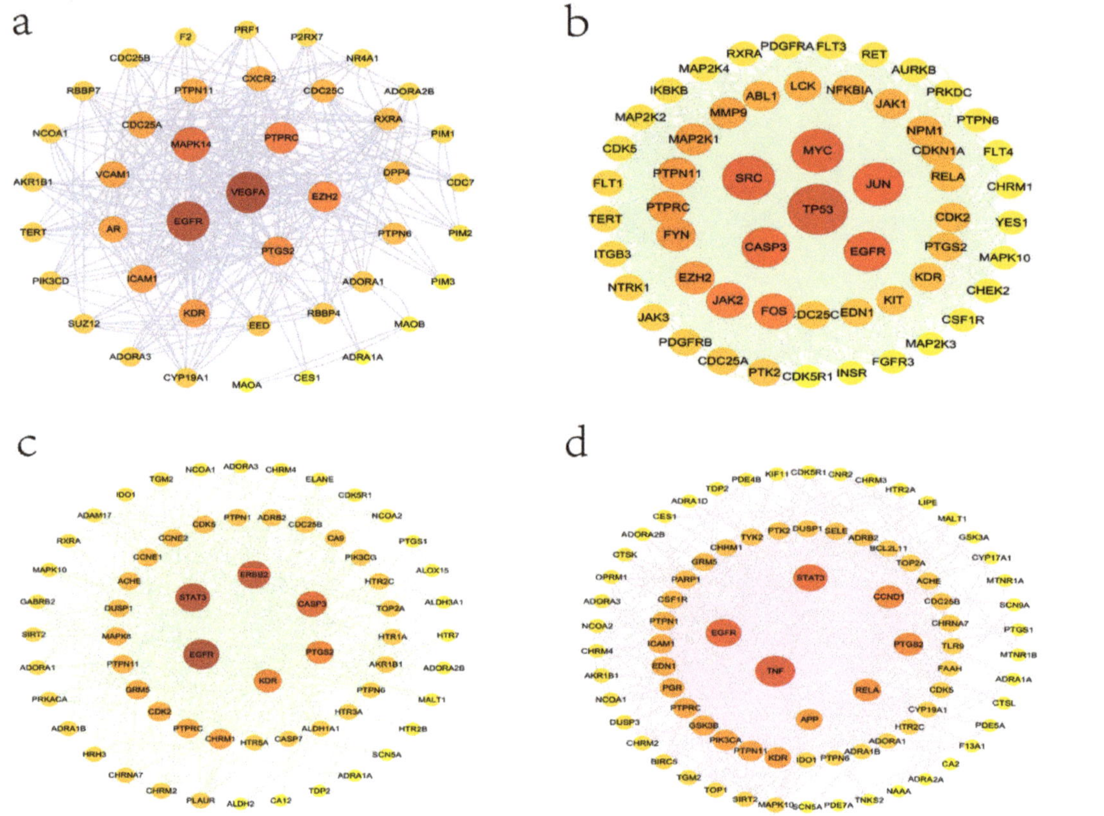

Figure 5. Protein network analysis of four Tanshinone components ((**a**): Tanshinone Ir; (**b**): Tanshinone IIA; (**c**): Dihydrotanshinone I; (**d**): Cryptotanshinone).

Finally, our results show that the target of TsIIA is significantly more than the other three components. Among them, cellular tumor antigen p53 (TP53), myc proto-oncogene protein (MYC), transcription factor AP-1 (JUN), Src, Caspase-3 (CASP3), and EGFR play a key role in the anti-prostate cancer process of TsIIA, followed by CYT, which has more targets than the other two components. EGFR, TNF, STAT3, prostaglandin G/H synthase 2 (PTGS2,), Transcription factor p65 (RELA), and other targets are the key targets of CYT, The second is DHTI, STAT3, receptor tyrosine-protein kinase erbB-2 (ERBB2), CASP3, EGFR, PTGS2, etc. are the key targets of DHTI, and finally, TsI, Vascular endothelial growth factor A(VEGFA), EGFR, MAPK14, protein tyrosine phosphatase receptor type C (PTPRC), enhancer of zeste homolog 2 (EZH2), etc. are the key targets. These key targets are essential for various biological processes of prostate cancer, and these components participate in regulating multiple signaling pathways.

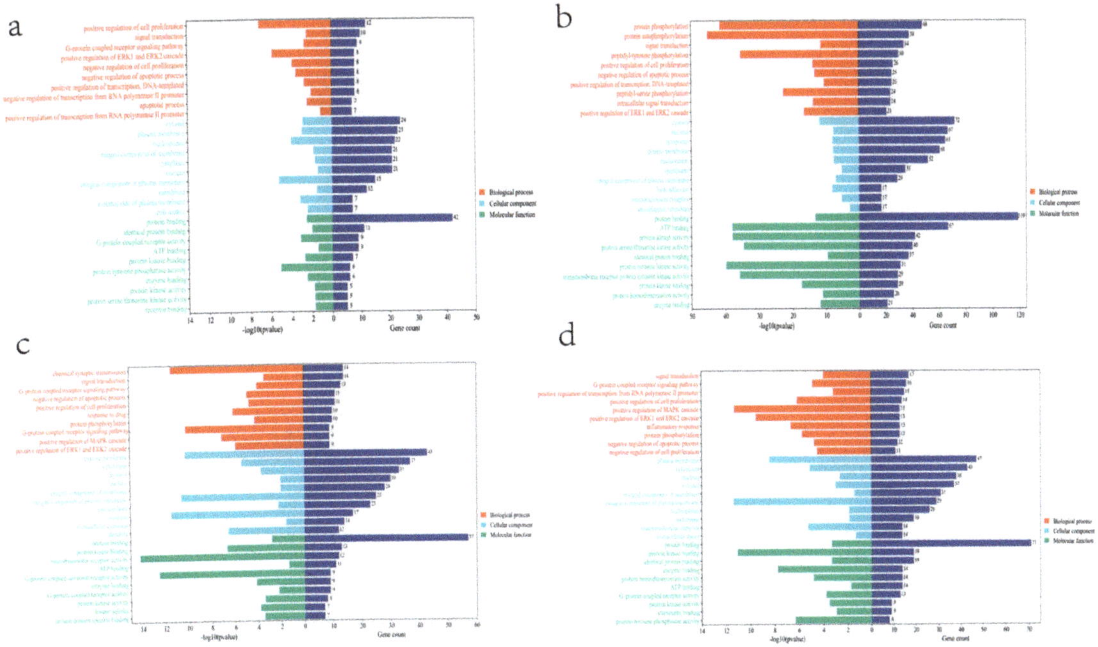

Figure 6. Go enrichment analysis of four components of Tanshinone((**a**): Tanshinone Ir; (**b**): Tanshinone IIA; (**c**): Dihydrotanshinone I; (**d**): Cryptotanshinone).

Secondly, our results also show that the biological processes of the four Tanshinone components mainly occur in the cell and participate in the activation and binding of a series of cell receptors and cascade downstream signaling pathways. KEGG analysis shows that PI3K Akt signaling pathway, MAPK signaling pathway, Ras signaling pathway, and rap signaling pathway play a key role in the anti-prostate cancer process of Tanshinone, which is consistent with previous studies, These pathways have significant significance for the metastasis, progression, and angiogenesis of prostate cancer. In addition, as mentioned above, Tanshinone has a significant effect on the regulation of immune pathways. we note that the four Tanshinone components have a regulatory effect on the PD-1/PD-L1 signaling pathway, T cell-related pathways, and immune helper cells and related factors mediated signaling pathways. Although these results are not in our screening results, they are statistically different (p-value < 0.05). This is consistent with the protein network analysis, which may have more significant significance for immunotherapy-insensitive prostate cancer. In addition, our results also show that Tanshinone has a regulatory effect on microRNAs in prostate cancer cells, and these small molecules are also essential for tumor survival and metastasis. In conclusion, our results and the existing laboratory data show that Tanshinone can inhibit the metastasis, invasion, and progression of prostate cancer through multiple targets and pathways. However, the current research is limited. Therefore, more research should be carried out in the future to further clarify the relevant mechanisms and molecular pathways of Tanshinone against prostate cancer, and more attention should be paid to the bioavailability and toxicological experiments of Tanshinone.

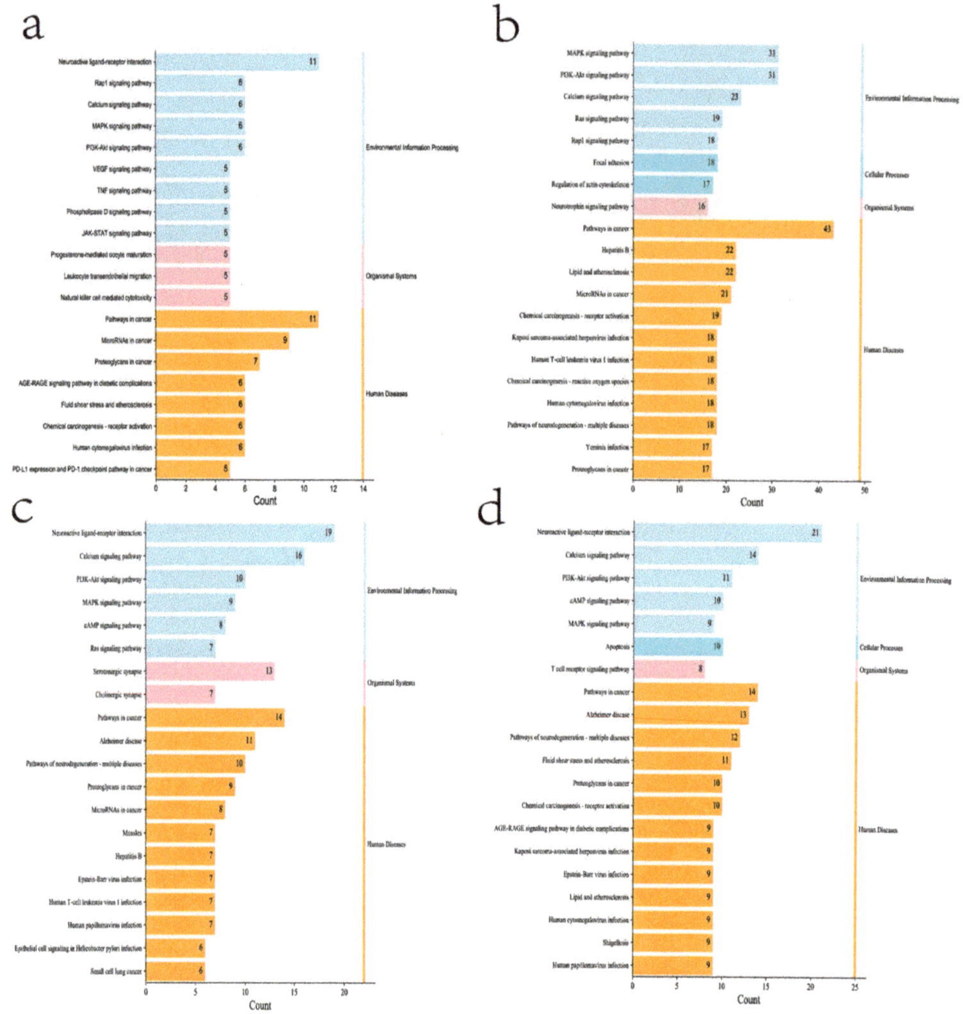

Figure 7. KEGG enrichment analysis of four components of Tanshinone ((**a**): Tanshinone Ir; (**b**): Tanshinone IIA; (**c**): Dihydrotanshinone I; (**d**): Cryptotanshinone).

Author Contributions: K.T. conceptualized the review, analyzed the data, and helped to write the manuscript. W.L., T.H., S.X., B.C., Y.Y. and W.Z. helped to write the manuscript and prepared the figures. All authors have read and agreed to the published version of the manuscript.

Funding: This study was supported by the National Natural Science Fund of China (81660263), Science and Technology Fund Project of Guizhou Health Commission (gzwkj2021–211), and Doctoral Fund of Affiliated Hospital of Guiyang Medical College, Guizhou Province, China (C-2012-6).

Acknowledgments: Thanks all the research participants of this study. This study was supported by the National Natural Science Fund of China (81660263), Science and Technology Fund Project of Guizhou Health Commission (gzwkj2021-211), and Doctoral Fund of Affiliated Hospital of Guiyang Medical College, Guizhou Province, China (C-2012-6).

Conflicts of Interest: The authors declare no conflict of interest.

References

1. Siegel, R.L.; Miller, K.D.; Jemal, A. Cancer statistics, 2020. *CA Cancer J. Clin.* **2020**, *70*, 7–30. [CrossRef] [PubMed]
2. Pernar, C.H.; Ebot, E.M.; Wilson, K.M.; Mucci, L.A. The Epidemiology of Prostate Cancer. *Cold Spring Harb. Perspect Med.* **2018**, *8*, a030361. [CrossRef] [PubMed]
3. Daniyal, M.; Siddiqui, Z.A.; Akram, M.; Asif, H.M.; Sultana, S.; Khan, A. Epidemiology, etiology, diagnosis and treatment of prostate cancer. *Asian Pac. J. Cancer Prev.* **2014**, *15*, 9575–9578. [CrossRef]
4. Karantanos, T.; Corn, P.G.; Thompson, T.C. Prostate cancer progression after androgen deprivation therapy: Mechanisms of castrate resistance and novel therapeutic approaches. *Oncogene* **2013**, *32*, 5501–5511. [CrossRef]
5. Cattrini, C.; Castro, E.; Lozano, R.; Zanardi, E.; Rubagotti, A.; Boccardo, F.; Olmos, D. Current Treatment Options for Metastatic Hormone-Sensitive Prostate Cancer. *Cancers* **2019**, *11*, 1355. [CrossRef]
6. Singh, K.; Nassar, N.; Bachari, A.; Schanknecht, E.; Telukutla, S.; Zomer, R.; Piva, T.J.; Mantri, N. The Pathophysiology and the Therapeutic Potential of Cannabinoids in Prostate Cancer. *Cancers* **2021**, *13*, 4107. [CrossRef] [PubMed]
7. Pang, H.; Wu, L.; Tang, Y.; Zhou, G.; Qu, C.; Duan, J.-A. Chemical Analysis of the Herbal Medicine Salviae miltiorrhizae Radix et Rhizoma (Danshen). *Molecules* **2016**, *21*, 51. [CrossRef]
8. Jiang, Z.; Gao, W.; Huang, L. Tanshinones, Critical Pharmacological Components in Salvia miltiorrhiza. *Front. Pharmacol.* **2019**, *10*, 202. [CrossRef]
9. Kai, G.; Xu, H.; Zhou, C.; Liao, P.; Xiao, J.; Luo, X.; You, L.; Zhang, L. Metabolic engineering tanshinone biosynthetic pathway in Salvia miltiorrhiza hairy root cultures. *Metab. Eng.* **2011**, *13*, 319–327. [CrossRef]
10. Cao, W.; Wang, Y.; Shi, M.; Hao, X.; Zhao, W.; Wang, Y.; Ren, J.; Kai, G. Transcription Factor SmWRKY1 Positively Promotes the Biosynthesis of Tanshinones in Salvia miltiorrhiza. *Front. Plant Sci.* **2018**, *9*, 554. [CrossRef]
11. Lai, Z.; He, J.; Zhou, C.; Zhao, H.; Cui, S. Tanshinones: An Update in the Medicinal Chemistry in Recent 5 Years. *Curr. Med. Chem.* **2021**, *28*, 2807–2827. [CrossRef] [PubMed]
12. Fu, L.; Han, B.; Zhou, Y.; Ren, J.; Cao, W.; Patel, G.; Kai, G.; Zhang, J. The Anticancer Properties of Tanshinones and the Pharmaco-logical Effects of Their Active Ingredients. *Front Pharmacol.* **2020**, *11*, 193. [CrossRef]
13. Fang, Z.; Zhang, M.; Liu, J.-N.; Zhao, X.; Zhang, Y.-Q.; Fang, L. Tanshinone IIA: A Review of its Anticancer Effects. *Front. Pharmacol.* **2021**, *11*, 611087. [CrossRef]
14. Ma, Y.; Cui, G.; Chen, T.; Ma, X.; Wang, R.; Jin, B.; Yang, J.; Kang, L.; Tang, J.; Lai, C.; et al. Expansion within the CYP71D subfamily drives the heterocyclization of tanshinones synthesis in Salvia miltiorrhiza. *Nat. Commun.* **2021**, *12*, 685. [CrossRef]
15. Huang, X.; Jin, L.; Deng, H.; Wu, D.; Shen, Q.-K.; Quan, Z.-S.; Zhang, C.-H.; Guo, H.-Y. Research and Development of Natural Product Tanshinone I: Pharmacology, Total Synthesis, and Structure Modifications. *Front. Pharmacol.* **2022**, *13*, 920411. [CrossRef]
16. Gao, H.; Sun, W.; Zhao, J.; Wu, X.; Lu, J.J.; Chen, X.; Xu, Q.M.; Khan, I.A.; Yang, S. Tanshinones and diethyl blechnics with an-ti-inflammatory and anti-cancer activities from Salvia miltiorrhiza Bunge (Danshen). *Sci. Rep.* **2016**, *6*, 33720. [CrossRef]
17. Guo, J.; Ma, X.; Cai, Y.; Ma, Y.; Zhan, Z.; Zhou, Y.; Liu, W.; Guan, M.; Yang, J.; Cui, G.; et al. Cytochrome P450 promiscuity leads to a bifurcating biosynthetic pathway for tanshinones. *New Phytol.* **2016**, *210*, 525–534. [CrossRef]
18. Zhao, J.-L.; Zhou, L.-G.; Wu, J.-Y. Effects of biotic and abiotic elicitors on cell growth and tanshinone accumulation in Salvia miltiorrhiza cell cultures. *Appl. Microbiol. Biotechnol.* **2010**, *87*, 137–144. [CrossRef]
19. Song, M.; Hang, T.J.; Zhang, Z.; Chen, H.Y. Effects of the coexisting diterpenoid Tanshinones on the pharmacokinetics of Cryp-totanshinone and Tanshinone IIA in rat. *Eur. J. Pharm. Sci.* **2007**, *32*, 247–253. [CrossRef]
20. Chen, F.; Li, L.; Tian, D.-D. Salvia miltiorrhiza Roots against Cardiovascular Disease: Consideration of Herb-Drug Interactions. *BioMed Res. Int.* **2017**, *2017*, 9868694.
21. Hao, D.-C.; Xiao, P.-G. Impact of Drug Metabolism/Pharmacokinetics and their Relevance Upon Salviabased Drug Discovery. *Curr. Drug Metab.* **2017**, *18*, 1071–1084. [CrossRef]
22. Sun, J.; Yang, M.; Han, J.; Wang, B.; Ma, X.; Xu, M.; Liu, P.; Guo, D. Profiling the metabolic difference of seven tanshinones using high-performance liquid chromatography/multi-stage mass spectrometry with data-dependent acquisition. *Rapid Commun. Mass Spectrom.* **2007**, *21*, 2211–2226. [CrossRef]
23. Kim, D.H.; Paudel, P.; Yu, T.; Ngo, T.M.; Kim, J.A.; Jung, H.A.; Yokozawa, T.; Choi, J.S. Characterization of the inhibitory activity of natural tanshinones from Salvia miltiorrhiza roots on protein tyrosine phosphatase 1B. *Chem. Interact.* **2017**, *278*, 65–73. [CrossRef]
24. Wang, L.; Liu, A.; Zhang, F.-L.; Yeung, J.H.; Li, X.-Q.; Cho, C.-H. Evaluation and SAR analysis of the cytotoxicity of tanshinones in colon cancer cells. *Chin. J. Nat. Med.* **2014**, *12*, 167–171. [CrossRef]
25. Zhang, Z.; Zhang, J.; Jin, L.; Song, T.; Wu, G.; Gao, J. Tanshinone IIA Interacts with DNA by Minor Groove-Binding. *Biol. Pharm. Bull.* **2008**, *31*, 2342–2345. [CrossRef]
26. Li, Z.; Zou, J.; Cao, D.; Ma, X. Pharmacological basis of tanshinone and new insights into tanshinone as a multitarget natural product for multifaceted diseases. *Biomed. Pharmacother.* **2020**, *130*, 110599. [CrossRef]
27. Ashrafizadeh, M.; Zarrabi, A.; Orouei, S.; Saberifar, S.; Salami, S.; Hushmandi, K.; Najafi, M. Recent advances and future directions in anti-tumor activity of cryptotanshinone: A mechanistic review. *Phytotherapy Res.* **2021**, *35*, 155–179. [CrossRef]
28. Wu, Y.H.; Wu, Y.R.; Li, B.; Yan, Z.Y. Cryptotanshinone: A review of its pharmacology activities and molecular mechanisms. *Fitoterapia* **2020**, *145*, 104633. [CrossRef]
29. Zhang, W.; Liu, C.; Li, J.; Lu, Y.; Li, H.; Zhuang, J.; Ren, X.; Wang, M.; Sun, C. Tanshinone IIA: New Perspective on the Anti-Tumor Mechanism of a Traditional Natural Medicine. *Am. J. Chin. Med.* **2022**, *50*, 209–239. [CrossRef]

30. Gong, Y.; Li, Y.; Lu, Y.; Li, L.; Abdolmaleky, H.M.; Blackburn, G.L.; Zhou, J.-R. Bioactive tanshinones in Salvia miltiorrhiza inhibit the growth of prostate cancer cells in vitro and in mice. *Int. J. Cancer* **2011**, *129*, 1042–1052. [CrossRef]
31. Lee, H.-J.; Jung, D.-B.; Sohn, E.J.; Kim, H.H.; Park, M.N.; Lew, J.-H.; Lee, S.-G.; Kim, B.; Kim, S.-H. Inhibition of Hypoxia Inducible Factor Alpha and Astrocyte-Elevated Gene-1 Mediates Cryptotanshinone Exerted Antitumor Activity in Hypoxic PC-3 Cells. Evidence-Based Complement. *Altern. Med.* **2012**, *2012*, 390957. [CrossRef]
32. Wu, C.Y.; Yang, Y.H.; Lin, Y.Y.; Kuan, F.C.; Lin, Y.S.; Lin, W.Y.; Tsai, M.Y.; Yang, J.J.; Cheng, Y.C.; Shu, L.H.; et al. Anti-cancer effect of danshen and dihydroisoTanshinone I on prostate cancer: Targeting the crosstalk between macro-phages and cancer cells via inhibition of the STAT3/CCL2 signaling pathway. *Oncotarget* **2017**, *8*, 40246–40263. [CrossRef]
33. Termini, D.; Hartogh, D.J.D.; Jaglanian, A.; Tsiani, E. Curcumin against Prostate Cancer: Current Evidence. *Biomolecules* **2020**, *10*, 1536. [CrossRef]
34. Won, S.H.; Lee, H.J.; Jeong, S.J.; Lü, J.; Kim, S.H. Activation of p53 signaling and inhibition of AR mediate Tanshinone IIA induced G1 arrest in LNCaP prostate cancer cells. *Phytother Res.* **2012**, *26*, 669–674. [CrossRef]
35. Li, C.; Han, X.; Zhang, H.; Wu, J.; Li, B. The interplay between autophagy and apoptosis induced by tanshinone IIA in prostate cancer cells. *Tumor Biol.* **2016**, *37*, 7667–7674. [CrossRef]
36. Hou, L.-L.; Xu, Q.-J.; Hu, G.-Q.; Xie, S.-Q. Synergistic antitumor effects of tanshinone II A in combination with cisplatin via apoptosis in the prostate cancer cells. *Yao xue xue bao = Acta Pharm. Sin.* **2013**, *48*, 675–679. (In Chinese)
37. Yun, S.-M.; Jung, J.H.; Jeong, S.-J.; Sohn, E.J.; Kim, B.; Kim, S.-H. Tanshinone IIA Induces Autophagic Cell Death via Activation of AMPK and ERK and Inhibition of mTOR and p70 S6K in KBM-5 Leukemia Cells. *Phytotherapy Res.* **2014**, *28*, 458–464. [CrossRef]
38. Won, S.-H.; Lee, H.-J.; Jeong, S.-J.; Lee, E.-O.; Jung, D.-B.; Shin, J.-M.; Kwon, T.-R.; Yun, S.-M.; Lee, M.-H.; Choi, S.-H.; et al. Tanshinone IIA Induces Mitochondria Dependent Apoptosis in Prostate Cancer Cells in Association with an Inhibition of Phosphoinositide 3-Kinase/AKT Pathway. *Biol. Pharm. Bull.* **2010**, *33*, 1828–1834. [CrossRef]
39. Chiu, S.C.; Huang, S.Y.; Chen, S.P.; Su, C.C.; Chiu, T.L.; Pang, C.-Y. Tanshinone IIA inhibits human prostate cancer cells growth by induction of endoplasmic reticulum stress in vitro and in vivo. *Prostate Cancer Prostatic Dis.* **2013**, *16*, 315–322. [CrossRef]
40. Zhang, Y.; Won, S.H.; Jiang, C.; Lee, H.J.; Jeong, S.J.; Lee, E.O.; Zhang, J.; Ye, M.; Kim, S.H.; Lü, J. Tanshinones from Chinese medicinal herb Danshen (Salvia miltiorrhiza Bunge) suppress prostate cancer growth and AR signaling. *Pharm. Res.* **2012**, *29*, 1595–1608. [CrossRef]
41. Liu, W.; Zhou, J.; Geng, G.; Shi, Q.; Sauriol, F.; Wu, J.H. Antiandrogenic, Maspin Induction, and Antiprostate Cancer Activities of Tanshinone IIA and Its Novel Derivatives with Modification in Ring, A. *J. Med. Chem.* **2012**, *55*, 971–975. [CrossRef]
42. Yu, J.; Li, S.; Zeng, X.; Song, J.; Hu, S.; Cheng, S.; Chen, C.; Luo, H.; Pan, W. Design, synthesis, and evaluation of proliferation inhibitory activity of novel L-shaped ortho-quinone analogs as anticancer agents. *Bioorg. Chem.* **2021**, *117*, 105383. [CrossRef]
43. Yao, Y.; Li, H.-Z.; Qian, B.-J.; Liu, C.-M.; Zhang, J.-B.; Lin, M.-C. Crypotanshione reduces the expression of metadherin in DU145 prostate cancer cells. *Zhonghua nan ke xue = Natl. J. Androl.* **2015**, *21*, 782–787. (In Chinese)
44. Wu, C.-Y.; Hsieh, C.-Y.; Huang, K.-E.; Chang, C.; Kang, H.-Y. Cryptotanshinone down-regulates androgen receptor signaling by modulating lysine-specific demethylase 1 function. *Int. J. Cancer* **2012**, *131*, 1423–1434. [CrossRef]
45. Park, I.J.; Kim, M.J.; Park, O.J.; Park, M.G.; Choe, W.; Kang, I.; Kim, S.S.; Ha, J. Cryptotanshinone sensitizes DU145 prostate cancer cells to Fas(APO1/CD95)-mediated apoptosis through Bcl-2 and MAPK regulation. *Cancer Lett.* **2010**, *298*, 88–98. [CrossRef]
46. Xu, D.; Lin, T.H.; Li, S.; Da, J.; Wen, X.Q.; Ding, J.; Chang, C.; Yeh, S. Cryptotanshinone suppresses AR-mediated growth in androgen dependent and castration resistant prostate cancer cells. *Cancer Lett.* **2012**, *316*, 11–22. [CrossRef]
47. Zhang, Y.; Cabarcas, S.M.; Zheng, J.I.; Sun, L.; Mathews, L.A.; Zhang, X.; Lin, H.; Farrar, W.L. Cryptotanshinone targets tu-mor-initiating cells through down-regulation of stemness genes expression. *Oncol Lett.* **2016**, *11*, 3803–3812. [CrossRef]
48. Chen, W.; Luo, Y.; Liu, L.; Zhou, H.; Xu, B.; Han, X.; Shen, T.; Liu, Z.; Lu, Y.; Huang, S. Cryptotanshinone inhibits cancer cell prolif-eration by suppressing Mammalian target of rapamycin-mediated cyclin D1 expression and Rb phosphorylation. *Cancer Prev. Res.* **2010**, *3*, 1015–1025. [CrossRef]
49. Lin, T.H.; Lee, S.O.; Niu, Y.; Xu, D.; Liang, L.; Li, L.; Yeh, S.D.; Fujimoto, N.; Yeh, S.; Chang, C. Differential androgen deprivation therapies with anti-androgens casodex/bicalutamide or MDV3100/Enzalutamide versus anti-AR ASC-J9(R) Lead to promotion versus suppression of prostate cancer metastasis. *J. Biol. Chem.* **2013**, *288*, 19359–19369. [CrossRef]
50. Kim, E.J.; Kim, S.Y.; Kim, S.-M.; Lee, M. A novel topoisomerase 2a inhibitor, cryptotanshinone, suppresses the growth of PC3 cells without apparent cytotoxicity. *Toxicol. Appl. Pharmacol.* **2017**, *330*, 84–92. [CrossRef]
51. Shin, D.-S.; Kim, H.-N.; Shin, K.D.; Yoon, Y.J.; Kim, S.-J.; Han, D.C.; Kwon, B.-M. Cryptotanshinone Inhibits Constitutive Signal Transducer and Activator of Transcription 3 Function through Blocking the Dimerization in DU145 Prostate Cancer Cells. *Cancer Res.* **2009**, *69*, 193–202. [CrossRef] [PubMed]
52. Shin, E.A.; Sohn, E.J.; Won, G.; Choi, J.U.; Jeong, M.; Kim, B.; Kim, M.J.; Kim, S.H. Upregulation of microRNA135a-3p and death receptor 5 plays a critical role in Tanshinone I sensitized prostate cancer cells to TRAIL induced apoptosis. *Oncotarget* **2014**, *5*, 5624–5636. [CrossRef] [PubMed]
53. Chuang, M.-T.; Ho, F.-M.; Wu, C.-C.; Zhuang, S.-Y.; Lin, S.-Y.; Suk, F.-M.; Liang, Y.-C. 15,16-Dihydrotanshinone I, a Compound ofSalvia miltiorrhizaBunge, Induces Apoptosis through Inducing Endoplasmic Reticular Stress in Human Prostate Carcinoma Cells. Evidence-Based Complement. *Altern. Med.* **2011**, *2011*, 865435.

54. Wang, M.; Zeng, X.; Li, S.; Sun, Z.; Yu, J.; Chen, C.; Shen, X.; Pan, W.; Luo, H. A Novel Tanshinone Analog Exerts Anti-Cancer Effects in Prostate Cancer by Inducing Cell Apoptosis, Arresting Cell Cycle at G2 Phase and Blocking Metastatic Ability. *Int. J. Mol. Sci.* **2019**, *20*, 4459. [CrossRef]
55. Xu, D.; Lin, T.-H.; Zhang, C.; Tsai, Y.-C.; Li, S.; Zhang, J.; Yin, M.; Yeh, S.; Chang, C. The selective inhibitory effect of a synthetic tanshinone derivative on prostate cancer cells. *Prostate* **2012**, *72*, 803–816. [CrossRef]
56. Bae, W.J.; Choi, J.B.; Kim, K.S.; Ha, U.S.; Hong, S.H.; Lee, J.Y.; Hwang, T.-K.; Hwang, S.Y.; Wang, Z.-P.; Kim, S.W. Inhibition of Proliferation of Prostate Cancer Cell Line DU-145 in vitro and in vivo Using Salvia miltiorrhiza Bunge. *Chin. J. Integr. Med.* **2020**, *26*, 533–538. [CrossRef]
57. Lee, J.; Choi, B.Y.; Keum, Y.-S. Acetonitrile extract of Salvia miltiorrhiza Radix exhibits growth-inhibitory effects on prostate cancer cells through the induction of cell cycle arrest and apoptosis. *Oncol. Lett.* **2017**, *13*, 2921–2928. [CrossRef]
58. Qiu, S.; Granet, R.; Mbakidi, J.P.; Brégier, F.; Pouget, C.; Micallef, L.; Sothea-Ouk, T.; Leger, D.Y.; Liagre, B.; Chaleix, V.; et al. Delivery of Tanshinone IIA and α-mangostin from gold/PEI/cyclodextrin nanoparticle platform designed for prostate cancer chemo-therapy. *Bioorg. Med. Chem. Lett.* **2016**, *26*, 2503–2506. [CrossRef]
59. Zhang, K.; Liu, X.; Ravi, S.O.A.S.; Ramachandran, A.; Ibrahim, I.A.A.; Nassir, A.M.; Yao, J. Synthesis of silver nanoparticles (AgNPs) from leaf extract of Salvia miltiorrhiza and its anticancer potential in human prostate cancer LNCaP cell lines. *Artif. Cells Nanomed. Biotechnol.* **2019**, *47*, 2846–2854. [CrossRef]
60. Sun, G.; Sun, K.; Sun, J. Combination prostate cancer therapy: Prostate-specific membranes antigen targeted, pH-sensitive nanoparticles loaded with doxorubicin and tanshinone. *Drug Deliv.* **2021**, *28*, 1132–1140. [CrossRef]
61. Bates, S.; Bonetta, L.; MacAllan, D.; Parry, D.; Holder, A.; Dickson, C.; Peters, G. CDK6 (PLSTIRE) and CDK4 (PSK-J3) are a distinct subset of the cyclin-dependent kinases that associate with cyclin D1. *Oncogene* **1994**, *9*, 71–79.
62. Petroni, G.; Formenti, S.C.; Chen-Kiang, S.; Galluzzi, L. Immunomodulation by anticancer cell cycle inhibitors. *Nat. Rev. Immunol.* **2020**, *20*, 669–679. [CrossRef]
63. Kato, J.; Matsushime, H.; Hiebert, S.W.; Ewen, M.E.; Sherr, C.J. Direct binding of cyclin D to the retinoblastoma gene product (pRb) and pRb phosphorylation by the cyclin D-dependent kinase CDK4. *Genes Dev.* **1993**, *7*, 331–342. [CrossRef] [PubMed]
64. Gao, X.; Leone, G.W.; Wang, H. Cyclin D-CDK4/6 functions in cancer. *Adv. Cancer Res.* **2020**, *148*, 147–169. [PubMed]
65. Hernández-Monge, J.; Rousset-Roman, A.B.; Medina-Medina, I.; Olivares-Illana, V. Dual function of MDM2 and MDMX toward the tumor suppressors p53 and RB. *Genes Cancer* **2016**, *7*, 278–287. [CrossRef] [PubMed]
66. Liu, C.; Sun, H.N.; Luo, Y.H.; Piao, X.J.; Wu, D.D.; Meng, L.Q.; Wang, Y.; Zhang, Y.; Wang, J.R.; Wang, H.; et al. Cryptotanshinone induces ROS-mediated apoptosis in human gastric cancer cells. *Oncotarget* **2017**, *8*, 115398–115412. [CrossRef]
67. Pistritto, G.; Trisciuoglio, D.; Ceci, C.; Garufi, A.; D'Orazi, G. Apoptosis as anticancer mechanism: Function and dysfunction of its modulators and targeted therapeutic strategies. *Aging* **2016**, *8*, 603–619. [CrossRef]
68. Goldar, S.; Khaniani, M.S.; Derakhshan, S.M.; Baradaran, B. Molecular Mechanisms of Apoptosis and Roles in Cancer Development and Treatment. *Asian Pac. J. Cancer Prev.* **2015**, *16*, 2129–2144. [CrossRef]
69. Lambert, A.W.; Pattabiraman, D.R.; Weinberg, R.A. Emerging Biological Principles of Metastasis. *Cell* **2017**, *168*, 670–691. [CrossRef]
70. Erdogan, B.; Webb, D.J. Cancer-associated fibroblasts modulate growth factor signaling and extracellular matrix remodeling to regulate tumor metastasis. *Biochem. Soc. Trans.* **2017**, *45*, 229–236. [CrossRef]
71. Cai, T.; Santi, R.; Tamanini, I.; Galli, I.C.; Perletti, G.; Bjerklund Johansen, T.E.; Nesi, G. Current Knowledge of the Potential Links between Inflammation and Prostate Cancer. *Int. J. Mol. Sci.* **2019**, *20*, 3833. [CrossRef] [PubMed]
72. Archer, M.; Dogra, N.; Kyprianou, N. Inflammation as a Driver of Prostate Cancer Metastasis and Therapeutic Resistance. *Cancers* **2020**, *12*, 2984. [CrossRef] [PubMed]
73. Nikonova, A.S.; Astsaturov, I.; Serebriiskii, I.G.; Dunbrack, R.L., Jr.; Golemis, E.A. Aurora A kinase (AURKA) in normal and patho-logical cell division. *Cell Mol. Life Sci.* **2013**, *70*, 661–687. [CrossRef]
74. Dhiman, G.; Srivastava, N.; Goyal, M.; Rakha, E.; Lothion-Roy, J.; Mongan, N.P.; Miftakhova, R.R.; Khaiboullina, S.; Rizvanov, A.A.; Baranwal, M. Metadherin: A Therapeutic Target in Multiple Cancers. *Front. Oncol.* **2019**, *9*, 349. [CrossRef] [PubMed]
75. Manzoni, L.; Zucal, C.; Di Maio, D.; D'Agostino, V.G.; Thongon, N.; Bonomo, I.; Lal, P.; Miceli, M.; Baj, V.; Brambilla, M.; et al. Interfering with HuR–RNA Interaction: Design, Synthesis and Biological Characterization of Tanshinone Mimics as Novel, Effective HuR Inhibitors. *J. Med. Chem.* **2018**, *61*, 1483–1498. [CrossRef]
76. D'Agostino, V.; Lal, P.; Mantelli, B.; Tiedje, C.; Zucal, C.; Thongon, N.; Gaestel, M.; Latorre, E.; Marinelli, L.; Seneci, P.; et al. Dihydrotanshinone-I interferes with the RNA-binding activity of HuR affecting its post-transcriptional function. *Sci. Rep.* **2015**, *5*, 16478. [CrossRef]
77. Soares, J.; Keppler, B.R.; Wang, X.; Lee, K.-H.; Jarstfer, M.B. ortho-Quinone tanshinones directly inhibit telomerase through an oxidative mechanism mediated by hydrogen peroxide. *Bioorg. Med. Chem. Lett.* **2011**, *21*, 7474–7478. [CrossRef]
78. Liu, X.-D.; Fan, R.-F.; Zhang, Y.; Yang, H.-Z.; Fang, Z.-G.; Guan, W.-B.; Lin, D.-J.; Xiao, R.-Z.; Huang, R.-W.; Huang, H.-Q.; et al. Down-Regulation of Telomerase Activity and Activation of Caspase-3 Are Responsible for Tanshinone I-Induced Apoptosis in Monocyte Leukemia Cells in Vitro. *Int. J. Mol. Sci.* **2010**, *11*, 2267–2280. [CrossRef]
79. Zhang, S.; Duan, S.; Xie, Z.; Bao, W.; Xu, B.; Yang, W.; Zhou, L. Epigenetic Therapeutics Targeting NRF2/KEAP1 Signaling in Cancer Oxidative Stress. *Front Pharmacol.* **2022**, *13*, 924817. [CrossRef]

80. Chen, W.; Lu, Y.; Chen, G.; Huang, S. Molecular evidence of cryptotanshinone for treatment and prevention of human cancer. *Anti-Cancer Agents Med. Chem.* **2013**, *13*, 979–987. [CrossRef]
81. Tsegay, P.S.; Lai, Y.; Liu, Y. Replication Stress and Consequential Instability of the Genome and Epigenome. *Molecules* **2019**, *24*, 3870. [CrossRef]
82. Budakoti, M.; Panwar, A.S.; Molpa, D.; Singh, R.K.; Büsselberg, D.; Mishra, A.P.; Coutinho, H.D.M.; Nigam, M. Micro-RNA: The dar-khorse of cancer. *Cell Signal.* **2021**, *83*, 109995. [CrossRef] [PubMed]
83. Lin, X.; Qureshi, M.Z.; Romero, M.A.; Khalid, S.; Aras, A.; Ozbey, U.; Farooqi, A.A. Regulation of signaling pathways by tanshinones in different cancers. *Cell. Mol. Biol.* **2017**, *63*, 53–58. [CrossRef] [PubMed]
84. Teo, M.Y.; Rathkopf, D.E.; Kantoff, P. Treatment of Advanced Prostate Cancer. *Annu. Rev. Med.* **2019**, *70*, 479–499. [CrossRef]
85. Komura, K.; Sweeney, C.J.; Inamoto, T.; Ibuki, N.; Azuma, H.; Kantoff, P.W. Current treatment strategies for advanced prostate cancer. *Int. J. Urol.* **2018**, *25*, 220–231. [CrossRef] [PubMed]
86. Hu, T.; To, K.K.; Wang, L.; Zhang, L.; Lu, L.; Shen, J.; Chan, R.L.; Li, M.; Yeung, J.H.; Cho, C.H. Reversal of P-glycoprotein (P-gp) mediated multidrug resistance in colon cancer cells by cryptotanshinone and dihydrotanshinone of Salvia miltiorrhiza. *Phytomedicine* **2014**, *21*, 1264–1272. [CrossRef]
87. Tian, Q.T.; Ding, C.Y.; Song, S.S.; Wang, Y.Q.; Zhang, A.; Miao, Z.H. New Tanshinone I derivatives S222 and S439 similarly inhibit topoisomerase I/II but reveal different p53-dependency in inducing G2/M arrest and apoptosis. *Biochem. Pharmacol.* **2018**, *154*, 255–264. [CrossRef]
88. Assaraf, Y.G.; Brozovic, A.; Gonçalves, A.C.; Jurkovicova, D.; Linē, A.; Machuqueiro, M.; Saponara, S.; Sarmento-Ribeiro, A.B.; Xavier, C.P.R.; Vasconcelos, M.H. The multi-factorial nature of clinical multidrug resistance in cancer. *Drug Resist. Updates* **2019**, *46*, 100645. [CrossRef]
89. Li, H.; Wang, H.; Ma, Y.; Zhao, J. Clarithromycin combined with tanshinone for rhinosinusal and laryngeal radiation injury in patients with nasopharyngeal carcinoma after radiotherapy. *Nan Fang Yi Ke Da Xue Xue Bao* **2012**, *32*, 1168–1170. (In Chinese)
90. Li, K.; Liu, W.; Zhao, Q.; Wu, C.; Fan, C.; Lai, H.; Li, S. Combination of tanshinone IIA and doxorubicin possesses synergism and attenuation effects on doxorubicin in the treatment of breast cancer. *Phytotherapy Res.* **2019**, *33*, 1658–1669. [CrossRef]
91. Ketola, K.; Viitala, M.; Kohonen, P.; Fey, V.; Culig, Z.; Kallioniemi, O.; Iljin, K. High-throughput cell-based compound screen iden-tifies pinosylvin methyl ether and Tanshinone IIA as inhibitors of castration-resistant prostate cancer. *J. Mol. Biochem.* **2016**, *5*, 12–22. [PubMed]
92. Lin, L.-L.; Hsia, C.-R.; Hsu, C.-L.; Huang, H.-C.; Juan, H.-F. Integrating transcriptomics and proteomics to show that tanshinone IIA suppresses cell growth by blocking glucose metabolism in gastric cancer cells. *BMC Genom.* **2015**, *16*, 41. [CrossRef] [PubMed]
93. Yang, Y.; Cao, Y.; Chen, L.; Liu, F.; Qi, Z.; Cheng, X.; Wang, Z. Cryptotanshinone suppresses cell proliferation and glucose me-tabolism via STAT3/SIRT3 signaling pathway in ovarian cancer cells. *Cancer Med.* **2018**, *7*, 4610–4618. [CrossRef] [PubMed]
94. Zhu, L.; Zhu, X.; Wu, Y. Effects of Glucose Metabolism, Lipid Metabolism, and Glutamine Metabolism on Tumor Microenvironment and Clinical Implications. *Biomolecules* **2022**, *12*, 580. [CrossRef] [PubMed]
95. Pardo, J.C.; de Porras, V.R.; Gil, J.; Font, A.; Puig-Domingo, M.; Jordà, M. Lipid Metabolism and Epigenetics Crosstalk in Prostate Cancer. *Nutrients* **2022**, *14*, 851. [CrossRef]
96. Galbraith, L.; Leung, H.Y.; Ahmad, I. Lipid pathway deregulation in advanced prostate cancer. *Pharmacol. Res.* **2018**, *131*, 177–184. [CrossRef]
97. Stoykova, G.E.; Schlaepfer, I.R. Lipid Metabolism and Endocrine Resistance in Prostate Cancer, and New Opportunities for Therapy. *Int. J. Mol. Sci.* **2019**, *20*, 2626. [CrossRef]
98. Abd Wahab, N.A.; Lajis, N.H.; Abas, F.; Othman, I.; Naidu, R. Mechanism of Anti-Cancer Activity of Curcumin on Andro-gen-Dependent and Androgen-Independent Prostate Cancer. *Nutrients* **2020**, *12*, 679. [CrossRef]
99. Oeckinghaus, A.; Ghosh, S. The NF-kappaB family of transcription factors and its regulation. *Cold Spring Harb. Perspect Biol.* **2009**, *1*, a000034. [CrossRef]
100. Chi, N.; Tan, Z.; Ma, K.; Bao, L.; Yun, Z. Increased circulating myeloid-derived suppressor cells correlate with cancer stages, interleukin-8 and -6 in prostate cancer. *Int. J. Clin. Exp. Med.* **2014**, *7*, 3181–3192.
101. Maubach, G.; Feige, M.H.; Lim, M.C.; Naumann, M. NF-kappaB-inducing kinase in cancer. *Biochim. et Biophys. Acta* **2019**, *1871*, 40–49. [CrossRef] [PubMed]
102. Nadiminty, N.; Tummala, R.; Liu, C.; Lou, W.; Evans, C.P.; Gao, A.C. NF-κB2/p52:c-Myc:hnRNPA1 Pathway Regulates Expression of AR Splice Variants and Enzalutamide Sensitivity in Prostate Cancer. *Mol. Cancer Ther.* **2015**, *14*, 1884–1895. [CrossRef]
103. Jain, G.; Voogdt, C.; Tobias, A.; Spindler, K.D.; Möller, P.; Cronauer, M.V.; Marienfeld, R.B. IκB kinases modulate the activity of the AR in prostate carcinoma cell lines. *Neoplasia* **2012**, *14*, 178–189. [CrossRef] [PubMed]
104. Wang, F.; Ma, J.; Wang, K.S.; Mi, C.; Lee, J.J.; Jin, X. Blockade of TNF-α-induced NF-κB signaling pathway and anti-cancer therapeutic response of Dihydrotanshinone I. *Int. Immunopharmacol.* **2015**, *28*, 764–772. [CrossRef]
105. Ke, F.; Wang, Z.; Song, X.; Ma, Q.; Hu, Y.; Jiang, L.; Zhang, Y.; Liu, Y.; Zhang, Y.; Gong, W. Cryptotanshinone induces cell cycle arrest and apoptosis through the JAK2/STAT3 and PI3K/Akt/NFκB pathways in cholangiocarcinoma cells. *Drug Des. Devel. Ther.* **2017**, *11*, 1753–1766. [CrossRef] [PubMed]
106. He, J.; Han, S.; Li, X.X.; Wang, Q.Q.; Cui, Y.; Chen, Y.; Gao, H.; Huang, L.; Yang, S. Diethyl Blechnic Exhibits Anti-Inflammatory and Antioxidative Activity via the TLR4/MyD88 Signaling Pathway in LPS-Stimulated RAW264.7 Cells. *Molecules* **2019**, *24*, 4502.

107. Wang, X.; Guo, D.; Li, W.; Zhang, Q.; Jiang, Y.; Wang, Q.; Li, C.; Qiu, Q.; Wang, Y. Danshen (Salvia miltiorrhiza) restricts MD2/TLR4-MyD88 complex formation and signalling in acute myocardial infarction-induced heart failure. *J. Cell Mol. Med.* **2020**, *24*, 10677–10692. [CrossRef]
108. Gao, H.; Liu, X.; Sun, W.; Kang, N.; Liu, Y.; Yang, S.; Xu, Q.-M.; Wang, C.; Chen, X. Total tanshinones exhibits anti-inflammatory effects through blocking TLR4 dimerization via the MyD88 pathway. *Cell Death Dis.* **2017**, *8*, e3004. [CrossRef]
109. Zhou, L.-H.; Hu, Q.; Sui, H.; Ci, S.-J.; Wang, Y.; Liu, X.; Liu, N.-N.; Yin, P.-H.; Qin, J.-M.; Li, Q. Tanshinone II-A Inhibits Angiogenesis through Down Regulation of COX-2 in Human Colorectal Cancer. *Asian Pac. J. Cancer Prev.* **2012**, *13*, 4453–4458. [CrossRef]
110. Su, C.C. Tanshinone IIA decreases the migratory ability of AGS cells by decreasing the protein expression of matrix metalloproteinases, nuclear factor κB-p65 and cyclooxygenase-2. *Mol. Med. Rep.* **2016**, *13*, 1263–1268. [CrossRef]
111. Ching, M.M.; Reader, J.; Fulton, A.M. Eicosanoids in Cancer: Prostaglandin E2 Receptor 4 in Cancer Therapeutics and Immunotherapy. *Front Pharmacol.* **2020**, *11*, 819. [CrossRef]
112. Motolani, A.; Martin, M.; Sun, M.; Lu, T. Phosphorylation of the Regulators, a Complex Facet of NF-κB Signaling in Cancer. *Biomolecules* **2020**, *11*, 15. [CrossRef] [PubMed]
113. Shafi, A.A.; Yen, A.E.; Weigel, N.L. ARs in hormone-dependent and castration-resistant prostate cancer. *Pharmacol. Ther.* **2013**, *140*, 223–238. [CrossRef]
114. Aurilio, G.; Cimadamore, A.; Mazzucchelli, R.; Lopez-Beltran, A.; Verri, E.; Scarpelli, M.; Massari, F.; Cheng, L.; Santoni, M.; Montironi, R. AR Signaling Pathway in Prostate Cancer: From Genetics to Clinical Applications. *Cells* **2020**, *9*, 2653. [CrossRef] [PubMed]
115. Dai, C.; Heemers, H.; Sharifi, N. Androgen Signaling in Prostate Cancer. *Cold Spring Harb. Perspect Med.* **2017**, *7*, a030452. [CrossRef] [PubMed]
116. Knudsen, K.E. Hormone Whodunit: Clues for Solving the Case of Intratumor Androgen Production. *Clin. Cancer Res.* **2014**, *20*, 5343–5345. [CrossRef]
117. Stanbrough, M.; Bubley, G.J.; Ross, K.; Golub, T.R.; Rubin, M.A.; Penning, T.M.; Febbo, P.G.; Balk, S.P. Increased Expression of Genes Converting Adrenal Androgens to Testosterone in Androgen-Independent Prostate Cancer. *Cancer Res.* **2006**, *66*, 2815–2825. [CrossRef]
118. Yu, J.; Zhai, D.; Hao, L.; Zhang, D.; Bai, L.; Cai, Z.; Yu, C. Cryptotanshinone Reverses Reproductive and Metabolic Disturbances in PCOS Model Rats via Regulating the Expression of CYP17 and AR. Evidence-Based Complement. *Altern. Med.* **2014**, *2014*, 670743.
119. Ye, D.; Li, M.; Zhang, Y.; Wang, X.; Liu, H.; Wu, W.; Ma, W.; Quan, K.; Ng, E.H.Y.; Wu, X.; et al. Cryptotanshinone Regulates Androgen Synthesis through the ERK/c-Fos/CYP17 Pathway in Porcine Granulosa Cells. Evidence-Based Complement. *Altern. Med.* **2017**, *2017*, 5985703.
120. Sharifi, N. The 5α-androstanedione pathway to dihydrotestosterone in castration-resistant prostate cancer. *J. Investig. Med.* **2012**, *60*, 504–507. [CrossRef]
121. Pisolato, R.; Lombardi, A.; Vicente, C.; Lucas, T.; Lazari, M.; Porto, C. Expression and regulation of the estrogen receptors in PC-3 human prostate cancer cells. *Steroids* **2016**, *107*, 74–86. [CrossRef]
122. Wang, C.; Du, X.; Yang, R.; Liu, J.; Xu, D.; Shi, J.; Chen, L.; Shao, R.; Fan, G.; Gao, X.; et al. The prevention and treatment effects of tanshinone IIA on oestrogen/androgen-induced benign prostatic hyperplasia in rats. *J. Steroid Biochem. Mol. Biol.* **2015**, *145*, 28–37. [CrossRef] [PubMed]
123. Bonkhoff, H. Estrogen receptor signaling in prostate cancer: Implications for carcinogenesis and tumor progression. *Prostate* **2017**, *78*, 2–10. [CrossRef] [PubMed]
124. Kowalska, K.; Piastowska-Ciesielska, A.W. Oestrogens and oestrogen receptors in prostate cancer. *SpringerPlus* **2016**, *5*, 522. [CrossRef] [PubMed]
125. Hua, H.; Kong, Q.; Zhang, H.; Wang, J.; Luo, T.; Jiang, Y. Targeting mTOR for cancer therapy. *J. Hematol. Oncol.* **2019**, *12*, 71. [CrossRef] [PubMed]
126. Saxton, R.A.; Sabatini, D.M. mTOR Signaling in Growth, Metabolism, and Disease. *Cell* **2017**, *168*, 960–976, Erratum in *Cell* **2017**, *169*, 361–371. [CrossRef]
127. Nagaraj, N.S.; Singh, O.V.; Merchant, N.B. Proteomics: A strategy to understand the novel targets in protein misfolding and cancer therapy. *Expert Rev. Proteom.* **2010**, *7*, 613–623. [CrossRef]
128. Lv, C.; Zeng, H.-W.; Wang, J.-X.; Yuan, X.; Zhang, C.; Fang, T.; Yang, P.-M.; Wu, T.; Zhou, Y.-D.; Nagle, D.G.; et al. The antitumor natural product tanshinone IIA inhibits protein kinase C and acts synergistically with 17-AAG. *Cell Death Dis.* **2018**, *9*, 165. [CrossRef]
129. Deng, L.; Chen, L.; Zhao, L.; Xu, Y.; Peng, X.; Wang, X.; Ding, L.; Jin, J.; Teng, H.; Wang, Y.; et al. Ubiquitination of Rheb governs growth factor-induced mTORC1 activation. *Cell Res.* **2019**, *29*, 136–150. [CrossRef]
130. Tee, A.R.; Manning, B.D.; Roux, P.P.; Cantley, L.C.; Blenis, J. Tuberous sclerosis complex gene products, Tuberin and Hamartin, control mTOR signaling by acting as a GTPase-activating protein complex toward Rheb. *Curr. Biol.* **2003**, *13*, 1259–1268. [CrossRef]
131. Su, C.-C.; Chiu, T.-L. Tanshinone IIA decreases the protein expression of EGFR, and IGFR blocking the PI3K/Akt/mTOR pathway in gastric carcinoma AGS cells both in vitro and in vivo. *Oncol. Rep.* **2016**, *36*, 1173–1179. [CrossRef] [PubMed]

132. Wang, L.; Yu, Z.; Ren, S.; Song, J.; Wang, J.; Du, G. Metabolic reprogramming in colon cancer reversed by DHTS through regulating PTEN/AKT/HIF1α mediated signal pathway. *Biochim. et Biophys. Acta (BBA)-Gen. Subj.* **2018**, *1862*, 2281–2292. [CrossRef] [PubMed]
133. Gwinn, D.M.; Shackelford, D.B.; Egan, D.F.; Mihaylova, M.M.; Mery, A.; Vasquez, D.S.; Turk, B.E.; Shaw, R.J. AMPK Phosphorylation of Raptor Mediates a Metabolic Checkpoint. *Mol. Cell* **2008**, *30*, 214–226. [CrossRef] [PubMed]
134. Inoki, K.; Ouyang, H.; Zhu, T.; Lindvall, C.; Wang, Y.; Zhang, X.; Yang, Q.; Bennett, C.; Harada, Y.; Stankunas, K.; et al. TSC2 Integrates Wnt and Energy Signals via a Coordinated Phosphorylation by AMPK and GSK3 to Regulate Cell Growth. *Cell* **2006**, *126*, 955–968. [CrossRef]
135. Chen, W.; Pan, Y.; Wang, S.; Liu, Y.; Chen, G.; Zhou, L.; Zhang, C.; Ni, W.; Wang, A.; Lu, Y.; et al. Correction to: Cryptotanshinone activates AMPK-TSC2 axis leading to inhibition of mTORC1 signaling in cancer cells. *BMC Cancer* **2019**, *19*, 257. [CrossRef]
136. Parmigiani, A.; Nourbakhsh, A.; Ding, B.; Wang, W.; Kim, Y.C.; Akopiants, K.; Guan, K.-L.; Karin, M.; Budanov, A.V. Sestrins Inhibit mTORC1 Kinase Activation through the GATOR Complex. *Cell Rep.* **2014**, *9*, 1281–1291. [CrossRef]
137. Shorning, B.Y.; Dass, M.S.; Smalley, M.J.; Pearson, H.B. The PI3K-AKT-mTOR Pathway and Prostate Cancer: At the Crossroads of AR, MAPK, and WNT Signaling. *Int. J. Mol. Sci.* **2020**, *21*, 4507. [CrossRef]
138. Yen, J.H.; Huang, S.T.; Huang, H.S.; Fong, Y.C.; Wu, Y.Y.; Chiang, J.H.; Su, Y.C. HGK-sestrin 2 signaling-mediated autophagy contrib-utes to antitumor efficacy of Tanshinone IIA in human osteosarcoma cells. *Cell Death Dis.* **2018**, *9*, 1003. [CrossRef]
139. Liu, Z.; Chen, X.; Wang, Y.; Peng, H.; Wang, Y.; Jing, Y.; Zhang, H. PDK4 protein promotes tumorigenesis through activation of cAMP-response element-binding protein (CREB)-Ras homolog enriched in brain (RHEB)-mTORC1 signaling cascade. *J. Biol. Chem.* **2014**, *289*, 29739–29749. [CrossRef]
140. Tambe, Y.; Terado, T.; Kim, C.J.; Mukaisho, K.; Yoshida, S.; Sugihara, H.; Tanaka, H.; Chida, J.; Kido, H.; Yamaji, K.; et al. Antitumor activity of potent pyruvate dehydrogenase kinase 4 inhibitors from plants in pancreatic cancer. *Mol. Carcinog.* **2019**, *58*, 1726–1737. [CrossRef]
141. Carriere, A.; Romeo, Y.; Acosta-Jaquez, H.A.; Moreau, J.; Bonneil, E.; Thibault, P.; Fingar, D.C.; Roux, P.P. ERK1/2 phosphorylate Raptor to promote Ras-dependent activation of mTOR complex 1 (mTORC1). *J. Biol. Chem.* **2011**, *286*, 567–577. [CrossRef] [PubMed]
142. Carrière, A.; Cargnello, M.; Julien, L.-A.; Gao, H.; Bonneil, E.; Thibault, P.; Roux, P.P. Oncogenic MAPK Signaling Stimulates mTORC1 Activity by Promoting RSK-Mediated Raptor Phosphorylation. *Curr. Biol.* **2008**, *18*, 1269–1277. [CrossRef] [PubMed]
143. Thorpe, L.M.; Yuzugullu, H.; Zhao, J.J. PI3K in cancer: Divergent roles of isoforms, modes of activation and therapeutic targeting. *Nat. Rev. Cancer* **2015**, *15*, 7–24. [CrossRef] [PubMed]
144. Mendoza, M.C.; Er, E.E.; Blenis, J. The Ras-ERK and PI3K-mTOR pathways: Cross-talk and compensation. *Trends Biochem. Sci.* **2011**, *36*, 320–328. [CrossRef]
145. Chen, W.; Liu, L.; Luo, Y.; Odaka, Y.; Awate, S.; Zhou, H.; Shen, T.; Zheng, S.; Lu, Y.; Huang, S. Cryptotanshinone activates p38/JNK and inhibits Erk1/2 leading to caspase-independent cell death in tumor cells. *Cancer Prev. Res.* **2012**, *5*, 778–787. [CrossRef]
146. Su, C. Tanshinone IIA can inhibit MiaPaCa-2 human pancreatic cancer cells by dual blockade of the Ras/Raf/MEK/ERK and PI3K/AKT/mTOR pathways. *Oncol. Rep.* **2018**, *40*, 3102–3111. [CrossRef]
147. Liu, P.; Cheng, H.; Roberts, T.M.; Zhao, J.J. Targeting the phosphoinositide 3-kinase pathway in cancer. *Nat. Rev. Drug Discov.* **2009**, *8*, 627–644. [CrossRef]
148. Zhang, L.; Lin, W.; Chen, X.; Wei, G.; Zhu, H.; Xing, S. Tanshinone IIA reverses EGF- and TGF-β1-mediated epitheli-al-mesenchymal transition in HepG2 cells via the PI3K/Akt/ERK signaling pathway. *Oncol Lett.* **2019**, *18*, 6554–6562.
149. Luo, Y.; Song, L.; Wang, X.; Huang, Y.; Liu, Y.; Wang, Q.; Hong, M.; Yuan, Z. Uncovering the Mechanisms of Cryptotanshinone as a Therapeutic Agent Against Hepatocellular Carcinoma. *Front. Pharmacol.* **2020**, *11*, 1264. [CrossRef]
150. Shi, D.; Zhao, P.; Cui, L.; Li, H.; Sun, L.; Niu, J.; Chen, M. Inhibition of PI3K/AKT molecular pathway mediated by membrane es-trogen receptor GPER accounts for Cryptotanshinone induced antiproliferative effect on breast cancer SKBR-3 cells. *BMC Pharmacol. Toxicol.* **2020**, *21*, 32. [CrossRef]
151. Liu, J.J.; Liu, W.D.; Yang, H.Z.; Zhang, Y.; Fang, Z.G.; Liu, P.Q.; Lin, D.J.; Xiao, R.Z.; Hu, Y.; Wang, C.Z.; et al. Inactivation of PI3k/Akt signaling pathway and activation of caspase-3 are involved in Tanshinone I-induced apoptosis in myeloid leu-kemia cells in vitro. *Ann. Hematol.* **2010**, *89*, 1089–1097. [CrossRef] [PubMed]
152. Wang, X.; Xu, X.; Jiang, G.; Zhang, C.; Liu, L.; Kang, J.; Wang, J.; Owusu, L.; Zhou, L.; Zhang, L.; et al. Dihydrotanshinone I inhibits ovarian cancer cell proliferation and migration by transcriptional repression of PIK3CA gene. *J. Cell. Mol. Med.* **2020**, *24*, 11177–11187. [CrossRef] [PubMed]
153. Don, M.-J.; Liao, J.-F.; Lin, L.-Y.; Chiou, W.-F. Cryptotanshinone inhibits chemotactic migration in macrophages through negative regulation of the PI3K signaling pathway. *J. Cereb. Blood Flow Metab.* **2007**, *151*, 638–646. [CrossRef] [PubMed]
154. Liu, Y.; Lin, F.; Chen, Y.; Wang, R.; Liu, J.; Jin, Y.; An, R. Cryptotanshinone Inhibites Bladder Cancer Cell Proliferation and Promotes Apoptosis via the PTEN/PI3K/AKT Pathway. *J. Cancer* **2020**, *11*, 488–499. [CrossRef]
155. Ye, Y.-T.; Zhong, W.; Sun, P.; Wang, D.; Wang, C.; Hu, L.-M.; Qian, J.-Q. Apoptosis induced by the methanol extract of Salvia miltiorrhiza Bunge in non-small cell lung cancer through PTEN-mediated inhibition of PI3K/Akt pathway. *J. Ethnopharmacol.* **2017**, *200*, 107–116. [CrossRef]
156. Papa, A.; Pandolfi, P.P. The PTEN-PI3K Axis in Cancer. *Biomolecules* **2019**, *9*, 153. [CrossRef]

157. Geybels, M.S.; Fang, M.; Wright, J.L.; Qu, X.; Bibikova, M.; Klotzle, B.; Fan, J.-B.; Feng, Z.; Ostrander, E.A.; Nelson, P.S.; et al. PTEN loss is associated with prostate cancer recurrence and alterations in tumor DNA methylation profiles. *Oncotarget* **2017**, *8*, 84338–84348. [CrossRef]
158. Wise, H.M.; Hermida, M.A.; Leslie, N.R. Prostate cancer, PI3K, PTEN and prognosis. *Clin. Sci.* **2017**, *131*, 197–210. [CrossRef]
159. Hong, J.-Y.; Park, S.H.; Park, H.J.; Lee, S.K. Anti-proliferative Effect of 15,16-Dihydrotanshinone I Through Cell Cycle Arrest and the Regulation of AMP-activated Protein Kinase/Akt/mTOR and Mitogen-activated Protein Kinase Signaling Pathway in Human Hepatocellular Carcinoma Cells. *J. Cancer Prev.* **2018**, *23*, 63–69. [CrossRef]
160. Holz, M.K.; Ballif, B.A.; Gygi, S.P.; Blenis, J. mTOR and S6K1 mediate assembly of the translation preinitiation complex through dynamic protein interchange and ordered phosphorylation events. *Cell* **2005**, *123*, 569–580. [CrossRef]
161. Jeoung, N.H.; Jeong, J.Y.; Kang, B.S. Cryptotanshinone Prevents the Binding of S6K1 to mTOR/Raptor Leading to the Sup-pression of mTORC1-S6K1 Signaling Activity and Neoplastic Cell Transformation. *J. Cancer Prev.* **2021**, *26*, 145–152. [CrossRef]
162. Li, G.; Shan, C.; Liu, L.; Zhou, T.; Zhou, J.; Hu, X.; Chen, Y.; Cui, H.; Gao, N. Tanshinone IIA inhibits HIF-1α and VEGF expression in breast cancer cells via mTOR/p70S6K/RPS6/4E-BP1 signaling pathway. *PLoS ONE* **2015**, *10*, e0117440. [CrossRef]
163. Barrera-Vázquez, O.S.; Gómez-Verjan, J.C.; Magos-Guerrero, G.A. Chemoinformatic Screening for the Selection of Potential Senolytic Compounds from Natural Products. *Biomolecules* **2021**, *11*, 467. [CrossRef] [PubMed]
164. Zou, Z.; Tao, T.; Li, H.; Zhu, X. mTOR signaling pathway and mTOR inhibitors in cancer: Progress and challenges. *Cell Biosci.* **2020**, *10*, 31. [CrossRef] [PubMed]
165. Huang, L.Q.; Gao, W.; Zhou, Y.J. Application of synthetic biology to sustainable utilization of Chinese materia medica re-sources. *Yao Xue Xue Bao* **2014**, *49*, 37–43. (In Chinese)
166. Chen, M.; Cai, Y.; Zhang, W.; Chen, Z.; Shi, Z.; He, C. Recent insights into the biological activities and drug delivery systems of tanshinones. *Int. J. Nanomed.* **2016**, *11*, 121–130. [CrossRef] [PubMed]
167. Gao, W.; Hu, T.-Y.; Guo, J.; Lv, D.-M.; Dai, Z.-B.; Zhou, Y.-J.; Huang, L.-Q. Research progress of synthetic biology for tanshinones. *China J. Chin. Mater. Medica* **2015**, *40*, 2486–2491.
168. Zhou, Y.J.; Gao, W.; Rong, Q.; Jin, G.; Chu, H.; Liu, W.; Yang, W.; Zhu, Z.; Li, G.; Zhu, G.; et al. Modular pathway engi-neering of diterpenoid synthases and the mevalonic acid pathway for miltiradiene production. *J. Am. Chem. Soc.* **2012**, *134*, 3234–3241. [CrossRef]
169. Ma, X.H.; Ma, Y.; Tang, J.F.; He, Y.L.; Liu, Y.C.; Ma, X.J.; Shen, Y.; Cui, G.H.; Lin, H.X.; Rong, Q.X.; et al. The Biosynthetic Pathways of Tanshinones and Phenolic Acids in Salvia miltiorrhiza. *Molecules* **2015**, *20*, 16235–16254. [CrossRef]
170. Song, J.-J.; Fang, X.; Li, C.-Y.; Jiang, Y.; Li, J.-X.; Wu, S.; Guo, J.; Liu, Y.; Fan, H.; Huang, Y.-B.; et al. A 2-oxoglutarate-dependent dioxygenase converts dihydrofuran to furan in Salvia diterpenoids. *Plant Physiol.* **2022**, *188*, 1496–1506. [CrossRef]
171. Zhang, Y.; Jiang, P.; Ye, M.; Kim, S.-H.; Jiang, C.; Lü, J. Tanshinones: Sources, Pharmacokinetics and Anti-Cancer Activities. *Int. J. Mol. Sci.* **2012**, *13*, 13621–13666. [CrossRef] [PubMed]
172. Estolano-Cobián, A.; Alonso, M.M.; Díaz-Rubio, L.; Ponce, C.N.; Córdova-Guerrero, I.; Marrero, J.G. Tanshinones and their Deriva-tives: Heterocyclic Ring-Fused Diterpenes of Biological Interest. *Mini Rev. Med. Chem.* **2021**, *21*, 171–185. [CrossRef] [PubMed]
173. Huang, X.; Deng, H.; Shen, Q.K.; Quan, Z.S. Tanshinone IIA: Pharmacology, Total Synthesis, and Progress in Struc-ture-modifications. *Curr. Med. Chem.* **2022**, *29*, 1959–1989. [CrossRef]
174. Wang, M.; Liu, J.; Zhou, B.; Xu, R.; Tao, L.; Ji, M.; Zhu, L.; Jiang, J.; Shen, J.; Gui, X.; et al. Acute and sub-chronic toxicity studies of Danshen injection in Sprague-Dawley rats. *J. Ethnopharmacol.* **2012**, *141*, 96–103. [CrossRef]
175. Lan, Y.; Wang, B.; Wang, X.; Wang, T.; Wang, C.; Zhang, H.; Chen, J.; Mei, W. Evaluation of tanshinone IIA developmental toxicity in zebrafish embryos. *Molecules* **2017**, *22*, 660.
176. Wang, C.; Wang, T.; Lian, B.-W.; Lai, S.; Li, S.; Li, Y.-M.; Tan, W.-J.; Wang, B.; Mei, W. Developmental toxicity of cryptotanshinone on the early-life stage of zebrafish development. *Hum. Exp. Toxicol.* **2021**, *40*, S278–S289. [CrossRef]
177. Yang, L.-J.; Jeng, C.-J.; Kung, H.-N.; Chang, C.-C.; Wang, A.-G.; Chau, G.-Y.; Don, M.-J.; Chau, Y.-P. Tanshinone IIA isolated from Salvia miltiorrhiza elicits the cell death of human endothelial cells. *J. Biomed. Sci.* **2005**, *12*, 347–361. [CrossRef]

molecules MDPI

Review

Can Natural Products Targeting EMT Serve as the Future Anticancer Therapeutics?

Sirajudheen Anwar [1,2,*], Jonaid Ahmad Malik [3,4], Sakeel Ahmed [5], Verma Abhishek Kameshwar [6], Jowaher Alanazi [1,2], Abdulwahab Alamri [1,2] and Nafees Ahemad [7]

1 Department of Pharmacology and Toxicology, College of Pharmacy, University of Hail, Hail 81422, Saudi Arabia
2 Molecular Diagnostics Unit and Personalized Treatment, University of Hail, Hail 81422, Saudi Arabia
3 Department of Pharmacology and Toxicology, National Institute of Pharmaceutical Education and Research, Guwahati 781101, Assam, India
4 Department of Biomedical Engineering, Indian Institute of Technology Ropar, Rupnagar 140001, Punjab, India
5 Department of Pharmacology and Toxicology, National Institute of Pharmaceutical Education and Research, Ahmedabad 382355, Gujarat, India
6 Department of Pharmacology, Amrita School of Pharmacy, Amrita Vishwa Vidyapeetham, Kochi 641112, Kerala, India
7 School of Pharmacy, Monash University Malaysia, Jalan lagoon Selatan, Bandar Sunway, Petaling Jaya 47500, Selangor DE, Malaysia
* Correspondence: si.anwar@uoh.edu.sa

Abstract: Cancer is the leading cause of death and has remained a big challenge for the scientific community. Because of the growing concerns, new therapeutic regimens are highly demanded to decrease the global burden. Despite advancements in chemotherapy, drug resistance is still a major hurdle to successful treatment. The primary challenge should be identifying and developing appropriate therapeutics for cancer patients to improve their survival. Multiple pathways are dysregulated in cancers, including disturbance in cellular metabolism, cell cycle, apoptosis, or epigenetic alterations. Over the last two decades, natural products have been a major research interest due to their therapeutic potential in various ailments. Natural compounds seem to be an alternative option for cancer management. Natural substances derived from plants and marine sources have been shown to have anti-cancer activity in preclinical settings. They might be proved as a sword to kill cancerous cells. The present review attempted to consolidate the available information on natural compounds derived from plants and marine sources and their anti-cancer potential underlying EMT mechanisms.

Keywords: epithelial-mesenchymal transition; cancer EMT; natural chemical entities; cancer; anticancer therapy; chemotherapy

Citation: Anwar, S.; Malik, J.A.; Ahmed, S.; Kameshwar, V.A.; Alanazi, J.; Alamri, A.; Ahemad, N. Can Natural Products Targeting EMT Serve as the Future Anticancer Therapeutics? *Molecules* **2022**, *27*, 7668. https://doi.org/10.3390/molecules27227668

Academic Editors: Alessandra Ammazzalorso, Barbara De Filippis and Marialuigia Fantacuzzi

Received: 4 October 2022
Accepted: 1 November 2022
Published: 8 November 2022

1. Introduction

Cancer is the leading cause of death globally [1]. According to the global demographic characteristics, it is expected to increase by approximately >20 million by 2025 [2]. The treatment paradigm improved in the past decade with the advancement in cancer research. Breast cancer (BC), colorectal cancer (CRC), lung cancer (LC), and prostate cancer (PC) are the most common types of cancers [1,3]. Various cellular pathways are involved in cancer development and progression. Several drug candidates are approved to target these pathways for their management [4]. One reason behind drug resistance is the process of Epithelial-mesenchymal transition (EMT) involved in cancer progression. EMT is an extremely regulated physiological process that has a significant role in tissue repair and embryogenesis [5]. During EMT, the cells undergo multiple morphologic, biological, and genetic rearrangements, leading to their mesenchymal phenotypes [6]. EMT is pathologically associated with fibrosis and cancer, leading to their progression. EMT has been linked to the formation of invasive and cancer stem cells in carcinomas [7].

EMT is initiated by EMT activating transcription factors (EMT-TFs), including SNAIL (SNAI1) and SLUG (SNAI2), the basic helix–loop–helix factors TWIST1 and TWIST2. As proven for SNAIL, TWIST, Zinc figure E-box binding homeobox 1 (ZEB1), and Zinc figure E-box binding homeobox 2 (ZEB2), these features can repress epithelial genes like the E-cadherin-producing CDH1 by binding to E-Box in their cognate promoter regions. Simultaneously, EMT-TFs activate genes associated with a mesenchymal phenotype, such as Vimentin (VIM), Fibronectin 1 (FN1), and N-Cadherin (CDH2). Several activities, however, are not common and are carried out by separate EMT- transcription factors (TFs) due to differences in coding sequences or protein size and structure [8]. An overview of the EMT pathway is shown in Figure 1. In other words, EMT is a biotic mechanism in which epithelial cells become polarized.

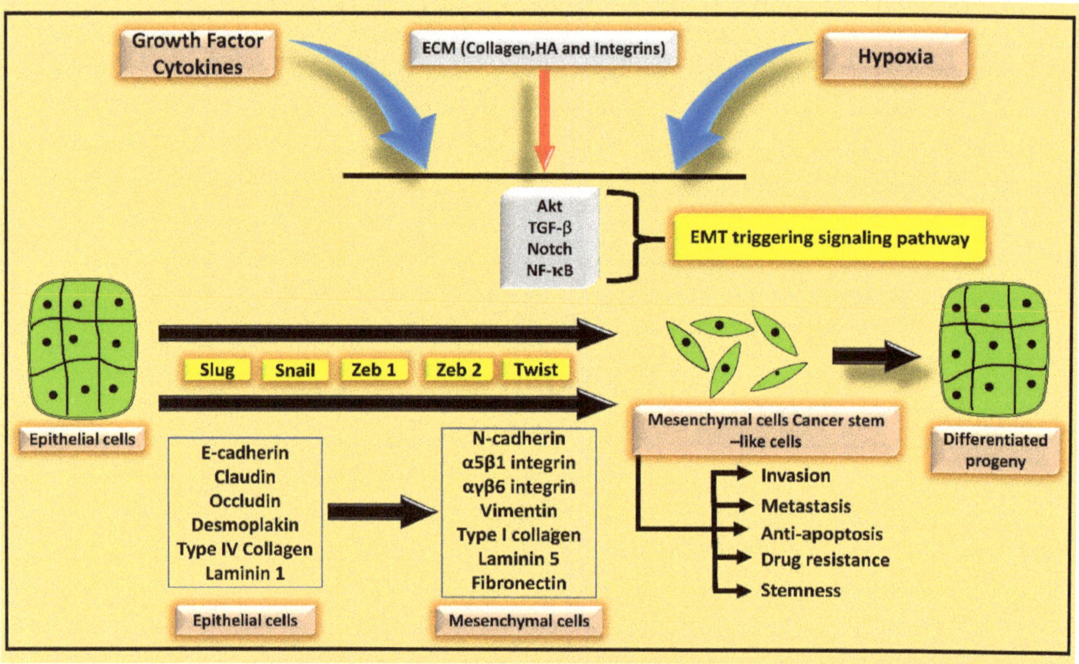

Figure 1. Hypoxia, growth factor, cytokines, and ECM activate the pathways that can trigger the EMT by activating EMT transcription factors (EMT-TFs), including SNAIL, SLUG, and the basic helix–loop–helix factors TWIST. As proven for SNAIL, TWIST, Zinc figure E-box binding homeobox 1 (ZEB1), and ZEB2, these features can repress epithelial genes like the E-cadherin-producing CDH1 by binding to E-Box in their cognate promoter regions. Simultaneously, EMT-TFs activate genes associated with a mesenchymal phenotype, such as Vimentin (VIM), Fibronectin 1 (FN1), and N-Cadherin (CDH2), etc. [8].

The heterogeneous mixture of cells like fibroblasts, endothelial cells, noncellular constituents, immune cells, extracellular matrix, cytokines, growth factors, and basement membrane is known as a tumor microenvironment (TME) [9]. EMT is essential for developing and initiating tumors and their recurrence and progression. In TME, the most abundant cells are cancer-associated fibroblasts (CAFs), which cross-talk with tumor cells, extracellular matrix (ECM), immune cells, and endothelial cells for cancer progression [9–13]. Several therapeutic agents are now being designed to target these CAFs [12,14]. Many natural agents have been identified to target CAF by altering the key signaling pathways, epigenetics, kinases, and enzymes. Targeting CAFs and altering the pathways affect cancer-stroma association in TME, resulting in decreased cancer progression. The natural compounds might have promised anti-cancer activity and are worth investigating against different tumors. The characteristic feature of carcinogenesis is ECM stiffness that supports the tumor cells. The crosslinking of ECM components like collagen with the tumor cells occurs via CAFs [15]. LOX-lysyl oxidase, the enzyme highly overexpressed in tumors derived from CAFs, acts as a collagen crosslinking initiator in several cancers like breast and gastric cancers, ultimately enhancing EMT, cell survival, invasion, drug resistance, and angiogenesis [16]. The ECM degrading enzymes like matrix metalloproteases (MMPs) and tissue inhibitors of metalloproteinase (TIMPs) inhibitors are altered by CAFs during angiogenesis and invasion, causing modulation of TME. The MMP2 and 9 are well investigated and highly associated with cancer growth and development [17,18]. The enzymes like metalloproteinases and disintegrin, associated with the MMPs super-family, are increased by CAFs, promoting cancer progression [19]. The CAFs also apply physical forces to pull out the epithelial basement membrane, causing the promotion of EMT in enzyme independent manner [20]. The CAFs promote EMT remolding and are promising therapeutic targets in halting EMT to prevent cancer metastasis. Natural compounds have proven to be the best alternatives to the current therapies against cancer. Many noteworthy examples are in front of us, where natural compounds have proven better than existing standard therapies against different ailments, such as cancer or infectious diseases. It is worth investigating the potential of natural compounds, whether from the marine, plant, or animal, against different types of cancers to find the solution for the growing deadly ailment in the world. Due to growing concerns regarding cancer metastasis, most therapies fail to cure, and the patients suffer greatly due to high toxicity. Cancer resistance is another challenge against current therapies, making cancer more complicated to manage. The natural compounds could be a game changer as anti-cancer therapy that specifically targets the EMT process and halts the process of cancer progression.

2. Cross-Talk between TGF-β and Other Signaling Pathways Mediating EMT

The signaling pathways cross-talk to form complex networks. Due to several cellular processes like apoptosis, differentiation, proliferation, and homeostasis, the Transforming growth factor β (TGF-β) cross-talk with various other signaling pathways during the EMT process (Figure 2) [21,22]. One of the mechanisms in which Akt activation and the phosphatase and tensin homolog (PTEN) dissociation from β-catenin are mainly responsible for the TGF-β mediated EMT process, where the displacement of β-catenin from adherent junctions occurs [23]. The other signaling pathway that cross-talks with TGF-β is Notch; Notch synergizes with TGF-β signals to enhance/inhibit its signaling activity depending on the input signal [21]. TGF-β signals activate the migration and inhibit the cell proliferation of endothelial cells. However, the Notch signals block the migration of bone morphogenetic protein (BMP) [24]. BMP stimulates the cell migration of endothelial cells; however, in the presence of Notch signaling, the migratory potential gets inhibited [24].

Interestingly, Notch signaling plays a crucial cross-talk in regulating migration by inducing gene expression. Notch dominates the BMP signaling; when the cell-to-cell contact is not there, endothelial cells are not in contact with the nearby cells to migrate until the new cell-to-cell attachment is set [21,24]. The TGF-β requires Notch signaling for the growth arrest in the epithelium; over thirty percent of the genes induced by TGF-β require Notch signaling [25]. The classy EMT marker, the TGF-β, also cross-talks with several other signaling pathways like Extracellular signal-regulating kinase (Erk), c-Jun N-terminal kinase (JNK), and p38. Erk, JNK, and p38 are indirectly regulating the TGF-β during EMT. However, TGF-β activates MAPK and Erk1/2 signaling pathways [26]. The cross-talk of TGF-β versus EGF signaling is the reason for activating Smad-dependent signaling and MAPK-mediated Erk1/2 [27]. The nuclear translocation of MAPK mediated by TGF-β is downregulated by the MAPK-Erk pathway that mediates nuclear exclusion and phosphorylation of Smad-2/3 [27]. During the initiation of EMT, the Akt and PTEN are also regulated by TGF-β. In addition, TGF-β cross-talk with ErbB signaling during the EMT development of breast cancer [28]. The TGF-β also regulates the phosphoinositide 3-kinase (PI3k)-Akt signaling pathways. Akt's activity increases due to the induction of TGF-β-mediated functional activities like cell migration, epithelial to mesenchymal shift, cell survival, and cell growth [27–29]. Human epidermal growth factor receptor 2 (HER2)/RAS opposes the TGF-β-induced programmed cell death and cell arrest; however, it promotes migratory and invasive activities of TGF-β [30]. The EMT-associated cross-talk is validated by pharmacological inhibition of insulin-like growth factor-1R (IGF-1R), which prevents TGF-β-mediated EMT protein signatures [31]. The cross-talk of different pathways involved in EMT is demonstrated in Figure 2.

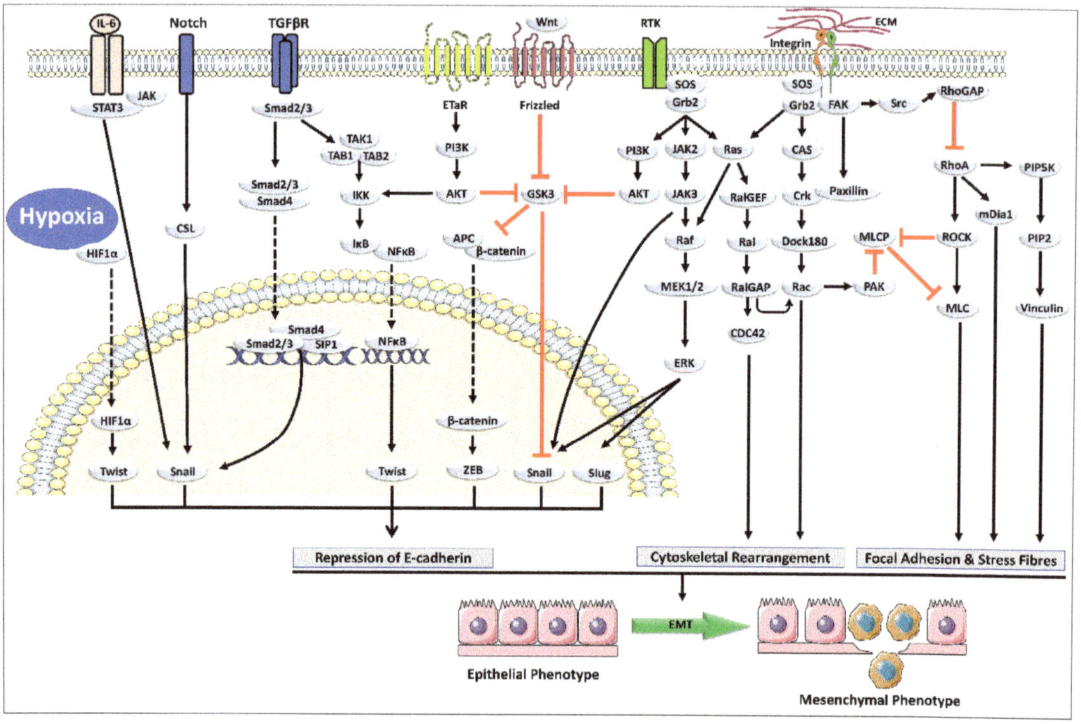

Figure 2. Illustrates the different pathways involved in initiating epithelial-mesenchymal transition (EMT) [32].

3. Natural Chemical Agents as Potential Leads against Cancer

Among approved chemotherapeutic medications, 80% are bioactive natural compounds [33,34]. 70% of disease conditions, including cancer, are treated with the help of natural products [35]. The natural compounds induce cytotoxicity by targeting various oncogenic signaling [36]. Several marine-derived metabolites show anti-cancer activity in preclinical and clinical settings [37]. Marine-derived compounds include sulfated polysaccharides, sterols, carotenoids, and chitosan. Sulfated polysaccharides and carotenoids have effectively worked against cancer, acquired immune deficiency syndrome (AIDS), CVDs, and other acute and chronic disorders [35]. Various effective marine-derived compounds are summarized in Table 1. Plants, bacteria, animals, insects, and marine life are some of the key sources of natural chemicals with pharmacological and cytotoxic actions such as anti-proliferative, anti-angiogenic, apoptosis-generating, necrosis-inducing, and anti-inflammatory [38]. Secondary metabolites (Alkaloids, tannins, saponins, flavonoids, steroids) are molecules produced by plants at very minute levels that are therapeutically beneficial in various illnesses [39]. Animals and insects are also rich suppliers of enzymes with various pharmacological applications. Researchers have recently focused on natural substances to investigate their possible use in cancer treatment with lesser side effects. Still, they have only identified a few molecules with clinical efficacy demonstrated in Table 2 [40]. Compounds with anti-proliferative, anti-inflammatory, anti-angiogenic, and apoptotic-inducing properties can treat cancer and reduce the side effects of conventional cancer chemotherapy. They also have a high potential for future use as anti-cancer drugs.

Natural products can offer new hope in fighting EMT and increase therapeutic options worldwide. Drugs of natural origin, like traditional and Chinese medicine, are currently being investigated for various ailments [41]. The cost-effectiveness and richness of good therapeutic efficacy and safety were natural compounds' true and popular features, considering them promising candidates against cancer [42]. The drugs against cancer at present share 1/3rd position share against cancer, meaning it is important to investigate more drugs from the natural origin against cancer [43]. Natural compounds have a high level of rigidity, enhancing the protein cross-talk more than synthetic drugs. They have diversity and versatile structure complexity, a unique natural feature making them the right candidates against cancer [43,44]. The signaling pathways that are responsible for cancer cell survival and TME maintenance are being halted by many natural compounds. The natural compounds have a comprehensive role in inhibiting tumor progression by blocking the survival pathways involved in EMT [9]. Many drugs have been used along with natural compounds, producing efficacious outcomes like decreasing drug resistance and toxicity [42,45]. Natural products can remold the TME [41]. Here we will show various candidates of natural origin demonstrating pharmacological activities against EMT and its associated factors.

Table 1. Marine and plants-derived compounds for anti-cancer activity.

Sr. No	Drug Product	Source (Marine Origin)	Mechanism of Action	Indication	FDA Status	Reference
			Marine Source			
1	Eribulin mesylate	Sponge *Halichondria okadai*	Keeps the cytoskeleton's growth cycle away from core aggregates tubulin	Metastatic breast cancer	Approved (Spain)	[46]
2	Brentuximab Vedotin	Sea hare *Dollabella Auricularia/* cyanobacteria	Cell cycle arrest from G2 to M phase	Hodgkin lymphoma	Approved (USA.)	[47]
3	Cytarabine, Ara-C	Sponge *Cryptotheca crypta*	Inhibition of DNA Synthesis	Acute lymphoblastic leukemia	Approved (USA.)	[46]
4	Halichondramide (HCA)	Marine sponge *Chondrosia corticata*	Phosphatase of regenerating liver-3 (PRL-3) and its downstream signaling pathway are suppressed.	Prostate Cancer	Approved	[48]

Table 1. *Cont.*

Sr. No	Drug Product	Source (Marine Origin)	Mechanism of Action	Indication	FDA Status	Reference
			Plant Source			
4	Ixabepilone	*Soragium cellulosum*	Cell-cycle arrest and apoptosis-inducer	Hand-foot syndrome	Approved	[49]
5	Romidepsin	*Chromobacterium violaceum*	Histone deacetylase inhibitors	Hematological toxicities like anemia	Approved	[50]
6	Podophyllotoxins	*Podophyllum (Berberidaceae)*	Inhibit the polymerization of tubulin, arresting the cell cycle in the metaphase	Ovarian cancer, immunosuppressive ability	Approved	[51]
7	Ligustrazine	Rhizome of *Ligusticum wallichii.*	Inhibit SK-OV-3 and OVCAR-3 cell viability, proliferation, migration, and invasion.	Ovarian cancer	Approved	[52]

Table 2. Potential NCEs with therapeutic effects against cancer.

Sr. No	NCE.	Source	Mechanism and Outcomes	Method of Validation	Potential Use	Reference
1	Oregonin	*Alnus sibirica (AS)*	Anti-proliferative activity, Inhibition of NF-κB, induction of apoptosis, DNA Methylation	MTT Assay, Western blotting, Flow, methylation-specific PCR, cytometry	Prostate cancer	[53]
2	Hirsutenone					
3	Hirsutanonol					
4	Chelerythrine chloride	*Chelidonium majus and Macleaya cordata*	cytotoxicity and anti-proliferative activity	Cell viability assays	NSCLC.	[39]
5	Thioholgamide	*Streptomyces* sp. *MUSC 136T.*	Caspase 3/7 Activation, membrane permeability	MTT assay	Colon, breast, liver, and lung cancers	[54]
6	7-deoxy-trans-dihydronarciclasin	*Scadoxus pseudocaulus*	Apoptosis inducer	Cytotoxicity assay	Follicular lymphoma	[55]
7	4-(4-hydroxy-3-methoxyphenyl) curcumin		Anti-proliferative, apoptosis-inducing	MTT assay, Western blotting analysis	Hepatic, colon, chronic myeloid leukemia, and lung cancer	[56–58]

4. Potential NCE to Target EMT

4.1. *Artemisinin (ATM)*

ATM is a sesquiterpene lactone isolated from sweet, warm wood, *Artemisia annua.* It is an antimalarial agent to treat multidrug-resistant *falciparum malaria* strains, mediated by producing organic peroxides [59]. ATM also has potent anti-cancer activity against CRC, BC, gastric cancer (GC), and cervix cancer (CC). Its anti-carcinogenic action is similar to antimalarial action in that free iron cleaves its endoperoxide bridge, releasing free radicals that cause cytotoxicity. ATM's low toxicity and high specificity for cancer cells led to its development as an anti-cancer molecule. Dihydroartemisinic acid (DHA), an ATM derivative, reduced inflammation in a rat arthritis model by downregulating Interleukin-6 (IL-6). Additionally, DHA has anti-cancer properties. It can induce apoptosis in leukemic cells via noxa-mediated mechanisms [60].

Moreover, it inhibits GC cell invasion, migration, and proliferation by inhibiting the activation of phosphoinositide 3-kinase/protein kinase B and SNAIL. According to Sun et al., DHA's anti-inflammatory and anti-cancer activities are mediated via microRNAs (miRNAs). DHA, for example, inhibits inflammation in vascular smooth muscle cells by regulating the miR-376b-3p/KLF pathway. The Jumonji and AT-rich interactive domain2 (ARID-2)/miR-7/miR-34a pathway inhibit prostate cancer cells by downregulating AXL tyrosine. In laryngeal cancer, miRNAs, in particular, play a function in EMT. For example, miR-217 inhibits EMT while miR-10b promotes it. miR-130b-3p is a tumor suppressor because it inhibits laryngeal cancer development, angiogenesis, migration, and invasion [61]. FoxM1, a member of the conserved forkhead box transcription factor family, is involved in cell cycle regulation, DNA damage repair, and apoptosis and has been associated with the development of breast, pancreas, and liver carcinomas. Nandi et al. hypothesized that FoxM1 was a critical inhibitory target of ATM in hepatocellular carcinoma (HCC) and that FoxM1 may play a role in the cell cycle triggered by DHA ATM-inhibited HCC cell survival and proliferation by attenuating FoxM1 and its transcription targets and interfering with FoxM1 trans-activation [62].

4.2. *Strychnine/Brucine*

Brucine is an alkaloid related to strychnine obtained from the *Strychnic Nux-vomica* tree. It has analgesic, anti-cancer, anti-inflammatory, antioxidant, and anti-venom properties [63]. In vitro, it inhibits the proliferation of Hela and K562 cell lines. Brucine also showed anti-metastasis action in MDA-MB-231 and Hs578-T-cells and inhibited invasive capacity and adhesion of MDA-MB-231 and Hs578-T-cells Matrigel, and preventing mRNA of E-cadherin, catenin, VIM, FN1, MMP-2, and MMP-9 in MDA-MB-231 cells [64]. These data collectively suggest that brucine might be a potential anti-cancer molecule; in vivo studies are still needed to confirm its anti-cancer potential.

4.3. *Eugenol*

A polypropanoid group of compounds is found in seeds of many plants, such as cloves, cinnamon, nutmeg, and bay leaves. It has antioxidant, anti-bacterial, anti-inflammatory, and anti-cancer activity and is widely used as a cosmetic, perfume, and culinary ingredient. It has anti-cancer potential due to its ability to increase reactive oxygen species (ROS) formation and apoptotic action, increase Cyt C's release, and inhibit the EMT process, limiting the cells' ability to metastasize [65]. It has shown anti-cancer activity against malignancies, including leukemia, lung, colon, colorectal, skin, gastric, breast, cervical, and prostate cancer, through the processes described below in Table 3.

Table 3. Mechanisms of Eugenol for anti-apoptotic in various cancers.

Type of the Tumor	Study Type	Effective Dose	Mechanism	References
Lung cancer	In vitro	1000 μM	Decrease cycloxygenase-2 activity, which leads to cell cycle arrest in the S phase followed by cell death	[66]
Colon cancer	In vitro	800 μM	Boosts the cytotoxic effects of cisplatin and doxorubicin synergistically.	[67]
Gastric cancer	In vitro	Low conc.	Inhibits cancer growth by upregulating preinvasive and angiogenic molecules and favoring apoptosis via the mitochondrial pathway via altering Bcl-2 family proteins.	[68]
Cervical cancer	In vitro	50–200 μM	Prevents the cell cycle and causes apoptosis, and inhibits DNA synthesis.	[69]
Breast cancer	In vitro	2 μM	Suppresses breast cancer-related oncogenes by downregulating E2F1 and its downstream anti-apoptotic target	[70]

4.4. *Resveratrol*

Resveratrol (RES) chemically trihydroxy stilbene is a polyphenol in grapes, berries, peanuts, and wine. RES has been shown to have cardioprotective, anti-inflammatory, and anti-aging effects. Studies also suggest that it also has anti-cancer properties. Moreover, RES has a regulatory role in EMT and the hedgehog (Hh) signaling pathway, which is critical for vertebrate development, homeostasis, and cancer. Hh is abnormally activated in breast, prostate, and pancreatic cancer (PC) and has a role in metastasis and invasion of GC via induction of the EMT. Hence, Hh signaling pathway is the center of attraction for anti-cancer activity. RES suppresses the Hh pathway, thus inhibiting cancer invasion and metastasis.

Moreover, RES has also been shown to block the Hh signaling pathway and EMT in malignancies [71]. A study proved that RES inhibited EMT in Glioblastoma (GBM) cells, as evidenced by morphological changes in the RES-treated G.B.M. cells. RES also inhibits EMT-mediated migration and invasion of GBM cells and EMT-induced stem cell-like properties in GBM cells [72]. A TGF-β/Smad signaling pathway is associated with the proliferation, differentiation, and migration of the cells and promotes results in invasion and metastasis. RES inhibited the penetration and metastasis by EMT-induced phosphorylation of Smad2 and Smad3 in a dose-dependent manner, suggesting the function of RES on EMT is related to Smad-dependent signaling [72].

4.5. *Polyphyllin 1*

Polyphyllin 1 (PP 1) demonstrated its anti-cancer activity via its apoptotic action and several pathways effectively against various cancers. Polyphyllin I induces apoptosis in HepF-2-Cells, and neural progenitor cells (NPC) cell lines [73]. The natural herb Paris polyphylla makes PP1 and has anti-cancer properties against various malignancies, including drug-resistant tumors. Paris polyphylla was recently found to inhibit CRC cells by activating autophagy and improving the efficiency of chemotherapy (Doxorubicin). By decreasing CIP2A/PP2A/Akt signaling, PP1 also reduced cisplatin-resistant GC cells. Liu et al. demonstrated that PP 1 has potent anti-cancer action on human non-small cell lung cancer (NSCLC) mediated by CHOP stabilization. PP1 induces ROS, and ER stress inhibits unfolded protein response (UPR) in cancer cells, subsequently increasing the levels of CHOP Via, accelerating CHOP gene expression. The UPR chaperone GRP78, restrained by PP1, is the main mechanism for CHOP stabilization [74].

4.6. *Paeoniflorin (PF)*

Paeoniflorin (PF) is a monoterpene glycoside derived from the root of *Paeonia lactiflora*. In the past, this plant's roots were utilized in eastern medicine for pain, muscle spasms, inflammation, menstruation dysfunction, and degenerative illnesses for a long time [75–78]. Studies indicated that PF inhibits tumor growth, invasion, and metastasis in vivo and in vitro. In hypoxia-induced EMT in MDA-MB-231 BC cells, PF treatment resulted in a considerable increase in E-cadherin levels and a drop in CDH2 and Vimentin levels in the cells. Subsequently, it suppressed the EMT process by altering the expression of HIF-1, which is involved in hypoxia-driven EMT [79]. The hippo pathway plays a significant role in the progression of GC. This pathway is said to be dysregulated and thus contributes to gastric oncology and metastasis. Two important factors, yes associated protein (YAP1) and Transcriptional coactivator with PDZ-binding motif (TAZ), produce their metastatic effect via crosslinking with Notch, TGF-β, and Wnt/ β-catenin in GC. In GC, PF exerts its anti-cancer effect via regulation of the hippo signaling pathway and downregulating the effect of TAZ [80]. Further, there is a need to explore its potential in other cancers.

4.7. *Halicondramine*

Halicondramine (HCA) is a trisoxazole-containing macrolide from the marine sponge Chondrosia corticata [81]. It possesses antifungal and cytotoxic properties. It also has anti-proliferative activity against cancerous cells [82,83]. Modulation of the EMT is a key target for their action. Treatment with HCA significantly reduced the expression of MMP2 and 9, and CDH2. On the contrary, E-cadherin expression was significantly increased. HCA also inhibits the expression of PRL-3, a metastasis-associated marker, and PI3 kinase subunits p85 and p110 (PRL-3's downstream targets). These findings imply that HCA inhibits EMT in human adenocarcinoma prostate cancer cells by modulating PRL-3 and downstream targets, such as PI3 kinase [48].

4.8. Ligustrazine

Ligustrazine (LSZ) is obtained from the rhizome of *Ligusticum wallichii* [84]. LSZ is shown to have anti-inflammatory, anti-fibrotic, antioxidant activity, and tumor-suppressing properties in numerous cancers, including LC, GC, BC, and melanoma [85]. LSZ showed anti-proliferative and anti-metastatic action [6]. LSZ increased E-cadherin expression while decreasing the mesenchymal indicators CDH2 and VIM expression. LSZ inhibits EMT in SK-OV-3 cells via modulating miR-211 expression [86].

4.9. Fucoidan

The Fucoidan (FC) is a polysaccharide obtained from brown seaweeds and has shown anti-proliferative action on BC cells, such as 4T1 and MDA-MB-231. It also lowered metastatic lung nodules in female Balb/c mice with 4T1 xenografts. The TGFRs molecular network is critical in controlling EMT in cancer cells. It was observed that FC efficiently reverses TGFR-induced EMT morphological alterations, increases epithelial markers, decreases mesenchymal markers and transcriptional repressor expression Twist, Snail, and Slug. Furthermore, fucoidan suppresses migration and invasion during EMT, implying that TGFR-mediated signaling is involved in BC cells [87].

4.10. Penisuloxazin A

Penisuloxazin A (PNSA) is a fungal mycotoxin that belongs to a new epipolythiodiketopiperazines (ETPs) possessing a rare 3H-spiro[benzofuran-2,2′-piperazine] ring system. PNSA prevented MDA-MB-231 cell adhesion to coated Matrigels containing several ECM components. Furthermore, after PNSA therapy, there is a transition from spindle-shaped or polygonal mesenchymal to flat polygonal epithelial-like cell morphology. These suggest that PNSA can prevent EMT in MDA-MB-231 cells [88]. PNSA is also considered a potent heat shock protein 90 (HSP90) inhibitor, a well-known N-terminal inhibitor binding to the ATP pocket of HSP90 in preventing BC cell metastasis. Multiple signaling pathways critical for cancer cell proliferation and metastasis can be disrupted by inhibiting HSP90 [89].

4.11. Sophocarpine

Sophocarpinr (SC) is one of the most active components of *Sophora alopecuroides* L, a tetracyclic quinolizidine alkaloid. SC has shown various pharmacological actions, including immunoregulatory, anti-inflammatory, and anti-nociceptive [90]. SC has also been shown to preserve heart function from ischemic reperfusion by inhibiting NF-kB and reducing hepatocyte steatosis via activation of the AMPK signaling pathway. Furthermore, in head and neck squamous cell carcinoma (HNSCC) cells, SC has shown anti-proliferative and anti-metastatic by inhibiting dicer-catalyzed miR-21 maturation and activation of the p38MAPK signaling pathway. SC also reduced the HNSCC tumor's growth in vivo by reversing the EMT in cancer cells. In UM-SCC-22B and UM-SCC-47 cells, SC treatment reduced the expression of the Ki-67 and VIM while increasing E-cadherin's expression [91]. These findings suggest that SC could be a promising lead drug for HNSCC.

4.12. Renieramycin M

Renieramycin M (RM) (22-Boc-Gly-RM), produced by *Xestospongia sp.*, is a semi-synthetic amino ester derivative of the bistetrahydroisoquinoline alkaloid. Studies suggested RM-mediated inhibition of anchorage-independent development and sensitization of detachment-induced cell death in human lung cancer cells [92]. A semi-synthetic derivative of RM with a hydroquinone amino ester extension was synthesized to retain cytotoxicity with increase cancer selectivity [93]. It hinders the phosphorylation of FAK and Akt molecules, which upregulate TIMP2 and TIMP3 and downregulate MMPs expression.

The inhibition of the p-FAK/p-Akt signal also marks the downregulation of CDH2 and Rac1-GTP and the upregulation of E-cadherin, where the regulation of cytoskeleton regulatory protein (Rac1-GTP), MMP-associated molecules (TIMP2, TIMP3) [94]. The mechanism of action of RM is demonstrated in Figure 3.

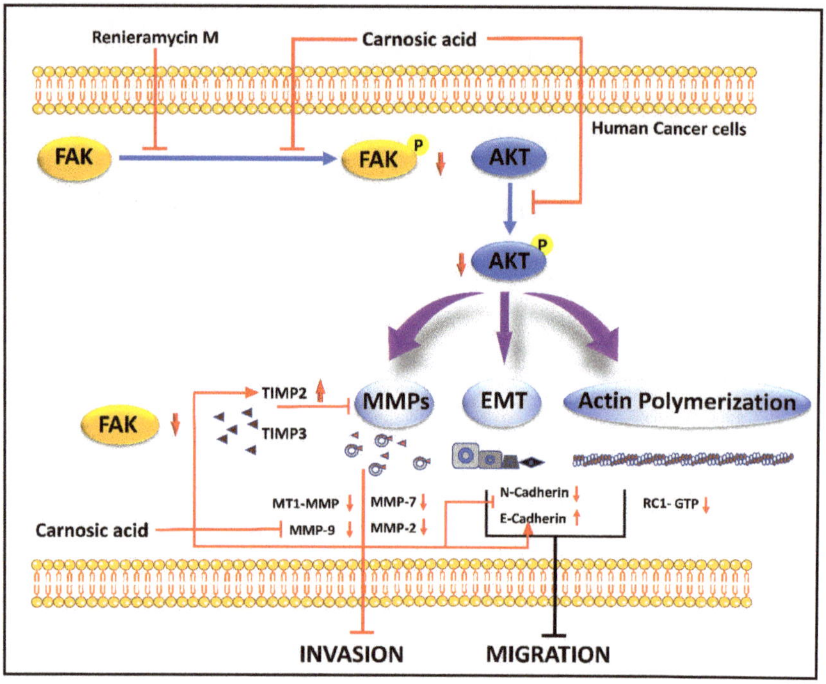

Figure 3. Inhibition of the FAK/AKT signaling pathway and subsequently decrease EMT markers, CDH2 MMPs, etc., and increases epithelial marker, E-cadherin, which reduces cell invasion and migration by Renieramycin M and Carnosic Acid [94,95].

4.13. Luteolin

Luteolin (LT) (3,4,5,7-tetrahydroxy flavone) is a flavonoid in many plants including broccoli, carrots, perilla leaves, seeds, and celery. It possesses anti-allergy, anti-inflammatory, anti-cancer, antioxidant, and anti-microbial properties [96–98]. In various cancers (including lung, GBM, BC, CRC, PC), LT inhibits cell proliferation and tumor growth, promotes cancer cell apoptosis and cell cycle arrest, reduces drug resistance, and reduces cancer cell invasiveness and metastasis [99]. LT can also stop EMT from occurring, shrinking in the cytoskeleton, increasing the expression of E-cadherin, and decreasing the expression of CDH2, Snail, and VIM [100]. LT inhibits the Smad 2/3 pathway and the Wnt/-catenin pathway by inhibiting the synthesis of Snail and Slug by downregulating the production of β-catenin. Doing so prevents metastasis by upregulating CDH2, Zo 1, and claudin 1 and downregulating CDH2, fibronectin, VIM, and MMP-2 [99,101]. The mechanism of the action of LT is demonstrated in Figure 4.

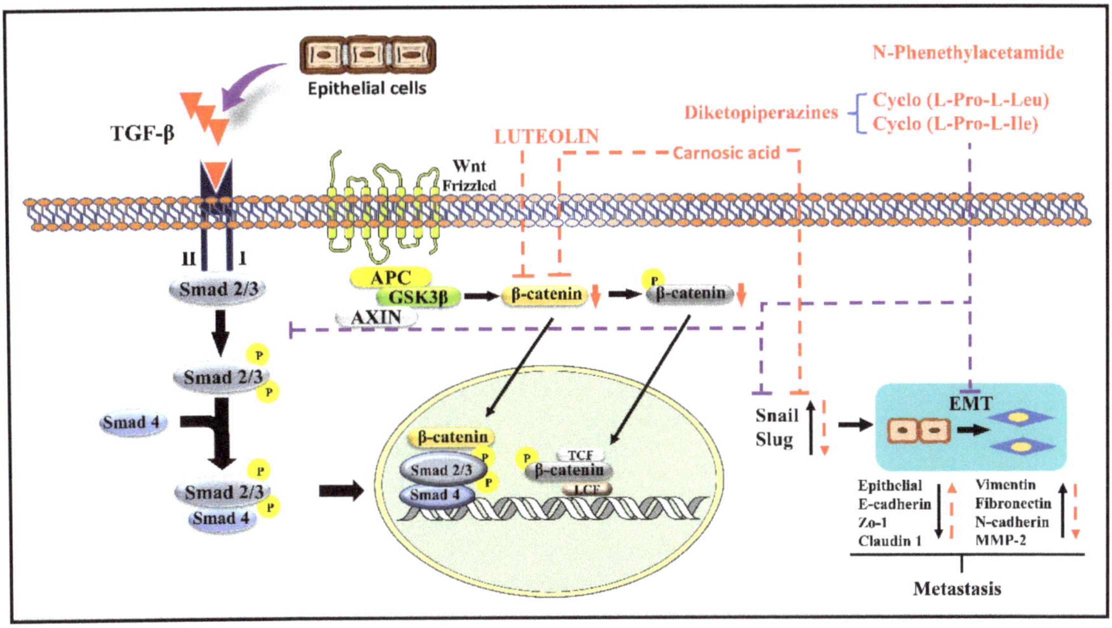

Figure 4. Possible mechanisms of luteolin, Carnosic acid, and N-Phenethylacetamide inhibit EMT via different pathways [94,95].

4.14. Carnosic Acid

Carnosic acid (CA), a polyphenolic diterpene found in rosemary (*Rosmarinus officinalis*), has anti-cancer, anti-viral, and anti-inflammatory activities. CA suppresses cancer cell migration and proliferation while lowering vascular endothelial growth factor expression. In leukemia and CRC cells, CA also causes cell cycle arrest at the G2/M phase by downregulating cyclin expression and has been shown to trigger apoptotic cell death in human NB and PrC cells [102]. CA inhibits EMT and cell migration in B16F10 cells in a dose-dependent manner. It prevents Src/AKT phosphorylation and, therefore, activation. It decreases the secretion of uPAc, MMP-9, and TIMP-1, whereas it increases the secretion of TIMP-2 and has no effect on the secretion of MMP-2 and plasminogen activator inhibitor-1 (PAI-1). It is also responsible for the decrease in the expression of Snail and Slug but does not affect the expression of Twist in B16F10 melanoma cells [95]. The mechanism of action of CA is demonstrated in Figures 3 and 4.

4.15. N-Phenethylacetamide

N-Phenethylacetamide (NPA) is found in the *Aquamarina Sp.* (MC085). Three compounds, two diketopiperazines [cyclo(L-Pro-L-Leu) (1) and cyclo(L-Pro-L-Ile) (2), and one NPA (3)] isolated with anti-cancer activity. By altering TGF-induced E.M.T., NPA inhibits the TGF/Smad pathway and suppresses A549 cell metastasis. It prevents Snail and Slug expression by inhibiting Smad 2/3 phosphorylation. It also suppresses Snail and Slug, which upregulates the epithelial markers E-cadherin, Zo-1, and claudin-1 while downregulating VIM, FN1, CDH2, and MMP-2 expression, preventing metastasis [101]. The mechanism of NPA is shown in Figure 4.

4.16. α-Solanine

α-Solanin (AS), a steroidal glycoalkaloid obtained from nightshade (Solanum nigrum Linn.), suppresses tumor cell growth and causes apoptosis in colon, liver, cervical, lymphoma, and stomach cancer cells. However, the mechanism by which it blocks cancer cell metastasis remains unknown. An animal model of BC induces cell death and inhibits cell proliferation and angiogenesis, resulting in chemotherapeutic actions [103,104]. It also increases E-cadherin expression, reducing VIM expression and cell invasion, which inhibits EMT. It also decreases extracellular inducer of matrix metalloproteinase (EMMPRIN), MMP-2, and MMP-9, increasing Cysteine-rich protein with Kazal motifs (RECK), TIMP-1, and TIMP-2 mRNA expression levels. It downregulated the phosphorylation of Akt, ERK1/2, and PI3K. Furthermore, it increases tumor suppressor miR-138 expression while decreasing oncogenic miR-21 expression [6,105].

4.17. Baicalein, Wogonin (WG), and Oroxylin-A (ORA)

Baicalein (BAI), wogonin (WG), and oroxylin-A (ORA) are present in a plant, namely *Scutellaria baicalensis* [105]. It has been reported that the extract of *Scutellaria baicalensis* has anti-tumor activity. A study reported that using the combination of BAI (65.8%), WG (21.2%), and ORA (13.0%) compounds against A549 lung adenoma cancer cells inhibited the EMT process significantly [105]. The Total Flavonoid Aglycones Extract (TFAE) isolated from *Scutellaria baicalensis* has shown inhibition against tumors by inducing apoptosis, mainly BAI, WG, and ORA [106]. It was reported that the TFAE of *Scutellaria baicalensis* has inhibited the EMT of A549 cells via PI3K/AKT-TWIST1 axis [105].

4.18. Coptidis Rhizoma

It was reported that the extract of Coptidis Rhizoma (CR) could inhibit the EMT process via the TGF-β signaling pathway [107]. It has been shown that 30% ethanol extract of Coptidis Rhizoma can inhibit cell migration and invasion via blocking E-cadherin and decreasing expression of vimentin, Snail, and ZEB2 [107]. It has a potential anti-metastatic effect and can be a candidate against cancer. The different pathways and proteins targeted by all natural products discussed in the present review are summarized in Figure 5.

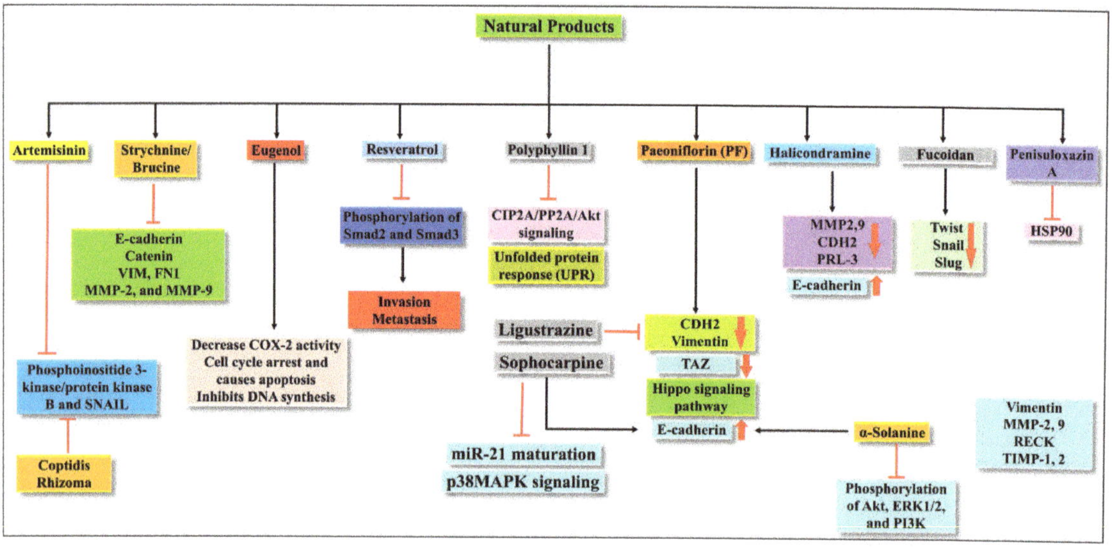

Figure 5. Illustration of the different pathways targeted by the natural products discussed in the present review.

5. Advantages of Targeting EMT

EMT is recognized as playing a key role in developing cancer, metastasis, and chemotherapy resistance, and its crucial roles throughout cancer progression have recently been discovered and investigated. Although there is still debate about whether EMT causes cancer metastasis, its importance in cancer chemoresistance is becoming more widely recognized, with many EMT-related signaling pathways implicated in cancer cell chemoresistance [39]. Targeted cancer treatments have been an emerging field in the recent decade. Several monoclonal antibody therapies and small chemicals, particularly kinase inhibitors, have been discovered/synthesized and undergo clinical trials with improved anti-cancer effectiveness. While many targeted therapeutic medications demonstrated encouraging preliminary clinical outcomes, such as enhanced overall survival, a significant percentage of patients who received targeted therapy acquired drug resistance following long-term treatment [108]. As a result, cancer drug resistance will determine the success of forthcoming targeted treatment medications. Drug resistance can be caused by various mechanisms, including drug efflux, drug metabolism, and drug target mutations [1,109]. The function of EMT in cancer therapy resistance has recently been explored. In the early 1990s, a relationship between EMT and cancer cell treatment resistance was proposed. Heckford et al. discovered that EMT occurred in two Adriamycin-resistant MCF-7 cells and vinblastine-resistant ZR-75-B cells [110]. Attempts have been devoted to targeting the ABC transporters to overcome drug resistance [111,112]. When it became obvious that EMT plays a critical role in drug resistance, scientists began exploring drugs targeting EMT to overcome drug resistance. Gupta et al. created EMT cells using E-cadherin shRNA and used this cell line to develop CSC-selective small molecule inhibitors. Using high-throughput screening, they discovered an antibiotic named Salinomycin that eliminated breast CSCs preferentially [113]. Salinomycin also reduced EMT caused by doxorubicin exposure and improved doxorubicin sensitivity in HCC cells [114]. It inhibited the expression and operation of drug efflux pumps in BC cells, resulting in a considerable reduction in doxorubicin resistance [115]. In addition to Salinomycin, several minor pharmacologic inhibitors of EMT have been discovered and tested in vitro and in vivo cancer treatment resistance models. Mocetinostat, a histone deacetylase (HDAC) inhibitor that restored miR-203 and decreased ZEB1 (EMT-TF) expression, reversed EMT in drug-resistant cancer cells and sensitized them to the chemotherapeutic agent docetaxel [116]. Curcumin, a component of curry, was discovered to sensitize 5-fluorouracil-resistant colorectal cancer cells via inhibiting EMT via miRNA [117]. According to Namba et al., EMT mediated by the Akt/GSK3/Snail1 pathway was a critical signaling event in acquiring gemcitabine resistance in PC cells. The anti-viral zidovudine inhibited these signaling pathways, restoring gemcitabine sensitivity in cancer cells. Co-administered zidovudine with gemcitabine reduced tumor growth and prevented cancer cells from establishing the EMT phenotype in mice with a gemcitabine-resistant pancreatic tumor xenograft [118]. Oncologists have recently focused on metformin since it has anti-cancer and chemopreventive qualities independent of anti-hyperglycemic effects [119,120]. Hirsch et al. later discovered that metformin targets BCSCs [121]. According to follow-up studies, metformin lowers CSCs by targeting EMT Metformin triggered transcriptional re-programming of BCSCs by lowering major EMT-TFs such as SNAIL2, Twist1, and ZEB1, according to Vazquez-Martin and colleagues [121]. Metformin has been shown to prevent EMT in lung cancer by inhibiting the IL-6/STAT3 axis in lung adenocarcinoma [122]. Although the direct molecular target of metformin in suppressing EMT is unknown, the Stimulation of AMPK may play a significant role in the drug's anti-EMT activity [123,124]. Metformin is being studied in over 200 human clinical studies for cancer therapy because of its possible CSC, anti-cancer properties, and favorable safety profile [125]. As a result, targeting EMT has been viewed as a unique strategy for combating cancer treatment resistance. In addition to the small compounds that have been created, a lot of pharmacological screening is being done to find new EMT inhibitors. Chua et al. created an EMT spot migration recognition method that can be utilized for high-content screening to screen small molecule EMT inhibitors that target certain growth factors. Scientists could undertake high throughput screening of small compounds utilizing enhanced screening platforms thanks to advancements in EMT and CSC biology [126]. Aref et al. also created a microfluidic device that mimics the 3D tumor microenvironment by including tumor cell spheroids and an adjacent endothelial monolayer. This approach is very beneficial in identifying EMT medicines active in a complex in vivo tumor microenvironment with several cell kinds interacting [127,128]. As a result, targeting EMTs with the natural chemical entity is viewed as a unique and innovative approach to combating cancer treatment resistance.

6. Targeting EMT Process by Molecular Docking (MD)

MD is a promising approach for estimating the interaction between biological molecules, such as proteins and ligands [129,130]. In the last decade, MD has emerged as a promising tool in identifying lead molecules against different ailments. MD is applied to cancer stem cells (CSC) associated metabolic and signaling pathways. Different metabolic pathways participate in CSC survival concerning cancer progression and alterations [130]. This is why metabolic re-programming is considered one of the cancer symbols [131].

Natural products are considered the grounds of multi-targeting molecules. Alkaloids, a class of natural producers, are one of the promising molecules that have the strength to combat CSCs via MD [130,131]. The drugs like salasonine and tylophorine have shown that they altered the Hedgehog (Hh) pathways and exerted anti-cancer effects on CSCs [130,131]. The targeting of overexpressed receptors in cancer tissues has demonstrated anti-cancer potential by natural products earlier through MD and experimental approaches [130,131]. It is reported that natural products represent a rich source of therapeutically active compounds which can interact with numerous cellular targets and minimize the side effects [132]. MD may help us find the natural lead molecules against the EMT process. Different receptors play a role in the EMT process, so it will be more important to screen out natural compounds against those receptors to find lead molecules.

7. Future Prospective

EMT has long been suspected of contributing to cancer therapy resistance. It became clear when scientists observed strong parallels in gene expression profiles and marker expression between EMT cells and CSCs. The resistance of CSCs against pharmacotherapy is a major challenge and poses a significant threat to cancer patients. The pathways involved in EMT have been deciphered by scientists, and have developed several methodologies to investigate the phenotypes in EMT. These understandings form the basis for drug screening against EMT-mediated cancer. The miRNA and some chemical agents demonstrate inhibitory activity against EMT, but no currently available miRNAs in clinical settings can solve this problem. So natural compounds showing good results can be the game changers in mitigating the EMT process. Several small chemical agents have been discovered to help drug-resistant cancer cells targeting EMT become more chemo-sensitive. Many of these, including Ligustrazine Penisuloxazin A, Halichondramide, Sophocarpine, Fucoidan, and Diketopiperazines, were investigated in human clinical trials with standard chemotherapies or targeted treatments.

Furthermore, EMT inhibitors' long-term safety is unknown. This is especially true if EMT inhibitors activate the MET pathway, which has been linked to cancer metastasis. Moreover, studies need to be conducted to investigate the link of EMT with different pathways involved in Cancers. There is a need to develop nanoformulations targeting the cancerous to avoid off-target side effects. Moreover, with the advancement of the compounds screening assays, more novel natural compounds need to be explored to find a more potent EMT inhibitor. Novel in vitro and in vivo approaches should be developed to reduce translational failure [133].

8. Conclusions

The part of EMT-MET in cancer cell dispersion and distant metastasis has been acknowledged. Recent research suggests that EMT may not be required for cancer cell metastasis despite its importance in chemoresistance. However, this is controversial because of the EMT phenotype's variability and adaptability. Only a fraction of EMT populations may be controlled by Fsp1. Finally, EMT is a critical cancer cell characteristic contributing to medication resistance. Inhibitors of this biological mechanism will be suitable "partners" for chemotherapy or targeted therapy medications, allowing current cancer therapies to achieve better clinical outcomes. Natural products play a dynamic role in controlling the process of EMT in cancer; many assays have been performed to prove their activity. EMT is a progression where cells can lose their epithelial properties like E-cadherin and a few more and gain mesenchymal properties like CDH2, VIM, FN1, etc. EMT has long been investigated for its involvement in cancer treatment resistance and metastasis. Assay techniques to analyze EMT phenotypic and drug screening have been created based on a better knowledge of natural chemicals and critical signaling pathways in EMT. Natural compounds that downregulate EMT phenotype and, as a result, drug resistance and metastasis have been identified, allowing scientists to discover natural compounds as EMT inhibitors capable of improving chemosensitivity of drug-resistant cancer cells while inhibiting metastasis. However, additional research is needed to fully comprehend the significance of EMT in cancer treatment resistance, cell proliferation, invasion, metastasis, and natural chemicals and their involvement in blocking EMT.

Author Contributions: Conceptualization: S.A. (Sirajudheen Anwar) and J.A.M.; Methodology: J.A.M. and S.A. (Sirajudheen Anwar); Software: S.A. (Sakeel Ahmed); Validation: J.A.M., S.A. (Sakeel Ahmed) and S.A. (Sirajudheen Anwar). Writing—original draft preparation: J.A.M., V.A.K. and S.A. (Sakeel Ahmed); Review and editing: S.A. (Sirajudheen Anwar), J.A., A.A. and N.A.; project administration: S.A. (Sirajudheen Anwar); Funding acquisition: S.A. (Sirajudheen Anwar). All authors have read and agreed to the published version of the manuscript.

Funding: This research has been funded from Research Deanship in University of Ha'il—Saudi Arabia through project number MDR-22 031.

Institutional Review Board Statement: Not applicable.

Informed Consent Statement: Not applicable.

Data Availability Statement: Not applicable.

Acknowledgments: Authors extend their appreciation to project fund from Research Deanship in University of Ha'il—Saudi Arabia through project number MDR-22 031.

Conflicts of Interest: Authors do not have any conflict of interest, personal or financial.

Sample Availability: Not applicable.

References

1. Malik, J.A.; Ahmed, S.; Jan, B.; Bender, O.; Al Hagbani, T.; Alqarni, A.; Anwar, S. Drugs repurposed: An advanced step towards the treatment of breast cancer and associated challenges. *Biomed. Pharmacother.* **2021**, *145*, 112375. [CrossRef] [PubMed]
2. Ferlay, J.; Soerjomataram, I.; Dikshit, R.; Eser, S.; Mathers, C.; Rebelo, M.; Parkin, D.M.; Forman, D.; Bray, F. Cancer incidence and mortality worldwide: Sources, methods and major patterns in GLOBOCAN 2012. *Int. J. Cancer* **2015**, *136*, E359–E386. [CrossRef] [PubMed]
3. Ferlay, J.; Steliarova-Foucher, E.; Lortet-Tieulent, J.; Rosso, S.; Coebergh, J.W.W.; Comber, H.; Forman, D.; Bray, F. Cancer incidence and mortality patterns in Europe: Estimates for 40 countries in 2012. *Eur. J. Cancer* **2013**, *49*, 1374–1403. [CrossRef] [PubMed]
4. Sanchez-Vega, F.; Mina, M.; Armenia, J.; Chatila, W.K.K.; Luna, A.; La, K.C.C.; Dimitriadoy, S.; Liu, D.L.; Kantheti, H.S.; Saghafinia, S.; et al. Oncogenic Signaling Pathways in The Cancer Genome Atlas. *Cell* **2018**, *173*, 321–337.e310. [CrossRef]
5. Kalluri, R.; Weinberg, R.A. The basics of epithelial-mesenchymal transition. *J. Clin. Investig.* **2009**, *119*, 1420–1428. [CrossRef]
6. Avila-Carrasco, L.; Majano, P.; Sánchez-Toméro, J.A.; Selgas, R.; López-Cabrera, M.; Aguilera, A.; González-Mateo, G.T. Natural Plants Compounds as Modulators of Epithelial-to-Mesenchymal Transition. *Front. Pharmacol.* **2019**, *10*, 715. [CrossRef]
7. Gundamaraju, R.; Lu, W.; Paul, M.K.; Jha, N.K.; Gupta, P.K.; Ojha, S.; Chattopadhyay, I.; Rao, P.V.; Ghavami, S. Autophagy and EMT in cancer and metastasis: Who controls whom? *Biochim. Biophys. Acta-Mol. Basis Dis.* **2022**, *1868*, 166431. [CrossRef]
8. Brabletz, S.; Schuhwerk, H.; Brabletz, T.; Stemmler, M.P. Dynamic EMT: A multi-tool for tumor progression. *EMBO J.* **2021**, *40*, e108647. [CrossRef]
9. Chiu, K.-J.; Chiou, H.-Y.C.; Huang, C.-H.; Lu, P.-C.; Kuo, H.-R.; Wang, J.-W.; Lin, M.-H. Natural Compounds Targeting Cancer-Associated Fibroblasts against Digestive System Tumor Progression: Therapeutic Insights. *Biomedicines* **2022**, *10*, 713. [CrossRef]
10. Chen, Y.; McAndrews, K.M.; Kalluri, R. Clinical and therapeutic relevance of cancer-associated fibroblasts. *Nat. Rev. Clin. Oncol.* **2021**, *18*, 792–804. [CrossRef]

11. Biffi, G.; Tuveson, D.A. Diversity and Biology of Cancer-Associated Fibroblasts. *Physiol. Rev.* **2021**, *101*, 147–176. [CrossRef] [PubMed]
12. Chen, X.; Song, E. Turning foes to friends: Targeting cancer-associated fibroblasts. *Nat. Rev. Drug Discov.* **2019**, *18*, 99–115. [CrossRef] [PubMed]
13. Liao, Z.; Tan, Z.W.; Zhu, P.; Tan, N.S. Cancer-associated fibroblasts in tumor microenvironment—Accomplices in tumor malignancy. *Cell. Immunol.* **2019**, *343*, 103729. [CrossRef] [PubMed]
14. Ermakov, M.S.; Nushtaeva, A.A.; Richter, V.A.; Koval, O. Cancer-associated fibroblasts and their role in tumor progression. *Vavilov J. Genet. Breed.* **2022**, *26*, 14–21. [CrossRef] [PubMed]
15. Nissen, N.I.; Karsdal, M.; Willumsen, N. Collagens and Cancer associated fibroblasts in the reactive stroma and its relation to Cancer biology. *J. Exp. Clin. Cancer Res.* **2019**, *38*, 115. [CrossRef]
16. Wang, T.-H.; Hsia, S.-M.; Shieh, T.-M. Lysyl Oxidase and the Tumor Microenvironment. *Int. J. Mol. Sci.* **2016**, *18*, 62. [CrossRef]
17. Najafi, M.; Farhood, B.; Mortezaee, K. Extracellular matrix (ECM) stiffness and degradation as cancer drivers. *J. Cell. Biochem.* **2019**, *120*, 2782–2790. [CrossRef]
18. Tune, B.X.J.; Sim, M.S.S.; Poh, C.L.; Mac Guad, R.; Woon, C.K.; Hazarika, I.; Das, A.; Gopinath, S.C.B.; Rajan, M.; Sekar, M.; et al. Matrix Metalloproteinases in Chemoresistance: Regulatory Roles, Molecular Interactions, and Potential Inhibitors. *J. Oncol.* **2022**, *2022*, 3249766. [CrossRef]
19. Mochizuki, S.; Ao, T.; Sugiura, T.; Yonemura, K.; Shiraishi, T.; Kajiwara, Y.; Okamoto, K.; Shinto, E.; Okada, Y.; Ueno, H. Expression and Function of a Disintegrin and Metalloproteinases in Cancer-Associated Fibroblasts of Colorectal Cancer. *Digestion* **2020**, *101*, 18–24. [CrossRef]
20. Glentis, A.; Oertle, P.; Mariani, P.; Chikina, A.; El Marjou, F.; Attieh, Y.; Zaccarini, F.; Lae, M.; Loew, D.; Dingli, F.; et al. Cancer-associated fibroblasts induce metalloprotease-independent cancer cell invasion of the basement membrane. *Nat. Commun.* **2017**, *8*, 924. [CrossRef]
21. Lindsey, S.; Langhans, S.A. Crosstalk of Oncogenic Signaling Pathways during Epitheliala€"Mesenchymal Transition. *Front. Oncol.* **2014**, *4*, 358. [CrossRef]
22. Peng, D.; Fu, M.; Wang, M.; Wei, Y.; Wei, X. Targeting TGF-β signal transduction for fibrosis and cancer therapy. *Mol. Cancer* **2022**, *21*, 104. [CrossRef]
23. Yu, M.; Trobridge, P.; Wang, Y.; Kanngurn, S.; Morris, S.M.; Knoblaugh, S.; Grady, W.M. Inactivation of TGF-β signaling and loss of PTEN cooperate to induce colon cancer in vivo. *Oncogene* **2014**, *33*, 1538–1547. [CrossRef]
24. Holderfield, M.T.; Hughes, C.C. Crosstalk Between Vascular Endothelial Growth Factor, Notch, and Transforming Growth Factor-β in Vascular Morphogenesis. *Circ. Res.* **2008**, *102*, 637–652. [CrossRef]
25. Niimi, H.; Pardali, K.; Vanlandewijck, M.; Heldin, C.-H.; Moustakas, A. Notch signaling is necessary for epithelial growth arrest by TGF-β. *J. Cell Biol.* **2007**, *176*, 695–707. [CrossRef]
26. Bhaskaran, N.; Souchelnytskyi, S. Systemic analysis of TGFβ proteomics revealed involvement of Plag1/CNK1/RASSF1A/Src network in TGFβ1-dependent activation of Erk1/2 and cell proliferation. *Proteomics* **2008**, *8*, 4507–4520. [CrossRef] [PubMed]
27. Guo, X.; Wang, X.-F. Signaling cross-talk between TGF-β/BMP and other pathways. *Cell Res.* **2009**, *19*, 71–88. [CrossRef] [PubMed]
28. Kretzschmar, M.; Doody, J.; Timokhina, I.; Massague, J. A mechanism of repression of TGFbeta / Smad signaling by oncogenic Ras. *Genes Dev.* **1999**, *13*, 804–816. [CrossRef]
29. Zhang, W.-J.; Luo, C.; Huang, C.; Pu, F.-Q.; Zhu, J.-F.; Zhu, Z.-M. PI3K/Akt/GSK-3β signal pathway is involved in P2X7 receptor-induced proliferation and EMT of colorectal cancer cells. *Eur. J. Pharmacol.* **2021**, *899*, 174041. [CrossRef]
30. Ueda, Y.; Wang, S.; Dumont, N.; Yi, J.Y.; Koh, Y.; Arteaga, C.L. Overexpression of HER2 (erbB2) in Human Breast Epithelial Cells Unmasks Transforming Growth Factor β-induced Cell Motility. *J. Biol. Chem.* **2004**, *279*, 24505–24513. [CrossRef] [PubMed]
31. Vazquez-Martin, A.; Cufí, S.; Oliveras-Ferraros, C.; Torres-Garcia, V.Z.; Corominas-Faja, B.; Cuyàs, E.; Bonavia, R.; Visa, J.; Martín-Castillo, B.; Barrajón-Catalán, E.; et al. IGF-1R/epithelial-to-mesenchymal transition (EMT) cross-talk suppresses the erlotinib-sensitizing effect of EGFR exon 19 deletion mutations. *Sci. Rep.* **2013**, *3*, srep02560. [CrossRef] [PubMed]
32. Imodoye, S.O.; Adedokun, K.A.; Muhammed, A.O.; Bello, I.O.; Muhibi, M.A.; Oduola, T.; Oyenike, M.A. Understanding the Complex Milieu of Epithelial-Mesenchymal Transition in Cancer Metastasis: New Insight Into the Roles of Transcription Factors. *Front. Oncol.* **2021**, *11*, 4360. [CrossRef]
33. Newman, D.J.; Cragg, G.M. Natural products as sources of new drugs from 1981 to 2014. *J. Nat. Prod.* **2016**, *79*, 629–661. [CrossRef]
34. Aware, C.B.; Patil, D.N.; Suryawanshi, S.S.; Mali, P.R.; Rane, M.R.; Gurav, R.G.; Jadhav, J.P. Natural bioactive products as promising therapeutics: A review of natural product-based drug development. *S. Afr. J. Bot.* **2022**. [CrossRef]
35. Dongare, P.N.; Motule, A.S.; More, M.P.; Patinge, P.A.; Bakal, R. An overview on anti-cancer drugs from marine source. *World J. Pharm. Res.* **2021**, *10*, 950–956. [CrossRef]
36. Nobili, S.; Lippi, D.; Witort, E.; Donnini, M.; Bausi, L.; Mini, E.; Capaccioli, S. Natural compounds for cancer treatment and prevention. *Pharmacol. Res.* **2009**, *59*, 365–378. [CrossRef]
37. Newman, D.J.; Cragg, G.M. Marine-Sourced Anti-Cancer and Cancer Pain Control Agents in Clinical and Late Preclinical Development. *Mar. Drugs* **2014**, *12*, 255–278. [CrossRef] [PubMed]
38. Park, S.-H.; Kim, M.; Lee, S.; Jung, W.; Kim, B. Therapeutic Potential of Natural Products in Treatment of Cervical Cancer: A Review. *Nutrients* **2021**, *13*, 154. [CrossRef]

39. Heng, W.S.; Cheah, S.-C. Chelerythrine Chloride Downregulates β-Catenin and Inhibits Stem Cell Properties of Non-Small Cell Lung Carcinoma. *Molecules* **2020**, *25*, 224. [CrossRef]
40. El-Adl, K.; Sakr, H.M.; Yousef, R.G.; Mehany, A.B.; Metwaly, A.M.; Elhendawy, M.A.; Radwan, M.M.; ElSohly, M.A.; Abulkhair, H.S.; Eissa, I.H. Discovery of new quinoxaline-2(1H)-one-based anticancer agents targeting VEGFR-2 as inhibitors: Design, synthesis, and anti-proliferative evaluation. *Bioorganic Chem.* **2021**, *114*, 105105. [CrossRef]
41. Park, S.-A.; Surh, Y.-J. Modulation of tumor microenvironment by chemopreventive natural products. *Ann. New York Acad. Sci.* **2017**, *1401*, 65–74. [CrossRef]
42. Sauter, E.R. Cancer prevention and treatment using combination therapy with natural compounds. *Expert Rev. Clin. Pharmacol.* **2020**, *13*, 265–285. [CrossRef]
43. Chamberlin, S.R.; Blucher, A.; Wu, G.; Shinto, L.; Choonoo, G.; Kulesz-Martin, M.; McWeeney, S. Natural Product Target Network Reveals Potential for Cancer Combination Therapies. *Front. Pharmacol.* **2019**, *10*, 557. [CrossRef]
44. Atanasov, A.G.; Zotchev, S.B.; Dirsch, V.M.; Supuran, C.T. Natural products in drug discovery: Advances and opportunities. *Nat. Rev. Drug Discov.* **2021**, *20*, 200–216. [CrossRef]
45. Dasari, S.; Njiki, S.; Mbemi, A.; Yedjou, C.G.; Tchounwou, P.B. Pharmacological Effects of Cisplatin Combination with Natural Products in Cancer Chemotherapy. *Int. J. Mol. Sci.* **2022**, *23*, 1532. [CrossRef]
46. Pereira, R.B.; Evdokimov, N.M.; Lefranc, F.; Valentaõ, P.; Kornienko, A.; Pereira, D.M.; Andrade, P.B.; Gomes, N.G.M. Marine-derived anti-cancer agents: Clinical benefits, innovative mechanisms, and new targets. *Mar. Drugs* **2019**, *17*, 329. [CrossRef] [PubMed]
47. Saeed, A.F.; Su, J.; Ouyang, S. Marine-derived drugs: Recent advances in cancer therapy and immune signaling. *Biomed. Pharmacother.* **2021**, *134*, 111091. [CrossRef]
48. Shin, Y.; Kim, G.D.; Jeon, J.-E.; Shin, J.; Lee, S.K. Antimetastatic Effect of Halichondramide, a Trisoxazole Macrolide from the Marine Sponge Chondrosia corticata, on Human Prostate Cancer Cells via Modulation of Epithelial-to-Mesenchymal Transition. *Mar. Drugs* **2013**, *11*, 2472–2485. [CrossRef] [PubMed]
49. Sarici, F.; Aksoy, S. Efficacy and safety of ixabepilone monotherapy and ixabepilone-capecitabine combination in patients with heavily pretreated metastatic breast cancer. *Int. J. Hematol. Oncol.* **2021**, *31*, 85–91. [CrossRef]
50. Mehta-Shah, N.; Lunning, M.A.; Moskowitz, A.J.; Boruchov, A.M.; Ruan, J.; Lynch, P.; Hamlin, P.A.; Leonard, J.; Matasar, M.J.; Myskowski, P.L.; et al. Romidepsin and lenalidomide-based regimens have efficacy in relapsed/refractory lymphoma: Combined analysis of two phase I studies with expansion cohorts. *Am. J. Hematol.* **2021**, *96*, 1211–1222. [CrossRef] [PubMed]
51. Shah, Z.; Gohar, U.; Jamshed, I.; Mushtaq, A.; Mukhtar, H.; Zia-Ui-Haq, M.; Toma, S.; Manea, R.; Moga, M.; Popovici, B. Podophyllotoxin: History, Recent Advances and Future Prospects. *Biomolecules* **2021**, *11*, 603. [CrossRef] [PubMed]
52. Zhang, C.; Guan, D.; Jiang, M.; Liang, C.; Li, L.; Zhao, N.; Zha, Q.; Zhang, W.; Lu, C.; Zhang, G.; et al. efficacy of leflunomide combined with ligustrazine in the treatment of rheumatoid arthritis: Prediction with network pharmacology and validation in a clinical trial. *Chin. Med.* **2019**, *14*, 26. [CrossRef] [PubMed]
53. Seonu, S.-Y.; Kim, M.-J.; Yin, J.; Lee, M.-W. *Alnus sibirica* Compounds Exhibiting Anti-Proliferative, Apoptosis-Inducing, and *GSTP1* Demethylating Effects on Prostate Cancer Cells. *Molecules* **2021**, *26*, 3830. [CrossRef]
54. Dahlem, C.; Siow, W.X.; Lopatniuk, M.; Tse, W.K.F.; Kessler, S.M.; Kirsch, S.H.; Hoppstädter, J.; Vollmar, A.M.; Müller, R.; Luzhetskyy, A.; et al. Thioholgamide A, a New Anti-Proliferative Anti-Tumor Agent, Modulates Macrophage Polarization and Metabolism. *Cancers* **2020**, *12*, 1288. [CrossRef] [PubMed]
55. Laure, A.; Pagning, N.; Tamokou, J.; Muhammad, B.T.; Ngnokam, D.; Azefacktapondjou, L.; Ali, M.S.; Hameed, M.W. Potential anti-proliferative effects of chemical constituents and hemisynthetic derivatives from Scadoxus pseudocaulus (Amarillydaceae). *Afr. Health Sci.* **2020**, *20*, 469–475. [CrossRef]
56. Deng, Y.; Chen, C.; Xiao, Z.; Huang, X.; Xu, J. Enhanced anti-hepatoma effect of a novel curcumin analog C086 *via* solid dispersion technology. *Drug Deliv.* **2020**, *27*, 927–937. [CrossRef] [PubMed]
57. Wu, L.; Yu, J.; Chen, R.; Liu, Y.; Lou, L.; Wu, Y.; Huang, L.; Fan, Y.; Gao, P.; Huang, M.; et al. Dual Inhibition of Bcr-Abl and Hsp90 by C086 Potently Inhibits the Proliferation of Imatinib-Resistant CML Cells. *Clin. Cancer Res.* **2015**, *21*, 833–843. [CrossRef]
58. Chen, C.; Liu, Y.; Chen, Y.; Xu, J. C086, a novel analog of curcumin, induces growth inhibition and down-regulation of NF?B in colon cancer cells and xenograft tumors. *Cancer Biol. Ther.* **2011**, *12*, 797–807. [CrossRef]
59. Anibogwu, R.; De Jesus, K.; Pradhan, S.; Pashikanti, S.; Mateen, S.; Sharma, K. Extraction, Isolation and Characterization of Bioactive Compounds from *Artemisia* and Their Biological Significance: A Review. *Molecules* **2021**, *26*, 6995. [CrossRef]
60. Zhao, X.; Zhong, H.; Wang, R.; Liu, D.; Waxman, S.; Zhao, L.; Jing, Y. Dihydroartemisinin and its derivative induce apoptosis in acute myeloid leukemia through Noxa-mediated pathway requiring iron and endoperoxide moiety. *Oncotarget* **2015**, *6*, 5582–5596. [CrossRef]
61. Sun, Y.; Lu, X.; Li, H.; Li, X. Dihydroartemisinin inhibits IL-6-induced epithelial–mesenchymal transition in laryngeal squamous cell carcinoma via the miR-130b-3p/STAT3/β-catenin signaling pathway. *J. Int. Med Res.* **2021**, *49*, 030006052110094. [CrossRef]
62. Nandi, D.; Cheema, P.S.; Singal, A.; Bharti, H.; Nag, A. Artemisinin Mediates Its Tumor-Suppressive Activity in Hepatocellular Carcinoma Through Targeted Inhibition of FoxM1. *Front. Oncol.* **2021**, *11*, 751271. [CrossRef]
63. Lu, L.; Huang, R.; Wu, Y.; Jin, J.-M.; Chen, H.-Z.; Zhang, L.-J.; Luan, X. Brucine: A Review of Phytochemistry, Pharmacology, and Toxicology. *Front. Pharmacol.* **2020**, *11*, 377. [CrossRef]

64. Li, M.; Li, P.; Zhang, M.; Ma, F. Brucine suppresses breast cancer metastasis via inhibiting epithelial mesenchymal transition and matrix metalloproteinases expressions. *Chin. J. Integr. Med.* **2018**, *24*, 40–46. [CrossRef]
65. Fathy, M.; Fawzy, M.A.; Hintzsche, H.; Nikaido, T.; Dandekar, T.; Othman, E.M. Eugenol exerts apoptotic effect and modulates the sensitivity of HeLa cells to cisplatin and radiation. *Eur. J. Mol. Clin. Med.* **2020**, *7*, 3979. [CrossRef] [PubMed]
66. Fangjun, L.; Zhijia, Y. Tumor suppressive roles of eugenol in human lung cancer cells. *Thorac. Cancer* **2018**, *9*, 25–29. [CrossRef]
67. Petrocelli, G.; Farabegoli, F.; Valerii, M.; Giovannini, C.; Sardo, A.; Spisni, E. Molecules Present in Plant Essential Oils for Prevention and Treatment of Colorectal Cancer (CRC). *Molecules* **2021**, *26*, 885. [CrossRef] [PubMed]
68. Manikandan, P.; Murugan, R.S.S.; Priyadarsini, R.V.; Vinothini, G.; Nagini, S. Eugenol induces apoptosis and inhibits invasion and angiogenesis in a rat model of gastric carcinogenesis induced by MNNG. *Life Sci.* **2010**, *86*, 936–941. [CrossRef] [PubMed]
69. Kurnia, P.H.; Bachtiar, E.A.; Ria, Q.F.; Fadhil, F.; Anita, D. Eugenol isolated from Syzygium aromaticum inhibits HeLa cancer cell migration by altering epithelial-mesenchymal transition protein regulators. *J. Appl. Pharm. Sci.* **2021**, *11*, 49–53. [CrossRef]
70. Al-Sharif, I.; Remmal, A.; Aboussekhra, A. Eugenol triggers apoptosis in breast cancer cells through E2F1/survivin down-regulation. *BMC Cancer* **2013**, *13*, 600. [CrossRef]
71. Gao, Q.; Yuan, Y.; Gan, H.-Z.; Peng, Q. Resveratrol inhibits the hedgehog signaling pathway and epithelial-mesenchymal transition and suppresses gastric cancer invasion and metastasis. *Oncol. Lett.* **2015**, *9*, 2381–2387. [CrossRef] [PubMed]
72. Song, Y.; Chen, Y.; Li, Y.; Lyu, X.; Cui, J.; Cheng, Y.; Zheng, T.; Zhao, L.; Zhao, G. Resveratrol Suppresses Epithelial-Mesenchymal Transition in GBM by Regulating Smad-Dependent Signaling. *BioMed Res. Int.* **2019**, *2019*, 1321973. [CrossRef]
73. Ahmad, B.; Rehman, S.U.; Azizullah, A.; Khan, M.F.; Din, S.R.U.; Ahmad, M.; Ali, A.; Tahir, N.; Azam, N.; Gamallat, Y.; et al. Molecular mechanisms of anticancer activities of polyphyllin VII. *Chem. Biol. Drug Des.* **2021**, *97*, 914–929. [CrossRef] [PubMed]
74. Liu, M.-M.; Zhu, M.-L.; Dong, R.-F.; Zhang, C.; Yang, L.; Kong, L.-Y.; Xia, Y.-Z. Polyphyllin I promotes cell death via suppressing UPR-mediated CHOP ubiquitination and degradation in non-small cell lung cancer. *Chin. J. Nat. Med.* **2021**, *19*, 255–266. [CrossRef]
75. Chen, Y.; Wu, K.; Wood, W.G. Paeonia lactiflora Extract Attenuating Cerebral Ischemia and Arterial Intimal Hyperplasia Is Mediated by Paeoniflorin via Modulation of VSMC Migration and Ras MEK/ERK Signaling Pathway. *Evid.-Based Complement. Altern. Med.* **2013**, *2013*, 482428.
76. Wang, X.; Feng, S.; Wang, Y.; Chen, N.; Wang, Z. Phytomedicine Paeoniflorin: A neuroprotective monoterpenoid glycoside with promising anti-depressive properties. *Phytomedicine* **2021**, *90*, 153669. [CrossRef] [PubMed]
77. Zhang, L.; Wei, W. Anti-inflammatory and immunoregulatory effects of paeoniflorin and total glucosides of paeony. *Pharmacol. Ther.* **2019**, *207*, 107452. [CrossRef]
78. Ji, Y.; Dou, Y.-N.; Zhao, Q.-W.; Zhang, J.; Yang, Y.; Wang, T.; Xia, Y.-F.; Dai, Y.; Wei, Z.-F. Paeoniflorin suppresses TGF-β mediated epithelial-mesenchymal transition in pulmonary fibrosis through a Smad-dependent pathway. *Acta Pharmacol. Sin.* **2016**, *37*, 794–804. [CrossRef]
79. Zhou, Z.; Wang, S.; Song, C.; Hu, Z. Paeoniflorin prevents hypoxia-induced epithelial–mesenchymal transition in human breast cancer cells. *OncoTargets Ther.* **2016**, *9*, 2511–2518. [CrossRef]
80. Niu, K.; Liu, Y.; Zhou, Z.; Wu, X.; Wang, H.; Yan, J. Antitumor Effects of Paeoniflorin on Hippo Signaling Pathway in Gastric Cancer Cells. *J. Oncol.* **2021**, *2021*, 4724938. [CrossRef]
81. Chill, L.; Yosief, T.; Kashman, Y. Halichondramine, a New Tetracyclic Bipiperidine Alkaloid from the Marine Sponge *Halichondria* sp. *J. Nat. Prod.* **2002**, *65*, 1738–1741. [CrossRef] [PubMed]
82. Halim, H.; Chunhacha, P.; Suwanborirux, K.; Chanvorachote, P. Anticancer and antimetastatic activities of renieramyein M, a marine tetrahydroisoquinoline alkaloid, in human non-small cell lung cancer cells. *Anti-Cancer Res.* **2011**, *31*, 193–201.
83. Bae, S.Y.; Kim, G.D.; Jeon, J.-E.; Shin, J.; Lee, S.K. Anti-proliferative effect of (19Z)-halichondramide, a novel marine macrolide isolated from the sponge Chondrosia corticata, is associated with G2/M cell cycle arrest and suppression of mTOR signaling in human lung cancer cells. *Toxicol. Vitr.* **2013**, *27*, 694–699. [CrossRef]
84. Chen, J.; Wang, W.; Wang, H.; Liu, X.; Guo, X. Combination treatment of ligustrazine piperazine derivate DLJ14 and adriamycin inhibits progression of resistant breast cancer through inhibition of the EGFR/PI3K/Akt survival pathway and induction of apoptosis. *Drug Discov. Ther.* **2014**, *8*, 33–41. [CrossRef] [PubMed]
85. Xie, H.-J.; Zhao, J.; Zhuo-Ma, D.; Zhan-Dui, N.; Er-Bu, A.; Tsering, T. Inhibiting tumour metastasis by DQA modified paclitaxel plus ligustrazine micelles in treatment of non-small-cell lung cancer. *Artif. Cells Nanomed. Biotechnol.* **2019**, *47*, 3465–3477. [CrossRef] [PubMed]
86. Zhang, H.; Ding, S.; Xia, L. Ligustrazine inhibits the proliferation and migration of ovarian cancer cells via regulating miR-211. *Biosci. Rep.* **2021**, *41*, BSR20200199. [CrossRef]
87. Hsu, H.-Y.; Lin, T.-Y.; Hwang, P.-A.; Tseng, L.-M.; Chen, R.-H.; Tsao, S.-M.; Hsu, J. Fucoidan induces changes in the epithelial to mesenchymal transition and decreases metastasis by enhancing ubiquitin-dependent TGF receptor degradation in breast cancer. *Carcinogenesis* **2012**, *34*, 874–884. [CrossRef]
88. Loh, C.Y.; Chai, J.Y.; Tang, T.F.; Wong, W.F.; Sethi, G.; Shanmugam, M.K.; Chong, P.P.; Looi, C.Y. The E-Cadherin and N-Cadherin Switch in Epithelial-to-Mesenchymal Transition: Signaling, Therapeutic Implications, and Challenges. *Cells* **2019**, *8*, 1118. [CrossRef]
89. Zhang, A.; Qi, X.; Du, F.; Zhang, G.; Li, D.; Li, J. PNSA, A Novel C-Terminal Inhibitor of HSP90, Reverses Epithelial–Mesenchymal Transition and Suppresses Metastasis of Breast Cancer Cells In Vitro. *Mar. Drugs* **2021**, *19*, 117. [CrossRef] [PubMed]

90. Gao, Y.; Li, G.; Li, C.; Zhu, X.; Li, M.; Fu, C.; Li, B. Anti-nociceptive and anti-inflammatory activity of sophocarpine. *J. Ethnopharmacol.* **2009**, *125*, 324–329. [CrossRef]
91. Liu, W.; Zhang, B.; Chen, G.; Wu, W.; Zhou, L.; Shi, Y.; Zeng, Q.; Li, Y.; Sun, Y.; Deng, X.; et al. Targeting miR-21 with Sophocarpine Inhibits Tumor Progression and Reverses Epithelial-Mesenchymal Transition in Head and Neck Cancer. *Mol. Ther.* **2017**, *25*, 2129–2139. [CrossRef] [PubMed]
92. Prateep, A.; Sumkhemthong, S.; Karnsomwan, W.; De-Eknamkul, W.; Chamni, S.; Chanvorachote, P.; Chaotham, C. Avicequinone B sensitizes anoikis in human lung cancer cells. *J. Biomed. Sci.* **2018**, *25*, 32. [CrossRef] [PubMed]
93. Chamni, S.; Sirimangkalakitti, N.; Chanvorachote, P.; Suwanborirux, K.; Saito, N. Chemistry of renieramycins. Part 19: Semi-syntheses of 22-O-amino ester and hydroquinone 5-O-amino ester derivatives of renieramycin M and their cytotoxicity against non-small-cell lung cancer cell lines. *Mar. Drugs* **2020**, *18*, 418. [CrossRef] [PubMed]
94. Oo, Y.; Nealiga, J.Q.L.; Suwanborirux, K.; Chamni, S.; Ecoy, G.A.U.; Pongrakhananon, V.; Chanvorachote, P.; Chaotham, C. 22-O-(N-Boc-l-glycine) ester of renieramycin M inhibits migratory activity and suppresses epithelial–mesenchymal transition in human lung cancer cells. *J. Nat. Med.* **2021**, *75*, 949–966. [CrossRef]
95. Park, S.Y.; Song, H.; Sung, M.-K.; Kang, Y.-H.; Lee, K.W.; Park, J.H.Y. Carnosic Acid Inhibits the Epithelial-Mesenchymal Transition in B16F10 Melanoma Cells: A Possible Mechanism for the Inhibition of Cell Migration. *Int. J. Mol. Sci.* **2014**, *15*, 12698–12713. [CrossRef]
96. Chung, J.G.; Wu, L.T.; Chang, S.H.; Lo, H.H.; Hsieh, S.E.; Li, Y.C. Inhibitory Actions of Berberine on Growth and Arylamine N-Acetyltransferase Activity in Strains of Helicobacter Pylori from Peptic Ulcer Patients. *Int. J. Toxicol.* **1999**, *18*, 35–40. [CrossRef]
97. Lin, Y.; Shi, R.; Wang, X.; Shen, H.-M. Luteolin, a Flavonoid with Potential for Cancer Prevention and Therapy. *Curr. Cancer Drug Targets* **2008**, *8*, 634–646. [CrossRef]
98. Chen, C.-Y.; Peng, W.-H.; Tsai, K.-D.; Hsu, S.-L. Luteolin suppresses inflammation-associated gene expression by blocking NF-κB and AP-1 activation pathway in mouse alveolar macrophages. *Life Sci.* **2007**, *81*, 1602–1614. [CrossRef]
99. Lin, D.; Kuang, G.; Wan, J.; Zhang, X.; Li, H.; Gong, X.; Li, H. Luteolin suppresses the metastasis of triple-negative breast cancer by reversing epithelial-to-mesenchymal transition via downregulation of β-catenin expression. *Oncol. Rep.* **2016**, *37*, 895–902. [CrossRef]
100. Imran, M.; Rauf, A.; Abu-Izneid, T.; Nadeem, M.; Shariati, M.A.A.; Khan, I.A.; Imran, A.; Orhan, I.E.E.; Rizwan, M.; Atif, M.; et al. luteolin, a flavonoid, as an anticancer agent: A review. *Biomed. Pharmacother.* **2019**, *112*, 108612. [CrossRef]
101. Lee, M.J.; Kim, G.J.; Shin, M.-S.; Moon, J.; Kim, S.; Nam, J.-W.; Kang, K.S.; Choi, H. Chemical Investigation of Diketopiperazines and N-Phenethylacetamide Isolated from *Aquimarina* sp. MC085 and Their Effect on TGF-β-Induced Epithelial–Mesenchymal Transition. *Appl. Sci.* **2021**, *11*, 8866. [CrossRef]
102. D'Alesio, C.; Bellese, G.; Gagliani, M.C.; Aiello, C.; Grasselli, E.; Marcocci, G.; Bisio, A.; Tavella, S.; Daniele, T.; Cortese, K.; et al. Cooperative antitumor activities of carnosic acid and Trastuzumab in ERBB2+ breast cancer cells. *J. Exp. Clin. Cancer Res.* **2017**, *36*, 154. [CrossRef] [PubMed]
103. Lin, K.; Lin, C.; Kuo, S.; Lai, J.; Wang, Y.; You, H.; Hsu, M.; Chen, C.; Shiu, L. Carnosic acid impedes cell growth and enhances anti-cancer effects of carmustine and lomustine in melanoma. *Biosci. Rep.* **2018**, *38*, BSR20180005.
104. Shen, K.-H.; Liao, A.C.-H.; Hung, J.-H.; Lee, W.-J.; Hu, K.-C.; Lin, P.-T.; Liao, R.-F.; Chen, P.-S. α-Solanine Inhibits Invasion of Human Prostate Cancer Cell by Suppressing Epithelial-Mesenchymal Transition and MMPs Expression. *Molecules* **2014**, *19*, 11896–11914. [CrossRef] [PubMed]
105. Cao, H.-J.; Zhou, W.; Xian, X.-L.; Sun, S.-J.; Ding, P.-J.; Tian, C.-Y.; Tian, F.-L.; Jiang, C.-H.; Fu, T.-T.; Zhao, S.; et al. A Mixture of Baicalein, Wogonin, and Oroxylin-A Inhibits EMT in the A549 Cell Line via the PI3K/AKT-TWIST1-Glycolysis Pathway. *Front. Pharmacol.* **2022**, *12*, 4171. [CrossRef]
106. Wang, Y.; Cao, H.-J.; Sun, S.-J.; Dai, J.-Y.; Fang, J.-W.; Li, Q.-H.; Yan, C.; Mao, W.-W.; Zhang, Y.-Y. Total flavonoid aglycones extract in Radix scutellariae inhibits lung carcinoma and lung metastasis by affecting cell cycle and DNA synthesis. *J. Ethnopharmacol.* **2016**, *194*, 269–279. [CrossRef] [PubMed]
107. Kang, Y.-H.; Wang, J.-H.; Lee, J.-S.; Lee, N.-H.; Son, C.-G. Coptidis Rhizoma Suppresses Metastatic Behavior by Inhibiting TGF-β-Mediated Epithelial-Mesenchymal Transition in 5-FU-Resistant HCT116 Cells. *Front. Pharmacol.* **2022**, *13*, 2336. [CrossRef] [PubMed]
108. Juchum, M.; Günther, M.; Laufer, S.A. Fighting cancer drug resistance: Opportunities and challenges for mutation-specific EGFR inhibitors. *Drug Resist. Updat.* **2015**, *20*, 12–28. [CrossRef] [PubMed]
109. Malik, J.A.; Jan, R.; Ahmed, S.; Anwar, S. Breast Cancer Drug Repurposing a Tool for a Challenging Disease. In *Drug Repurposing-Molecular Aspects and Therapeutic Applications*; IntechOpen: London, UK, 2022. [CrossRef]
110. Sommers, C.L.; Heckford, S.E.E.; Skerker, J.M.; Worland, P.; Torri, J.A.; Thompson, E.W.; Byers, S.W.; Gelmann, E.P. Loss of epithelial markers and acquisition of vimentin expression in adriamycin- and vinblastine-resistant human breast cancer cell lines. *Cancer Res.* **1992**, *52*, 5190–5197.
111. Lancet, J.E.E.; Baer, M.R.; Duran, G.E.; List, A.; Fielding, R.; Marcelletti, J.F.; Multani, P.S.S.; Sikic, B.I. A phase I trial of continuous infusion of the multidrug resistance inhibitor zosuquidar with daunorubicin and cytarabine in acute myeloid leukemia. *Leuk. Res.* **2009**, *33*, 1055–1061. [CrossRef]

112. Kühnle, M.; Egger, M.; Müller, C.; Mahringer, A.; Bernhardt, G.; Fricker, G.; König, B.; Buschauer, A. Potent and Selective Inhibitors of Breast Cancer Resistance Protein (ABCG2) Derived from the *p*-Glycoprotein (ABCB1) Modulator Tariquidar. *J. Med. Chem.* **2009**, *52*, 1190–1197. [CrossRef]
113. Gupta, P.B.; Onder, T.T.; Jiang, G.; Tao, K.; Kuperwasser, C.; Weinberg, R.A.; Lander, E.S. Identification of Selective Inhibitors of Cancer Stem Cells by High-Throughput Screening. *Cell* **2009**, *138*, 645–659. [CrossRef]
114. Zhou, Y.; Liang, C.; Xue, F.; Chen, W.; Zhi, X.; Feng, X.; Bai, X.; Liang, T. Salinomycin decreases doxorubicin resistance in hepatocellular carcinoma cells by inhibiting the β-catenin/TCF complex association via FOXO3a activation. *Oncotarget* **2015**, *6*, 10350–10365. [CrossRef]
115. Hermawan, A.; Wagner, E.; Roidl, A. Consecutive salinomycin treatment reduces doxorubicin resistance of breast tumor cells by diminishing drug efflux pump expression and activity. *Oncol. Rep.* **2015**, *35*, 1732–1740. [CrossRef]
116. Meidhof, S.; Brabletz, S.; Lehmann, W.; Preca, B.; Mock, K.; Ruh, M.; Schüler, J.; Berthold, M.; Weber, A.; Burk, U.; et al. ZEB 1-associated drug resistance in cancer cells is reversed by the class I HDAC inhibitor mocetinostat. *EMBO Mol. Med.* **2015**, *7*, 831–847. [CrossRef] [PubMed]
117. Toden, S.; Okugawa, Y.; Jascur, T.; Wodarz, D.; Komarova, N.L.; Buhrmann, C.; Shakibaei, M.; Boland, C.R.; Goel, A. Curcumin mediates chemosensitization to 5-fluorouracil through miRNA-induced suppression of epithelial-to-mesenchymal transition in chemoresistant colorectal cancer. *Carcinogenesis* **2014**, *36*, 355–367. [CrossRef] [PubMed]
118. Namba, T.; Kodama, R.; Moritomo, S.; Hoshino, T.; Mizushima, T. Zidovudine, an anti-viral drug, resensitizes gemcitabine-resistant pancreatic cancer cells to gemcitabine by inhibition of the Akt-GSK3β-Snail pathway. *Cell Death Dis.* **2015**, *6*, e1795. [CrossRef] [PubMed]
119. Tomimoto, A.; Endo, H.; Sugiyama, M.; Fujisawa, T.; Hosono, K.; Takahashi, H.; Nakajima, N.; Nagashima, Y.; Wada, K.; Nakagama, H.; et al. metformin suppresses intestinal polyp growth in ApcMin/+ mice. *Cancer Sci.* **2008**, *99*, 2136–2141. [CrossRef] [PubMed]
120. Jiralerspong, S.; Palla, S.L.; Giordano, S.H.; Meric-Bernstam, F.; Liedtke, C.; Barnett, C.M.; Hsu, L.; Hung, M.-C.; Hortobagyi, G.N.; Gonzalez-Angulo, A.M. Metformin and Pathologic Complete Responses to Neoadjuvant Chemotherapy in Diabetic Patients With Breast Cancer. *J. Clin. Oncol.* **2009**, *27*, 3297–3302. [CrossRef]
121. Hirsch, H.A.; Iliopoulos, D.; Tsichlis, P.N.; Struhl, K. Metformin Selectively Targets Cancer Stem Cells, and Acts Together with Chemotherapy to Block Tumor Growth and Prolong Remission. *Cancer Res.* **2009**, *69*, 7507–7511. [CrossRef]
122. Zhao, Z.; Cheng, X.; Wang, Y.; Han, R.; Li, L.; Xiang, T.; He, L.; Long, H.; Zhu, B.; He, Y. Metformin Inhibits the IL-6-Induced Epithelial-Mesenchymal Transition and Lung Adenocarcinoma Growth and Metastasis. *PLoS ONE* **2014**, *9*, e95884. [CrossRef]
123. Qu, C.; Zhang, W.; Zheng, G.; Zhang, Z.; Yin, J.; He, Z. Metformin reverses multidrug resistance and epithelial–mesenchymal transition (EMT) via activating AMP-activated protein kinase (AMPK) in human breast cancer cells. *Mol. Cell. Biochem.* **2013**, *386*, 63–71. [CrossRef] [PubMed]
124. Chou, C.-C.; Lee, K.-H.; Lai, I.-L.; Wang, D.; Mo, X.; Kulp, S.K.; Shapiro, C.L.; Chen, C.-S. AMPK Reverses the Mesenchymal Phenotype of Cancer Cells by Targeting the Akt–MDM2–Foxo3a Signaling Axis. *Cancer Res.* **2014**, *74*, 4783–4795. [CrossRef] [PubMed]
125. Lv, J.; Shim, J.S. Existing drugs and their application in drug discovery targeting cancer stem cells. *Arch. Pharmacal Res.* **2015**, *38*, 1617–1626. [CrossRef] [PubMed]
126. Chua, K.-N.; Sim, W.-J.; Racine, V.; Lee, S.-Y.; Goh, B.C.; Thiery, J.P. A Cell-Based Small Molecule Screening Method for Identifying Inhibitors of Epithelial-Mesenchymal Transition in Carcinoma. *PLoS ONE* **2012**, *7*, e33183. [CrossRef] [PubMed]
127. Aref, A.R.R.; Huang, R.Y.-J.; Yu, W.-M.; Chua, K.N.; Sun, W.; Tu, T.-Y.; Bai, J.; Sim, W.-J.; Zervantonakis, I.; Thiery, J.P.; et al. Screening therapeutic EMT blocking agents in a three-dimensional microenvironment. *Integr. Biol.* **2013**, *5*, 381–389. [CrossRef] [PubMed]
128. Bai, J.; Tu, T.-Y.; Kim, C.; Thiery, J.P.; Kamm, R.D. Identification of drugs as single agents or in combination to prevent carcinoma dissemination in a microfluidic 3D environment. *Oncotarget* **2015**, *6*, 36603–36614. [CrossRef]
129. Alamri, A.; Rauf, A.; Khalil, A.A.; Alghamdi, A.; Alafnan, A.; Alshammari, A.; Alshammari, F.; Malik, J.A.; Anwar, S. In Silico Screening of Marine Compounds as an Emerging and Promising Approach against Estrogen Receptor Alpha-Positive Breast Cancer. *BioMed Res. Int.* **2021**, *2021*, 9734279. [CrossRef] [PubMed]
130. Arjmand, B.; Hamidpour, S.K.; Alavi-Moghadam, S.; Yavari, H.; Shahbazbadr, A.; Tavirani, M.R.; Gilany, K.; Larijani, B. Molecular Docking as a Therapeutic Approach for Targeting Cancer Stem Cell Metabolic Processes. *Front. Pharmacol.* **2022**, *13*, 768556. [CrossRef] [PubMed]
131. Jagust, P.; De Luxán-Delgado, B.; Parejo-Alonso, B.; Sancho, P. Metabolism-Based Therapeutic Strategies Targeting Cancer Stem Cells. *Front. Pharmacol.* **2019**, *10*, 203. [CrossRef]
132. Taylor, W.F.; Jabbarzadeh, E. The use of natural products to target cancer stem cells. *Am. J. Cancer Res.* **2017**, *7*, 1588–1605. [PubMed]
133. Anwar, S.; Saleem, H.; Khurshid, U.; Ansari, S.Y.; Alghamdi, S.; Al-Khulaidi, A.W.A.; Malik, J.A.; Ahemad, N.; Awadh Ali, N.A. Comparative phytochemical composition, oleuropein quantification, antioxidant and cytotoxic properties of Olea europaea L. leaves. *Nat. Prod. Res.* **2022**. [CrossRef] [PubMed]

cancers

MDPI

Review

Natural Products and Small Molecules Targeting Cellular Ceramide Metabolism to Enhance Apoptosis in Cancer Cells

Farjana Afrin [1], Sameena Mateen [1], Jordan Oman [1], James C. K. Lai [1], Jared J. Barrott [2] and Srinath Pashikanti [1,*]

1 Biomedical and Pharmaceutical Sciences, Kasiska Division of Health Sciences, College of Pharmacy, Idaho State University, Pocatello, ID 83209, USA; farjanaafrin@isu.edu (F.A.); sameenamateen@isu.edu (S.M.); jordanoman@isu.edu (J.O.); jameslai@isu.edu (J.C.K.L.)

2 Cell Biology and Physiology, College of Life Sciences, Brigham Young University, Provo, UT 84602, USA; jared_barrott@byu.edu

* Correspondence: pashsrin@isu.edu; Tel.: +1-208-282-3837

Simple Summary: Ceramide and associated enzymes play a substantial role in cell function such as in cell proliferation, differentiation, and apoptosis processes. Knowing the enzymatic pathway and targeting particular enzymes from that pathway can lead to a very successful therapeutic outcome. As such, this review is focused on the elaboration of the natural products and small inhibitor molecules that can target important enzymes such as ceramidase and ceramide synthase that participate in the central lipid ceramide pathway, as well as the outcome when those pathways are disturbed during disease progression. In addition, this paper also discusses cancer that is associated with the imbalance of ceramide enzymes.

Abstract: Molecular targeting strategies have been used for years in order to control cancer progression and are often based on targeting various enzymes involved in metabolic pathways. Keeping this in mind, it is essential to determine the role of each enzyme in a particular metabolic pathway. In this review, we provide in-depth information on various enzymes such as ceramidase, sphingosine kinase, sphingomyelin synthase, dihydroceramide desaturase, and ceramide synthase which are associated with various types of cancers. We also discuss the physicochemical properties of well-studied inhibitors with natural product origins and their related structures in terms of these enzymes. Targeting ceramide metabolism exhibited promising mono- and combination therapies at preclinical stages in preventing cancer progression and cemented the significance of sphingolipid metabolism in cancer treatments. Targeting ceramide-metabolizing enzymes will help medicinal chemists design potent and selective small molecules for treating cancer progression at various levels.

Keywords: natural products and related small molecules; sphingolipids; ceramide; ceramide synthase; anticancer therapies

Citation: Afrin, F.; Mateen, S.; Oman, J.; Lai, J.C.K.; Barrott, J.J.; Pashikanti, S. Natural Products and Small Molecules Targeting Cellular Ceramide Metabolism to Enhance Apoptosis in Cancer Cells. *Cancers* **2023**, *15*, 4645. https://doi.org/10.3390/cancers15184645

Academic Editors: Barbara De Filippis, Marialuigia Fantacuzzi and Alessandra Ammazzalorso

Received: 6 August 2023
Revised: 8 September 2023
Accepted: 11 September 2023
Published: 20 September 2023

1. Introduction

Sphingolipids (SLs) are key modulators of physiological processes including the cell cycle, apoptosis, angiogenesis, stress, and inflammation [1]. Among SLs, ceramides (Cers) and sphingosine-1-phosphate (S1P) are the most studied (Figure 1) and often exert opposing biological functions. Cancer cells show a shift in the balance between proapoptotic ceramide (Cer) and cancer-promoting S1P. This phenomenon is associated with pancreatic cancer progression and poor therapeutic outcomes [2,3]. Biochemical dysregulation of SL metabolism can be used as a biomarker and prognostic factor in pancreatic cancer [4–6]. Further studies suggest that Cer generation and accumulation are critical determinants facilitating apoptosis in pancreatic cancer cells in response to cytotoxic agents, including gemcitabine (GMZ) [7], which highlights the significance of manipulating these pathways to overcome resistance of pancreatic cancer to current therapies. Cer and its biosynthetic derivatives are important to rapidly dividing cells such as cancer cells because Cer is a basic unit of stable lipid membranes that supports transmembrane functionality and integrity [8].

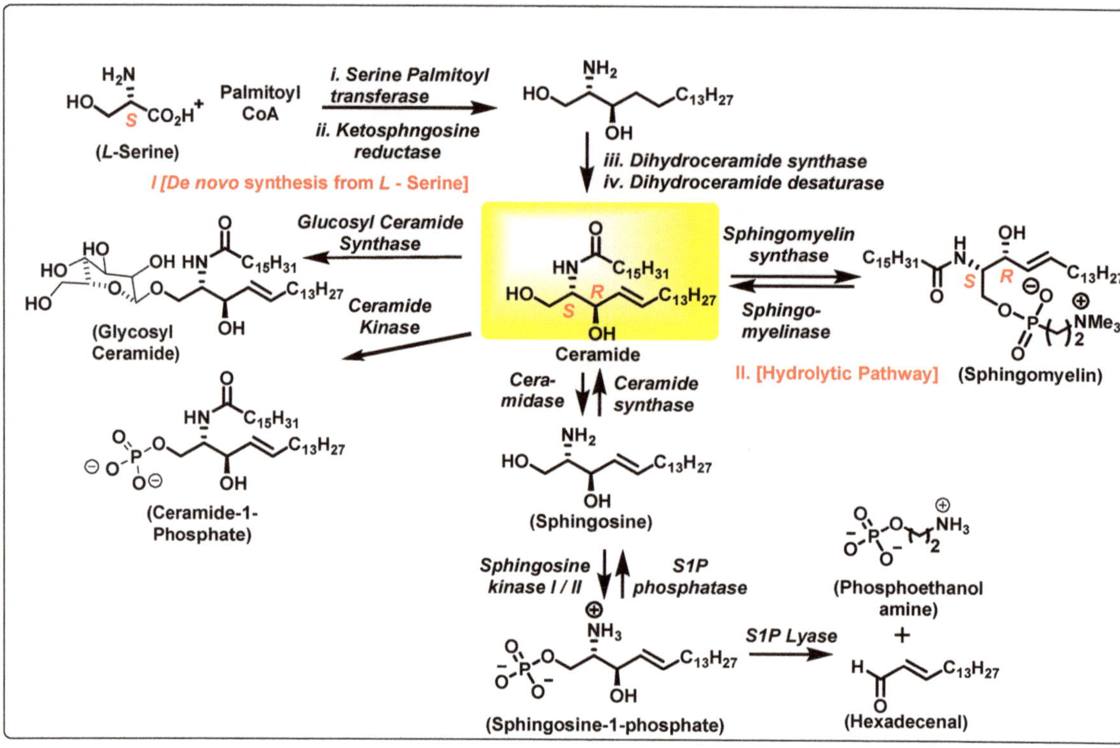

Figure 1. Ceramide biosynthesis and metabolism pathway.

The polarity in the structure of SLs makes them a basic unit of a membrane or vesicle. These are biosynthesized not only in the mammalian system but also in other eukaryotic and prokaryotic organisms, and in marine plants. Most notable are the ones that are secondary metabolites from fungi. The metabolites from fungi are a survival strategy in the ecosystem of vertebrates [9]. These secondary metabolites are a source of hits for medicinal chemistry approaches towards developing drugs involving sphingolipid biochemistry. This review is focused on ceramide-metabolizing enzymes, which have the capacity to control ceramide flux. Most of these natural products have attracted the attention of research groups with the aim of accomplishing total synthesis, as well as others that perform SAR studies. Some of these have resulted in the identification of small molecule hits. A list of natural products and small molecules for each of the ceramide-metabolizing enzymes, as well as their clinical relevance, is provided in the following sections. The synthesis of small molecules targeting these enzymes strengthened the application of a chiral pool strategy involving diastereoselective and enantioselective syntheses. Fingolimod, an FDA-approved medication, is used for treating relapsing forms of multiple sclerosis. Fingolimod was developed from the fungal metabolite myriocin. Fingolimod has a structural resemblance to sphingosine. Miglustat is another FDA-approved medication targeting glucosylceramide synthase. Miglustat is prescribed to treat Gaucher disease [10]. Miglustat has a structural resemblance to the enzyme substrate. These properties have encouraged academia and the pharma industry to probe these pathways further in recent years.

Given the broad biological significance of SLs, this review has focused on updating the knowledge of medicinal chemistry approaches used to increase cellular Cer levels. The pharmacological goal is to inhibit enzymatic functions that increase cytotoxic Cer, thus inducing cellular apoptosis. Knowledge of the pathway and its associated enzymes paves the way for identifying medicinal chemistry approaches targeting these enzymes, which could help overcome chemotherapy-resistant cancer cells by exploring combination therapies that target the Cer metabolism pathway. A brief discussion about the effect of the natural products, small molecules, on the catalysis of these enzymes is also discussed.

2. The Ceramide Biosynthesis Pathway

Central to SLs is Cer, which constitutes the hydrophobic backbone of all complex SLs (e.g., glycosphingolipids (GS), sphingomyelin (SM), cerebrosides, and gangliosides) and structurally consists of a fatty acyl of variable chain lengths bound to an amino group of a sphingoid base. The fatty acyl chains are, in general, saturated or monounsaturated and can contain an OH group linked to C-2 or to the terminal carbon atom (α- and ω-hydroxy fatty acids, Figure 1). Among ceramide-containing SLs, those containing long (C16–20) and very long (C22–24) acyl chains are the most abundant in mammalian cells, but Cers with longer acyl chains (C26–36) are also found in epidermal keratinocytes and male germ cells during their differentiation and maturation [8].

Cer is biosynthesized starting from L-serine in the de novo synthetic pathway (Figure 1). Cer biosynthesis involves cellular serine palmitoylation using the cofactor-activated palmitoyl CoA by serine palmitoyl transferase, resulting in 3-keto sphingosine. This is a rate-determining step in the biosynthesis of SLs. A cellular enantioselective reduction in the ketone catalyzed by ketosphingosine reductase allows the required 1,2 *anti*-amino alcohol system to be formed. N-palmitoylation of ketosphingosine followed by desaturation results in the trans-alkene Cer. The structural and stereochemical core of Cer has the inherent chirality of *L*-serine, N-palmitoylation, and lipophilic alkyl chain modifications. There are different types of Cers based on the side chain substitutions on the polar head group—both N-alkyl and the alkyl side chains.

The Cer metabolic pathway is very dynamic and can result in various SLs being synthesized to accommodate cellular needs and enhance cell signaling pathways. Cer-metabolizing enzymes are cell fate specific and expressed based on the physiological role of the cell. Cancer cells tend to upregulate enzymes that promote the production of SLs and cell membrane stability. The remainder of this review will highlight the importance of six different classes of SL-metabolizing enzymes: ceramidase, sphingosine kinase (SK), sphingomyelin synthase (SMS), 3-ketosphinganine reductase, dihydroceramide desaturase, and ceramide synthases.

3. Ceramidase

Ceramidases (CDases) are a group of ceramide-metabolizing enzymes that hydrolyze Cer to produce sphingosine. Sphingosine is then further metabolized into S1P by SK1 or SK2. In humans, there are five known CDases genes. The CDases expressed by these genes can be divided into three categories depending on the pH required for their optimal catalytic activity: (i) acid ceramidase (encoded by the *ASAH1* gene), (ii) neutral ceramidase (encoded by the *ASAH2* gene), and (iii) alkaline ceramidase (encoded by the *ACER1*, *ACER2*, and *ACER3* genes) [11].

3.1. Acid Ceramidase

Acid ceramidase (AC)/*ASAH1* is also called N-acylsphingosine amidohydrolase. AC has a molecular weight of 50 kDa and requires a pH of 4.2–4.3 for its optimal activity [12]. Under these acidic conditions, the byproduct, sphingosine amine, exits as an ammonium species providing the active site tolerance for this charged functional group. The 3D crystal structure of AC is generated using EzCADD utilizing PDB file (Figure 2) [13,14]. After performing EZ pocket calculation, one of the binding pockets is shown with Cys143 [13].

AC hydrolyzes the amide bond in unsaturated ceramides with C6–C16 acyl chains [15]. It is mainly localized in lysosomes and maintains intralysosomal Cer homeostasis [16]. AC is expressed ubiquitously and has a higher expression in the heart and kidneys [17]. The K_M value of AC was determined to be 389 to 413 μM by using ^{14}C-labeled and BODIPY-conjugated C-12 Cer substrate, N-lauroylsphingosine [18]. An SL activator protein, Saposin D, is responsible for the enzymatic activity of AC, as evidenced by the Cer accumulation that occurs in the absence of Saposin D [19]. Further studies narrated the activator protein Saposin D having binding interactions with the polar head group of monomeric SL, embedded in intracellular lysosomal membrane, in close proximity to AC in order to perform catalysis [14,20]. This model shows evidence of a multimeric complex lipid–protein interactions for AC catalysis. The altered function of a mutated AC, the overexpression of normal AC, and the dysregulation of activity of AC have highlighted the importance of its role in SL metabolism. The dysregulation of AC is associated with a wide range of diseases, thereby suggesting that AC could be an attractive therapeutic target for drug discovery.

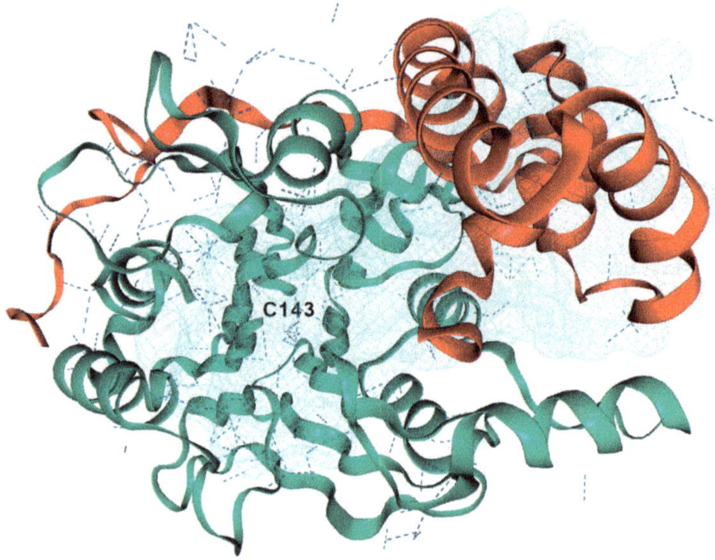

Figure 2. 3D crystal structure of human acid ceramidase (ASAH1, aCDase). PDB ID: 5U7Z. Chain A is red, chain B is teal, and dashed lines indicate hydrogen bonding. The active site is located near Cys143 and a binding pocket near the active site was generated using ezPocket with fconv at 89.4, −3.53, and 203.26 (x, y, z), respectively.

3.2. *Role of AC in Pathological Conditions*

Lysosome architecture involves the basic unit, SL. Both Farber disease (FD) and spinal muscular atrophy with progressive myoclonic epilepsy (SMA-PME) are rare lysosomal storage disorders. They are caused by a missense mutation in the *ASAH1* gene resulting in the absence or decrease in the AC enzyme. There have been fewer than 200 cases of FD and SMA-PME. With no cure for AC deficiency, gene therapy and enzyme replacement therapy is under development [21]. *Asah1* knockout in mice results in embryonic lethality [22]. Examples of AC inhibitors are shown in Figure 3. All the inhibitors exhibit a polar head group with a lipophilic tail. The calculated logP is congruent with the observation that these molecules are more lipophilic. AC is implicated in several cancers, as discussed below.

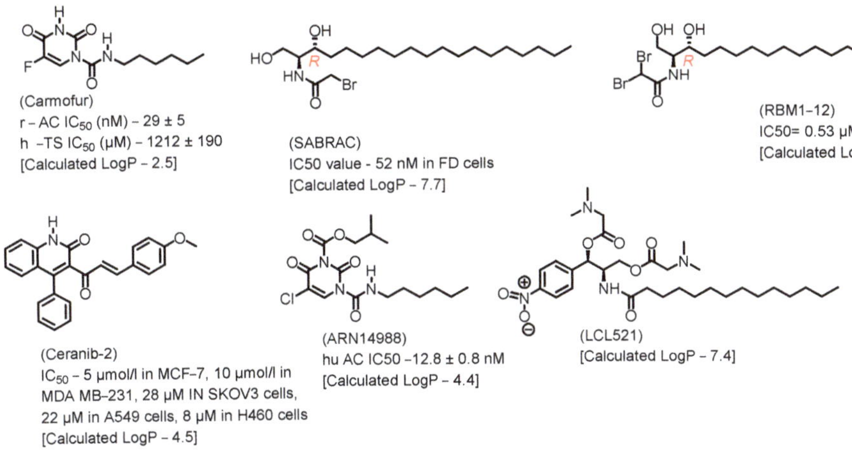

Figure 3. Examples of AC inhibitors.

3.2.1. Prostate Cancer (PC)

The role of AC in tumor proliferation and resistance to treatment has been studied in depth in regard to PC. PC cells develop resistance by upregulating AC. Clonogenicity and cytotoxicity assays confirm that radio sensitization can be established by the genetic downregulation of AC with small interfering RNA (siRNA). Also, the radiation-induced AC upregulation creates cross-resistance to chemotherapy. The use of the small molecule AC inhibitor, LCL385, sensitizes primary prostatic carcinoma cell line (PPC-1) cells to radiation [23]. In addition, the same cell line preferentially upregulates AC, resulting in increased radiation resistance and proliferation. The use of an AC inhibitor, LCL521, acts as a radiosensitizer preventing relapse [24]. This was validated with immunohistochemical studies in these tissues, where higher levels of AC were observed after radiation treatment failure than in irradiation-naïve cancer, intraepithelial neoplasia, or benign tissue.

In addition, AC inhibition prevented relapse in an animal xenograft model by producing radio sensitization. Higher IHC expression of AC in primary PCs is associated with a more advanced disease stage. In a model derived from PC-3 cells, the highly tumorigenic, metastatic, and chemo-resistant PC-3/Mc clone expressed higher levels of AC than the non-metastatic PC-3/S clone. Stable knockdown of *ASAH1* in PC-3/Mc cells resulted in an accumulation of Cer, a reduction in clonogenic potential, and the inhibition of tumorigenesis and lung metastases [25]. Treatment of DU-145 cells with the AC inhibitor LCL204, a lysosomotropic analog of B13, induces apoptosis in a cathepsin-dependent manner. Upon treatment with this inhibitor, destabilization of membranous lysosomes and the release of lysosomal proteases into the cytosol lead to mitochondria depolarization and caspase activation, resulting in apoptosis [26]. Both PC-3 and DU 145 are hormone-refractory human PC cell lines. In both of these cell lines, combination treatment with fenretinide (4-HPR), a ceramide-generating anticancer agent, and DM102, a novel synthetic AC inhibitor, resulted in a considerable decrease a cell viability and the combination therapy was more effective than either treatment alone. In the PC-3 cell line, the treatment induces apoptosis through ROS generation. However, another AC inhibitor, *N*-oleoylethanolamine (NOE), in combination with 4-HPR, does not result in synergistic activity [27]. In another study using PPC1 and DU145 PC cells, AC overexpression was shown to result in increased lysosomal density and autophagy and increased expression of the motor protein KIF5B, contributing to lysosomal stability. AC overexpression, in addition to increasing radiation and chemotherapy resistance, increases stress resistance. Although increased lysosomal density in these cells makes them more sensitive to therapeutic agents targeting lysosomes, the overexpression of AC provides a new therapeutic target [28].

3.2.2. Head- and Neck Cancer (HNC)

AC was overexpressed in four of six primary tumor tissues and six of nine cell lines in HNC. AC also contributed to decreased cisplatin sensitivity. Pharmacological (with N-oleoyl-ethanolamine) or genetic (with short hairpin RNA) inhibition of AC enhanced cisplatin-induced HNC cell death by increasing Cer and activating other proapoptotic proteins [29]. In mouse squamous cell carcinoma SCCVII, the inhibition of AC with the small molecule inhibitor LCL521 significantly decreased the survivability after photodynamic therapy by effectively restricting regulatory T lymphocytes and myeloid-derived suppressor cell activity [30]. The combination of photodynamic therapy and dasatinib also decreases SCCVII cell survivability by decreasing AC, leading to increased Cer activating caspase-3-induced apoptosis [31]. In SCC-1, overexpression of AC increased the resistance to Fas-induced cell death, which was reversible using specific AC siRNA. The AC inhibitor LCL 204 sensitizes HNSCC cell lines to Fas-induced apoptosis both in vitro and in a xenograft model in vivo, providing an option for combination therapy [32].

3.2.3. Melanoma

The largest organ of the human body, the skin, has a very complex structure with four main layers. SLs are found throughout each layer, and maintain the functions of this organ. AC expression is significantly higher in normal human melanocytes and proliferative melanoma cell lines, compared with other skin cells (keratinocytes and fibroblasts) and non-melanoma cancer cells. Melanoma cells exhibit lower amounts of Cer by downregulating the de novo synthesis pathway. The AC inhibitor ARN14988 in combination with 5-Fluoro Uracil increases cytotoxicity in the proliferative melanoma cell lines by increasing Cer and reducing S1P levels [33]. In human A375 melanoma cells, dacarbazine (DTIC) decreases ACdase activity through reactive-oxygen-species-dependent activation of cathepsin B-mediated degradation of the enzyme. Downregulating AC expression increased Cer level and sensitivity to DTIC, providing a therapeutic tool for the treatment of metastatic melanoma [34]. The deletion of *ASAH1* in human A375 melanoma cells using CRISPR-Cas9-mediated gene editing showed a significantly greater accumulation of long-chain saturated Cers that are substrates for AC in *ASAH1*-null cells. The cells lose the ability to undergo self-renewal [35]. Our hypothesis on this observation correlates with Cer flux and its function.

3.2.4. Myeloid Leukemia

Primary acute myeloid leukemia (AML) cells have a higher expression of AC, which is essential for AML blast survival. In AML cell lines, increased levels of AC induced a higher expression of antiapoptotic Mcl-1 protein, increased S1P, and decreased Cer. Treatment with the AC inhibitor, LCL204, induces Cer accumulation and decreases Mcl-1. The overall survival of C57BL/6 mice engrafted with leukemic C1498 cells increased significantly with LCL204 treatment, while the treatment significantly decreased the disease burden in NSG mice engrafted with primary human AML cells [36]. IFN regulatory factor 8 (IRF8) is a key transcription factor for myeloid cell differentiation. Without IRF8, hematopoietic cells in human myeloid leukemia patients rapidly proliferate and remain undifferentiated. Thus, acting as a tumor suppressor by promoting cell differentiation, IRF8 expression is frequently lost in myeloid leukemias. One of the repressive transcriptional targets of IRF8 is AC; consequently, as IRF8 is lost, AC expression increases, solidifying its role as a tumor suppressor. In chronic myelogenous leukemia (CML), overexpression of IRF8 repressed AC expression, resulting in C16 Cer accumulation and increased sensitivity of CML cells to FasL-induced apoptosis. AC expression is significantly higher in cells derived from IRF8-deficient mice. In these cells, inhibition of AC activity or application of exogenous Cer sensitizes the cells to FasL-induced apoptosis [37].

3.2.5. Non-Small Cell Lung Cancer (NSCLC)

In NSCLC cells with acquired resistance to ChoKα inhibitors, these cells also display increased levels of *ASAH1*. Inhibition of AC synergistically sensitizes lung cancer cells to the antiproliferative effect of ChoKα inhibitors, which opens up a new therapeutic option for combinatorial treatments of ChoKα inhibitors and AC inhibitors [38].

3.2.6. Breast Cancer

Higher expression of AC has been observed in ER-positive and luminal-A-like breast cancer. High expression of AC in invasive breast cancer is associated with improved prognosis and reduced incidence of recurrence in preinvasive ductal carcinoma in situ (DCIS) [39]. The effect of AC inhibitors (DM102 and NOE) in combination with C6-Cer (C6-cer), a cell-permeable analog of Cer, has been studied in three different breast cancer cell lines MDA-MB-231, MCF-7, and BT-474 cells. Although as single agents, both C6-cer and DM102 are moderately cytotoxic, their combination induced synergistic decreases in viability. In MDA-MB-231 cells, apoptosis is induced by caspase 3/7 activation and poly (ADP-ribose) polymerase (PARP) cleavage. In the same cell line, C6-cer/DM102 increases ROS levels and results in mitochondrial membrane depolarization. Furthermore, the C6-cer/DM102 combination is antagonistic in BT-474 cells, suggesting different molecular mechanisms being cell-type-specific. AC expression is correlated to the human epidermal growth factor receptor 2 (HER2) status [40]. Another study shows that an AC inhibitor, ceranib-2, induces apoptosis in MDA-MB-231 and MCF-7 by activating stress-activated protein kinase/c-Jun N-terminal kinase and mitogen-activated protein kinase apoptotic pathways by inhibiting the antiapoptotic pathway [41]. Ceranib-2 exhibits similar effects in PC cell lines too [42].

3.2.7. Ovarian Cancer (OC)

In an immunohistochemical analysis study of 112 OC patients, low AC expression has been correlated with tumor progression. This analysis contradicts the concept of AC being a cancer progression promoter, suggesting AC is involved in alternative pathways in different cancers, which requires further investigation [43].

3.2.8. Hepatobiliary Cancers

AC is downregulated using the chemotherapeutic agent daunorubicin in human (HepG2) and mouse (Hepa1c17) hepatoma cell lines, as well as in primary cells from murine liver tumors, but not in cultured mice. Genetic (small interfering RNA) or pharmacological inhibition of AC with *N*-oleoylethanolamine (NOE) sensitized the cell lines to daunorubicin-induced cell death, preceded by structural mitochondrial changes, stimulation of reactive oxygen species generations and cytochrome *c* release followed by caspase-3 activation. In vivo siRNA treatment targeting AC reduced tumor growth in liver tumor xenografts of HepG2 cells and enhanced daunorubicin therapy, providing a potential therapeutic target for liver cancer [44].

The key chemotherapeutic agent in pancreatic cancer, gemcitabine, exhibits different efficacy due to polymorphism in the expression of enzymes that regulate its metabolism [41,45]. Deoxycytidine kinase (dCK), which phosphorylates gemcitabine, activates the drug, while cytidine deaminase (CDA) inactivates gemcitabine by deamination [6]. In MIA PaCa-2 and PANC-1 pancreatic cancer cell lines, the novel Cer analog, AL6, inhibits cell growth, induces apoptosis, and synergistically enhances the cytotoxic activity of gemcitabine. AL6 also increases the gene expression of the gemcitabine-activating enzyme deoxycytidine kinase (dCK), improving the efficacy of gemcitabine. This study suggests the use of AL6 and gemcitabine combination therapy for pancreatic cancer [45].

3.2.9. Colon Cancer

Colorectal adenocarcinoma tissues have higher *ASAH1* expressions when compared with the adjacent normal colonic mucosa. In HCT116 colon cancer cells, there is an inverse correlation between the AC expression and the p53 functional activity. Inhibition of AC using carmofur in HCT116 CELLS significantly increased the antiproliferative, proapoptotic, antimigratory, and anticlonogenic effects of oxaplatin [46]. In the human colon cancer cell line, the AC inhibitor ceranib-2 increases apoptosis by increasing *ASAH1* mRNA expression and reducing *TNFR1* expression [47].

4. Sphingosine Kinase

Sphingosine-1-phosphate (S1P) is a bioactive SL that regulates the growth, survival, and migration of several cell types. S1P is a ligand for five transmembrane G-protein-coupled receptors, S1P1-5, and for several intracellular targets such as histone deacetylases 1 and 2 [48]. Cellular biosynthesis of S1P occurs through phosphorylation of Sphingosine (Sph) catalyzed by SKs. Sphingosine, an effector molecule is biosynthesized by ceramidase activity on the central lipid Cer. SKs exist in two isoforms, SK1 and SK2, encoded by unlinked genes.

The crystal structure of SK1 from the Protein Data Bank is shown in Figure 4, and was generated using ezCADD [13,49]. The active site has the ligand D-erythro-sphingosine. Using ezCADD computer modelling software, we have identified the surrounding amino acids around this ligand. The polar head group is closer to Asp341 and Asp178. The lipophilic tail portion is surrounded by nonpolar amino acids [13]. Pharmacologically, Cer and Sph are associated with growth arrest and apoptosis. On the contrary, S1P is associated with prosurvival roles [50]. SKs and S1P have been implicated in a variety of disease states including cancer [51,52], sickle cell disease [53,54], atherosclerosis [55,56], asthma [57,58], diabetes, fibrosis [59], etc.

Although SK1 and SK2 share a high degree of homology, they differ in size, localization, distribution, and intracellular roles [60,61]. While double-knockout studies in mice suggest that SKs are the sole source of S1P, some functional redundancy exists, as SK1 or SK2 null mice are viable and fertile [62].

The biological significance of SKs has encouraged academia and pharmaceutical companies to target SKs for their therapeutic value. Initial drug discovery efforts resulted in SK1 potent inhibitors, complimented by the availability of the SK1 crystal structure. Based on a Protein Data Bank search, no crystal structure for SK2 has been reported. Potent, selective SK2 inhibitors have been developed through homology modeling of SK1. Competitive inhibition strategies have been reported, and strategies aimed toward competitive inhibition remain a focus. Shown in Figure 5 are the representative SK 2 inhibitors with moderate potency and selectivity. ABC294640 was the first SK2 inhibitor with K_i 10 μM [63] that has been deployed in a variety of disease models, which include ulcerative colitis [64] Crohn's disease [65] ischemia/reperfusion injury [66] osteoarthritis [65] colon cancer [67] and colorectal cancer [68]. However, ABC294640 has recently been reported to have an off-target effect of acting as a tamoxifen-like molecule with the estrogen receptor [69]. A recent study has shown that the sensitivity of BRAFV600E mutant colon cancer cells to Vemurafenib can be increased by reducing the AKT-mediated expression of nucleophosmin and translationally controlled tumor protein [70]. This study highlights the significance of sphingolipid biochemistry and targeting multiple pathways in combination in order to achieve effective cancer therapies. ABC294640 was the first SK2 inhibitor, and when utilizing this as a biological probe, several outcomes were reported in terms of S1P-mediated signaling. For example, mitophagy-mediated apoptosis was unraveled in a multiple myeloma cell line [71]. Other inhibitors, namely SG-12 [72], ®-FTY720-OMe [73], K145 [74], and VT-ME6 [75] exhibited optimal potency and selectivity. K145 has a lipophilic phenoxy ether with a polar head group exhibiting structural similarity to R-FTY720-OMe. K145 is an SK2 inhibitor under investigation for treating leukemia.

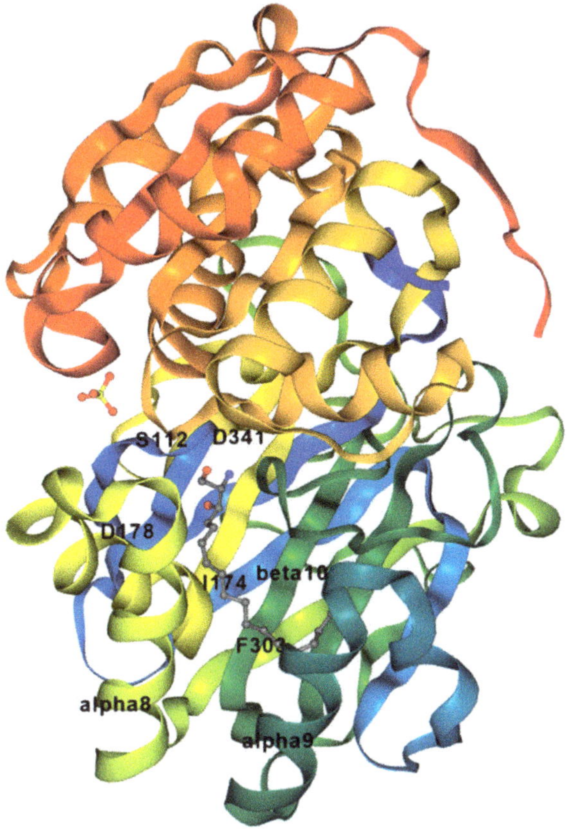

Figure 4. Crystal structure of Sphingosine Kinase 1. PDB ID: 3VZB. Protein is shown in rainbow color scheme, the ligand D-*erythro* sphingosine is shown in element color scheme with gray, red, and blue for carbon, oxygen, and nitrogen, respectively, and sulfur ion is also shown in crystal structure with element color scheme yellow for sulfur. Active site is located near α8 and 9 helix and β10 sheet.

Based on structure–activity relationship (SAR) studies, isoform-selective SK2 inhibitors with improved potency and half-life in mice were developed. These inhibitors include SLR080811, [76] SLP120701, [77] SLM6031434, [78] SLC5091592 [79], and VT 20dd [80] and are depicted in Figure 6. SLR080811, with a Ki of 13.3 μM and 1.3 μM for SK1 and SK2, respectively, is under study for colorectal cancers with resistance to 5-fluorouracil. [76]. An important finding from these studies was the observation of elevated S1P levels in the mice upon pharmacological inhibition of SK2. Extensive SAR studies of SLR080811 resulted in an azetidine, SLP120701, with an improved half-life of 8 hours in mice [77]. Modifications in the tail region further improved SK2 selectivity as seen with the analog SLM6031434 [78], and a lipophilic-tail-substituted naphthalene-oxy analog, as seen with SLC5091592 [79]. These analogs showed improved SK2 selectivity and potency, comparable to second-generation SK2 inhibitors presented in Figure 6.

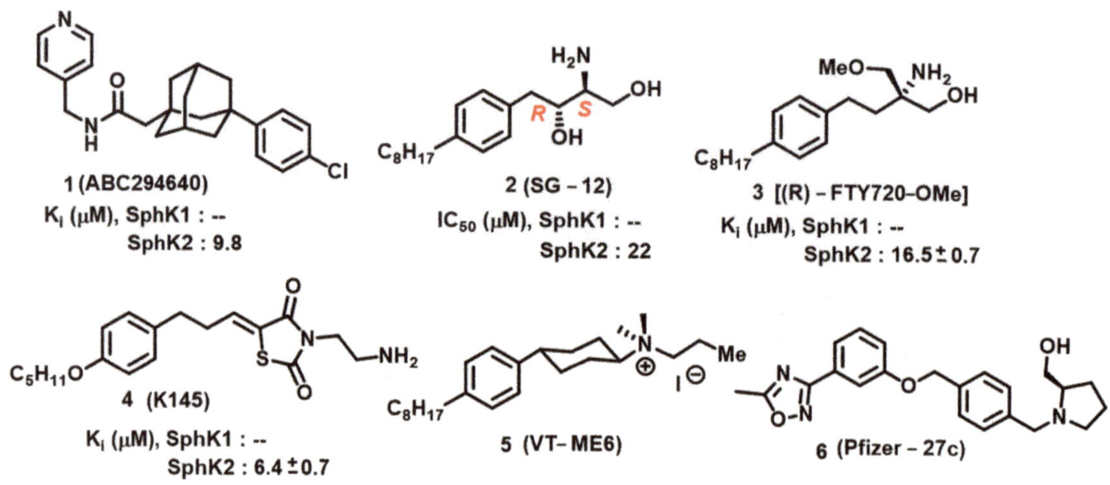

Figure 5. Sphingosine Kinase 2 inhibitors.

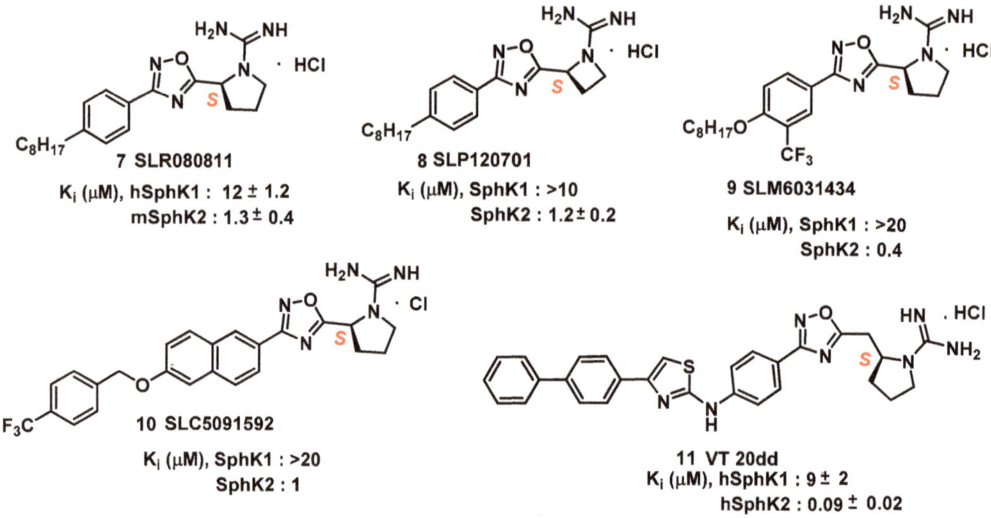

Figure 6. Other Sphingosine Kinase inhibitors.

As evidenced, sphingosine kinase tail regions can be modified to improve kinase specificity and selectivity. This statement is highlighted by a study that took scaffold of aminothiazole and developed the SK2 inhibitor 20dd (Figure 6). 20dd demonstrated improved potency, selectivity, and in vivo outcomes [80]. A PubMed search for probes of the anticancer potential for these analogs has not been reported so far, but with favorable pharmacological features such as selectivity and specificity towards SKs, further exploration into 20dd and its analogs is warranted.

5. Sphingomyelin Synthase

Sphingomyelin Synthase (SMS) is responsible for generating SM and diacylglycerol (DAG) by transferring the phosphocholine from phosphatidylcholine onto the primary hydroxyl group of Cer [81,82]. Thus, SMS is also biologically important as it regulates the levels of Cer and DAGs, resulting in bioactive lipids [83]. In the de novo synthesis pathway,

Cer biosynthesis starts with L-serine and palmitoyl CoA to give 3-Ketosphinganine, which then undergoes a series of enzymatic reactions to yield Cer on the cytoplasmic side of the endoplasmic reticulum (ER) membrane. Cer is then transferred to the Golgi compartment in a non-vesicle way by the Cer transfer protein (CERT). There, SMS transfers the phosphocholine headgroup from phosphatidylcholine to Cer, yielding SM and DAG. The SM produced in this step is then sorted into cell membranes by either vesicle traffic or protein-facilitated transportation [84]. It is noteworthy that SM is the basic component of lipid rafts. Lipid rafts are important microdomains of cell membranes that provide a platform for many receptors and transport proteins. The SMS gene family consists of three members—sphingomyelin synthase 1 (*SGMS1*), sphingomyelin synthase 2 (*SGMS2*), and sterile alpha motif domain containing 8 (*SAMD8*), which encode their respective proteins: SMS1, SMS2, and SMS-related protein (SMSr). Even though SMSr displays high homology with SMS1 and SMS2, it does not have any SM synthase activity [82]. SMS1 and SMS2 are localized in the trans-Golgi network, where SM is synthesized from Cer, which is transported from the ER to the Golgi by the CERT [1]. SMSs are present in all tissues, and SMS1 is the principal contributor to the SMS activity in most cells. Both isoforms share 57% of sequential identity and are conserved in mammals [82]. In SMS1, a sterile alpha motif (SAM) is present, which takes part in protein–protein interactions, and which is not present in SMS2. SMSs contain six transmembrane regions with both N- and C-termini exposed into the cytosol.

Biological Significance of Sphingomyelin Synthase

The formation of SM is essential for cell growth and survival. In a mouse lymphoid cell line deficient in SM synthase activity, loss of SMS activity halted cell growth in serum-free conditions, which could, however, be restored by supplemental exogenous SM or heterologous expression of SMS1 [85]. Different studies have correlated the up- and downregulation of SM synthase activity to mitogenic and proapoptotic signaling in different mammalian cell types [86–88]. Although the cellular pathway for the effects of SMS is unclear, it can exert its effect through the following mechanisms: (1) SM accumulation in the plasma membrane, and its affinity for sterols, contributes to the rigidity of the cell membrane; and (2) SM accumulation in the plasma membrane acts as a source of a number of other SLs, which are catalyzed by acidic or neutral sphingomyelinases (SMases) [89,90]. Cer, sphingosine, and sphingosine 1-phosphate are all potential SM metabolites and have proven to be significant regulators of cellular functions like cell proliferation, differentiation, and apoptosis [2,91,92]. The microdomain formation of SM in the Golgi apparatus plays a role in the sorting process of different SLs [93]. SM synthesis can act as a source of DAG in the trans-Golgi network, thus facilitating the protein kinase D recruitment leading to the formation of transport carrier proteins [94]. SM synthesis regulates the cellular levels of both the proapoptotic factor Cer and the mitogenic factor DAG, directly impacting cell proliferation [88,95]. Some of the SMS inhibitors are natural products which originate from the marine environment; these molecules and their synthetic analogs resemble SMS substrates and are depicted in Figure 7.

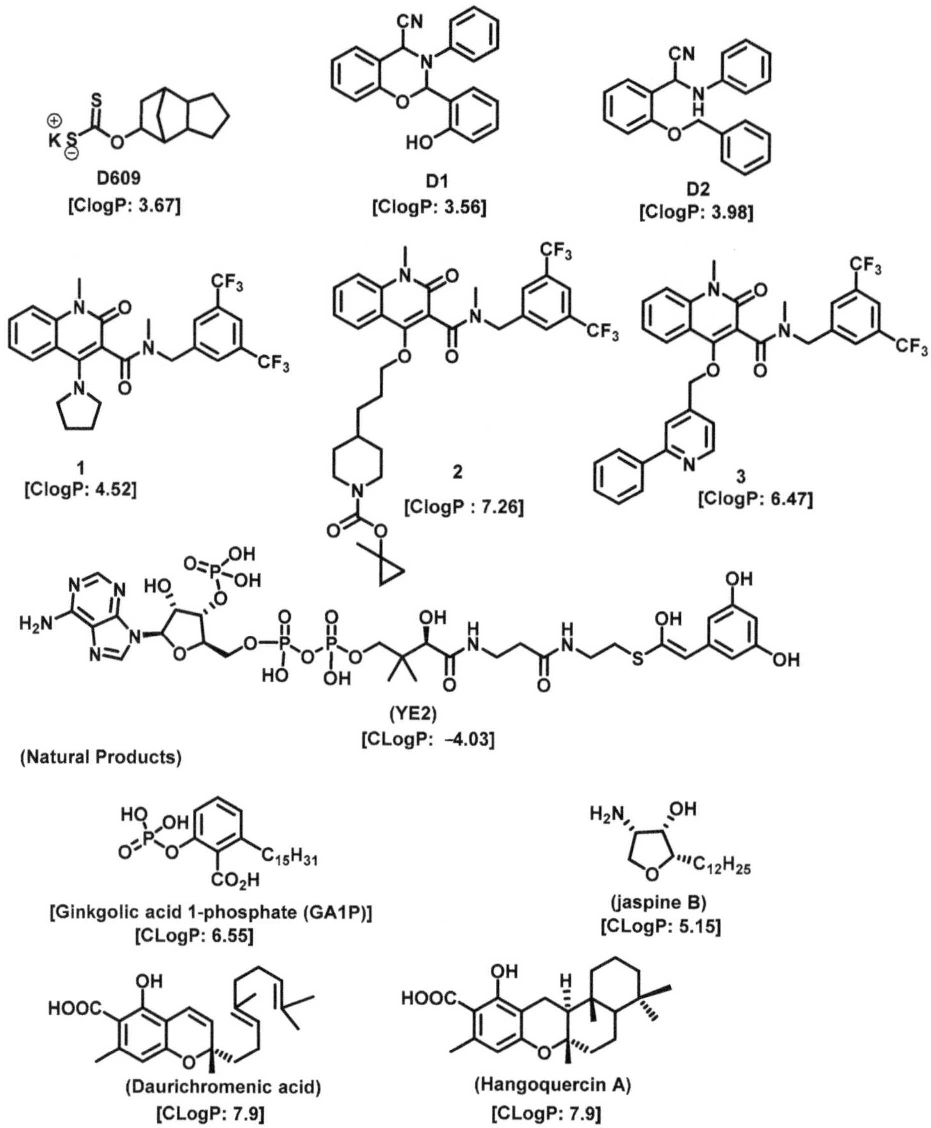

Figure 7. Sphingomyelin Synthase inhibitors.

6. 3-Ketosphinganine Reductase

3-Ketosphinganine reductase (KSR) mediates the reduction of ketosphinganine into sphinganine (Sa). In certain cancer cells (HGC27, T98G, and U87MG), 3-ketosphinganine (KSa) and its deuterated analog at C4 (d2KSa) are metabolized to produce high levels of dihydrosphingolipids [96]. Although the function of KSR has been studied in yeast and plants, the role in human pathology lacks supportive findings.

7. Dihydroceramide Desaturase

Dihydroceramide Δ4-desaturase (DES) is the member of the desaturase family which converts the dihydrosphingosine backbone within ceramide into a sphingosine backbone [97]. The first step is utilizing molecular oxygen to introduce a hydroxyl group into the C4 position of the dihydrosphingosine backbone, which is then followed by a dehydration reaction producing a double bond in the C4–C5 position of dihydroceramide, with the aid of NADPH [98–100]. The only difference between dihydroceramide and Cer is that Cer has a *trans* double bond at the C4–C5 position. In mammals, two gene isoforms named *DES1* and *DES2* have been identified [101]. The *DES1* gene contains multiple transmembrane domains, and a recent study shows that it requires myristoylation on its N-terminus for full activity [101,102]. DES1 is localized in the ER membrane where it has access to newly synthesized dihydroceramide species [97]. 4-hydroxyceramide is an intermediate reaction product in the conversion of dihydroceramide to ceramide, which is also known as phytoceramide. In plants and yeast, it is the predominant ceramide species. In mammals, DES1 is found in all tissues and only converts dihydroceramide species into fully desaturated Cer, whereas DES2 is capable of creating either phytoceramide or ceramide from dihydroceramide precursors [103,104]. DES2 is highly expressed in skin, intestines, and kidneys [103]. The deletion of *DES1* and *DES2* shifts the SL synthesis pathway toward the SL, lacking the double bonds introduced by DES1 and DES2, such as dhS1P, dhSph, dhsphingomyelin (dhSM), and especially DhCer [105]. In *Des1*$^{-/-}$ mice, the inability to form Cer leads to highly elevated dihydroceramide, low levels of Cer, multi-organ dysfunction, and failure to thrive [106]. Cer has signaling properties that are distinct from dihydroceramide and phytoceramide, suggesting that most cells have evolved to recognize Cer as a more significant determinant for initiating a cellular response [107].

7.1. Role of Dihydroceramides in Various Diseases

7.1.1. DhCer in Brain Diseases

Increased DhCer levels have been observed after hypoxia and subarachnoid hemorrhage [108,109]. Both studies suggest the involvement of DhCer in the mechanisms of disease in oxygen deprivation states such as stroke. Altered DhCer levels have also been noted in studies related to certain neuronal diseases such as leukodystrophia [110], Alzheimer's [111], and Huntington's disease (HD) [112]. The association of DhCer with the progression of degenerative brain diseases and other brain-related diseases makes it a potential target as a biomarker or diagnostic tool.

7.1.2. DhCer in Cardiovascular Disease

DhCers were found to be increased in both human atherosclerotic plaques and rat models of hypercholesterolemia [113,114]. DhCer also correlates with the release of macrophage inflammatory protein 1β (MIP-1β). However, the role of DhCer in plaque stability is debatable, because the extracellular addition of DhCer to human aortic smooth muscle cells did not cause apoptosis, whereas the addition of Cer did [115]. Apart from these studies, increased DhCer levels have been found in patients with rheumatoid arthritis [116] and in doxorubicin-induced cardiac toxicity [117]. All these studies suggest the role of DhCer as a marker for cardiac pathology.

7.1.3. DhCer in Cancer Therapy

As Cer has been studied for its apoptotic property, in most of these studies, DhCer has been considered as a precursor to Cer [114,118,119]. Some studies have focused on DhCer's potential role in cancer cell autophagy [120–122] in cancer-induced bone pain [123], and in cell cytotoxicity [124]. The fluctuation in the DhCer and Cer levels in cancer cells seems to differ according to the site of origin of the cancer. For example, in cancerous tissue of human endometrial cells, the level of DhCer was increased 3- to 4.6-fold, and Cer and S1P were increased 1.6- to 1.9-fold [125]; whereas in melanoma cells, DhCers and Cers were significantly lowered compared with non-malignant melanocytes [33]. Recent studies have focused on the gatekeeper enzyme dihydroceramide desaturase 1 (DES1), a new target for cancer therapy, for a better understanding of the pathological effects of DhCer in cancer. DES1 performs desaturation resulting in olefinated functionality in Cer.

4-HPR-fenretinide, a DES1 inhibitor, is currently being studied for different types of cancers including peripheral T-cell lymphomas and solid tumors. In SMS-KCNR neuroblastoma cells, 4-HPR-fenretinide directly inhibits DES1 with an IC_{50} of 2.32 μM. Inhibition of SK sensitizes cells to 4-HPR-fenretinide's cytotoxic effects due to an increased level of DhCers [126]. The possible interaction between 4-HPR-fenretinide's inhibition of DES1 and SK activity has been supported by a few other studies [122,127–129]. In cancer cell lines like HEK293, MCF 7, A549, and SMS-KCNR cells, oxidative stress can also inhibit DES1, which is followed by an increased level of DhCers [130]. Increasing the exogenous DhCer levels induced autophagy in T98G, U87MG glioblastoma cells [121], and DU145 cells [120] and reduced proliferation in castration-resistant PC cells [131]. In the human gastric cancer cell line, HGC-27, DhCers exerted autophagic effects when DES1 was inhibited by XM462 and resveratrol, resulting in higher levels of DhCer [122]. DhCer only induced autophagy when the de novo SL biosynthesis pathway was altered; in studies where both DhCers and Cers levels were increased, apoptosis occurred instead of autophagy [132]. DES1 assisted with the advancement of metastasis in PC cells [133] and esophageal carcinoma, possibly through increased cyclin D1 expression as a result of NF-κB activation [134]. These studies suggest the potential of increasing DhCer levels to increase autophagy and inhibiting metastasis through DES1 inhibition as promising targets for cancer therapy. A list of DES1 inhibitors that consist of natural products and related molecules that resemble SL structures, are shown in Figures 8 and 9, respectively [103].

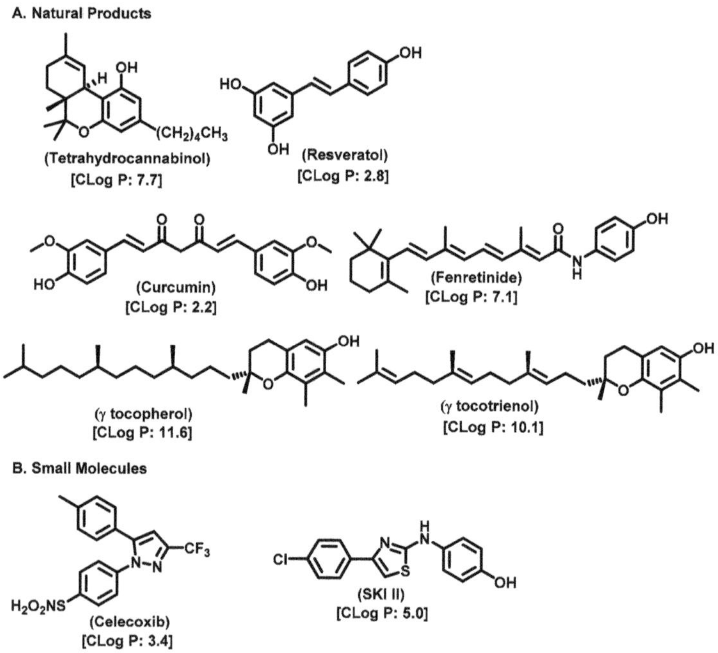

Figure 8. Natural products and small molecules of non-Sphingolipid analogs reported as dihydroceramide desaturase inhibitors.

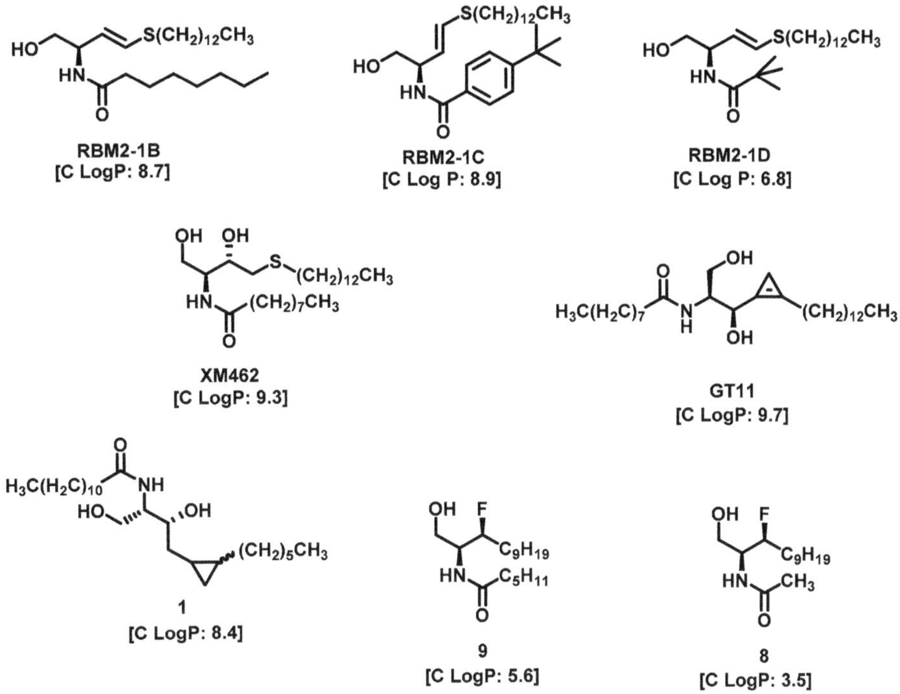

Figure 9. Chemical structure of sphingolipid analogs reported as dihydroceramide desaturase inhibitors.

8. (Dihydro)ceramide Synthase

Dihydrosphingosine (DHSph) is further acylated by six different (dihydro)ceramide synthases. In mammals, six distinct (dihydro)ceramide synthases, abbreviated as CerS1-6, have been identified and are encoded by six distinct genes [135,136]. In SL metabolism, no other step has as many genes devoted to it as (dihydro)ceramide synthesis, suggesting that each different CerS has distinct functions.

9. Ceramide Synthases

Ceramide synthases are a group of enzymes which play a central role in SL metabolism by catalyzing the formation of Cers from sphingoid bases and acyl-CoA substrates. So far, six CerSs (CerS1–CerS6) have been identified and each of them has a unique characteristic which will be discussed below.

9.1. Ceramide Synthase 1

Studies have shown Ceramide Synthase 1 (CerS1) to prefer stearoyl CoA as a substrate for producing the long-chain C18-ceramide [137]. In humans, CerS1 expression has been detected in glioblastoma cells [138], lung cells [138], and brain tissue [137]. Studies have shown an upregulated expression of CerS1 in the anterior cingulate cortex in post-mortem brain tissue from Parkinson's disease patients [139]. In Parkinson's disease patients, the C16:0-, C18:0-, C20:0-, C22:0-, and C24:1-ceramides concentration level is elevated in plasma, indicating the involvement of other CerS isoforms in the development of the disease [140]. CerS1 is also linked to the autoimmune disorder multiple sclerosis, a neuronal disease characterized by the demyelination of neurons. In the spontaneous relapse-remitting EAE (experimental autoimmune encephalomyelitis), CerS1 expression in the lumber spinal cord is decreased [141]. CerS1 is also associated with the development of obesity. In liver microsomes of high-fat, diet-induced obese (DIO) mice, an upregulation of CerS1 expression is shown due to a high-fat diet [142].

CerS1 has been identified to play a role in the pathogenesis of head- and neck squamous cell carcinoma (HNSCC). Studies have substantiated correlations between reduced C18-ceramide in HNSCC tumors and increased lymphovascular invasion, nodal metastasis, and higher tumor stages [143]. In A549 human lung adenocarcinoma cells, C18-Cer that is generated by overexpressed CerS1 represses the promoter activity of human telomerase reverse transcriptase (hTERT) [143]. Human breast tumors exhibit increased CerS1 mRNA levels when compared with normal breast tissue, and this was correlated with poor prognosis of the patients [144]. In human colorectal cancer (CRC) tissue compared with nontumor colonic tissue, elevated CerS1 mRNA levels were observed; however, this was accompanied by a reduction in C18-ceramide levels [145].

In neuroblastoma cells, CerS1 downregulation results in ER stress and proapoptotic signaling [146]. In human glioma tissue, C18-ceramide levels are lower than in control tissue, and overexpression of CerS1 or exogenous C18-ceramide triggers ER stress, lethal autophagy, and cell death in glioma cell lines [147]. These studies stipulate that CerS1 and its product C18-ceramide can exhibit antiproliferative effects in different cancer cell lines and tissues.

9.2. *Ceramide Synthase 2*

Ceramide Synthase 2 (CerS2) utilizes C20–C26 acyl CoA species and is responsible for long-chain ceramide species [148]. CerS2 has a substrate specificity towards C20:0-, C22:0-, C24:0-, C24:1-, and C26:0-acyl-CoAs. Its KM towards sphinganine is 4.8 ± 0.4 μM. In humans, CerS2 is expressed in the kidneys, liver, brain, heart, placenta, and lungs, and in breast tissue, skeletal muscle, testis, intestines, and adipose tissue [148–151]. This broad and quantitatively strong tissue distribution of CerS2 indicates its prominent role among the CerS isoforms and the importance of CerS2-derived long-chain Cers for basal cellular SL metabolism. Due to its wide distribution and distinct genomic features, the *CERS2* gene has been described as a potential housekeeping gene in mammalian cells. The CerS2 protein is localized in the ER.

CerS2 is strongly associated with the development of multiple sclerosis. In the experimental autoimmune encephalomyelitis (EAE) model, *CerS2* knockdown has a protective effect, possibly due to an impaired migration of neutrophils into the CNS [152]. In the spontaneous relapse-remitting EAE mouse model, *CerS2* expression decreased in the lumbar spinal cord [141]. CerS2 is also linked to the chronic neurodegenerative Alzheimer's disease. In an Alzheimer's disease model, there was increased expression of CerS2 in brain tissue, which led to apoptosis in glial cells [153]. In progressive myoclonic epilepsy (PME) patients, heterozygous deletions of *CerS2* in fibroblasts have been observed, which suggests that a reduced *CerS2* level led to PME development [154]. CerS2 plays a significant role in CNS development and pathological conditions.

Several studies have supported the role of CerS2 as a tumor suppressor protein and in maintaining cell- and tissue integrity. In human HCC tissue, a low expression of CerS2 correlates with tumor progression and poor prognosis [155]. In breast cancer patients, inverse relationships between CerS2 expression and tumor progression, lymph node metastasis, and HER2 expression were discovered [156]. CerS2 overexpression inhibits proliferation and triggers cell cycle arrest and apoptosis in a p21/p53-dependent manner in papillary thyroid cancer cells [157]. A decreased level of CerS2 inhibits tumor growth and metastasis in meningioma, [158] bladder cancer [159–161], and PC [162,163].

9.3. *Ceramide Synthase 3*

CerS3 prefers middle- and long-chain acyl CoAs and generates C18:0-ceramide and longer-chain Cers [164,165]. In human tissue, CerS3 is expressed in keratinocytes, and shows high expression in the kidneys and liver with moderate expression in the brain, heart, skeletal muscle, placenta, and lungs [166,167].

Mutation of *CerS3* has been reported as a reason for autosomal recessive congenital ichthyosis (ARCI), a keratinization disorder [168]. CerS3 mRNA is reduced to 70% in these patients' skin. Another study supported this cause by showing a splice mutation in CerS3 leading to a reduced number of very long chain Cers in the skin, which are essential for epidermal differentiation, an essential process for the maintenance of epidermal barrier function [164,169]. There are a lack of data on CerS3 expression in cancer, possibly due to a restricted expression of CerS3 in the mammalian body, the limited availability of specific antibodies, and the lethality of *CerS3* knockout mice. One study reported decreased *CerS3* mRNA levels in human breast tumors compared with normal breast tissue. CerS3 is the only ceramide synthase which is downregulated compared with significantly upregulated CerS2, 4, 5, and 6 [144].

9.4. Ceramide Synthase 4

Ceramide Synthase 4 (CerS4) exhibits a substrate specificity towards C18:0- and C20:0-acyl-CoAs. In humans, it is expressed in kidney tissue (renal papillae, medulla, and cortex) [170] and breast tissue [151].

In an Alzheimer's disease mouse model, upregulation of CerS4 expression and increased C20:0- and C24:0-ceramide in the hippocampal brain tissue was observed [148,153]. In human liver cancer tissue, CerS4 is upregulated at the mRNA- and protein level and promotes liver cancer cell proliferation associated with NF-κB signaling [166,171]. In human breast cancer tissue, there is higher *CerS4* mRNA expression compared with healthy breast tissue [151]. *CerS4* expression is higher in estrogen receptor (EsR)-positive tumors than in EsR-negative tumors [172]. It is possible that the increase in the ceramide synthesis by CerS and other CerSs might promote breast and colorectal cancer cell growth through a disturbed cellular SL homeostasis. Moreover, breast cancer patients with higher mRNA expression of *CerS4*, along with *CerS1* and *CerS5*, show a worse prognosis than those with low *CerS* expression levels [144].

9.5. Ceramide Synthase 5

Ceramide Synthase 5 (Cers5) prefers palmitoyl CoA as substrate, generates predominantly C16-ceramide species [173], and is expressed in human lung, [150] kidney (renal papillae, medulla, and cortex) [170], and breast tissue [151]. The KM towards sphinganine is 1.8 ± 0.4 μM and is expressed in the moth ER and nucleus. A study has shown a mild upregulation of *CerS5* in the lumber spinal cord in the spontaneous relapse-remitting EAE mice model [141]. In addition, *CerS5* mRNA expression is elevated in patient-derived colorectal cancer (CRC) tissue in comparison to normal colonic mucosa [174–176], and *CerS5* can be used as a marker for CRC [176]. Another study where data from a reverse-phase protein microarray using epithelium-enriched, human CRC tissue samples were used revealed that high CerS5 protein expression is associated with the autophagy-regulating protein signaling network, in contrast to low CerS5 levels that are associated with an apoptosis-related proteomic network [177]. In human neuroglioma tissue, elevated expressions of *CerS5* mRNA and protein levels were observed when compared with normal nervous ganglion tissue [178]. These studies suggest the correlation between high CerS5 expression and tumor cell proliferation and cancer progression in CRC, breast cancer, and other malignancies.

9.6. Ceramide Synthase 6

Ceramide Synthase 6 (CerS6) has a substrate specificity for C14:0- and C16:0 acyl-CoAs and its KM towards sphinganine is about 2.0 ± 0.6 μM. It is mainly localized at the ER. In humans, it is expressed in kidney (renal papillae, medulla, and cortex) [170] and breast tissue [151].

Increased *CerS6* expression is observed in neutrophils isolated from blood [152] and in macrophages and astroglia in the lumbar spinal cord [179] in a progressive, chronic experimental autoimmune encephalomyelitis (EAE) mouse model. In spontaneous relapse-remitting EAE, overexpression of *CerS6* in macrophages was observed [141].

When comparing with corresponding healthy tissues, an abnormal higher CerS6 level is observed in colorectal cancer (CRC) [174,175] and breast cancer [144,151,180,181]. Also, CerS6 expression is higher in estrogen receptor (EsR)-positive breast tumors than in EsR-negative tumors [151,172,182]. A similar kind of pattern was observed in gastric cancer. CerS6 overexpression corelates with poor patient survival and *CerS6* knockdown decreases proliferation, migration, and invasion of gastric cancer cells. The proposed mechanism is the downregulation of the suppressor of cytokine signaling 2 (SOCS2) by overexpressed *CerS6*, leading to the activation of JAK-STAT signaling, followed by enhanced expression of genes involved in cell cycle progression (cyclins A and B) and metastasis (MMP-2 and -9) [183,184].

10. Natural Product Inhibitors and Their Analogs

To provide a review of inhibitors targeting ceramide-metabolizing enzymes, representative natural products and small molecules were discussed for each enzyme. Several of these analogs have been tested in vitro and in vivo. Table 1 summarizes these molecules.

Table 1. Summary of some of the selected inhibitors targeting ceramide-metabolizing enzymes and their mechanism of action.

Enzyme	Inhibitors	Mechanism of Action and Binding Characteristics	Ref #
Acid Ceramidase	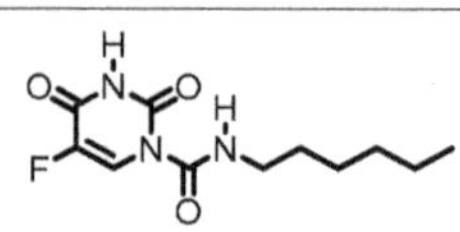 (Carmoflur)	Carmoflur decreases the growth of glioblastoma cell lines and cells isolated from glioblastoma-patient-derived xenografts. It covalently binds to the active site of ASAH1 to inhibit its function, resulting in increased C14:0, C16:0, and C18:0 ceramide.	[185]
Acid Ceramidase	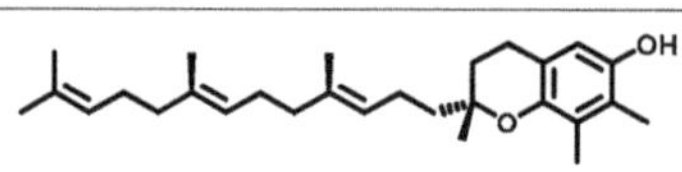 (Fenretinide)	Fenretinide treatment results in a cellular ceramide increase in tumor cells. The MOA involves ROS accumulation, cytochrome C release from mitochondrial membrane resulting in mitochondrial membrane depolarization, and cell apoptosis.	[186]
Sphingomyelin synthase	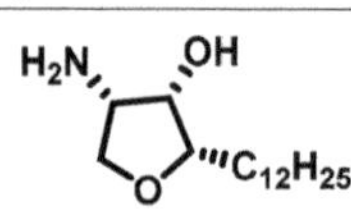 (jaspine B)	In vitro studies in cancer cells demonstrated that mitochondrial membrane bound cytochrome C release, resulting in apoptosis.	[187]
Sphingosine Kinase	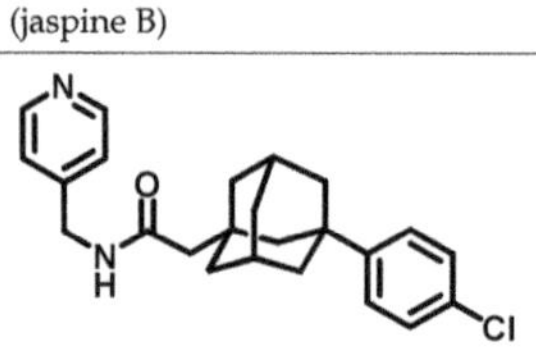 (ABC294640)	Sphingosine Kinase II specific competitive inhibitor. SphKII binding models suggest ABC294640 binding in a J-channel of the active site.	[188]
Sphingosine Kinase II	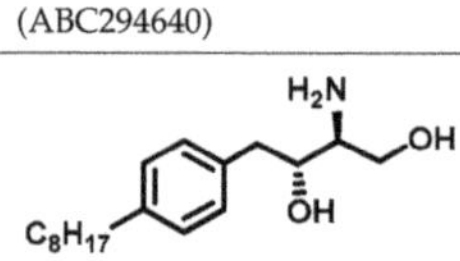 (SG-12)	SG-12 is a synthetic analogue of sphingosine that acts as an SKII inhibitor. It induces apoptosis via phosphorylation by SKII.	[72]

Table 1. *Cont.*

Enzyme	Inhibitors	Mechanism of Action and Binding Characteristics	Ref #
Sphingosine Kinase II	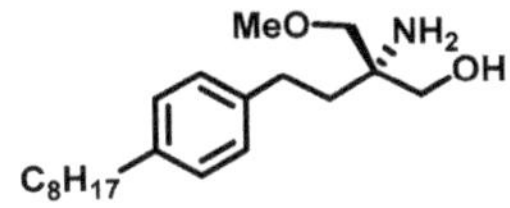 (FTY720-OMe)	(*R*)-FTY720-OMe helps block DNA synthesis and actin rearrangement induced by sphingosine 1-phosphate (S1P) in MCF-7 breast cancer cells. It can also reduce sphingosine kinase 2 (SK2) expression and prevent DNA synthesis in HEK 293 cells.	[73]
Sphingosine Kinase II	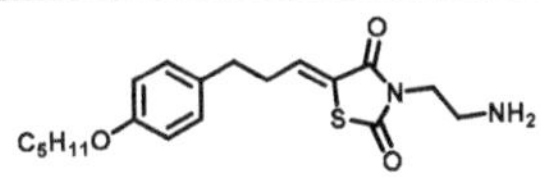 (K145)	Apoptotic effects in U937 cells, possibly through inhibition of the phosphorylation of downstream RK and Akt signaling pathways.	[74]
Sphingosine Kinase I	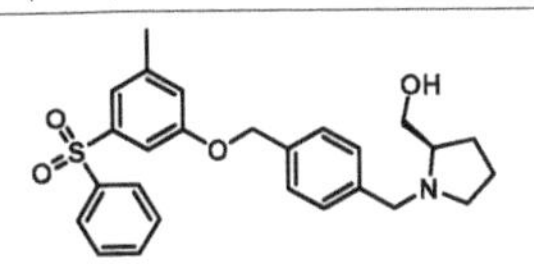 (PF—543)	Despite being SK1 selective, PF-543 demonstrates poor anticancer activity in several cancer cells.	[189]
Dihydroceramide desaturase	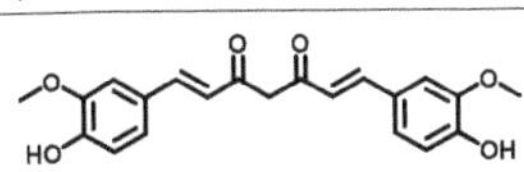 (Curcumin)	In a model of lipid trafficking impairment in C6 glial cells, curcumin stimulated ceramide synthesis by increasing the intracellular concentration of ceramide-dihydroceramide.	[190]
Dihydroceramide desaturase	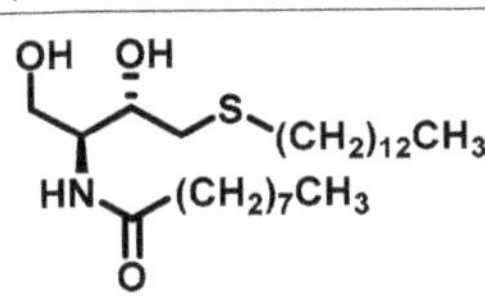 (XM462)	Inhibition studies in rat liver microsomes proved XM462 as mixed type inhibitor by a dose dependent inhibition of DES1.	[191]
Dihydroceramide desaturase	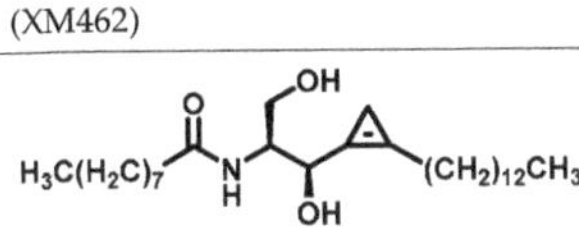 (GT11)	A Cyclopropene ring mimics the ceramide double bond, the natural 2*S*,3*R* stereochemistry, a free hydroxyl group, amide, and alkyl chains.	[191]

11. Conclusions

Fingolimod and Miglustat are FDA-approved medications related to the biochemistry of endogenous SLs. Targeting enzymes involved in SL biosynthesis, metabolism, and catabolism show promising hits for drug discovery efforts based on sphingolipidomics. Currently, there are several molecules in clinical studies that push our understanding of the SL biology in several disease states, mainly cancer. As discussed, a functional lipid raft is made of SLs. Small molecules and biologics targeting the signaling proteins embedded in these lipid rafts and the relevance of these proteins in terms of sphingolipid flux is fertile for future investigations. So far, the strategies aimed at increasing cellular Cer have opened up an avenue for perturbing cellular ceramide biosynthesis and metabolism. Of the several hallmarks of cancer that promote chemoresistance, targeting Cer-metabolizing enzymes appears to be a promising drug target. The molecular objective is to increase cellular Cer, and this has opened a new avenue of targeting resistant cancers based on membrane trafficking. Using a combination approach along with FDA-approved regimens has promising applications.

Author Contributions: Conceptualization, F.A., S.M. and S.P.; resources, S.P., J.C.K.L. and J.J.B.; writing—original draft preparation, F.A., S.M., J.O., J.C.K.L., J.J.B. and S.P.; writing—review and editing, F.A., S.M., J.O., J.C.K.L., J.J.B. and S.P.; visualization, F.A., S.M., J.O., J.C.K.L., J.J.B. and S.P.; supervision, S.P.; funding acquisition, S.P. All authors have read and agreed to the published version of the manuscript.

Funding: This research was supported, in part, by funds from Biomedical and Pharmaceutical Sciences, College of Pharmacy, Idaho State University; the National Science Foundation (NSF) MRI grant CHE-2019074; the American Association of Colleges of Pharmacy NIA award—2023; the Office of Research—ISU (LIGS33); the Pardee Foundation Grant; and the Institute for Modeling Collaboration and Innovation, University of Idaho, COBRE: P20GM104420 for chemdraw software, INBRE Program NIH grant number P20GM103408 (National Institute of General Medical Sciences).

Institutional Review Board Statement: Not applicable.

Informed Consent Statement: Not applicable.

Data Availability Statement: Not applicable.

Acknowledgments: We wish to thank Apurbha Dutta, School of Pharmacy, The University of Kansas, and Webster L. Santos, Chemistry Department, Virginia Tech, for their continued intellectual support in sphingolipid biochemistry; collaborator Ali Aghazadeh Habashi; and Amy E. Bryant, Marvin K. Schulte, and Kavita Sharma, Biomedical and Pharmaceutical Sciences, Idaho State University, Pocatello, ID, for their interest and support. The authors apologize to those investigators whose publications were not mentioned in this review due to space limitations.

Conflicts of Interest: The authors declare no conflict of interest.

Abbreviations

SL	Sphingolipid
S1P	Sphingosine-1-phosphate
CDases	Ceramidases
AC	Acid ceramidase
AML	Acute myeloid leukemia
HNC	Head- and Neck Cancer
SMS	Sphingomyelin synthase
DES	Dihydroceramide desaturase
DHSph	Dihydrosphingosine
CerS	Ceramide synthase
GMZ	Gemcitabine
FD	Farber disease
siRNA	Small interfering RNA
PPC-1	Primary prostatic carcinoma cell line
NOE	*N*-oleoylethanolamine
DTIC	Dacarbazine
IRF8	IFN regulatory factor 8
NSCLC	Non-Small Cell Lung Cancer
DCIS	Ductal carcinoma in situ
HER2	Human Epidermal Growth Factor Receptor 2
OC	Ovarian cancer
dCK	Deoxycytidine kinase
CDA	Cytidine deaminase
CERT	Ceramide transfer protein
KSR	3-Ketosphinganine reductase

References

1. Adada, M.; Luberto, C.; Canals, D. Inhibitors of the Sphingomyelin Cycle: Sphingomyelin Synthases and Sphingomyelinases. *Chem. Phys. Lipids* **2016**, *197*, 45–59. [CrossRef] [PubMed]
2. Ogretmen, B.; Hannun, Y.A. Biologically Active Sphingolipids in Cancer Pathogenesis and Treatment. *Nat. Rev. Cancer* **2004**, *4*, 604–616. [CrossRef] [PubMed]

3. Beckham, T.H.; Elojeimy, S.; Cheng, J.C.; Turner, L.S.; Hoffman, S.R.; Norris, J.S.; Liu, X. Targeting Sphingolipid Metabolism in Head and Neck Cancer: Rational Therapeutic Potentials. *Expert. Opin. Ther. Targets* **2010**, *14*, 529–539. [CrossRef] [PubMed]
4. Zhao, X.; Sun, B.; Zhang, J.; Zhang, R.; Zhang, Q. Short-Chain C6 Ceramide Sensitizes AT406-Induced Anti-Pancreatic Cancer Cell Activity. *Biochem. Biophys. Res. Commun.* **2016**, *479*, 166–172. [CrossRef]
5. Beckham, T.H.; Lu, P.; Jones, E.E.; Marrison, T.; Lewis, C.S.; Cheng, J.C.; Ramshesh, V.K.; Beeson, G.; Beeson, C.C.; Drake, R.R.; et al. LCL124, a Cationic Analog of Ceramide, Selectively Induces Pancreatic Cancer Cell Death by Accumulating in Mitochondria. *J. Pharmacol. Exp. Ther.* **2013**, *344*, 167–178. [CrossRef]
6. Peters, G.J.; van der Wilt, C.L.; van Moorsel, C.J.A.; Kroep, J.R.; Bergman, A.M.; Ackland, S.P. Basis for Effective Combination Cancer Chemotherapy with Antimetabolites. *Pharmacol. Ther.* **2000**, *87*, 227–253. [CrossRef]
7. Modrak, D.E.; Leon, E.; Goldenberg, D.M.; Gold, D.V. Ceramide Regulates Gemcitabine-Induced Senescence and Apoptosis in Human Pancreatic Cancer Cell Lines. *Mol. Cancer Res.* **2009**, *7*, 890–896. [CrossRef]
8. Castro, B.M.; Prieto, M.; Silva, L.C. Ceramide: A Simple Sphingolipid with Unique Biophysical Properties. *Prog. Lipid Res.* **2014**, *54*, 53–67. [CrossRef]
9. Delgado, A.; Fabriàs, G.; Casas, J.; Abad, J.L. Natural Products as Platforms for the Design of Sphingolipid-Related Anticancer Agents. *Adv. Cancer Res.* **2013**, *117*, 237–281.
10. Pineda, M.; Walterfang, M.; Patterson, M.C. Miglustat in Niemann-Pick Disease Type C Patients: A Review. *Orphanet J. Rare Dis.* **2018**, *13*, 140. [CrossRef]
11. Hannun, Y.A.; Obeid, L.M. Many Ceramides. *J. Biol. Chem.* **2011**, *286*, 27855–27862. [CrossRef]
12. Schulze, H.; Schepers, U.; Sandhoff, K. Overexpression and Mass Spectrometry Analysis of Mature Human Acid Ceramidase. *Biol. Chem.* **2007**, *388*, 1333–1343. [CrossRef]
13. Tao, A.; Huang, Y.; Shinohara, Y.; Caylor, M.L.; Pashikanti, S.; Xu, D. EzCADD: A Rapid 2D/3D Visualization-Enabled Web Modeling Environment for Democratizing Computer-Aided Drug Design. *J. Chem. Inf. Model.* **2019**, *59*, 18–24. [CrossRef]
14. Gebai, A.; Gorelik, A.; Li, Z.; Illes, K.; Nagar, B. Structural Basis for the Activation of Acid Ceramidase. *Nat. Commun.* **2018**, *9*, 1621. [CrossRef] [PubMed]
15. Mao, C. Ceramidases: Regulators of Cellular Responses Mediated by Ceramide, Sphingosine, and Sphingosine-1-Phosphate. *Biochim. Et Biophys. Acta (BBA)-Mol. Cell Biol. Lipids* **2008**, *1781*, 424–434. [CrossRef] [PubMed]
16. Gatt, S. Enzymatic Hydrolysis of Sphingolipids. I. Hydrolysis and Synthesis of Ceramides by an Enzyme from Rat Brain. *J. Biol. Chem.* **1966**, *241*, 3724–3730. [CrossRef] [PubMed]
17. Li, C.-M.; Park, J.-H.; He, X.; Levy, B.; Chen, F.; Arai, K.; Adler, D.A.; Disteche, C.M.; Koch, J.; Sandhoff, K.; et al. The Human Acid Ceramidase Gene (ASAH): Structure, Chromosomal Location, Mutation Analysis, and Expression. *Genomics* **1999**, *62*, 223–231. [CrossRef] [PubMed]
18. He, X.; Okino, N.; Dhami, R.; Dagan, A.; Gatt, S.; Schulze, H.; Sandhoff, K.; Schuchman, E.H. Purification and Characterization of Recombinant, Human Acid Ceramidase. *J. Biol. Chem.* **2003**, *278*, 32978–32986. [CrossRef]
19. Azuma, N.; Obrien, J.S.; Moser, H.W.; Kishimoto, Y. Stimulation of Acid Ceramidase Activity by Saposin D. *Arch. Biochem. Biophys.* **1994**, *311*, 354–357. [CrossRef]
20. Schuette, C.G.; Pierstorff, B.; Huettler, S.; Sandhoff, K. Sphingolipid Activator Proteins: Proteins with Complex Functions in Lipid Degradation and Skin Biogenesis. *Glycobiology* **2001**, *11*, 81R–90R. [CrossRef]
21. Yu, F.P.S.; Amintas, S.; Levade, T.; Medin, J.A. Acid Ceramidase Deficiency: Farber Disease and SMA-PME. *Orphanet J. Rare Dis.* **2018**, *13*, 121. [CrossRef]
22. Li, C.-M.; Park, J.-H.; Simonaro, C.M.; He, X.; Gordon, R.E.; Friedman, A.-H.; Ehleiter, D.; Paris, F.; Manova, K.; Hepbiloikler, S.; et al. Insertional Mutagenesis of the Mouse Acid Ceramidase Gene Leads to Early Embryonic Lethality in Homozygotes and Progressive Lipid Storage Disease in Heterozygotes. *Genomics* **2002**, *79*, 218–224. [CrossRef] [PubMed]
23. Mahdy, A.E.; Cheng, J.C.; Li, J.; Elojeimy, S.; Meacham, W.D.; Turner, L.S.; Bai, A.; Gault, C.R.; McPherson, A.S.; Garcia, N.; et al. Acid Ceramidase Upregulation in Prostate Cancer Cells Confers Resistance to Radiation: AC Inhibition, a Potential Radiosensitizer. *Mol. Ther.* **2009**, *17*, 430–438. [CrossRef]
24. Cheng, J.C.; Bai, A.; Beckham, T.H.; Marrison, S.T.; Yount, C.L.; Young, K.; Lu, P.; Bartlett, A.M.; Wu, B.X.; Keane, B.J.; et al. Radiation-Induced Acid Ceramidase Confers Prostate Cancer Resistance and Tumor Relapse. *J. Clin. Investig.* **2013**, *123*, 4344–4358. [CrossRef] [PubMed]
25. Camacho, L.; Meca-Cortés, Ó.; Abad, J.L.; García, S.; Rubio, N.; Díaz, A.; Celià-Terrassa, T.; Cingolani, F.; Bermudo, R.; Fernández, P.L.; et al. Acid Ceramidase as a Therapeutic Target in Metastatic Prostate Cancer. *J. Lipid Res.* **2013**, *54*, 1207–1220. [CrossRef] [PubMed]
26. Holman, D.H.; Turner, L.S.; El-Zawahry, A.; Elojeimy, S.; Liu, X.; Bielawski, J.; Szulc, Z.M.; Norris, K.; Zeidan, Y.H.; Hannun, Y.A.; et al. Lysosomotropic Acid Ceramidase Inhibitor Induces Apoptosis in Prostate Cancer Cells. *Cancer Chemother. Pharmacol.* **2008**, *61*, 231–242. [CrossRef]
27. Gouazé-Andersson, V.; Flowers, M.; Karimi, R.; Fabriás, G.; Delgado, A.; Casas, J.; Cabot, M.C. Inhibition of Acid Ceramidase by a 2-Substituted Aminoethanol Amide Synergistically Sensitizes Prostate Cancer Cells to N-(4-Hydroxyphenyl) Retinamide. *Prostate* **2011**, *71*, 1064–1073. [CrossRef]

28. Turner, L.S.; Cheng, J.C.; Beckham, T.H.; Keane, T.E.; Norris, J.S.; Liu, X. Autophagy Is Increased in Prostate Cancer Cells Overexpressing Acid Ceramidase and Enhances Resistance to C6 Ceramide. *Prostate Cancer Prostatic Dis.* **2011**, *14*, 30–37. [CrossRef]
29. Roh, J.-L.; Park, J.Y.; Kim, E.H.; Jang, H.J. Targeting Acid Ceramidase Sensitises Head and Neck Cancer to Cisplatin. *Eur. J. Cancer* **2016**, *52*, 163–172. [CrossRef]
30. Korbelik, M.; Banáth, J.; Zhang, W.; Saw, K.M.; Szulc, Z.M.; Bielawska, A.; Separovic, D. Interaction of Acid Ceramidase Inhibitor LCL521 with Tumor Response to Photodynamic Therapy and Photodynamic Therapy-Generated Vaccine. *Int. J. Cancer* **2016**, *139*, 1372–1378. [CrossRef]
31. Separovic, D.; Breen, P.; Boppana, N.B.; Van Buren, E.; Joseph, N.; Kraveka, J.M.; Rahmaniyan, M.; Li, L.; Gudz, T.I.; Bielawska, A.; et al. Increased Killing of SCCVII Squamous Cell Carcinoma Cells after the Combination of Pc 4 Photodynamic Therapy and Dasatinib Is Associated with Enhanced Caspase-3 Activity and Ceramide Synthase 1 Upregulation. *Int. J. Oncol.* **2013**, *43*, 2064–2072. [CrossRef]
32. Elojeimy, S.; Liu, X.; Mckillop, J.C.; El-Zawahry, A.M.; Holman, D.H.; Cheng, J.Y.; Meacham, W.D.; Mahdy, A.E.; Saad, A.F.; Turner, L.S.; et al. Role of Acid Ceramidase in Resistance to FasL: Therapeutic Approaches Based on Acid Ceramidase Inhibitors and FasL Gene Therapy. *Mol. Ther.* **2007**, *15*, 1259–1263. [CrossRef] [PubMed]
33. Realini, N.; Palese, F.; Pizzirani, D.; Pontis, S.; Basit, A.; Bach, A.; Ganesan, A.; Piomelli, D. Acid Ceramidase in Melanoma. *J. Biol. Chem.* **2016**, *291*, 2422–2434. [CrossRef]
34. Bedia, C.; Casas, J.; Andrieu-Abadie, N.; Fabriàs, G.; Levade, T. Acid Ceramidase Expression Modulates the Sensitivity of A375 Melanoma Cells to Dacarbazine. *J. Biol. Chem.* **2011**, *286*, 28200–28209. [CrossRef] [PubMed]
35. Lai, M.; Realini, N.; La Ferla, M.; Passalacqua, I.; Matteoli, G.; Ganesan, A.; Pistello, M.; Mazzanti, C.M.; Piomelli, D. Complete Acid Ceramidase Ablation Prevents Cancer-Initiating Cell Formation in Melanoma Cells. *Sci. Rep.* **2017**, *7*, 7411. [CrossRef] [PubMed]
36. Tan, S.-F.; Liu, X.; Fox, T.E.; Barth, B.M.; Sharma, A.; Turner, S.D.; Awwad, A.; Dewey, A.; Doi, K.; Spitzer, B.; et al. Acid Ceramidase Is Upregulated in AML and Represents a Novel Therapeutic Target. *Oncotarget* **2016**, *7*, 83208–83222. [CrossRef]
37. Hu, X.; Yang, D.; Zimmerman, M.; Liu, F.; Yang, J.; Kannan, S.; Burchert, A.; Szulc, Z.; Bielawska, A.; Ozato, K.; et al. IRF8 Regulates Acid Ceramidase Expression to Mediate Apoptosis and Suppresses Myelogeneous Leukemia. *Cancer Res.* **2011**, *71*, 2882–2891. [CrossRef]
38. Ramirez de Molina, A.; de la Cueva, A.; Machado-Pinilla, R.; Rodriguez-Fanjul, V.; Gomez del Pulgar, T.; Cebrian, A.; Perona, R.; Lacal, J.C. Acid Ceramidase as a Chemotherapeutic Target to Overcome Resistance to the Antitumoral Effect of Choline Kinase α Inhibition. *Curr. Cancer Drug Targets* **2012**, *12*, 617–624. [CrossRef]
39. Sänger, N.; Ruckhäberle, E.; Györffy, B.; Engels, K.; Heinrich, T.; Fehm, T.; Graf, A.; Holtrich, U.; Becker, S.; Karn, T. Acid Ceramidase Is Associated with an Improved Prognosis in Both DCIS and Invasive Breast Cancer. *Mol. Oncol.* **2015**, *9*, 58–67. [CrossRef]
40. Flowers, M.; Fabriás, G.; Delgado, A.; Casas, J.; Abad, J.L.; Cabot, M.C. C6-Ceramide and Targeted Inhibition of Acid Ceramidase Induce Synergistic Decreases in Breast Cancer Cell Growth. *Breast Cancer Res. Treat.* **2012**, *133*, 447–458. [CrossRef]
41. Vethakanraj, H.S.; Sesurajan, B.P.; Padmanaban, V.P.; Jayaprakasam, M.; Murali, S.; Sekar, A.K. Anticancer Effect of Acid Ceramidase Inhibitor Ceranib-2 in Human Breast Cancer Cell Lines MCF-7, MDA MB-231 by the Activation of SAPK/JNK, P38 MAPK Apoptotic Pathways, Inhibition of the Akt Pathway, Downregulation of ERα. *Anticancer Drugs* **2018**, *29*, 50–60. [CrossRef]
42. Kus, G.; Kabadere, S.; Uyar, R.; Kutlu, H.M. Induction of Apoptosis in Prostate Cancer Cells by the Novel Ceramidase Inhibitor Ceranib-2. *Vitr. Cell Dev. Biol. Anim.* **2015**, *51*, 1056–1063. [CrossRef] [PubMed]
43. Hanker, L.C.; Karn, T.; Holtrich, U.; Gätje, R.; Rody, A.; Heinrich, T.; Ruckhäberle, E.; Engels, K. Acid Ceramidase (AC)—A Key Enzyme of Sphingolipid Metabolism—Correlates With Better Prognosis in Epithelial Ovarian Cancer. *Int. J. Gynecol. Pathol.* **2013**, *32*, 249–257. [CrossRef] [PubMed]
44. Morales, A.; París, R.; Villanueva, A.; Llacuna, L.; García-Ruiz, C.; Fernández-Checa, J.C. Pharmacological Inhibition or Small Interfering RNA Targeting Acid Ceramidase Sensitizes Hepatoma Cells to Chemotherapy and Reduces Tumor Growth In Vivo. *Oncogene* **2007**, *26*, 905–916. [CrossRef]
45. Giovannetti, E.; Leon, L.G.; Bertini, S.; Macchia, M.; Minutolo, F.; Funel, N.; Alecci, C.; Giancola, F.; Danesi, R.; Peters, G.J. Study of Apoptosis Induction and Deoxycytidine Kinase/Cytidine Deaminase Modulation in the Synergistic Interaction of a Novel Ceramide Analog and Gemcitabine in Pancreatic Cancer Cells. *Nucleosides Nucleotides Nucleic Acids* **2010**, *29*, 419–426. [CrossRef] [PubMed]
46. Klobučar, M.; Grbčić, P.; Pavelić, S.K.; Jonjić, N.; Visentin, S.; Sedić, M. Acid Ceramidase Inhibition Sensitizes Human Colon Cancer Cells to Oxaliplatin through Downregulation of Transglutaminase 2 and B1 Integrin/FAK−mediated Signalling. *Biochem. Biophys. Res. Commun.* **2018**, *503*, 843–848. [CrossRef]
47. Baspinar, M.; Ozyurt, R.; Kus, G.; Kutlay, O.; Ozkurt, M.; Erkasap, N.; Kabadere, S.; Yasar, N.F.; Erkasap, S. Effects of Ceranib-2 on Cell Survival and TNF-Alpha in Colon Cancer Cell Line. *Bratisl. Med. J.* **2017**, *118*, 391–393. [CrossRef]
48. Hait, N.C.; Allegood, J.; Maceyka, M.; Strub, G.M.; Harikumar, K.B.; Singh, S.K.; Luo, C.; Marmorstein, R.; Kordula, T.; Milstien, S.; et al. Regulation of Histone Acetylation in the Nucleus by Sphingosine-1-Phosphate. *Science* **2009**, *325*, 1254–1257. [CrossRef]
49. Wang, Z.; Min, X.; Xiao, S.-H.; Johnstone, S.; Romanow, W.; Meininger, D.; Xu, H.; Liu, J.; Dai, J.; An, S.; et al. Molecular Basis of Sphingosine Kinase 1 Substrate Recognition and Catalysis. *Structure* **2013**, *21*, 798–809. [CrossRef]

50. Spiegel, S.; Milstien, S. The Outs and the Ins of Sphingosine-1-Phosphate in Immunity. *Nat. Rev. Immunol.* **2011**, *11*, 403–415. [CrossRef]
51. Kunkel, G.T.; Maceyka, M.; Milstien, S.; Spiegel, S. Targeting the Sphingosine-1-Phosphate Axis in Cancer, Inflammation and Beyond. *Nat. Rev. Drug Discov.* **2013**, *12*, 688–702. [CrossRef]
52. Truman, J.-P.; García-Barros, M.; Obeid, L.M.; Hannun, Y.A. Evolving Concepts in Cancer Therapy through Targeting Sphingolipid Metabolism. *Biochim. Et Biophys. Acta (BBA)-Mol. Cell Biol. Lipids* **2014**, *1841*, 1174–1188. [CrossRef]
53. Lemaire, M. WANTED: Natural-Born Sickler. *Sci. Transl. Med.* **2014**, *6*, 240ec101. [CrossRef]
54. Zhang, Y.; Berka, V.; Song, A.; Sun, K.; Wang, W.; Zhang, W.; Ning, C.; Li, C.; Zhang, Q.; Bogdanov, M.; et al. Elevated Sphingosine-1-Phosphate Promotes Sickling and Sickle Cell Disease Progression. *J. Clin. Investig.* **2014**, *124*, 2750–2761. [CrossRef]
55. Balakumar, P.; Kaur, T.; Singh, M. Potential Target Sites to Modulate Vascular Endothelial Dysfunction: Current Perspectives and Future Directions. *Toxicology* **2008**, *245*, 49–64. [CrossRef] [PubMed]
56. Machida, T.; Hamaya, Y.; Izumi, S.; Hamaya, Y.; Iizuka, K.; Igarashi, Y.; Minami, M.; Levi, R.; Hirafuji, M. Sphingosine 1-Phosphate Inhibits Nitric Oxide Production Induced by Interleukin-1β in Rat Vascular Smooth Muscle Cells. *J. Pharmacol. Exp. Ther.* **2008**, *325*, 200–209. [CrossRef]
57. Sorrentino, R.; Bertolino, A.; Terlizzi, M.; Iacono, V.M.; Maiolino, P.; Cirino, G.; Roviezzo, F.; Pinto, A. B Cell Depletion Increases Sphingosine-1-Phosphate–Dependent Airway Inflammation in Mice. *Am. J. Respir. Cell Mol. Biol.* **2015**, *52*, 571–583. [CrossRef]
58. Price, M.M.; Oskeritzian, C.A.; Falanga, Y.T.; Harikumar, K.B.; Allegood, J.C.; Alvarez, S.E.; Conrad, D.; Ryan, J.J.; Milstien, S.; Spiegel, S. A Specific Sphingosine Kinase 1 Inhibitor Attenuates Airway Hyperresponsiveness and Inflammation in a Mast Cell–Dependent Murine Model of Allergic Asthma. *J. Allergy Clin. Immunol.* **2013**, *131*, 501–511.e1. [CrossRef]
59. Pyne, N.J.; Dubois, G.; Pyne, S. Role of Sphingosine 1-Phosphate and Lysophosphatidic Acid in Fibrosis. *Biochim. Et Biophys. Acta (BBA)-Mol. Cell Biol. Lipids* **2013**, *1831*, 228–238. [CrossRef] [PubMed]
60. Maceyka, M.; Sankala, H.; Hait, N.C.; Le Stunff, H.; Liu, H.; Toman, R.; Collier, C.; Zhang, M.; Satin, L.S.; Merrill, A.H.; et al. SphK1 and SphK2, Sphingosine Kinase Isoenzymes with Opposing Functions in Sphingolipid Metabolism. *J. Biol. Chem.* **2005**, *280*, 37118–37129. [CrossRef] [PubMed]
61. Neubauer, H.A.; Pitson, S.M. Roles, Regulation and Inhibitors of Sphingosine Kinase 2. *FEBS J.* **2013**, *280*, 5317–5336. [CrossRef] [PubMed]
62. Mizugishi, K.; Yamashita, T.; Olivera, A.; Miller, G.F.; Spiegel, S.; Proia, R.L. Essential Role for Sphingosine Kinases in Neural and Vascular Development. *Mol. Cell Biol.* **2005**, *25*, 11113–11121. [CrossRef] [PubMed]
63. French, K.J.; Zhuang, Y.; Maines, L.W.; Gao, P.; Wang, W.; Beljanski, V.; Upson, J.J.; Green, C.L.; Keller, S.N.; Smith, C.D. Pharmacology and Antitumor Activity of ABC294640, a Selective Inhibitor of Sphingosine Kinase-2. *J. Pharmacol. Exp. Ther.* **2010**, *333*, 129–139. [CrossRef] [PubMed]
64. Maines, L.W.; Fitzpatrick, L.R.; French, K.J.; Zhuang, Y.; Xia, Z.; Keller, S.N.; Upson, J.J.; Smith, C.D. Suppression of Ulcerative Colitis in Mice by Orally Available Inhibitors of Sphingosine Kinase. *Dig. Dis. Sci.* **2008**, *53*, 997–1012. [CrossRef]
65. Maines, L.W.; Fitzpatrick, L.R.; Green, C.L.; Zhuang, Y.; Smith, C.D. Efficacy of a Novel Sphingosine Kinase Inhibitor in Experimental Crohn's Disease. *Inflammopharmacology* **2010**, *18*, 73–85. [CrossRef]
66. Shi, Y.; Rehman, H.; Ramshesh, V.K.; Schwartz, J.; Liu, Q.; Krishnasamy, Y.; Zhang, X.; Lemasters, J.J.; Smith, C.D.; Zhong, Z. Sphingosine Kinase-2 Inhibition Improves Mitochondrial Function and Survival after Hepatic Ischemia–Reperfusion. *J. Hepatol.* **2012**, *56*, 137–145. [CrossRef]
67. Chumanevich, A.A.; Poudyal, D.; Cui, X.; Davis, T.; Wood, P.A.; Smith, C.D.; Hofseth, L.J. Suppression of Colitis-Driven Colon Cancer in Mice by a Novel Small Molecule Inhibitor of Sphingosine Kinase. *Carcinogenesis* **2010**, *31*, 1787–1793. [CrossRef]
68. Xun, C.; Chen, M.-B.; Qi, L.; Tie-Ning, Z.; Peng, X.; Ning, L.; Chen, Z.-X.; Wang, L.-W. Targeting Sphingosine Kinase 2 (SphK2) by ABC294640 Inhibits Colorectal Cancer Cell Growth In Vitro and In Vivo. *J. Exp. Clin. Cancer Res.* **2015**, *34*, 94. [CrossRef]
69. Antoon, J.W.; White, M.D.; Meacham, W.D.; Slaughter, E.M.; Muir, S.E.; Elliott, S.; Rhodes, L.V.; Ashe, H.B.; Wiese, T.E.; Smith, C.D.; et al. Antiestrogenic Effects of the Novel Sphingosine Kinase-2 Inhibitor ABC294640. *Endocrinology* **2010**, *151*, 5124–5135. [CrossRef]
70. Grbčić, P.; Eichmann, T.O.; Kraljević Pavelić, S.; Sedić, M. The Sphingosine Kinase 2 Inhibitor ABC294640 Restores the Sensitivity of BRAFV600E Mutant Colon Cancer Cells to Vemurafenib by Reducing AKT-Mediated Expression of Nucleophosmin and Translationally-Controlled Tumour Protein. *Int. J. Mol. Sci.* **2021**, *22*, 10767. [CrossRef]
71. Wu, J.; Fan, S.; Feinberg, D.; Wang, X.; Jabbar, S.; Kang, Y. Inhibition of Sphingosine Kinase 2 Results in PARK2-Mediated Mitophagy and Induces Apoptosis in Multiple Myeloma. *Curr. Oncol.* **2023**, *30*, 3047–3063. [CrossRef]
72. Hara-Yokoyama, M.; Terasawa, K.; Ichinose, S.; Watanabe, A.; Podyma-Inoue, K.A.; Akiyoshi, K.; Igarashi, Y.; Yanagishita, M. Sphingosine Kinase 2 Inhibitor SG-12 Induces Apoptosis via Phosphorylation by Sphingosine Kinase 2. *Bioorg. Med. Chem. Lett.* **2013**, *23*, 2220–2224. [CrossRef]
73. Lim, K.G.; Sun, C.; Bittman, R.; Pyne, N.J.; Pyne, S. (R)-FTY720 Methyl Ether Is a Specific Sphingosine Kinase 2 Inhibitor: Effect on Sphingosine Kinase 2 Expression in HEK 293 Cells and Actin Rearrangement and Survival of MCF-7 Breast Cancer Cells. *Cell Signal* **2011**, *23*, 1590–1595. [CrossRef] [PubMed]
74. Liu, K.; Guo, T.L.; Hait, N.C.; Allegood, J.; Parikh, H.I.; Xu, W.; Kellogg, G.E.; Grant, S.; Spiegel, S.; Zhang, S. Biological Characterization of 3-(2-Amino-Ethyl)-5-[3-(4-Butoxyl-Phenyl)-Propylidene]-Thiazolidine-2,4-Dione (K145) as a Selective Sphingosine Kinase-2 Inhibitor and Anticancer Agent. *PLoS ONE* **2013**, *8*, e56471. [CrossRef] [PubMed]

75. Raje, M.R.; Knott, K.; Kharel, Y.; Bissel, P.; Lynch, K.R.; Santos, W.L. Design, Synthesis and Biological Activity of Sphingosine Kinase 2 Selective Inhibitors. *Bioorg. Med. Chem.* **2012**, *20*, 183–194. [CrossRef] [PubMed]
76. Kharel, Y.; Raje, M.; Gao, M.; Gellett, A.M.; Tomsig, J.L.; Lynch, K.R.; Santos, W.L. Sphingosine Kinase Type 2 Inhibition Elevates Circulating Sphingosine 1-Phosphate. *Biochem. J.* **2012**, *447*, 149–157. [CrossRef] [PubMed]
77. Patwardhan, N.N.; Morris, E.A.; Kharel, Y.; Raje, M.R.; Gao, M.; Tomsig, J.L.; Lynch, K.R.; Santos, W.L. Structure−Activity Relationship Studies and in Vivo Activity of Guanidine-Based Sphingosine Kinase Inhibitors: Discovery of SphK1- and SphK2-Selective Inhibitors. *J. Med. Chem.* **2015**, *58*, 1879–1899. [CrossRef]
78. Kharel, Y.; Morris, E.A.; Congdon, M.D.; Thorpe, S.B.; Tomsig, J.L.; Santos, W.L.; Lynch, K.R. Sphingosine Kinase 2 Inhibition and Blood Sphingosine 1-Phosphate Levels. *J. Pharmacol. Exp. Ther.* **2015**, *355*, 23–31. [CrossRef]
79. Congdon, M.D.; Kharel, Y.; Brown, A.M.; Lewis, S.N.; Bevan, D.R.; Lynch, K.R.; Santos, W.L. Structure–Activity Relationship Studies and Molecular Modeling of Naphthalene-Based Sphingosine Kinase 2 Inhibitors. *ACS Med. Chem. Lett.* **2016**, *7*, 229–234. [CrossRef]
80. Childress, E.S.; Kharel, Y.; Brown, A.M.; Bevan, D.R.; Lynch, K.R.; Santos, W.L. Transforming Sphingosine Kinase 1 Inhibitors into Dual and Sphingosine Kinase 2 Selective Inhibitors: Design, Synthesis, and in Vivo Activity. *J. Med. Chem.* **2017**, *60*, 3933–3957. [CrossRef]
81. Futerman, A.H.; Stieger, B.; Hubbard, A.L.; Pagano, R.E. Sphingomyelin Synthesis in Rat Liver Occurs Predominantly at the Cis and Medial Cisternae of the Golgi Apparatus. *J. Biol. Chem.* **1990**, *265*, 8650–8657. [CrossRef]
82. Huitema, K.; van den Dikkenberg, J.; Brouwers, J.F.H.M.; Holthuis, J.C.M. Identification of a Family of Animal Sphingomyelin Synthases. *EMBO J.* **2004**, *23*, 33–44. [CrossRef]
83. Albi, E.; Lazzarini, R.; Magni, M.V. Reverse Sphingomyelin-Synthase in Rat Liver Chromatin. *FEBS Lett.* **2003**, *549*, 152–156. [CrossRef]
84. Taniguchi, M.; Okazaki, T. The Role of Sphingomyelin and Sphingomyelin Synthases in Cell Death, Proliferation and Migration—From Cell and Animal Models to Human Disorders. *Biochim. Et Biophys. Acta (BBA)-Mol. Cell Biol. Lipids* **2014**, *1841*, 692–703. [CrossRef]
85. Yamaoka, S.; Miyaji, M.; Kitano, T.; Umehara, H.; Okazaki, T. Expression Cloning of a Human CDNA Restoring Sphingomyelin Synthesis and Cell Growth in Sphingomyelin Synthase-Defective Lymphoid Cells. *J. Biol. Chem.* **2004**, *279*, 18688–18693. [CrossRef]
86. Luberto, C.; Hannun, Y.A. Sphingomyelin Synthase, a Potential Regulator of Intracellular Levels of Ceramide and Diacylglycerol during SV40 Transformation. *J. Biol. Chem.* **1998**, *273*, 14550–14559. [CrossRef]
87. Riboni, L.; Viani, P.; Bassi, R.; Giussani, P.; Tettamanti, G. Basic Fibroblast Growth Factor-Induced Proliferation of Primary Astrocytes. *J. Biol. Chem.* **2001**, *276*, 12797–12804. [CrossRef]
88. Hannun, Y.A.; Obeid, L.M. The Ceramide-Centric Universe of Lipid-Mediated Cell Regulation: Stress Encounters of the Lipid Kind. *J. Biol. Chem.* **2002**, *277*, 25847–25850. [CrossRef]
89. Wiegmann, K.; Schütze, S.; Machleidt, T.; Witte, D.; Krönke, M. Functional Dichotomy of Neutral and Acidic Sphingomyelinases in Tumor Necrosis Factor Signaling. *Cell* **1994**, *78*, 1005–1015. [CrossRef]
90. Adam-Klages, S.; Adam, D.; Wiegmann, K.; Struve, S.; Kolanus, W.; Schneider-Mergener, J.; Krönke, M. FAN, a Novel WD-Repeat Protein, Couples the P55 TNF-Receptor to Neutral Sphingomyelinase. *Cell* **1996**, *86*, 937–947. [CrossRef]
91. Spiegel, S.; Milstien, S. Sphingosine-1-Phosphate: An Enigmatic Signalling Lipid. *Nat. Rev. Mol. Cell Biol.* **2003**, *4*, 397–407. [CrossRef] [PubMed]
92. Taniguchi, M.; Okazaki, T. Role of Ceramide/Sphingomyelin (SM) Balance Regulated through "SM Cycle" in Cancer. *Cell. Signal.* **2021**, *87*, 110119. [CrossRef]
93. Holthuis, J.C.M.; Pomorski, T.; Raggers, R.J.; Sprong, H.; Van Meer, G. The Organizing Potential of Sphingolipids in Intracellular Membrane Transport. *Physiol. Rev.* **2001**, *81*, 1689–1723. [CrossRef] [PubMed]
94. Baron, C.L.; Malhotra, V. Role of Diacylglycerol in PKD Recruitment to the TGN and Protein Transport to the Plasma Membrane. *Science* **2002**, *295*, 325–328. [CrossRef] [PubMed]
95. Hampton, R.Y.; Morand, O.H. Sphingomyelin Synthase and PKC Activation. *Science* **1989**, *246*, 1050. [CrossRef]
96. Ordóñez, Y.F.; González, J.; Bedia, C.; Casas, J.; Abad, J.L.; Delgado, A.; Fabrias, G. 3-Ketosphinganine Provokes the Accumulation of Dihydroshingolipids and Induces Autophagy in Cancer Cells. *Mol. Biosyst.* **2016**, *12*, 1166–1173. [CrossRef]
97. Cadena, D.L.; Kurten, R.C.; Gill, G.N. The Product of the MLD Gene Is a Member of the Membrane Fatty Acid Desaturase Family: Overexpression of MLD Inhibits EGF Receptor Biosynthesis. *Biochemistry* **1997**, *36*, 6960–6967. [CrossRef]
98. Geeraert, L.; Mannaerts, G.P.; Van Veldhoven, P.P. Conversion of Dihydroceramide into Ceramide: Involvement of a Desaturase. *Biochem. J.* **1997**, *327*, 125–132. [CrossRef]
99. Michel, C.; van Echten-Deckert, G.; Rother, J.; Sandhoff, K.; Wang, E.; Merrill, A.H. Characterization of Ceramide Synthesis. *J. Biol. Chem.* **1997**, *272*, 22432–22437. [CrossRef]
100. Savile, C.K.; Fabriàs, G.; Buist, P.H. Dihydroceramide Delta(4) Desaturase Initiates Substrate Oxidation at C-4. *J. Am. Chem. Soc.* **2001**, *123*, 4382–4385. [CrossRef]
101. Beauchamp, E.; Goenaga, D.; Le Bloc'h, J.; Catheline, D.; Legrand, P.; Rioux, V. Myristic Acid Increases the Activity of Dihydroceramide Δ4-Desaturase 1 through Its N-Terminal Myristoylation. *Biochimie* **2007**, *89*, 1553–1561. [CrossRef]

102. Ternes, P.; Franke, S.; Zähringer, U.; Sperling, P.; Heinz, E. Identification and Characterization of a Sphingolipid Δ4-Desaturase Family. *J. Biol. Chem.* **2002**, *277*, 25512–25518. [CrossRef] [PubMed]
103. Casasampere, M.; Ordoñez, Y.F.; Pou, A.; Casas, J. Inhibitors of Dihydroceramide Desaturase 1: Therapeutic Agents and Pharmacological Tools to Decipher the Role of Dihydroceramides in Cell Biology. *Chem. Phys. Lipids* **2016**, *197*, 33–44. [CrossRef]
104. Mizutani, Y.; Kihara, A.; Igarashi, Y. Identification of the Human Sphingolipid C4-Hydroxylase, HDES2, and Its up-Regulation during Keratinocyte Differentiation. *FEBS Lett.* **2004**, *563*, 93–97. [CrossRef] [PubMed]
105. Siddique, M.M.; Bikman, B.T.; Wang, L.; Ying, L.; Reinhardt, E.; Shui, G.; Wenk, M.R.; Summers, S.A. Ablation of Dihydroceramide Desaturase Confers Resistance to Etoposide-Induced Apoptosis In Vitro. *PLoS ONE* **2012**, *7*, e44042. [CrossRef] [PubMed]
106. Holland, W.L.; Brozinick, J.T.; Wang, L.-P.; Hawkins, E.D.; Sargent, K.M.; Liu, Y.; Narra, K.; Hoehn, K.L.; Knotts, T.A.; Siesky, A.; et al. Inhibition of Ceramide Synthesis Ameliorates Glucocorticoid-, Saturated-Fat-, and Obesity-Induced Insulin Resistance. *Cell Metab.* **2007**, *5*, 167–179. [CrossRef] [PubMed]
107. Hannun, Y.A.; Obeid, L.M. Principles of Bioactive Lipid Signalling: Lessons from Sphingolipids. *Nat. Rev. Mol. Cell Biol.* **2008**, *9*, 139–150. [CrossRef]
108. Testai, F.D.; Kilkus, J.P.; Berdyshev, E.; Gorshkova, I.; Natarajan, V.; Dawson, G. Multiple Sphingolipid Abnormalities Following Cerebral Microendothelial Hypoxia. *J. Neurochem.* **2014**, *131*, 530–540. [CrossRef]
109. Testai, F.D.; Xu, H.-L.; Kilkus, J.; Suryadevara, V.; Gorshkova, I.; Berdyshev, E.; Pelligrino, D.A.; Dawson, G. Changes in the Metabolism of Sphingolipids after Subarachnoid Hemorrhage. *J. Neurosci. Res.* **2015**, *93*, 796–805. [CrossRef]
110. Edvardson, S.; Yi, J.K.; Jalas, C.; Xu, R.; Webb, B.D.; Snider, J.; Fedick, A.; Kleinman, E.; Treff, N.R.; Mao, C.; et al. Deficiency of the Alkaline Ceramidase ACER3 Manifests in Early Childhood by Progressive Leukodystrophy. *J. Med. Genet.* **2016**, *53*, 389–396. [CrossRef]
111. Mielke, M.M.; Haughey, N.J.; Bandaru, V.V.R.; Weinberg, D.D.; Darby, E.; Zaidi, N.; Pavlik, V.; Doody, R.S.; Lyketsos, C.G. Plasma Sphingomyelins Are Associated with Cognitive Progression in Alzheimer's Disease. *J. Alzheimer's Dis.* **2011**, *27*, 259–269. [CrossRef] [PubMed]
112. Di Pardo, A.; Basit, A.; Armirotti, A.; Amico, E.; Castaldo, S.; Pepe, G.; Marracino, F.; Buttari, F.; Digilio, A.F.; Maglione, V. De Novo Synthesis of Sphingolipids Is Defective in Experimental Models of Huntington's Disease. *Front. Neurosci.* **2017**, *11*, 698. [CrossRef] [PubMed]
113. González-Peña, D.; Checa, A.; de Ancos, B.; Wheelock, C.E.; Sánchez-Moreno, C. New Insights into the Effects of Onion Consumption on Lipid Mediators Using a Diet-Induced Model of Hypercholesterolemia. *Redox Biol.* **2017**, *11*, 205–212. [CrossRef] [PubMed]
114. Maeng, H.J.; Song, J.-H.; Kim, G.-T.; Song, Y.-J.; Lee, K.; Kim, J.-Y.; Park, T.-S. Celecoxib-Mediated Activation of Endoplasmic Reticulum Stress Induces de Novo Ceramide Biosynthesis and Apoptosis in Hepatoma HepG2 Cells. *BMB Rep.* **2017**, *50*, 144–149. [CrossRef] [PubMed]
115. Edsfeldt, A.; Dunér, P.; Ståhlman, M.; Mollet, I.G.; Asciutto, G.; Grufman, H.; Nitulescu, M.; Persson, A.F.; Fisher, R.M.; Melander, O.; et al. Sphingolipids Contribute to Human Atherosclerotic Plaque Inflammation. *Arter. Thromb. Vasc. Biol.* **2016**, *36*, 1132–1140. [CrossRef]
116. Fang, L.; Mundra, P.A.; Fan, F.; Galvin, A.; Weir, J.M.; Wong, G.; Chin-Dusting, J.; Cicuttini, F.; Meikle, P.; Dart, A.M. Plasma Lipidomic Profiling in Patients with Rheumatoid Arthritis. *Metabolomics* **2016**, *12*, 136. [CrossRef]
117. Ji, R.; Chang, J.Y.; Liao, X.; Zhang, X.; Kennel, P.; Castillero, E.; Brunjes, D.; Akashi, H.; Homma, S.; Goldberg, I.; et al. Abstract 17320: Inhibition of Ceramide Synthesis Preserves Cardiac Function and Increases Survival in Doxorubicin-Induced Cardiomyopathy. *Circulation* **2015**, *132*, A17320. [CrossRef]
118. Park, M.A.; Mitchell, C.; Zhang, G.; Yacoub, A.; Allegood, J.; Häussinger, D.; Reinehr, R.; Larner, A.; Spiegel, S.; Fisher, P.B.; et al. Vorinostat and Sorafenib Increase CD95 Activation in Gastrointestinal Tumor Cells through a Ca^{2+}-*De Novo* Ceramide-PP2A-Reactive Oxygen Species–Dependent Signaling Pathway. *Cancer Res.* **2010**, *70*, 6313–6324. [CrossRef]
119. Gencer, E.B.; Ural, A.U.; Avcu, F.; Baran, Y. A Novel Mechanism of Dasatinib-Induced Apoptosis in Chronic Myeloid Leukemia; Ceramide Synthase and Ceramide Clearance Genes. *Ann. Hematol.* **2011**, *90*, 1265–1275. [CrossRef]
120. Zheng, W.; Kollmeyer, J.; Symolon, H.; Momin, A.; Munter, E.; Wang, E.; Kelly, S.; Allegood, J.C.; Liu, Y.; Peng, Q.; et al. Ceramides and Other Bioactive Sphingolipid Backbones in Health and Disease: Lipidomic Analysis, Metabolism and Roles in Membrane Structure, Dynamics, Signaling and Autophagy. *Biochim. Et Biophys. Acta (BBA)-Biomembr.* **2006**, *1758*, 1864–1884. [CrossRef]
121. Casasampere, M.; Ordóñez, Y.F.; Casas, J.; Fabrias, G. Dihydroceramide Desaturase Inhibitors Induce Autophagy via Dihydroceramide-Dependent and Independent Mechanisms. *Biochim. Et Biophys. Acta (BBA)-Gen. Subj.* **2017**, *1861*, 264–275. [CrossRef]
122. Signorelli, P.; Munoz-Olaya, J.M.; Gagliostro, V.; Casas, J.; Ghidoni, R.; Fabriàs, G. Dihydroceramide Intracellular Increase in Response to Resveratrol Treatment Mediates Autophagy in Gastric Cancer Cells. *Cancer Lett.* **2009**, *282*, 238–243. [CrossRef]
123. Grenald, S.A.; Doyle, T.M.; Zhang, H.; Slosky, L.M.; Chen, Z.; Largent-Milnes, T.M.; Spiegel, S.; Vanderah, T.W.; Salvemini, D. Targeting the S1P/S1PR1 Axis Mitigates Cancer-Induced Bone Pain and Neuroinflammation. *Pain* **2017**, *158*, 1733–1742. [CrossRef]
124. Holliday, M.W., Jr.; Cox, S.B.; Kang, M.H.; Maurer, B.J. C22:0- and C24:0-Dihydroceramides Confer Mixed Cytotoxicity in T-Cell Acute Lymphoblastic Leukemia Cell Lines. *PLoS ONE* **2013**, *8*, e74768. [CrossRef]

125. Knapp, P.; Baranowski, M.; Knapp, M.; Zabielski, P.; Błachnio-Zabielska, A.U.; Górski, J. Altered Sphingolipid Metabolism in Human Endometrial Cancer. *Prostaglandins Other Lipid Mediat.* **2010**, *92*, 62–66. [CrossRef] [PubMed]
126. Illuzzi, G.; Bernacchioni, C.; Aureli, M.; Prioni, S.; Frera, G.; Donati, C.; Valsecchi, M.; Chigorno, V.; Bruni, P.; Sonnino, S.; et al. Sphingosine Kinase Mediates Resistance to the Synthetic Retinoid N-(4-Hydroxyphenyl)Retinamide in Human Ovarian Cancer Cells. *J. Biol. Chem.* **2010**, *285*, 18594–18602. [CrossRef]
127. Noack, J.; Choi, J.; Richter, K.; Kopp-Schneider, A.; Régnier-Vigouroux, A. A Sphingosine Kinase Inhibitor Combined with Temozolomide Induces Glioblastoma Cell Death through Accumulation of Dihydrosphingosine and Dihydroceramide, Endoplasmic Reticulum Stress and Autophagy. *Cell Death Dis.* **2014**, *5*, e1425. [CrossRef] [PubMed]
128. Valsecchi, M.; Aureli, M.; Mauri, L.; Illuzzi, G.; Chigorno, V.; Prinetti, A.; Sonnino, S. Sphingolipidomics of A2780 Human Ovarian Carcinoma Cells Treated with Synthetic Retinoids. *J. Lipid Res.* **2010**, *51*, 1832–1840. [CrossRef] [PubMed]
129. Wang, H.; Maurer, B.J.; Liu, Y.-Y.; Wang, E.; Allegood, J.C.; Kelly, S.; Symolon, H.; Liu, Y.; Merrill, A.H., Jr.; Alfred, H.; et al. N-(4-Hydroxyphenyl)Retinamide Increases Dihydroceramide and Synergizes with Dimethylsphingosine to Enhance Cancer Cell Killing. *Mol. Cancer Ther.* **2008**, *7*, 2967–2976. [CrossRef]
130. Idkowiak-Baldys, J.; Apraiz, A.; Li, L.; Rahmaniyan, M.; Clarke, C.J.; Kraveka, J.M.; Asumendi, A.; Hannun, Y.A. Dihydroceramide Desaturase Activity Is Modulated by Oxidative Stress. *Biochem. J.* **2010**, *427*, 265–274. [CrossRef]
131. Venant, H.; Rahmaniyan, M.; Jones, E.E.; Lu, P.; Lilly, M.B.; Garrett-Mayer, E.; Drake, R.R.; Kraveka, J.M.; Smith, C.D.; Voelkel-Johnson, C. The Sphingosine Kinase 2 Inhibitor ABC294640 Reduces the Growth of Prostate Cancer Cells and Results in Accumulation of Dihydroceramides In Vitro and In Vivo. *Mol. Cancer Ther.* **2015**, *14*, 2744–2752. [CrossRef]
132. Hernández-Corbacho, M.J.; Canals, D.; Adada, M.M.; Liu, M.; Senkal, C.E.; Yi, J.K.; Mao, C.; Luberto, C.; Hannun, Y.A.; Obeid, L.M. Tumor Necrosis Factor-α (TNFα)-Induced Ceramide Generation via Ceramide Synthases Regulates Loss of Focal Adhesion Kinase (FAK) and Programmed Cell Death. *J. Biol. Chem.* **2015**, *290*, 25356–25373. [CrossRef]
133. McNair, C.; Urbanucci, A.; Comstock, C.E.S.; Augello, M.A.; Goodwin, J.F.; Launchbury, R.; Zhao, S.G.; Schiewer, M.J.; Ertel, A.; Karnes, J.; et al. Cell Cycle-Coupled Expansion of AR Activity Promotes Cancer Progression. *Oncogene* **2017**, *36*, 1655–1668. [CrossRef]
134. Zhou, W.; Ye, X.-L.; Sun, Z.-J.; Ji, X.-D.; Chen, H.-X.; Xie, D. Overexpression of Degenerative Spermatocyte Homolog 1 Up-Regulates the Expression of Cyclin D1 and Enhances Metastatic Efficiency in Esophageal Carcinoma Eca109 Cells. *Mol. Carcinog.* **2009**, *48*, 886–894. [CrossRef] [PubMed]
135. Pewzner-Jung, Y.; Ben-Dor, S.; Futerman, A.H. When Do Lasses (Longevity Assurance Genes) Become CerS (Ceramide Synthases)? *J. Biol. Chem.* **2006**, *281*, 25001–25005. [CrossRef] [PubMed]
136. Lahiri, S.; Lee, H.; Mesicek, J.; Fuks, Z.; Haimovitz-Friedman, A.; Kolesnick, R.N.; Futerman, A.H. Kinetic Characterization of Mammalian Ceramide Synthases: Determination of K(m) Values towards Sphinganine. *FEBS Lett.* **2007**, *581*, 5289–5294. [CrossRef] [PubMed]
137. Venkataraman, K.; Riebeling, C.; Bodennec, J.; Riezman, H.; Allegood, J.C.; Sullards, M.C.; Merrill, A.H.; Futerman, A.H. Upstream of Growth and Differentiation Factor 1 (Uog1), a Mammalian Homolog of the Yeast Longevity Assurance Gene 1 (LAG1), RegulatesN-Stearoyl-Sphinganine (C18-(Dihydro)Ceramide) Synthesis in a Fumonisin B1-Independent Manner in Mammalian Cells. *J. Biol. Chem.* **2002**, *277*, 35642–35649. [CrossRef]
138. Sridevi, P.; Alexander, H.; Laviad, E.L.; Pewzner-Jung, Y.; Hannink, M.; Futerman, A.H.; Alexander, S. Ceramide Synthase 1 Is Regulated by Proteasomal Mediated Turnover. *Biochim. Et Biophys. Acta (BBA)-Mol. Cell Res.* **2009**, *1793*, 1218–1227. [CrossRef]
139. Abbott, S.K.; Li, H.; Muñoz, S.S.; Knoch, B.; Batterham, M.; Murphy, K.E.; Halliday, G.M.; Garner, B. Altered Ceramide Acyl Chain Length and Ceramide Synthase Gene Expression in Parkinson's Disease. *Mov. Disord.* **2014**, *29*, 518–526. [CrossRef]
140. Mielke, M.M.; Maetzler, W.; Haughey, N.J.; Bandaru, V.V.R.; Savica, R.; Deuschle, C.; Gasser, T.; Hauser, A.-K.; Gräber-Sultan, S.; Schleicher, E.; et al. Plasma Ceramide and Glucosylceramide Metabolism Is Altered in Sporadic Parkinson's Disease and Associated with Cognitive Impairment: A Pilot Study. *PLoS ONE* **2013**, *8*, e73094. [CrossRef]
141. Eberle, M.; Ebel, P.; Wegner, M.-S.; Männich, J.; Tafferner, N.; Ferreiros, N.; Birod, K.; Schreiber, Y.; Krishnamoorthy, G.; Willecke, K.; et al. Regulation of Ceramide Synthase 6 in a Spontaneous Experimental Autoimmune Encephalomyelitis Model Is Sex Dependent. *Biochem. Pharmacol.* **2014**, *92*, 326–335. [CrossRef]
142. Cinar, R.; Godlewski, G.; Liu, J.; Tam, J.; Jourdan, T.; Mukhopadhyay, B.; Harvey-White, J.; Kunos, G. Hepatic Cannabinoid-1 Receptors Mediate Diet-Induced Insulin Resistance by Increasing de Novo Synthesis of Long-Chain Ceramides. *Hepatology* **2014**, *59*, 143–153. [CrossRef] [PubMed]
143. Karahatay, S.; Thomas, K.; Koybasi, S.; Senkal, C.E.; ElOjeimy, S.; Liu, X.; Bielawski, J.; Day, T.A.; Gillespie, M.B.; Sinha, D.; et al. Clinical Relevance of Ceramide Metabolism in the Pathogenesis of Human Head and Neck Squamous Cell Carcinoma (HNSCC): Attenuation of C18-Ceramide in HNSCC Tumors Correlates with Lymphovascular Invasion and Nodal Metastasis. *Cancer Lett.* **2007**, *256*, 101–111. [CrossRef] [PubMed]
144. Moro, K.; Kawaguchi, T.; Tsuchida, J.; Gabriel, E.; Qi, Q.; Yan, L.; Wakai, T.; Takabe, K.; Nagahashi, M. Ceramide Species Are Elevated in Human Breast Cancer and Are Associated with Less Aggressiveness. *Oncotarget* **2018**, *9*, 19874–19890. [CrossRef] [PubMed]
145. Zhao, L.; Spassieva, S.D.; Jucius, T.J.; Shultz, L.D.; Shick, H.E.; Macklin, W.B.; Hannun, Y.A.; Obeid, L.M.; Ackerman, S.L. A Deficiency of Ceramide Biosynthesis Causes Cerebellar Purkinje Cell Neurodegeneration and Lipofuscin Accumulation. *PLoS Genet.* **2011**, *7*, e1002063. [CrossRef]

146. Vanni, N.; Fruscione, F.; Ferlazzo, E.; Striano, P.; Robbiano, A.; Traverso, M.; Sander, T.; Falace, A.; Gazzerro, E.; Bramanti, P.; et al. Impairment of Ceramide Synthesis Causes a Novel Progressive Myoclonus Epilepsy. *Ann. Neurol.* **2014**, *76*, 206–212. [CrossRef]
147. Wang, Z.; Wen, L.; Zhu, F.; Wang, Y.; Xie, Q.; Chen, Z.; Li, Y. Overexpression of Ceramide Synthase 1 Increases C18-Ceramide and Leads to Lethal Autophagy in Human Glioma. *Oncotarget* **2017**, *8*, 104022–104036. [CrossRef]
148. Laviad, E.L.; Albee, L.; Pankova-Kholmyansky, I.; Epstein, S.; Park, H.; Merrill, A.H.; Futerman, A.H. Characterization of Ceramide Synthase 2. *J. Biol. Chem.* **2008**, *283*, 5677–5684. [CrossRef]
149. Pan, H.; Qin, W.-X.; Huo, K.-K.; Wan, D.-F.; Yu, Y.; Xu, Z.-G.; Hu, Q.-D.; Gu, K.T.; Zhou, X.-M.; Jiang, H.-Q.; et al. Cloning, Mapping, and Characterization of a Human Homologue of the Yeast Longevity Assurance Gene LAG1. *Genomics* **2001**, *77*, 58–64. [CrossRef]
150. Petrache, I.; Kamocki, K.; Poirier, C.; Pewzner-Jung, Y.; Laviad, E.L.; Schweitzer, K.S.; Van Demark, M.; Justice, M.J.; Hubbard, W.C.; Futerman, A.H. Ceramide Synthases Expression and Role of Ceramide Synthase-2 in the Lung: Insight from Human Lung Cells and Mouse Models. *PLoS ONE* **2013**, *8*, e62968. [CrossRef] [PubMed]
151. Schiffmann, S.; Sandner, J.; Birod, K.; Wobst, I.; Angioni, C.; Ruckhäberle, E.; Kaufmann, M.; Ackermann, H.; Lötsch, J.; Schmidt, H.; et al. Ceramide Synthases and Ceramide Levels Are Increased in Breast Cancer Tissue. *Carcinogenesis* **2009**, *30*, 745–752. [CrossRef]
152. Barthelmes, J.; de Bazo, A.M.; Pewzner-Jung, Y.; Schmitz, K.; Mayer, C.A.; Foerch, C.; Eberle, M.; Tafferner, N.; Ferreirós, N.; Henke, M.; et al. Lack of Ceramide Synthase 2 Suppresses the Development of Experimental Autoimmune Encephalomyelitis by Impairing the Migratory Capacity of Neutrophils. *Brain Behav. Immun.* **2015**, *46*, 280–292. [CrossRef]
153. Wang, G.; Silva, J.; Dasgupta, S.; Bieberich, E. Long-Chain Ceramide Is Elevated in Presenilin 1 (PS1M146V) Mouse Brain and Induces Apoptosis in PS1 Astrocytes. *Glia* **2008**, *56*, 449–456. [CrossRef]
154. Mosbech, M.; Olsen, A.S.B.; Neess, D.; Ben-David, O.; Klitten, L.L.; Larsen, J.; Sabers, A.; Vissing, J.; Nielsen, J.E.; Hasholt, L.; et al. Reduced Ceramide Synthase 2 Activity Causes Progressive Myoclonic Epilepsy. *Ann. Clin. Transl. Neurol.* **2014**, *1*, 88–98. [CrossRef] [PubMed]
155. Ruan, H.; Wang, T.; Yang, C.; Jin, G.; Gu, D.; Deng, X.; Wang, C.; Qin, W.; Jin, H. Co-Expression of LASS2 and TGF-B1 Predicts Poor Prognosis in Hepatocellular Carcinoma. *Sci. Rep.* **2016**, *6*, 32421. [CrossRef] [PubMed]
156. Fan, S.; Niu, Y.; Tan, N.; Wu, Z.; Wang, Y.; You, H.; Ke, R.; Song, J.; Shen, Q.; Wang, W.; et al. LASS2 Enhances Chemosensitivity of Breast Cancer by Counteracting Acidic Tumor Microenvironment through Inhibiting Activity of V-ATPase Proton Pump. *Oncogene* **2013**, *32*, 1682–1690. [CrossRef] [PubMed]
157. Zeng, F.; Huang, L.; Cheng, X.; Yang, X.; Li, T.; Feng, G.; Tang, Y.; Yang, Y. Overexpression of LASS2 Inhibits Proliferation and Causes G0/G1 Cell Cycle Arrest in Papillary Thyroid Cancer. *Cancer Cell Int.* **2018**, *18*, 151. [CrossRef] [PubMed]
158. Ke, R.-H.; Wang, Y.; Mao, Y.; Zhang, J.; Xiong, J. Decreased Expression of LASS2 Is Associated with Worse Prognosis in Meningiomas. *J. Neurooncol.* **2014**, *118*, 369–376. [CrossRef]
159. Wang, H.; Wang, J.; Zuo, Y.; Ding, M.; Yan, R.; Yang, D.; Ke, C. Expression and Prognostic Significance of a New Tumor Metastasis Suppressor Gene LASS2 in Human Bladder Carcinoma. *Med. Oncol.* **2012**, *29*, 1921–1927. [CrossRef]
160. Wang, H.; Zhang, W.; Zuo, Y.; Ding, M.; Ke, C.; Yan, R.; Zhan, H.; Liu, J.; Wang, J. MiR-9 Promotes Cell Proliferation and Inhibits Apoptosis by Targeting LASS2 in Bladder Cancer. *Tumor Biol.* **2015**, *36*, 9631–9640. [CrossRef]
161. Chen, Y.; Wang, H.; Xiong, T.; Zou, R.; Tang, Z.; Wang, J. The Role of LASS2 in Regulating Bladder Cancer Cell Tumorigenicity in a Nude Mouse Model. *Oncol. Lett.* **2017**, *14*, 5149–5156. [CrossRef] [PubMed]
162. Xu, X.; You, J.; Pei, F. Silencing of a Novel Tumor Metastasis Suppressor Gene LASS2/TMSG1 Promotes Invasion of Prostate Cancer Cell in Vitro through Increase of Vacuolar ATPase Activity. *J. Cell. Biochem.* **2012**, *113*, 2356–2363. [CrossRef] [PubMed]
163. Xu, X.; Liu, B.; Zou, P.; Zhang, Y.; You, J.; Pei, F. Silencing of LASS2/TMSG1 Enhances Invasion and Metastasis Capacity of Prostate Cancer Cell. *J. Cell. Biochem.* **2014**, *115*, 731–743. [CrossRef] [PubMed]
164. Mizutani, Y.; Kihara, A.; Igarashi, Y. LASS3 (Longevity Assurance Homologue 3) Is a Mainly Testis-Specific (Dihydro)Ceramide Synthase with Relatively Broad Substrate Specificity. *Biochem. J.* **2006**, *398*, 531–538. [CrossRef] [PubMed]
165. Levy, M.; Futerman, A.H. Mammalian Ceramide Synthases. *IUBMB Life* **2010**, *62*, 347–356. [CrossRef]
166. Cai, X.-F.; Tao, Z.; Yan, Z.-Q.; Yang, S.-L.; Gong, Y. Molecular Cloning, Characterisation and Tissue-Specific Expression of Human LAG3, a Member of the Novel Lag1 Protein Family. *DNA Seq.* **2003**, *14*, 79–86. [CrossRef]
167. Mizutani, Y.; Kihara, A.; Chiba, H.; Tojo, H.; Igarashi, Y. 2-Hydroxy-Ceramide Synthesis by Ceramide Synthase Family: Enzymatic Basis for the Preference of FA Chain Length. *J. Lipid Res.* **2008**, *49*, 2356–2364. [CrossRef]
168. Eckl, K.-M.; Tidhar, R.; Thiele, H.; Oji, V.; Hausser, I.; Brodesser, S.; Preil, M.-L.; Önal-Akan, A.; Stock, F.; Müller, D.; et al. Impaired Epidermal Ceramide Synthesis Causes Autosomal Recessive Congenital Ichthyosis and Reveals the Importance of Ceramide Acyl Chain Length. *J. Investig. Dermatol.* **2013**, *133*, 2202–2211. [CrossRef]
169. Radner, F.P.W.; Marrakchi, S.; Kirchmeier, P.; Kim, G.-J.; Ribierre, F.; Kamoun, B.; Abid, L.; Leipoldt, M.; Turki, H.; Schempp, W.; et al. Mutations in CERS3 Cause Autosomal Recessive Congenital Ichthyosis in Humans. *PLoS Genet.* **2013**, *9*, e1003536. [CrossRef]
170. Marsching, C.; Rabionet, M.; Mathow, D.; Jennemann, R.; Kremser, C.; Porubsky, S.; Bolenz, C.; Willecke, K.; Gröne, H.-J.; Hopf, C.; et al. Renal Sulfatides: Sphingoid Base-Dependent Localization and Region-Specific Compensation of CerS2-Dysfunction. *J. Lipid Res.* **2014**, *55*, 2354–2369. [CrossRef]

171. Chen, J.; Li, X.; Ma, D.; Liu, T.; Tian, P.; Wu, C. Ceramide Synthase-4 Orchestrates the Cell Proliferation and Tumor Growth of Liver Cancer in Vitro and in Vivo through the Nuclear Factor-KB Signaling Pathway. *Oncol. Lett.* **2017**, *14*, 1477–1483. [CrossRef] [PubMed]
172. Ruckhäberle, E.; Rody, A.; Engels, K.; Gaetje, R.; von Minckwitz, G.; Schiffmann, S.; Grösch, S.; Geisslinger, G.; Holtrich, U.; Karn, T.; et al. Microarray Analysis of Altered Sphingolipid Metabolism Reveals Prognostic Significance of Sphingosine Kinase 1 in Breast Cancer. *Breast Cancer Res. Treat.* **2008**, *112*, 41–52. [CrossRef] [PubMed]
173. Riebeling, C.; Allegood, J.C.; Wang, E.; Merrill, A.H.; Futerman, A.H. Two Mammalian Longevity Assurance Gene (LAG1) Family Members, Trh1 and Trh4, Regulate Dihydroceramide Synthesis Using Different Fatty Acyl-CoA Donors. *J. Biol. Chem.* **2003**, *278*, 43452–43459. [CrossRef] [PubMed]
174. Chen, L.; Chen, H.; Li, Y.; Li, L.; Qiu, Y.; Ren, J. Endocannabinoid and Ceramide Levels Are Altered in Patients with Colorectal Cancer. *Oncol. Rep.* **2015**, *34*, 447–454. [CrossRef]
175. Jang, S.; Park, W.; Min, H.; Kwon, T.; Baek, S.; Hwang, I.; Kim, S.; Park, J. Altered MRNA Expression Levels of the Major Components of Sphingolipid Metabolism, Ceramide Synthases and Their Clinical Implication in Colorectal Cancer. *Oncol. Rep.* **2018**, *40*, 3489–3500. [CrossRef]
176. Kijanka, G.; Hector, S.; Kay, E.W.; Murray, F.; Cummins, R.; Murphy, D.; MacCraith, B.D.; Prehn, J.H.M.; Kenny, D. Human IgG Antibody Profiles Differentiate between Symptomatic Patients with and without Colorectal Cancer. *Gut* **2010**, *59*, 69–78. [CrossRef]
177. Fitzgerald, S.; Sheehan, K.M.; Espina, V.; O'Grady, A.; Cummins, R.; Kenny, D.; Liotta, L.; O'Kennedy, R.; Kay, E.W.; Kijanka, G.S. High CerS5 Expression Levels Associate with Reduced Patient Survival and Transition from Apoptotic to Autophagy Signalling Pathways in Colorectal Cancer. *J. Pathol. Clin. Res.* **2015**, *1*, 54–65. [CrossRef]
178. Jiang, Z.; Li, F.; Wan, Y.; Han, Z.; Yuan, W.; Cao, L.; Deng, Y.; Peng, X.; Chen, F.; Fan, X.; et al. LASS5 Interacts with SDHB and Synergistically Represses P53 and P21 Activity. *Curr. Mol. Med.* **2016**, *16*, 582–590. [CrossRef]
179. Schiffmann, S.; Ferreiros, N.; Birod, K.; Eberle, M.; Schreiber, Y.; Pfeilschifter, W.; Ziemann, U.; Pierre, S.; Scholich, K.; Grösch, S.; et al. Ceramide Synthase 6 Plays a Critical Role in the Development of Experimental Autoimmune Encephalomyelitis. *J. Immunol.* **2012**, *188*, 5723–5733. [CrossRef]
180. Erez-Roman, R.; Pienik, R.; Futerman, A.H. Increased Ceramide Synthase 2 and 6 MRNA Levels in Breast Cancer Tissues and Correlation with Sphingosine Kinase Expression. *Biochem. Biophys. Res. Commun.* **2010**, *391*, 219–223. [CrossRef]
181. Makoukji, J.; Raad, M.; Genadry, K.; El-Sitt, S.; Makhoul, N.J.; Saad Aldin, E.; Nohra, E.; Jabbour, M.; Sangaralingam, A.; Chelala, C.; et al. Association between CLN3 (Neuronal Ceroid Lipofuscinosis, CLN3 Type) Gene Expression and Clinical Characteristics of Breast Cancer Patients. *Front. Oncol.* **2015**, *5*, 215. [CrossRef] [PubMed]
182. Ruckhäberle, E.; Holtrich, U.; Engels, K.; Hanker, L.; Gätje, R.; Metzler, D.; Karn, T.; Kaufmann, M.; Rody, A. Acid Ceramidase 1 Expression Correlates with a Better Prognosis in ER-Positive Breast Cancer. *Climacteric* **2009**, *12*, 502–513. [CrossRef] [PubMed]
183. Uen, Y.-H.; Fang, C.-L.; Lin, C.-C.; Hseu, Y.-C.; Hung, S.-T.; Sun, D.-P.; Lin, K.-Y. Ceramide Synthase 6 Predicts the Prognosis of Human Gastric Cancer: It Functions as an Oncoprotein by Dysregulating the SOCS2/JAK2/STAT3 Pathway. *Mol. Carcinog.* **2018**, *57*, 1675–1689. [CrossRef] [PubMed]
184. Minamoto, S.; Ikegame, K.; Ueno, K.; Narazaki, M.; Naka, T.; Yamamoto, H.; Matsumoto, T.; Saito, H.; Hosoe, S.; Kishimoto, T. Cloning and Functional Analysis of New Members of STAT Induced STAT Inhibitor (SSI) Family: SSI-2 and SSI-3. *Biochem. Biophys. Res. Commun.* **1997**, *237*, 79–83. [CrossRef]
185. Dementiev, A.; Joachimiak, A.; Nguyen, H.; Gorelik, A.; Illes, K.; Shabani, S.; Gelsomino, M.; Ahn, E.-Y.E.; Nagar, B.; Doan, N. Molecular Mechanism of Inhibition of Acid Ceramidase by Carmofur. *J. Med. Chem.* **2019**, *62*, 987–992. [CrossRef]
186. Mody, N.; Mcilroy, G.D. The Mechanisms of Fenretinide-Mediated Anti-Cancer Activity and Prevention of Obesity and Type-2 Diabetes. *Biochem. Pharmacol.* **2014**, *91*, 277–286. [CrossRef]
187. Salma, Y.; Lafont, E.; Therville, N.; Carpentier, S.; Bonnafé, M.-J.; Levade, T.; Génisson, Y.; Andrieu-Abadie, N. The Natural Marine Anhydrophytosphingosine, Jaspine B, Induces Apoptosis in Melanoma Cells by Interfering with Ceramide Metabolism. *Biochem. Pharmacol.* **2009**, *78*, 477–485. [CrossRef]
188. Pashikanti, S.; Foster, D.J.; Kharel, Y.; Brown, A.M.; Bevan, D.R.; Lynch, K.R.; Santos, W.L. Sphingosine Kinase 2 Inhibitors: Rigid Aliphatic Tail Derivatives Deliver Potent and Selective Analogues. *ACS Bio Med. Chem. Au* **2022**, *2*, 469–489. [CrossRef]
189. Pyne, S.; Adams, D.R.; Pyne, N.J. Sphingosine Kinases as Druggable Targets. In *Lipid Signaling in Human Diseases*; Springer: Cham, Switzerland, 2018; pp. 49–76.
190. García-Seisdedos, D.; Babiy, B.; Lerma, M.; Casado, M.E.; Martínez-Botas, J.; Lasunción, M.A.; Pastor, Ó.; Busto, R. Curcumin Stimulates Exosome/Microvesicle Release in an in Vitro Model of Intracellular Lipid Accumulation by Increasing Ceramide Synthesis. *Biochim. Et Biophys. Acta (BBA)-Mol. Cell Biol. Lipids* **2020**, *1865*, 158638. [CrossRef]
191. Munoz-Olaya, J.M.; Matabosch, X.; Bedia, C.; Egido-Gabás, M.; Casas, J.; Llebaria, A.; Delgado, A.; Fabriàs, G. Synthesis and Biological Activity of a Novel Inhibitor of Dihydroceramide Desaturase. *ChemMedChem* **2008**, *3*, 946–953. [CrossRef]

MDPI
St. Alban-Anlage 66
4052 Basel
Switzerland
www.mdpi.com

MDPI Books Editorial Office
E-mail: books@mdpi.com
www.mdpi.com/books

www.ingramcontent.com/pod-product-compliance
Lightning Source LLC
Chambersburg PA
CBHW061451220926
51850CB00004B/64
* 9 7 8 3 0 3 6 5 9 7 4 6 1 *